T0156219

Eighth Edition

POLICY & POLITICS

in Nursing and Health Care

Diana J. Mason, PhD, RN, FAAN
Consultant and Journalist
Senior Policy Service Professor
Center for Health Policy and Media Engagement
School of Nursing
George Washington University
Washington, DC
Professor Emerita
Hunter-Bellevue School of Nursing
City University of New York
New York, New York

Elizabeth Dickson, PhD, RN
Assistant Professor
College of Nursing
Center for Participatory Research
University of New Mexico
Albuquerque, New Mexico

Monica R. McLemore, PhD, RN, MPH, FAAN
Associate Professor
Family Health Care Nursing
Clinician-Scientist
Advancing New Standards in Reproductive Health (ANSIRH)
University of California, San Francisco
San Francisco, California

G. Adriana Perez, PhD, RN, CRNP, ANP-BC, FAAN, FGSA
Assistant Professor of Nursing
Family and Community Health
School of Nursing
Senior Fellow
Leonard Davis Institute of Health Economics
University of Pennsylvania
Philadelphia, Pennsylvania

ELSEVIER

Elsevier
3251 Riverport Lane
St. Louis, Missouri 63043

POLICY & POLITICS IN NURSING AND HEALTH CARE ISBN: 978-0-323-55498-5

Senior Content Strategist: Sandra Clark
Content Development Manager: Lisa Newton
Publishing Services Manager: Julie Eddy
Book Production Specialist: Clay S. Broeker
Design Direction: Maggie Reid

Printed in the United States of America

Last digit is the print number: 9 8 7 6 5 4 3 2 1

ABOUT THE EDITORS

DIANA J. MASON, PhD, RN, FAAN, is Senior Policy Service Professor at the Center for Health Policy and Media Engagement, George Washington University School of Nursing; and Professor Emeritus, Hunter-Bellevue School of Nursing, City University of New York. She is the Deputy Program Director for the International Council of Nurses' Global Nursing Leadership Institute, which prepares nurse leaders around the world to shape global, regional, and national policies to improve the health of populations. She is a past President of the American Academy of Nursing, former Editor-in-Chief of the *American Journal of Nursing*, and producer and moderator of a community radio program on health and health policy since 1985. She has served as the only health professional on the National Advisory Committee for Kaiser Health News since its inception in 2009. She blogs on policy for *HealthCetera* and *JAMA News Forum*. Dr. Mason is the principal investigator on a replication of the 1998 *Woodhull Study on Nurses and the Media* published in 2018 in the *Journal of Nursing Scholarship* and an additional analysis of journalists' experiences with using nurses as sources in health news stories published in the *American Journal of Nursing*.

Dr. Mason is a member of the Board of Directors of the Primary Care Development Corporation, a nonprofit Community Development Financial Institution focused on building the nation's capacity for primary care; and of Public Health Solutions, New York City's largest public health organization that focuses on improving the health of vulnerable families. She chairs the National Advisory Board of the Center for Health and Social Care Integration at Rush University Medical Center and is Facilitator and Co-Chair of the Catskills Addiction Coalition. She served as a member of the National Academies of Science, Engineering and Medicine Committee for the report on *Integrating Social Needs Care into the Delivery of Health Care to Improve the Nation's Health*, and she co-chaired the Josiah Macy Foundation invitational conference and report on *Registered Nurses: Partners in Transforming Primary Care*.

The recipient of numerous awards for leadership, dissemination of science, writing, education, policy, and advocacy, Dr. Mason is a fellow of the American Academy of Nursing and the New York Academy of Medicine, from which she received the Academy Medal for Distinguished Contributions in Health Policy in 2019. She received a BSN from West Virginia University, an MSN from St. Louis University, a PhD from New York University, an honorary Doctorate of Science from West Virginia University, and an honorary doctorate of humane letters from Long Island University.

ELIZABETH DICKSON, PhD, RN, is an Assistant Professor at the University of New Mexico, College of Nursing in Albuquerque, New Mexico and a fellow of the Robert Wood Johnson Foundation Nursing and Health Policy Collaborative. Dr. Dickson's public health experience spans local, county, state, and federal public health agencies, with foci on maternal-child health, childhood immunizations, tuberculosis management, STD/HIV prevention, family planning, and school health programs in California, Arizona, and New Mexico.

Dr. Dickson's program of research focuses on the intersection of adolescent health, health education, school health and education policy, and school nursing. She serves on the Board of Directors for the New Mexico Alliance for School Based Health Care and multiple state and local community advisory boards for projects focused on improving LGBTQ adolescent health and health education. Dr. Dickson testified before legislative health and education committees regarding her research on sexual health education in secondary schools. Her research collaboration includes the University of New Mexico Center for Participatory Research, where she serves as co-investigator for NIH/NINR-supported research exploring community-based participatory research within academic and community partnerships.

Dr. Dickson received a BS in business management from California State University, Sacramento, an MSN from Samuel Merritt College, Oakland, California, and a PhD in nursing from the University of New Mexico.

MONICA R. McLEMORE, PhD, MPH, RN, FAAN is an associate professor in the Family Health Care Nursing Department, a research scientist with Advancing New Standards in Reproductive Health, and a member of the Bixby Center for Global Reproductive Health. Her program of research is focused on understanding reproductive health and justice. She has published 49 peer-reviewed articles, op-eds, and commentaries, and her research has been cited in the *Huffington Post*, Lavender Health, two amicus briefs to the Supreme Court of the United States, and a National Academies of Science, Engineering, and Medicine report. Her work has appeared in publications such as *Dame* magazine, Politico, and ProPublica/NPR, and she made a voice appearance in Terrance Nance's HBO series *Random Acts of*

Flyness. She is an elected member of the governing council for Sexual and Reproductive Health (SRH) section of the American Public Health Association and became chair-elect of the SRH section at the 2018 annual meeting. She is a recipient of the 2015 teaching award from the American College of Nurse Midwives and one of 10 Culture of Health, Breakthrough Leaders in Nursing—a program of the Robert Wood Johnson Foundation, AARP, and the Center to Champion Nursing in America. She currently serves on the board of Centering Health Care International. In 2018 Dr. McLemore received the Person of the Year Award from the Abortion Care Network, and she was inducted as a fellow of the American Academy of Nursing in 2019.

G. ADRIANA PEREZ, PhD, RN, CRNP, ANP-BC, FAAN, FGSA, is an Assistant Professor of Nursing and Senior Fellow at the Leonard Davis Institute of Health Economics at the University of Pennsylvania, School of Nursing. Her program of research focuses on the development and testing of theory-based community interventions to promote cardiovascular health and cognitive health in older Latinos. Current studies are funded by the National Institutes of Health/National Institute of Nursing Research Supplement to Promote Diversity in Health Related Research Program and the Penn Center for Improving Care Delivery for the Aging, National Institute on Aging. She was selected as a Congressional/Health and Aging Policy Fellow (2011-2013) supported by the Atlantic Philanthropies and Centers for Disease Control and Prevention.

Dr. Perez is a Fellow of the American Academy of Nursing and the Gerontological Society of America (GSA). She has served as Chair of the Academy's Expert Panel on Aging; Chair of the Public Policy Committee for the National Association of Hispanic Nurses; member of the UnitedHealth Group External Clinician Advisory Board; and appointed board member for the American Organization of Nurse Leaders. Dr. Perez received the GSA 2018 Senior Service America, Senior Scholar Award for Research Related to Disadvantaged Older Adults. She is a board-certified Adult Nurse Practitioner at Mercy LIFE, providing community-based long-term care for diverse, frail elders who reside in North Philadelphia.

Dr. Perez grew up in Yuma, Arizona, near the United States–Mexico border. She received her BSN, MS Adult Nurse Practitioner, and PhD from Arizona State University, College of Nursing & Health Innovation. She received the Patricia G. Archbold Predoctoral Scholarship and Claire M. Fagin Postdoctoral Fellowship from the John A. Hartford Foundation, National Hartford Center for Gerontological Nursing Excellence.

Dawn Marie Adams, DNP, ANP Cert, MSN, BSN
Director
Office of Integrated Health
Department of Behavioral Health and Developmental Services
Richmond, Virginia
Adjunct Professor
Old Dominion University
Norfolk, Virginia
Delegate
House, Virginia General Assembly
Richmond, Virginia

Susan L. Adams, PhD, BSN, MSN
Associate Professor
Betty Irene Moore School of Nursing
University of California, Davis
Sacramento, California

Gale Adcock, BSN, MSN
Representative, District 41
North Carolina House of Representatives
Raleigh, North Carolina
Chief Health Officer
SAS Institute
Cary, North Carolina

Lucia Judith Alfano, RN, MA
Assistant Professor of Nursing
Division of Nursing
Concordia College
Bronxville, New York

Carmen Alvarez, PhD, MSN, BSN
Assistant Professor
Community–Public Health
Johns Hopkins University School of Nursing
Baltimore, Maryland

Angela Amar, PhD, RN
Dean
School of Nursing
University of Nevada, Las Vegas
Las Vegas, Nevada

Amy L. Anderson, RN, DNP, CNE
Assistant Professor of Professional Practice
Harris College of Nursing and Health Sciences
Texas Christian University
Fort Worth, Texas

Rhonda Anderson, RN, BS, MPA, DNSc(h)
Consultant Healthcare
RMA Consulting
Scottsdale, Arizona
Consultant/Surveyor
Medical Travel
Global Healthcare Accreditation
Palm Beach Gardens, Florida

Susan Apold, PhD, ANP-BC, AGNP, FAAN, FAANP
Dean
School of Health Sciences and Nursing
Concordia College
Bronxville, New York

Debra A. Banks, RN, BSN, MSN
Clinical Nurse Director of Neurosurgery
University of New Mexico Health Sciences Center
Albuquerque, New Mexico

Kenya V. Beard, EdD, MSN, BS
Associate Professor of Nursing
City University of New York
Dix Hills, New York

Mary L. Behrens, MS, BS, FNP-BC, FAANP
President
Wyoming Center for Nursing
Casper, Wyoming
Board Member/Nursing
University of Wisconsin
Madison, Wisconsin

Susan I. Belanger, PhD, RN, MA, NEA-BC
Interim SVP Mission Integration and System Ethicist
Covenant Health
Tewksbury, Massachusetts

Laurie S. Benson, BSN
Executive Director
Nurses on Boards Coalition
Washington, DC

Virginia Trotter Betts, RN, MSN, JD, FAAN
President and Chief Executive Officer
Health Futures, Inc.
Nashville, Tennessee

Mary Blankson, DNP, APRN, FNP-C
Chief Nursing Officer
Community Health Center, Inc.
Middletown, Connecticut

Linda Burnes Bolton, RN, DrPH, FAAN
Senior Vice President
Cedars-Sinai Health System
Los Angeles, California

Patricia K. Bradley, PhD, RN, MSN, FAAN
Associate Professor
Fitzpatrick College of Nursing
Villanova University
Villanova, Pennsylvania

Sherl Brand, RN, BSN
Senior Vice President
Strategic Solutions
CareCentrix
Hartford, Connecticut

Andrea Brassard, PhD, FNP-BC, FAANP, FAAN
Senior Strategic Policy Advisor
Center to Champion Nursing in America
AARP of Washington, DC
Bowie, Maryland

Andrea Uitti Bresnahan, RN, MSN, DNP
Associate Director of Programs and Services
Florida Center for Nursing
University of Central Florida
Orlando, Florida

Toby Bressler, PhD, RN, OCN
Director of Nursing for Oncology and Clinical Quality
Oncology Nursing
Mount Sinai Health System
Associate Professor of Medical Oncology
Icahn School of Medicine at Mount Sinai
New York, New York

Lori Brierley
Director of Communications
First District Health Unit
Minot, North Dakota

Edie Brous, BSN, MS, MPH, JD
Nurse Attorney
Edith Brous, Esq. PC
New York, New York

Loretta Jackson Brown, PhD, BSN, MSN
Senior Health Communication Specialist
National Center for Injury Prevention and Control
Centers for Disease Control and Prevention
Atlanta, Georgia

Mary Lou Brunell, RN, MSN
Executive Director
Healthcare Workforce Research Initiative
University of Central Florida
Orlando, Florida

Kelly Buettner-Schmidt, PhD
Associate Professor
School of Nursing
North Dakota State University
Fargo, North Dakota

Pamela Z. Cacchione, PhD, CRNP, BC, FGSA, FAAN
Ralston House Term Chair of Gerontological Nursing
School of Nursing
Senior Fellow
Leonard Davis Institute of Health Economics
University of Pennsylvania
Nurse Scientist
Penn Presbyterian Medical Center
Philadelphia, Pennsylvania

Peggy L. Chinn, PhD, RN, FAAN
Professor Emerita
Nursing
University of Connecticut
Storrs, Connecticut

Mary Ann Christopher, RN, MSN, FAAN
Vice President, Clinical Operations and Transformation
Horizon Blue Cross Blue Shield of New Jersey
Newark, New Jersey

Carey S. Clark, PhD, RN, AHN-BC, FAAN
Associate Professor of Nursing
University of Maine at Augusta
Denmark, Maine

Sean P. Clarke, RN, PhD, FAAN
Executive Vice Dean and Professor
Rory Meyers College of Nursing
New York University
New York, New York

Jake Coffey, MA, MPH
Director of Advocacy
National Alliance on Mental Illness
Nashville, Tennessee

Sally S. Cohen, PhD, RN, FAAN
Clinical Professor
Rory Meyers College of Nursing
New York University
New York, New York

Heide Cygan, BSN, DNP
Assistant Professor of Community, Systems, and Mental Health
Rush University College of Nursing
Chicago, Illinois

Nadia Campos de Andrade, RN, MSN, AGACNP-BC, PhD candidate
Community, Global and Public Health
Johns Hopkins School of Nursing
Baltimore, Maryland

Catherine M. Dentinger, MS, MPH
Captain
Division of Parasitic Diseases and Malaria, U.S. President's Malaria Initiative
Centers for Disease Control and Prevention
Antananarivo, Madagascar

Michele Diaz, RN, MS
PhD Nursing Student of Community Health Systems
University of California, San Francisco
San Francisco, California

Toni DiChiacchio, DNP
Assistant Dean, Faculty Practice, Community Engagement and Health Policy
School of Nursing
West Virginia University
Morgantown, West Virginia

Elizabeth Dickson, PhD, RN
Assistant Professor
College of Nursing
Center for Participatory Research
University of New Mexico
Albuquerque, New Mexico

Sita M. Diehl, MSSW
Principal
Sita Diehl Consulting, LLC
Madison, Wisconsin

Patricia D'Antonio, PhD, RN, FAAN
Professor of Nursing
Family and Community Health
School of Nursing
University of Pennsylvania
Philadelphia, Pennsylvania

Regina S. Eddie, PhD, BS, MS
Assistant Professor
School of Nursing
Northern Arizona University
Flagstaff, Arizona

Esther Emard, RN, MSN, MSLIR
Instructor
School of Nursing
George Washington University
Washington, DC

Robin Dawson Estrada, PhD, RN, CPNP-PC
Assistant Professor and Director, Smart Start Nursing Program
College of Nursing
University of South Carolina
Columbia, South Carolina

Pamela Stewart Fahs, PhD
Professor and Associate Dean
Decker School of Nursing
Binghamton University
Binghamton, New York

Julie Fairman, PhD
Nightingale Professor in Honor of Nursing Veterans
Biobehavioral Health Sciences
University of Pennsylvania
Philadelphia, Pennsylvania

Nina R. Fekaris, RN, MS, BSN, NCSN
President
National Association of School Nurses
Silver Springs, Maryland

Margaret Mary Flinter, PhD, MSN
Senior Vice President and Clinical Director
Executive Leadership
Senior Research Scientist
Weitzman Institute
Community Health Center (CHC), Inc.
Middletown, Connecticut

Mary Foley, PhD, RN
Clinical Faculty
Department of Physiology
University of California, San Francisco
San Francisco, California

Renee S. Frauendienst, BSN
Public Health Division Director and CHS Administrator
Human Services of Stearns County
St. Cloud, Minnesota

Eileen K. Fry-Bowers, PhD, JD
Associate Professor
Hahn School of Nursing and Health Science
University of San Diego
San Diego, California

Beth Gharrity Gardner, PhD
Research Associate
Department of Social Sciences—Political Sociology and
    Social Policy
Humboldt University
Berlin, Germany

Catherine Alicia Georges, RN, EdD, FAAN
Professor and Chairperson
Nursing
Lehman College
Bronx, New York

Rosemary Gibson, MSc
Author of *The Treatment Trap*
Senior Adviser
The Hastings Center
Garrison, New York

Barbara Glickstein, RN, MPH, MS
Founder
Barbara Glickstein Strategies
New York, New York

Zil Garner Goldstein, BA, BSN, MSN
Assistant Professor of Medical Education
Infectious Disease
Clinical Program Director
Center for Transgender Medicine and Surgery
Mount Sinai Health System
New York, New York

Alexia E. Green, PhD, RN
Visiting Professor and Robert Wood Johnson Foundation
    Nursing and Health Policy Collaborative Project
    Director
College of Nursing
University of New Mexico
Albuquerque, New Mexico
Professor and Dean Emerita
School of Nursing
Texas Tech University Health Sciences Center
Lubbock, Texas

Bethany Hall-Long, PhD, MSN, BSN
Professor
School of Health Sciences
University of Delaware
Newark, Delaware
Lt. Governor
State of Delaware
Dover, Delaware

Kimberly J. Harper, RN, MS, FAAN
Chief Executive Officer
Indiana Center for Nursing
Indianapolis, Indiana
Chairman of the Board
Nurses on Boards Coalition
Washington, DC

Susan B. Hassmiller, PhD, RN, FAAN
Senior Adviser for Nursing
Robert Wood Johnson Foundation
Director
Future of Nursing: Campaign for Action
Princeton, New Jersey

Jennifer Hatzfeld, PhD
Executive Director
TriService Nursing Research Program
Uniformed Services University of the Health Sciences
Bethesda, Maryland

Katie Huffling, RN, MS, CNM
Executive Director
Alliance of Nurses for Healthy Environments
Mount Rainier, Maryland

Lauren M. Inouye, RN, MPP
Vice President
Public Policy and Government Affairs
Council of Graduate Schools
Washington, DC

Jean Johnson, PhD, RN, FAAN
Dean Emerita and Professor
School of Nursing
George Washington University
Washington, DC

Jane Clare Joyner, JD, MSN
Attorney
Office of the Solicitor
Department of Labor
Washington, DC

Florence Kariuki, BSN, MHA
Clinical Design Lead
Healthcare Management and Transformation
Horizon Blue Cross Blue Shield of New Jersey
Newark, New Jersey

Deirdre E. Kearney, MSN
Nurse Director
Lovelace Westside Hospital
Albuquerque, New Mexico

David M. Keepnews, PhD, RN, JD, NEA-BC, FAAN
Professor
School of Nursing
George Washington University
Washington, DC

Mary Beth Kingston, RN, MSN
Chief Nursing Officer
Administration
Advocate Aurora Health
Milwaukee, Wisconsin

Amy R. Kolwaite, BSN, MS, MPH
Nurse Epidemiologist
International Infection Control Program
Division for Healthcare Quality Promotion
Centers for Disease Control and Prevention
Atlanta, Georgia

Mary Jo Kreitzer, PhD, RN, FAAN
Director
Earl E. Bakken Center for Spirituality and Healing
Professor
School of Nursing
University of Minnesota
Minneapolis, Minnesota

Rebecca (Rice) Bowers Lanier, EdD, MSN, MPH
President
B2L Consulting
Richmond, Virginia

Kathryn Laughon, PhD, RN, FAAN
Associate Professor
School of Nursing
University of Virginia
Charlottesville, Virginia

Ramon Lavandero, MA, MSN, FAAN
Senior Strategic Adviser and Organizational Historian
American Association of Critical-Care Nurses
Aliso Viejo, California
Clinical Associate Professor
School of Nursing
Yale University
West Haven, Connecticut

Roberta Proffitt Lavin, PhD, FNP-BC, FAAN
Professor and Executive Associate Dean of Academic
    Programs
College of Nursing
University of Tennessee
Knoxville, Tennessee

Katarzyna Lessard, JD, MSN, BSN, BA
Assistant Professor of Nursing
Quinnipiac University
North Haven, Connecticut

Sandra B. Lewenson, RN, EdD, FAAN
Professor
Lienhard School of Nursing—Graduate
Pace University
Pleasantville, New York

Maria LoGrippo, PhD, MSN, RN
Assistant Professor and Director of RN to BS
Nursing
Rutgers University
Westfield, New Jersey

Grant R. Martsolf, PhD, RN, MPH, FAAN
Professor
Department of Acute and Tertiary Care
University of Pittsburgh
Adjunct Policy Researcher
RAND Corporation
Pittsburgh, Pennsylvania

Diana J. Mason, PhD, RN, FAAN
Senior Policy Service Professor
Center for Health Policy and Media Engagement
School of Nursing
George Washington University
Washington, DC
Professor Emerita
Hunter-Bellevue School of Nursing
Hunter College
New York, New York

Donna Mazyck, MS, BSN
Executive Director
National Association of School Nurses
Silver Spring, Maryland

Ruth McDermott-Levy, PhD, MPH, MSN
Associate Professor and Director
Center for Global and Public Health
M. Louise Fitzpatrick College of Nursing
Villanova University
Villanova, Pennsylvania

Monica R. McLemore, PhD, RN, MPH, FAAN
Associate Professor
Family Health Care Nursing
Clinician-Scientist
Advancing New Standards in Reproductive Health (ANSIRH)
University of California, San Francisco
San Francisco, California

DeAnne K. Hilfinger Messias, PhD, RN, FAAN
Professor
College of Nursing and Women's and Gender Studies
University of South Carolina
Columbia, South Carolina

Clair Millet, DNP, MN, BSN
Director
Continuing Nursing Education and Faculty Development
School of Nursing
Louisiana State University Health Sciences Center
New Orleans, Louisiana

Gina Miranda-Diaz, DNP, MSN, MPH, BSN
Former Director and Health Officer
Health Department
Union City Town Hall
Union City, New Jersey
Associate Professor
Felician University
Lodi, New Jersey

Wanda Montalvo, PhD
Executive Director
Jonas Nursing and Veterans Healthcare
School of Nursing
Columbia University
Staten Island, New York

Carolyn Montoya, PhD, MSN, BSN
Associate Dean of Clinical Affairs
College of Nursing
University of New Mexico
Albuquerque, New Mexico

Mary Muhlbradt
Community Relations Coordinator
Marketing and Community Relations
Trinity Health
Minot, North Dakota

Erica Mumm, RN, DNP
Clinical Assistant Professor of Nursing
Quinnipiac University
Hamden, Connecticut

Carole R. Myers, PhD, MSN, BS
Professor
College of Nursing
University of Tennessee
Knoxville, Tennessee

Len M. Nichols, PhD
Professor of Health Policy and Director
Center for Health Policy Research and Ethics
George Mason University
Fairfax, Virginia

Eileen T. O'Grady, PhD, RN, NP
Founder
The School of Wellness
Eileen O'Grady Wellness Coaching, LLC
McLean, Virginia

Ellen Frances Olshansky, PhD, RN, WHNP-BC, FAAN
Professor Emerita
Sue and Bill Gross School of Nursing
Founding Director
Program in Nursing Science
University of California, Irvine
Irvine, California

Freida H. Outlaw, PhD, RN, MSN, FAAN
Executive Academic Program Consultant
Substance Abuse Mental Health Services Administration
American Nurses Association, Minority Fellowship
    Program
Silver Spring, Maryland

Danielle Howa Pendergrass, DNP, APRN, WHNP-BC
President
Access to Care
Eastern Utah Women's Health, LLC
Price, Utah

G. Adriana Perez, PhD, RN, CRNP, ANP-BC, FAAN, FGSA
Assistant Professor of Nursing
Family and Community Health
School of Nursing
Senior Fellow
Leonard Davis Institute of Health Economics
University of Pennsylvania
Philadelphia, Pennsylvania

Lynn Price, JD, MSN, MPH
Professor Emerita
Quinnipiac University
Hamden, Connecticut

Joyce A. Pulcini, PhD, RN, PNP-BC, FAAN, FAANP
Professor
School of Nursing
George Washington University
Washington, DC

Betty Rambur, PhD, RN, FAAN
Routhier Endowed Chair for Practice and Professor
    of Nursing
College of Nursing
University of Rhode Island
Kingston, Rhode Island

Susan C. Reinhard, PhD, RN, FAAN
Senior Vice President
Public Policy Institute
AARP
Washington, DC

Beth L. Rodgers, PhD, RN, FAAN
Professor and Chair
Adult Health and Nursing Systems
School of Nursing
Virginia Commonwealth University
Richmond, Virginia

Carol A. Romano, PhD, RN, FACMI, FAAN
Dean and Professor
Graduate School of Nursing
Uniformed Services University of the Health Sciences
Bethesda, Maryland

Nicole Rouhana, PhD, FNP-BC, CNM
Director of Graduate Nursing Programs
Decker School of Nursing
Binghamton University
Binghamton, New York

Carol F. Roye, RN, EdD, MS
Associate Dean for Faculty Scholarship
College of Health Professions
Pace University
Pleasantville, New York

Maria Elena Ruiz, PhD, RN, FNP-BC
Associate Adjunct Professor
School of Nursing
Faculty Affiliate
Chicano Studies Research Center
University of California, Los Angeles
Los Angeles, California

Sandra Whitley Ryals, MS, BSN, RN
Board Member
ANA-PAC Board of Trustees
Silver Spring, Maryland
Former State Agency Director
Virginia Department of Health Professions
Richmond, Virginia

Donna Sabella, PhD, MEd, MSN, PMHNP-BC
Seedworks Endowed Associate Professor of Nursing
University of Massachusetts, Amherst
Amherst, Massachusetts

Barbara J. Safriet, BA, JD, LLM
Resident Professor of Health Law and Policy
Lewis and Clark Law School
Portland, Oregon

Bonnie R. Sakallaris, PhD, RN
Vice President
Optimal Healing Environments
Thought Leadership and Innovation Foundation
McLean, Virginia
Adjunct Faculty
School of Nursing
George Washington University
Washington, DC

Jane E. Salvage, BA, MSc
Independent Consultant
Lewes, United Kingdom

Chelsea Savage, RN, DNP, MSHA, BA, CPHRM
Professional Liability Investigator
VCU Health
Richmond, Virginia

Hillary Schneller, JD
Staff Attorney
U.S. Legal Program
Center for Reproductive Rights
New York, New York

Mary Jean Schumann, DNP, MBA, CPNP-PC, FAAN
Associate Professor
School of Nursing
George Washington University
Washington, DC

Casey R. Shillam, PhD, RN
Dean
School of Nursing
University of Portland
Portland, Oregon

Joanne Spetz, PhD
Professor
Philip R. Lee Institute for Health Policy Studies
Associate Director for Research
Healthforce Center
University of California, San Francisco
San Francisco, California

Caroline Stephens, PhD, RN, GNP-BC, FAAN
Associate Professor
Department of Community Health Systems
School of Nursing
University of California, San Francisco
San Francisco, California

Sheila Cox Sullivan, PhD, RN
Director of Research EBP and Analytics
Office of Nursing Services
Department of Veterans Affairs, Central Office
Washington, DC

Susan Swider, PhD
Professor
Community, Systems, and Mental Health Nursing
Rush University
Chicago, Illinois

Kathleen E. Sykes, MA
Senior Advisor for Aging and Environmental Health (Retired)
Office of Research and Development
U.S. Environmental Protection Agency
Washington, DC

Carol R. Taylor, PhD, RN, MSN
Professor of Nursing and Medicine and Senior Clinical Scholar
Kennedy Institute of Ethics
Georgetown University
Washington, DC

Clifton P. Thornton, RN, MSN, BSN, BS, CNMT, CPNP
Pediatric Nurse Practitioner
Sidney Kimmel Comprehensive Cancer Center
Johns Hopkins University School of Medicine
Baltimore, Maryland

Valerie Tobin, RN, MS, PMHCNS-BC
PhD Student
College of Nursing
Rush University
Advanced Practice Nurse
Howard Brown Health
Chicago, Illinois

Linda M. Valentino, RN, MSN, NEA-BC
Vice President of Nursing Operations
Mount Sinai Hospital
New York, New York

Tener Goodwin Veenema, PhD, RN, MPH, MS, FAAN
Professor
Acute and Chronic Care
Johns Hopkins School of Nursing
Baltimore, Maryland

Laura M. Wagner, PhD, RN
Associate Professor
Community Health Systems
School of Nursing
University of California, San Francisco
San Francisco, California

Joanne Warner, PhD, BA, MA
Dean Emerita
School of Nursing
University of Portland
Portland, Oregon

Karin Elisabeth Warner, DNP, MS, MA
Professor, Acute and Tertiary Care
University of Pittsburgh
Pittsburgh, Pennsylvania

Deborah Washington, PhD, RN
Director of Diversity
Nursing and Patient Care Services
Massachusetts General Hospital
Boston, Massachusetts

Dorinda L. Welle, PhD
Assistant Professor
College of Nursing
University of New Mexico
Albuquerque, New Mexico

Kristi K. Westphaln, PhD, RN, CPNP-PC
Postdoctoral Fellow
Department of Pediatrics
School of Medicine
Case Western Reserve University
Cleveland, Ohio

Jill F. White, PhD, MEd, MHPol
Professor Emerita
Faculty of Nursing and Midwifery
University of Sydney
Sydney, Australia

Rita Wray, RN, BC, MBA, FAAN
Founder and Chief Executive Officer
Wray Enterprises, Inc.
Brandon, Mississippi

Heather M. Young, PhD, RN
Professor and Dean Emerita
Betty Irene Moore School of Nursing
University of California, Davis
Sacramento, California

Sarah Stover Filer Zollweg, BSN
Nurse Health Educator
Health Risk Reduction Services
University of Michigan
Ann Arbor, Michigan

REVIEWERS

Karen E. Alexander, PhD, RN, CNOR
Assistant Professor and Director
RN-BSN Program
Nursing—Clinical Health and Applied Sciences
University of Houston, Clearlake-Pearland
Pearland, Texas

Tammy Bryant, RN, MSN, Certification in Gerontology
Program Chair and Associate of Science in Nursing
Southern Regional Technical College
Thomasville, Georgia

Kathleen M. Burke, PhD, RN
Assistant Dean in Charge of Nursing and Professor of Nursing
Adler Center of Nursing Excellence
Ramapo College of New Jersey
Mahwah, New Jersey

Debrayh Gaylle, RN, MS, EdD
Assistant Professor of Nursing
San Jose State University
San Jose, California

Claudia M. Grobbel, RN, DNP, CNL
Associate Professor
School of Nursing
Oakland University
Rochester Hills, Michigan

Barbara Knopp, RN, MSN
Director of Nursing Programs
Edgecombe Community College
Rocky Mount, North Carolina

CONTENTS

UNIT 3 Policy and Politics in the Government

UNIT 4 Policy and Politics in the Workplace and Workforce

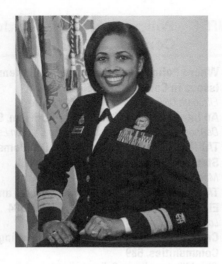

Our nation has made great progress in improving the health of its people over the last century, as have other nations. Many people assume it's because we have built a highly technological health care system that is able to provide the latest in diagnostic and treatment services. However, since 2015, our rates of maternal mortality have increased while life expectancy at birth has decreased. Racial and ethnic health disparities persist and are reflected in these two indicators of the health of the nation.

We know that improvements in nutrition, sanitation, seatbelt use, vaccinations, and other factors have been drivers of improvements in the nation's health, and these factors are shaped by public policies. Social determinants of health are again receiving the attention they deserve from local communities and the nation. However, more needs to be done, and the nation's nurses can and must be leaders in calling for health and social policies that will promote the health of communities, whether through economic development; quality education; reduction of crime and trauma; access to affordable and nutritious foods; preventing addictions to nicotine, opioids, and other substances; prevention of the spread of infectious diseases, including HIV; or other "upstream" measures.

As the Principal Deputy Assistant Secretary for Health in the U.S. Public Health Service, after serving as Acting U.S. Surgeon General and Deputy U.S. Surgeon General, I'm keenly aware of the important role that nurses can play in promoting the health of our nation. You don't have to be Acting Surgeon General to do so! Even if you're working in acute care, you see the effects of unhealthy lifestyles and communities on the lives of individuals and families and can provide a voice to move organizations and communities to address social determinants. And how healthy is the community in which you live? Think about what would happen to this nation if every nurse became a local or regional leader in creating public policies that will foster health.

Policy & Politics in Nursing and Health Care is the classic book for helping nurses to understand how policymaking and politics work, to acquire tools for shaping these policies, and to learn about contemporary issues related to health and social policy. The importance of this book in developing the next generation of nurse leaders in policy cannot be overstated, but it's not the only tool you'll need. Honing your policy and political skills requires action. I'm doing what I can to be a leader and hope that you will join me in being the nurse leaders our nation needs.

Rear Admiral Sylvia Trent-Adams, PhD, RN, FAAN

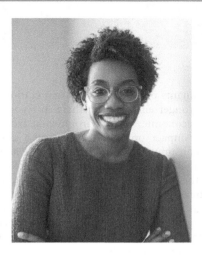

Growing up in Naperville, Illinois, being a Girl Scout was part of my identity. I remember being a young girl and taking the pledge "to help people at all times." I couldn't have predicted how that would play out into a future career of service, continuing from a Girl Scout to a nurse, and then to serving my community as a member of the House of Representatives.

During a swimming lesson when I was 8 years old, I discovered I had a heart condition, supraventricular tachycardia, which occasionally prevents my heart from maintaining a normal rhythm. I saw my Girl Scout pledge come to life through the providers who helped me during my initial treatment. They made a lasting impression on me and inspired me to pursue nursing so I could help people too. I went to the University of Michigan for my nursing degree and completed a joint Master's degree in nursing and public health from Johns Hopkins University in Baltimore.

My path to policy was forged during my undergraduate years in nursing school when I took a course on nursing politics that changed my life and motivated me to engage in policy work. So, I took my personal experience as a patient as well as my nursing education and training to work for the Obama Administration as a Senior Advisor in the Department of Health and Human Services, assisting in public health emergencies like the Ebola epidemic in 2014 and the water crisis in Flint, Michigan in 2016.

Serving in the Obama Administration and later working to implement the Affordable Care Act helped solidify my values and fed my passion to make quality health care more affordable for American families. Shortly after I left the Administration, I knew I wanted to continue that work, and I decided to run for Congress. In January 2019, I was sworn in as the first woman and the first person of color to represent my community, and as one of only two nurses to serve in the 116th Congress. Since my very first day, I've been fighting to advance policies that expand access to health care and improve the health of individuals, families, and communities like the one I represent in Illinois.

Whether serving as health care providers, community leaders, or even policymakers, nurses across this country are in a position to boldly lead. In partnership with the Robert Wood Johnson Foundation, The National Academies of Science, Engineering, and Medicine (formerly the Institute of Medicine) will be launching a new study, *The Future of Nursing 2020-2030*. This groundbreaking publication will build on the first *Future of Nursing* report to outline the role of nurses in creating a culture of healthy people and neighborhoods. The new study will examine the role of nurses in building healthy communities through a holistic approach that considers issues like training, care delivery, and solutions to address disparities.

The country needs new leaders who can make progress on the issues that matter to our communities, and there is no one better than nurses to lead the way. Our patients, their families, and their communities are counting on us. This book serves as a guide to policy and politics in nursing and health care. I was proud to be one of the contributors in the sixth edition of this classic book, and I know that the eighth edition will inspire many nurses, nursing students, faculty, and researchers to develop their knowledge and skills in using policy to promote the nation's health.

Representative Lauren Underwood, MSN, MPH, RN

PREFACE

As the prior edition of *Policy & Politics in Nursing and Health Care* (seventh edition) was going to press, the Patient Protection and Affordable Care Act (ACA) had become the law of the land. Despite significant progress in reducing the nation's number of people who are uninsured or underinsured, subsequent changes in our political landscape brought changes to the ACA that have undermined, instead of strengthened, the law. Once again, our nation seems poised to have the worst record of any developed nation on access to health care, the quality of much of that care, and the health of the population.

The 2016 elections brought a significant change in federal leadership, followed by a midterm election that saw an unprecedented number of women running for office at local, state, and national levels. More women were elected to the House of Representatives than ever before, including a registered nurse, Lauren Underwood (see the Foreword by Representative Underwood). During a time when science is too easily dismissed or discounted, nurses' voices are crucial to shape evidence-based policies that improve the quality of health care, improve access to that care, and promote the health of individuals, families, and communities.

Because we live in politically polarizing times, we thought it important to be explicit with the values and assumptions that we shared in developing this edition:

1. *Health care is a right, not a privilege.* We know the scientific evidence and have witnessed firsthand what happens when people don't have access to health care. They die prematurely, are disabled unnecessarily, lose jobs, go into bankruptcy, and struggle to provide for themselves and their families. The United States is the only developed nation that fails to ensure that all of its people have access to health care, and our outcomes for the uninsured and the communities in which they live show it, including having a compromised workforce.

2. *Health disparities persist in American society and must be reduced.* The United States is the only developed nation in which longevity of the population is decreasing and maternal mortality is increasing. This is particularly true for people of color and those living in poverty. A healthy nation focuses on all of its people, not just on those already advantaged.

3. *Social factors play a larger role in shaping the health of families and communities.* Although the seventh edition of the book incorporated a focus on the social

determinants of health, the current edition places an even stronger emphasis on them in recognition that social, economic, and environmental factors have a greater impact on health than health care. Health care's consumption of approximately 18% of the U.S. gross domestic product is undermining efforts to promote the health of families and communities rather than treating preventable illnesses—and at a very high price in humanistic and monetary terms. We believe that, regardless of where a nurse works (whether acute care, long-term care, school health, or other setting), all of us must be leaders in embracing a population health perspective that incorporates these other factors in our daily work.

4. *Nurses are the most trusted profession by the public and must live up to this honor by leading change in the communities where we live, work, play, and learn.* This is a value expressed by contributing authors throughout the current edition of *Policy & Politics in Nursing and Health Care.* There are myriad examples of nurses leading change in health and social policies to improve health, and we have incorporated some of them here. We encourage readers to seek out other examples in your own communities, health care settings, the policy world, and elsewhere. *The Future of Nursing 2020-2030* is underway as we go to press and is expected to highlight nurses' roles in building a culture of health and addressing social determinants of health, and recommend that more of us step up to be leaders in this space. Florence Nightingale, Harriet Tubman, and Lillian Wald are nurses from our history whose work illustrates that such leadership is part of our legacy. We issue the challenge to all readers to advance their work and continue in their footsteps.

This book reflects these assumptions in most chapters, but not all. We did not seek to invite only contributors who might agree with our assumptions. Rather, we expected them to provide the evidence for their positions and recommendations.

This eighth edition of *Policy & Politics in Nursing and Health Care* aims to help nurses explore the problems that impede health in our nation and globally, learn the best evidence available about policy options that are likely to successfully address these problems, and develop their political and policy acumen. As with prior editions, the book's target audience is novice to expert—whether undergraduate, masters or doctoral students, or practicing nurses. Some chapters provide the basics of policymaking and politics, whereas others delve more deeply into the nuances of specific policy matters and political strategy. We have placed a stronger emphasis on the implications of the issues discussed for advanced practice nurses, including those pursuing or holding the doctorate of nursing practice (DNP). The DNP was designed to prepare nurses as clinical leaders who could develop evidence-based approaches to improving the health of specific populations, and policy *is* a population health intervention. However, we maintain that every nurse has a social responsibility to shape public and private policies to promote health.

Although the book is organized around a framework, it is not designed to be read only from start to finish. Rather, we encourage readers to explore the table of contents and search for those topics about which they want to learn more. We hope the book will guide nursing students and nurses who are policy novices throughout their journey of engagement in the world of policy and politics.

WHAT'S NEW IN THE EIGHTH EDITION?

This edition continues the almost 35-year approach of prior editions that have led others to describe the book as a "classic" in nursing literature. However, classics become stagnant if not refreshed. A new team of editors has brought a fresh perspective to this edition. The order of authorship on the cover does not reflect effort; rather, the editing of this book was truly a team effort.

Central to the changes in this edition are:

- Updates on the ACA and its implementation, its impact on nursing and the health of people, the role of politics in our health care system, and the need for further policy reforms.
- As noted previously, the importance of addressing upstream factors or social determinants of health is a major theme.
- In response to the mistrust of science and facts in some circles, authors have provided more depth and breadth to the evidence that undergirds policy issues and potential responses, with the understanding that evidence is necessary, but often not sufficient, for policy change.
- New and updated Taking Action chapters provide real-life examples of nurses' activism. For example, the Taking Action on Removing APRN Regulatory Barriers in West Virginia can serve as a case study on political strategy when in a polarized political environment.
- All of the chapters have been updated. For example, the chapter on media provides greater depth on the

political context of media in our times to help readers to understand how to use media in credible ways. Other chapters have been significantly revised by new authors, with fresh perspectives on topics such as:

- Primary care
- Nursing education
- Using research to advance health and social policies
- Highlights of the ACA, with implications for nurses and other health professionals
- The politics of advanced practice nursing
- Ethical dimensions of policy and politics
- Patient engagement
- Overtreatment
- Women's reproductive health
- Public health
- Emergency preparedness
- Developing families
- Nurses in boardrooms
- Quality and safety in health care
- Nurses' work environments
- The intersection of technology and health care
- Community-based organizations addressing health
- School nursing
- American Indian/Alaska Native policy issues

USING THE EIGHTH EDITION

Using the book as a course text. Faculty will find content in this book that will enhance learning experiences in policy, leadership, community activism, administration, research, health disparities, and other key issues and trends of importance to courses at every educational level. Many of the chapters will help students in clinical courses understand the dynamics of the health system. Students will find chapters that assist them in developing new skills, building a broader understanding of nursing leadership and influence, and making sense of the complex business and financial forces that drive many actions in the health system. In particular, the Taking Action chapters provide examples of nurses taking on real-world policy challenges. The book presents an in-depth view of the issues that impact nurses and suggests a variety of opportunities for nurses to engage in the policy issues about which they care deeply.

Using the book in government activities. The unit on policy and politics in the government includes content that will benefit nurses considering running for elective office, seeking a political appointment, and learning to lobby elective officials about health care issues.

Using the book in the workplace. Policy problems and political issues abound in nursing workplaces. This book offers critical insights into how to effectively resolve problems and influence workplace policy as well as how to develop politically astute approaches to making changes in the workplace.

Using the book in professional organizations. Organizations use the power of numbers. The unit on associations and interest groups will help groups determine strategies

for success and how to capitalize on working with other groups through coalitions.

Using the book in community activism. With an expanded focus on community advocacy and activism, readers will find information they need to effectively influence policy solutions to problems in their local communities, along with global perspectives.

ACKNOWLEDGMENTS

In every edition of this book, the co-editors have expressed their sincere gratitude to the many authors who have contributed their time and expertise to write a chapter out of a commitment to furthering the education of nurses and other health professionals on policy and politics. This edition is no exception. We are grateful for the thoughtful contributions of more than 120 authors and hope that readers will learn from them.

We are also grateful for the enduring contributions and imprint of the prior co-editors of this book that have made it the leading resource in its field. Susan Talbott was the co-editor on the first edition; Mary Chaffee on the fourth through sixth editions; Judith Leavitt on the second through sixth editions; and Frieda Outlaw, Eileen O'Grady, and Deborah Gardner on the seventh edition. We hope that they are pleased with the continued development of the book.

We owe a huge debt of thanks to Bryan Jackson, the book's editorial manager for this edition. He tracked our work, kept the co-editors moving along, coordinated our communications, and was simply amazingly organized. He did all of this while a student, working multiple jobs, and always being a supportive voice. Bryan, we are grateful for your superb work.

We also acknowledge the continuing support of Elsevier and the editorial team that worked with Sandra Clark and Lisa Newton. We are indebted to Clay Broeker, an extraordinary production manager who has worked on the last four editions of the book. Thank you, Clay, for your continued commitment to excellence in publishing.

Each of us has some special people to acknowledge.

Diana Mason

First, I am incredibly grateful to this new team of co-editors who as mid-career colleagues are unafraid to question the book's longstanding approaches and assumptions. They also worked superbly well as a team. This and their vision for nursing and health in our nation give me hope for nursing's future. I also want to acknowledge my husband, James Ware, for his continued support of my long days of work on this book and to my loving dog, Ricky, for his tolerance of walks delayed or missed.

Elizabeth Dickson

I would like to thank my husband, Jeff, and sons, T. and J., whose continued love, patience, and unconditional support leaves me speechless—words seem to fail me every time I try to express my gratitude. My deepest respect and thanks to our friends, family, and community that surround and support us. To Diana, thank you for opening this door for us to join you on this adventure; and to Monica, Adriana, and Bryan—this incredible group of colleagues—thank you for your hard work and dedication.

Monica R. McLemore

I would like to thank Diana Mason for the opportunity to work with these incredibly brilliant scholars and colleagues—it has been an experience of a lifetime. I also give thanks to the ancestors who make my existence possible. Finally, I am extremely thankful to my partner James and his careful support and stewardship of Aife (the dog) and Bella and Catness (the cats), as well as the kittens Brutus and Sirius, while I wrestled with fulfilling my tasks while standing on the shoulders of the previous editorial team.

G. Adriana Perez

I am honored to have worked with such dynamic scholars. Diana Mason, I appreciate you and the opportunity you have given us to learn from you and each other. I thank my family for inspiring me—my mother who came to this country as a young immigrant in pursuit of a better life and grandmother who was a nurse in Mexico. I am grateful to the love of my life, Nick, for always making me laugh. Gracias to my research participants, patients, and students for reminding me that in order to fully achieve a healthier future for all, we must link our research to practice and policy.

1

Frameworks for Action in Policy and Politics

Diana J. Mason, Elizabeth Dickson, Monica R. McLemore,
and G. Adriana Perez

"The most common way people give up their power is by thinking they don't have any."

Alice Walker

When Lauren Underwood was a young girl, she found out that she had supraventricular tachycardia for which she was treated. The health professionals who provided her initial treatment so inspired Underwood that she became a registered nurse. She is one of millions of Americans with a preexisting condition that made health insurance inaccessible for many people before the Affordable Care Act (ACA). Prior to that landmark legislation that reduced the number of people who were uninsured by 20 million (Kaiser Family Foundation [KFF], 2018), insurance companies could have either denied Underwood coverage or charged so much for a health plan that it would be unaffordable. After the 2016 elections, President Donald Trump and a Republican-controlled Congress renewed efforts to roll back the ACA under campaign promises to "repeal and replace Obamacare." A number of executive and legislative actions were taken to undo key features of the law, among them proposals to get rid of protections for people with preexisting conditions. At a community meeting hosted by the League of Women Voters, Congressman Randy Hultgren (R-IL), Underwood's congressional representative at the time, promised he would only support legislation repealing Obamacare that protected coverage for people with preexisting conditions. He then proceeded to vote for the 2017 American Healthcare Act that included ending the preexisting condition protections. Underwood was in the audience and decided to act. She ran for Congress.

As a Black nurse from Illinois who lived in a Republican-dominated congressional district, Underwood conducted a grassroots campaign that took her to some all-White neighborhoods and households that may never have considered voting for a person of color for their congressional representative. Underwood spoke directly to the benefits of the ACA, first as a nurse who had seen what happens to people who do not have health insurance and cannot afford care; and second, as a former special adviser to the U.S. Department of Health and Human Services during the Obama administration. She showed that she understood the issues that people cared about (health care, including mental health; jobs; and family) and was skilled in interacting with people.

Against the odds, Underwood defeated six Democratic men in the primary elections and then became the public face of the dramatic 2018 midterm elections in which Democrats took back control of the U.S. House of Representatives. She is regarded as one of the smart, new women leaders in our federal government and joins fellow nurses Eddie Bernice Johnson (D-TX), the first nurse to be elected to Congress; and Karen Bass (D-CA), a member of Congress since 2011. She follows another nurse, Diane Black (R-TN), who lost her bid for reelection in 2018.

These nurses are not alone in serving in important policymaking positions:

- Dawn Adams won another race-against-the-odds for Virginia's state assembly (see Chapter 43);
- Bethany Hall-Long became the Lieutenant-Governor of Delaware after serving for a number of years in the state's legislature (see Chapter 47);
- Rear Admiral Sylvia Trent-Adams served as the nation's Acting Surgeon General in the first year of the Trump Administration and then as Deputy Surgeon General (see Chapter 44 and the Foreword);
- Mary Wakefield was appointed by President Barak Obama to be the Acting Deputy Secretary of Health and Human Services after heading up its Health Resources and Services Administration;
- Erin Murphy has served in the Minnesota legislature and ran for Governor in 2018.

It seems that some nurses have awakened to their potential for shaping and leading the development of health and social policies in their own communities, states, and the nation. However, serving in an elected or appointed political office is not the only way to influence the development and implementation of health policy. The work that nurses do every day—the care and advocacy for patients, their families, and communities—and the lives we live, along with the places we work, play, and love, are shaped by local, state, and national policies. The forces of policy that form our lives as constituents and nurses are real—policy is being made around us constantly, in Washington, DC, in our state capitols, and in our local city halls. It is time for us to seize the opportunities for shaping our worlds. This chapter provides a foundation for learning how policy and its political context can be advanced to promote the health of individuals, families, communities, and nations.

FOCUS ON POLICY: WHAT POLICY?

Many nurses and others in health care often think of policy as "health policy" or "health care policy." The ACA is an example of a major federal policy that aimed to improve people's access to health care, particularly through providing affordable health coverage for essential services. However, access to coverage does not necessarily mean access to care, nor does it ensure a healthy population. Health care access means having the ability to receive the right type of care, when needed, at an affordable price.

The U.S. health care system is grounded in expensive, high-tech acute care that does not produce the desired health outcomes we ought to have and want and too often damages instead of heals. Despite spending more per person on health care than any other nation, the United States performs worse than other nations on most indicators of quality, efficiency, access, and other organizational performance measures (Papanicolas, Woskie, & Jha, 2018; Schneider, et al., 2017), and preventable medical errors are estimated to be the third leading cause of death in the country (Makary & Daniel, 2016). The nation also ranks at the bottom on certain health outcomes, including life expectancy at birth for both men and women, infant mortality rate, mortality rates for suicide and cardiovascular disease, and the prevalence of diabetes and obesity in children (National Research Council, 2013).

THE AFFORDABLE CARE ACT

The ACA included elements to change this picture by focusing on creating more value in health care, improving care coordination, expanding access to coverage or health insurance, and reforming how we pay for care. Fig. 1.1 illustrates these four cornerstones. The ACA aimed to move the health care system in the direction of keeping people out of hospitals, in their own homes and communities, with an emphasis on wellness, health promotion, and better management of chronic illnesses. In addition, it included provisions to hold hospitals and other health care organizations accountable for both their spending and outcomes.

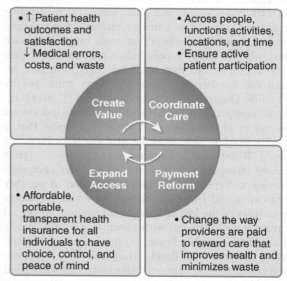

Fig. 1.1 Four cornerstones of reform. (From O'Grady, E. T., & Johnson, J. [2013]. Health policy issues in changing environments. In A. Hamric, C. Hanson, D. Way, & E. O'Grady [Eds.], *Advanced practice nursing: An integrative approach* [5th ed.]. St. Louis, MO: Elsevier Saunders.)

The ACA is arguably the most significant piece of social legislation passed in the United States since the enactment of Medicare and Medicaid in 1965 (see Chapter 18 for a detailed discussion of the ACA). Implementation continues to be a vexing process that requires tweaking, much as the Social Security Act did when it was passed in 1965 (Social Security Administration, n.d.). But the ACA became a political flashpoint, defining the ideologies of U.S. political parties. Democrats committed to the law but called for refining it, whereas Republicans overtook the House of Representatives in 2012 with calls for "repealing and replacing Obamacare." The public remained largely uninformed and misinformed about the legislation; 3 years after its passage, 4 out of 10 Americans were still unaware of many of its provisions and unsure that the ACA had become law (KFF, 2013). When the Trump Administration began to use executive orders to scale back and reverse regulations for implementing the ACA, the public became confused about whether the ACA and Obamacare were the same thing. Most of those who now had health coverage under the ACA wanted to keep their insurance but did not realize that this was Obamacare (Dropp & Nyhan, 2017). Confusion is likely to continue as attacks on the ACA persist. In 2018 a federal court in Texas ruled that the ACA was unconstitutional, a decision that was reviewed by the Fifth Circuit Court of Appeals and may go to the Supreme Court. In 2019, the U.S. Department of Justice said that it would support the Texas court's decision, despite the department's usual practice of defending federal laws.

UPSTREAM FACTORS: SOCIAL DETERMINANTS OF HEALTH

Promoting health requires more than a high-performing health care system (Tilden et al., 2018). First and foremost, health is created where people live, love, work, learn, worship, and play. It is becoming clear that one's health status may be more dependent on one's zip code than on one's genetic code (Graham, 2016). Geographic analyses of race and ethnicity, income, and health status repeatedly show that financial, racial, and ethnic inequities persist (Marmot & Allen, 2014). There are multiple ways in which exposure to structural racism has been shown to harm the physical, social, and economic health of individuals, families, and communities (Bailey et al., 2017). More so, the health of individuals and families is severely compromised in communities where good education, nutritious foods, safe places to exercise, and well-paying jobs are scarce (Artiga & Hinton, 2018). Creating a healthier nation requires that we address "upstream factors"—the broad range of issues, other than health care, that can undermine or promote health—also known as "social determinants of health" (World Health Organization [WHO], n.d.). Upstream factors promoting health include safe environments, adequate housing, economically thriving communities with employment opportunities, access to affordable and healthful foods, and models for addressing conflict through dialogue rather than violence (Fig. 1.2). The

Economic stability	Neighborhood and physical environment	Education	Food	Community and social context	Health care system
Employment	Housing	Literacy	Hunger	Social integration	Health coverage
Income	Transportation	Language	Access to healthy options	Support systems	Provider availability
Expenses	Safety	Early childhood education		Community engagement	Provider linguistic and cultural competency
Debt	Parks	Vocational training		Discrimination	
Medical bills	Playgrounds	Higher education		Stress	Quality of care
Support	Walkability				
	Zip code/ geography				

Health outcomes
Mortality, morbidity, life expectancy, health care expenditures, health status, functional limitations

Fig. 1.2 Social determinants of health. (From Artiga, S., & Hinton, E. [2018]. *Beyond health care: The role of social determinants in promoting health and health equity. Henry J Kaiser Family Foundation.* Retrieved from www.kff.org/disparities-policy/issue-brief/beyond-health-care-the-role-of-social-determinants-in-promoting-health-and-health-equity/.)

key to reducing and eliminating health disparities, which disproportionately affect racial and ethnic minorities, is to provide effective interventions that address upstream factors both from within and outside of health care systems.

There is growing recognition that even the health care system has to change its model from one that is strictly biomedical to one that recognizes that health is in large part determined by psychosocial factors (Adler et al., 2016). How does someone with diabetes successfully manage their condition if they are homeless, without refrigeration for insulin or access to healthy food or safe parks for physical activity? A focus on such factors is essential for economic and moral reasons. Even in the most affluent nations, those living in poverty have substantially shorter life expectancies and experience more illness than those who are wealthy, resulting in high costs in human and financial terms (Khullar & Chokshi, 2018). However, most of the focus on reducing disparities, including socioeconomic ones, has been on health policy that addresses access, coverage, cost, and quality of care once the individual has entered the health care system—despite the fact that most health care problems begin long before people seek medical care (Williams et al., 2008). Thus changing our nation's poor performance on health care and the health of its people requires knowledge about the political aspects of the social determinates of health. Political aspects of the social determinants of health appear in Box 1.1.

The ACA began to carve out a role for the health care system in addressing upstream factors. For example, the law requires that nonprofit hospitals do more to demonstrate a "community benefit" to maintain their federal tax breaks than they have had to do in the past. Hospitals must conduct a community health assessment, develop a community health improvement plan, and partner with others to implement it. This aligns with a growing emphasis on population health: the health of a group, whether defined by a common disease or health problem or by geographic or demographic characteristics (Felt-Lisk & Higgins, 2011). This focus on the health of populations within their respective communities is key for all health care organizations.

To improve the health of the U.S. population *and* reduce health care costs, we must build in to the health care system better ways to address social determinants of health and to enhance health promotion and wellness, disease prevention, and chronic care management—all essential components of primary care (Wagner, 1998; Starfield, 1998; Rowe et al., 2016). Nurses are critical to this shift from disease care to preventing illnesses, promoting health, and coordinating health care. A 2017 report by the Josiah Macy, Jr. Foundation called for a more robust, primary care

---

BOX 1.1 Political Aspects of the Social Determinants of Health

- The health of individuals and populations is determined significantly by social factors.
- The social determinants of health produce great inequities in health within and between societies.
- The poor and disadvantaged experience worse health than the rich, have less access to care, and die younger in all societies.
- The social determinants of health can be measured and described.
- The measurement of the social determinants provides evidence that can serve as the basis for political action.
- Evidence is generated and used in a continuous cycle of evidence production, policy development, implementation, and evaluation.
- Evidence of the effects of policies and programs on inequities can be measured and can provide data on the effectiveness of interventions.
- Evidence regarding the social determinants of health is insufficient to bring about change on its own; political will combined with evidence offers the most powerful strategy to address the negative effects of the social determinants.

Adapted from National Institute for Health and Clinical Excellence. (2007). *The social determinants of health: Developing an evidence base for political action. Final report to the World Health Organization Commission on the Social Determinants of Health.* Lead authors: J. Mackenbach, M. Exworthy, J. Popay, P. Tugwell, V. Robinson, S. Simpson, T. Narayan, L. Myer, T. Houweling, L. Jadue, and F. Florenza.

---

system, one that builds its capacity by using registered nurses—and not just advanced practice registered nurses (APRNs)—as care team leaders who practice at the top of their education and training, with a responsibility for these foci (Bodenheimer & Mason, 2017).

For decades, nurses have led changes in health promotion and health care delivery but without naming or measuring their activities. However, there are notable exceptions to this invisibility. The American Academy of Nursing's *Raise the Voice Campaign* (American Academy of Nursing, n.d.) has identified nurses who have developed innovative models of care for which there are good clinical and financial outcome data. Known as "Edge Runners," these nurses have demonstrated that nursing's emphasis on care coordination, health promotion, patient- and family-centeredness, and the community context of care provides evidence-based models that can help to transform the health care system (Mason, Jones, Roy, Sullivan, & Wood, 2015). Many also address social determinants of health (Martsolf, Sloan, Villarruel, Sullivan, & Mason, 2018). Some of these models of care were included as programs to scale up under the ACA: transitional care, the Living Independent for Elders; home visitation programs for high-risk pregnant women (Nurse-Family Partnership); and nurse-managed health centers (NMHCs).

Consider the 11th Street Family Health Services, a federally qualified NMHC located in an underserved neighborhood in North Philadelphia. Public health nurse Patricia Gerrity, a faculty member at Drexel University School of Nursing and founder of 11th Street, recognized that the leading health problems in this community were diabetes, obesity, heart failure, and depression. Working with a community advisory group, Gerrity focused on addressing access to nutrition as an "upstream factor" to improve the health of those living in the community. With no supermarket in the neighborhood until 2011, she invited area farmers to the neighborhood to provide a farmers' market, created a community vegetable garden maintained by the local youth, and invited area residents to attend nutrition classes on culturally relevant, healthy cooking. Subsequently under the leadership of nurse Roberta Waite and endowed as the Stephen and Sandra Sheller 11th Street Family Health Services, it is leading the way as one of more than 200 NMHCs in the United States that have improved clinical and financial outcomes by addressing the needs of individuals, families, and communities (American Academy of Nursing, n.d., b; Martsolf, Sloan, Mason, Sullivan, & Villarruel, 2017). Although the ACA authorized continued support for NMHCs, the law did not mandate funding and Congress did not appropriate funding for them (see Chapter 31 for a more detailed discussion of NMHCs and primary care.)

The ACA did not go far enough in shifting attention from acute care to promoting the health of communities and populations. Another approach to this shift is that of "health in all policies," the idea that policymakers consider the health implications of social and economic policies that focus on other sectors, such as education, community development, tax codes, and housing (Rudolph et al., 2013). As health professionals who focus on the family and community context of the patients they serve, nurses can raise questions about the potential health impact of public policies in every environment in which they work.

The Quadruple Aim

In 2008, Don Berwick and his colleagues at the Institute for Healthcare Improvement (IHI) first described the *Triple Aim* of a value-based health care system (Berwick, Nolan, & Whittington, 2008): (1) improving population health, (2) improving the patient experience of care, and (3) reducing per capita costs. This framework aligned with the ACA and later was modified to be the Quadruple Aim to include the dimension of clinician and staff satisfaction in recognition that "care of the patient requires care of the provider" (Bodenheimer & Sinsky, 2014).

The Quadruple Aim represents a balanced approach: by examining a health care delivery problem from all four dimensions, health care organizations and society can identify system problems and direct resources to activities that can have the greatest impact. Looking at each of these dimensions in isolation prevents organizations from discovering how a new objective—for instance, decreasing readmission rates to improve quality and reduce costs—could negatively impact the aim of population health, as scarce community resources are directed to acute care transitions and unintentionally shifted away from prevention activities. Solutions must also be evaluated from these four interdependent dimensions. The Quadruple Aim compels delivery systems and payers to broaden their focus on acute and highly specialized care toward more integrated care, including primary and preventive care (McCarthy & Klein, 2010).

The IHI (n.d.) identified these components of any approach seeking to achieve the Triple Aim:
- a focus on individuals and families
- a redesign of primary care services
- population health management
- a cost-control platform
- system integration and execution

Note that these address the goal of creating a high-performing health care system but do not focus on geographic communities or social determinants per se. However, these two concepts can be incorporated into the Quadruple Aim of improving the health of populations and reducing health care costs (Billioux, Verlander, Anthony, & Alley, 2017).

The success of the nursing profession's continued evolution will hinge on its ability to address the Quadruple Aim by taking on new roles, more creatively engaging with patients, and stepping into executive and leadership roles in every sector of heath care, society, and government. Nurses must do this work from an interprofessional context, leading efforts to break down health professions' silos and hierarchies and keeping the patient and family at the center of care.

NURSING AND HEALTH AND SOCIAL POLICY

Health policy affects every nurse's daily practice. Indeed, health policy determines who gets what type of health care, when, how, from whom, and at what cost. The study of health policy is an indispensable component of professional development in nursing, whether it is undertaken to advance a healthier society, promote a safer health care system, or support nursing's ability to care for people with equity and skill. Just as Florence Nightingale understood that health policy held the key to improving the health of the poor and the military, so are today's nurses needed to create compelling cases and actively influence better health policies at every level of governance—as Congresswoman Lauren Underwood understood. With national attention focused on how to transform health care in ways that produce better outcomes and reduce health care costs, nursing has an unprecedented opportunity to provide proactive and visionary leadership. But will we do so?

A 2018 study found that nurses were cited as sources in only 2% of health news stories and never in stories on policy (Mason et al., 2018). In a companion study, health journalists attributed this invisibility, in part, to nurses' reluctance to respond to requests for interviews, nursing journals' failure to promote the important research they publish, and nursing associations being largely invisible to newsrooms (Mason, Glickstein, & Westphaln, 2018). However, the journalists pointed out that they, their newsrooms, and the public relations staff in health care organizations and universities are biased about women, nurses, and positions of authority in health care. As the largest health care profession and one that remains comprised predominantly of women, nursing has great potential power but faces social barriers that persist amid societal inaccuracies about nurses' expertise and roles. The #MeToo movement may help to make such biases visible and help to ameliorate them, but nurses have to be proactive in changing them.

The Institute of Medicine's (IOM, now National Academy of Medicine) landmark report, *The Future of Nursing: Leading Change, Advancing Health* (2011), noted that nurses are essential for transforming health and health care in the nation. The report called for nurses to be leaders in redesigning health care and to be at all decision-making tables on health and health care. An interim evaluation of progress made on the report's recommendations found evidence of progress but noted that more attention needed to be given to developing nurses' leadership skills (National Academies of Science, Engineering, and Medicine, 2016). This is certainly the case in the policy arena, although the examples of nurse leaders in policy that we have cited provide encouragement and role models for us all.

POLICY AND THE POLICY PROCESS

What do we mean by policy? *Policy* has been defined as the authoritative decisions made in the legislative, executive, or judicial branches of government intended to influence the actions, behaviors, or decisions of citizens (Longest, 2010). However, that definition limits its application to sectors outside of government. For example, health care organizations set policy that affects employees, patients, and even surrounding communities (e.g., by closing a neighborhood clinic or buying property for hospital expansion). Thus a broader definition of *policy* is "a relatively stable, purposive course of action or inaction followed by an actor or set of actors in dealing with a problem or matter of concern" (Anderson, 2015, p. 6).

Public policy is policy crafted by governments. When the intent of a public policy is to influence health or health care, it is a *health policy. Social policies* identify courses of action to deal with social problems. All are made within a dynamic environment and a complex policymaking process. *Private policies* are those made by nongovernmental entities, whether health care organizations, insurers, or others. Indeed, there is growing recognition that policies set by health care organizations and insurers, for example, can limit APRN practice even in states that have removed laws requiring physician supervision or collaboration. A hospital can limit what registered nurses and APRNs do as long as the organization does not call for nurses to practice beyond the state's scope-of-practice policy.

Policies are crafted everywhere, from small towns to Capitol Hill. States use policies to specify requirements for health professions' licensure, to set criteria for Medicaid eligibility, and to require immunization for public university students, for example. Hospitals use policies to direct when visitors may visit patients, to manage staffing, and to respond to disasters. Public schools use state policies to specify who may administer medications to schoolchildren and what may be sold from a school vending machine. Towns, cities, and other municipalities use policies to manage public water, to define who may run for office, and to decide if residents may keep exotic pets.

In a capitalist economy such as that of the United States, private markets can control the production and consumption of goods and services, including health care. The government often "intervenes" with policies when private markets have failed to achieve desired public objectives. But when is it necessary for the government to intercede? Broadly speaking, in the current U.S. political system, the divide between liberal and conservative political parties is a fundamental disagreement about the degree to which government can and should solve problems (Kelly, 2004) in education, national security, the environment, and nearly every other aspect of public life (see Chapter 6 on Political Philosophy and Chapter 37 on Policy and Politics in Government). The American political landscape is continuously shifting, as public mood shifts with new members of Congress being elected and senior members wanting to stay in office.

Longest (2010) describes two types of public policies the government develops:

- *Allocative policies* provide benefits to a distinct group of individuals or organizations, at the expense of others, to achieve a public objective (this is also referred to as the *redistribution of wealth*). The enactment of Medicare in 1965 was an allocative policy that provided health benefits to older adults using federal funds (largely from middle- and high-income taxpayers).
- *Regulatory policies* influence the actions, behavior, and decisions of individuals or groups to ensure that a public objective is met. The Health Insurance Portability and Accountability Act (HIPAA) of 1996 regulates health care privacy or how individually identifiable health information is managed by users, as well as other aspects of health records.

Policymaking is an often-unpredictable dance that requires a high degree of political competence. Our system is based on continuous policy modification—incremental change is exceedingly more likely than revolutionary change. However, there are exceptions; once in a generation, a large social program is passed, such as Medicare and Medicaid in the 1960s and the ACA in 2010.

FORCES THAT SHAPE HEALTH AND SOCIAL POLICY

Some of the most prominent forces that shape health policy appear in Fig. 1.3.

Values

Values undergird proposed and adopted policies and influence all political and policymaking activities. Public policies reflect a society's values and also its conflicts in values. A policy reflects which values are given priority in a specific decision (Kraft & Furlong, 2017). Once framed, a policy reveals the underlying values that shaped it. Different people value different things, and when resources are finite, policy choices ultimately bring a disadvantage to some groups;

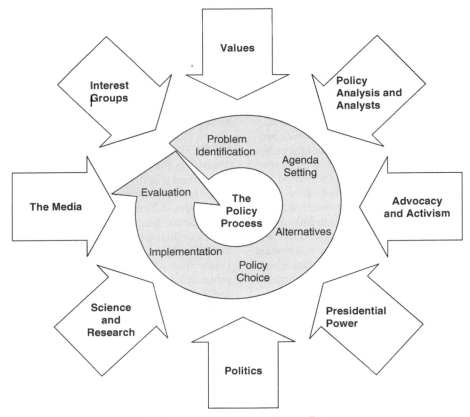

Fig. 1.3 The forces that shape policy.

some will gain something from the policy, and some will lose. To support or oppose a policy requires value judgments (Majone, 1992). Conflicts between values were apparent throughout the debates on the ACA. For example, despite a strong contingent of advocates for a government-run, non-profit insurance option that would compete with private insurers, the insurance industry opposed it, as did others who saw it as an increase in government control, and it was not included in the law but continued to be discussed during the Democratic 2020 presidential campaign.

Politics

Politics is the use of relationships and power to gain ascendancy among competing stakeholders to influence policy and the allocation of scarce resources. Because inevitably there are competing interests for scarce resources, policy-making is done within a political context.

The definition of politics contains several important concepts. *Influencing* indicates that there are opportunities to shape the outcome of a process. *Allocation* means that decisions are being made about how to distribute resources. *Scarce* implies the limits to available resources and that all parties probably cannot have all they want. Finally, *resources* are usually considered to be financial but could also include human resources (personnel), time, or physical space such as offices.

Engaging in the political context of policymaking includes knowing the positions of key stakeholders and political parties, as well as the electoral process, public opinion, the influence of media coverage, and more (see Chapter 8 for a discussion of political analysis and strategies). Understanding politics is an invitation not to misuse power, people, or information but rather align the health of the public with the interest of the policymaker. For example, a congresswoman may have run her campaign focused on improving the economy. She may not have linked the rising obesity epidemic as a threat to the larger macroeconomy and American productivity. Nurses are able to link obesity to the economy by describing the catastrophic direct and indirect costs of the obesity epidemic and how it is making the United States less competitive in a global market. This is a way for nurses to use their power to create more urgency about the most pressing public health issues.

Science and Research

The information age has created an emphasis on evidence-based practice and policies, but we seem to be in danger of living in a world that eschews evidence. Scientific findings play a powerful role in the first step of the policy process: getting attention to particular problems and moving them to the policy agenda. Research can also be valuable in defining the size and scope of a problem and substantiating

policy recommendations. This can help to obtain support for a proposed policy and in lobbying for support of it. Evidence should be used to inform policy debates and shape policy choices to help ensure that the solution will be effective.

The role of evidence in the policymaking process cannot be overstated, and it is not enough to determine if policies are supportive or punitive—it is necessary to understand policies in context. In other words, in some circumstances, policies may be supported by good evidence such as screening for alcohol and tobacco use during pregnancy, which could potentially mitigate poor outcomes; however, unintended consequences can result if not informed by context (Subbaraman et al., 2018). Pregnant people delay prenatal care if they believe screening for alcohol and tobacco will result in criminalization of themselves or loss of their children (Roberts et al., 2012). Thus it is important that both policies and their implementation be informed by rigorous evidence.

That said, evidence is essential but may not be sufficient to advance policies. As Haskins and Margolis (2014) note, when policy is made, politics and values often surpass rigorous, well-collected data, as well as dominate the conversations about what is considered evidence. This has been apparent in recent debates over two long-standing policy issues: climate change and childhood vaccinations. Despite evidence showing that humans are contributing to devastating changes in the earth's climate or that childhood vaccinations do not cause autism, debates about these issues continue to affect whether policies are or are not adopted to address the problems.

Policy Analysis and Analysts

Analysis is the examination of an object or a process to understand it better. Policy analysis uses various methods to assess a problem and determine possible solutions. This encourages deliberate critical thinking about the causes of problems, identifies the ways a government or other groups could respond, evaluates alternatives, and determines the most desirable policy choice (see Chapter 7 on The Policy Process). Policy analysts are individuals who, with professional training and experience, analyze problems and weigh potential solutions. Citizens can also use policy analysis to better understand a problem, alternatives, and potential implications of policy choices (Kraft & Furlong, 2017).

Advocacy and Activism

Patient advocacy has long been a central role for nurses. Nurses bring their expertise as advocates to a larger scale by working in policy and politics. Nursing's Social Policy Statement (American Nurses Association [ANA], 2010), a document that defines nursing and its social contract, endorses advocacy through policy as a professional responsibility. Political activism may be associated with protests but has grown to include additional diverse and effective strategies such as blogging, arguing evidence to support policy choices, and garnering media attention in sophisticated ways. See Chapter 3 for more on advocacy.

Interest Groups and Lobbyists

Interest groups advocate for policies that are advantageous to their membership (see Chapter 66 on interest groups and Chapter 40 on lobbying). Groups often employ lobbyists to advocate on their behalf and their power cannot be underestimated. The Center for Responsive Politics tracks spending on campaigns and lobbying by individuals and organizations (www.opensecrets.org). Data from the center shows that, in 2018, $2.59 billion was spent lobbying in the United States, down from a high of $3.51 billion in 2010; and there were 11,272 registered lobbyists, down from a high of 14,826 in 2007. Of all industry sectors, health care ranked first in spending on lobbying, at $421.5 million. For organizations representing the health professions, the National Council of State Boards of Nursing spent more on lobbying than any other nursing organization ($555,000) in 2018 but ranked 30th overall. The ANA ranked fourth among nursing organizations ($333,676), although it spent $1.6 million in 2017. The American Medical Association spent more than $15 million in 2018 and ranked first among all health professions organizations.

The Media

The power of media is demonstrated in political and issue campaigns, whether through paid political advertisements or the "talking heads" on "news" programs that present polarized views. The aim is to deliver messages that resonate with the values and emotions of a target audience to support or oppose a candidate or proposed policy. The strategic use of media is imperative in today's cacophony of information. Gaining the attention of a target audience is power. Persuading that audience to behave the way you want is ultimate power.

In this information age, nurses must proactively use media to influence policy and make themselves available to speak with journalists about policy matters. However, as noted earlier, nurses have not always been eager to enter the media spotlight (see Chapter 12 on using media as a policy and political tool), particularly when it comes to talking with journalists. Social media is a tool for influencing policymakers and provides nurses with an opportunity to control their message.

The Power of Presidents and Other Leaders

The president embodies the power of the executive branch of government and is the only person elected to represent the entire nation within the federal government. As the most visible government official, the role of the president is able to propel issues to the top of the nation's policy agenda. Although the president and White House staff cannot introduce legislation, they can set policy agendas for Congress, working through the congressional representatives of their political party, as well as provide draft legislation and legislative guidance. Whether the president's legislative policy priorities are at the top of the congressional agenda will depend on whether the president's political party holds the majority of seats in Congress. The president can also issue executive orders when they do not have congressional support for policy change.

Theoretically, the three branches of government serve as a check-and-balance system to ensure the principles of democracy are upheld and that the interests of the citizens in the republic are equitably represented. For health policy, the role and power of the office of the president and the executive branch of the U.S. government cannot be overstated in terms of setting the tone, providing the vision, and engaging the public in determining effective health policies that ensure that all individuals can function as full citizens in society.

THE FRAMEWORK FOR ACTION

Nursing has a covenant with the public. The profession's practice laws, standards, and ethics have roots in its history of activism for social justice. A social contract with society demands professional responsibility. Thus every nurse must continuously consider the policy context of our daily practice in any setting. The solutions to today's most intractable health care problems, including perverse payment mechanisms, deeply disturbing social injustice, and shocking ethnic and racial disparities, are not simple to solve. However, according to the annual Gallup poll (Brenan, 2018), the public regards nurses' "honesty and ethical standards" more highly than those of any other profession. This public trust places a moral imperative on nurses to vigorously engage in influencing policy. Nurses work where policies are implemented; we see policies close up wherever we care for their patients and can actively work to change the unintended consequences we witness. This imperative requires us to expand our involvement in policy decisions at the institutional, community, state, federal, or international realm and is not restricted to any one setting.

The Framework for Action (Fig. 1.4) illustrates that nurses operate in four spheres: government, workplace,

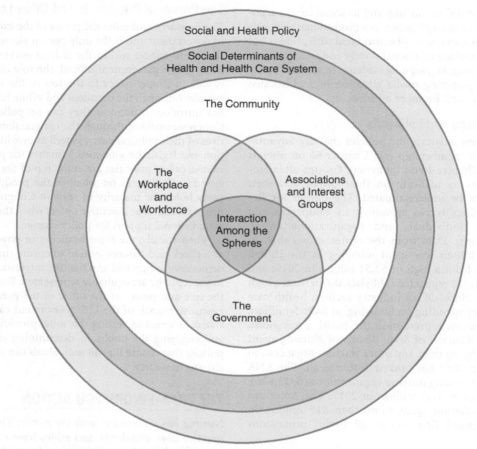

Fig. 1.4 A framework: Spheres of influence for action. Nurses need to work in multiple spheres of influence to shape health and social policy. Policies are designed to remedy problems in the health system and to address social determinants of health; both of which aim to improve health.

interest groups (including professional organizations), and community to influence policies that affect health and health care and core/social determinants of health. The focus in all spheres is on health, to represent that optimal health is viewed as the goal of nursing's policy efforts. Optimal health (whether for the individual patient, family, a population, or community) is the central focus of the political and policy activity described in this book. This focus makes it clear that the ultimate goal for advancing nursing's interests must be to promote the public's health.

Nursing embraces a broad definition of health that aligns with WHO (1948): "Health is a state of complete physical, mental and social well-being and not merely the absence of disease or infirmity." It incorporates the concept of positive health, not just ill health. This definition

requires a focus on social determinants of health and creating communities that thrive economically, have safe environments, and use resources to ensure that their members have access to good nutrition and other elements that can promote health.

The four spheres of influence provide a visual medium for understanding the policy arena but are not discrete silos. Policy can be shaped in more than one sphere at a time, and action in one sphere can influence others. For example, to achieve greater access to care for the uninsured, nurses may work in their own organization to alter policy to increase access to services. They may also use political strategies in the media, such as blogging or being interviewed on television, to express their support for better access to care. They may work with a professional association or an interest group to communicate their views to policymakers. Additional context (the who, what, where, when, and why of nursing's policy influence) is provided in Fig. 1.5.

The Government

Government action and policy affect lives from birth until death. It funds prenatal care, inspects food, controls the safety of toys and cars, operates schools, builds highways, and regulates what is transmitted on airwaves. It provides for the common defense; supplies fire and police protection; and gives financial assistance to the poor, aged, and others who cannot maintain a minimal standard of living. The government responds to disaster, subsidizes agriculture, and licenses funeral homes.

Although most U.S. health care is provided in the private sector, much is paid for and regulated by the government. So, how the government crafts health policy is extremely important (Weissert & Weissert, 2019). Government plays a significant role in influencing nursing and nursing practice. States determine the scope of professional activities considered to be nursing, with notable exceptions of the military, veterans' administration, and Indian health service. Federal and state governments determine who is eligible for care under specific benefit programs and who can be reimbursed for providing care. Sometimes government provides leadership in defining problems for both the public and private sectors to address. There are more than a dozen House and Senate committees and subcommittees that shape policy on health, and many more committees address social problems that affect health. In the House of Representatives, the Congressional Nursing Caucus, an informal, bipartisan group of legislators who have declared their interest in helping nurses, lobbies for federal funding for nursing education.

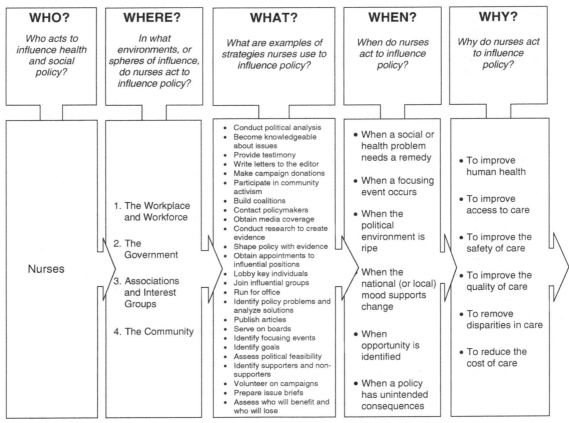

Fig. 1.5 The who, what, where, when, and why of nursing's policy influence.

Abraham Lincoln's description of a "government of the people, by the people, for the people" (Lincoln, 1863) captures the intricate nature of the relationship of government and its people. There are many ways nurses can influence policymaking in the government sphere at local, state, and federal levels of government. Examples include:

- Obtaining appointment to influential government positions
- Serving in federal, state, and local agencies
- Serving as elected officials
- Working as paid lobbyists
- Communicating positions to policymakers
- Providing testimony at government hearings
- Participating in grassroots efforts, such as rallies, to draw attention to problems

The Workforce and Workplace

Nurses work in a variety of settings: hospitals, clinics, schools, private sector firms, government agencies, military services, research centers, nursing homes, and home health agencies. All of these environments are political ones; resources are finite, and nurses must work in each to influence the allocation of organizational resources. Policies guide many activities in the health care workplaces where nurses are employed. Many that affect nursing and patient care are internal organizational policies such as staffing policies, clinical procedures, and patient care guidelines. External policies are operative in the health care workplace also; for example, state laws regulating nursing licensure. Federal laws and regulations are evident in the nursing workplace such as Occupational Health and Safety Administration regulations regarding worker protection from bloodborne pathogens.

Policy influences the size and composition of the nursing workforce. The ACA authorized increased funding for scholarships and loans for nursing education, potentially augmenting existing workforce programs funded under Title VII and Title VIII of the Public Health Service Act. The nongovernmental Commission on Graduates of Foreign Nursing Schools is authorized by the federal government to protect the public by ensuring that nurses and other health care professionals educated outside the United States are eligible and qualified to meet U.S. licensure, immigration, and other practice requirements (Commission on Graduates of Foreign Nursing Schools, 2009). The National Council of State Boards of Nursing is a not-for-profit organization that brings together state boards of nursing to act on matters of common interest affecting the public's health, safety, and welfare, including the development of licensing examinations in nursing (National Council of State Boards of Nursing, 2009). These are just a few examples of the external forces that shape workforce and workplace policy.

Associations and Interest Groups

Professional nursing associations have played a significant role in influencing practice. Many associations have legislative or policy committees that advocate policies supporting their members' practice and advance the interests of their patient populations. Working with a group increases the effectiveness of advocacy, provides for the sharing of resources, and enhances networking and learning. In fact, these associations can be excellent training grounds for novice nurses to learn about policy and political action (see Chapter 4).

When nursing organizations join forces through coalitions, their influence can be multiplied. For example, the Nurses on Boards Coalition (www.nursesonboardscoalition.org) is a group of national nursing organizations, schools of nursing, health care organizations, and other strategic partners to work on *The Future of Nursing* report's recommendation to increase nurse appointments to commissions, task forces, boards, and other entities. See Chapter 49 for more on the Coalition.

Nurses can be influential, not just in nursing associations, but by working with other interest groups such as the American Public Health Association or the Sierra Club. Some interest groups have a broad portfolio of policy interests, whereas others focus on one disease (e.g., National Breast Cancer Coalition) or one issue (e.g., driving while intoxicated, the primary focus of Mothers Against Drunk Driving). Interest groups have become powerful players in policy debates; those with large funding streams are able to shape public opinion with media advertisements.

The Community

A limited number of nurses will have the opportunity to influence policy at the highest levels of government, but extensive opportunities exist for nurses to influence health and social policy in communities. Nursing has a rich history of community activism with remarkable examples provided by leaders such as Lillian Wald, Harriet Tubman, and Ruth Lubic. This legacy continues today with the community advocacy efforts of nurses such as Lucia Alfano, Gina Miranda-Diaz, Danielle Pendergrass, and one of this book's editors (McLemore) who were designated by the Campaign for Action as "Breakthrough Leaders in Nursing" (see Chapters 78, 29, and 13 for the stories of Alfano, Miranda-Diaz, and McLemore). Others stories throughout this book highlight the leadership of nurses in their communities (for example, see Chapters 75 and 76).

A community is a group of people who share something in common and interact with one another, who may exhibit a commitment to one another or share a geographic boundary (see Chapter 73). A community may be a neighborhood, a city, an online group with a common interest, or a faith-based network. Nurses can be influential in communities by identifying problems, strategizing with others, mobilizing support, and advocating change. In residential communities (such as towns, villages, and urban districts), there are opportunities to serve in positions that influence policy, whether planning boards, civic organizations, and parent-teacher associations, or other group.

POLICY AND POLITICAL COMPETENCE

Competence is being adequately prepared or qualified to perform a specific role. It encompasses a combination of knowledge, skills, and behaviors that improve performance. Nurses are often reluctant to become involved in policy because of the "politics." Political skill has a bad reputation; for some, it conjures up thoughts of manipulation, self-interested behavior, and favoritism. Although "playing politics" is not generally considered to be a compliment, true political skill is critical in health care leadership, advocating for others, and shaping policy. It is simply not possible to succeed in any decision-making arena by ignoring the political realm. Ferris, Davidson, and Perrewe (2010) consider political skill to be the ability to understand others and to use that knowledge to influence others to act in a way that supports one's objectives. They identify political skill in four components:

1. *Social astuteness:* Skill at being attuned to others and social situations; ability to interpret one's own behaviors and the behavior of others.

2. *Interpersonal influence:* Convincing personal style that influences others featuring the ability to adapt behavior to situations and be pleasant and productive to work with.

3. *Networking ability:* The ability to develop diverse networks of people and position oneself to create and take advantage of opportunities.

4. *Apparent sincerity:* The display of high levels of integrity, authenticity, sincerity, and genuineness (pp. 9–12).

In most cases, policymakers are generalists who make decisions on a broad range of issues. Nurses can have a profound impact on policymaking by using their knowledge to frame and define health policy alternatives. Influencing policy at all levels requires a strong set of interpersonal skills, integrity, and knowledge. Political competency, at either the individual or the organizational level, can be defined by three main elements: deep knowledge, political antennae, and power (O'Grady & Johnson, 2013) (Fig. 1.6).

- *Deep knowledge* requires freely sharing expertise and gaining the knowledge you need from others. Subject-matter expertise without knowledge of policy and its processes is a doomed strategy. Deep knowledge involves knowing the viewpoints of others, including the opposition, and having a clear message and data ready to support your position and neutralize opposition.

- *Political antennae* means the ability to scan the environment and identify opportunities to offer solutions to policy problems. These problems should focus not just on nursing but on broader health and health care issues. Having political antennae requires active listening to

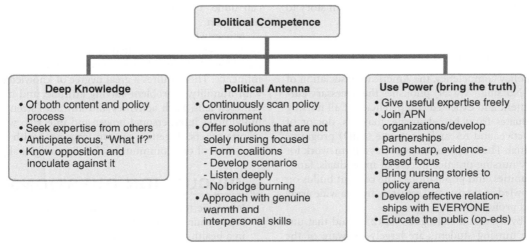

Fig. 1.6 Political competencies. *APN,* Advanced practice nursing. (From O'Grady, E. T., & Johnson, J. [2013]. Health policy issues in changing environments. In A. Hamric, C. Hanson, D. Way, & E. O'Grady [Eds.], *Advanced practice nursing: An integrative approach* [5th ed.]. St. Louis, MO: Elsevier Saunders.)

understand policymaker's values and motives, and compose messages and responses to fit their political objectives. It also requires avoiding bridge-burning in relationships. Political and policy disagreements require a response of genuine warmth, a quality that can go a long way in building trust. Learning how to navigate differences and agreeing to disagree without being disagreeable are important political skills.

• *Power* is the ability to act to achieve a goal. In the policy process, this means recognizing the policymakers with power, who is on which congressional committee, and who are the thought-leaders in the community. Creating coalitions with individuals and groups with similar goals is an important way nurses can augment their policymaking power. Most importantly, an individual nurse can claim power by being knowledgeable, articulate, and having an "elevator speech" that can spark interest in a policymaker or staff member.

Application of power requires raising one's awareness about what is true and what is false. Being grounded in truth, such as knowing the value of human caring and the role that nursing can have on individuals and populations, is a form of personal integrity that leads to power. To be effective in the policy arena, nurses must have a sharp focus on the evidence, not emotion. Advancing nursing's policy agenda through such a use of power demands that we drop nursing parochialism and focus on problem solving. Nursing *parochialism* is when a nurse is in a problem-solving context (policy meeting) and offers up only the solution of "nurses" as the remedy to every problem. Parochialism is an approach that narrows options and interests and appears self-serving. However, bringing nurses' stories to the policy arena is a powerful way to pair the human story to the scientific evidence.

NURSING ESSENTIALS

To ensure policy competency, the American Association of Colleges of Nursing (AACN) publishes the necessary curriculum content and expected competencies of all nursing school graduates from baccalaureate, master's, doctor of nursing practice, and research doctorate (PhD) programs they credential. These documents serve as a framework for 21st century nursing practice in care of individuals, families, communities, and populations. The content builds on nursing knowledge, theory, and research, from a wide array of fields and professions.

A study by Byrd and colleagues (2012) found that undergraduate nursing students are largely unaware of the importance of political activity for nurses. After participating in a robust and active public policy learning activity, students measured high on a political astuteness scale. This

study suggests that political skills can be learned when presented with relevance to nursing and used to hone skills such as inquiry, critical thinking, and complex problem solving. These results highlight the importance of increasing students' awareness of how to participate in the political process, as well as encouraging their participation in student and professional organizations.

For each level of nursing education—bachelors, master's, and doctorate (DNP and PhD)—there are clear expectations that nursing graduates will have policy competency (AACN, n.d.; 2010). It is expected that DNP graduates are able to design, implement, and advocate health policies that improve the health of populations. In addition, a DNP graduate integrates these practice experiences with two additional skill sets: the ability to analyze the policy process and the ability to engage in politically competent action (AACN, 2006).

CONCLUSION

Corralling the political power of the 4 million registered nurses in the United States (ANA, 2018) can occur when individual nurses join, support, and fully engage with their professional nursing organizations. More than any other effort to date, *The Future of Nursing* report (IOM, 2011) brought nurses together to engage across associations and educational institutions and, with new community partners, to change policy such as state laws and regulations that limit full practice authority for APRNs. Many of the recommendations direct policy changes resonant with nurses and a new *The Future of Nursing 2030* report by the National Academy of Medicine promises to broaden the recommendations to incorporate how nurses can build a culture of health in our communities and our nation.

Nurses who effectively use power are a sought-after and valued asset. They are invited to the table and are not only asked back but invited to more tables with ever-expanding influence. This requires a great degree of knowledge, along with humility, a problem-solving attitude, and a patient-centered lens. Such activities and attitudes strengthen an individual's interpersonal power and integrity, which can inspire others. Together, we can improve health care and the health of our communities, locally and globally.

DISCUSSION QUESTIONS

1. What are the most pressing health care problems you see in your community? How can you frame that issue in a health policy context?
2. Can you identify areas in your own political competence that require growth? What do you need to learn to be more effective?

3. Why has nursing made policy and political competence such a strong part of the nursing curriculum and role development?

REFERENCES

Adler, N., Cutler, D., Fielding, J.E., Galea, S., Glymour, M.M., Koh, H.K., & Satcher, D. (2016). *Addressing social determinants of health and health disparities: A vital direction for health and health care.* NAM Perspectives. Discussion Paper, National Academy of Medicine, Washington, DC. Retrieved from https://nam.edu/wp-content/uploads/2016/09/Addressing-Social-Determinants-of-Health-and-Health-Disparities.pdf.

American Academy of Nursing. (n.d., a). *Raise the voice.* Retrieved from www.aannet.org/raisethevoice.

American Academy of Nursing. (n.d., b). *Edge runners: The eleventh street family health service.* Retrieved from www.aannet.org/edge-runners–eleventh-street-family-health-services.

American Association of Colleges of Nursing. (2006). *The essentials of doctoral education for advanced nursing practice.* Retrieved from www.aacn.nche.edu/publications/position/DNPEssentials.pdf.

American Association of Colleges of Nursing [AACN]. (2010). *The research-focused doctoral program in nursing: Pathways to excellence.* Retrieved from www.aacnnursing.org/Portals/42/Publications/PhDPosition.pdf.

American Association of Colleges of Nursing [AACN]. (n.d.). *Essentials.* Retrieved from www.aacnnursing.org/Education-Resources/AACN-Essentials.

American Nurses Association [ANA]. (2010). *Nursing's social policy statement: The essence of the profession.* (3rd ed.) Washington, DC: American Nurses Association.

American Nurses Association. (2018). *About ANA.* Retrieved from www.nursingworld.org/ana/about-ana/.

Anderson, J. E. (2015). *Public policymaking* (8th ed.). Farmington Hills, MI: Cengage Learning.

Artiga, S. & Hinton, E. (2018). *Beyond health care: The role of social determinants in promoting health and health equity.* Retrieved from www.kff.org/disparities-policy/issue-brief/beyond-health-care-the-role-of-social-determinants-in-promoting-health-and-health-equity/.

Bailey, Z. D., Krieger, N., Agénor, M., Graves, J., Linos, N., & Bassett, M. T. (2017). Structural racism and health inequities in the USA: evidence and interventions. *The Lancet, 389*(10077), 1453-1463.

Berwick, D., Nolan, T., & Whittington, J. (2008). The Triple Aim: Care, health, and cost. *Health Affairs, 27*(3), 759–769. Retrieved from content.healthaffairs.org/content/27/3/759.full.

Billioux, A., Verlander, K., Anthony, S., & Alley, D. (2017). *Discussion paper: Standardized screening for health-related needs in clinical settings: The Accountable Health Communities Screening Tool.* National Academy of Medicine. Retrieved from https://nam.edu/standardized-screening-for-health-related-social-needs-in-clinical-settings-the-accountable-health-communities-screening-tool.

Bodenheimer, T. & Mason, D.J. (2017). *Registered nurses: Partners in transforming primary care: Proceedings of a conference on preparing registered nurses for enhanced roles in primary care.* New York: Josiah Macy, Jr. Foundation. Retrieved from http://macyfoundation.org/docs/macy_pubs/Macy_Monograph_Nurses_2016_webPDF.pdf.

Bodenheimer, T. & Sinsky, C. (2014). From Triple to Quadruple Aim: Care of the patient requires care of the provider. *Annals of Family Medicine, 12*(6), 573-576. Retrieved from www.annfammed.org/content/12/6/573.full.

Brenan, M. (2018). *Nurses again outpace other professions for honesty, ethics.* Retrieved from https://news.gallup.com/poll/245597/nurses-again-outpace-professions-honesty-ethics.aspx.

Byrd, M.E., Costello, J., Gremel, K., Schwager, J., Blanchette, L., & Malloy, T.E. (2012). Political astuteness of baccalaureate nursing students following an active learning experience in health policy. *Public Health Nursing, 29*(5), 433–443.

Commission on Graduates of Foreign Nursing Schools. (2009). *Commission on graduates of foreign nursing schools: Mission and history.* Retrieved from www.cgfns.org.

Dropp, K., & Nyhan, B. (2017). *One third don't know that Obamacare is the ACA.* Retrieved from www.nytimes.com/2017/02/07/upshot/one-third-dont-know-obamacare-and-affordable-care-act-are-the-same.html.

Felt-Lisk, S., & Higgins, T. (2011). *Exploring the promise of population health management programs to improve health: Mathematica policy research issue brief.* Retrieved from www.mathematica-mpr.com/publications/PDFs/health/PHM_brief.pdf.

Ferris, G., Davidson, S., & Perrewe, P. (2010). *Political skill at work: Impact on work effectiveness.* Boston, MA: Nicholas Brealey Publishing.

Haskins, R., & Margolis, G. (2014). *Show me the evidence: Obama's fight for rigor and results in social policy.* Washington, DC: Brookings Institution Press.

Institute for Healthcare Improvement. (n.d.). *The Triple Aim: IHI Triple Aim initiative.* Retrieved from www.ihi.org/Engage/Initiatives/TripleAim/Pages/default.aspx.

Institute of Medicine. (2011). *The future of nursing: Leading change, advancing health.* Washington, DC: National Academies Press. Retrieved from www.iom.edu/nursing.

Kaiser Family Foundation. (2018). *Key facts about the uninsured population.* Retrieved from www.kff.org/uninsured/fact-sheet/key-facts-about-the-uninsured-population/.

Kaiser Family Foundation [KFF]. (2013). *Kaiser health tracking poll: August 2013.* Retrieved from kff.org/health-reform/poll-finding/kaiser-health-tracking-poll-august-2013.

Kelly, N. (2004). Does politics really matter? Policy and government's equalizing influence in the United States. *American Politics Research, 32*(3), 264–284.

Khullar, D., & Chokshi, D.A. (2018). Health, income, & poverty: Where we are and what could help. *Health Affairs.* Retrieved from www.healthaffairs.org/do/10.1377/hpb20180817.901935/full/.

Kraft, M., & Furlong, S. (2017). *Public policy: Politics, analysis, and alternatives* (6th ed.). Washington, DC: CQ Press.

Lincoln, A. (1863). *Gettysburg Address*. Retrieved from www.ourdocuments.gov/doc.php?flash=old&doc=36.

Longest, B. (2010). *Health policymaking in the United States* (5th ed.). Chicago, IL: Health Administration Press.

Majone, G. (1992). *Evidence, argument, and persuasion in the policy process*. New Haven, CT: Yale University Press.

Makary, M. & Daniels, M. (2016). Medical error—The third leading cause of death in the U.S. *British Medical Journal*, 353, i2139. Retrieved from www.bmj.com/content/353/bmj.i2139.

Marmot, M. & Allen, J. (2014). Social determinants of health equity. *American Journal of Public Health*, 104(Suppl 4), S517-S519.

Martsolf, G., Sloan, J., Mason, D.J., Sullivan, C., & Villarruel, A. (2017). *RAND Report: Nurse-designed models of care and culture of health: Three case studies*. Santa Monica, CA: RAND Corporation.

Martsolf, G., Sloan, J., Villarruel, A., Sullivan, C., & Mason, D.J. (2018). Promoting a culture of health through cross-sector collaborations. *Health Promotion Practice*, 19(5), 784-791.

Mason, D.J., Jones, D., Roy, C., Sullivan, C., & Wood, L. (2015). Commonalities of nurse-designed models of health care. *Nursing Outlook*, 63(2015), 540-553.

Mason, D.J., Glickstein, B., & Westphaln, K. (2018). Journalists' experiences with using nurses as sources in health news stories. *American Journal of Nursing*, 118(10), 42-50.

Mason, D.J., Nixon, L., Glickstein, B. Han, S., Westphaln, K., & Carter, L. (2018). The Woodhull study revisited: Nurses' representation in health news media twenty years later. *Journal of Nursing Scholarship*, 50(6), 695-704.

McCarthy, D., & Klein, S. (2010). *The Triple Aim journey: Improving population health and patients' experience of care, while reducing costs*. Retrieved from www.commonwealthfund.org/Publications/Case-Studies/2010/Jul/Triple-Aim-Improving-Population-Health.aspx.

National Academies of Sciences, Engineering, and Medicine. (2016). *Assessing progress on the Institute of Medicine report: The future of nursing*. Washington, DC: The National Academies Press. Retrieved from www.nap.edu/download/21838.

National Council of State Boards of Nursing. (2009). *National Council of State Boards of Nursing—About NCSBN*. Retrieved from www.ncsbn.org/about.htm.

National Research Council. (2013). *U.S. health in international perspective: Shorter lives, poorer health*. Retrieved from www.nap.edu/catalog.php?record_id=13497.

O'Grady, E.T., & Johnson, J. (2013). Health policy issues in changing environments. In A. Hamric, C. Hanson, D. Way, & E. O'Grady (Eds.), *Advanced practice nursing: An integrative approach* (5th ed.). St. Louis, MO: Elsevier Saunders.

Papanicolas, I., Woskie, L.R., & Jha, A.K. (2018). Health care spending in the United States and other high-income countries. *JAMA*. 319(10), 1024-1039.

Roberts, S. & Nuru-Jeter, A. (2012). Universal screening for alcohol and drug use and racial disparities in child protective services reporting. *Journal of Behavioral Health Services Research*, 39(1):3-16.

Rowe, J., Rizzo, V., Kricke, G.S., Krajci, K., Rodriguez-Morales, G., Newman, M., & Golden, R. (2016). The ambulatory integration of the Medical and Social (AIMS) model: A retrospective evaluation. *Social Work in Health Care*, 55(5), 347-361.

Rudolph, L., Caplan, J., Ben-Moshe, K., & Dillon, L. (2013). *Health in all policies: A guide for state and local governments*. Retrieved from www.phi.org/uploads/files/Health_in_All_Policies-A_Guide_for_State_and_Local_Governments.pdf.

Schneider, E.C., Sarnak, D.O., Squires, D., Shah, A., & Doty, M.M. (2017). *Mirror, mirror: International comparisons reflect flaws and opportunities for better U.S. health care*. Retrieved from https://interactives.commonwealthfund.org/2017/july/mirror-mirror/.

Social Security Administration. (n.d.). *Legislative history*. Retrieved from www.ssa.gov/history/law.html.

Starfield, B. (1998). *Primary care: Balancing health needs, services, and technology*. New York: Oxford University Press.

Subbaraman, M.S., Thomas, S., Treffers, R., Delucchi, K., Kerr, W.C., Martinez, P., & Roberts, S. (2018). Associations between state-level policies regarding alcohol use among pregnant women, adverse birth outcomes, and prenatal care utilization: Results from 1972 to 2013 Vital Statistics. *Alcoholism: Clinical and Experimental Research*. [Epub ahead of print].

Tilden, V., Cox, K., Moore, J., & Naylor, M. (2018). Strategic partnerships to address adverse social determinants of health: Redefining health care. *Nursing Outlook*, 66(3), 233–236.

Wagner, E.H. (1998). Chronic disease management: What will it take to improve care for chronic illness? *Effective Clinical Practice*, 1(1), 2–4.

Weissert, C., & Weissert, W. (2019). *Governing health—The politics of health policy* (5th ed.). Baltimore, MD: Johns Hopkins University Press.

Williams, D.R., Costa, M.V., Odunlami, A.O., & Mohammed, S.A. (2008). Moving upstream: How interventions that address the social determinants of health can improve health and reduce disparities. *Journal of Public Health Management and Practice*, 14(Suppl.), S8–S17.

World Health Organization. (1948). *Preamble to the Constitution of the World Health Organization*. Retrieved from www.who.int/about/definition/en/print.html.

World Health Organization. (n.d.). *Social determinants of health*. Retrieved from www.who.int/social_determinants/en/.

2

Historical Perspective on Policy, Politics, and Nursing

Patricia D'Antonio, Julie Fairman, and Sandra B. Lewenson

"Reform can be accomplished only when attitudes are changed."

Lillian Wald

In 1893, Lillian Wald, then a young medical student, visits the sick mother of a poor and vulnerable New York City family. What she sees—a young mother struggling to recover in a ramshackle tenement, with little access to fresh air and healthy food—and what she does—leaving medical school and returning to nursing because she believed nurses could have a greater impact—changes her life (Wald, 1915). She and her nursing school colleague, Mary Brewster, establish the Henry Street Settlement House in New York City's lower east side. Like many reformers in the late 19th century, Wald and Brewster believed that only by living in impoverished, immigrant communities could they effect meaningful change in the city's housing, sanitation, nutrition, and educational policies. However, Wald takes her vision one step further. She establishes the Visiting Nurse Service at the Henry Street Settlement (D'Antonio, 2010). At a time when the best in health care centered on the home, she decides that those most vulnerable would have the best in nursing care when ill at home and they would also have the best in health promotion and disease prevention; these families would learn from visiting nurses how to keep themselves healthy in the face of the infectious diseases rampant at the time. In addition, these visiting nurses would respond to calls from the families in the community just as she would respond to the calls from physicians. Turning her vision into a reality took hard work and strategic partnerships with insurance companies, donors, schools, and the New York City's Department of Health. However, she prevails—and changes the structure of the U.S. health care system. What come to be known as public health nurses remain central to developing programs addressing public health efforts to promote health and prevent disease. Wald's skill lay in her ability to harness the support of those in power.

Recognizing the strength of coalitions to enact change, Wald, along with her colleagues at the settlement house and other nurse leaders, participated in the establishment of the National Organization of Public Health Nursing in 1912, creating an organization to control the standards and practice of public health nurses. She created coalitions, such as that with the American Red Cross, when concerned about the need for access of care in rural communities (Lewenson, 2015), and she knew how to procure the financial resources from private foundations and donors to support many of her public health initiatives. Her success lay in creating coalitions that first identified problems, then found the right resources, and effected successful solutions by making the issues ones that the public "owns."

Why should anyone care about one story about one famous nurse? Because the issues that Wald and her colleagues set out to address remain central to the current debates about how to get the best in health care to vulnerable and dispossessed individuals, families, communities, and populations. Rates of infectious diseases are again climbing in the United States and across the globe, adding to the increasingly recognized and growing burden of non-infectious diseases. Even though its fate is uncertain at the time of this writing and it was an imperfect vehicle, major policy initiatives such as the Affordable Care Act (ACA) promised and did increase access to health care, improved quality, and attempted to contain costs by shifting the focus from acute care hospitals to homes, communities, and primary care sites. The ACA privileged health promotion and disease prevention in ways unprecedented since the early 1920s, but as is wont to happen, politics, rather than evidence, reshaped the debate after the 2016 election. Remembering Wald's story shows that nurses have been, and will continue to be, active participants in health policy debates from the home to the national level and in turning ideas into reality but that their actions will always be part and process of the political system.

Stories create the foundation upon which policies move forward or fail, but the reason for exploring the intersections of history and health policy transcends simply knowing stories. Examining points at these intersections allows for a richer understanding of the possibilities and the problems that resonate in health policy deliberations. The distance of time as one studies change over time, the core of historical methods, allows a different view of the tensions existing between public and private spheres of influence, community needs and professional prerogatives, best evidence, and political power. This chapter uses historical case studies, looking to the past to find themes, ideas, and actions that can provide tools for considering future policy deliberations and actions.

"NOT ENOUGH TO BE A MESSENGER"

Buoyed by the success of public health initiatives like Wald's, public health officials returned from rebuilding post–World War I Europe to implement a bold new vision in the United States. The turn toward health care, in addition to illness care, was one of the hallmark characteristics of the "new public health" of the 1920s. If the prewar public health agenda of reformers like Wald focused on the ill individual and environment, then the postwar agenda would focus on the individual alone and how that individual could experience even greater health through the practices of personal hygiene, mental hygiene, and social hygiene. Its centerpiece was the "periodic medical examination"—now being urged for women as well as children. Public health leadership was well aware that cancer and degenerative heart disease were emerging as leading causes of death, and they urged nurses to preach to patients to demand, and physicians to provide, examinations that would detect susceptibility to these diseases or identify them when there were still treatment options. They also recognized that routine prenatal examinations that identified and treated medical problems offered the best hope of decreasing appallingly high rates of maternal mortality and launched campaigns that urged mothers and fathers to see pregnancy as akin to a disease and not as a normal phenomenon (D'Antonio, 2014). The problem lay in convincing the public.

In New York City, the focus of this section and the epicenter of both the public health and nursing worlds, public health leadership in the city turned to nurses to deliver this message. This decision seemed self-evident. Public health nurses had long considered themselves and had been considered by others as the "connecting link" between patients and physicians, between and among institutions, and between scientific knowledge and its implementation in the homes they visited. They became the centerpiece of the city's "demonstration projects," an envisioned mix of different types of public and private partnerships that would test ways of delivering this message that were carefully coordinated for efficiencies, cost-effectiveness, and high quality.

Public health nursing leaders in New York City believed that the turn toward health, particularly that of mothers and young children, would define their professional identity and disciplinary independence to a broader community. Health work with mothers and young children had been part of their traditional practices; and, as men were more likely to have periodic medical examinations associated with the purchase of life insurance policies and employment, women and young children seemed particularly vulnerable. In 1921, with funds from an anonymous donor, a small group of White New York City public health nurses, some also involved in the demonstration projects, launched The Citizen's Health Protective Society in the middle-class Manhattanville section of the city. This would be a self-sustaining insurance program that promised prenatal care for mothers, attendance at a medically supervised childbirth if delivered at home, and nine visits for all mothers in the postpartum period. It also promised health supervision of babies and preschool children and bedside nursing if sick at home. Do you want, it queried in handouts to families in Manhattanville, a carefully selected White, middle-class community, a self-supporting nursing and health service for $6 per year for an individual and $16 per year for families of three or more? Manhattanville did not. The Society moved to a more promising location at 134 Street and Amsterdam Avenue. This community remained uninterested as well. The Society closed in 1924. Families appreciated health work, but they would pay only for illness care. They would not pay for nursing health care (Maternity Center Association, 1924).

Public health nurses in the city's demonstration projects had more success. These nurses, similar to progressive urban colleagues throughout the country, went one step farther than their health education mandate. They used their experiences in the demonstration projects to move to identifying families as their practice domain. They built knowledge that bridged the biologic sciences that supported their public health practices with the new social sciences that buttressed their work with families. However, this practice brought them out of bounded disciplinary interests and into a place at the center of not only their own but also others' agendas. Foundations, families, physicians, and other public health workers all had particular ideas about what nurses should and could do as they delivered their messages of health.

This placed the demonstration project nurses squarely in the middle of escalating tensions among New York City's Department of Health, the private agencies who delivered home health care, and the Rockefeller Foundation and Milbank Memorial Fund who provided the financing, over who controlled the public health agenda. The private or (as they referred to themselves) voluntary agencies and philanthropies publicly ceded control to the official agency that the Departments of Health represented, but privately they constantly sought ways to turn the Department of Health toward their priorities. In New York City, both the private agencies and Rockefeller Foundation and the Milbank Memorial Fund believed public health nurses were key to this process. Indeed, the involvement of the city's public health nurses in the demonstration projects operating in the East Harlem section of the city had been a central element in the Rockefeller Foundation's support. It could not be a true demonstration of care control, the Foundation believed, unless it involved the city's own public health nurses who ran clean milk and infant welfare stations and who implemented programs of case finding, case holding, and case control of tuberculosis and other infectious diseases. In addition, it could not be a true maternal-child nursing service without the support of the city's school nurses who worked with those older than 6 years. The Foundation's policy, in the United States and abroad, was one of working only through governmental public health authorities to ensure the sustainability of its initiatives. It hoped to use a consolidated private and public health nursing system in East Harlem to ultimately do the same in New York City (D'Antonio, 2014).

However, the public health nursing leaders of the city's demonstration projects never persuaded the various heads of the New York City's Department of Health to let its nurses join any of their projects. The Department of Health maintained that its nurses were official agents of the city with real police power that it hoped they would rarely use; it needed to maintain control of their practices. The Department of Health had its own agenda for its nurses. It wanted to position them as representatives of a new public health message clothed in tact and sympathy rather than, as in the past, the bearer of quarantine placards and sanitary citations.

More importantly, the nurses involved in the health demonstration projects had shared no investment with their supporting philanthropies in involving the city's own public health nurses. Because, in the end, they won what they themselves wanted. By the end of the formal demonstration period in 1928, both private and public health nurses in New York City—not the physicians who had done so in the past—supervised the independent practices of other public health nurses. This was a substantive achievement. Public health nurses employed by New York City finally gained control of their own nursing practices.

At the same time, nurses in the demonstration projects thrived in their missions of service to mothers and young children and of research on the most pressing issues in public health nursing. It launched a program that continued a long-standing nursing mission to provide bedside nursing to sick residents in their own homes. It also strengthened its outreach to pregnant women, encouraging medically supervised births preferably in hospitals and providing both prenatal and postpartum care in homes. It started new health education services for preschool children. It also began sustained research projects about the organization of public health nursing work, particularly that situating generalized nursing as the standard for urban public health nursing. In addition, in 1928, in response to the needs of the discipline for more advanced clinical education, it recast itself as a postgraduate training site for public health nursing students in New York, from around the nation and from international sites of Rockefeller Foundation philanthropy (D'Antonio, 2013).

New York City's health demonstration projects eventually established what are currently the norms for primary, pregnancy, dental, and pediatric care. However, this change came almost painfully slowly through the day-to-day work of public health nurses going door to door, street to street, school to school, and neighborhood to neighborhood preaching the gospel of good health to those without access to the resources that class, race, ethnicity, and financial stability provided to others. As importantly, however, it came through the efforts of families to first incorporate and then to normalize these messages of health by removing them from stigmatizing sites of health and social welfare (in which the public health nurses were located) and placing them within the schools that the community embraced. The nurses in New York City's health demonstration projects slowly moved from understanding their role as bringing "medicine and a message" of middle-class values to immigrant families they wished to assimilate, to conceiving it as one of being "more than just a messenger" as they sought to serve as embodiments of a new emphasis on sound mental and physical health. Support for public health nursing did decline in the 1930s as nurses painfully realized that it was "not enough to be a messenger," but the decline was less about no longer serving families who needed to assimilate, as other historians have suggested. The decline was as much about families taking responsibility for their health (D'Antonio, 2014).

New York City's public health nurses were also working in a context increasingly dominated by the rise in hospitals and their outpatient clinics where families increasingly sought health care. However, the nurses in New York City's demonstration projects paid little attention to warnings about the implications of these new clinical sites for public health practice. They steadfastly maintained the site of their practices to that place where it could be most effectively and independently exercised: with cooperative families in their own homes, in the clinics the nurses controlled, and in the classrooms they created. Despite their commitment to maternal-child health initiatives, this narrow focus allowed them to professionally ignore one of the most pressing public health issues in the city—and indeed the United States—in the early 1930s: the newly rising rates of maternal mortality attributed by both the New York Academy of Medicine and the Maternity Center Association to poor obstetric practices in hospitals that women were increasingly choosing as sites of their infants' births. These nurses could not see or take responsibility for solving problems that lay inside public health policies but outside of their defined disciplinary purviews and sites of practice (D'Antonio, 2014).

BRINGING TOGETHER THE PAST FOR THE PRESENT: WHAT WE LEARNED FROM HISTORY

Generations later, a different group of constituents gathered to consider a new agenda for nursing in the 21st century that would situate patient care, rather than professional self-interest, at the forefront. In 2009 the Robert Wood Johnson Foundation (RWJF) in collaboration with the then Institute of Medicine (IOM) (currently the National Academy of Medicine) commissioned a new study charged with developing recommendations for reconceptualizing nursing practice and education (see Chapter 71). The committee appointed by the IOM was indicative of the changing health care political landscape and reflected the multiple stakeholders and thought leaders who were or would be partners with nurses to improve patient care. The committee was very diverse in age, profession, political leanings, and race/ethnicity and included consumer representation. The 6 nurses on the 18-member committee all came from diverse backgrounds and served as a contrast to the dominance of White women in the profession seen in the demonstration projects and public health leadership of the 1920s and 1930s. The pivotal role of foundations had changed: they now shared influence with multiple stakeholders such as the federal government, pharmaceutical corporations, consumer groups, and the insurance industry. These groups were now critical players in shaping the scope of nursing practice. In ways unthinkable in the 1920s and 1930s, consumers of nursing care played pivotal roles.

The final report, *The Future of Nursing: Leading Change, Advancing Health*, and its recommendations reflected the diversity of the committee and the stakeholders as well as the political landscape of health reform being debated as the committee deliberated (IOM, 2011). The report and the actions taken since, particularly by the Campaign for Action (https://campaignforaction.org), an initiative of the AARP and the RWJF, have provided the foundation for policy change through the development of state action coalitions and nationally based coalitions such as Nurses on Boards (https://campaignforaction.org/issue/promoting-nursing-leadership/). This national and state-based call for action, rather than the small demonstration projects of the early 20th century, may also reflect the changing role of philanthropies, as well as the power of new media to shape the policy message.

The first recommendation that nurses should practice to the fullest extent of their knowledge and skills links the story of the New York public health nurses to the nurses of the present. The conceptualization of the role of the public health nurses with families and communities, as well as their aims and efforts to fully incorporate their skills and knowledge into their practice, reflects historic continuities of nursing practice over the past century. This continuity resonated strongly with the public, professional organizations, and federal and state governments. Since the report was issued, nine states have removed practice barriers to allow nurse practitioners to practice independently and numerous other states are expanding their practice acts (https://campaignforaction.org). At the national level, retail clinics, health care service sites in drug stores, and big box stores typically staffed with nurse practitioners are growing in number and popularity, and nurse-managed health centers are recognized by many health systems as a practice model that can provide access to high-value care for people with limited resources (Brooks Carthon et al., 2016; Fairman et al., 2011). In general, policymakers and the public still see nurses—but now nurse practitioners rather than, as in the past, public health nurses—as a viable and valuable policy solution to the current primary care provider shortage and misdistribution. However, this recognition does not always translate to policy change.

Health policy researcher Debra Stone notes that there is no strict dichotomy between reason and power and between policy and politics (Stone, 2001). The IOM's *The Future of Nursing* report placed nurses at the center of a perfect storm of these forces and reflected the political, economic, and social context that propelled both professional and public interests (IOM, 2011). The report recommendations were also strategically shaped to position the patient as the focus of care within a reformed health system, and the history of both public health nurses and nurse practitioners is a reminder of the importance of public need when public disciplinary interests are articulated. History is also a reminder that sometimes small, piecemeal changes or events can be the springboard for larger policy issues at the right time and place.

When thinking about the policy levers that drive our health care system, we can look to history as a way of providing perspective and for pulling apart the power dynamics that drive policymaking. Our examples demonstrate how the IOM report placed nurse practitioners, just as the Public Health Department and the Rockefeller Foundation situated the earlier public health nurses, as policy solutions for improving the health care of the nation at a particular time and place. Our histories show that policymaking is untidy; we want it to be rational, but "reasoned analysis is necessarily political. It always involves choices to include things and exclude others and to view the world in a particular way when other visions are possible" (Stone, 2001, p. 378). The public health nurses of the 1920s and 1930s were perhaps not as facile at understanding this reality or not as skilled at thriving within an environment when the political alliances were flexible and shifting, but they did adjust. These are important lessons to learn and remember. Currently, as we try to reformulate our health care system to be more accessible, efficient, and inclusive, policymakers are making choices about providers and services. Nurse practitioners are part of policy solutions as seen through the norming of retail clinics and nurse-managed health centers. However, they need to remember that strategic alliances shift, that new stakeholders emerge, and that future policy decisions may not always be rational, but they will always be political. New political stakeholders, as we have seen since the 2016 election, will have the power to reshape health care according to their own alliances. Nurses will have to necessarily develop strategies to be part of the process in a very different policy environment. How nurses and their organizations are able to influence and challenge new directions will have a critical impact on the health of individuals, families, and communities.

There are both historical continuities and differences in the stories of public health nurses of the 1920s and 1930s and the growing appeal of nurse practitioners nowadays to policymakers and stakeholders. The ability to build coalitions and partnerships is as critical nowadays as it was in the 1920s and 1930s. In the early 1960s, when nurse Loretta Ford and physician Henry Silver serendipitously found they shared common interests of providing better care to rural poor families, they knew physician manpower was unavailable and that the nurse with additional skills and knowledge could provide the needed level of care. The United States was suffering from a primary care shortage

similar to the current shortage. Although they published their model early, they were not alone in coming to these conclusions. Nurse Barbara Resnick and physician Charles Lewis in Kansas City in the mid-1960s were also situating nurses as the solution to patient dissatisfaction with the lack of continuity of care in their university outpatient clinics. Although models like these were part of larger changes occurring where physicians were in short supply or nurses initiated their own practices, individual and sporadic efforts such as these were not enough to drive changes in policy even when analytic reasoning indicated their effectiveness. Nurse practitioners lacked a unified coalition to move their interest forward (e.g., to change restrictive state practice regulations and payment structures), and they lacked interested groups and partners outside of nursing to help broaden their appeal. Although individual physicians were supportive, organized medicine was not (Fairman, 2011).

Having data is important, as the public health nurses understood, but, as Stone (2001) also argued, politics may trump data. Data supporting the value and quality of nurse practitioner services began appearing in the early 1970s. A meta-analysis of 1970s-era studies of nurse practitioner effectiveness done by the Congressional Office of Technology Assessment documented their effectiveness in 1984. Although powerful in its scope and innovation, this study did not stimulate the interests of lawmakers at the state and federal levels, who could have used the data to develop a reasoned policy analysis. Although professional nursing did have lobbyists working on professional issues, the organizations were more focused on workplace issues than broader policies and were not mature or flexible enough to work together as a larger, powerful group until the late 1970s. Organized medicine was indeed "organized" and had powerful lobbies and leadership that kept its message simple and consistent and one that would be replayed for decades. The message was that physicians were the only safe providers because of their longer and more intensive education; yet, their position actually lacked data. This message, particularly from the American Medical Association, continues.

Another lesson learned from the public health nurse narrative that resonates nowadays is the importance of the creation of bridges between the community and the health system. In the late 1970s, professional nursing organizations such as the American Nurses Association (ANA) seized a strategic opportunity to reformulate their policy agenda. Building on the growing body of studies that indicated high patient satisfaction and clinical effectiveness of nurse practitioners as providers, and a growing strategic and political movement that situated the patient as the focus of professional legitimacy, the ANA built policy positions that situated nurse practitioners as normative providers for groups of patients such as older adults, children, and healthy adults. A deceptively strong and influential patient movement was also beginning to support nurse practitioner–provided care. Although patient support was unorganized and lacked a single leader, patients across the country showed their appreciation by returning for follow-up visits and bringing in their family and neighbors. The ANA effectively built upon the momentum patients provided to begin to form coalitions and work more effectively with the nascent nurse practitioner organizations to generate more powerful policy positions and partnerships.

We also learn from history that sometimes coalitions are not enough to move the policy levers. Even as nurses built coalitions and patients became their advocates through the 1980s and 1990s, there were pieces missing. For example, medical organizations influential in the policy arena did not offer nurses large-scale support. Most physician organizations were not interested in partnerships and still held strong political capital at the state and national levels. Individual physicians certainly supported nurse practitioners in their own practices, but much of organized medicine did not see them as independent providers or partners.

Organized medicine could situate nurses in this way because it still had enormous political power and resources, but physicians' cultural authority has now been challenged. Fraud and payment scandals and the exposing of physicians' relationships with pharmaceutical companies generated public skepticism during a time of patient empowerment movements and civil and women's rights movements. As historians Beatrix Hoffman and Nancy Tomes (2011) noted, patients reinvented "new terms for themselves—consumers, clients, citizens, and survivors—in their search to be heard in the health care arena" (p. 2) and exercised greater control over their care. In their search, patients found nurse practitioners qualified and value-based providers, educated and willing to see the patient as the "source of control" as the IOM report *Crossing the Quality Chasm* posited (IOM, 2001).

The stories of nurse practitioners and public health nurses are also connected by the ability to thrive and continue negotiations within a slow and subtle policy process. Incremental change occurred in health policy at the turn of the 21st century, although this was not a naturally rational or progressive movement. One of the ways this transformation can be illustrated is by the shift in the language defining who could provide care and receive payment. Many stakeholders worked over decades to bring about these changes. These categories are politically constructed worldviews, bestowing advantages and disadvantages. The change in language signified the slowly occurring power shift and the power of professional nursing and its allies to renegotiate the boundaries of patient care. Federal legislation began to include the term "provider" instead of "physician," or the more inclusive phrase "physicians and nurses." Medicare recognized nurse practitioners as primary care providers, although the states still maintain their regulatory authority to allow or not allow full scope of practice.

Another lesson learned is that coalitions must be flexible and ready to change. As the power dynamics in health care started to shift, nurse practitioners gained new partners and support. Since the 1980s, the Federal Trade Commission produced advocacy letters declaring restrictive practice acts anticompetitive and against the interests of consumers. Their activity in this area accelerated in the first decade of the 21st century. The AARP, the largest consumer group in the world, had nurses in key leadership positions to steer the organization, which developed policy positions that supported nurse practitioners. As medicine was becoming more corporatized and less patient centric, the public began rating nurses as the most trusted health professional in Gallup polls, with the exception of 2001, when firefighters topped the list (Gallup, n.d.). Policymaker recognition of the high cost of physician education and the viability of nurse practitioners as a reasonable and faster option to provider supply growth was supported by reports by the Rand Health Foundation and the National Governors Association.

Even so, nurse practitioners have not always been part of the policy solutions, even when evidence of their contributions to the primary care shortage existed. The 2012 Graduate Nurse Education Demonstration Project (https://innovation.cms.gov/initiatives/gne/) funded by the Centers for Medicare and Medicaid Services illustrated the ability of the nursing schools involved to produce more primary care nurse practitioners if Title XVIII funds (which fund medical training only) were allocated to nurse practitioner training. Although the Demonstration Project was seen as a success, building more capacity in medical education continues to be the traditional policy strategy, even as it became harder and harder to attract physicians into primary care. Shifting alliances and priorities at the federal level will require deftness and political savvy the nursing profession must develop.

By the time the IOM's *The Future of Nursing* report was published in 2011, patient support, coalition building, and new partnerships had more effectively positioned nurse practitioners to be a consistent part of the policy process. Although the IOM report might have served as the spark, it was nested in both the policies and politics of the past century, as well as the context surrounding health reform debates occurring in Congress. A litany of factors including rising health care costs, a shifting focus from specialty to primary care, and a shortage of primary care providers created a demand for new and more efficient models of care. Nurses gained willing and energetic partners in the public media and with the patients they served. A large private foundation, RWJF, leveraged its long-term interest in nursing to support the IOM report and will also support a follow-up study in 2020. Other new partners came forward; in particular, the Association of American Medical Colleges showed courage and strength by supporting nurse practitioners in press releases and policy statements. The nursing profession as a driver of policy change had come of age. It developed coalitions across nursing professional organizations that were focused on policy, and it developed new partnerships with powerful organizations outside of nursing that saw nursing's value while creating new opportunities and connections with nursing to both influence policymakers and drive policy change.

CONCLUSION

The two stories—about public health nurses shaping health outcomes of immigrant populations during the early 20th century and about the evolving policy support (via the IOM report) for nurse practitioners—show how health care policies and politics, perhaps even more than nurses' work, shape the delivery of care and the outcomes sought. An important lesson is that nurses are not a homogenous group. For the public health nurses, the day-to-day politics between and among professionals and the various private and public enterprises that offer health care options, especially to vulnerable populations, have typically directed their focus on more traditional methods of providing care rather than seeking nursing as part of the solution to the delivery of primary health care. Yet, the value public health nurses brought to community and population health argue for nurses to participate in policymaking and to advocate their inclusion in health care solutions. For nurse practitioners, history is a reminder of how they gained policy momentum amid the shifting weights of reasoning and power and with the growing power of consumer movements. New coalitions will have to be formed as political ideology changes. Learning to participate effectively while continuing to maintain the values of patient advocacy and equity in a reframed health care arena with shifting values and priorities will be a critical journey. Both stories illustrate how messy policymaking can be, how alliances can be tenuous while understanding the value of coalitions and partnerships as stabilizing agents in uncertain policy environments. History provides

rich data that can help nurses to advocate the role this profession holds as part of a larger solution to improve health care in the United States.

DISCUSSION QUESTIONS

1. What types of alliances exist, and what types need to be cultivated to affect change in your own areas of nursing practice?
2. What are the problems and/or the possibilities in developing cross-disciplinary, as well as public and private, alliances to effect change?
3. What type of historical evidence can be used to support nursing's political advocacy in providing primary health care?
4. Explore the advocacy efforts Lillian Wald, public health nurses in urban and rural settings, and nurse practitioners used to effect change in health care.

REFERENCES

Brooks Carthon, M.J., Wiltse, K., Altares Sarik, D. & Fairman, J.A. Effective strategies for achieving scope of practice reform in Pennsylvania. *Policy, Politics and Nursing Practice, 17*(2), 99-102.

D'Antonio, P. (2010). *American nursing: A history of knowledge, authority and the meaning of work.* Baltimore, MD: Johns Hopkins University Press.

D'Antonio, P. (2013). Cultivating constituencies: The story of the East Harlem Nursing and Health Service, 1928–1941. *American Journal of Public Health, 103*(6), 988–996.

D'Antonio, P. (2014). Lessons learned: Nursing and health demonstration projects in New York City, 1920-1935. *Policy, Politics and Nursing Practice, 14*(3–4), 133–141.

Fairman, J. (2011). Patients and the rise of the nurse practitioner profession. In B. Hoffman, N. Tomes, R. Grob, & M. Schlesinger (Eds.), *Patients as policy actors* (pp. 215–230). New Brunswick, New Jersey: Rutgers University Press.

Fairman, J., Rowe, J., Hassmiller, S., & Shalala, D. (2011). Broadening the scope of nursing practice. *New England Journal of Medicine, 364*(3), 193–196.

Gallup. (n.d.). *Honesty/ethics in professions.* Retrieved from www.gallup.com/poll/1654/Honesty-Ethics-Professions.aspx.

Institute of Medicine. (2001). *Crossing the quality chasm: A new health system for the 21st century.* Washington, DC: National Academy Press.

Institute of Medicine. (2011). *The future of nursing: Leading change, advancing health.* Washington, DC: The National Academies Press.

Lewenson, S.B. (2015). Town and country nursing: Community participation and nurse recruitment. In J. Kirchgessner & A. Keeling (Eds.), *Nursing rural America* (pp. 1–19). New York: Springer.

Maternity Center Association. (1924). Columbia University Health Sciences Center, Box 52, Folder 2.

Stone, D. (2001). *Policy paradox: The art of political decision making* (revised ed.). New York: Norton.

Tomes, N., & Hoffman, B. (2011). Introduction: Patients as policy actors. In B. Hoffman, N. Tomes, R. Grob, & M. Schlesinger (Eds.), *Patients as policy actors*. New Brunswick, NJ: Rutgers.

Wald, L. D. (1915). *The house on Henry Street*. New York: Henry Holt and Company.

ONLINE RESOURCES

American Association for the History of Nursing
www.aahn.org
The Future of Nursing: Campaign for Action
https://campaignforaction.org
Learning Historical Research
www.williamcronon.net/researching/
Nursing History and Health Care
www.nursing.upenn.edu/nhhc/Pages/Welcome.aspx

3

Advocacy in Nursing and Health Care

Susan Apold[a]

"Advocacy is a dish best served coordinated."

Suzanne Miyamoto, Nurses in Washington Internship speech, 2014

The word *advocacy* is defined as "the act or process of supporting a cause or proposal." It is derived from the Latin "advocatus," meaning "legal counselor." Labonte (1994) describes advocacy as influencing public policy. Within that context, it is the active support for causes, individuals, and groups, particularly those who are unable to voice arguments or positions on their own behalf.

Advocacy has not always been an explicit expectation of the professional nurse; however, the early writings of Nightingale reflected her commitment to health, healing, and acting in the best interests of patients. The rise of consumerism in the 1970s made explicit the role of the nurse as a patient advocate. Currently, the very definition of nursing in the 21st century addresses the role of the nurse as advocate (Table 3.1). This chapter will explore nurses' responsibility to advocate for policies that address access to health care, health promotion, disease prevention, and issues that affect health.

EVOLUTION OF NURSING'S ADVOCACY ROLE

Nurses have a long history of advocating on behalf of and alongside patients, families, and communities to promote health, equality, and justice. The nursing profession also has staunchly advocated for itself in an effort to provide patients with the essential work of nurses.

For example, Nightingale's advocacy is foundational to modern nursing practice. Her staunch devotion to human rights drove her advocacy for quality patient

care, outcome-based interventions, respect for the relationship between the environment and the patient, and the role of education in preparing qualified women to provide patient care.

Dorothea Dix advocated for the dignity and care of patients suffering from psychiatric illness and advocated for humane treatment of the mentally ill. She influenced state and federal legislatures and helped to craft laws that protected the "insane" and "mentally disturbed." She petitioned Pope Pius IX to consider the plight of institutionalized people.

Beginning in the 1980s, Loretta Ford recognized the need for children to have quality primary care and identified nurses as a resource to provide access to such care. Ford is responsible for developing the role of the nurse practitioner (NP) and advocating that nurses practice to the full extent of their education and licenses.

Currently, the nurse's role as advocate is codified in the profession's definition and principles. Nursing belongs to society and exists because of an identified social need—the need for "careers" of health, wellness, and illness. The profession is charged by society for providing this service in every situation in which nursing is needed. For this reason, nurses have a professional and moral imperative to use their voices to present the unique and essential perspective of nursing at every forum where nursing and health care is discussed. *Nursing's Social Policy Statement: The Essence of the Profession* (American Nurses Association [ANA], 2010) outlines nursing's accountability to society and identifies nursing's leadership role in essential health-related issues. This leadership implies advocating for health as a human

---

[a]This chapter adapts some content developed by Chad Priest from the chapter on advocacy published in the prior edition of this book.

TABLE 3.1 Profession of Nursing's Imperative to Engage in Advocacy	
Document	**Exemplars of Language Regarding the Role of Nurses in Advocacy**
Definition of Nursing	"Nursing is the protection, promotion, and optimization of health and abilities; prevention of illness and injury; alleviation of suffering through the diagnosis and treatment of human response; and advocacy in the care of individuals, families, communities, and populations" (American Nurses Association [ANA], 2010).
ANA Code of Ethics	Provision 2: "The nurse promotes, advocates for, and protects the rights, health, and safety of the patient" (ANA, 2015).
The Essentials of Baccalaureate Education for Professional Nursing Practice	"Baccalaureate Generalist nurses are providers of direct and indirect care. In this role, nurses are patient advocates and educators . . . Baccalaureate generalist nurses are members of the profession and in this role are advocates for the patient and the profession . . . . As advocates for high quality care for all patients, nurses are knowledgeable and active in the policy processes defining healthcare delivery and systems of care" (American Association of Colleges of Nursing [AACN], 2008, pp. 8 and 9).
The Essentials of Master's Education in Nursing	Standard VI: Health Policy and Advocacy: "Recognizes that the master's prepared nurse is able to intervene at the system level through the policy development process and to employ advocacy strategies to influence health and health care" (AACN, 2011, p. 5).
The Essentials of Doctoral Education for Advanced Nursing Practice	Standard V: Health Care Policy for Advocacy in Health Care: " . . . the DNP graduate is able to design, implement and advocate for health care policy that addresses issues of social justice and equity in health care" (AACN, 2006, p. 13).
International Council of Nurses (ICN) Code of Ethics for Nurses	"The nurse shares with society the responsibility for initiating and supporting action to meet the health and social needs of the public, in particular those of vulnerable populations . . . The nurse advocates for equity and social justice in resource allocation, access to health care and other social and economic services" (ICN, 2012, p. 2).

right, providing for strategies to promote health and prevent disease, advocating for expansion of health care access, and identifying and delivering resources and strategies that will enable all members of society to access health care and be able to live healthy lives (ANA, 2010).

Advocacy is a prominent theme in myriad documents that govern and describe nursing practice and education (see Table 3.1). Nurses' role as advocates transcends the traditional bedside action and advocacy for an individual patient. It has expanded to influencing public and private sector policies that pertain to health, including advocating for what communities need to be healthy.

The role of the nurse as advocate has evolved over the years, from performing nursing functions adequately and safely to advocating for issues of social justice. It is a central tenet of nursing practice throughout the world (Hanks, 2013; Vaartio et al., 2006).

Early in the history of the profession, nurses advocated that the best interests of patients were served by supporting the actions and decisions of physicians and promoting confidence in the health care system—such as it was. Instructional books from the early period of the profession characterized the nurse as a warrior in the battle against disease and illness, glamorizing a life of "toil and discipline" in which nurses pledged loyalty to their physician leaders. Nurses were explicitly taught that loyalty to the physician equated with faithfulness to the patient (Priest, 2016; Winslow, 1984). The Florence Nightingale Pledge of 1893 included: "With loyalty will I endeavor to aid the physician in his work and devote myself to the welfare of those committed to my care" (Florence Nightingale

Pledge, n.d.). Patient advocacy was nursing's responsibility only in so far as that advocacy was promoted as loyalty to the physician and his decision making.

In 1929 a new graduate nurse, Lorenza Somera, was given an order by a surgeon to administer cocaine instead of *procaine* injections to a tonsillectomy patient (Priest, 2016; Winslow, 1984). Somera loyally carried out the physician's order, resulting in the death of the patient. Although it was clear that the physician had erred in ordering the incorrect medication, he was acquitted of all charges while Somera was found guilty of manslaughter for failing to question the orders of the physician. The Somera case sparked worldwide protests from nurses and served to push nursing toward independent practice and accountability. It was also one of many events that led to a reconceptualization of the dominant nursing metaphor from loyalty to physicians to advocacy for patients.

A contemporary public demonstration of a nurse advocating for her patient that led to policy change occurred in July, 2017, when registered nurse (RN) Alex Wubbles was arrested for refusing to allow police officers from drawing blood on a patient without the patient's consent. Wubbles' primary allegiance and responsibility was to the patient. Her false arrest resulted in a settlement of $500,000 with both the University and State of Utah. Wubbles will continue to advocate for patients because she will be donating half of that settlement to a campaign that will provide Utah citizens with free body camera footage of any encounter with the police. The law firm that represented Wubbles agreed to provide free legal services to support this initiative. As a result of this incident, in 2018, the University of Utah Medical Center revised its policies to continue to support the rights of its patients and nurses' responsibility to advocate for those rights (Stevens, 2017).

Professional advocacy involves nurses championing issues that support the profession (e.g., safe staffing, nurses' health, healthy work environments). *Issues advocacy* involves the role of the profession in championing social, economic, legal, and environmental factors that influence the health of the population. Nurses can and should also engage in *political advocacy*—the active engagement in the political process through activities such as voting, campaigning for candidates running for office, donating to a political action committee (PAC), and lobbying and educating elected officials about important issues.

Nurses have played a role in advocating for a variety of social reform issues influencing health, including smoke-free environments, calorie and restaurant labeling, and protections in the work environment (Ezeonwu, 2015; Johnson et al., 2012; Nagelhout et al., 2014). Every nursing organization engages in both professional and issues advocacy. For example:

- The ANA (2018) "... believes that advocacy is a pillar of nursing. Nurses instinctively advocate for their patients, in their workplaces, and in their communities; but legislative and political advocacy is no less important to advancing the profession and patient care." The ANA gives voice to the profession at state and federal levels and advocates for issues such as reducing gun violence, environmental safety, and promotion of policies that support access to care for all Americans.
- The American Association of Nurse Practitioners (AANP) supports patients, issues, and the profession through their advocacy work in removing legislative barriers to practice for NPs. It has been successful in expanding scope of practice for NPs in 22 states and the District of Columbia (AANP, 2018). In addition, the AANP participated in changes in the payment schedule for health care providers and influencing Medicare reform.
- In 2018 the American Academy of Nursing (2018) released a statement in opposition to a policy which separated children from their parents at the United States border. That same year, the National Association of Pediatric Nurse Practitioners (NAPNAP) released a position statement opposing border separation of children and parents (NAPNAP, 2018).
- The Nursing Community Coalition brings more than 60 nursing organizations together in pursuit of professional and issues advocacy. In 2018 more than 40 nursing organizations urged President Trump and Congress to make high-quality, affordable health care a top priority policy initiative.

MODELS OF NURSING ADVOCACY

A number of nursing theorists have developed models of nursing advocacy (Ezeonwu, 2015). Curtain (1979) proposed a theory of human advocacy and used the concept of "advocate" to describe the philosophical foundation and ideal of nursing. In this model, advocacy does not refer to "legal advocacy" or even "health advocacy" but human advocacy. The role of the nurse is to be a human advocate. This does not necessarily mean intervening on a patient's behalf but advocating for the patient's humanity. Curtain believes that illness wounds patients and robs them of their humanity. The nurse assumes the role of advocate by healing the wounds of "loss of independence," "loss of freedom," and "loss of ability to make informed decisions." In this early theory of advocacy, the nurse is not specifically called upon to act or support a cause, provide a patient with a voice, or influence public policy, but to prevent a loss of humanity.

Gadow (1983) proposed a theory of existential advocacy that requires humans to be "authentic" or self-directed.

The nurse becomes an existential advocate by "participating with the patient in determining the personal meaning which the experience of illness, suffering, or dying is to have for that individual" (p. 97). Kohnke's functional model of advocacy (1978) focuses on patient choice. In this model of advocacy, the nurse provides the patient with important information, determines that the patient understands that information, and then supports the patient's right to make the best decision for himself/herself even if the nurse disagrees with it. In 1989 Fowler proposed a broader theory of nursing advocacy: advocacy for social justice. This theory includes the role of nurse as patient advocate not only at the bedside but within health care facilities and throughout society.

Bu and Jezewski (2007) built upon all of these theories and proposed a unified theory of advocacy with three basic tenets: "(a) safeguarding patients' autonomy, (b) acting on behalf of patients, and (c) championing social justice in provision of health care" (p. 104). Contemporary models of advocacy address patient needs *and* the nurse's role in advocating for all issues that pertain to the health of patients, including advocacy for the nursing profession.

PREPARING NURSES FOR THEIR ROLE AS ADVOCATES

Although advocacy is viewed by nurses and the public alike as a major role for the nurse, very little is done to formally prepare nurses for this role. Nursing curriculums at the undergraduate and graduate levels do not make explicit the skill set necessary to advocate effectively. Advocacy is primarily learned after graduation in practice settings and often by observing other nurses acting as advocates (Foley et al., 2002; Hanks, 2008).

Advocacy often involves conflict, and it always involves communication. It requires sophisticated leadership skills, including emotional intelligence, self-awareness, relationship management, team building, conflict management, interprofessional collaboration, problem solving and sensitivity, effective communication skills, and use of influence (Tomajan, 2012). Nursing education must provide students at all levels of education with this knowledge and these skills. This includes using role-playing scenarios on advocacy and examining advocacy behaviors in clinical experiences. Curriculums need to identify advocacy mentors for students to consult when advocacy issues arise. These mentors can be found in clinical settings and in nursing organizations.

The literature supports experiences and characteristics that are common to nurses who advocate for patients and who seek advocacy opportunities in their practices. Altun and Ersoy (2003) reported that nurses who had ethics courses or who were taught ethics were more likely to engage in advocacy behavior. Others have shown that nurses' advocacy behaviors are linked with higher levels of education (Hanks, 2010; Kubsch, Sternard, Hovarter, & Matzke, 2003). Nurse educators can use this information to design curriculums that address students' development of advocacy skills through opportunities such as lobby day activities, patient advocacy days, and structured class debates. This education should include practicing nurses and students.

Advocacy education also requires a discussion about what advocacy "feels" like. Serving in an advocacy role takes courage. An advocate is often called upon to speak truth to authority and stand in the tension of an opposing point of view. Cultivating that courage requires conversations about the affective dimension of advocacy: the physical, emotional, and psychological energy needed to advocate effectively.

OVERCOMING BARRIERS TO ADVOCACY

Hanks' (2007) concept analysis of barriers to advocacy suggests that powerlessness, fear of punishment, conflicts of interest, and lack of institutional support are major reasons why nurses do not engage in advocacy.

As a predominantly female profession, nursing has never been considered powerful. Women's voices are not considered to be as powerful as the voices of men. Nurses have difficulty advocating for themselves, and the consequences of oppressed group behavior (lateral violence, infighting, incivility) continue to be prevalent even 35 years after Roberts (1983) first used Freire's (1968) theory of oppressed group behavior to describe nursing's relative powerlessness. Members of oppressed groups fear their oppressors and are angry at them. When that fear and anger are internalized, the oppressed come to believe that they are inferior, powerless, and unable to unify enough to gain power in their own right within the system. This reality, coupled with a history that valued and encouraged subservience, obedience, and unquestioning loyalty to physicians and health care institutions, contributes mightily to the image of the nurse as powerless and not influential. Although nurses do appear to engage in advocacy activities when confronted with the well-being of their individual patients, they are less inclined to engage in the long-term organized advocacy necessary for social justice.

Nurses also fear retribution. Although much has been done to protect employees from retaliation for "whistleblowing," advocacy requires risk taking and no small measure of courage. Nurses—in reality, anyone who advocates on behalf of another—can experience punishment, demotion, and labeling. Advocacy can disrupt relationships in employment and policymaking settings.

Overcoming the Barriers

Little research has been done to identify the characteristics of nurses who are successful advocates, but it appears that nurses who have a good self-concept, strong values, confidence, and a positive professional identity are more likely to take risks in the name of advocating for patients, communities, and the profession (Panticuff, 1989). Forums in which to share stories of successes and failures in advocacy and their impact on future advocacy activities can be motivating to novice and experienced nurses alike.

Building on her work—oppressed group behavior in nursing—Roberts (2000, 2015) posits that a strong sense of professional identity is necessary to engage in leadership and advocacy work. This identity is developed over time. It begins with early career acceptance of the role and status of the professional nurse; connection with other nurses through participation on committees and in professional organizations; synthesis of professional experiences leading to a positive view of nursing; and ultimately, commitment to create change and advocate for issues of social justice. Nursing curriculums, professional organizations and nursing leaders can use this model to foster a strong professional identity in pursuit of overcoming barriers to advocacy.

The Institute of Medicine Report (2011), *The Future of Nursing*, provides nurses at all levels and types of practice with a mandate to find and use individual voices and the collective voice of the profession in pursuit of advocacy work. Likely the most important report on nursing in our time, it looks to the profession to fill "new expanded roles in a redesigned health care system." However, this is not possible, without the voices of nurses raised up not in fear but in unity to make health care more equitable, accessible, and compassionate.

Nursing executives can build a culture of advocacy, one in which nurses and all members of the health care team engage in routine advocacy for patients, nurses, the profession of nursing, and public policies that affect health. Engaging in advocacy must become both an expectation and routine behavior. When nurses are encouraged, as part of their professional responsibility, to attend to social and economic factors that influence health and then advocate for policies that promote a culture of health, nurses will have an increased comfort level with raising their voices for patients at the bedside and society as a whole.

LIVED EXPERIENCE OF ADVOCACY

Hanks' (2008) qualitative work on the lived experience of advocacy identifies three themes: nurses experience with advocacy (speaking out and speaking for patients; being compelled to act on the unmet needs of patients); experiences with outcomes of advocacy (fulfillment and frustration; the change in the patient); and educational preparation for the advocacy role (primarily learned on the job; confidence gained through experience).

The lived experience of three nationally recognized nurse leaders are included here as exemplars of successful nursing advocacy experiences.

Patient Advocacy

Janis Sunderhaus, RN, is the President and Chief Executive Officer of Health Partners of Western Ohio, a Federally Qualified Health Center she established in 2003. With 12 locations in Western Ohio, these clinics provide medical, pediatric, dental, behavioral health service, substance abuse, pharmacy, and social services. Sunderhaus discusses the reality that the actual in-the-moment experience of advocating for patients is not taught in school and is often not encouraged by nurses. Advocating for patients requires nurses to "stick your neck out" and "stand between the patient and someone else." She recalls a time in the 1980s, when she worked on an infectious disease unit with patients who had all sorts of infections that no one understood. She asked a resident for orders for pain medication for a patient who was a sex worker and was in agony from herpes throughout her entire gastrointestinal system. The resident declined to give her pain medication because he wanted to "keep an eye on the disease progression." Sunderhaus saw a patient with whom she had a shared humanity. Her view of her patients was consistent with Curtain's perspective that nurses advocate for patients' humanity. When the medication was not forthcoming, Sunderhaus called the resident's attending physician at his home on "football Sunday." Janis recalls that it was a singularly unpleasant position to be in. "I was afraid, I was shaking, I really didn't want to have to do this. I was uncomfortable, but it had to be done. I had to be that patient's voice." Sunderhaus adds, "And you know what? It's like that every time." As nurses continue through their careers, it becomes easier, but it is also easier when nurses aggressively participate in building a culture of advocacy so that "doing the right thing" is expected behavior. "That way," she says, "you don't have to fight every single time."

Professional Advocacy

Donald Gardenier was a Peace Corps volunteer in Patagonia before becoming a nurse. A National Health Service Corps Scholar, he worked to place primary care providers in underserved areas. Gardenier had ample opportunity to advocate for his patients throughout his career. He makes the case that it is the nurse's job to get what the patient needs and then give it to him or her. He subscribes to

Kohnke's model of functional advocacy. Gardenier sought an opportunity to disseminate his clinical work more widely and use organized nursing to make that happen. He recounts, "I didn't know anything about this type of work, but I did it anyway, because it had to be done." Specifically, Gardenier participated in the merger of two nursing organizations into one to leverage the numbers and create a unified position that one large organization would bring to the political table. "I didn't always know the exact right course of action, but I was always confident that this work had to be done for the profession because our profession is about our patients." Gardenier recalls moments of conflict and discomfort, along with the awareness that these were necessary for a final positive outcome.

Political Advocacy

Denise Link is an NP and political activist who began practicing as an NP before the role's title and scope had been legally defined. During her first year of practice providing health services to underserved women, Link's clinic received a communication from the State Attorney General's office saying that, although the performance of a Pap test was within the scope of practice of an RN, use of a speculum to perform a pelvic examination was not. Understanding that if she could not use a speculum, she could not complete an exam, she says that she became a "political activist that day. I was not going to deprive my patients' access to care because of some poorly thought out regulation. I realized that if I wanted to make changes to my practice, it had to be in the political arena." And so it began for Link. She says, "I understood my power and I was not afraid to use it." She joined professional organizations at the local, state, and national levels. She used her voice in state capitols and on Capitol Hill in Washington, D.C. Link did not approach advocacy with trepidation or lack of knowing what to do because she came from a family of political activists. She had a voice early in her career, and she used it politically to provide her patients with the access and quality that they deserve.

Advocacy on behalf of the public's health can be extremely rewarding. Nurses are in a unique position to be advocates for health.

DISCUSSION QUESTIONS

1. What examples have you seen of nurses advocating for the health of populations, including through workplace or political action? What made these nurses effective advocates?
2. What experience do you have as an advocate for health in your workplace, a professional organization, or government? How did it feel? Were you successful? What are the barriers you experienced and how did you overcome these? What would you do differently?

REFERENCES

Altun, I., & Ersoy, N. (2003). Undertaking the role of patient advocate: A longitudinal study of nursing students. *Nursing Ethics, 10*(5), 462–471.

American Academy of Nursing. (2018). *Separation of children from their parents increases likelihood of toxic stress.* Retrieved from https://higherlogicdownload.s3.amazonaws.com/AANNET/c8a8da9e-918c-4dae-b0c6-6d630c46007f/UploadedImages/docs/Press%20Releases/2018/2018-Academy_Statement_on_Separation_of_Children-Parents_at_Border__1_.pdf.

American Association of Colleges of Nursing (2006). *The essentials of doctoral education for advanced nursing practice.* Washington, DC: AACN.

American Association of Colleges of Nursing (2008). *The essentials baccalaureate nursing education for professional nursing practice.* Washington, DC: AACN.

American Association of Colleges of Nursing (2011). *The essentials of master's education in nursing.* Washington, DC: AACN.

American Association of Nurse Practitioners. (2018). *State practice environment.* Retrieved from www.aanp.org/advocacy/state/state-practice-environment.

American Nurses Association. (2010). *Nursing's social policy statement: The essence of the profession.* Silver Spring, MD: ANA.

American Nurses Association. (2015). *Code of ethics for nurses with interpretive statements.* Silver Spring, MD: ANA.

American Nurses Association. (2018). *Advocacy.* Retrieved from www.nursingworld.org/practice-policy/advocacy/.

Bu, X., & Jezewski, M.A. (2007). Developing a mid-range theory of patient advocacy through concept analysis. *Journal of Advanced Nursing, 57*(1), 101–110.

Curtain, L. (1979). The nurse as advocate: A philosophical foundation for nursing. *Advances in Nursing Science, 1*(3), 1–10.

Ezeonwu, M. (2015). Community health nursing advocacy: A concept analysis. *Journal of Community Health Nursing, 32,* 115–128.

Florence Nightingale Pledge. (n.d.). *Vanderbilt nurse.* Retrieved from www.vanderbilt.edu/vanderbiltnurse/2010/11/florence-nightingale-pledge/.

Foley, B.J., Minick, P., & Kee, C. (2002). How nurses learn advocacy. *Journal of Nursing Scholarship, 34*(2), 181–186.

Fowler, M. D. (1989). Social advocacy. *Heart & Lung: The Journal of Critical Care, 18*(1), 97–99.

Freire, P. (1968). *Pedagogy of the oppressed.* New York: Bloomsbury Publishing.

Gadow, S. (1983). *Existential advocacy. Philosophical foundations of nurse-patient relationship.* Boston, MA: Allyn and Bacon.

Hanks, R. G. (2007). Barriers to nursing advocacy: A concept analysis. *Nursing Forum, 42*(4), 171–177.

Hanks, R.G. (2008). The lived experience of nursing advocacy. *Nursing Ethics, 15*(4), 468–477.

Hanks, R.G. (2010). The medical-surgical nurse perspective of advocate role. *Nursing Forum, 45*(2), 97–107.

Hanks, R.G. (2013). Social advocacy: A call for nursing action. *Pastoral Psychology, 62*(1), 163–173.

Institute of Medicine. (2011). *The future of nursing: Leading change, advancing health.* Washington, DC: National Academies Press. Retrieved from http://books.nap.edu/openbook.php?record_id=12956&page=R1.

International Council of Nurses. (2012). *The ICN code of ethics for nurses.* Geneva, Switzerland: ICN.

Johnson, D.B., Payne, E.C., McNeese, M.A., & Allen, D. (2012). Menu-labeling policy in King County, Washington. *American Journal of Preventive Medicine, 43*(3S2), S130–S135. Retrieved from http://dx.doi.org/10.1016/j.amepre.2012.05.014.

Kohnke, M.F. (1978). The nurse's responsibility to the consumer. *American Journal of Nursing, 78*(3), 440–442.

Kubsch, S., Sternard, M., Hovarter, R., & Matzke, V. (2003). A holistic model of advocacy: Factors that influence its use. *Complementary Therapy in Nursing Midwifery, 10,* 37–45.

Labonte, R. (1994). Health promotion and empowerment: Reflections on professional practice. *Health Education Quarterly, 21*(2), 253–268.

Nagelhout, G.E., Wolfson, T., Zhuang, Y.L., Gamst, A., Willemsen, M.C., & Zhu, S.H. (2014). Population support before and after the implementation of smoke-free laws in the United States: Trends from 1992 to 2007. *Nicotine & Tobacco Research, 17*(3), 350–355.

National Association of Pediatric Nurse Practitioners. (2018). *NAPNAP statement opposing the border separation of children and families.* Retrieved from www.napnap.org/napnap-statement-opposing-border-separation-children-and-parents.

Nursing Community Coalition. (2018). *Letter to Congress.* Retrieved from www.napnap.org/sites/default/files/userfiles/about/Nursing%20Letter%20in%20Support%20of%20Children%27s%20Health.pdf.

Panticuff, J. (1989). Infant suffering and nurse advocacy. *Nursing Clinics of North America, 24,* 987–997.

Priest, C. (2016). Frameworks for action in policy and politics. In D. Mason, D. Gardner, F. Outlaw, & E. O'Grady (Eds.), *Policy & politics in nursing and health care* (7th ed., pp. 25–38). St. Louis: Elsevier.

Roberts, S.J. (1983). Oppressed group behavior: Implications for nursing. *Advanced in Nursing Science, 5*(4), 21–30.

Roberts, S.J. (2000). Development of a positive professional identity: Liberating oneself from the oppressor within. *Advances in Nursing Science, 22*(4): 71–82.

Roberts, S.J. (2015). Lateral violence in nursing: A review of the past three decades. *Nursing Science Quarterly, 28*(1), 36–41.

Stevens, M. (2017, November 2). Arrested nurse settles with Salt Lake City and University for $500,000. *The New York Times.* Retrieved from www.nytimes.com/2017/11/02/us/utah-nurse-settlement.html.

Tomajan, K. (2012, January 31). Advocating for nurses and nursing. *OJIN: The Online Journal of Issues in Nursing, 17*(1), Manuscript 4. Retrieved from http://ojin.nursingworld.org/MainMenuCategories/ANAMarketplace/ANAPeriodicals/OJIN/TableofContents/Vol-17-2012/No1-Jan-2012/Advocating-for-Nurses.html.

Vaartio, H., Leino-Kilpi, H., Salantera, S., & Suominen, T. (2006). Nursing advocacy: How is it defined by patients and nurses, what does it involve and how is it experienced? *Scandinavian Journal of Caring Sciences, 20*(3), 282–292.

Winslow, G.R. (1984). From loyalty to advocacy: A new metaphor for nursing. *Hastings Center Report, 14*(3), 32–40.

4

Learning the Ropes of Policy and Politics

Wanda Montalvo[a]

"We should always have three friends in our lives. One who walks ahead who we look up to and follow; one who walks besides us, who is with us every step of our journey; and then, one who we reach back for and bring along after we've cleared the way."

Michelle Obama

Every politically active person, from U.S. presidents to chief executive officers, *learned* the political and policy skills that catapulted them into positions of power and responsibility. Nurses arrive in those positions in a similar fashion—these are learnable skills. Although one can learn about the policy process and political analysis through formal education, it is only through the lived experience and practice that one can apply what has been learned to become influencers of policy. Finding politically savvy mentors who can teach, believe in, and support us; celebrate our successes; and help us to learn from our failures is key.

Students new to politics, as well as experienced nurses, have unlimited ways to expand their knowledge and involvement. To improve one's skills and stimulate one's interest, conceptual frameworks help the intangible to be perceptible (see Chapter 1) and to help identify windows of opportunity to engage in policy. Nurses can become significant participants and leaders in the multiplayer process of policymaking because it is nonlinear with multiple entry points. The first step is to decide how much energy and time one is willing to devote.

POLITICAL CONSCIOUSNESS RAISING: THE "AHA" MOMENT

How does one get started? Many find that there is a defining moment when the old ways of reacting to issues of injustice, inequality, or powerlessness no longer work. It is the moment when a person realizes that an issue or problem is caused by failures in the system. For instance, lack of support staff on an acute care unit may be related to decreased reimbursement rates rather than an uncaring hospital administration. Disruptions in funding and eligibility for Medicaid and Medicare determine whether a low-income neighbor is able to access health care, as was evident in states that chose not to expand their Medicaid programs under the Affordable Care Act. Disparities in health outcomes may be due, in part, to health policies. Policies do not emerge in a vacuum but occur because of bargaining between contending groups shaped by institutional and political "rules of the game." Realizing that a problem may be caused by a policy failure is a critical first step toward becoming part of the policy solution. This is political consciousness raising and an "aha" moment. It is the adrenaline rush that urges, "Something must be done—and I need to become involved."

Until that defining moment, nurses may feel frustrated, angry, or hopeless. When the "aha" moment hits, they begin to understand that they can and must influence those who make the laws and regulations that create the inequities. Nurses then recognize the personal nature of policy issues ("the personal is political"). When nurses collectively accept

---

[a]This chapter includes updates from previous editions of the book by Andréa Sonenberg, Judith K. Leavitt, Janet Y. Harris, Mary W. Chaffee, and Connie Vance.

that they are capable of providing solutions to address the inadequacies of the health care system, the profession becomes political. The result is that individual nurses and the profession become empowered to act. Feeling empowered is essential to true advocacy (Sessler-Branden, 2012).

Being politically active as a nurse is grounded in the role of *advocacy*. Florence Nightingale saw nursing in all of its forms as advocacy—a "calling" that required nurses to look for and act in ways to be world citizens for the sake of human health (Dossey et al., 2005). Through her grounded theory research, Sessler-Branden (2012) identified this far-reaching definition of advocacy: "a dynamic process through which the nurse engages in a set of actions with broadly stated goals ultimately affecting a desired change at any level of patient care, health care systems and/or health policy." Chapter 3 provides a more extensive discussion of advocacy.

GETTING STARTED

Nurses appear on the Gallup poll as the highest ranked profession for honesty and ethical standards for 16 years (Brenan, 2018), yet the medical profession remains a dominant voice and influencer of health policy (Catallo, Spalding, Haghiri-Vijeh, 2014). Only by self-activation to engage with a policy or social justice issue will nurses know whether their actions contributed to a policy shift related to issues such as scope of practice or women's reproductive health. Remember, political skills can be learned and refined over time to influence any platform (e.g., workplace, school, local, state, or federal policy), so do not be discouraged. Politics requires the kind of communication skills and knowledge nurses use to persuade patients to collaborate in self-care or get out of bed after abdominal surgery. Nurses are health care experts who can speak knowledgeably about what patients and communities need. See Box 4.1 for some ideas to get started.

Nurses benefit from learning the components of political skill. Ferris (2007) defined four distinct components of political skill:

- *Social astuteness:* Individuals possessing political skill are astute observers of others and keenly attuned to diverse social situations. They comprehend social interactions and accurately interpret their behavior; they are able to discern the situation and are self-aware.
- *Interpersonal influence:* Politically skilled individuals have a subtle and convincing personal style that exerts a powerful influence to persuade those around them. They are able to strategically modify their behavior to different persons in different settings.
- *Networking ability:* Individuals with strong political skill are adept at developing and building partnerships

---

BOX 4.1   Getting Started

Remember, policy work includes efforts at your work site, school, local community board, or place of worship. Here are some ways to get started:

- Visit the American Nurses Association website (www.nursingworld.org) and select a template from the Advocacy Toolkit and email, call, or write a letter to legislator.
- Visit the *Future of Nursing* Campaign for Action (www.campaignforaction.org) and connect with local state action coalition.
- Participate in a political rally by simply marching and holding up a sign. Let your voice be heard!
- Attend a local community board meeting to observe local political and civic leaders discuss local issues and set local policy. Consider adding your nursing expertise by volunteering to join a workgroup.
- Volunteer to join an employer-sponsored committee (e.g., governance, quality, workforce).
- Employers like hospitals and universities offer platforms for bi-directional learning related to governance or health policy to help build knowledge (Waddell, Audette, DeLong, Brostoff, 2016).
- Take a course to increase political awareness within or outside of nursing.
- To develop policy-networking skills, ask a person with relationships with policymakers for an introduction.
- Attend local community events and become a familiar face to a policymaker. Use Twitter to promote nursing's expertise and tag the presenters.
- You are the expert! Do not assume the policymaker or staffer fully understands the core issue. Share your knowledge to help educate people and influence decision-makers.
- Write letters to the editor or op-ed and acknowledge policymakers who support your issue.
- Follow policymakers on social media and help promote and support issues of interest.
- Learn strategies on how to increase your influence. Listen to RNFMRadio episode #239 *Increase Your Influence and Authority* (http://rnfmradio.com/episode239/).

---

with diverse networks of people for beneficial alliances and coalitions.

- *Apparent sincerity:* Politically skilled individuals appear to others as possessing high levels of integrity, authenticity, sincerity, and genuineness. This dimension of political skill strikes at the very heart of whether or not influence attempts will be successful because it focuses on the perceived intentions. If actions are not interpreted as manipulative or coercive, individuals high in

LEARNING THE ROPES	PARTICIPATING IN DEMOCRACY	INFLUENCING AND ADVOCATING	USING ADVANCED POLITICAL SKILLS
• Get a mentor • Educate self about policy and politics • Read and consider health care and social issues • Get an internship • Read, listen to, and discuss the news and current issues • Network with other nurses • Participate in nursing legislative events • Learn about advocacy and activism • Study policy • Strengthen communication skills (written and verbal) • Attend educational programs or camps • Learn the structure of governments • Identify your elected representatives • Learn the scope of influence of groups with authority (e.g., local board of health, organizational groups, congressional committees) • Join policy and advocacy groups on professional social networking sites	• Volunteer on a political campaign • Vote • Explain political views to others • Learn about political candidates and their views • Participate in voter registration activities • Sign petitions • Post candidates' signs on your property or vehicle • Weigh pros and cons of political positions • Join a political party • Research the status of a bill • Serve as a volunteer poll worker on election day	• Post opinions on blogs • Participate in professional organization's legislative activities • Write op-eds and letters to editors of newspapers and other media • Express opinions via social media (e.g., Twitter) • Speak at public hearings • Cultivate a relationship with elected representatives • Respond to "action alerts" sent out by professional organizations • Participate in rallies and protests • Network with opinion leaders (local organizers, business owners, and others) • Support a political candidate (go door-to-door, attend meetings, make calls) • Express opinions to elected officials via letter, e-mail, call, or visit • Make financial contributions to political action committees • Hold a house party fundraiser for a candidate • Participate in community meetings	• Run for elective office • Obtain a political appointment • Serve as a paid political staff member • Provide expert testimony • Hold a media event • Host television, radio, or other media broadcasts • Write a newspaper column • Serve as a policy analyst • Obtain an appointment to a board or committee • Serve as a speechwriter • Participate in political surveys and polling • Manage a political campaign • Become a lobbyist • Publish articles on health care issues and solutions • Provide an interview with the media

Fig. 4.1 The Spectrum of Political Competencies and examples of activities.

apparent sincerity inspire trust and confidence from those around them.

The Spectrum of Political Competencies (Fig. 4.1) demonstrates the breadth and variety of political and policy competencies ranging from novice to more sophisticated levels, including running for elective office. Initial experiences in activism and advocacy as a student are available through the National Student Nurses Association (NSNA) Health Policy and Advocacy Committee. Participating in lobby days and observing skilled lobbyists negotiate with policymakers are great ways to sharpen one's political skills. At these events, nurse lobbyists and citizen activists serve as role models to nurses and students by exhibiting effective networking strategies and influencer behaviors while lobbying policymakers on specific legislation. These activists (Fig. 4.2) also provide the inspiration and vision for what can be done if nurses work together toward shared goals. This is real-life learning, and it is a highly effective and practical way of developing political awareness and know-how.

MENTOR ADVANTAGE

Emerging nurse leaders seeking to advance their careers and develop political skills should secure a mentoring relationship. Mentoring is a vehicle for developing political skill and contextual knowledge, part of a critical set of competencies used throughout a protégé's career. Stewart (1996) defines mentoring in nursing as a teaching-learning process acquired through personal experience within a one-to-one, reciprocal relationship between two individuals diverse in age, personality, life cycle, professional status, and/or credentials. Mentoring provides the protégé with opportunities for coaching, friendship, role modeling, challenging assignments, and sponsorship (Bunkers, 2018). Mentoring should be continuous, goal directed, and under

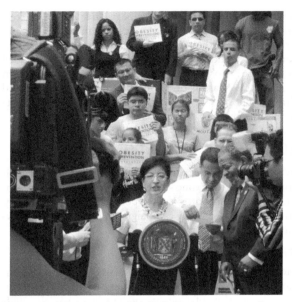

Fig. 4.2 Wanda Montalvo, RN, PhD, leads a press conference asking the New York City Council to support the Childhood Obesity Initiative.

the aegis of a capable person who can be a trusted teacher and counselor (Vance & Olson, 1998). The characteristics of successful mentors include being trustworthy, an active listener, accessible, and able to support the protégé's professional development (Green & Jackson, 2014).

Effective mentors are able to share life experiences and wisdom, identify the protégé's strengths and limitations, and provide critical feedback to support career and political skill development. A study among nurses who either possessed a doctoral degree (PhD or DNP) or were a candidate for the degree revealed that the mentoring functions of advocacy, career development, learning facilitation, and friendship correlated with political skill development in the protégé (Montalvo & Bryne, 2016). Compared with nonmentored individuals, productive mentoring relationships result in the protégé gaining increased visibility, self-efficacy, access to new social networks, and greater career mobility (Peiser, Ambrose, Burke, & Davenport, 2017). These gains include research productivity, career development, and improved leadership skills. Furthermore, mentoring has a positive influence on the development of relationships, work culture, and collaboration (Hafsteinsdottir, vand der Zwaag, & Schuurmans, 2017).

The protégé must be mindful and respectful of the mentor's time, proactively prepare and schedule meetings with the mentor, and be open to mentor feedback (Straus, 2013).

Mentors should be on the lookout for emerging nurse leaders to identify a protégé with a similar cognitive style to facilitate effective communication and relationship building (Armstrong, Allinson, & Hayes, 2002). Alternately, peer-to-peer mentoring opens additional opportunities to access support and expand one's thinking by interacting with colleagues, seeking input, and sharing gained wisdom as a collective, not just one mentee (McBride, Campbell, Woods, & Manson, 2017).

Finding a Mentor

To find a mentor, it is important to determine what you would like to learn or in what area of politics and policy you would like to be involved. Start with self-reflection, and write down your areas of strength and areas of self-improvement. Consider the political and policy skills you want to develop. This will help you to think about the type of qualities you are searching for in a mentor.

Leverage your networks to identify people whom you have noticed, heard, or read about who are activists in your area of interest. Good sources for finding mentors are nursing associations, schools of nursing, professional organizations, local governmental offices, and local political organizations and campaigns. You can contact the person directly or ask a colleague to help with an introduction. Make clear why you think the person, whether in or outside of nursing, would be a good mentor. Tell them what you want to learn and why you would like them to assist you. Protégés and mentors benefit from holding each other accountable, so consider establishing a mentoring contract with agreed goals and timeframe to help clarify expectations of the relationship (Montalvo & Bryne, 2016). See Table 4.1 for an example of what to include in a contract. The important criteria for a mentor are knowledge and an interest in you. Remember to give the relationship time to develop, be honest about expectations, and recognize that the mentor-protégé relationship is reciprocal as you learn from each other.

Collective Mentoring

Learning politics is not a solitary activity. Every nurse should assume responsibility for actively mentoring others as they refine their repertoire of skills and deepen their involvement. Reciprocal collective mentoring is extremely effective in expanding the political power of the profession and its members.

Inherent in this form of mentoring is the development of networks of people who are active in policy and who take responsibility for expanding the networks. Nurses in these networks should develop strategies for mentoring political neophytes and identify nurses in nontraditional careers such as entrepreneurs, nonprofit agencies, military,

TABLE 4.1	Sample Mentoring Contract
Goals	What do you hope to accomplish? Learn new skills, expand social network, meet and engage legislative staff, join a community board.
Strategy for achieving goal?	Help to plan committee meeting and observe process, participate in research, publish, write policy brief or op-ed.
Meeting frequency	Discuss frequency, duration, and method of meeting (e.g., in-person at office, offsite, video, phone call). Agree to keep sensitive issues confidential.
Duration of mentoring relationship	Formal can vary from 6 to 12 months or longer with informal mentoring lasting longer. A formal mentoring contract can be set for 12 months. As long as both parties feel comfortable with the productivity and progress, mentorship may continue and eventually transition to a collegial peer-to-peer relationship.
Plan on evaluating mentorship relationship	Protégé and mentor need to discuss how progress and goals will be evaluated and outcomes accomplished (e.g., paper, active policy engagement, writing a blog or op-ed, presenting at conference).

or philanthropy (Wall, 2013). Networking opportunities exist among political leaders in professional associations. Many state nursing associations are successfully reaching out to collectively mentor hundreds of nursing students through lobby days in national and state capitols. Nursing students and practicing nurses have many opportunities to experience collective mentoring with leaders and peers in organizations such as the NSNA, Graduate Nursing Student Academy, American Nurses Association (ANA), American Organization for Nursing Leadership (AONL) , minority nursing associations, specialty and state nursing associations, and volunteer health-related organizations. In addition, local political parties, community organizations, and the offices of elected officials offer mentored experiences in lobbying, policy development, media contacts, fundraising, and the political process.

In the workplace, one can learn from health professionals who serve as leaders on influential committees. At

Boston Children's Hospital, the Legislative Action Interest Group (LAIG) developed a policy forum to engage and bridge strategies between nursing, department of patient care services, and Office of Government Relations (Waddell et al., 2016). Hospital nurses interested in participating in a legislative hearing or public listening session received direct support from LAIG leaders to prepare oral or written testimony.

EDUCATIONAL OPPORTUNITIES

Whatever your educational and political goals, there is something for everyone—from continuing education programs to graduate programs in political science and policy, from workshops run by campaign organizations to fellowships and conferences.

Programs in Schools of Nursing

Health policy is one of the "essentials" of nursing education at the baccalaureate, master's, and DNP levels (American Association of Colleges of Nursing [AACN], 2008, 2010, 2018a, 2018b). Some schools of nursing are developing DNP or PhD programs that focus on policy. Nursing programs also offer healthy policy courses as either core requirements or electives.

Degree Programs and Courses in Public Health, Public Administration, and Public Policy

College and university departments of public health, political science, political administration, and others offer policy tracks, programs, and courses that are widely available at the baccalaureate, master's, and doctoral levels. These are easily accessible through online catalogs.

Continuing Education

Annual conferences on health policy are offered by academic institutions, professional associations, and health policy organizations. Other conferences will have a health policy track or session. Monitor websites and your state nursing association's meeting announcements for offerings. Search the internet using *health policy meeting*, *health policy conference*, or *health care meeting* as search terms.

Workshops

A quick, intensive, and participatory approach is to take a 1- or 2-day workshop in politics, campaigning, or policy from political or educational institutions. At the state and national level, political parties host campaign workshops, as do other nonpartisan groups. The Nurse in Washington

Internship (NIWI) sponsored by The Nursing Organizations Alliance (The Alliance) is a 2.5-day experience (www.nursing-alliance.org).

Learning by Doing

There are many ways to obtain valuable practical experience in health policy and politics, from volunteerism to internships to self-study programs.

Internships and Fellowships. Internships and fellowships provide great learning experiences. These practical placements offer valuable mentoring and networking opportunities to refine skills with knowledgeable leaders. Summer or year-long internships may be arranged for credit in an academic program or through local, state, and federal legislative bodies and in government agencies. Professional associations like the ANA offers a year-long mentored experience called American Nurses Advocacy

Institute (*www.nursingworld.org*). Organizations such as the Robert Wood Johnson Foundation, the American Academy of Nursing (AAN), state policy centers, and others offer internships or fellowships in policy. The Health and Policy in Aging Program is an opportunity for learning about aging policy in Washington, DC (www.healthandagingpolicy.org).

Volunteer Service. A great way to learn the ropes of politics is to volunteer to work on a political campaign, including of nurses such as Alana Cueto. Candidates for elective office at all levels of government welcome volunteers who donate time and energy. Building relationships through volunteer service is a critical part of learning and educating policymakers of nursing's expertise (Fig. 4.3).

Professional Association Activities. Professional nursing associations offer volunteer opportunities that lead

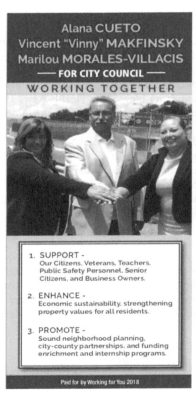
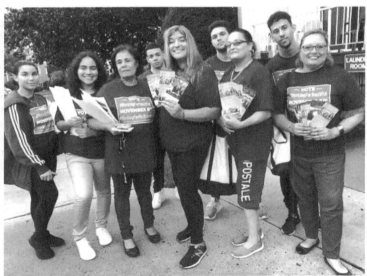

Fig. 4.3 Alana Cueto, MSN, RN, *(right)* with Marilou Villacis, LPN, and Vincent Makinsky in their 2018 political campaign in Perth Amboy, New Jersey. Cueto enlisted the support of nurse colleagues in her campaign for City Council.

to rich educational, mentoring, and networking experiences. Multiple organizations offer tool kits, training materials, legislative briefs, and mentoring around policy issues of concern to their membership. Associations like the Academy Health, American Public Health Association, the American Cancer Society, and the American Heart Association have strong advocacy and legislative programs. Check their websites for volunteer opportunities.

Internet Discussion Boards and Other Resources. Numerous sites offer pathways for engagement across various policy topics to expand learning and social networking opportunities. Join a professional networking site, such as LinkedIn to identify and join relevant discussion groups. Be broadminded about what groups discuss health policy; they range from local policy to global health groups. Professional organizations often post legislative agendas on their webpage with user-friendly links to generate letters to one's legislators.

Self-Study

The value of reading and self-directed learning help to improve one's understanding of policy and politics. The Politics & Ideas (www.politicsandideas.org) offers webinars and frameworks to help improve use of knowledge for policymaking. Many types of literature, such as eBooks, podcasts, and university websites, exist covering diverse interests related to policy.

Professional Journals. Many professional nursing, health care, and social sciences journals include updates on current political issues. Some are wholly focused on policy and politics (e.g., *Policy, Politics, & Nursing Practice; Health Affairs*); others publish regular political and policy content (e.g., *American Journal of Nursing, Nursing Outlook, Nursing Economics, Journal of the American Medical Association [JAMA]*).

Organizational Newsletters. Join listservs to receive organizational newsletters, both professional and interest group, that feature health policy–related columns.

Books. Browse through the political science, government, or current events sections of your favorite bookstore, and you are likely to find a goldmine. Search for the words *politics, policy,* or *health policy,* and see what piques your interest.

Newspapers. Major metropolitan newspapers offer political analysis of national, regional, and local politics. Those recognized for in-depth political reporting on health issues include the *Washington Post* (www.washingtonpost.com), the *New York Times* (www.nytimes.com), the *Los Angeles Times* (www.latimes.com), and the *Wall Street Journal* (www.wsj.com).

Television and Social Media. Network and cable news programs and television news-magazines address political issues and government activities. The ultimate viewing experience for politicos is C-SPAN, due to the wealth of information about the democratic process, without editing, commentary, or analysis (www.c-span.org/networks/). As a public service created by the U.S. cable television industry, constituents can access the live gavel-to-gavel proceedings, debates, and decisions of the U.S. House of Representatives and the U.S. Senate. The integration of social media platforms such as Twitter allow interest groups to interact directly and participate in televised stories and discussions. Social media facilitates communication among individuals to advocate on topics of concern, share expertise, and disseminate ideas (Bressler & Caceres, 2018). Follow health trends by Kaiser Health News (https://khn.org/ and @KHNews).

Radio. Radio continues to be a rich source of political information and debate on AM, FM, and satellite radio stations such as:
- National Public Radio (NPR) (www.npr.org) also offers podcasts and the blog Shots Health News (www.npr.org/sections/health-shots/) for researched in-depth reporting.
- C-SPAN Radio offers public affairs commercial-free programming 24 hours a day, accessed through the radio or the internet (www.c-span.org).
- Liberal and conservative political radio programs that serve as forums to debate hot political topics. Check your local radio program website for airtime and station.

Internet. An all-you-can-eat political buffet exists on the internet, a diverse universe ranging from well-substantiated journalism to blogs with absolutely no quality control. Nurses must learn to be savvy and use trustworthy platforms to promote our presence and expert knowledge (see Chapter 12).

FELLOWSHIP EXPERIENCE

As a short-term professional development opportunity, a policy fellowship provides a structured lived experience with mentoring in a safe learning environment. The experience gained is dependent on the program's format and use of project assignments, policy networking, writing, and analysis to develop practical policy skills.

The Jonas Health Policy Scholars program of the AAN provided Teresa Hagan Thomas, PhD, RN, and Emerson Ea, PhD, RN, FAAN, with an opportunity to "learn the ropes" via a robust mentored fellowship. They had access to a cadre of experienced nurse leaders able to guide their policy skill development via participation on expert panels, coauthored briefs, white papers, policy networking, and mentoring. As a lived experience, they managed multiple projects and participated in meetings and work teams to facilitate the execution of policy strategies.

Thomas participated on AAN's Women's Health Expert Panel to promote evidence-based policies related to sexual and reproductive health care. During her fellowship, several state and national movements proposed limiting access to women's health care services. The expert panel used a plethora of policy strategies to address these movements. For example, the expert panel submitted an Amicus Brief in support of safe services and equal access on abortion care and authored a position statement in support of safe, evidence-based care for women (Taylor et al., 2017). An abundance of policy networking opportunities gave Thomas access to multistakeholder groups. Thomas learned strategies on how to respond swiftly to disruptive policies using a "rapid response" protocol. They also trained local grassroots advocates with guidance on how to use social media and write op-eds for public online and print publications. Mentors provided expert guidance and supported her in participating in these policy processes and products. Thomas learned what it takes to not only publish policy analyses but also how to execute the work required for promoting evidence-based health policy, engaging stakeholders, and mobilizing grassroots actions. The fellowship gave her an attractive and competitive skill set that she highlighted during her subsequent job search. As an academic researcher, she has worked with colleagues to revise the DNP-level health policy course at her school to help students learn about health policy and actively engage in local, state, and national health policy efforts.

The AAN fellowship experience of Dr. Emerson Ea began with the AAN Cultural Competence and Health Equity Expert Panel, whose mission is to advance cultural competency that leads to a measurable impact on health disparities. Ea assisted in the development of policy products that aligned with the strategic priorities of the Academy and provided him with invaluable knowledge and experience. He witnessed first hand how evidence is translated into policy—a fluid and iterative process that requires continuous dialogue and refinement. As part of his mentoring experience, he learned how an extensive search of the literature helps to inform policy brief development and how his clinical and personal experience informed strategy—an experience both rewarding and empowering. Subsequently, Ea worked as a community leader, advocating for health equity for the Filipino population in New York City. In 2017 he assumed the position of Chair-elect of Kalusugan Coalition, a multidisciplinary community-based organization representing the New York and New Jersey area to promote cardiovascular health among Filipinos. Leveraging the skills gained during his policy fellowship, he worked with Filipino restaurants in the New York City area to adopt nutrition-related policies to improve cardiovascular health among Filipinos. As a partner of New York University Center for the Studies of Asian American Health, the Kalusugan Coalition led efforts to educate, train, and engage workers of Filipino restaurants to promote healthy food options among restaurant customers—an effort to promote incremental policy changes at the grassroots level. In addition, his work as a Policy Scholar at the AAN included significant contributions to a position statement on the health of migrants, refugees, and displaced persons adopted by the International Council of Nurses in 2018.

Nurses have limitless opportunities from all educational levels and experience to learn policy and political skills to improve health for individuals and populations.

DISCUSSION QUESTIONS

1. Create a one-page plan for your own learning about policy and politics.
2. Give examples of four opportunities for learning by doing.
3. List three places you can look for a mentor.

REFERENCES

American Association of Colleges of Nursing. (2008). *The essentials of baccalaureate education for professional nursing practice.* Washington, DC: AACN. Retrieved from www.aacn.nche.edu/education-resources/BaccEssentials08.pdf.

American Association of Colleges of Nursing. (2010). *The research-focused doctoral program in nursing pathways to excellence.* Washington, DC: AACN. Retrieved from www.aacn.nche.edu/education-resources/PhDPosition.pdf.

American Association of Colleges of Nursing. (2018a). *The essentials of doctoral education for advanced nursing practice.* Washington, DC: AACN. Retrieved from www.aacnnursing.org/DNP/DNP-Essentials.

American Association of Colleges of Nursing. (2018b). *The essentials of master's education for advanced practice nursing.* Washington, DC: AACN. Retrieved from www.aacnnursing.org/Teaching-Resources/Tool-Kits/Masters.

Armstrong, S.J., Allinson, C.W., & Hayes, J. (2002). Formal mentoring systems: An examination of the effects of mentor/

protégé cognitive styles on the mentoring process. *Journal of Management Studies, 39*(8), 1111–1137.

Brenan, M. (2018). *Nurses again outpace other professions for honesty, ethics.* Retrieved from https://news.gallup.com/poll/245597/nurses-again-outpace-professions-honesty-ethics.aspx.

Bressler, T., & Caceres, B.A. (2018). Get a seat at the virtual table. *Nursing Economics, 36*(1), 49-50.

Bunkers, S. & Hegge, M. (2018). Mentoring: The giving of blessings. *Nursing Science Quarterly, 31*(4), 319-324.

Catallo, C., Spalding, K., & Haghiri-Vijeh, R. (2014). Nursing professional organizations: What are they doing to engage nurses in health policy? *Sage Open, 4*(4), 1–9.

Dossey, B., Slanders, L., Beck, D.M., & Attewell, A. (2005). *Florence Nightingale today: Healing, leadership, global action.* Silver Spring, MD: ANA.

Ferris, G.R. (2007). Political skill in organizations. *Journal of Management, 33*(3), 290–320.

Green, J., & Jackson, D. (2014). Mentoring: Some cautionary notes for the nursing profession. *Contemporary Nurse, 47*(1-2), 79-87.

Hafsteinsdóttir, T.B., van der Zwaag, A.M., & Schuurmans, M.J. (2017). Leadership mentoring in nursing research, career development and scholarly productivity: A systematic review. *International Journal of Nursing Studies, 75*, 21–34.

Institute of Medicine. (2011). *The future of nursing: Leading change, advancing health.* Washington, DC: National Academies Press.

International Council of Nurses. (2018). *The health of migrants, refugees and displaced persons.* Retrieved from www.icn.ch/sites/default/files/inline-files/ICN%20PS%20Health%20of%20migrants%2C%20refugees%20and%20displaced%20persons.pdf.

McBride, A.B., Campbell, J., Woods, N.F., & Manson, S.M. (2017). Building a mentoring network. *Nursing Outlook, 65*(3), 305–314.

Montalvo, W., & Byrne, M.W. (2016). Mentoring nurses in political skill to navigate organizational politics. *Nursing Research and Practice.* [Epub.]

Peiser, G., Ambrose, J., Burke, B., & Davenport, J. (2017). The role of the mentor in professional knowledge development across four professions. *International Journal of Mentoring and Coaching in Education, 7*(1), 2–18.

Sessler-Branden, P. (2012). *The nurse as advocate: A grounded theory perspective.* (Doctoral dissertation.) Vanderbilt University. Retrieved from https://eric.ed.gov/?id=ED552771.

Stewart, B.M. (1996). An evolutionary concept analysis of mentoring in nursing. *Journal of Professional Nursing, 12*(5), 311–321.

Straus, S.E. (2013). Characteristics of successful and failed mentoring relationships: A qualitative study across two academic health centers. *Academic Medicine, 88*(1), 82–89.

Taylor, D., Olshansky, E.F., Woods, N., Johnson-Mallard, V., Safriet, B.J., & Hagan, T. (2017). Position statement: Political interference in sexual and reproductive health research and health professional education. *Nursing Outlook, 65*(2), 242–245.

Vance, C., & Olson, R.K. (1998). *The mentor connection in nursing.* New York: Springer Publishing Company.

Waddell, A., Audette, K., DeLong, A., & Brostoff, M. (2016) A hospital-based interdisciplinary model for increasing nurses' engagement in legislative advocacy. *Policy, Politics, & Nursing Practice, 17*(1), 15–23.

Wall, S. (2013). Nursing entrepreneurship: motivators, strategies and possibilities for professional advancement and health system change. *Nursing Leadership, 26*(2), 29–40. Retrieved from https://era.library.ualberta.ca/items/bd716de0-6eb3-4cbb-9476-b84a3be10625/view/20f9a2c6-24cc-461e-b1ef-ecca4082f524/NL_2013_26_2.pdf.

ONLINE RESOURCES

American Association of Colleges of Nursing Grassroots Liaisons
www.aacnnursing.org/Policy-Advocacy/Get-Involved/State-Grassroots-Liaisons
American Nurses Association Practice and Policy
www.nursingworld.org/practice-policy
C-SPAN
www.c-span.org
Henry Kaiser Family Foundation
https://kff.org
Kaiser Health News
https://khn.org
Robert Wood Johnson Foundation Policy
www.rwjf.org/en/topics/rwjf-topic-areas/health-policy.html

5

TAKING ACTION: Just Say Yes: Learning to Move Beyond the Fear

Chelsea Savage

"When I dare to be powerful, to use my strength in the service of my vision, then it becomes less and less important whether I am afraid."

Audre Lorde

When I was growing up, the government gave my single mother, brother, and myself much-needed help. We struggled and survived at times through welfare, Section 8 housing, food stamps, and free lunches. When I was married with three stepchildren and one child of my own, I again was grateful for the assistance I found in Medicaid when giving birth to my daughter; Women, Infants, and Children (WIC) Food and Nutrition Service; Pell grants to continue my education; the Children's Health Insurance Program (CHIP) for health care for my children; and food stamps.

But I was raised in an abusive religious cult. We kept ourselves separate from the world by our dated dresses, our belief as the "chosen," and emphasis on the apocalypse. Women were "keepers of the home" only, and children were kept from school. I was lucky enough to get a 6th grade education and later taught myself enough to get my General Education Diploma. Between the ages of 13 and 15, I was allowed to volunteer at our local hospital. This sparked my interest in nursing. I did not get my nursing degree until I was 26. As a nurse, I saw so much suffering that I could not close my eyes to it, so I supported politics that I felt would supply help to the need I saw.

My commitment to social justice began in 2007 in Richmond, Virginia, as a Fellow for "Hope in the Cities," a program sponsored by Initiatives of Change, USA (www.us.iofc.org/) that focuses on building trust through honest conversations on race, reconciliation, and responsibility. From the rich discussions I had with diverse individuals and groups, I developed an ability to look for and understand the story of the "other" and to use this in conversations to facilitate peace and understanding. We walked the slave trail in Richmond and stood in front of monuments to the confederacy while listening to the pain they evoked. Learning how to accept divergent realities through deep conversation has served me well in the political arena where differences can collide or lead to more creative policy solutions to current problems. Three things created opportunities that led to my running for political office: my passion for social justice, my mentors, and an insatiable curiosity that propelled me to venture into uncharted territories.

MENTORS, PASSION, AND CURIOSITY

I was finishing a fellowship in Health Law when Shirley Gibson, a mentor and then president of the Virginia Organization of Nurse Executives, asked me to chair the Legislative Committee for the organization. I said yes, and, within a couple of weeks, I was networking with leaders in the state and leading advocacy on health issues. I was one of the representatives of several diverse nursing organizations that comprised the Legislative Coalition of Virginia Nurses (LCVN), founded in part by one of my mentors, Becky Bowers-Lanier, a well-regarded nursing leader in health policy, and Sallie Eissler, a pediatric nurse practitioner. They decided LCVN needed a succession plan: I was elected Chair of LCVN.

As chair of LCVN, as well as Assistant Commissioner of Government Affairs for the Virginia Nurses Association (VNA), I met with policymakers and campaign managers for the governor's race; created legislative platforms that outlined succinctly our legislative priorities; assisted with the passage of the Virginia Indoor Clean Air

Act that banned smoking in public places; and fought for a raise in nursing school faculty salaries to address the nursing shortage. Sally was also head of the Political Action Committee for the VNA and a political junkie. She suggested I learn about politics in Virginia by applying to the Sorensen Institute Political Leaders Program (PLP) through the University of Virginia. PLP focused on building political networks and learning to function in the system. Because of my connections though PLP, in 2012 I was tapped to be Co-Chair for Nurses for Obama in Virginia, with a mission of educating the public on the Affordable Care Act (ACA). Radio interviews and newspaper articles followed.

I was aware that, if you are not careful, working publicly on behalf of candidates in an election year can create problems with your employer and problems with nonpartisan nursing professional organizations. However, a colleague advised me that nurses are certainly able to wear more than one hat. I could be a supporter of the ACA and even President Obama as an individual nurse, but it was up to me to make it clear I was not representing the views of my employer or my professional association.

By a stroke of luck, I attended the Virginia Democratic Women's Caucus and happened to sit at the table with the board of Emerge Virginia (www.emergeva.org/home), an organization that teaches Democratic women how to run for office and mentors them along the way. I told them I was a PLP fellow. They immediately said, "You have to do our program. PLP teaches you about politics, but we teach you how to run for office." It was during this women's caucus meeting that I had my first awe-struck moment. All the women who were running for office were asked to stand up, and I remember looking at them in amazement wondering what kind of character and fortitude could create these women. I could never do that.

The following year, I heard from Emerge Virginia, asking me to put in an application for the 2016 class. I felt too busy in my personal life at the time and asked that they keep me in mind for the next year, the class of 2017. And they did.

My life's motto has always been to say "yes" to opportunities. After the 2016 elections, Emerge Virginia was inundated with applications. I was not sure I would get in, but I interviewed and was accepted. The one thing I knew I wanted from my time at Emerge was to stop being afraid. I was so tired of being afraid to speak up. I had media training but was still fearful of political action that was unsolicited, such as knocking on doors and making phone calls on behalf of a candidate. I wanted to expand who I was as a person to include someone who could connect intentionally and purposefully with my community. Emerge Virginia was going to help me do so.

In January of 2017, my Emerge class was given a tour of the Capitol and met with the governor, legislators, and leaders in the Democratic Caucus. Being on the periphery of the political scene as a health policy advocate for more than 10 years made this somewhat perfunctory for me until one meeting that was pivotal. Our class met with the leaders of the Virginia House Democratic Caucus to discuss some of the nuts and bolts of running. I listened and then threw out a question. "What kind of handicap does being gay give me if I run for office?" To my surprise the answer was "None! It is a good thing!" I was not expecting that answer. This was Virginia. It was not until Emerge Virginia Executive Director Julie Copland sent out an email to our class asking for candidates to run sooner rather than later in the house races, that a switch was flipped in me. I was no longer that girl looking at the chasm that separated me and those women candidates for office standing in the Democratic Women's Caucus meeting in 2014. Why? Because Julie Copland asked me. She asked me with the authority of a woman who knows what it takes to be a candidate, who has run campaigns, and who would have my back if I stepped up. That was all I needed.

RUNNING FOR OFFICE

Mentors Becky and Sally always asked, "When are you going to run for office?" I would laugh but thought, "Maybe when I am grayer with an unquestionable resume of political experience." But I knew now was the "perfect storm," the perfect time to run, and I could not say no. My capstone project for my Doctorate in Nursing Practice was a qualitative study on the lived experiences of nurse health policy advocates (Savage, 2015). Over and over I heard my subjects describe that the reason they were active in health policy advocacy was because of the counterculture movements in the late 1960s and 1970s. They participated in consciousness-raising groups, women meeting in living rooms and creating change. Now, another political movement was happening in the country, and I was going to be part of it.

The *first* indicator of a perfect storm was at the Henrico County Democratic Committee Meeting right after I announced I was running. There were probably 250 to 300 people in a meeting that usually could barely bring out 25 to 50. The *second* indicator was at the newly formed advocacy group, the Liberal Women of Chesterfield County. Again, there were 250 or more people and BABIES! That's right—young mothers and children were there. I had never seen this kind of political participation! The *third* indicator was the realization that the duration of this participation in politics would not be short. The new president kept saying and doing things that continually stoked political action.

So I said "yes" to the executive director and deputy executive director for the Virginia House Democratic Caucus, who then reviewed the arduous process of becoming a candidate. They told me I would be doing this on my own with minimal help, using only the funds I could raise. But I was not alone. Emerge Virginia was there to teach me during my campaign and provide encouragement and support. I was still on my own, and I was not the perfect candidate. I was a mom who was too shy to sell her own daughter's Girl Scout cookies—and now I was going to run for office and raise thousands of dollars!

The first real step after all the documents were signed and turned in was to get a direct mail company. I hired an amazing firm that not only did my direct mail, they also were excellent strategists that helpfully did not charge a fee for their advice, only what it cost for the direct mail, which would come much later in my campaign. Then I had to find a campaign manager.

When I entered the world of campaign managers for the state house I found myself in a sort of "twilight zone" where my universe was to be smoothly set in order and expeditiously run by young people in their early 20s. I realized the skills of these political operatives only as I saw them unfold every day in my campaign (Fig. 5.1). I had an amazing campaign manager named Brian Robinson-Gallagher. He researched donors, had perfect advice, and

got along well with my direct mail company. I will never forget the day in my campaign when I ran by his apartment to pick up my next batch of fundraising calls that he had researched. He actually had to sit in the parking lot beside my car because he had been knocking on doors for me 7 hours straight and could not stand. The bond the candidate forms and that I formed with Brian was and is phenomenal—and, boy, did I need his support.

The phone calls terrified me, as did the door knocking. Cold calling potential donors and asking for ridiculous sums of money are the requirements to the tune of 2 hours a night. The goal was to call the potential donor and, after a couple seconds talking about your campaign, make the ask. My favorite ask was, "I was wondering if you could support my campaign in any way, whatever you can give . . ." Big fail! The proper way to make an ask is, "I would love it if you could make a $150 donation to my campaign . . ." and silence. No back peddling—you sit there and wait. It is harder than it may seem. The first fundraising circle for a candidate is their personal contacts. I never ask my friends for anything and knew this was going to be hard. I thought maybe I would get $200. Instead, I got thousands. My friends and acquaintances, anyone who had the fortune of being my Facebook friend, gave and then gave again.

My first hurdle, though, was the door knocking. To get my name on the ballot I needed 125 signatures. My campaign director was able to give me the addresses of constituents who would be more likely to vote Democratic, but I lived in the same house for almost 13 years and did not know the names of my neighbors. I had to make myself walk up the steps of an unknown house, knock on the door, and, if owners were home and answered their door, ask them for their signature. This was a big deal for me.

One of my classmates in Emerge Virginia was running for town council. Because I had been at my campaign a month or so before her, she asked for advice on how to knock on doors, nursing the same fears and shyness that I had. "This is what I do," I told her. "I actually visualize myself carrying my quivering soul up the sidewalk, driveway, and front steps of the house then I knock on the door. When the door is opened, you have to say something. I got my stump speech down to three talking points that I could make either 30 seconds or 20 minutes long depending on the situation."

Like saying yes to running for office, I said yes to phone calling and knocking on doors. This was my goal from the beginning—to break out of the prison of my own fears. Now I tell women who are thinking of running for office, "Run scared, if you have too. Don't wait to feel up to it. You

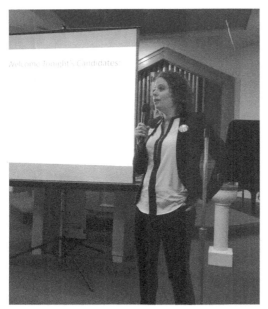

Fig. 5.1 Chelsea Savage, RN, DNP, speaking at a campaign event.

can physically make that phone call, you can physically

knock on that door, your mind will follow, and you will get stronger. Don't ever let fear keep you from your potential. Say yes."

I lost the Democratic nomination, coming out second in a field of four, but I am so happy I said "yes" to that experience. The question everyone asks: "Will you run again?" I don't know. I might. I know I do want to keep throwing away old templates and being open to all forms of "yes"

opportunities as a responsible citizen of my community and the nursing profession.

REFERENCES

Savage, C.L. (2015). *The lived experiences of nurse health policy advocates.* (Unpublished doctoral dissertation). American Sentinel University, Aurora, Colorado.

6

A Primer on Political Philosophy

Beth L. Rodgers and Sally S. Cohen

> *"If I were to attempt to put my political philosophy tonight into a single phrase, it would be this: Trust the people."*
>
> **Adlai Stevenson**

Terminology and ideas related to political thought are showing up in conversations in all sorts of venues. Consumers of popular media, scientists reading scholarly work, and people in the course of their everyday lives often comment on ideas and positions using a variety of labels and terminology to characterize their thoughts or to label the ideas of others. It is important to understand some of the major concepts and traditions from political philosophy. This is particularly important as it provides a way to get beyond what can seem confrontational, to dissect various positions in an effort both to understand and to evoke action. Nurses need to be mindful of the ideologic, philosophic, and political themes that structure contemporary health policy debates. Such knowledge can enhance the ability of nurses to develop strategies that consider political and ideologic perspectives, many of which are not always evident but nonetheless often drive political deliberations and outcomes. This foundational understanding of political philosophy then informs discussion regarding the role of the state, the evolution of major political ideologies, and an examination of how the crucial issues, such as race and gender, influence political thought and action.

POLITICAL PHILOSOPHY

Political philosophers examine, analyze, and search for answers to fundamental questions about the state and its moral and ethical responsibilities. They ask questions such as, "What constitutes the state?," "What rights and privileges should the state protect?," "What laws and regulations should be implemented?," and "To what extent should government control people's lives?" Political philosophy encompasses the goals, rules, or behaviors that citizens, states, and societies ought to pursue. It is closely related to legal and moral philosophy as all three involve discussion of values, the distinctions between right and wrong, and the "distribution of the burdens and benefits, with legal philosophy specifically addressing legal regulations on rights, responsibilities, and opportunities" (Reiff, 2018, p. 70).

From another perspective, political philosophy addresses two issues. The first is about the distribution of material goods, rights, and liberties. The second issue pertains to the possession and determination of political power. It includes such questions as, "Why do others have rights over me?," "Why do I have to obey laws that other people developed and with which I disagree?," and "Why do the wealthy often have more power than the majority?" (Wolff, 1996). Reiff (2018) provides a contemporary perspective on the enduring question of the nature of political philosophy by pointing out that it "should be about how we can better understand the nature and potential of social cooperation and how we can use that understanding to improve the arrangements under which we live" (p. 69). Although political philosophy sometimes can seem detached from real life, it can help with understanding basic questions about human nature, the role of government, the place for regulation, the provision of services to meet basic needs, and other critical questions about the organization of human existence.

The "doctrines" of political philosophy have strong historical roots; yet, they continue to be integral to "our most basic outlooks and attitudes that are still alive and very much with us" (Smith, 2012, p. 4). Although "there are no permanent answers" to the questions that political philosophers ask, their questions endure over centuries, with disagreement within and across eras regarding issues such as justice, rights, freedom, authority, and what constitutes a good citizen or a good person (Smith, 2012).

Political philosophy is a normative discipline; it tries to establish how people ought to be, as expressed through regulations or laws. It involves making judgments about the world rather than simply describing or observing people and society. Political philosophers attempt to explain what is right, just, or morally correct. It is a constantly evolving discipline, prompting us to think about how concerns and questions can have different answers over time. The "proper subject of political philosophy is political action" (Smith, 2012, p. 5). This refers to political action aimed at changing or improving the status quo, or action aimed at preserving it, so that it does not become worse.

For nurses, political philosophy offers ways of analyzing and working with situations that arise in practice, policy, organizational, and community settings. For example, it helps to determine how far government authorities may go in regulating nursing practice. It offers ways of understanding complex ethical situations—such as end-of-life care, the use of technology in clinical settings, and reproductive health—when there is no clear answer regarding what constitutes the rights of individuals, clinicians, government officials, or society at large. Political philosophy offers normative ways of addressing such situations by focusing on the relationships among individuals, government, and society. Finally, political philosophy enables nurses to think about their roles as members of society, organizations, and health care delivery settings in attempting to attain important health policy goals, such as reducing the number of people without health care coverage and eliminating disparities among ethnic groups.

THE STATE

The idea of the *state* is key to understanding political philosophy. In political philosophy (and political science), the state does not refer to one of the 50 states of the United States. Rather, it is a "particular kind of social group" (Shively, 2014, p. 18). The state arose from the notion that people cannot rule at their will. As Andrew Levine (2002) explained, "Few, if any, human groupings have persisted for very long without authority relations of some kind" (p. 6). The *modern state is* a highly organized, government entity that influences many aspects of everyday lives (Shively, 2014). It typically refers to the "governing apparatus that makes and enforces rules" (Shively, 2014, p. 64). Therefore, the terms *state* and *government* may be interchangeable. It is the role of the state (or government) in health policy issues—such as licensure of health professionals and institutions, financing care, ensuring adequate environmental quality, protecting against

bioterrorist attacks, and subsidizing care—that is important for nurses in their professional practice and personal lives. Usually people think of national governments as the modern state. However, local and geographic state governments also assume important roles in protecting individuals, regulating trade, and ensuring individual rights and well-being. In distinguishing between a nation and a state, note that a state is a political entity "with sovereignty," meaning it has responsibility for the conduct of its own affairs. In contrast, a nation is "a large group of people who are bound together, and recognize a similarity among themselves, because of a common culture" (Shively, 2014, p. 57). A common theme of current conversation about policy and politics in the United States is how much authority and sovereignty belongs to the national government, and how much should be under the control of other geographically bounded entities.

Despite these distinctions, the terms *state* and *nation* may overlap in common parlance because government leaders often appeal to the "emotional attachment of people in their nation" in building support for the legal entity of a *state* (Shively, 2014, p. 58). Few would dispute that the political culture of the United States is different from that of other countries. Historically, the social context of the United States has taken pride in the sense of individualism, a laissez-faire approach to government and economics, and a strong belief in the rights of individuals. Policy analysts often point to the unique political culture as an explanation for why U.S. social policy deviates from that of other countries. An example is the difficulty in establishing any type of national health insurance program. The Affordable Care Act (ACA) may have been considered progress in this regard, but it still relied on a combination of private and public initiatives, while most other developed countries have strong, state-sponsored health care insurance (Canada) or delivery systems (United Kingdom).

Individuals and the State

The idea of the state exists to capture the notion that people need some form of organization and rules to prevent chaos and disorder. Free will is an important idea when talking about human behavior; however, most philosophers will argue that free will either must have, or inherently does have, limits particularly in reference to its interface with the free will of others who may be on a different path. The state is the mechanism for imposing some degree of order or control while recognizing the fact that the thing being ordered involves an array of individuals. Numerous philosophers have addressed this delicate relationship between individuals and the state, and a few of the more significant contributors to shaping our ideas of this relationship are described in the following sections.

Thomas Hobbes (1588–1679). Hobbes helped to shape ideas regarding the relationship between individuals and the state with his emphasis on a "social contract" which claims, "individuals in a hypothetical state of nature would choose to organize their political affairs" (Levine, 2002, p. 18). As Shively (2014) succinctly explained, "Of their free wills, by a cooperative decision, the people set up a power to dominate them for the common good" (p. 47). Hobbes's theory was important in establishing governance and authority, without which people would live in a natural condition of chaos. To avoid such situations, according to Hobbes, people living in communities voluntarily establish rules by which they abide.

John Locke (1632–1704). Locke, a British political philosopher who greatly influenced liberal thinkers, including the writers of the U.S. Constitution, emphasized the importance of individual rights in relationship to the state. For Locke, individual rights were more important than state power, and states exist to protect the "inalienable" rights afforded mankind. One of the premises of Locke's theories is that people should be free from coercive state institutions. Moreover, the rights inherent in such freedom are different from the legal rights established by governmental authority under a Hobbesian contract. They are basic to the nature of humanity.

Jeremy Bentham (1748–1832). Bentham, heralded as the father of classic utilitarianism, asserted that individuals and governments strive to attain pleasure over pain. When applying this principle to governments, the primary interest of a community is its pleasure, good, or happiness. The interests of the community must include the interests of the individual, thus this same principle applies to individual good or pleasure (Bentham, 1789/1907) and "requires us to maximize the greatest happiness of the greatest number in the community" (Shapiro, 2003, p. 19). Instead of relying on natural law, Bentham favored the establishment of legal systems "enforced by the sovereign" (Shapiro, 2003, p. 19). Bentham's utilitarianism has become foundational to many contemporary theories in economics, political science, bioethics, and other disciplines.

The tension between individual rights and the role of the state is inherent in many health policy discussions. For example, consider substance use. Although individuals have the "right" to smoke tobacco and drink alcohol and one might argue that the state should protect individuals' rights to do so, such freedoms may interfere with others' rights to fresh air and freedom from harm (e.g., from second-hand smoke inhalation or from incidents related to alcohol use). The state has a legitimate role to intervene, but the challenge lies in finding the right balance between the rights of individuals on both sides of the issue and balancing them with the rights of the state. These debates

also can raise questions about the nature of the individual, or personhood, which may be invoked in policy discussion related to contraception and embryonic stem cell research.

Political Ideologies

Contemporary conversations involve a lot of terminology and labels about policy positions that can evoke emotional response in many cases, and often the terminology is not applied accurately. Discussion of political philosophy needs clear definitions for different ideologies and the terminology used to characterize diverse viewpoints.

A political ideology is a "set of ideas about politics, all of which are related to one another and that modify and support each other" (Shively, 2014, p. 23). Political ideologies are characterized by distinctive views on the organization and functioning of the state. They help people to analyze and make decisions about complex, political issues and provide a way for policymakers to convince others that their position on an issue will advance the public good. Three major political ideologies, liberalism, socialism, and conservatism, originated with 18th- and 19th-century European philosophers and are the basis of political deliberations and policies throughout the world (Shively, 2014). The terms and definitions of *liberalism* and *conservatism* have evolved over time and are not necessarily consistent with the ideologies as they currently exist. In addition, ideology may vary across topics (such as social conservatism and fiscal conservatism), and other variations occur over time, leading to the use of "neo-" and "post-" to distinguish versions. Nevertheless, it is critical to appreciate the origins of these ideologies so that the nuances in their rhetoric and their role in health policy can be fully understood. Major points of each of these ideologies are provided in Box 6.1.

Liberalism

American political thought was greatly influenced by 18th-century European liberalism and the political thinking of Hobbes, Locke, and others. Liberalism relies on the notion that members of a society should be able to "develop their individual capacities to the fullest" (Shively, 2014, p. 29). People also must be responsible for their actions and must not be dependent on others.

John Stuart Mill (1806–1873). Mill, a British political philosopher, published an influential essay "On Liberty" (1859) that is foundational to modern liberal thinking. Mill was committed to individual rights and freedom of thought and expression but not unconditionally. He based his work on Locke's philosophies, tempered by Bentham's utilitarian philosophy.

Mill contended that individuals were sovereign over their own bodies and minds but could not exert such

BOX 6.1 Comparison of Dominant Political Philosophies

Liberalism	Conservatism	Socialism
• Individuals should be able to develop fully as individuals • Emphasizes individual rights and freedom of thought and expression (but not without limits) • Individuals have control over own bodies and minds, but not to extent of harming others • Democracy as ideal form of government, allowing everyone to participate and express views freely • Government protections against abuse of power	• Historically: Those in power have responsibility to help those not in power • Contemporary form: Opposes rapid and fundamental change but advocates for decreased federal involvement in all matters, reduced tax burden, traditional social values, and transfer of authority to the geographic states • Preference for tradition, stability, and structure • Patterns of power that are predictable	• Government should protect workers for negative situations and conditions • Equality regardless of role or status • Economy supports the good of all • Concept of a common good • Lack of individual ownership • Lack of privatization • Centralized government in control

sovereignty if it harmed others. A leading, contemporary political philosopher and political scientist, Ian Shapiro, applied Mill's balancing of individual rights with his "harm principle" as follows: "... although sanitary regulations, workplace safety rules, and the prevention of fraud coerce people and interfere with their liberty, such policies are acceptable because the legitimacy of the ends they serve is 'undeniable'" (Shapiro, 2003, p. 60).

Conservatism

Although liberals call for changing the existing social and political order, conservatives counter with a preference for stability and structure. Conservatism often is traced to origins following the French Revolution, when it began to develop as a distinguishable ideology. British Parliamentarian Edmund Burke often is regarded as the originator of modern conservatism. In his seminal text, *Reflections on the Revolution in France* (1790/1890), Burke argued for a return to prerevolution ideas and the stability that preceded the revolutionary period, referring to the revolution and instability as the loss of a compass (p. 87). Although several variations of conservative ideology have evolved throughout history, including the attribution of the term "conservative" to some communist groups in the 1980s, conservatism generally favors tradition and stability in the guidance of human existence.

Guided by the notion that government had a responsibility to provide structured assistance to others, 19th-century European conservatives, especially in Great Britain and Germany, developed many programs that featured government support to the disadvantaged (e.g., unemployment assistance and income subsidies). They accepted welfare policies that were foundational to the revival of Europe after World War II. They have been major players in contemporary European politics, especially in Great Britain, offering a synergy with American conservatism.

Socialism

Socialism grew out of dissatisfaction with liberalism by many in the working class. Unable to prosper under liberalism, which relied on individual capacities, socialists looked to the state for policies to protect workers from sickness, unemployment, unsafe working conditions, and other situations.

Karl Marx, the German philosopher (1818–1883), is widely considered the originator of socialism. For Marx, individuals could improve their situation only by identifying with their economic class. The 19th-century Industrial Revolution had created the working class, which, according to Marx, was oppressed by capitalists who used workers for their profits. According to Marx, only revolution could relieve workers of their oppression. Socialism arose to equalize access to resources through more centralized control. The collective nature of socialism is in contrast to the primacy of private property that characterizes capitalism. Additional tenets of socialism are provided in Box 6.1.

Communism and Democratic Socialism. Socialism originated and proliferated in Europe toward the end of the 19th and into the early 20th centuries when it split into two ideologies, communism and democratic socialism. In 1917, communists, under the leadership of V. I. Lenin, took over the Russian Empire and formed a socialist state, the Union of Soviet Socialist Republics (USSR). Lenin and his communist followers believed in revolution as the only way to advance socialism and achieve total improvement in workers' conditions. In contrast, democratic socialists were more willing to work with government institutions, participate in democracies, and "settle for partial improvements for workers, rather than holding out for total change" (Shively, 2014, p. 38). Between 1989 and 1991, communist regimes in Eastern Germany, the USSR, and throughout Eastern Europe collapsed. In their quest for economic and political change, the new Eastern European governments have turned to democracy, democratic socialism, capitalism, and other economic and political models.

Currently, only a handful of countries (e.g., Cuba, China, North Korea, Vietnam) are under communist rule. Socialists, especially democratic socialists, have prevailed in Scandinavia and Western Europe. They have been instrumental in advancing the modern welfare state in those countries and elsewhere around the world (Shively, 2014). Because of the widely varying forms of socialism, including promarket socialism, deep scrutiny is needed before applying this label to a specific political viewpoint.

Contemporary Conservatism and Liberalism

Contemporary political conservatism grew in popularity in United States in the late 20th century. It is similar to classic conservatism but differs in that contemporary conservatives oppose a strong government role in assisting the disadvantaged, and oppose rapid, fundamental change. They call for devolution of responsibility for health and other social issues from the federal government to state authorities, a diminished presence of government in all aspects of policy, a reduced tax burden, and the importance of traditional social values. Many political observers point to the 1980 election of President Ronald Reagan as a turning point for the rise of contemporary American conservatism.

In contrast, liberals today support an expanded government role to help people who need income support, health care coverage, child care assistance, vocational guidance, tuition, and other aspects of social policy. The Great Society programs of President John F. Kennedy and Lyndon B. Johnson in the 1960s and early 1970s boosted American liberal policies. Among the highlights of the Great Society initiatives were the enactment of Medicare, Medicaid, and Head Start. These federal government initiatives were founded on the importance of the state helping the disadvantaged through government-sponsored programs. They are in line with traditional liberal philosophies, described previously, which support the notion that individuals should be given equal opportunities to pursue their inalienable rights. Such rights include their health and welfare, broadly defined, even though the right to health care is not a legal one under the U.S. Constitution.

Although much discussion tends to place liberal and conservative views as extremes, most people's views lie somewhere in between. Moreover, many organizations take policy positions on health care and other issues that are in concert with a certain ideologic perspective but may deviate from those positions on other matters. Considering the diversity of existing thought, decision making may benefit from collective discussion that supports optimal outcomes rather than a win or lose of one perspective over another.

GENDER AND RACE IN POLITICAL PHILOSOPHY

In the postmodern era of philosophy, scholars noted traditional philosophy failed to represent the voices of numerous groups. Two perspectives that were notably absent were those based on gender and race. More recently, the perspective of class has emerged to introduce new ideas, leading to the evolution of political ideologies of division along a variety of lines, both obvious and subtle.

Gender emerges in political philosophy as a particular policy viewpoint, as well as an emphasis on the treatment of people of different genders. Feminist political philosophy emphasizes politics as a social contract, and rejection of the contract as being necessarily male-centered. Pateman (2018) noted that the social contract fails to recognize the unique needs of women and, instead, tends to subjugate them to the concerns of the males who formulated earlier ideas of political philosophy.

Feminism, as a political philosophy, ranges from a call for consideration of women's perspectives to radical feminism and may be extended to rejection of the heterosexual norm (MacKinnon, 2007). Democratic feminism, a variant of democratic theory, argues for an egalitarian foundation in which there are "norms of equality and symmetry" and "open debate" is possible (Benhabib, 1996, p. 70). This theory in political philosophy is related to "deliberative democratic theory," which focuses on deliberation in the process of decision making. Democratic feminists would argue that deliberation must include diverse perspectives, including those of women, to be effective.

One drawback to feminist political philosophy is that it can divide people based on gender. Someone's identity is not merely female or male but is connected with ethnicity, socioeconomic status, work role, family structure, sexual orientation, and other related factors. Consequently, a focus on gender as a key point in political philosophy fails to recognize the intricate interplay of the various facets that constitute identity and the phenomenon referred to as intersectionality (Crenshaw, 1989). Failure to recognize the intersection of these aspects contributes to fractured identities and polarization as various individuals are more easily reconceptualized as "other" (Bradley, 2016).

Building on the initial release of Carol Pateman's *Sexual Contract*, Mills (1997) identified the "Racial Contract" as another example of how traditional approaches to political philosophy overlooked the realities of most of the world's population of people of color, which includes Black people, Native Americans, people of Asian origin, and millions of others who are non-White in ancestry. Mills (1997) explained that the "social contract tradition," which is essential for much of "Western political theory," was a contract that White men had written and intended only to apply to themselves (p. 3).

THE WELFARE STATE

The welfare state refers to the "share of the economy devoted to government social expenditures" (Hacker, 2002, pp. 12–13). According to the Organization for Economic Co-operation and Development (OECD) (2018) statistics, the United States ranks below the midpoint in social expenditures as a percentage of gross domestic product (GDP) compared with other developed countries. In health expenditures, it consistently ranks higher than all other countries used for comparison purposes. However, the portion funded by government is not proportionately increased in comparison (OECD, 2018).

The cornerstone of the U.S. welfare system is the 1935 U.S. Social Security Act, which established the Social Security program, welfare, federal maternal and child health programs, and other important initiatives to ameliorate the devastation of the Great Depression. Occasionally, social security is erroneously referred to as an "entitlement," although it is not a welfare program. As approximately 24% of the federal budget, this would provide a faulty inflation of the amount of funding going toward "welfare" (Pew Research Center, 2017).

Types of Welfare States

The phrase "welfare state" often is used as if it were a description of a static entity; rather, there are multiple variations of welfare states across the United States and internationally. There are many different types of welfare states, based on the division of responsibilities for social services between public and private sectors and the role of a central government authority. The most well-known categorization is Esping-Andersen's (1990) description of three types of welfare state: social-democratic, corporatist, and liberal. Although this categorization encompasses all aspects of social policy, Aspalter (2011) further emphasizes the origin of support, as well as its duration across the life span.

In social-democratic welfare states (e.g., Scandinavian countries), most social programs are publicly administered and relatively few privately sponsored social benefits are offered. These countries have "pursued a welfare state that would promote an equality of the highest standards" (Esping-Andersen, 1990, p. 27).

Corporatist welfare states are typically the Western European nations (e.g., France, Italy, and Germany), where social rights and status differentials have endured and affected social policies. These countries grant social rights to many but primarily provide state interventions when family capacities fail.

Liberal welfare states include the United States, Canada, and Australia, where privately sponsored benefits dominate. Among liberal welfare states, the United States is distinctive for its large percentage of social spending in the form of privately sponsored benefits. Welfare and other social benefits are highly stigmatized, and the state encourages market involvement as much as possible (Esping-Andersen, 1990).

POLITICAL PHILOSOPHY AND IMPLICATIONS FOR NURSES

How might nurses apply these concepts of political philosophy to their involvement in health politics and policy? Nurses are participants in the larger society and need to be aware of the context, trends, and policies that affect their lives and the lives of others in their community. Nurses bring a unique perspective to policy discussions, with expertise and experience related to social issues, community well-being, and health care. Regardless of partisan preference, nurses can participate in the ideologic and political debates that shape health policy and the lives of others in their communities. Everyone has perspectives on the role of government and individual's rights, with regard to certain policies, and this includes a political ideology and policy positions. Understanding one's own perspective is essential to engaging in conversation with others who may hold similar or widely disparate views. That knowledge can be used as the basis for advocating for policies that have the potential to improve health and patient outcomes and in understanding the perspectives of others.

When engaging in political deliberations, listen to the rhetoric that others use and identify the underlying political and philosophical threads. Use similar language based on sound knowledge when you meet with policymakers, or use written texts to advance your positions. Box 6.2 provides cases of how ideology influences policy choice.

The relationship between nursing and the state has yet to be carefully explored. There are many aspects of nursing's political history that remain untapped and that warrant closer examination of how the profession has interacted with state structures in the policy process. Whether working with public officials, strategizing to create links between policy and practice, or studying the role of the state in policies pertaining to nursing, political philosophy is the foundation of thought and action. It can be a lively

---

BOX 6.2   Ideology and Policy Options: Case Examples

Uninsured Americans

1. Ideology that government role should be minimal leads to increased emphasis on individual accountability (conservatism). Policy options favor incentives for health savings accounts, tax credits, and other policies that support individual action.

2. Ideology that the state has an obligation to ensure basic level of care and access leads to creation or support of government-run programs (socialism). Policy options favor expansion of government programs such as Medicare, Medicaid, and Children's Health Insurance Program (CHIP) for those lacking insurance.

Motorcycle Helmet Use

1. Ideology that promoting a peaceful and orderly society is important and control of personal action is warranted if necessary for the good of society (Hobbesian or Social Contract framework, idea of common good). Policy options favor laws and enforcement requiring helmets to decrease burden on society.

2. Ideology that motorcyclists have the right to decide for themselves whether or not they wear helmets (liberal). Policy option favors no helmet law and promotion of individual choice.

---

aspect of nurses' strategic thinking in linking policy, politics, and practice.

DISCUSSION QUESTIONS

1. When meeting a nursing delegation from 10 different countries, how might you use political philosophy to explain the U.S. health care system (access, quality, and financing), the role of the U.S. welfare state, and the position of national nursing organizations on related issues?

2. Consider certain groups that have been excluded from mainstream political philosophy: what do you see nursing's individual and collective role in ensuring that they receive the same benefits and privileges as people from other groups?

REFERENCES

Aspalter, C. (2011). The development of ideal-typical welfare regime theory. *International Social Work, 54*(6), 735–750.

Benhabib, S. (1996). *Democracy and difference: Contesting the boundaries of the political.* Princeton, NJ: Princeton University Press.

Bentham, J. (1907). *An introduction to the principles of morals and legislation.* Oxford: Clarendon Press. (Original work published 1789).

Burke, E. (1890). *Reflections on the revolution in France.* (F.G. Selby, ed.). London: Macmillan. (Original work published 1790.)

Bradley, H. (2016). *Fractured identities: Changing patterns of inequality.* Malden, MA: Polity.

Crenshaw, K. (1989). Demarginalizing the intersection of race and sex: A Black feminist critique of antidiscrimination doctrine, feminist theory and antiracist politics. *University of Chicago Legal Forum, 1*(8), 139–168. Retrieved from http://chicagounbound.uchicago.edu/uclf/vol1989/iss1/8.

Esping-Andersen, G. (1990). *The three worlds of welfare capitalism.* Princeton, NJ: Princeton University Press.

Hacker, J.S. (2002). *The divided welfare state: The battle over public and private social benefits in the United States.* New York: Cambridge University Press.

Levine, A. (2002). *Engaging political philosophy from Hobbes to Rawls.* Malden, MA: Blackwell Publishers.

MacKinnon, C.A. (2007). *Women's lives, men's laws.* Cambridge, MA: Harvard University Press.

Mills, C.W. (1997). *The racial contract.* Ithaca, NY: Cornell University Press.

Organisation for Economic Co-Operation and Development (OECD). (2018). *OECD data: Selected indicators for the United States.* Retrieved from https://data.oecd.org/united-states.htm.

Pateman, C. (2018). *The sexual contract.* Stanford, CA: Stanford University Press.

Pew Research Center (2017). *What does the federal government spend your tax dollars on? Social insurance programs, mostly.* Retrieved from www.pewresearch.org/fact-tank/2017/04/04/what-does-the-federal-government-spend-your-tax-dollars-on-social-insurance-programs-mostly/.

Reiff, M.R. (2018). Twenty-one statements about political philosophy: An introduction and commentary on the state of the profession. *Teaching Philosophy, 41*(1), 65–115.

Shapiro, I. (2003). *The moral foundations of politics.* New Haven: Yale University Press.

Shively, W.P. (2014). *Power and choice: An introduction to political science* (14th ed.). New York: McGraw-Hill.

Smith, S.B. (2012). *Political philosophy.* New Haven: Yale University Press.

Wolff, J. (1996). *An introduction to political philosophy.* Oxford, UK: Oxford University Press.

ONLINE RESOURCES

Open courses on political philosophy, such as this one offered by Professor Stephen B. Smith at Yale University, including short lectures on YouTube

https://oyc.yale.edu/political-science/plsc-114

Internet Encyclopedia of Philosophy

www.iep.utm.edu

The Policy Process

Eileen T. O'Grady

> *"There are three critical ingredients to democratic renewal and progressive change in America: good public policy, grassroots organizing and electoral politics."*

Paul Wellstone

Nurses can more strategically and effectively influence policy if they have a clear understanding of the policymaking process. Conceptual models can help to organize and interpret information by depicting complex ideas in a simplified form; to this end, political scientists have developed a number of conceptual models to explain the highly dynamic process of policymaking. This chapter reviews two of these conceptual models.

HEALTH POLICY AND POLITICS

Health policy encompasses the political, economic, social, cultural, and social determinants of individuals and populations and attempts to address the broader issues in health and health care (see Box 7.1 for policy definitions). A clear understanding of the points of influence to shape policy is essential and includes framing the problem itself. For example, if nurses working in a nurse-managed clinic are troubled by staff shortages or long patient waits, they may be inclined to see themselves as the solution by working longer hours and seeing more patients. Defining and framing the problem is the first step in the policy process and involves assessing its history, patterns of impact, resource allocation, and community needs. Broadening and framing the problem to influence or educate stakeholders at the local, state, or federal level could include advocating for better access or funding for nursing workforce development (see Box 7.1).

The next step is to bring the problem to the attention of those who have the power to implement a solution. Other key factors to consider include generating public interest, the availability of viable policy solutions, the likelihood

that the policy will serve most of the people at risk in a fair and equitable fashion, and consideration of the organizational, community, societal, and political viability of the policy solution.

Public interest is a fascinating dynamic that is particularly important to influencing policy agendas at the community and broader policy levels. Public awareness is often necessary for political action to take place and for the policy process to be initiated. For example, trends associated with health behaviors (e.g., the increased rates of childhood obesity, drunk driving, smoking, or gun violence), whether gradual or resulting from a crisis situation, can all shift public perception and open a policy debate. Research consistently shows that a wide range of social and economic factors affect health, although this broader causality is beginning to be understood by the public. For example, a poll of rural Americans found that 57% think opioid addiction is a serious and urgent problem in their community, with 49% personally knowing someone who has struggled with opioid addiction. Twenty-five percent said it was the most urgent health problem facing their communities, followed by cancer (12%) and access to care (11%); 64% said solutions were better long-term jobs, improving the quality of local schools, and access to health care (Harvard T.H. Chan School of Public Health, 2018).

As public knowledge increases, trends become increasingly objectionable to some members of society, which propels them to seek solutions. For example, the rate of deaths caused by drunk driving resulted in strict nationwide drunk driving laws, and research on the impact of

BOX 7.1   Policy Definitions

Policy is authoritative decision making related to choices about goals and priorities of the policymaking body. In general, policies are constructed as a set of regulations (public policy), practice standards (workplace), governance mandates (organizations), ethical behavior (research), and ordinances (communities) that direct individuals, groups, organizations, and systems toward the desired behaviors and goals.

Health policy is the authoritative decisions made in the legislative, judicial, and executive branches of government that are intended to direct or influence the actions, behaviors, and decisions of others (Longest, 2016).

Policy analysis is the investigation of an issue including the background, purpose, content, and effects of various options within a policy context and their relevant social, economic, and political factors (Dye, 2016).

second-hand smoking led to the near-universal ban on smoking in shared open spaces.

When people have a strong sense that the status quo is unacceptable, they begin to organize in a predicable fashion, leading to actions such as forming coalitions or establishing a nonprofit organization. To move policy agendas forward, organizations must mature and build the resources needed to be effective in the policy realm.

Interest groups, such as trade associations and political action committees, can stimulate a shift from awareness of a policy issue to action, wherein people work collectively to find solutions. Professional nursing organizations serve as an interest group for nurses, not only to explore issues about the advancement of nursing but also to focus on societal issues such as reforming health care, informing the public of emerging diseases and health threats, and addressing health disparities.

Identifying and framing a problem is the first step, but it is also necessary to identify potential solutions. For example, concerns were raised in Washington State about the ability of insured workers to access health care in rural areas. This resulted in a delay in workers returning to work, as well as insufficient reporting of injuries. Because nurse practitioners (NPs) had been restricted in performing some of the functions related to certifying worker disability compensation, worker access to these providers was underused. As a result, the Washington State legislature enacted a pilot program to allow NPs to expand their scope of practice to include serving as attending providers for injured workers. Despite some stakeholder concerns, subsequent analysis of

the pilot program established that it was both effective and an efficient use of resources (Sears & Hogg-Johnson, 2009). A policy that will solve the problem is dependent on a thorough analysis of the problem itself and the viable, evidence-based policy options.

Fairness and equity are primary values that inspire nurses and others to participate in the policy process. Fawcett and Russell (2001) consider the equity of a policy as the extent to which it allows the benefits and burdens of nursing practice to be equally distributed to all—in particular, equal access to health services. For many nurses, advocating for fairness and equity is an application of patient advocacy, especially when human rights and health disparities are at stake. As noted in Chapter 1, social determinants of health illustrate that, in addition to individual choices, there are important environmental factors beyond the control of the individual that require collective action if health and health care are to be accessible for all.

Political viability also must be considered. Policy that is considered desirable to both politicians and stakeholders will have the best chance of passage. For example, public concerns about health effects from exposure to second-hand smoke have been communicated to policymakers many times. Although policymakers may want to take action to protect the public from tobacco smoke in public places, the pressure from tobacco companies for policymakers not to act has been equally powerful. As a result, public policy related to second-hand smoking languished for years in many states. However, when local communities in these states changed their ordinances to restrict smoking in public, there was increased pressure on state legislators to take action.

UNIQUE ASPECTS OF U.S. POLICYMAKING

The United States stands out from peer nations for having one of the most complicated health care delivery and finance systems in the world. It has a highly decentralized delivery "system" that also includes a mix of public and private payers and no single entity, authority, or government agency is ultimately responsible for health care. All of these facts lead to a convoluted patchwork of decision making, causing health care policy in the United States to be a highly complex and politically polarizing process. The current health care structure reflects policy decisions from the values of society, including residual policies from the colonial era. The U.S. Constitution does not specifically mention health care, but the preamble indicates that the federal government should "promote the general welfare." This lies at the heart of the current political debate between the Democrat and Republican Parties regarding the role of the federal government in health care.

Federalism is the system of government in which power is divided between a central authority (federal) and constituent political units (state governments). This division of power and authority, although purposely designed by the founding fathers, is the source of much tension, acrimony, and complexity in U.S. policymaking. Medicare, Medicaid, and Children's Health Insurance Program (CHIP) are examples of federally driven policies that create a partnership with states to administer health care under federal guidance. Meanwhile, regulation of health professionals, private health insurance coverage, and long-term care policies have long been the domain of the individual states. This complexity between the state and federal spheres illuminates the fragmented and seemingly chaotic approach to solving health care problems in the United States.

Many aspects of the original Affordable Care Act (ACA, 2010) protect states' rights to choose the degree to which they carry out some of its most important provisions, such as creating health exchanges to expand access to care. This built-in flexibility of the ACA allows states to experiment with local solutions because, for example, what works in Fargo may not work in Manhattan. The ACA escalated tensions between federal mandates and states' rights, as evidenced by the Supreme Court's role in settling the dispute resulting from the multistate lawsuit challenging the constitutionality of the ACA's mandate that every citizen purchase health insurance. In 2012 the Supreme Court upheld the individual mandate as a federal law that states must accept, and it ruled that the expansion of the Medicaid program was constitutional. But, it also protected states' rights by ruling that states cannot be penalized if they choose not to participate in the expansion (O'Connor & Jackson, 2012).

The trend to allow states increased flexibility in recent decades adds complexity to health policymaking and amplifies the need for nurses to understand the policymaking process. Nurses must be knowledgeable of the structure and players of policymaking so that decision-making bodies are targeted appropriately. For example, there have been incidences of nurses who have approached federal legislators to persuade them to increase funding for school nursing, unaware that school nursing is entirely a local or state issue.

The U.S. Constitution gives the federal government the power to block state laws when it chooses to do so. As noted earlier, state governments have authority to regulate health professionals as part of their charge to protect the public; although this is not in the Constitution, it has been the case since the formation of the nation (Safriet, 1992). This status quo is no longer appropriate because new forms of remote care delivery can render geographic boundaries irrelevant. Federalism is intended to create and sustain a highly decentralized locus of authority and is one of the most important dynamics in U.S. policymaking. This decentralized dynamic also, however, makes health care delivery systems complicated and difficult to reform.

Incrementalism refers to policymaking that proceeds slowly by degrees and is the way that most policymaking proceeds. Within the U.S. Constitution, the three branches of government (executive, legislative, and judicial) are designed deliberately to prevent one person or group from obtaining dictatorial powers. The disadvantage of this "checks and balances" structure is that it is very difficult for comprehensive policy reforms to succeed.

Once in a generation there is a major reform in U.S. health policy: for example, Social Security in the 1930s; Medicare and Medicaid in 1965; CHIP in the 1990s; and the ACA in 2010. However, most health policy reform in the United States has been incremental. The U.S. system empowers political players who represent a minority viewpoint to block the actions of the majority, resulting in paralysis. This was illustrated in 2013, 3 years after the ACA was signed into law, when members of the House of Representatives shut down the government for 16 days (at an estimated cost of $24 billion) in an attempt to defund some of the provisions of the ACA.

Policies in the United States are far easier to stop and obstruct than pass and implement. Policymaking is largely a process of continuous fine-tuning of what already exists. A good example of incrementalism is the policy toward gays in the military. In the early 1990s it was highly controversial to implement the "don't ask, don't tell" mandate that allowed gays to serve. By the early 2000s, public opinion on homosexuality shifted dramatically, and the military currently accepts individuals with this sexual orientation. Twenty-five years after "don't ask, don't tell," public acceptance of same-sex couples was evident by the 2015 Supreme Court ruling on marriage equality, making it legal for gays to marry.

Lindblom (1979) first described the concept of incrementalism in the early 1950s. When policymakers face a highly complex, theoretical, or resource-intensive decision and lack the time, capacity, or understanding to analyze all of the various policy options, they may limit themselves to a set of particular strategies instead of tackling the problem holistically. Policy solutions may be restricted to a set of familiar policy options that align with the status quo and lack a thorough evidence base. Therefore incrementalism, although effective in limiting the power of any one person, group, or branch of government, also creates a process that is neither proactive, goal-oriented, nor ambitious; it ossifies timely policy and limits innovation (Weiss & Woodhouse, 1992). There are examples of policy change that are revolutionary in nature, often born out of social movements, a crisis or new technology. The "Me Too" movement is creating revolutionary policy change very rapidly and is highly disruptive of the status quo. What is one day acceptable becomes unacceptable over a matter of weeks, forcing organizations of every type to review and generate policy around sexual misconduct. There are clear downsides to these rapid changes, because systems do not have time to adapt and generate sensible policies.

CONCEPTUAL BASIS FOR POLICYMAKING

Two different yet complementary models from political scientists illustrate how the seemingly chaotic policymaking process has a form, rhythm, and predictability.

Kingdon's Policy Streams Model

Kingdon (1995) proposed a policy streams model to reflect the issue of "policy looking for a problem." He described three streams of policy activity: the *problem stream*, the *policy stream*, and the *political stream*. These three streams must align to move through the open policy window at the same time (also referred to as the Garbage Can Model because the three streams must make their way through a minefield of debris). The problem must come to the attention of the policymaker, it must have a menu of viable policy solution options, and it must occur in the right political circumstances.

The *problem stream* describes the complexities in focusing policymakers on one specific problem out of many. For example, early in the process of developing the language for health reform legislation, policymakers engaged in a long process to define exactly which problems associated with the U.S. health care system should be included in a legislative package. Driving the problem stream are values, so access could be framed as a free market versus social justice issue. Values tend to have a stronger emotional component attached to them so that part of the challenge is the lack of agreement about which problems are the most urgent and require legislation. Some believe that cost is the biggest problem, others want to limit health reform to malpractice reform, and some want to improve access to care or quality. Until the problem is adequately defined, appropriate policy solutions cannot be identified.

The *policy stream* describes policy goals and the ideas of those in policy subsystems, such as researchers, congressional committee members and staff, agency officials, and interest groups. Ideas in the policy stream disseminate through policy circles in search of problems. Some nursing policy proposals have not clearly aligned with a timely problem stream, such as pushing to get school-based registered nurses (RNs) in every school in the country at a time when there are severe state budget cuts and teacher walkouts due to low pay. The solution proposed must be hitched to an identifiable, timely, and urgent problem.

The third stream, the *political stream*, describes factors in the political environment that influence the policy agenda, such as an economic recession, special interest media, or pivotal political power shifts. The political circumstances that push problems to the top of the policy agenda need a high degree of public importance and a low degree of stakeholder conflict around the proposed solutions. A great deal of stakeholder conflict weakens the possibility that the policy window will open.

If these three conditions occur at the same time, a policy window opens and progress can be made on the issue. Kingdon (1995) sees these streams as moving constantly; waiting for a window of opportunity to open through couplings of any two streams—particularly when one is the political stream—creates new opportunities for policy change. However, such opportunities are time limited: if change does not occur while the window is open, the problems and options will not be addressed.

For example, although health reform was a high priority for newly elected President Obama in 2009, the economic crisis and recession became a powerful political stream bringing to bear a major debate about how escalating health care costs were making the United States less competitive in the global marketplace. The movement of U.S. jobs overseas and the recession were linked to out-of-control health care costs and the need to reform health care; thus a policy window was opened.

Longest's Policy Cycle Model

Health policy is a cyclical process. Longest (2016) mapped out an interrelated model to capture how U.S. policymaking works. It is a continuous, highly dynamic cycle that captures the incrementalism inherent in U.S. governmental decision making (Fig. 7.1). In its simplest form, there are three phases to the policy process: a *policy formulation phase*, a *policy implementation phase*, and a *policy modification phase*. Each phase contains a set of actions and activities that produce outcomes or products that influence the next stage. Although simple in design, this model is deceptively complex. Defining the policy problem with adequate clarity so that it gains the attention of policymakers and stakeholders is challenging—each policy problem has many solutions and competitors seeking a place on the policy agenda. The importance of framing and agenda setting is underscored by Doreatha Brande's (1893 to 1948) quote, "A problem clearly stated is a problem half solved."

Policy formulation includes all the activities that are involved in policymaking, including those activities that inform the legislators. It is in this phase that nurses can

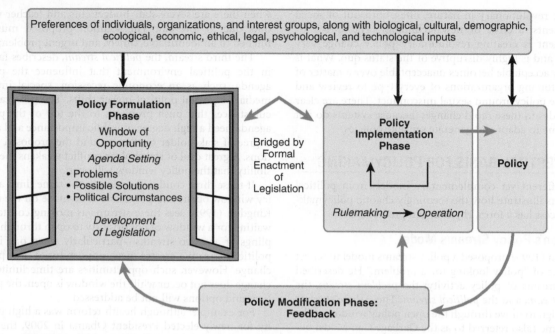

Preferences of individuals, organizations, and interest groups, along with biological, cultural, demographic, ecological, economic, ethical, legal, psychological, and technological inputs

Policy Formulation Phase

Window of Opportunity

Agenda Setting

- Problems
- Possible Solutions
- Political Circumstances

Development of Legislation

Bridged by Formal Enactment of Legislation

Policy Implementation Phase

Rulemaking ⟶ *Operation*

Policy

Policy Modification Phase: Feedback

Fig. 7.1 Longest's policy framework. (Redrawn from Longest, B. [2016]. *Health policymaking in the United States* [6th ed.]. Chicago: Health Administration Press.)

serve as a knowledge source to legislators in helping to frame problems by bringing nursing stories and patient narratives to illustrate how health problems play out with individual constituents/populations. The most effective time to influence legislation is before it is drafted, so that nurses can help to frame the issues to align with their desire for policy outcomes that are patient centered.

Policy implementation comprises the rule-making phase of policy development. The legislative branch passes the law to the executive branch, which is charged with implementation. This includes adding specificity to the law and may also include, for example, defining "the health care provider" to include advanced practice nurses (provider-neutral terminology). The writing of rules after legislation is passed is a crucial and often overlooked aspect of policy-making (see Chapter 39 on Legislation and Regulation). At this juncture, nurses with appropriate expertise can monitor and influence how the rules are written. Once written, federal regulations are published in the daily Federal Register for 60 days to receive public comment. States have similar regulatory processes.

Stakeholder groups can exert enormous influence during the implementation phase (Regulations.gov, 2013). When strong letter-writing campaigns are used, the rule-making agency may be forced to publish those comments

and make adjustments according to their volume and scientific rigor. It is not unusual for the intent of a policy to get lost in the translation to program development. This rule-making phase is an important leverage point for nurses to closely monitor and respond to regulations through grassroots campaigns.

Two important aspects of American democracy are at play during the public comment phase: (1) informed citizenry—the democratic process only works if its citizenry is informed; and (2) government is not all-knowing—the government acknowledges it does not hold all of the expertise; it must solicit that expertise from the public (Regulations.gov, 2013). An example of rulemaking that limited nursing occurred in 2013 when the Georgia legislature revised its scope of practice law for nurses. The law had many benefits for advanced practice registered nurses (APRNs), but the state's executive branch made the rules and regulations more restrictive than they were before the legislation was passed. The restrictions caused many APRNs to continue to work under the old scope of practice that was less restrictive (Center to Champion Nursing in America, 2010).

Policy modification allows all previous decisions to be revisited and modified. Policies that were initially pertinent may become inappropriate over time. Almost all policies have unintended consequences, which is why many stakeholders seek to modify policies continuously. Policies may negatively impact the population in myriad unexpected ways. Examples of unintended consequences include the following:

- The Health Insurance Portability and Accountability Act (HIPAA) was created to protect privacy but wreaks havoc when hospital staff are prevented from sharing by phone with family members any information about the status of their gravely ill, out-of-state college-age daughter.
- Information technology designed to capture high-quality data during clinical visits has created an unsatisfying intrusion into the patient-provider relationship.
- Placing caps on Medicare drug benefits to rein in costs has created an uptick in preventable hospital admissions as a result of patients not having access to medicine.

NURSES' COMPETENCE IN THE POLICYMAKING PROCESS

To effectively influence the policymaking process, nurses must successfully analyze the process and influence it with a high degree of political competence. Policy development that is dominated by public interest generally follows a course of action that is based on data, information, and community values and addresses a solution to an actual or potential problem. It tends to be practical decision making. Stakeholder coalitions that promote the public's interest can exert enormous influence in shaping health policy.

An example of a provider interest group with a focus on the public interest is the National Association of Pediatric Nurse Practitioners (NAPNAP), which identified childhood obesity as an organizational priority. It participated in a wide range of governmental committees, interviews on news media, and development of clinical practice guidelines, as well as created culturally appropriate resources for parents. Pediatric NPs have effectively participated in a range of policy endeavors to address the alarming childhood obesity epidemic (NAPNAP, 2015). They have published their strongly worded, far-reaching *Position Statement on the Prevention and Identification of Overweight and Obesity in the Pediatric Population* that recommends policy solutions, clinical solutions, and public awareness campaigns (Box 7.2).

BOX 7.2 Example of a Position Statement: NAPNAP Position Statement on Immunizations

The National Association of Pediatric Nurse Practitioners (NAPNAP) supports the timely and complete immunization of all infants, children, adolescents, and adults in an attempt to maximize the health and well-being of all people. Routine childhood immunizations prevent as many as 3 million deaths per year. In addition, 1.5 million deaths per year could be avoided if global vaccination efforts continue to improve (World Health Organization, 2017).

During the past two decades, immunization exemptions have steadily risen until the 2012–2013 school year, when the rate of immunization exemptions plateaued. Still, immunization exemptions corrode community immunity provided by population-based vaccination programs, and this warrants careful and continued monitoring to prevent vaccine-preventable disease outbreaks in the United States (Omer, Porter, Allen, Salmon, & Bednarczyk, 2018).

The Centers for Disease Control and Prevention (CDC) Committee on Infectious Diseases and the Advisory Committee on Immunization Practices annually review and recommend routine vaccination to prevent 17 vaccine preventable diseases (CDC, 2015, 2018b). In concert with the American Academy of Pediatrics, NAPNAP recognizes the importance of timely vaccinations for children and strongly encourages parents to adhere to the recommended immunization schedule as the best way to protect their children and community from vaccine-preventable infectious diseases (American Academy of Pediatrics, 2018).

NAPNAP considers nurse practitioners (NPs) to be in the best position to inform parents of the scientific and evidence-based foundation of the current immunization recommendations. This education must include the most current scientific evidence related to vaccine safety, risk, and benefits. Parents should know how to find the most current, correct, and evidence-based resources. Conversely, they must be informed about sources and dangers of misinformation. Using a nonjudgmental approach, NPs are compelled to inform parents about the risks of not vaccinating their children as recommended by the evidence.

NAPNAP expects NPs to be skillful clinicians and encourages NPs to become identified as leaders in the health and safety of children and families. NPs must remain knowledgeable about the ever-changing science of vaccination and recommendations for immunizations. Promoting vaccines should be done at the individual, local, state, national,

Continued

BOX 7.2   Example of a Position Statement: NAPNAP Position Statement on Immunizations—cont'd

and international levels. NPs are encouraged to participate on employer, hospital, school, local, state, and national committees that address immunization policies and practices, including advocating for increased funding for vaccines.

In an effort to ensure that all pediatric populations are protected against vaccine-preventable illness and remain healthy, NAPNAP affirms that NPs and other pediatric health care providers must do the following.

1. Ensure access to timely immunization for all children.
2. Avoid any and all missed opportunities to vaccinate.
3. Consider every health care encounter as a means to review immunization records, educate parents about immunization safety and efficacy, and vaccinate as needed.
4. Acknowledge the ultimate goal of immunizing children in a timely fashion is to maximize the health of each individual child.
5. Encourage and enable parents and caregivers to critically evaluate vaccine information.
6. Recommend parents, caregivers, and other adults to remain compliant with recommended immunizations for their age and risk group in order to protect children in their care.
7. Distribute the evidence-based CDC Vaccine Information Statements (VISs) for each recommended vaccine to parents and caregivers at every immunization encounter (CDC, 2018a).
8. Ensure adherence to immunization schedules by utilizing electronic health records, statewide vaccine registries, and recall systems to promote continued development of these systems.
9. Remain knowledgeable via local or national immunization groups, educational programs or conferences, evidence-based research articles, and peer-reviewed journals.
10. Immediately incorporate changes in immunization policies, recommendations, and practices into daily practice (Kroger, Duchin, & Vazquez, 2017).
11. Provide complete, accurate, and culturally sensitive educational programs about immunizations to the public, childcare centers, schools, and community groups, including information on benefits, safety, evidence-based quality resources, and the importance of active and timely participation in immunization programs.
12. Utilize news, social media, and other applicable communication methods to influence and direct the conversation regarding immunization safety, efficacy, and necessity.

13. Utilize quality improvement principles to evaluate immunization practices for the purpose of improving compliance with recommended immunization practices and educating members of the health care team.
14. Lead policy change in states to eliminate nonmedical exemptions for school entry.
15. Actively participate on local, state, and national committees, advisory groups, and other venues that impact policies concerning childhood immunization practices.
16. Support any local, state, or federal legislation that aims to keep childhood immunizations available, accessible, and affordable for all children regardless of social or economic status or the type of health insurance.
17. Serve as immunization expert on local, regional, or national committees to support the safety and efficacy of childhood immunization programs.
18. Advocate for an integrated national immunization infrastructure to ensure the supply and delivery of vaccines, maintenance of coverage rates, outbreak control, and immunization education (Groom et al., 2015).
19. Understand the responsibility to report adverse outcomes following any immunization to the Vaccine Adverse Event Reporting System (VAERS; CDC, 2017) and the purpose of the Vaccine Injury Compensation Program (VICP; U.S. Department of Health and Human Services, Health Resources and Services Administration, 2018).
20. Keep informed of the incidence of vaccine-preventable diseases in your area, and be proficient in the ability to diagnose the illness.
21. In the event of vaccine-preventable disease diagnosis, encourage parents to keep children with vaccine-preventable disease at home from school and out of public settings for the duration of the outbreak as recommended by state and national guidelines (Aronson & Shope, 2016).

In summary, NAPNAP is an organization whose mission is to empower pediatric nurse practitioners, pediatricfocused advanced practice registered nurses, and their interprofessional partners to enhance child and family health through leadership, advocacy, professional practice, education, and research and is committed to the health and wellbeing of all children and their families. NAPNAP recognizes the immense benefits of immunizations for children and the community alike. NAPNAP encourages NPs, as well as other pediatric health care providers, to consistently assess patient immunization status, limit missed opportunities to vaccinate, support immunization programs, and promote community awareness of the value of immunization of all children. NPs are compelled to be informed clinicians, skilled communicators, strong leaders, advocates, and champions for evidence-based immunization programs. It is the position of NAPNAP that NPs and elected leaders at the local, state, and federal levels support legislative efforts to appropriate funds for comprehensive immunization delivery, for a national immunization registry, and to maintain the VAERS and VICP programs.

The National Association of Pediatric Nurse Practitioners would like to acknowledge the following members from the Immunization Special Interest Group (SIG) for their contribution to this statement: Lacey Eden, MS, NP-C; Cheryl Cairns, DNP, CPNP, RN, APN; Karlen E. Luthy, DNP, FNP-C, FAAN, FAANP; and Mary Koslap-Petraco, DNP, PPCNP-BC, CPNP, FAANP.

References

American Academy of Pediatrics. (2018). *Immunization schedules for 2018.* Itasca, IL: Author. Retrieved from https://redbook. solutions.aap.org/SS/Immunization_Schedules.aspxcdc.

Aronson, S.S. & Shope, T.R. (2016). *Managing infectious disease in child care and schools* (4th ed.). Elk Grove Village, IL: American Academy of Pediatrics. Retrieved from http://ebooks. aappublications.org/content/managing-infectious-diseases-inchild-care-and-schools-4th-ed.

Centers for Disease Control and Prevention. (2015). *Epidemiology and prevention of vaccine-preventable diseases.* Atlanta, GA: Author. Retrieved from www.cdc.gov/vaccines/pubs/pinkbook/genrec.html.

Centers for Disease Control and Prevention. (2017). *Vaccine adverse event reporting system (VAERS).* Atlanta, GA: Author. Retrieved from www.cdc.gov/vaccinesafety/ensuringsafety/monitoring/vaers/index.html.

Centers for Disease Control and Prevention. (2018a). *Instructions for using Vaccine Information Statements.* Atlanta, GA: Author. Retrieved from www.cdc.gov/vaccines/schedules/hcp/adult.html.

Centers for Disease Prevention and Control. (2018b). *Recommended immunization schedule for children and adolescents aged 18 years or younger, United States, 2018.* Atlanta, GA: Author. Retrieved from www.cdc.gov/vaccines/schedules/hcp/child-adolescent.html.

Groom, H., Hopkins, D.P., Pabst, L.J., Morgan, J.M., Patel, M., Calonge, N., . . . & Community Preventive Services Task Force. (2015). Immunization information systems to increase vaccination rates: A community guide systematic review. *Journal of Public Health Management and Practice, 21,* 227–248.

Kroger, A.T. Duchin, J., & Vazquez, M. (2017). *General best practice guidelines for immunizations. Best practice guidelines for immunization of the Advisory Committee for Immunization Practice (ACIP).* Atlanta, GA: Centers for Disease Control and Prevention. Retrieved from www.cdc.gov/vaccines/hcp/aciprecs/general-recs/downloads/general-recs.pdf.

Omer, S.B., Porter, R.M., Allen, K., Salmon, D.A., & Bednarczyk, R.B. (2018). Trends in Kindergarten rates of vaccine exemption and state-level policy, 2011–2016. *Open Forum Infectious Diseases, 5*(2), 1–6.

U.S. Department of Health and Humans Services, Health Resources and Services Administration. (2018). *National vaccine injury compensation program.* Rockville, MD: Author. Retrieved from www.hrsa.gov/vaccine-compensation/index.html.

World Health Organization. (2017). *Immunization coverage.* Geneva, Switzerland: Author. Retrieved from www.who.int/news-room/fact-sheets/detail/immunization-coverage.

From NAPNAP position statement on Immunizations. *Journal of Pediatric Health Care, 32*(6), A9–A11. Retrieved from www. jpedhc.org/article/S0891-5245(18)30378-X/pdf. Reprinted with permission of the *Journal of Pediatric Health Care.*

Longest (2016) has identified best practices that leaders of advocacy organizations undertake to promote their health-related mission. Once the organization makes policy influence a priority, a governmental relations (or affairs) team is formed (or a firm is contracted) to do the work. If these teams are competent, they can transform the effectiveness of the organizations by giving the CEO (and/or board of directors) anticipatory guidance. The ability of organizations to anticipate lead time and direct resources appropriately is the key function of a strong public policy team. This anticipatory approach moves maturing organizations away from reacting to policy changes and toward strategic leadership. Effective advocacy organizations are continuously analyzing the environment, primarily looking out (not in) at the ever-changing political landscape.

Professional nursing organizations (e.g., the American Academy of Nursing, the American Nurses Association, and many nursing specialty groups) are concerned not only with public policy that impacts the health of all people but also with policy that impacts nurses and the practice of nursing. These organizations, individually and collectively, support policies that are in the best interest of their members.

Engaging in Policy Analysis

Issue analysis is similar to the nursing process: it is necessary to clearly identify the problem (including the context of the problem, alternatives for resolution and the consequences of each, along with specific criteria for evaluating the alternatives) and recommend the optimal solution. Issue papers or policy briefs provide the mechanism to do this. These identify the underlying issue and stakeholders and specify solutions along with their positive and negative consequences. Issue papers help to clarify arguments in support of a position, recognize the arguments of the opposition, and lay out the evidence or lack thereof for an issue and potential solutions.

A one-page, "leave-behind" position statement provides a summary for the policymaker to read and gain a grasp of the issue quickly. A standard format for a policy brief includes summary of the issue, background information, analysis of alternatives, a recommendation for action, references, and personal contact information (Box 7.3).

BOX 7.3   Example of a Policy Brief: The American Academy of Nursing. Elder Justice: Preventing and Intervening in Elder Mistreatment Policy Brief

Introduction

In the United States, as many as 1 in 10 older adults and 47% of persons with dementia living at home experience some form of mistreatment (Institute of Medicine [IOM], 2014). Elder mistreatment results in diminished well-being and quality of life and violates the rights of older adults to be safe and free from violence. Elder mistreatment can occur anywhere—in the home, in care and residential facilities, and in the community. It can also be malignantly contagious within settings and families and across the lifespan (Dong, 2012). With the rapid growth of the U.S. population of older adults, now estimated to reach 84 million by the year 2050 (Ortman, Velkoff, & Hogan, 2014), the issue of elder mistreatment is a major national health concern.

The American Academy of Nursing's Strategic Goal #3 (2014–2017)—to lead change to improve health and healthcare and drive policy—is especially related to this issue. Health care professionals in regular contact with vulnerable older adults—including the nation's 3 million nurses—are in an ideal position to identify and report suspected cases of mistreatment; they are, however, among the least likely to do so (Schmeidel, Daly, Rosenbaum, Schmuch, & Jogerst, 2012). This policy brief summarizes some of the most relevant information in the field of elder mistreatment and recommends partnered action by health professions organizations and other stakeholders to promote elder justice and improve overall health and well-being of this vulnerable group.

Background

The successful legislation of the Elder Justice Act in 2010 as a part of the Patient Protection and Affordable Care Act (United States. Congress. Senate. Committee on Finance, 2006) has done much to accelerate nationally the deserved attention that elder mistreatment in all of its forms demands. Unfortunately, to date, no funds have been appropriated by Congress to carry out the important provisions of this Act or its earlier iteration (Older Americans Act Amendments of 2006, October 17, 2006) related to direct services, education or policy and resource development for elder justice. The American Academy of Nursing is committed to justice for all individuals and especially those who are frail, disadvantaged, and potentially incapable of defending themselves in the presence of elder mistreatment. Two of the Academy's special interest groups—Aging and Psychiatric, Mental Health & Substance Abuse—stand ready to bring to bear their collective resources and talents to help address this serious and potentially fatal syndrome.

There is currently no overarching theory or conceptual framework for elder mistreatment, although several borrowed from other fields (Ecological Model, Sociocultural Model, Cycle of Violence Theory, Life Course Perspective as examples) have been used (IOM, 2013). And, while there is no universally accepted definition, the Elder Justice Roadmap Project (Connolly, Brandl, & Brekman, 2014) has defined it broadly as physical, sexual, or psychological abuse, as well as neglect, abandonment, and financial exploitation of an older person by another person or entity, that occurs in any setting (e.g., home, community, or facility), either in a relationship where there is an expectation of trust and/or when an older person is targeted based on age or disability. Elder justice recognizes an older person's rights and his or her ability to be free of abuse, neglect, and exploitation. The Elder Justice Act defines elder justice activities as "efforts to prevent, detect, treat, intervene in, and prosecute elder abuse, neglect, and exploitation and to protect elders with diminished capacity while maximizing their autonomy" (United States Congress Senate Committee on Finance, 2006).

A number of risk factors for elder mistreatment and its subsequent health outcomes create opportunities for prevention or intervention. These include increased physical dependency of frail elders on caregivers; fewer family members living in the same geographic region or caregivers being elderly or impaired themselves; substance abuse, cognitive impairment and mental illness among

BOX 7.3 Example of a Policy Brief: The American Academy of Nursing. Elder Justice: Preventing and Intervening in Elder Mistreatment Policy Brief—cont'd

caregivers and/or the mistreated as well as poverty, age, race, functional disability, frailty, loneliness and low education (Fulmer, 2013). For the elder, the experience of mistreatment itself, in any of its forms, often also results in behavioral health symptoms including depression, risk of suicide, anxiety, cognitive dysfunction, and sleep difficulty; self-treatment with drugs and alcohol; injuries and morbidities resulting in higher use of emergency department, hospital and nursing home services, and greater mortality (Dong, 2014). Thus, elder mistreatment is not only harmful to individuals, but is also detrimental to social, legal, and health systems (Vognar & Gibbs, 2014).

There is growing interest in and commitment to the prevention and treatment of elder mistreatment among national agencies and institutes whose collaboration could achieve greater impact. The recent release of the Elder Justice Roadmap (Connolly et al., 2014), developed with support from the Department of Justice (DOJ) and the Department of Health and Human Services (HHS), provides impetus and guidance for advancing strategic policy, practice, education, and research initiatives that can help move forward components of the recently enacted Elder Justice Act and recommendations from the IOM's 2013 Forum on Global Violence workshop (2014). Furthermore, the 2015 White House Conference on Aging (WHCoA) has identified four themes, of which Elder Justice is one. Elder justice is also a priority area for the American Academy of Nursing which has a broad and deep reach in national policy and can play a critical role in helping to advance the recommendations from these initiatives. All nurses and other health professional groups must capitalize on the opportunities created by these recent initiatives to contribute to the national conversation. Their input and feedback can help shape the aging policy landscape through a variety of mechanisms, including listening sessions, regional forums, social media, and the WHCoA website. In addition, they can help to educate legislators and their policy staff by sharing this policy brief.

Recommendations

Health professionals, and especially nurses, play an extraordinarily important role in the advancement of our understanding of and response to the complex phenomenon of elder mistreatment. As the largest professional health care workforce, nurses serve at the frontline in the prevention, assessment, and management of elder mistreatment. Partnered organizational support of efforts related to prevention, recognition and treatment, education and training, and research will make important inroads in solving this critical problem. The following recommendations align with those found in the Elder Justice Roadmap (Connolly et al., 2014).

Prevention

Nurses and other health professionals should support elder mistreatment prevention by aligning with existing efforts to shore up community-based networks and resources that buttress and sustain older adults and their families. Programs currently gaining momentum include Age Friendly Communities and the Village Movement, both aimed at enhancing safe and healthy aging-in-place.

The Academy Recommends

- Encouragement of all health professionals, including nurses, to use opportunities like social media, online resources, and public service messaging to combat ageism and raise the public's awareness of elder mistreatment and its severity, identifying high-risk situations and the need to intervene before mistreatment arises or escalates.
- Engagement of state and Area Agency on Aging efforts to provide supports, improve awareness of at-risk elders, and facilitate effective preventive resources.
- Heightened attention to needs of underserved, isolated, or vulnerable populations at highest risk for mistreatment, e.g., a partnership with National Indigenous Elder Justice Initiative housed at the University of North Dakota's Center for Rural Health, among others.
- Increased awareness of the activities and products of the International Network for the Prevention of Elder Abuse, a nongovernmental organization affiliated with the United Nations.
- Better preparation of older adults and adult children who will take care of their aging parents through public awareness and caregiver education and training.

Recognition and Treatment

Health professions societies and academies should advocate broader use of efforts to recognize and intervene in elder mistreatment. These include integrated care models (IOM, 2012), routine screening, and use of related evidence-based intervention models.

The Academy Recommends

- A campaign to encourage nurses and others in primary care settings to ask privately—of every client age 65 and older—the screening question, "Do you feel safe at home?"

Continued

BOX 7.3   Example of a Policy Brief: The American Academy of Nursing. Elder Justice: Preventing and Intervening in Elder Mistreatment Policy Brief—cont'd

- Expansion of Medicare/Medicaid reimbursement to better cover screening and basic first level mental health services by primary care provider staff. This will enhance inclusion of routine screening for mistreatment, substance use and mental health problems as part of the annual Medicare health promotion visit.
- Recognition by the National Quality Forum of elder mistreatment assessment as a quality indicator across healthcare settings, thus enhancing adoption of the practice.
- Advocacy for scaling up use in primary care settings of depression and substance use intervention models that work, such as IMPACT or SBIRT.
- Support for the Administration on Aging (AoA)'s National Center on Elder Abuse (NCEA) to heighten awareness and serve as a resource for policy makers, social service and health care practitioners, the justice system, researchers, advocates, and families.

Education and Training

The Health Resources and Services Administration, in concert with the AoA's National Center for Elder Abuse, should convene a group to determine key training models and materials that would address attention to mistreatment in clinical practice and make recommendations for health sciences curricula and continuing education. This collaborative effort will also enhance broad-based learning for advocates, caregivers, community leaders, financial services industry personnel, and legal/law enforcement workers, as well as health care professionals and social service providers.

The Academy Recommends

- Interprofessional training to address ageism, mistreatment and behavioral health at pre- and post-professional levels.
- Mandatory continuing education for nurses on elder abuse, similar to the recent National Council of State Boards of Nursing requirement for child abuse education; this model could also be used by other health professions.
- A requirement by the National Academies of Practice that all distinguished practitioners have an awareness of and plan for addressing all forms of family violence, including elder mistreatment.
- Contribute, use, disseminate, and review training materials for the Elder Abuse Training Repository of the NCEA, a national resource center dedicated to the provision of information to professionals and the public,

technical assistance, and training to state and community-based organizations.

Research

The National Institute for Nursing Research, in partnership with the National Institute on Aging, the Substance Abuse and Mental Health Services Administration and the Department of Justice together with its Elder Justice Steering Committee and nongovernmental funding agencies, should establish guidelines for setting priorities and securing funding to advance a RESEARCH AND PROGRAM EVALUATION AGENDA that addresses recommendations from the Elder Justice Roadmap.

The Academy Recommends

- Prioritization of research on elder mistreatment in all its forms, as this emphasis is crucial to fostering quality of life for older adults and a just and healthier society.
- Strategic promotion of prevention research priorities and evaluation strategies identified in the Elder Justice Roadmap, as well as Adult Protective Services intervention studies and recruitment to the elder justice field researchers with expertise in studying prevention.
- Assurance that critical research foci include epidemiology of this multidimensional and complex problem, especially psychological abuse.
- Demonstration of effectiveness of preventive, early recognition, surveillance, intervention (including legal), and rehabilitative programs in diverse individuals, including those with cognitive impairment, across settings.
- Inclusion of projects that result in recommendations for promoting and protecting resilience, mental health and coping and that empower older people, their families, and their communities.

Acknowledgment

This policy brief was prepared by the Expert Panel on Aging and the Psychiatric, Mental Health & Substance Abuse Expert Panel on behalf of the American Academy of Nursing. We gratefully recognize Terry Fulmer, PhD, RN, FAAN, Lois Evans, PhD, RN, FAAN, Kitty Buckwalter, PhD, RN, FAAN, Marie Boltz, PhD, RN, CRNP, FAAN, and Tara Cortes PhD, RN, FAAN, for their contributions in authoring this policy brief.

References

Connolly, M.-T., Brandl, B., & Brekman, R. (2014). *Elder justice roadmap report*. Washington, DC: U.S. Department of Justice.

BOX 7.3 **Example of a Policy Brief: The American Academy of Nursing. Elder Justice: Preventing and Intervening in Elder Mistreatment Policy Brief—cont'd**

Dong, X. (2012). *Elder abuse and the contagion of violence: One size doesn't fit all.* Washington, DC: Institute of Medicine.

Dong, X. (2014). Elder abuse: research, practice, and health policy: The 2012 GSA Maxwell Pollack Award lecture. *The Gerontologist, 54,* 153–162

Fulmer, T. (2013). Mistreatment of older adults. In S. Durso, & G. Sullivan (Eds.). *Geriatric review syllabus: A core curriculum in geriatric medicine* (8th ed., pp. 104–108). New York: American Geriatrics Society.

Institute of Medicine. (2012). *The mental health and substance use workforce for older adults: In whose hands?* Washington, DC: National Academies Press.

Institute of Medicine. (2014). *Forum on global violence prevention: Elder abuse and its prevention* (pp. 59–66). Washington, DC: National Research Council.

Older Americans Act Amendments of 2006, Public Law 109–365 (October 17, 2006).

Ortman, J.M., Velkoff, V.A., & Hogan, H. (2014). *An aging nation: The older population in the United States* (Current Population Reports). Washington, DC: U.S. Census Bureau.

Schmeidel, A.N., Daly, J.M., Rosenbaum, M.E., Schmuch, G.A., & Jogerst, G.J. (2012). Healthcare professionals' perspectives on barriers to elder abuse detection and reporting in primary care settings. *Journal of Elder Abuse & Neglect, 24,* 17–36

United States Congress Senate Committee on Finance. (2006). *Elder Justice Act: Report (to accompany S.2010).* Washington, DC: U.S. GPO.

Vognar, L. & Gibbs, L.M. (2014). Care of the victim. *Clinics in Geriatric Medicine, 30,* 869–880.

From Elder justice: Preventing and intervening in elder mistreatment. *Nursing Outlook, 63*(5), 610–613. Retrieved from www.nursingoutlook.org/article/S0029-6554(15)00256-0/fulltext. Reprinted with permission of the American Academy of Nursing.

Infusing the Evidence Base into Health Policy

Data and research are highly valuable in understanding a health policy issue and in developing a solution to the problem. It is assumed that health policy driven by an evidence base will link the evidence, policy solution, and the significance of the situation. However, evidence may support opposing views of a policy solution. For example, will expanding access to care for the poor increase or decrease costs? There is evidence that supports both sides of this policy debate, and the cost shifting currently in place for most delivery systems makes it difficult to ascertain which view is correct—or which values are most important.

Another barrier to crafting policy is that there can be a lack of clarity about the evidence that is needed. Nurses generally understand that evidence-based practice is based on science. However, there is a hierarchy of what constitutes evidence from scientific inquiry that ranges from systematic review, randomized controlled trials, cohort studies, case-control studies, cross-sectional surveys, case reports, expert opinion, and anecdotal information (Glasby & Beresford, 2006). This hierarchy can make it difficult to reach an agreement among stakeholders, policymakers, and the public about what evidence is appropriate and most valuable for health policy. New evidence may need to be developed before one can move ahead with a policy recommendation; this may include evidence informed by input from community stakeholders. Although policymaking is dependent on good data and evidence about what works, data and evidence may not be enough to outweigh the influence of the political environment.

Policy-Relevant Research

Despite the debate over what constitutes evidence and which evidence is relevant for health policy, health services research (HSR) can be very effective in developing policy options. HSR is a far broader form of research than clinical research in that it is a multidisciplinary field of scientific inquiry that looks at how people gain access to health care, how much care costs, and what happens to patients as a result of this care. The main goals of HSR are to identify the most effective ways to deliver high-quality, cost-effective, safe care across systems (Agency for Healthcare Research and Quality [AHRQ], 2013). These include issues such as the restructuring of health services, human resource use in health care settings, primary care design, patient safety and quality, and patient outcomes. For example, Linda Aiken's work on safe staffing (Aiken, 2007; Aiken et al., 2002), Mary Naylor's work on transitions in care for older adults (Naylor et al., 2004), and Mary Mundinger's work on the use of NPs (Mundinger et al., 2000) are widely cited in policy literature. There has been an increase in comparative effectiveness research, which uses a design to inform decisions about Medicare. It uses a range of data sources to compare the costs and harms of various treatment decisions and is commonly used to study the cost effectiveness of drugs, medical devices, and surgical procedures.

CONCLUSION

Goethe wrote, *"Everything is hard before it is easy,"* and it underscores the importance of going after meta-causes of problems in our health care system. Nurses should seize opportunities to be active in all policy arenas to assure that solutions improve the health of people. In addition to lobbying policymakers, nurses can run for elective office at all levels of government; nurses serve in policy research roles; as policy analysts within professional nursing or patient advocacy organizations and health care institutions and within state or federal agencies; and as staff to policymakers. Nursing leaders have had considerable impact on policy from their leadership positions in organizations such as AARP, the National Academy of Medicine, and the Health Services and Resources Administration. Such involvement in health policy is a natural extension of nurses' role as advocate.

DISCUSSION QUESTIONS

1. Identify a problem you face regularly in your clinical setting. Next, identify how this problem could be framed as a policy issue.
2. The Kingdon and Longest models help us to interpret how policy works. Select one model and apply it to a policy issue you care about.
3. Name three actions you and your peers could do to strengthen nursing's influence in the policy process?

REFERENCES

Agency for Healthcare Research and Quality. (2013). *An organizational guide to building research capacity*. Retrieved from www.ahrq.gov/funding/training-grants/hsrguide/hsrguide.html.

Aiken, L. (2007). Supplemental nurse staffing in hospitals and quality of care. *Journal of Nursing Administration, 37*, 335–342.

Aiken, L., Clarke, S., Sloane, D., Sochalski, J., & Silber, J. (2002). Hospital nurse staffing and patient mortality, nurse burnout, and job dissatisfaction. *JAMA, 288*(16), 1987–1993.

Center to Champion Nursing in America. (2010). *Access to care and advanced practice nurses: A review of Southern U.S. practice laws*. AARP Public Policy Institute. Retrieved from https://campaignforaction.org/resource/access-care-advanced-practice-nurses-review-southern-us-practice-laws/.

Dye, R. (2016). *Understanding public policy* (15th ed.). New York: Pearson.

Fawcett, J., & Russell, G. (2001). A conceptual model of nursing and health policy. *Policy, Politics, & Nursing Practice, 2*(2), 108–116.

Glasby, J., & Beresford, P. (2006). Who knows best? Evidence-based practice and the service user contribution. *Critical Social Policy, 26*(1), 268–284.

Harvard T.H., & Chan School of Public Health. (2018). *Life in rural America*. NPR/Robert Wood Johnson Foundation/Harvard School of Public Health. Retrieved from www.rwjf.org/en/library/research/2018/10/life-in-rural-america.html.

Kingdon, J.W. (1995). *Agendas, alternatives, and public policies*. Boston: Little, Brown.

Lindblom, C. (1979). Still muddling, not yet through. *Public Administration Review, 39*(6), 517–526.

Longest, B. (2016). *Health policymaking in the United States* (6th ed.). Chicago: Health Administration Press.

Mundinger, M., Kane, R., Lenz, E., Totten, A., Tsai, W., Cleary, P., . . . & Shelanski, M. (2000). Primary care outcomes in patients treated by nurse practitioners or physicians: A randomized trial. *JAMA, 283*, 59–68.

National Association of Pediatric Nurse Practitioners. (2015). *Position statement on childhood obesity*. Retrieved from www.jpedhc.org/article/S0891-5245(15)00152-2/fulltext.

Naylor, M., Brooten, D., Campbell, R., Maislin, G., McCauley, K., & Schwartz, J. (2004). Transitional care of older adults hospitalized with heart failure: A randomized, controlled trial. *Journal of the American Geriatric Society, 52*(7), 675–684.

O'Connor, M., & Jackson, W. (2012). Analysis: U.S. Supreme Court upholds the Affordable Care Act: Roberts rules? *The National Law Review*. Retrieved from www.natlawreview.com/article/analysis-us-supreme-court-upholds-affordable-care-act-roberts-rules.

Regulations.gov. (2013). *eRulemaking program* [website to enable citizens to search, view and comment on regulations issued by the US Government]. Retrieved from www.regulations.gov/#!aboutProgram.

Safriet, B. (1992). Health care dollars and regulatory sense: The role of advanced practice nursing. *Yale Journal on Regulations, 417*, 442–445.

Sears, J., & Hogg-Johnson, S. (2009). Enhancing the policy impact of evaluation research: A case study of nurse practitioner role expansion in a state workers' compensation system. *Nursing Outlook, 57*(2), 99–106.

Weiss, A., & Woodhouse, E. (1992). Reframing incrementalism: A constructive response to the critics. *Policy Sciences, 25*, 255–273.

ONLINE RESOURCES

The Campaign to Promote Civic Education
www.new.civiced.org/programs/promote-civics
The Center for Responsive Politics: Open Secrets
www.opensecrets.org

8

Political Analysis and Strategies

Mary Foley[a]

"The difficult can be done immediately, the impossible takes a little longer."

Unknown author, Army Corps of Engineers motto, World War II

The knowledge and expertise of nurses regarding health and health care are critical to the political process and the development of health policy. However, the word *politics* often evokes negative emotions, and many nurses may not feel inclined to get involved. Nonetheless, nurses have the skills to be active participants in the political arena for a number of reasons. First, nurses are skilled at assessment, and being engaged in the political process involves analysis of the relevant issues and their background and importance. Second, nurses understand people, and in order to understand an issue, it is critical to know who is affected and who is involved in trying to solve the problem. Finally, nurses are relationship builders, and the political process involves the development of partnerships and networks to solve problems. As skilled communicators, nurses have the ability to work with other professionals, patients, families, and their communities to solve health care problems that affect their patients and the health care system. Nurses have much to offer in the political process and need to develop skills in political analysis and strategy to truly make a difference.

WHAT IS POLITICAL ANALYSIS?

Political analysis is the process of examining an issue and understanding the key factors and people that might potentially influence a policy goal. It involves the analysis of

government and organizations, both public and private; people and their behavior; and the social, political, historical, and economic factors surrounding the policy. It also includes the identification and development of strategies to attain or defeat a policy goal. Political analysis involves multiple components, or steps.

Identification of the Issue

The first step in conducting a political analysis is to identify and describe the issue or problem. Identifying and framing the issue involves asking who, what, when, where, and how questions to gather sufficient information to lay the groundwork for developing an appropriate response to the issue. Start with what you know about the issue:

- What is the issue?
- Is it my issue and can I solve it?
- When did the issue first occur, is it a new or old problem?
- Is this the real issue, or merely a symptom of a larger one?
- Does it need an immediate solution, or can it wait?
- Is it likely to go away by itself?
- Can I risk ignoring it?

Beware of issue rhetoric that is either too narrowly defining an issue in a technical way, or defining the issue too broadly in a societal way (Bardach, 2012). Decide what is missing from what you know about the issue and gather additional information:

- Why does the problem exist?
- Who is causing the problem?
- Who is affected by the issue?
- How significant is the issue?
- What additional information is needed?
- What are the gaps in existing data?

[a]This chapter updates a chapter originally developed by Susan Talbott, Diana Mason, Judy Leavitt, Sally Cohen, and Ellen-Marie Whelan and draws substantially upon their excellent work.

Don't cut corners or overlook the importance of this step in the political analysis, as a well-defined issue is important to the whole process as is identifying and defining the right issue. The way a problem is defined has considerable impact on the number and type of proposed solutions (Fairclough, 2013). The challenge for those seeking to get policymakers to address particular issues (e.g., poverty, the underinsured, or unacceptable working conditions) is to define the issue in ways that will prompt decision makers to take action. This requires careful crafting of messages so that calls for solutions are clearly justified. This is known as framing the issue. In the workplace, framing may entail linking the problem to one of the institution's priorities or to a potential threat to its reputation, public safety, or financial standing. For example, inadequate nurse staffing could be linked to increases in rates of morbidity and mortality, outcomes that can increase costs and jeopardize an institution's reputation and future business.

It is important not to confuse symptoms, causes, or solutions with issues. Sometimes what appears to be an issue is not. For example, proposed mandatory continuing-education for nurses is not an issue; rather, it is a possible solution to the challenge of ensuring the competency of nurses. After an analysis of the issue of clinician competence, one might establish a goal that includes legislating mandatory continuing education. The danger of framing issues as solutions is that it can limit creative thinking about the underlying issue and leave the best solutions uncovered.

Context of the Issue

The second part in the political analysis process is to do a situational analysis by examining the context of the problem. This analysis should include, at a minimum, an examination of the social, cultural, ethical, political, historical, and economic contexts of the problem. Several questions can guide you in analyzing the background of the issue:

- What are the social, cultural, ethical, political, historical, and economic factors that are creating or contributing to this problem?
- What are the background and root causes of each of these factors?
- Are these factors constraining or facilitating a solution to the problem?
- Are there other environmental obstacles affecting this issue?

It is important to be as thorough as possible at this stage and to consider whether the source of the information is verifiable and impartial. It is also important to understand any opposing views.

When assessing the political context, nurses need to clarify which level of government (federal, state, or local) or organization is responsible for a particular issue. Scope of practice is a good example. Although typically defined by the states, there are examples where the federal government has superseded the state's authority, such as in the Veteran's Administration and the Indian Health Service. Nurses also need to know which branch of government (legislative, executive, or judicial) has primary jurisdiction over the issue at a given time. Although there is often overlap among these branches, nurses will find that a particular issue falls predominantly within one branch.

Knowledge of past history of an issue can provide insight into the positions of key public officials so that communications with those individuals and strategies for advancing an issue can be developed accordingly. For example, if it is known that a particular legislator has always questioned the ability of advanced practice registered nurses (APRNs) to practice independently, then that individual may need stronger emphasis on the evidence about the quality and value of APRNs to support legislation allowing direct billing of APRNs under Medicare.

This type of context analysis is also applicable to the workplace or community organization. Regardless of the setting, assessing the history of the issue would include identifying who has responsibility for decision making for a particular issue; which committees, boards, or panels have addressed the issue in the past; the organizational structure; and the chain of command.

At an institutional level, once the relevant political forces in play have been identified, the formal and informal structures and the functioning of those structures need to be analyzed. The formal dimensions of the entity can often be assessed through documents related to the organization's mission, goals, objectives, organizational structure, bylaws, annual reports (including financial statement), long-range plans, governing body, committees, and individuals with jurisdiction. The informal dimensions of the organization, such as personal relationships and personal communication networks that could be positive or negative, are more difficult to analyze but need to be understood to get a full picture of the context of the issue.

One final example in the analysis of the context of the issue is worth mentioning. Does the entity use parliamentary procedure? Parliamentary procedure provides a democratic process that carefully balances the rights of individuals, subgroups within an organization, and the membership of an assembly. The basic rules are outlined in Robert's Rules of Order (*www.rulesonline.com*). Whether in a legislative session or the policymaking body of large organizations, one must know parliamentary procedure to develop a political strategy to get an issue passed or rejected. There have been many issues that have failed or passed because of insufficient knowledge of rule-making.

Political Feasibility

The third part of a political analysis is to analyze the political feasibility of solving an issue. There are several ways to conduct a political feasibility analysis. A simple analysis is conducting a force field analysis (Lewin, 1951) to identify the barriers and facilitators to making change to solve the issue. The force field analysis asks you to think critically about the issue and the forces affecting it by creating a two-column chart. One column lists the restraining forces, or all of the reasons that preserve the status quo and any reasons why the issue should stay the same. The second column lists the driving forces, or forces that are pushing the issue to change. This exercise requires that the whole picture is considered and provides a list of the important factors that surround the issue.

A second option is to use John Kingdon's (2010) model of public policymaking (see Chapter 7). Kingdon proposes three streams or processes that affect whether an issue gets on the political agenda; the problem stream is where people agree on an issue or problem, collect data about the issue, and share the definition of problem; the policy stream is characterized by discussion and proposal of policy solutions for the issue; and the political stream is when public mood and political will exists to want to address the issue. Kingdon's model explains that an issue gets on the political agenda only when the three streams couple or converge and a window of opportunity is thereby created. This analysis provides consideration of what needs to happen for the issue to advance to the public policy agenda, including an analysis of the policy and political factors.

The Stakeholders

Stakeholders are those parties who have influence over the issue, are directly influenced by it, or could be mobilized to care about it. In some cases, the stakeholders are obvious. For example, nurses are stakeholders on issues such as staffing ratios. In other situations, one can develop potential stakeholders by helping them to see the connections between the issue and their interests. Other individuals and organizations can be stakeholders when it comes to staffing ratios. Among them are employers (i.e., hospitals, nursing homes), payers (i.e., insurance companies), legislators, other health care professionals, and consumers.

The role of consumers cannot be underestimated. In the political arena, these are the constituents and therefore the voters, and they can wield tremendous power over an issue and its solution. In many cases, nurses are advocates and work on behalf of stakeholders, such as the patients who are affected by the care they receive. Nursing has increasingly realized the potential of consumer power in moving forward nursing and health care issues. For example, a consumer advocacy organization such as AARP possesses significant lobbying power. When nurses wanted to advance the idea of a Medicare Graduate Nursing Education (GNE) benefit, similar to the Medicare Graduate Medical Education funding to hospitals for the clinical training of interns and residents, AARP championed the proposal because it views the nursing shortage as a threat to its members' ability to access health care. GNE was included in the Affordable Care Act (ACA) as a pilot project.

In commencing a stakeholder analysis, it is important to evaluate the relationships you, or others in your group, have with key stakeholders. Look at the connections with possible stakeholders throughout your organization, community, places of worship, or businesses. Consider the following when doing a stakeholder analysis:

- Who are the stakeholders on this issue?
- Which of these stakeholders are potential supporters or opponents?
- Can any of the opponents be converted to supporters?
- What are the values, priorities, and concerns of the stakeholders?
- How can these be tapped in planning political strategy?
- Do the supportive stakeholders reflect the constituency that will be affected by the issue?

For example, as states expand coverage of health services through the state's Medicaid program, it is vital to have those who now qualify let their policymakers know how important the issue is for them and to share their personal stories of how this insurance coverage has made a difference. Yet stakeholders who are recipients of the services are too often not identified as vital for moving an issue forward. Nurses, as direct caregivers, have an important role in ensuring that recipients of services are included as stakeholders; especially when bringing issues to elected officials.

Economics and Resources

An effective political strategy must take into account the resources that will be needed to address an issue successfully. Resources include money, time, connections, and intangible resources, such as creative solutions. The most obvious resource is money, which must be considered when defining the issue and getting it recognized or on the public agenda. Thus, before launching an initiative to champion an issue, it is necessary to determine the resources that will be necessary, how much it will cost, who will bear those costs, the source of the money, and what value will be achieved from the outlay of the resources. It is critical to fully examine, despite the initial financial outlay, the potential for cost savings it may produce. It could be helpful to know how budgets are formulated for a given organization, professional group, or government agency. What is the budget process? How much money is allocated to a particular cost center or budget line? Who decides how the funds will be used? How is the use of funds evaluated? How might an individual or group influence the budget process?

Money is not the only resource to evaluate. Sharing available resources, such as space, people, expertise, and in-kind services, may be best accomplished through a coalition. It may require a mechanism for each entity to contribute a specific amount or to tally their in-kind contributions such as office space for meetings; use of a photocopier, telephone, or other equipment; and use of staff to assist with production of brochures and other communications. Other cost considerations include publicity efforts such as printing materials, paying for postage, and accessing electronic communications.

Values Assessment

Every political issue should prompt discussions about values. Values underlie the responsibility of public policymakers to be involved in the regulation of health care. In particular, calls for extending the reach of government in the regulation of health care facilities imply that one accepts this as a proper role for public officials, rather than as a role of market forces and the private sector. Thus electoral politics affect the policies that may be implemented. An analysis that acknowledges how congruent nurses' values are with those of individuals in power can affect the success of advancing an issue. There are issues that would be considered morality issues—those that primarily revolve around ideology and values, rather than costs and distribution of resources. Among well-publicized morality issues are abortion, stem cell research, and immigration. However, most issues that are not classified as morality issues still require an assessment of the values of supporters and their opponents.

Any call for government support of health care programs implies a certain prioritization of values: Is health more important than education, or jobs, or military action in the Middle East? Elected officials must always make choices among competing demands. And their choices reflect their values, the needs and interests of their constituents, and their financial supporters such as large corporations. Similarly, nurses' choice of issues on the political agenda reflects the profession's values, political priorities, and ways to improve health care.

Although nurses may value a range of health and social programs, legislators review issues within the context of demands from all of their constituencies. When an issue is discussed, it is critical to link the issue to the problem it may solve. It is also important to make sure issues are framed to show how they will help the public at large and not just the nursing profession. For example, when a request for increased funding for nursing education is made, linking this request to the need to alleviate the nursing shortage or to increase the number of nurses necessary for successful implementation of health care reform would be important.

Networks and/or Coalitions

Although individuals develop political skill and expertise, it is the influence of networks and coalitions or like-minded groups that wields power most effectively. It is critical to the political analysis process to evaluate what networks or coalitions exist that are involved with the issue.

Too often nurses become concerned about a particular issue and try to change it without help from others. In the public arena particularly, an individual is rarely able to exert adequate influence to create long-term policy change. For instance, many APRNs have tried to change state Nurse Practice Acts to expand their authority. As well intentioned as the policy solutions may be, they will likely fail unless nurses can garner the support of other powerful stakeholders such as members of the state board of nursing, the state nurses association, physicians, and consumer advocacy groups. Such stakeholders often hold the power to either support or oppose the policy change. (See Chapter 75 for a discussion of building coalitions.)

Power

Effective political strategy requires an analysis of the power of proponents and opponents of a particular solution. Power is one of the most complex political and sociological concepts to define and measure. It is critical to be aware of the sources of power, regardless of setting or issue, to understand how influence happens and to build your own sources of power for leadership in the political process.

Power can be a means to an end, or an end in itself. Power also can be actual or potential. Many in political circles depict the nursing profession as a potential political force considering the millions of nurses in this country and the power they could wield if more nurses participated in politics and policy formation. Any discussion of power and nursing must acknowledge the inherent issues of hierarchy and power imbalance that arise from the long-standing relationships between nurses and physicians. Some of nurses' discomfort with the concept of power may also arise from the inherent nature of "gender politics" within the profession. Male or female, gender affects every political scenario that involves nurses. Working in a predominantly female profession means that nurses are accustomed to certain norms of social interactions (Tannen, 2001). In contrast to nursing, the power and politics of public policymaking typically are male dominated, although women are steadily increasing their ranks as elected and appointed government officials. Moreover, many male and female public officials have stereotypic images of nurses as women who lack political savvy. This may limit officials' ability to view nurses as potential political partners. Therefore, nurses need to be sensitive to gender issues that may affect, but certainly not prevent, their political success.

Any power analysis must include reflection on one's own power base. Power can be obtained through a variety of sources such as those listed in Box 8.1 (Benner, 1984; French & Raven, 1959; Raven, 1965). An analysis of the extent of one's power using these sources can provide direction on how to enhance that power. Although the individual may hold expert power, it will be limited if one attempts to go it alone. An individual nurse may not have sufficient power to champion an issue through the legislative or regulatory process, but a network, coalition, or alliance of nurses or nursing organizations can wield significant power to move an issue to the public agenda and to successfully solve it.

Consider the nursing organization that is seeking to secure legislative support for a key piece of legislation. It can develop a strategy to enhance its power by finding a highly

---

BOX 8.1   Sources of Power

1. **Legitimate (or positional) power** is derived from a belief that one has the right to power to make decisions and to expect others to follow them. It is power obtained by virtue of an organizational position rather than personal qualities, whether from a person's role as the chief nurse officer or the state's governor.
2. **Reward power** is based on the ability to compensate another and is the perception of the potential for rewards or favors as a result of honoring the wishes of a powerful person. A clear example is the supervisor who has the power to determine promotions and pay increases.
3. **Expert power** is based on knowledge, skills, or special abilities, in contrast to positional power. Benner (1984) argues that nurses can tap this power source as they move from novice to expert practitioner. It is a power source that nurses must recognize is available to them. Policymakers are seldom experts in health care; nurses are.
4. **Referent power** is based in identification or association with a leader or someone in a position of power who is able to influence others and commands a high level of respect and admiration. Referent power is used when a nurse selects a mentor who is a powerful person, such as the chief nurse officer of the organization or the head of the state's dominant political party. It can also emerge when a nursing organization enlists a highly regarded public personality as an advocate for an issue it is championing.
5. **Coercive power** is based on the ability to punish others and is rooted in real or perceived fear of one person by another. For example, the supervisor who threatens to fire those nurses who speak out is relying on coercive power, as is a state commissioner of health who threatens to develop regulations requiring physician supervision of nurse practitioners.
6. **Information power** results when one individual has (or is perceived to have) special information that another individual needs or desires. For example, this source of power can come from having access to data or other information that would be necessary to push a political agenda forward. This power source underscores the need for nurses to stay abreast of information on a variety of levels: in one's personal and professional networks, immediate work situation, community, and the public sector, as well as in society. Use of information power requires strategic consideration of how and with whom to share the information.
7. **Connection power** is granted to those perceived to have important and sometimes extensive connections with individuals or organizations that can be mobilized. For example, the nurse who attends the same church or synagogue as the president of the home health care agency, knows the appointments secretary for the mayor, or is a member of the hospital credentialing committee will be accorded power by those who want access to these individuals or groups.
8. **Persuasion power** is based in the ability to influence or convince others to agree with your opinion or agenda. It involves leading others to your viewpoint with data, facts, and presentation skills. For example, a nurse is able to persuade the nursing organization to sponsor legislation or regulation that would benefit the health care needs of her specialty population. It may be the right thing to do, but the nurse uses her skills of persuasion for her own personal or professional agenda.
9. **Empowerment** arises from any or all of these types of power, shared among the group. Nurses need to share power and recognize that they can build the power of colleagues or others by sharing authority and decision making. Empowerment can happen when the nurse manager on a unit uses consensus building when possible instead of issuing authoritative directives to staff or when a coalition is formed and adopts consensus building and shared decision making to guide its process.

regarded, high-profile individual to be its spokesperson with the media (referent power), by making it known to legislators that their vote on this issue will be a major consideration in the next election's endorsement decisions (reward or coercive power), or by having nurses tell the media stories that highlight the problem the legislation addresses (expert power). A longer-range power-building strategy would be for the nursing organizations to extend their connections with other organizations by signing onto coalitions that address broader health care issues and expanding connections with policymakers by attending fundraisers for key legislators (connection power); getting nurses into policymaking positions (legitimate power); hiring a government affairs director to help inform the group about the nuances of the legislature (information power); using consensus building within the organization to enhance nurses' participation and activities (empowerment), or, finally, by identifying a legislative champion for the issue who could garner the use of several power bases at once.

Goals and Proposed Solutions

Typically there is more than one solution to an issue and each option differs with regard to cost, practicality, and duration. These are the policy options. The political analysis of the issue involves the context of the issue, stakeholders, values, power, and what is politically feasible. By identifying the goal, and developing and analyzing possible solutions, nurses will acquire further understanding of the issue and what is possible for an organization, workplace, government agency, or professional organization to undertake. There needs to be a full understanding of the big picture and where the issue fits into that vision. For example, if nurses want the federal government to provide substantial support for nursing education, they need to understand the constraints of federal budgets and the demands to invest in other programs, including programs that benefit nurses and other health care professionals. Moreover, support for nursing education can take the form of scholarships, loans, tax credits, aid to nursing schools, or incentives for building partnerships between nursing schools and health care delivery systems. Each option presents different types of support, and nurses would need to understand the implications of the alternatives before asking for federal intervention.

The amount of money and time needed to address a particular issue also needs to be taken into account. Are there short-term and long-term alternatives that nurses want to pursue simultaneously? Is there a way to start off with a pilot or demonstration program with clear paths to expansion? How might one prioritize various solutions? What are the tradeoffs that nurses are willing to make to obtain the stated political goals?

Such questions need to be considered in developing a political strategy.

POLITICAL STRATEGIES

Once a political analysis is completed, it is necessary to develop a plan that identifies activities and strategies to achieve the policy goals. The development and implementation of a political strategy to solve an issue requires that there is a tightly framed message, an aligned common purpose or goal, and a well-defined target audience. Messaging is critical to the development of a political strategy. Nurses need to be able to communicate with policymakers, other health care leaders, and the public and may sometimes use social media for messaging to advise on institutional and public policy.

Look at the Big Picture

It is human nature to view the world from a personal standpoint, focusing on the people and events that influence one's daily life. However, developing a political strategy requires looking at the larger environment. This can provide a more objective perspective and increase nurses' credibility as broad-minded visionaries, looking beyond personal needs.

In the heat of legislative battles and negotiations, it is easy to get distracted. However, the successful advocate is the one who does not lose sight of the big picture and is willing to compromise for the larger goal. It is critical for nurses to frame their policy work in terms of improving the health of patients and the broader health delivery system, rather than a singular focus on the profession.

Do Your Homework

We can never have all the information about an issue, but we need to be sufficiently prepared before we advocate. Usually it is unlikely to know beforehand when a particular policy will be acted on; nonetheless, it is not sufficient to claim ignorance when confronted with questions that should be answered. However, if one has done everything possible to prepare and is asked to supply information that is not anticipated, it is reasonable and preferable to indicate that one does not know the answer. The information should then be obtained as soon as possible and distributed to the policymaker who requested it. Remember not to let perfection be the enemy of good; gather the requested information, and present it as clearly and simply as possible.

Some of the ways to be adequately prepared are provided in Box 8.2.

Read Between the Lines

It is as important to be aware of the way one conveys information as it is to provide the facts. When legislators say

---

BOX 8.2   **Being Prepared for Political Advocacy**

Here are some ways to ensure that you're prepared for advocacy around a specific issue. Conducting a full political analysis will inform your preparation strategy.

- Clarify your position on the problem, your goal in pursuing the issue, and possible solutions.
- Gather information and data, and search the clinical and policy literature.
- Prepare documents to describe and support the issue.
- Assess the power dynamics of the stakeholders.
- Assess your own power base and ability to maneuver in the political arena.
- Plan a strategy, and assess its strengths and weaknesses.
- Prepare for the opposition.
- Line up support.

---

they think your issue is important, it does not necessarily mean that they will vote to support it. A direct question, such as "Will you vote in support of our bill?," needs to be asked of policymakers to know their position. Communication theory notes that the overt message is not always the real message (Gerston, 2010). Some people say a lot by what they choose not to disclose. What is not being said? Are there hidden agendas that the stakeholders are concerned about? When framing the issue, know the hidden agendas and covert messages. Be careful to make the issue as clear as possible and test it on others to be certain that reading between the lines conveys the same message as the overt rhetoric.

In God We Trust, All Others Bring Data

This quote is attributed to W. Edwards Deming (Hastie, Tibshirani, & Friedman, 2011) who developed principles for managers to transform business effectiveness through the application of statistical methods. He suggested that by presenting data to workers, they can see the outcomes or intended results of their work and make improvements to meet goals. This quote resonates in today's current heath care environment in that it requires measurement and data reporting by most health care organizations, by many health care professionals, and at all levels of practice, including the institutional, local, state, and national. Data are important to the political analysis process and again during strategy development to move an issue through the policy process. Decision makers are often dissatisfied with their ability to get or understand the data needed to make good policy decisions. They need an interpretation of the data in a form that is understandable and useable for their

purposes. Nurses are skilled are interpreting and reporting data in the clinical setting and as researchers and consumers of clinical research. A nurse can make himself or herself valuable to a policymaker by preparing a report of the important points on an issue under consideration that translates data into concise information.

Money Talks

Follow the money and understand the flow of funds within a private health care organization/system or the public sector. Money is important in both the public and private sectors, and the more money you have, the more powerful you appear to others, whether the money is revenue, profits, or donations. In the political arena, special interest groups, such as professional organizations (for example, the American Nurses Association), solicit money from their members and spend it to maintain a presence in Washington, DC, and 50 state capitals through political action committees (PACs). Other organizations, such as labor unions, trade associations, and some large corporations, also make donations to influence the agenda in Washington and the state capitals. One other type of influential group is the "527 committees" that get their name from the Internal Revenus Service (IRS) code section that governs their existence. These 527 committees are advocacy issue groups that are outside the mainstream of special interest groups and corporate America. They may have ties to some of the other groups, but they have less stringent rules to follow on the use of money and how it influences the political process.

These advocacy groups hire professional advocates or lobbyists to monitor the policy and political environments and influence elected and appointed officials on issues of importance to their special interest group. Even though money is important to have and can be very influential, the problem with money in politics is who is spending the money, what they are asking for in return, and how that affects the allocation of public resources.

Communication Is 20% *What* You Say and 80% *How* You Say It and to Whom

Using the power that results from personal connections can be an important strategy in moving a critical issue forward. In the example of APRN reimbursement, the original legislation that gave some APRNs Medicare reimbursement was greatly facilitated by the fact that the chief of staff for the Senate Majority Leader was a nurse. Or consider the nurse who is the neighbor and friend of the secretary to the chief executive officer (CEO) in the medical center. This nurse is more likely to gain access to the CEO than will someone who is unknown to either the secretary or the CEO. Building relationships and partnerships and networking are important long-term strategies for increasing influence but can also be short-term strategies.

Equally important is the way the message is framed and conveyed to stakeholders. We have often been told: it's not what you say but how you say it. When delivering the message, learn to use strong, affirmative language to describe nursing practice. Use the rhetoric that incorporates lawmakers' lingo and the buzzwords of key proponents. This requires having a sense of the values of the target audiences, whether they are legislators, regulators, hospital administrators, community leaders, or the consumer public. Stakeholders appreciate a succinct and framed message that is responsive to the values and concerns of your supporters or opponents. For example, during health reform discussions, APRNs framed their issue in terms of quality of care and cost savings. Since the nation continues to be concerned about the amount of money spent on health care, the message of reducing costs without compromising quality resonated with the Administration, Members of Congress, insurers, employers, and the public alike. How you convey your message involves developing rhetoric or catchy phrases that the media might pick up on and perpetuate. Nurses need to develop their effectiveness in accessing and using the media, an essential component of getting the issue on the public's agenda.

Learn and use good communication techniques—in particular, use a persuasive and assertive communication style that focuses on the facts and the data, and limits any emotional appeals to stories that illustrate the human impact of the problem. As discussed above, it is important to develop a message that is important to your target audience.

And finally, don't be afraid to toot your own horn. Don't assume that your good work will be recognized or valued by others. If nursing is leading an initiative or has generated the research evidence to support the issue, present the evidence to the policymakers and let them know what has been studied or found to be effective, and inform them that nurses led the work.

You Scratch My Back and I'll Scratch Yours

Developing networks involves keeping track of what you have done for others and not being afraid to ask a favor in return. Often known as quid pro quo (literally, something for something), it is the way political arenas work in both public and private sectors. Leaders expect to be asked for help and know the favor will be returned. Because nurses interface with the public all the time, they are in excellent positions to assist, facilitate, or otherwise do favors for people. Too often, nurses forget to ask for help from those whom they have helped and who would be more than willing to return a favor. Consider the lobbyist for a state

nurses' association who knew that the chair of the Senate public health and welfare committee had a grandson who was critically injured in a car accident. She visited the child several times in the hospital, spoke with the nurses on the unit, and kept the legislator informed about his grandson's progress and assured him that the boy was well cared for. When the boy recovered, the legislator was grateful and asked the lobbyist what he could do to move her issue. Interchanges like this occur every day and create the basis for quid pro quo.

Strike While the Iron Is Hot

The timing of an issue will often make a difference in terms of a successful outcome. A well-planned strategy may fail because the timing is not good. An issue may languish for some period because of a mismatch in values, concerns, or resources but then something may change to make an issue ripe for consideration. The passage of the ACA is a good example. President Obama knew from studying the history of legislation in this country that the best chance of passing sweeping legislation was in the early years of a presidential term. Once elected, with both the U.S. House of Representatives and the U.S. Senate under the control of the Democratic Party, the president knew that the only hope of passing comprehensive health care reform would be if it became his priority within his first year.

United We Stand, Divided We Fall

The achievement of policy goals can be accomplished only if supporters demonstrate a united front. Collective action is almost always more effective than individual action. Collaboration through networking, alliances, and coalition building can demonstrate broad support for an issue.

A 2010 Gallup poll of health care leaders found that the lack of a united front by national nursing organizations was viewed as a major reason why nursing's influence on health care reform would not be significant (Khoury, Blizzard, Moore, & Hassmiller, 2011). To maximize nursing's political potential, we must look for opportunities to reach consensus or remain silent in the public arena on an issue that is not of paramount concern.

Sometimes diverse groups can work together on an issue of mutual interest, even though they are opponents on other issues. Public and private interest groups that identify with nursing's issues can be invaluable resources for nurses. They often have influential supporters or may have research information that can help nurses move an issue forward.

The Best Defense Is a Good Offense

A successful political strategy is one that tries to accommodate the concerns of the opposition. It requires disassociating from the emotional context of working with opponents and is the first step in principled negotiating. A person who is skillful at managing conflict will be successful in politics. The saying that politics makes strange bedfellows arose out of the recognition that long-standing opponents can sometimes come together around issues of mutual concern, but it often requires creative thinking and a commitment to fairness to develop an acceptable approach to resolving an issue.

It is also important to anticipate problems and areas for disagreement and be prepared to counter them. When the opposition is gaining momentum and support, it can be helpful to develop a strategy that can distract attention from the opposition's issue or that can delay action. For example, one state nurses' association continually battles the state medical society's efforts to amend the Nurse Practice Act in ways that would restrict nurses' practice and provide for physician supervision. Nurses have become concerned about the possibility of passage during a year when the medical society's influence with the legislature was high. A key strategy to deal with this specific example is to develop coalitions and alliances to work with other health provider organizations engaged in similar battles with the physicians (e.g., optometrists, pharmacists) to monitor the current environment and be vigilant if changes arise. With this type of strategy in place, the physician groups will know that there would be a large coalition to deal with if any changes are proposed.

In developing a good defense, arm yourself with data and information about the issue. Be sure to understand how the issue fits in to either the organization's current priorities or other important public agenda items. Know the supporters and opponents of the issue. Many groups maintain voting records of legislators on their key legislative agenda priorities. Finally, learning as much as you can about current public agenda items and organizational priorities is critical to being an informed health care professional. Visit your professional organization websites, including NursingWorld.org, the online home of the American Nurses Association. Also, the websites of specialty nursing organizations can provide valuable up-to-date information on the key issues facing the profession and health care in general.

Don't Make Enemies and Don't Burn Bridges

To burn one's bridges is to cut off any potential future support or collaboration with a person or organization. Because nursing or even health care is such a small world, it is critically important not to burn bridges, no matter how tempted you might be! Building bridges rather than burning them is a much smarter option for the future. It is critical to handle tricky political maneuvers with care and finesse. Everyone has experienced a sound defeat at some stage, and the person who can congratulate the winner and move on to learn from the experience will thrive.

Rome Was Not Built in a Day

It is important to remember that it takes a long time to do important work, to create something long lasting and sustainable. This is very true when referring to influence in the political process, whether it is governmental or organizational. It is often reported that it feels like the arguments have been going on for years, but policy successes will not happen immediately. It will take the involvement of many workers or volunteers and countless meetings, going through the political analysis of an issue and pursuing a political strategy to find a policy solution. It is critical not to overestimate the importance of that building process nor underestimate the importance of adding another brick.

DISCUSSION QUESTIONS

1. When you are attempting to undertake a political analysis of an issue, one of the key questions to continually ask during the process is: "In this political [or social or economic] climate, can we get this done?" How would you evaluate the barriers that arise from climate or context or timing on a specific issue of interest?
2. For the same issue, who are the stakeholders and how could they be used in a political analysis that might be different from their use in political advocacy?
3. What are the political strategies that could leverage facilitators and constraints into political momentum to move the issue forward?

REFERENCES

Bardach, E. (2012). *A practical guide for policy analysis* (4th ed.). Washington, DC: CQ Press.

Benner, P. (1984). *From novice to expert.* Menlo Park, CA: Addison-Wesley.

Fairclough, N. (2013). *Critical discourse analysis: The critical study of language.* New York: Routledge Press.

French, J., & Raven, B. (1959). The basis of social power. In D. Cartwright (Ed.), *Studies in social power* (pp. 150–167). Ann Arbor, MI: University of Michigan Press.

Gerston, L.N. (2010). *Public policymaking: Process and principles.* Armonk, NY: M.E. Sharpe.

Hastie, T., Tibshirani, R., & Friedman, J. (2011). *The elements of statistical learning* (2nd ed.). New York: Springer.

Khoury, C., Blizzard, R., Wright Moore, L., & Hassmiller, S. (2011). National leadership from bedside to boardroom: A Gallup national survey of opinion leaders. *Journal of Nursing Administration, 41*(7/8), 299–305.

Kingdon, J. (2010). *Agendas, alternatives and public policies* (2nd ed.). (Longman Classics in Political Science). New York: Pearson.

Lewin, K. (1951). *Field theory in social science.* New York: Harper and Row.

Raven, B.H. (1965). Social influence and power. In I.D. Steiner and M Fishbein.(Eds.), *Current studies in social psychology* (pp 371-382). New York: Holt, Rinehart, Winston.

Tannen, D. (2001). *Talking from 9 to 5: Women and men at work* (reprint ed.). New York: William Morrow Paperbacks.

ONLINE RESOURCES

American Association of Colleges of Nursing
www.aacn.nche.edu/government-affairs/AACNPolicyHandbook_2010.pdf
American Nurses Association's Take Action
www.nursingworld.org/shortcut-rnaction/
American Organization of Nurse Executives
http://advocacy.aone.org
National League for Nursing
www.nln.org/advocacy-public-policy/overview

9

Communication and Conflict Management in Health Policy

Karin Elisabeth Warner

"I never saw an instance of one or two disputants convincing the other by argument."

Thomas Jefferson

The goal of this chapter is to shape a better understanding of the necessity and power of conflict, and provide some tools for successfully working through policy issues where there may be at least two opposing sides. I will reframe how we might look at conflict so our approach *through* it results in successful negotiating and maneuvering through conversations about things we care about. What human factors lead to conflict? How does understanding Maslow's Hierarchy of Needs help us in our interactions with others? The chapter presents two models for policy formulation and guidelines for having strategic conversations and dialogue.

UNDERSTANDING CONFLICT

What is it about the human condition that brings about conflict? Like it or not, it is an inherent part of interactions between people that can spark creativity and lead to better performance (Kendall, 2016), awareness of different views, or sides of issues—leading to more thorough policy analysis and better policy decisions. We need to understand the origins of conflict if we are to effectively maneuver through policy issues, situations, meetings, dilemmas, and life—with an appreciation of unique individual perspectives, a quintessential part of our human condition.

Maslow's Hierarchy of Needs

In early publications on human motivations, Maslow (Fig. 9.1) describes physiological motivators as drivers of our behavior, such that if any of our *basic* physiological needs are not met, we seek out fulfillment of those needs, disregarding all others (Green, 2000). He and others have

written much surrounding this issue, but the bottom line is that if *one* of our basic needs are not met (i.e., food, clothing, shelter, safety, and security), generally, all of the other faculties that *could* be cultivated lie *dormant*. So how does this relate to conflict, policymaking, and to *advocacy*?

As long as we are human, we *will* have differences and misunderstandings. We *will* have conflict, as it grows out of individual views and perceptions. Disagreement arises from differing views of the world: what *is*, what *should be*, and *what should be done about it*. We can use knowledge to learn through conflict and make the world a better place. *Advocacy* was born through conflict. The goal, then, is to understand what is motivating the actions and beliefs of those who see things differently than you, and try to appreciate those views and seek a common understanding. The very position we hold so ardently is formed with only the knowledge and perceptions in life that *we have experienced*. We need to develop the skills of listening with an *open mind* in order to *understand other points of view*. We need to be open to learn and appreciate the position others have taken on an issue. It may change our view—or at least will inform us with knowledge to make better assessments and judgments about actions to take.

A STRATEGIC COMMUNICATION FRAMEWORK

When discussing an issue where you anticipate differing views, there are key people that you need to talk to in order to gain support for your interests. It is important to identify who those people are and prepare for effective dialogue, especially if it is important to persuade them to take

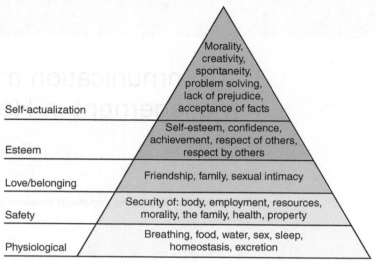

Fig. 9.1 Maslow's Hierarchy of Needs.

a different position than the one they currently hold. The Tretler Cloud (Fig. 9.2) is a useful tool to use when preparing for these discussions.

The Tretler Cloud, created by David Tretler (2014) at the U.S. National War College, is a very practical tool to identify areas to be considered when advocating for *or against* a particular policy or action. In addition, this framework is useful for assessing and appreciating the environment that policymakers are working in—which will surely affect how your information is received by them, and if it can *or will be* persuasive. For example, from its beginning, the Trump administration was very focused on domestic matters, how foreign countries participate in trade with us, and the perception of "fairness" (or not) in trade balance toward the United States—notwithstanding our nation's participation in trade policies that have been in place for many years. Those administrative perceptions led to decisions on interaction (tariffs and restrictions on trade) with other countries. How will your key policymaker be affected (or not) by the position of the current Administration on matters of interest to you? This assessment of the external environment within which the policies and decisions are made is important to monitor and appreciate, as they are fluid and will change as events occur and decisions are made. There are concurrent secondary and tertiary effects of decisions made, and these will affect the strategic intent of positions held by those in power. We have to be skillful in appreciating the current political environment and be able to assess multiple possible collateral effects of policy decisions made by decision makers that may impact our interests and thus the feasibility of gaining their support for the policy issue of interest.

Assessing the Strategic Environment

To use the Tretler Cloud, we need to first seek understanding of other views on the matter of interest, and accept that there will likely be many. Each of the other views are formed uniquely by individual life experiences, closely held beliefs and biases—as are ours. This acknowledgment of differences in point of view and perspective is critical. So, to effectively communicate and advocate for select policies, it is helpful to have an understanding of the strategic environment surrounding the issue.

Several key questions need to be asked when assessing the strategic environment of any issue:

- **What is the problem?**
- **What are the interests?** And of whom; there are usually many sides.
- **What are the threats?**
- **What are the opportunities?**
- **What assumptions do you have about this issue?** Remember that your assumptions are made based on your current knowledge and world view.
- **What are the constraints?**
- **What is the domestic situation?** (Leadership views, public support, current trends, or others issues having bearing on this issue)
- **What are the international conditions**—or conditions of a state, nation, committee, unit, area, outside factors affecting the issues, and so forth?

Woven through these questions is an assessment of the WAYS, ENDS, MEANS, and the RISK and COSTS of the alternatives proposed for solving the problem. For each alternative that you have proposed, there is a desired END

Strategy framework

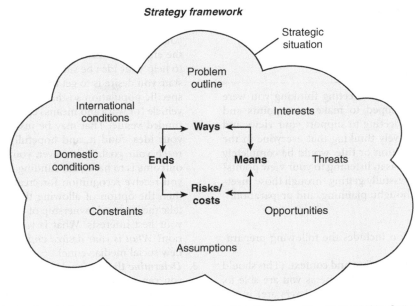

Fig. 9.2 Tretler Cloud Model. (From Dr. David Tretler, Strategy Professor, The National War College Lecture, March 2014.)

or OUTCOME that must be defined. Working backward from the END or desired OUTCOME, how or by what WAYS and MEANS do you propose to reach that end? The MEANS are the *capabilities available* to use to reach your desired outcome or end, and the WAYS are the *actions or strategies* you develop to use through those means.

For each alternative proposed, what is the anticipated COST (in pursuing that outcome through your stated ways and means)? What RISK do you foresee and to whom or what institutions or agendas in the short term and in the long term? The risk should be objectively assessed, and this is a critical part of your assessment of the strategic environment.

By using a tool such as the Tretler Cloud, your mind is trained to assess issues with discipline that will enlighten and inform so you can develop a successful strategy *through* the conflict to produce an acceptable outcome wherever possible. Part of this process involves constantly scanning the environment and readjusting the strategy as needed. Most strategies as written never make it out of the board room—things change in the contextual environment before they can be fully executed, so that awareness must be understood upfront. This means we have to plan and reassess, be agile with the strategy, and be willing to modify the ways and means to reach the objective goal at any time.

Contributing to this strategic and environmental assessment model is appreciation of how policy formulation actually does occur. One of my favorite models is the Garbage Can Model of policy formulation, which was adapted for the formulation of public policy by John Kingdon (1984). Kingdon describes how the policy process begins as a "policy primeval soup," in which specialists try out their proposals for policies in many different ways. They may introduce bills, write speeches, draft testimony or give speeches. These ideas or solutions are floated and come in contact with other proposals. Or they may fold into other ideas or be revised, only to be floated again, waiting for the separate streams of problems, policies, and politics to come together at a critical time to enable a coupling within the swirling of "garbage" in the garbage can. This resulting "coupling" is how public policies are created (see Chapter 7 on the policy process for more on Kingdon's model).

How do the environment, timing, assumptions, domestic, and international conditions flow to create opportunities for policy change, and how do they impact the various policy streams? As Kingdon (1995) describes, when these policy streams collide, this creates a window of opportunity for advocates—for or against policy issues—to *act*.

As you are assessing the strategic environment and understand how the policy streams may be interacting with the participants and the opportunities that are present, how can you behave *effectively* through this process to achieve your interests?

THE STRATEGY FOR EFFECTIVE COMMUNICATION

Have you ever walked into a meeting thinking you were fully prepared and equipped to make your points and persuade those in the meeting to support your views and recommendations—naively thinking that everyone in the room, regardless of position or title, would be completely objective and without bias in listening to your view points? I know I have. But successfully getting through those meetings requires careful thought, planning, and preparation.

Preparing

Strategic communication includes the following preparatory steps (1 to 5).

1. *Analyze* **the strategic situation and context.** (This should sound familiar.) With as much time as you are able to, determine who your audience is (or players are) in the meeting. Do some homework to understand what positions they bring into the meeting. Google them and read their corporate or academic profile. What do they stand for? What are their values, beliefs, and interests? What have they written about? What relative competitive advantage do they have? How are they perceived by various stakeholders, including others in attendance at the meeting? What are the relationships among others in the meeting?

2. *Define* **the ends.** What is the goal you want to attain? What are *your* interests—*your* desired end state? Is it changing, introducing, or ending a policy? Gaining support for an initiative? Whatever your goal, clearly identify the interests, link them to well-defined goals and objectives, and identify the perceived threats to accomplishing the goals and possible opportunities that could be present in the meeting. (Refer back to the *Tretler Cloud*; this should all start making sense as we pull it together.) Let's look at a specific example to illustrate what is meant here. For example, assume you have created and done a successful pilot on a targeted social media venue that, if fully funded and deployed, would benefit a specific segment of the population and provide much needed support and access to health care delivery that has not been provided before. This new intervention could save lives, and that outcome is really important to you as a health care professional. You need funding to get this new idea deployed, and you find interest from a well-funded source for pursuing the idea. But through meeting with the potential funding source, you discover that, in order to receive funding to continue developing your great idea, you have to take the back seat and allow the money to be given to another entity. The other organization will "take over" and continue your work. You will still be *leading* the actual work of the effort, but their organization will own the funding to help your idea be successful and deployed. If the end state you desire is to get this idea funded and out to the specific population so that you can save lives, then the vehicle (or ways and means) could be through this well-funded venue. That may be just fine, as they will take your idea, fund it, and hopefully drive the success to reach your goal. If, however, your desired end state or outcome is to have your funding come *directly to you* so you receive recognition for creation of this great idea, then the option of allowing the well-funded venue to take the lead and ownership of your work may not be in your best interests. What is *your interest* in this situation? *What is your desired end state or outcome* for this new social media venue?

3. *Determine* **the means.** How feasible (or *likely*) is it that you can accomplish your goal(s)? How will you do it? What tools or methods do you have to influence the policy change, or outcome of the meeting? Do you have compelling data? Is it the right data? Were you measuring the right things to make your points? Do you have a forum to present your views and compelling data to the group? Are you talking with the *right* influencers? Who holds the power to make a decision? Using the previous example as a discussion point, the means of getting this health care idea supported requires funding, so a funding source and marketing the idea is the means. But the *way* in which this happens is part of your strategy formulation.

4. *Formulate* **the ways.** Orchestrate the means or capabilities in ways that will help you achieve your goals. Be agile, and adapt your plan as needed. Remember that knowledge is power! You have to know and understand the political leaders, influencers, and know who they represent and report to, as well as formal and informal alliances that have been built around the issue you are interested in. What has been tried or done before that worked? What did not work? Do you know why? Who has been effective in blocking progress in this area before? How did they do it, and why are they so against the issue? Again, going back to the previous example mentioned in *Defining the Ends* above, the *way* to get your great health care idea funded and deployed, in order to reach your target population and save lives, may very well be to go through this funding source you have identified, instead of having the funding come directly to you. There are many *alternate ways and means* to reach a goal or objective.

5. *Assess.* Part of your plan should be doing a cost-benefit analysis, even if just a cursory one. What are the secondary

or tertiary effects or unintended consequences of what you are proposing? Will there be long-term effects that you had not considered? Can you quantify that cost (or time or personnel)? Are there other ways you may be able to achieve your goal that could bring the others along? Be open for new ideas. This is where the diversity of your team is so important. There is strength in the diversity of thought that can lead to innovative ways (and means) to accomplish a goal (desired end state). Ensure you are surrounding yourself with individuals who have different experiences and disciplines than you. The lens through which *they* see the world will be different than yours, which is what you want.

Now that you have pulled your background information together, have identified the players, and have an idea about the strategy for the meeting, let's talk about having *strategic conversations* (Salacuse, 2006) and then the skills for *negotiating* (Ury, 1991).

Strategic Conversations

What is a strategic conversation? These are conversations between leaders where you are not just exchanging information, but the purpose is to *change behaviors or attitudes* of others in desired way (Salacuse, 2006). This is critical in policymaking. Strategic conversations are competitive because both sides are trying to advance their own interests. To be successful in these conversations, leaders have to *anticipate* and take into account the interests, goals, and desires of others. If we have done a thorough environmental assessment using the Tretler Cloud, we will be able to anticipate possible actions of others and be able to plan our strategies and conversations around those possibilities. There are key principles for strategic conversations among leaders (Salacuse, 2006):

1. Clearly state, define and stay focused on your goal or interests.
2. Appeal to and shape the interests of the other person, as identified during preparation for the conversation.
3. Frame the issue in a way they can understand.
4. Seek mutual agreement on the goal of the conversation or negotiation.
5. Bargain. Is there a way to give and take to meet mutual goals? (Remember that this involves *listening*!)
6. Mobilize social pressure by third parties or the web of relationships.
7. Anticipate the possible actions of the other person; "look ahead and work back" (p. 52).
8. Generate options together through dialogue (again, really listen to the other views).
9. Evaluate options using a fair process.
10. Decide and gain commitment for the decision.

Once you engage in strategic conversation using the background information gained from your preparatory work to understand the issues and where the key players stand, you can begin the fluid process of negotiation.

Negotiation

William Ury (1991) has written thoughtfully about "negotiating your way from confrontation to cooperation," and having real *dialogue* is a key part of this (Isaacs, 1999).

Preparing. As we have previously discussed, preparing is the most important first step. Using a tool like the Tretler Cloud, provides a disciplined way to identify your interests, and the interests of those you are seeking to influence, as well as other factors that may affect individual positions.

Identifying the Interests of both sides is the next step in negotiation. Can you put yourself in the shoes of those with different views? How are they seeing the issue, and what factors have affected this view for them?

Identifying Suitable Options is the third step. Are you able to come up with other solutions besides the one you currently have? Be open to new suggestions, where there may be possibilities to accomplish your intent and theirs as well.

Establish Standards. By turning the selection process into a fair way to select the choice, it is no longer a contest of wills between opposing sides. If the differing sides can agree to standards within which to select the best choice, there is a good likelihood of reaching a mutually acceptable decision. These standards should be established at the outset.

Identify Alternatives. "The purpose of negotiation is not always to reach agreement . . . (but) to explore whether you can satisfy your interests better through an agreement than you could by pursuing your best alternative to a negotiated agreement (BATNA)" (Ury, 1991, p. 21). What is *your* BATNA or "walk away" alternative? What option do you have before negotiation takes place that, if things don't go well, you already have a course of action that you can live with? *That* is your BATNA. If you know in advance that your BATNA really isn't very good, then it's in your best interest to work very hard to come to a negotiated agreement.

Consider again the example from above. If the goal of your great idea is to get the device to reach the intended audience, and you need funding to get it done—although you would like the funding to come to *you*—you may not be able to negotiate successfully to that end. There may be rules, funding requirements, or other factors that preclude that from being a viable option. If you accept before entering into the meeting that you will allow the funding for your work to be given to another "front" organization to be able to reach the desired population with your idea, then this would be your BATNA.

GENERAL RULES FOR SUCCESSFUL PERSONAL INTERACTIONS

Even when having challenging discussions, we should seek to build rapport and relationships—not enemies. We should have real *dialogue*. Isaacs (1999) defines dialogue as a "conversation with a center, not sides," where the aim is to reach a base of shared meaning that helps to coordinate and align our actions and values. In addition, he states that "dialogue is a conversation in which *people think together in relationship*. Thinking *together* implies that you no longer take your own position as final. You relax your grip on certainty and listen to the possibilities that result simply from being in relationship with others—possibilities that might not otherwise have occurred" (p. 19). This is hard to do, initially, because most have us have not been trained to be aware of our own interactive behavior in conversations that may actually *hinder* effective communication. During interactions with others, the only person you can control is yourself. By practicing the art of dialogue, your ability to listen and consider other views may put the other individuals at ease, change the course of events, and surprise all of you with an outcome that had not been considered possible.

CHALLENGES

So you are practicing this art of listening and dialogue, but the other individuals or group of people you are meeting with are not reciprocating. They won't listen and don't let you bring up counterarguments. They assert their position forcefully, and attack you and your ideas. Then what do you do? How do you negotiate through that scenario? If you have done your homework, you will already have a sense of what the goals, interests, and factors affecting those you are meeting with are, and you may have a good sense of what their bottom line is. Don't show all your cards—and watch your own personal behavior. There is no way to win a disagreement by acting out. We have seen this human behavior, even in our professional work environments. So, with that knowledge going into the meeting, you should already have at hand *your* BATNA. Depending on how the meeting goes, you should already know what the minimal walk-away goal is.

In summary, conflict is inevitable in policymaking, but there are approaches to help you assess the strategic environment surrounding your issues of interest, shape and align your strategy to have successful dialogue about those areas of interest, and navigate through negotiations where the interests of different individuals are not aligned.

DISCUSSION QUESTIONS

1. How can you apply the Tretler Cloud for Strategy Formulation to a policy issue of interest to you?
2. Can you think of examples of how advocacy been born out of a conflict situation related to policy?
3. Should negotiation be a part of every conflict or communication resolution?

REFERENCES

Green, C. (2000). Maslow, A. (1943). A theory of human motivation. *Psychological Review, 50*, 370-396. Retrieved from https://psychclassics.yorku.ca/maslow/motivation.htm.

Isaacs, W. (1999). *Dialogue and the art of thinking together.* New York: Doubleday. New York: Doubleday.

Kendall, B. (2016, February). *How not to deal with conflict.* Retrieved from www.opp.com/en/Knowledge-centre/Blog: https://www.opp.com/en/Knowledge-centre/Blog/2016/February/How-not-to-deal-with-conflict.

Kingdon, J. (1984). *Agendas, alternatives, and public policies.* Ann Arbor, MI: Harper Collins.

Kingdon, J. (1995). *Agendas, alternatives, and public policies* (2nd ed.). New York: Harper Collins.

Salacuse, J. (2006). *Leading leaders. How to manage smart, talented, and powerful people.* New York: American Management Association.

Tretler, J. (2014). *The Tretler Cloud.* Lecture, National War College. Fort McNair, Washington, DC. Presented at the National War College, March 2014.

Ury, W. (1991). *Getting past no: Negotiating your way from confrontation to cooperation.* New York: Bantam.

ONLINE RESOURCES

Community Tool Box, Center for Community Health and Development at the University of Kansas
https://ctb.ku.edu/en/advocating-change
Negotiation and Dispute Resolution Resources, American Association of Nurse Anesthetists
www.aana.com/practice/state-law-and-practice/negotiation-and-dispute-resolution-resources

10

Research as a Political and Policy Tool

Lynn Price, Katarzyna Lessard, and Erica Mumm

"If politics is the art of the possible, research is surely the art of the soluble."

Sir Peter Medawar

That research has any nexus to politics or policy may strike one as curious, if not an outright oxymoron. Research, using any methodology, is carefully considered, designed, implemented, and interpreted. Politics is, well, messy. Policy emerges from political process and is often complex and messy in its own right. Yet research is a powerful lever in the world of politics and policymaking and has come to play an increasingly influential role in the crafting of both political messages and policy declarations in nursing and health care.

SO WHAT IS POLICY?

Policy is usually thought of as formal rules, set by Congress, state legislatures, or agencies at city, county, state, or federal levels. But it is also made by private entities. Clinics and hospitals have infection-control policies, visitation policies, and other rules pertaining to their work. Nursing schools have policies about student conduct and grading. Insurance companies create policies about how much of the physician's rate for services will be paid to nurse practitioners (NPs) and which prescription medications will be covered under a plan. Policymakers in both private and public venues look to evidence to inform decisions.

Research alone is not responsible for producing policy. The rules for the use of data are the same, but as the players change, so do considerations about research, how best to use findings, or even what research question to ask. One can think of this as the political ecology of policymaking, the many subtle and sometimes overt influences that surround the making of any policy.

WHAT IS RESEARCH WHEN IT COMES TO POLICY?

Research in policymaking venues involves quantitative and qualitative methodology. Although this includes the randomized controlled trial, systematic reviews and meta-analyses have recently become popular in advancing policy positions. These reviews distill and analyze quantitative data from the existing literature; the end product is a complete summary of evidence, efficient for both advocates and policymakers.

Data mining analyzes data collected from large data sets often from large health systems or government agencies. This marriage of data and health care policymaking has a long history (Almasalha et al., 2013; Cheung, Moody, & Cockram, 2002; Diers, 2007; Duffield, Diers, Aisbett, & Roche, 2009; Heslop, Gardner, Diers, & Poh, 2004; Khokhar et al., 2017). Using secondary data is challenging but rewarding given its immense scope in time and data points, compared with what most researchers can accomplish in traditional data collection (Trinh, 2018).

Other sources of data also contribute to the policymaking process. Reports from expert panels, foundations, and research agencies can carry great weight if introduced in the context of moving a policy issue forward. Op-ed pieces by experts and position papers generated by legislative staff or others can also be powerful. One must be wide open to sources when looking for evidence to support or oppose a policy position (Green, 2017).

In presenting data to policymakers, it behooves advocates to be short and to the point. Policymakers deal with a tremendous number of issues across economic, health, and social terrains. Maintaining focus on one's issue requires policy briefs that are short, identify the problem and the policy solution, and provide strategies recognizing both the evidence and the overall context in which policymakers act (Cairney & Kwiatkowski, 2017).

Narrative, the telling of a pertinent story to bring the issue to life, also has its place in the process (Mosley & Gibson, 2017). Extensive research into human thinking and decision-making indicates that narrative provides us with both cognitive and emotional content, both fundamental aspects of human thinking when forming opinions (World Bank, 2015).

THE CHEMISTRY BETWEEN RESEARCH AND POLICYMAKING

Research can be extremely useful in illuminating on a problem and nudging policymakers to action. Nursing has a distinguished lineage of nurses affecting policy through the use of data, from Nightingale's Crimean data, to American midwives' collection of practice data (Diers & Burst, 1983). Today, health care research examines the linkage of the health care puzzle pieces intricately intertwined in practice: delivery of care, providers, procedures, patients, families, cultures, and reimbursement. One consequence is a growing acknowledgement by non-nurse researchers of the role of nursing, particularly advanced practice nursing (Barnes et al., 2017; Leach et al., 2018).

USING RESEARCH TO CREATE, INFORM, AND SHAPE POLICY

Research rarely exists in a vacuum, particularly health services research. Cairney and Kwiatkowski (2017) argue that research design and dissemination should be used strategically and tactically. The Institute of Medicine's (IOM's) seminal 2011 report, *The Future of Nursing: Leading Change, Advancing Health*, exemplifies strategic thinking. This evidence-based report summarized the position of nursing in the U.S. health system and focused on the barriers nursing faced in implementing the full effect of the profession's capacity. As illustrated in Box 10.1, savvy health services researchers sought to amplify the IOM report message, with studies tactically aimed at questions policymakers might have about NP qualifications to step into full leadership within the health care system.

Each of the articles featured in Box 10.1 informs the greater conversation about advancing NP practice within the context of promoting full practice authority. As of 2018, nine additional states have granted full practice authority to NPs since the release of the recommendations (Campaign for Action, 2018). Furthermore, the U.S. Department of Veterans Affairs amended its regulations to

---

BOX 10.1   Evolution of Research Related to Advanced Practice Registered Nurses Full Practice Authority

The timeline below details the evolution of research related to nurse practitioner (NP) full practice authority.

- 2011—The Institute of Medicine publishes *The Future of Nursing*, recommending full, unrestricted practice for all U.S. NPs.
- 2011—Newhouse et al. publish a systematic review of previous research on the efficacy, safety, and acceptance of NPs.
- 2012—Newhouse et al. publish a systematic review of policy implications of unrestricted NP practice.
- 2013—Stanik-Hutt et al. publish a systematic review of NP and physician primary care outcomes.
- 2016—Perloff, DesRoches, & Buerhaus publish research comparing cost and outcomes of primary care provided by NPs and physicians.
- 2017—Woo, Lee, & Tam publish a systematic review of NPs care quality and outcomes, patient satisfaction, and cost in critical and emergency care settings.
- 2017—Barnes et al. publish an examination of the impact of various policies regulating practice and payment for NPs on clinical practice.
- 2017—Poghosyan & Carthon publish research on NP impact on reducing health disparities.
- 2018—Traczynski & Udalova publish research on the impact of NP unrestricted practice on care utilization and patient outcomes.

---

permit full practice authority for NPs effective in 2017 (Full Practice Authority for Advanced Practice Registered Nurses, 2017).

RESEARCH AND POLITICAL WILL

The key to moving any issue into the public or institutional eye is transforming it into a political issue; that is, casting the issue as problematic enough to make public or private policymakers want to fix it. Sometimes political leaders themselves offer the issue as important, as was the case with health care reform under the Obama administration. Other times, the issue comes to the fore because of particular news events, as with the increasing movement by teens to battle gun violence.

In 2012, the most politically influential mass shooting took place in Newtown, Connecticut, where 20 students and 6 teachers were killed. Although parental voices were strong following this horrific event, nothing changed regarding federal policy. As highlighted in Table 10.1, since

TABLE 10.1 Mass Shooting Events and Policy Outcomes

Date	Shooting Location	Deaths	Outcomes
2012	Sandy Hook Elementary School Newtown, CT (https://www.sandyhookpromise.org/)	27	Parent initiative *Sandy Hook Promise* initiated by parents; supported by Senator Murphy; no national policy initiative.
2013	Washington Navy Yard (Zapotosky, 2015)	12	Improved outcomes in methods of response; no national policy initiative.
2015	Emanuel African Methodist Episcopal Church, South Carolina (Archie & Paul, 2018)	9	Confederate flag has been removed from South Carolina capitol building and City of Charleston has apologized for its role in the slave trade; no national policy changes have been initiated.
2016	PULSE Nightclub Shooting (Hermann, Herszenhorn, & Lichtblau, 2016)	49	Sparks legislative discussion on banning sale of guns to people on terror watch list; Senator Reid of Nevada states, "It is shameful that the United States Senate has done nothing—nothing—to stop these mass shootings"; Brady campaign renews the call to impose tougher restrictions on high-powered rifles.
2017	Las Vegas Casino (Vasilogambros, 2018)	58	States look to ban bump stocks; enforcement of the law is difficult.
2018	Marjory Stoneham Douglas High Parkland, FL (Karimi & Yan, 2018; Witt, 2018)	17	Students around the country take part in walkouts; March For Our Lives initiative; Florida Governor Rick Scott initiates SB 7026 tightening gun control; Broward County School board calls on Congress to act.
2018	Tree of Life Synagogue, Pittsburg, PA (Smith & Almaguer, 2018)	11	Call for politicians to take action.

2012, there have been repeated mass shootings and the response in Washington remains stagnant, offering condolences but failing to take action.

Alter and Chan, in *Time* magazine (2018), did a cover feature on five Parkland Florida teen survivors of the mass shooting that took place in their high school on February 14, 2018. The Parkland Florida teen survivors' platform? To reframe the discussion away from the perspective of current elected officials who continue to support the National Rifle Association (NRA) and maintain the focus and conversation on the tragic deaths of mass-shooting victims. The #Never-Again and the "March for our Lives" movements are an example of an issue being brought to the front and center of policy conversations (Witt, 2018). The issue of gun violence is being forced upon policymakers, when policy discussions pertaining to gun violence have been ignored and glossed over. What policy solutions are these teens asking for? Most simplistically, universal background checks, digitalization of ATF records, and a ban on high-capacity magazines and assault weapons (Witt, 2018).

The Parkland, Florida teens' #NeverAgain movement has influenced change in their state: Florida recently adopted policies to ban bump stocks, impose waiting periods, raise the minimum age to buy a gun, and allow law enforcement to remove weapons from those with mental illness posing concern. In addition, businesses such as Delta Airlines, MetLife, and Dick's Sporting Goods have publicly cut ties with the NRA (Schick, 2018). These young up-and-coming voters are strategically poised: victims of a tragedy, near voting age, and savvy with social media. The question, however, lies in the potential for actual policy change. Will the United States maintain the status quo or take action for policy change? Perhaps the target audience is actually policy change within state law, following Florida's example.

The constraint to policy change, specifically related to gun law, lies in the policy issue of federal research dollars to study gun violence. Stark and Shah (2017) explain that there is limited research on gun violence despite the 30,000 deaths per year, the largest number of gun deaths in an industrialized nation. This lack of research initiative stems from the 1996 Congressional Appropriations Bill that states that the Centers for Disease Control and Prevention (CDC) cannot use funds that may result in data supporting the need for gun control: similar restrictions exist for the National Institutes of Health (NIH) (Kellerman & Rivara, 2013;

Rubin, 2016). In speaking to the need for research and the looming power of the NRA, physicians and health care professionals across the country initiated a public outcry campaign, #ThisIsOurLane, in response to the NRA implication that physicians should stay out of the gun control controversy. Taichman, Bornstein, and Laine (2018) explain the public health crisis resulting from gun violence and the responsibility that nurses and doctors have to speak out on the topic.

However, highlighting a problem and getting it on the agenda is not enough to advance policy in most instances. There must be enough political will to devote attention, time, and effort to solve the problem, particularly when the problem is pervasive or long-standing. As illustrated in Box 10.2, research can help move difficult policy issues forward (Fig. 10.1).

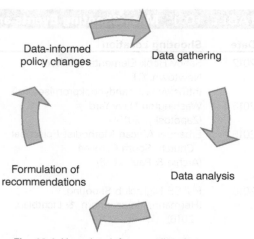

Fig. 10.1 How data informs policy change.

BOX 10.2   Data Drives Policy Reform—Massachusetts Response to the Opioid Epidemic

The Massachusetts response to the opioid crisis provides a compelling example of how strategic use of data can inform the policy conversation and sustain political will to tackle a complex problem.

Massachusetts enacted Chapter 55 of the Acts of 2015 (An Act Requiring Certain Reports for Opiate Overdoses), providing analysis of multiple government data sets across various agencies in connection with opioid overdoses in Massachusetts, and required a published report on the findings from the cross-agency analysis.

The Chapter 55 legislative report (Massachusetts Department of Public Health, 2016) detailed opioid use and overdose trends, providing recommendations to address the findings. Action plans from the Governor's Opioid Addiction Working Group (2017; 2018) detailed how these annual legislative reports have informed policy decisions. For example:

Report Finding: Individuals recently released from Massachusetts prisons were 56 times more likely to die from an opioid-related overdose than the general public.

Report Recommendation: Expand medication-assisted treatment (MAT) and overdose prevention services in correctional facilities. Prior to release, put in place access to post-incarceration medical care and substance use prevention and treatment.

Massachusetts Policy Impact: Massachusetts enacted Chapter 208 of the Acts of 2018 (an Act for Prevention and Access to Appropriate Care and Treatment of Addiction). This legislation includes provisions to expand access to MAT at correctional facilities and establish a pilot program for the delivery of MAT at five county correctional facilities.

This interplay of research, political will, and policymaking is neither a rational process, nor is it random. There are other reasons policymakers often do not jump readily toward change. Often very powerful and well-funded stakeholders (e.g., the NRA or organized medicine in one form or another) sit at the table where policy decisions are being made, and oppose any change. Their presence is a potent deterrent for policymakers to change their positions on an issue. Research, along with a compelling story, must engage legislators in advancing policy issues. As further profiled in Box 10.3, negative publicity and research data related to long wait times for veterans to access care within the Veteran's Health Administration (VA) served as a catalyst for the 2016 rule change granting advanced practice registered nurses (excluding nurse anesthetists) full practice authority within the VA system, irrespective of individual state restrictions.

Major policy change is most often incremental despite research supporting the change and frustrating to those who are advocating for new policy. However, continued research validating the need for change, demonstrating positive effects of the proposed policy changes and the lack of negative impact, are critical to build and can be extremely effective in the long run.

Research not only illuminates a policy problem and presents an intervention as the solution; it also has a vital role in creating an atmosphere conducive for policymakers to step up to the plate. This is especially true when the policy issue is likely to be controversial, as is the case with gun control. Research can enhance, perhaps even shape, the political climate in which change can occur; this is valuable insight for nursing as it continues to increase in political influence within policymaking circles.

BOX 10.3 Data Drives Policy Reform—Veteran Wait Times

- In April 2014, CNN broke a story on long wait times for veterans within the Veteran's Health Administration (VA) system and attributed veteran deaths to these wait times (Bronstein & Griffin, 2014). The VA faced harsh criticism as the story was widely reported in the news cycle.
- The VA Office of Inspector General (2014) conducted a comprehensive review of veteran wait times and found clinically significant delays in access to care.
- In August 2014, Congress enacted H.R. 3230 (Veterans Access, Choice, and Accountability Act of 2014) to address access to care issues by establishing and funding the Choice Program. The Choice Program allows veterans to receive care from non-VA providers in certain instances when such care is not readily available through the VA system.
- In 2015, the RAND Corporation conducted an independent assessment of the VA health care system pursuant to the Veterans Access, Choice, and Accountability Act of 2014. The assessment identified granting independent practice authority for all advanced practice registered nurses (APRNs) as one high-impact policy option for increasing access to care for veterans (Farmer, Hosek, & Adamson, 2016).
- In May 2016, the VA proposed a rule that would grant APRNs full practice authority (Advanced Practice Registered Nurses, 2016).
- During the comment period, the Federal Trade Commission submitted a memo in support of the proposed rule on grounds of improved access, cost containment, and expansion in innovation (Federal Trade Commission, 2016).
- In December 2016, the VA issued the final rule granting APRNs full practice authority to three APRN roles including nurse practitioners (NPs), concluding that standardization of full practice authority for APRNs would increase access and decrease wait times for veterans (Full Practice Authority for Advanced Practice Registered Nurses, 2017).

RESEARCH: NOT JUST FOR JOURNALS

Traditional research can be found in academic, peer-reviewed journals, but that is not necessarily the best place to propel data to support and shape policy. There is a large sea of "gray literature" that offers current-event data in a nontraditional way, including government reports, white papers (e.g., Commonwealth Fund, the Kaiser Family Foundation), policy reports, and print and social media. Gray literature data can direct the political climate, inspire advocacy groups, and serve as foundational platforms for transformative ideas (Lawrence, 2018). In addition, negative-result data are often not published through traditional scholarly journals because they are not as valued, interesting to the reader, or favored by publishers (Mlinarić, Horvat, & Smolcic, 2017). These data are available to policymakers and can inform policy debates and issues.

Artful dissemination in documentaries (television and movie) is another way research influences policy context by engaging the public (and policymakers) directly through visual and narrative data. Several recent documentaries have explored various aspects of the opioid epidemic and vividly brought the magnitude of the problem to life through stories showing the very personal impact of opioid addiction on individuals, families, and communities. Two such documentaries include Frontline's 2016 documentary *Chasing Heroin* and HBO's 2017 documentary *Warning: This Drug May Kill You*. The HBO documentary includes a segment on Purdue Pharma's OxyContin marketing practices. Numerous lawsuits have been filed by states and local governments against Purdue Pharma and other opioid manufacturers alleging that the misleading marketing practices and mischaracterization of available evidence by these companies contributed to the opioid crisis. Purdue Pharma issued a statement in early 2018 that its sales representatives would no longer promote opioids to prescribers (Purdue Pharma L.P., 2018). With the opioid epidemic in the public spotlight, other entities have also taken action aimed at curtailing the problem. The CDC issued opioid-prescribing guidelines for providers (Dowell, Haegerich, & Chou, 2016). Insurers such as Blue Cross Blue Shield have put into place restrictions on coverage of opioid prescriptions (Capital BlueCross, 2018). In direct response to the growing number of deaths from opioid overdose, some state legislatures have enacted naloxone access laws, such as Connecticut's Public Act No. 16-43 "An Act Concerning Opioids and Access to Overdose Reversal Drugs" (Davis & Carr, 2017).

There is much to consider in regards to research as a political and policy tool. Documentaries, negative results data, and the pull of the nation's political interests all contribute to moving policy forward on the political agenda. Nurses, at the frontlines of patient care and as the largest group of health care professionals, are strategically positioned to take action to use research as a political and policy tool. For example, make policymakers aware of the various types of research data available and help interpret the research outcomes. Nursing's role in bringing the best health care research to the policy table matters to patients, to policymakers, and for the delivery of meaningful health care for all.

DISCUSSION QUESTIONS

1. What contexts inform the crafting of policy?
2. When and how does research connect with policymaking?
3. You and your research team have concluded that the consistent use of vaping/marijuana by adolescents negatively impacts memory retention. Describe your strategy for bringing this to the attention of policymakers, such as your local school board or state legislators.

REFERENCES

Advanced Practice Registered Nurses, 81 Fed. Reg. 33,155 (May 25, 2016).

Almasalha, F., Xu, D., Kennan, G.M., Khokhar, A., Yao, Y., Chen, Y.C., . . . & Wilkie, D.J. (2013). Data mining nursing care plans of end-of-life patients: A study to improve healthcare decision making. *International Journal of Nursing Knowledge, 24*(1), 15–24.

Alter, C., & Chan, M. (2018, April). The young and the relentless. *The New Yorker, 191*(12), 24–32.

An Act Concerning Opioids and Access to Overdose Reversal Drugs, Conn. Pub. Act 16-043 (2016)

An Act for Prevention and Access to Appropriate Care and Treatment of Addiction, Chap. 208, 2018 Leg., 190th Sess. (Mass. 2018).

An Act Requiring Certain Reports for Opiate Overdoses, Chap. 55, 2015 (Mass. 2015).

Archie, A., & Paul, D. (2018, July 25). "The Emmanuel Nine": A tentative memorial for the victims of the Charleston church massacre. *Cable News Network.* Retrieved from www.cnn.com/2018/07/16/us/memorial-site-planned-for-charleston-church-shooting/index.html.

Barnes, H., Maier, C.B., Sarik, D.A., Germack, H.D., Aiken, L.H., & McHugh, M.D. (2017). Effects of regulation and payment policies on nurse practitioners' clinical practices. *Medical Care Research and Review, 74*(4), 431-451.

Bills, L. (Producer), Weiss, S. (Producer), & Peltz, P. (Director). (2017). *Warning: This drug may kill you* [video file]. Retrieved from www.hbo.com.

Bronstein, S., & Griffin, D. (2014). A fatal wait: Veterans languish and die on a VA hospital's secret list. *Cable News Network.* Retrieved from www.cnn.com/2014/04/23/health/veterans-dying-health-care-delays/index.html.

Cairney, P., & Kwiatkowski, R. (2017). How to communicate effectively with policymakers: Combine insights from psychology and policy studies. *Palgrave Communications, 3*, 1–8.

Campaign for Action. (2018). *State progress in removing barriers to practice and care* [infographic]. Retrieved from https://campaignforaction.org/resource/state-progress-removing-barriers-practice-care/.

Capital BlueCross (2018, March 22). *Capital BlueCross announces significant reduction in opioids dispensed following prescription limitations* [press release]. Retrieved from www.bcbs.com/press-releases/capital-bluecross-announces-significant-reduction-opioids-dispensed-following.

Cheung, R.B., Moody, L.E., & Cockram, C. (2002). Data mining strategies for shaping nursing and health policy agendas. *Policy, Politics, & Nursing Practice, 3*(3), 248–260. https://doi.org/10.1177/15254402003003009.

Davis, C., & Carr, D. (2017). State legal innovations to encourage naloxone dispensing. *Journal of the American Pharmacists Association, 57*(2), S180–S184.

Diers, D. (2007). Finding midwifery in administrative data systems. *Journal of Midwifery and Women's Health, 52*(2), 98–105.

Diers, D., & Burst, H.V. (1983). Effectiveness of policy-related research: Nurse-midwifery as a case study. *Journal of Nursing Scholarship, 15*(3), 68–74.

Dill, M.J., Pankow, S., Erikson, C., & Shipman, S. (2013). Survey shows consumers open to greater role for physician assistants and nurse practitioners. *Health Affairs, 32*(6), 1135–1142.

Dowell, D., Haegerich, T.M., & Chou, R. (2016). CDC guideline for prescribing opioids for chronic pain—United States, 2016. *MMWR Recommendations and Reports, 65*(1), 1–49. http://dx.doi.org/10.15585/mmwr.rr6501e1.

Duffield, C., Diers, D., Aisbett, C., & Roche, M. (2009). Churn: Patient turnover and case mix. *Nursing Economics, 27*(3), 185–191. Retrieved from www.nursingeconomics.net/cgi-bin/WebObjects/NECJournal.woa.

Farmer, C.M., Hosek, S.D., & Adamson, D.M. (2016). *Balancing demand and supply for veterans' health care: A summary of three RAND assessments conducted under the Veterans Choice Act* [research report]. Retrieved from www.rand.org/pubs/research_reports/RR1165z4.html.

Federal Trade Commission. (2016). *FTC staff comment to the Department of Veterans Affairs: Proposed rule regarding advanced practice registered nurses* [public comment]. Retrieved from www.ftc.gov/system/files/documents/advocacy_documents/comment-staff-ftc-office-policy-planning-bureau-competition-bureau-economics-department-veterans/v160013_staff_comment_department_of_veterans_affairs.pdf.

Full Practice Authority for Advanced Practice Registered Nurses, 38 CFR 17.415 (2017).

Gaviria, M. (Producer and Director) & Cohen, W. (Producer) (2016). *Chasing heroin* [video file]. Retrieved from www.pbs.org/wgbh/frontline/film/chasing-heroin/.

Governor's Opioid Addiction Working Group. (2017). *Governor's working group on opioids update: Action items* [PowerPoint slides]. Retrieved from www.mass.gov/files/documents/2017/11/15/2017-annual-update-action-items-gov-working-group.pdf.

Governor's Opioid Addiction Working Group. (2018). *Governor's opioid addiction working group: See the recommendations and action plans from the group* [web page]. Retrieved from www.mass.gov/lists/governors-opioid-addiction-working-group.

Green, J.F. (2017). Policy entrepreneurship in climate governance: Toward a comparative approach. *Environment and Planning C: Politics and Space, 35*(8), 1471-1482.

Hermann, P. & Herszenhorn, D.M. & Lichtblau, E. (2016, June 13). Orlando shooting reignites gun control debate in Congress. *The New York Times.* Retrieved from www.nytimes.com.

Heslop, L., Gardner, B., Diers, D., & Poh, B.C. (2004). Using clinical data for nursing research and management in health services. *Contemporary Nurse, 17*(1–2), 8–18.

Institute of Medicine. (2011). *The future of nursing: Leading change, advancing health.* Washington, DC: National Academies Press.

Karimi, F., & Yan, H. (2018). What's changed one month after the Parkland shooting? *Cable News Network.* Retrieved from www.cnn.com/2018/03/14/us/parkland-school-shooting-a-month-later/index.html.

Kellerman, A.L., & Rivara, F.P. (2013). Silencing the science on gun research. *Journal of the American Medical Association, 309*(6), 549-550.

Khokhar, A., Lodhi, M.K., Yao, Y., Ansari, R., Keenan, G., & Wilkie, D.J. (2017). Framework for mining and analysis of standardized nursing care plan data. *Western Journal of Nursing Resear* ch, 39(1), 20–41.

Lawrence, A. (2018). Influence seekers: The production of grey literature for policy and practice. *Information Services & Use, 37*(4), 389–403.

Leach, B., Gradison, M., Morgan, P., Everett, C., Dill, M.J., & Strand de Oliveira, J. (2018). Patient preference in primary care provider type. *Healthcare, 6,* 13–16.

Massachusetts Department of Public Health. (2016). *Legislative report: Chapter 55 opioid overdose study—September 2016* [legislative report]. Retrieved from www.mass.gov/service-details/chapter-55-overdose-report.

Mlinarić, A., Horvat, M., & Šupak Smolčić V. (2017). Dealing with the positive publication bias: Why you should really publish your negative results. *Biochemia Medica, 27*(3), 030201.

Mosley, J.E., & Gibson, K. (2017). Strategic use of evidence in state-level policymaking: Matching evidence type to legislative stage. *Policy Sciences, 50*(4), 697–719.

National Academies of Sciences, Engineering, and Medicine. (2016). *Assessing progress on the Institute of Medicine report the future of nursing.* Washington, DC: National Academies Press.

Newhouse, R.P., Stanik-Hutt, J., White, K.M., Johantgen, M., Bass, E.B., Zangaro, G . . . & Weiner, J.P. (2011). Advanced practice nurse outcomes 1990-2008: A systematic review. *Nursing Economics, 29*(5), 1–21. Retrieved from www.nursingeconomics.net/cgi-bin/WebObjects/NEC Journal.woa.

Newhouse, R.P., Weiner, J.P., Stanik-Hutt, J., White, K.M., Johantgen, M., Steinwachs, D., . . . & Bass, E.B. (2012). Policy implications for optimizing advanced practice registered nurse use nationally. *Policy, Politics & Nursing Practice, 13*(2), 81–89.

Perloff, J., DesRoches, C.M., & Buerhaus, P. (2016). Comparing the cost of care provided to Medicare beneficiaries assigned to primary care nurse practitioners and physicians. *Health Services Research* 51(4), 1407–1423.

Poghosyan, L., & Carthon, M.B. (2017). The untapped potential of the nurse practitioner workforce in reducing health disparities. *Policy, Politics, & Nursing Practice, 18*(2), 84–94.

Purdue Pharma L.P. (2018, February 9). *Purdue Pharma L.P. issues statement on opioid promotion* [press release]. Retrieved from www.purduepharma.com/news-media/2018/02/purdue-pharma-l-p-issues-statement-on-opioid-promotion/.

Rubin, R. (2016). Tale of 2 agencies: CDC avoids gun violence research but NIH funds it. *Journal of the American Medical Association, 315*(16), 1689-1691.

Schick, M. (2018). A look at all the companies that have cut ties with the NRA in the wake of the Parkland, Fla., shooting. *The Boston Globe.* Retrieved from www.thebostonglobe.com.

Smith, S., & Almaguer, M. (2018, October 28). Former Tree of Life synagogue rabbi calls for action after shooting. *National Broadcasting Company News.* Retrieved from www.nbcnews.com/news/us-news/former-tree-life-synagogue-rabbi-calls-action-after-shooting-n925321.

Stanik-Hutt, J., Newhouse, R.P., White, K.M., Johantgen, M., Bass, E.B., Zangaro, G., . . . & Weiner, J.P. (2013). The quality and effectiveness of care provided by nurse practitioners. *Journal for Nurse Practitioners, 9*(8), 492–500.

Stark, D.E., & Shah, N.H. (2017). Funding and publication of research on gun violence and other leading causes of death. *Journal of the American Medical Association, 317*(1), 84–85.

Taichman, D., Bornstein, S.S. & Laine C. (2018). Firearm injury prevention: AFFIRMing that doctors are in our lane. *Annals of Internal Medicine* (advance online publication).

Traczynski, J., & Udalova, V. (2018). Nurse practitioner independence, health care utilization, and health outcomes. *Journal of Health Economics, 58,* 90–109.

Trinh, Q-D. (2018). Understanding the impact and challenges of secondary data analysis. *Urologic Oncology, 36*(4), 163–164.

Veteran's Health Administration Office of Inspector General. (2014). *Veterans health administration: Review of alleged patient deaths, patient wait times, and scheduling practices at the Phoenix VA health care system* [investigative report]. Retrieved from www.va.gov/oig/pubs/vaoig-14-02603-267.pdf.

Vasilogambros, M. (2018). *So states ban bump stocks. Now how do they enforce the law?* [Stateline article]. Retrieved from www.pewtrusts.org/en/research-and-analysis/blogs/stateline/2018/05/18/so-states-ban-bump-stocks-now-how-do-they-enforce-the-law.

Veterans Access, Choice, and Accountability of 2014, H.R. 3230, 113th Cong. (2013-2014).

Wamsley, L. (2018, November 11). After NRA mocks doctors, physicians reply: "This is our lane." *National Public Radio.* Retrieved from www.npr.org/2018/11/11/666762890/after-nra-mocks-doctors-physicians-reply-this-is-our-lane.

Witt, E. (2018). How the survivors of Parkland began the never again movement. *The New Yorker.* Retrieved from www.newyorker.com.

Woo, B., Lee, J., & Tam, W. (2017). The impact of the advanced practice nursing role on quality of care, clinical outcomes, patient satisfaction, and cost in the emergency and critical care settings: A systematic review. *Human Resources for Health,* 15(63), 1–22.

World Bank. (2015). *World development report 2015: Mind, society, and behavior.* Washington, DC: World Bank.

Xue, Y., Ye, Z., Brewer, C., & Spetz, J. (2016). Impact of state nurse practitioner scope-of-practice regulation on health care delivery: Systematic review. *Nursing Outlook,* 64, 71–85.

Zapotosky, M. (2015, July 2). Lessons from 2013 navy yard killings helped guide much-improved response. *The Washington Post.* Retrieved from www.washingtonpost.com.

ONLINE RESOURCES

Kaiser Family Foundation: This site has a wealth of current information about American health care and reform efforts in the states and at the federal level
https://kff.org

Pew Research Center: This nonpartisan site conducts and compiles data-driven social science research
www.pewresearch.org

World Health Organization: This site is the leading voice for global health data and public health initiatives across the world
www.who.int/en/

11

Using Research to Advance Health and Social Policies for Children

Eileen K. Fry-Bowers and Kristi K. Westphaln[a]

"The true character of society is revealed in how it treats its children."

Nelson Mandela

Children are, indeed, the future, yet ensuring the health and well-being of American children and youth has never quite risen to the top of the U.S. political agenda of either political party. Policymakers, elected officials, and the public have yet to fully understand the connection between child well-being and societal welfare, but evidence reveals that the health of American children and youth is at serious risk. Consider that:

- The infant death rate in the United States is higher than that of most European countries (MacDorman, Matthews, Mohangoo, & Zeitlin, 2014).
- Nearly one in five American children aged 2 to 19 years is obese, with low-income children and children of color disproportionately affected (Centers for Disease Control and Prevention [CDC], 2018b).
- Youth aged 15 to 19 years are 82 times more likely to die from gun homicide than their peers in other developed nations (Thakrar, Forrest, Maltenfort, & Forrest, 2018).
- In some U.S. states, 10% (and as high as 15%) of children have no health insurance, reducing access to important preventive health care services (Kaiser Family Foundation, 2018).
- Nearly 13 million U.S. children live in families that struggle with food insecurity (Feeding America, 2018), and 2.5 million children (approximately 1 in 30) are homeless annually (American Institute for Research, 2018).
- The U.S. child poverty rate exceeds nearly all other Organization for Economic Co-operation and Development (OECD) countries (OECD, 2018), with nearly 3 million children living in families that live on less than $2 per day (Edin & Shaefer, 2015).

These startling statistics demand focused and sustained attention and an investment in health, education, housing, and other social policies to maximize child and youth development and well-being to build the human capital that will help the nation to move confidently into the future.

CHILDREN'S RIGHTS IN THE UNITED STATES

"Childhood" is a relatively new concept. Until the late 19th century, children, like wives, were regarded as property. At the turn of the century, children were expected to participate in the workforce, child morbidity and mortality were high, and few children had access to education. The progressive "child-saving" movement of the early 20th century advanced federal policies that addressed child health (including mandatory immunizations), child labor, delinquency, and poverty, and in 1938, Congress passed the Fair Labor Standards Act (FLSA) (see Table 11.1).

During the second half of the 20th century, reformers advocated for children's rights to self-determination or self-expression. Federal support for initiatives to advance children's health (e.g., Medicaid, Vaccination Assistance Act) and education (e.g., Elementary and Secondary Education Act, Head Start), as well as programs to ameliorate poverty among low-income families proliferated (e.g., Supplemental Food Programs for Women, Infants, and Children; Food Stamps). Court decisions such as *Brown v. Board of Education* (1954), *In re Gault* (1967), *Tinker v. de Moines Independent Community School District* (1969), and *Planned Parenthood v. Danforth* (1976), in which the Court

---

[a]This chapter updates a chapter originally developed by Louise Kahn, MSN, RN, Freida Hopkins Outlaw, PhD, RN, FAAN, and Sally S. Cohen, PhD, RN, FAAN.

TABLE 11.1 Timeline of Early 20th-Century Child Welfare Reforms	
1904	Formation of the National Child Labor Committee
1909	First White House Conference on the Care of Dependent Children
1913	Children's Bureau established within the U.S. Department of Labor
1916	Congress passes Keating-Owens Act
1918	Keating-Owens Act ruled unconstitutional (*Hammer v. Dagenhart*, 247 U.S. 251)
1920	Child labor reforms present in every state
1938	Congress passes Fair Labor Standards Act

recognized that children possess constitutional rights, ushered in a new era for the recognition of children's rights.

CHILDHOOD AS A DEVELOPMENTAL STAGE

Child development involves the biological, psychological, and socioemotional changes that occur between the prenatal period and the end of adolescence and entry into young adulthood. It is a continuous and sequential process yet unique to each child. Each stage is affected by preceding developmental experiences. Children develop best when they have secure relationships with caregivers, and development and learning occur within multiple social and cultural contexts.

A child's brain demonstrates impressive plasticity, as well as significant susceptibility. Brains exposed to different environmental events, including sensory stimuli, drugs, diet, hormones, or stress, can develop in very different ways (Kolb & Gibb, 2011). In fact, early childhood exposure to severe, prolonged, or repetitive adversity such as trauma, abuse, or neglect, coupled with inadequate nurturance or caregiving, can lead to permanent alterations in the structure and function within the brains of young children (Shonkoff et al., 2012) and may be linked to maladaptive coping and mood dysregulation, learning difficulties, loss of memory capacity, stress response hyperactivity, and physical disease, which may not become apparent until adulthood (Franke, 2014). In fact, Felitti and colleagues (1998) noted that adults exposed to adverse childhood experiences (ACEs; defined as exposures to violence [physical, emotional, sexual], neglect, social discrimination, disruptive family environments, parental mental health or substance abuse problems, parental incarceration, and or death of a parent) experienced higher rates of cardiovascular illness, diabetes, strokes, and cancer (Felitti et al., 1998).

Additional evidence suggests ACEs are associated with higher health costs across the life course and may contribute to health inequities (Merrick, Ford, Ports, & Guinn, 2018; Purewal et al., 2016). Although ACEs have the capacity to trigger or exacerbate negative health trajectories, exposures to positive health factors can mitigate their effects (Szilagyi & Halfon, 2015). Therefore optimally timed interventions during times of rapid brain development in childhood have the potential to alter the health outcomes from the individual to population-level aggregates.

CHILD WELL-BEING IN THE UNITED STATES

No comprehensive, agreed-upon indices exist to measure what constitutes child health or well-being. The National Research Council and the National Academy of Medicine regard health as composed of four domains: sociodemographic, psychological, behavioral, and contextual (community), which results in focus on health conditions (asthma, obesity); functional problems (attention deficits; hearing, vision, and communication problems); health potential (cognitive development); and birth-related characteristics (low birth weight) (Institute of Medicine and National Research Council, 2011). *Kids Count Data Report* (Annie E. Casey Foundation, 2018) and Child Trends (2018) both use other indicators of child well-being, such as markers of health care utilization (e.g., immunization rates, dental care) and health risk behaviors (HRBs; e.g., substance use, sexually transmitted infections). Because no single resource provides comprehensive information about the health status and well-being of U.S. children and adolescents, and existing data sources define and measure them differently, we are limited in our ability to identify, monitor, and address health disparities among children and adolescents, particularly over time. The use of common definitions and data elements and standardized data collection processes could reduce duplication, allow for comparisons across communities and time, and maximize use of resources and could be particularly useful for understanding preventable, ongoing, or serious health conditions in specific child populations or over time (Institute of Medicine and National Research Council, 2011).

By some measures though, children's physical health is the best that it has been in a century. However, whereas infectious disease was the primary threat to child health 100 years ago, social and environmental factors are key drivers of child well-being today, with noncommunicable conditions negatively impacting the health and development of children, as well as setting the stage for adult morbidity (Rosenbaum & Blum, 2015), and are endured most heavily by low-income children and children of color (Forum on Child and Family Statistics, 2018).

Although the leading causes of morbidity and mortality for American children older than 1 year of age are still preventable injuries such as falls, motor vehicle collisions, and drowning, children of all ages experience high rates of physical assault, negligence, and maltreatment, and mental and behavioral disorders in children are rising, as are the rates of homicide and suicide (CDC, 2018a). Current evidence suggests that approximately 30% of children younger than school aged are diagnosed with developmental delays or behavioral disorders, and 22% of adolescents are diagnosed with mental or behavioral health disorders that negatively impact their school performance (Halfon et al., 2014). In addition, HRBs account for a substantial portion of all health care costs, particularly for chronic illness (CDC, 2017). Factors that predict HRBs in child and youth populations intersect with sociodemographic factors associated with access, quality, and use of health care, health status, and health outcomes and contribute to health inequities, as well as serve as precursors to many common adult chronic health conditions (CDC, 2015).

POVERTY AND TOXIC STRESS

Children living in poverty are commonly exposed to environmental hazards, unsafe living conditions, unstable families, and poor nutrition (Shonkoff et al., 2012), with the accumulated burden exacting a detrimental toll on developmental milestones, school performance, activities of daily life, and health (Cheng, Emmanual, Levy, & Jenkins, 2015).

Approximately 15 million American children live in households below the federal poverty level (National Center for Children in Poverty, 2018). Poverty rates among Black, American Indian, and Latino children are two to three times higher than for Asian and White children (Kids Count Data Center, 2018). In addition, children living in a female-headed household are more likely to live in poverty than children in married-couple families, and more children aged 0 to 5 years live in poverty than older children (Forum on Child and Family Statistics, 2018). Despite small improvements following the recession, the poverty rate for all children younger than 18 years increased more than one-third (15.9% in 2000 to 20.7% in 2015) (Children's Defense Fund, 2017).

The current economic burden of childhood poverty in the United States is approximately $500 billion (Holzer et al., 2007), which does not include the long-term consequences to health and quality of life. Health disparities that originate in childhood can lead to adult chronic illnesses, with affected adults at risk for lost earnings, who may then have difficulty providing for their children, thus perpetuating the cycle (Carter, 2014).

CURRENT CHILD HEALTH POLICY

Children are typically covered by private insurance via employer-sponsored insurance (ESI) or publicly funded insurance via Medicaid or the Children's Health Insurance Program (CHIP). Approximately 49% of children are covered through parental ESI, whereas Medicaid and CHIP cover nearly 40% of children, 48% of children with special health care needs, and 40% of births nationwide. Medicaid is the largest provider of health insurance for children and adults in the United States and provides critical financial support for the nation's safety net of clinics, hospitals, and long-term care facilities serving the poor and uninsured (Turner, McKee, Chen, & Coursolle, 2017). Medicaid also supports school-based health centers (SBHCs) and school districts that provide medically necessary, educational support services to children with special health care needs under the Individuals with Disabilities Education Act (Pudaleski, 2017). Federal law requires all states participating in Medicaid to provide persons younger than 21 years of age with Early and Periodic Screening, Diagnostic, and Treatment (EPSTD) services. This includes more robust services than Medicaid alone, such as vision, hearing, and preventive dental services, which have improved health outcomes for generations of low-income children. Together, Medicaid and CHIP have driven down the rate of uninsured children from 14% in 1997 to 5.3% in 2015 (Artiga & Ubri, 2017).

Federal legislators have suggested instituting "block grants" or "per capita caps" for Medicaid to reduce the amount and variability of federal spending and incentivize states to reduce costs. These proposals eliminate the legal entitlement and guaranteed federal match for Medicaid, while allowing states greater flexibility to decide who and what to cover under Medicaid. Block grants or per capita grants would dramatically alter the structure of Medicaid and shift costs and risks to states, beneficiaries, and health care providers (Georgetown University, 2016). By capping the federal share of responsibility, states would have to determine how to spend the limited dollars and what essential services to cut. Consequently, states would not have the resources to respond to changing conditions and would be limited in their ability to address unanticipated growth in health care costs resulting from a public health crisis, such as a disaster, epidemic, or a new costly treatment option. Proposed changes to the current Medicaid financing structure could seriously impact populations who rely on its guaranteed benefits and raise the real possibility that vulnerable populations, such as children and their parents, people with disabilities, seniors, and many others, would have to compete for scarce health care dollars.

OPPORTUNITIES FOR IMPROVEMENT IN CHILD HEALTH POLICY

Key Considerations

Demographic trends involving American youth are shifting by race, ethnicity, family composition, and overall numbers. The U.S. Census Bureau projects that by 2060, more than one-third of children will identify as Hispanic, non-White, and the number of children who identify as two or more races will reach 11.3% of the total number of U.S. children (Vespa & Armstrong, 2018).

Moreover, whereas children represented approximately 23% of the U.S. population in 2016, that number is projected to decrease to 20% by 2050 (Myers, 2017). American birth rates and the subsequent available workforce are decreasing just as the baby boomer generation retires and life expectancy continues to rise. Stricter immigration policies also reduce the American labor force due to the loss of children from immigrant parents (Myers, 2017). These trends will eventually result in a critical shortage of both economic and caregiving resources for older adults. The ratio of working-age adults to older adults (the old-age dependency ratio) is anticipated to decrease from 3.5 to 1 in 2020 to 2.5 to 1 in 2060 (U.S. Census Bureau, 2018). The diminishing number of children suggests decreased future economic productivity, decreased financial contributions to social security and Medicare, and decreased number of caregivers to care for the rapidly growing aging population (Myers, 2017).

Improving Social Policies to Support Child Well-Being

Early investment in the social, environmental, and physical well-being of children leads to positive health trajectories and decreased health costs across the life course (Halfon et al., 2014). Unfortunately, both Republican and Democratic administrations share a history of underprioritizing children. For example, the 2018 federal budget offered by the executive branch proposed reducing federal outlays by approximately $4.2 trillion over the course of 10 years and reduced discretionary spending on children by $70 billion (Isaacs, Lou, & Hong, 2017). Compared with prior spending, the 2018 budget represented a 9% to 10% overall loss of federal spending toward children (Isaacs et al., 2017).

The loss of funding for children at the federal level impacts spending in the state, local, and research arenas. State and local policies dictate the majority of spending for health care, education, and income support (Myers, 2017). As such, states will need to reevaluate priorities, likely resulting in cuts to essential programs that benefit children and families. The skills of many working adults are determined by where they spend part or all of their childhood and where they receive health care and education, yet 40% of U.S.-born adults currently reside in a different state than where they were born (Myers, 2017). As a result, erosion of public investment in education, housing, and social and health services at local and state levels can have far-reaching consequences for the nation.

Although clinicians, advocates, and policymakers alike recognize that behavioral, social, and environmental conditions impact health, practical interventions to address these social determinants of health (SDOH) reside outside current payment and delivery mechanisms. Given that health outcomes are indeed influenced by agriculture, housing, education, transportation, and other sectors, and recognizing the inherent limitations in government funding, cross-sector partnerships are increasingly important levers for driving improvement in population health (Beers, Spencer, Moses, & Hamblin, 2018). "Collective impact" describes the intentional collaborative action by partners across community, government, philanthropy, and business sectors (Kania & Kramer, 2011). Collective impact initiatives take many forms but include five key elements (Box 11.1) and have been used across the nation to address readiness for kindergarten (Houston, TX), preterm birth (Fresno, CA), childhood asthma (Dallas, TX), and youth substance abuse (Staten Island, NY) (Box 11.2).

A second model, "pay-for-success," also known as social impact bonds or initiatives, turns the current health care service reimbursement payment mechanism on its head by incentivizing investment in SDOH (Galloway, 2014). Pay-for-success models involve the contracting of social services that tie payment for service delivery to achievement of measurable outcomes. Although an investor assumes the financial risk, they are repaid and receive an additional return on investment if the intervention succeeds (Galloway, 2014). Still novel in the United States, pay-for-success projects addressing child health are in various stages of development and implementation across the country (Box 11.3). No single policy, government or public entity, or private organization can address the complex social issues that impact child health. However, mindsets must shift, along with government policies and structures, for us to make progress on some of the persistent and intractable issues impacting child well-being.

BOX 11.1 Five Key Elements of Collective Impact

Common agenda. All participants possess a shared vision for change that includes a common understanding of the problem and a joint approach to solving it using agreed-upon actions.

Shared measurement systems. Participants agree to common method for consistently measuring and reporting data.

Mutually reinforcing activities. Each participant undertakes a specific set of activities and all of the differentiated activities are coordinated through a mutually reinforcing plan of action.

Continuous communication. Open and continuous communication is required to build trust, support mutual objectives, and create common motivation.

Backbone support organizations. A separate backbone support organization provides the administrative infrastructure, logistical skills, and leadership to serve the entire initiative.

Source: Kania, J., & Kramer, M. (2011, Winter). Collective impact. *Stanford Social Innovation Review*. Retrieved from https://ssir.org/articles/entry/collective_impact.

BOX 11.2 Examples of Collective Impact Initiatives

Early Matters, Houston, Texas

An education-focused collective impact initiative formed by more than 100 community leaders to address kindergarten readiness through a holistic approach that emphasized the roles of poverty, health, and family stress (www.early-mattershouston.org)

Fresno County Preterm Birth Collective Impact Initiative, Fresno, California

A collective impact initiative formed by stakeholders from hospitals, community clinics, nonprofits, funders, and local governments, supported by a local university performing the backbone function, to address prenatal health and education, care and support for pregnant women, and greater coordination of social and behavioral services (www.ptbifresno.org)

Health and Wellness Alliance, Dallas, Texas

A collective impact initiative formed by health care organizations, school districts, government agencies, social service nonprofits, and faith-based organizations, supported by the regional children's hospital as backbone, to identify strategies to address the social and environmental determinants of asthma (www.childrens.com/keeping-families-healthy/community-resources/family-education/health-and-wellness-alliance)

Tackling Youth Substance Abuse, Staten Island, New York

A collective impact initiative formed by community leaders, law enforcement agencies, educators, parents, teens, and medical professionals, with backbone support provided by a local philanthropic foundation to reduce the use of alcohol and prescription drugs and reduce unhealthy choices by youth (sipcw.org/tysa)

IMPLICATIONS FOR ADVOCACY, POLICY, AND RESEARCH

U.S. child health policy remains a patchwork of efforts at the federal, state, and local levels. The fragmentation of responsibility between families and these multiple layers of government seriously impedes efforts to develop a cogent, equitable, and comprehensive policy for U.S. children who live in very different places and have different access to resources. Children, by virtue of their developmental dependence, generally must rely on advocacy "by proxy" from parents, professionals, and public interest groups to speak on their behalf in the halls of Congress, the state legislature, and the voting booth. The challenge lies in engaging these children's advocates to work in a coordinated and consistent effort across policy domains to achieve evidence-based, sustainable policies that support child well-being.

Palfrey (2006) suggests that child health advocacy consists of four interconnected components: clinical advocacy, group advocacy, professional advocacy, and legislative advocacy. Only when these components come together in the

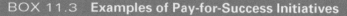

BOX 11.3   Examples of Pay-for-Success Initiatives

Example 1: Nurse-Family Partnership, South Carolina

Expands Nurse-Family Partnership services to an additional 3200 first-time, low-income mothers and children across the state.

Philanthropic funders include:

- BlueCross BlueShield of South Carolina Foundation ($3.5 million)
- The Duke Endowment ($8 million)
- The Boeing Company ($800,000)
- Greenville County, SC First Steps ($700,000)
- Laura and John Arnold Foundation ($491,000)
- Consortium of private funders ($4 million)

In addition, Medicaid will fund $13 million via a Medicaid Waiver.

The private philanthropic funding finances the expansion upfront and transfers risk away from the state government and South Carolina tax payers (www.nursefamilypartnership.org/public-policy/pay-for-success).

Example 2: Partnering for Family Success Program, County of Cuyahoga, Ohio

Delivers an intensive 12- to 15-month treatment program to 135 families over 5 years to reduce the length of stay in out-of-home foster care placement for children whose families are homeless.

A consortium of five funders have provided $4 million in upfront funding:

- The Reinvestment Fund ($1.575 million in loan funding at 5% interest)
- The George Gund Foundation ($1 million in loan funding at 2% interest for $725,000 and 0% interest for $275,000)
- Nonprofit Finance Fund ($325,000 in loan funding at 2% interest).
- The Cleveland Foundation ($750,000 in loan funding at 2% interest)
- Sisters of Charity Foundation of Cleveland (two recoverable grants of $75,000 and $200,000 in loan funding at 2% interest)

Cuyahoga County will repay funders only if program is proven to shorten length of stay in out-of-home foster care (www.thirdsectorcap.org/cuyahoga/).

context of political will and accountability can meaningful change occur. Advocates must acknowledge the tensions inherent in "children's issues," including the question: who is responsible for a child—the family or society? Developing a coherent vision is difficult under the best of circumstances, but political and ideologic polarization in recent years has crippled informed dialogue. Nevertheless, child health advocates must leverage evidence about the importance of investing in child policy and work to protect programs that have demonstrated success. This includes cultivating partnerships between public and private sectors, investing in relationships between health and educational systems, and considering innovative methods, such as a collective impact framework or a pay-for-success model, to make a meaningful impact on child and youth health and well-being.

DISCUSSION QUESTIONS

1. Discuss the connections among child health, educational achievement, and SDOH.

2. Define a children's policy problem, and describe how you might frame a social policy to ameliorate that problem.

3. How might nurses promote and implement public health approaches to children's mental health?

REFERENCES

American Institute for Research (2018). *National center on family homelessness*. Retrieved from www.air.org/center/national-center-family-homelessness.

Annie E. Casey Foundation. (2018). *Kids Count Data Center*. Retrieved from https://datacenter.kidscount.org/topics.

Artiga, S., & Ubri, P. (2017). *Key issues in children's health coverage*. Retrieved from: www.kff.org/medicaid/issue-brief/key-issues-in-childrens-health-coverage/.

Beers, A., Spencer, A., Moses, K., & Hamblin, A. (2018). *Promoting better health beyond health care*. Hamilton, NJ: Center for Health Care Strategies, Inc. Retrieved www.chcs.org/media/BHBHC_Report_053018.pdf.

Carter, B. (2014). Child poverty: Limiting children's life chances. *Journal of Child Health Care, 18*(1), 3-5.

Centers for Disease Control and Prevention. (2015). *CDC features: CDC releases youth risk behaviors survey results and trends report.* Retrieved from www.cdc.gov/features/yrbs/.

Centers for Disease Control and Prevention. (2017). *National center for chronic disease prevention and health promotion. Chronic disease overview.* Retrieved from www.cdc.gov/chronicdisease/overview/index.htm.

Centers for Disease Control and Prevention. (2018a). *National Center for Health Statistics: Leading causes of death, children 1–4, 5–14.* Retrieved from www.cdc.gov/nchs/fastats/child-health.htm.

Centers for Disease Control and Prevention. (2018b). *Prevalence of obesity among adults and youth: United States, 2015–2016.* Retrieved from www.cdc.gov/nchs/products/databriefs/db288.htm.

Cheng, T.L., Emmanual, M.A., Levy, D.J., & Jenkins, R.R. (2015). Child health disparities: What can clinicians do? *Pediatrics, 136*(5), 961–968.

Child Trends. (2018). *Child Trends.* Retrieved from www.childtrends.org.

Children's Defense Fund. (2017). *The state of America's children 2017.* Retrieved from www.childrensdefense.org/library/state-of-americas-children/2017-soac.pdf.

Edin, K.J., & Shaefer, H.L. (2015). *$2.00 a day. Living on almost nothing in America.* Boston, MA: Houghton Mifflin Harcourt.

Feeding America. (2018). *Child food insecurity.* Retrieved from www.feedingamerica.org/research/map-the-meal-gap/2016/2016-map-the-meal-gap-child-food-insecurity.pdf.

Felitti, V.J., Anda, R.F., Nordenberg, D., Williamson, D.F., Spitz, A.M., Edwards, V., . . . & Marks, J.S. (1998). Relationship of childhood abuse and household dysfunction to many of the leading causes of death in adults. The adverse childhood experiences (ACE) study. *American Journal of Preventive Medicine, 14*(4), 245–258.

Forum on Child and Family Statistics. (2018). *America's children: Key national indicators of well-being, 2017.* Retrieved from www.childstats.gov/americaschildren/.

Franke, H.A., (2014). Toxic stress: Effects, prevention and treatment. *Children, 1*(3), 390–402.

Galloway, I. (2014). Using pay-for-success to increase investment in the nonmedical determinants of health. *Health Affairs, 33*(11), 1897–1904.

Georgetown University Health Policy Institute, Center for Children and Families. (2016). *Medicaid's role for young children.* Retrieved from http://ccf.georgetown.edu/wp-content/uploads/2017/02/MedicaidYoungChildren.pdf.

Halfon, N., Larson, K., Lu, M., Tullis, E., & Russ, S. (2014). Life course health development: Past, present, and future. *Maternal and Child Health Journal, 18*(2), 344–365.

Holzer, H.J., Schanzenback, D.W., Duncan, G.J., & Judwig, J. (2007). *The economic costs of poverty in the United States: Subsequent effects of children growing up poor.* Washington, DC: Center for American Progress. Retrieved from https://cdn.americanprogress.org/wp-content/uploads/issues/2007/01/pdf/poverty_report.pdf.

Institute of Medicine and National Research Council. (2011). *Child and adolescent health and health care quality: Measuring what matters.* Washington, DC: The National Academies Press.

Isaacs, J.B., Lou, C., & Hong, A. (2017). *How would spending on children be affected by the proposed 2018 budget? A kids' share analysis of the President's 2018 budget.* Retrieved from www.urban.org/sites/default/files/publication/95306/spending_under_administration_budget_final3.pdf.

Kaiser Family Foundation. (2018). *Health insurance coverage of children 0-18.* Retrieved from www.kff.org/other/state-indicator/children-0-18/?currentTimeframe=0&sortModel=%7B%22colId%22:%22Location%22,%22sort%22:%22asc%22%7D.

Kania, J. & Kramer, M. (2011, Winter). Collective impact. *Stanford Social Innovation Review.* Retrieved from https://ssir.org/articles/entry/collective_impact.

Kids Count Data Center. (2018). *Children in poverty by race and ethnicity.* Retrieved from https://datacenter.kidscount.org/data/tables/44-children-in-poverty-by-race-and-ethnicity#detailed/1/any/false/870,573,869,36,868,867,133,38,35,18/10,11,9,12,1,185,13/324,323.

Kolb, B., & Gibb, R. (2011). Brain plasticity and behaviour in the developing brain. *Journal of the Canadian Academy of Adolescent Psychiatry, 20*(4), 265–276.

MacDorman, M.F., Matthews, T.J., Mohangoo, A.D., & Zeitlin, J. (2014). International comparisons of infant mortality and related factors: United States and Europe, 2010. *National Vital Statistics Report, 63*(5), 1–6.

Merrick, M.T., Ford, D.C., Ports, K.A., & Guinn, A.S. (2018). Prevalence of adverse childhood experiences from the 2011-2014 behavioral risk factor surveillance system in 23 states. *JAMA Pediatrics, 172*(11), 1038–1044.

Myers, D. (2017). *The new importance of children in America.* Retrieved from www.childrenshospitals.org/-/media/Files/CHA/Main/Research_and_Data/Pediatric_Health_Care_Trends/2017/the_new_importance_of_children_in_america_report_101217.pdf.

National Center for Children in Poverty. (2018). *Child poverty.* Retrieved from http://nccp.org/topics/childpoverty.html.

Organization for Economic Co-operation and Development. (2018). *Poverty rate (indicator).* Retrieved from https://data.oecd.org/inequality/poverty-rate.htm.

Palfrey, J. (2006). *Child health in America.* Baltimore, MD: The Johns Hopkins University Press.

Pudaleski, S. (2017). *Cutting Medicaid: A prescription to hurt the neediest kids.* Retrieved from http://aasa.org/uploadedFiles/Policy_and_Advocacy/Resources/medicaid.pdf.

Purewal, S.K., Bucci, M., Gutierrez Wang, L., Kadiatou, K., Silverio Marques, S., Oh, D., & Burke Harris, N. (2016). Screening for adverse childhood experiences (ACEs) in an integrated pediatric care model. *Zero to Three, 36*(3), 10–17.

Rosenbaum, S., & Blum, R. (2015). How healthy are our children? *The Future of Children, 25*(1), 11–34.

Shonkoff, J.P., Garner, A.S., Committee on Psychosocial Aspects of Child and Family Health, Committee on Early Childhood, Adoption, and Dependent Care, Section on Developmental and Behavioral Pediatrics, Siegel, B.S., . . . & Wood, D.L.

(2012). The lifelong effects of early childhood adversity and toxic stress. *Pediatrics, 129*(1), e232-e246.

Szilagyi, M., & Halfon, N. (2015). Pediatric adverse childhood experiences: Implications for life course trajectories. *Academic Pediatrics, 15*(5), 467–468.

Thakrar, A.P., Forrest, A.D., Maltenfort, M.G., & Forrest, C.B. (2018). Child mortality in the U.S. and 19 OECD comparator nations: A 50-year time-trend analysis. *Health Affairs, 37*(1).

Turner, W., McKee, C., Chen, A., & Coursolle, A. (2017). *What makes Medicaid, Medicaid? Services*. Retrieved from www.healthlaw.org/about/staff/wayne-turner/all-publications/what-makes-medicaid-medicaid-services#.WzgbeS2ZMyl.

United States Census Bureau. (2018). *Newsroom. Older people projected to outnumber children for first time in U.S. history*. Retrieved from www.census.gov/newsroom/press-releases/2018/cb18-41-population-projections.html.

Vespa, J., & Armstrong, D. M. (2018). *Demographic turning points for the United States: Population projections for 2020 to 2060.* Retrieved from www.census.gov/content/dam/Census/library/publications/2018/demo/P25_1144.pdf.

ONLINE RESOURCES

Adverse Childhood Events
www.cdc.gov/ace
Harvard Center for Developing Child
https://developingchild.harvard.edu/topics/science_of_early_childhood
Nurse Family Partnership
www.nursefamilypartnership.org
Systems of Care
www.childwelfare.gov/topics/management/reform/soc/

12

Using the Power of the Media to Influence Health Policy and Politics

Beth Gharrity Gardner, Diana J. Mason, Barbara Glickstein,
and Monica R. McLemore

"There is no more important struggle for American democracy than ensuring a diverse,
independent and free media. Free Press is at the heart of that struggle."

Bill Moyers

In 1997, the *Woodhull Study on Nursing and the Media: Health Care's Invisible Partner* found that nurses were used as sources in only 4% of health news stories published in leading print newspapers, news magazines, and trade publications like *Modern Health Care*. Twenty years later, the same publications cited nurses only 2% of the time (Mason et al., 2018c). Nurses were never sourced for stories on health policy. This dismal picture is an outgrowth of longstanding biases about women, nurses, and positions of authority in health care among journalists, newsrooms, public relations staff, and others (Mason, Glickstein, & Westphaln, 2018b). It is also the result of nurses and nursing organizations failing to be proactive in accessing and using media to advance their perspectives on policy. Interviews with health journalists revealed that nurses often shy away from journalists' requests for interviews. Furthermore, nursing organizations and journals are not reaching out to journalists on topics the journalists cover, including evidence-based policy issues.

It is time to change this picture. This chapter discusses the power and volatile context of media in today's world, particularly in the United States, and provides readers with tools to strategically use media to shape health and social policies.

MEDIA LANDSCAPE

"Fake news," "echo chambers," "filter bubbles," "alternative facts," "post-truth"—these are some of the buzzwords for describing the contemporary media environment and why people are falling for misinformation. Concerns about reliable sources of public information that are key to an informed citizenry and democracy are not new. We have known for a long time that the vision of a healthy democracy in which people make decisions based on factual information provided by mass media has never been realized; nor is it entirely realistic. This was true of American media before newspapers began institutionalizing professional, journalistic standards of objectivity and political independence in the 1920s; through the accelerated deregulation of media under President Reagan in the1980s; to the subsequent widespread proliferation of newer digital media in the 2000s (Berry & Sobieraj, 2014).

Debates over contemporary health care topics offer many instances when misinformation gained currency well before the 2016 presidential election raised alarms about deliberate information manipulation. For example, consider the dynamics that unfolded when the Affordable Care Act (ACA) was introduced in 2009. This health care reform proposal faced opposition from prominent conservatives who began circulating concerns and false claims about the proposal, including that its Independent Payment Advisory Board for determining Medicare spending would become a "death panel," denying life-saving care to sick, older, and disabled Americans (Nyhan, 2010).

The Obama administration, independent observers, and media fact-checkers alike debunked the myth of "death panels" that would pressure people to "end their lives sooner." Nonetheless, a great deal of publicity kept it alive, amplified by both these refutations and the endorsements of pundits across media channels, predominantly conservative cable news, talk radio, and online outlets

(Meirick, 2013). A month after Republican vice-presidential candidate, Sarah Palin's Facebook post denounced "Obama's 'death panels,'" the vast majority of Americans reported having heard the claim, and substantial segments of the public reported believing it or being uncertain about its veracity. Although the ACA was ultimately signed into law in 2010, disbelief about what the ACA actually entailed resulted in the Obama administration removing provisions for reimbursing counseling about end-of-life and advance directives (Leonard, 2015).

The story about the "death panels" likely gained traction among audiences because, for all its outrageousness, it was already somewhat familiar to them. On one hand, the "newsworthiness" of contentious rhetoric, and the sheer volume and retelling of claims—retweeting, sharing, recommending, (dis)liking—across diverse media outlets and without proper vetting made this style of storytelling familiar and appealing (Polletta & Callahan, 2017). On the other, part of a story's power comes from conveying normative points (i.e., "the moral of the story") and referring to familiar plotlines or protagonists people can easily identify (Polletta et al., 2011). The "death panels" myth accorded with similarly misleading and popularly accepted plotlines, including the Republican strategic narrative about liberal government overreach threatening American values of individualism and personal choice (Nyhan, 2010).

Popular stories about policy and politics, regardless of their accuracy, may become persuasive because they make complex, abstract issues seem engaging and concrete. One could substitute the fictive stories about the ACA for those about vaccines causing autism or less policy-oriented accounts, such as those about President Obama's birthplace. Although most of these examples call out conservatives' use of rhetoric, the game is played across the political spectrum from conservatives to liberals.

Several factors exacerbate the current spread of misinformation through media. First, political opinion news media (especially partisan commentary and "news analysis") are outpacing news and investigative journalism directed at balancing information and presenting facts in American media (Berry & Sobieraj, 2014; Polletta & Callahan, 2017). Second, people with little interest in politics can bypass the news entirely or tailor their exposure to information that fits their opinion (Sunstein, 2018). Third, public trust in the traditional institutions of authority and information vetting (e.g., public officials, democratic governance, and the news media) remains near historic lows (Pew Research Center [Pew], 2018b). Rumors and falsehoods can flourish under such conditions of ambiguity and uncertainty over reliable information. While both Republicans and Democrats continue to voice little or no confidence in public officials, when it comes to "trust and confidence" in news media and its watchdog role, the partisan divide is greater than ever (Pew, 2018b). Whether this is a cause or a consequence of "fake news," the rise of "infotainment," the weakening of traditional news organizations, or something else remains unclear. Conceivably, the door has been opened for opinion-based claims because they are more widely available, more engaging, and less prone to challenge than evidence-based claims.

Although this paints a rather grim picture, much is being done to address these issues and nurses can play a key role in doing so. The nursing profession is the most trusted profession almost every year in Gallup surveys of the public (Brenan, 2018). However, it will take a critical mass of nurses developing media competencies to gain comparable standing as credible advocates for health and social policy across media platforms.

WHAT IS THE MEDIA?

The media has never been a static institution. New communication technologies continue to develop and diffuse across an even wider swath of demographic groups in the United States. Various forms of information, including news, flow across televisions, personal computers, game consoles, and smartphones, as well as websites, including social media applications. Certain shifts in *newer* digital media use are more pronounced than others. Almost all adults (93%) get at least some of their news online, and 67% do so through social media (Gramlich, 2018). The most substantial increases in social media news use over the past few years have been driven by older, less educated, and non-White Americans (Pew, 2017). Social media use continues to be greatest among those between the ages of 13 and 24, but even the typical adult was following three social media sites in 2018 (Pew, 2018c).

Importantly, however, such statistics tend to obscure the interweaving of older, traditional offline broadcast media channels and outlets with newer online, social media channels. These more traditional, legacy media sources largely represent the 20th century field of journalism and news organizations that controlled news products and services from newsgathering, writing, and editorial selection, to press production and delivery. Although people are increasingly seeing news via newer, digital platforms, much of the news content still originates in traditional news media organizations—whether repackaged for the digital platform, given a new headline or image, or shared differently (Pew, 2017). For instance, Facebook does not yet produce its own news content. We need to keep these layers of content mediation or repackaging in mind and remember that television, news websites, radio, and (until 2018) newspapers were all more popular platforms for news consumption than social media (Shearer, 2018). Although traditional media can feed news to online platforms, online platforms are often what helps stories or headlines go viral. It is against this backdrop that "fake news"—inaccurate information that imitates legitimate news content in form but not in organizational intent or process—and its progenitors have parasitically benefitted from the "real news" ecosystem while undermining its credibility (Lazer et al., 2018). The power of social media in disseminating both accurate and inaccurate information cannot be underestimated.

Social Media

Since the Pew Research Center first began collecting data in 2012, Facebook has remained the primary social media platform for most Americans. Of the two-thirds (68%) of U.S. adults using Facebook, 74% access it daily and 67% get news there (Pew, 2018a). Despite Twitter's smaller user base, an even higher percentage of its users (71%) are exposed to news on the site (Pew, 2018a). Given social media's reach and ability to provide effective correction of health *mis*information (Vraga & Bode, 2017), it would seem that nurses would be leveraging these platforms to provide expert voices about research findings and health policy.

Unfortunately, existing guidelines (National Council of State Boards for Nursing, 2011) and instructions (Gennaro, 2015) for social media use by nurses have mainly been geared toward prevention of Health Insurance Portability and Accountability Act (HIPAA) violations and other negative injunctions, with few geared toward leveraging social media to advance nursing policy (Shattell et al., 2015d; Shattell et al., 2015b). However, there are ways for nurses to use social media to disseminate science, discuss essential topics that impact nursing, and educate the public about the importance of nursing in the provision of evidence-based care (Shattell et al., 2015a; Shattell et al., 2015c).

Overview of Social Media Platforms. The learning curve for social media has significantly decreased given the ubiquity of use and emerging similarities with other familiar websites and apps. See Table 12.1 for some basics about seven leading platforms in 2018.

By digitally mediating interpersonal networks, social media can serve as a vehicle to revise stereotypes that conceal the contributions of nurses and nursing to policy efforts. Social media is also a powerful tool for expanding the reach of individuals and professional organizations—particularly in the dissemination of key research findings that should inform policy development and implementation. Tweeting from conferences and meetings, for example, provides real-time content to attendees, provides opportunities

for wider engagement, and allows for the rapid alignment of policy statements. The scale and coordination advantages of social media can support nurses in wielding the collective power to make changes that benefit the patients, families, and communities we serve (Burton et al., 2017).

HOW DOES MEDIA MATTER?

As a premier forum for political communication, the media is a powerful resource for influencing political outcomes—from elections and getting policy issues on the public's agenda to specific actions by individual policymakers.

Shaping Elections

Social networking platforms have not yet established accountability mechanisms commensurate with those of traditional, mass media organizations (i.e., editorial judgment, fact-checking procedures, and reputational constraints). This disparity became particularly salient during and following the 2016 presidential election. Recent research on social media's role in spreading misleading information and public misperceptions about the election shows there is good reason to be concerned (Flynn, Nyhan, & Reifler, 2017; Jamieson, 2018). Some studies even suggest that people who use Facebook (or other social media) as a "major" source for news are more susceptible to disinformation (Allcott & Gentzkow, 2017; Silverman & Singer-Levine, 2016).

In the 3 months prior to the 2016 election, "fake news" versions of the top election stories on Facebook were liked or shared more often than accurate versions of election stories from the largest U.S. media outlets (Silverman, 2016). A series of investigations conducted by BuzzFeed News found that a significant portion of these viral, false election news stories originated on websites run by young men in Macedonia who were not advocating a political agenda; rather, they were just trying to earn a living through the advertising revenues such stories were producing for the politically-motivated actors spearheading the country's fake-news industry (Silverman et al., 2018). Prior to discovering they could make more money with politics, especially staunch conservative politics, these same content re-packagers were running health and beauty websites. This case underscores how the accuracy of information has little bearing on profitably in the current media system.

President Donald Trump's approach to mediated politics illustrates the power of social media in communicating more directly to audiences and circumventing traditional media filters. Trump has used Twitter almost daily but held fewer press conferences than his predecessors. According to

TABLE 12.1 Social Media Platforms

Platform	Year Established	Users	Purpose
Facebook	2004	2 billion worldwide	Connect people around the world based on personal relationships.
YouTube	2005	1.5 billion worldwide	Video sharing site that allows for live streaming of television and other events (owned by Google)
LinkedIn	2002	590 million worldwide	Social networking site to connect workers, employers, and jobseekers
Twitter	2006	336 million worldwide	Platform for rapid communication
Reddit	2005	330 million worldwide	Aggregated social news, web content, and discussion boards
Snapchat	2011	186 million worldwide and largest platform used by people under 35	App offers a "new kind of camera" that allows users to connect to friends and the world
Instagram	2010	77.5 million in United States	Photo-sharing site that allows for videos and stories (owned by Facebook)

The platforms included in the table were top ranked in 2018, with user data from Statista, the Statistics Portal. (2018). *Most famous social network sites worldwide as of April 2018, ranked by number of active users.* Retrieved from www.statista.com/statistics/272014/global-social-networks-ranked-by-number-of-users/.

journalist Neal Gabler (2016), "What FDR was to radio and JFK to television, Trump is to Twitter." Indeed, it is hard for people to forget the unsubstantiated messages Trump has tweeted both before and after taking office, which often feature attacks on reputable media sources as "fake news" or "the enemy of the people."

Getting on the Public's Agenda and Shaping Policy Debates

One of the most important roles the media plays is getting issues on public's and policymakers' agendas. How the media covers issue debates and the key players involved powerfully shapes which issues policymakers prioritize. For example, media coverage of people who died because they did not have health insurance to pay for treatment of cancer and other serious conditions helped to garner support for health care reform and the passage of the ACA. Once passed, opponents kept the "repeal and replace Obamacare" message in the media and on the public's agenda. Just the use of the term "Obamacare" to refer to the ACA created a misleading symbol of government overreach among people opposed to "big government" or Obama or the dependency implied in "care." Having set the agenda in these terms, once Republicans took control of Congress and the presidency in 2016 their attempts to cut all or key features of the ACA became potential realities.

Support for "repeal and replace Obamacare" waned as some people realized that "Obamacare" *was* the ACA and that repealing or cutting it might mean losing their health insurance. For example, Kentucky named their ACA insurance marketplace *Kynect* to dissociate it from Obamacare, which most Kentuckians disliked. Sarah Kliff (2016), a Vox reporter, found that although Kentucky's high rate of uninsured people declined by 60% under the ACA, 82% of its residents voted for Trump. Despite thinking Obamacare and the ACA were two different things, most people simply could not believe Trump would repeal it because so many people benefited from the ACA. They believed he would make it better.

Media coverage of nurses and the nursing profession can crucially influence health policy. The media's coverage of the scope of practice of advanced practice registered nurses (APRNs) is one important example. IOM's *The Future of Nursing* report (Institute of Medicine, 2011) recommended removing legal and regulatory barriers to APRNs' ability to practice to the top of their education and training without legally mandated collaboration or supervision by a physician. The media discussed this controversial issue in story after story with evidence documenting that APRNs provide care equal to or better than physicians, and the public was satisfied with the care provided by nurse practitioners and nurse midwives. Framed as an issue of access to care, "full practice authority" made it onto the agenda of state policymakers across the country.

WHO CONTROLS THE MEDIA?

The media landscape and who owns it used to be pretty straightforward. Through the 20th century, the owners of mass media were a powerful, exclusive club. The U.S. media system has entered a period of intense change; the boundaries between sectors are blurring, with power shifting into even fewer hands and those of the tech giants. The newspapers, broadcast networks, and magazines that were the main institutional home for journalism have faced economic crises and downsized their newsrooms; in some cities and towns, papers have folded altogether. The decimation of local newsrooms is among the catalysts in the rise of content makers and re-packagers seeking profit or political influence as opposed to the truth-seeking of most journalists.

The regulatory authority for broadcasting and telecommunication is the Federal Communications Commission (FCC), with five Commissioners appointed by the president and confirmed by the Senate. Although appointments are partisan, no more than three can be from a single political party. In 2017 the FCC voted to relax broadcast ownership rules that allowed a single corporation, Sinclair Broadcast Group, to purchase Tribune Media. Even though Tribune Media stopped the sale, Sinclair Broadcast Group and other large corporate media companies supported the FCC changes, arguing that they needed large scale ownership to reduce costs and increase audience reach. The FCC ruled with them, thereby removing the cross-ownership ban that previously kept TV stations from owning newspapers in the same market. Critics of the ruling noted it ended diversity in broadcasting and protections against anticompetitive practices, whereas proponents said it moved ownership rules into the digital age (Fung, 2017).

The reality is that the FCC changes have permitted media mergers, resulting in fewer companies owning more media outlets. In 1983, 90% of U.S. media were controlled by 50 companies; in 2018 most media are controlled by six companies (Rapp & Jenkins, 2018). The axis of concern with increased media concentration is that owners can advance their economic and political interests not only through wielding their concentrated power to influence media regulation but also through preferred policies in what will be presented, what consumer data will be collected, and how.

Despite this concentration in ownership, new forms of nonprofit, grant-funded news, and media fact-checking operations are proliferating to protect independent journalism. For example, ProPublica (propublica.org) is an investigative news operation that began with private funding from Herbert and Marion Sandler but has subsequently diversified its funding sources for reasons of sustainability and credibility. A number of initiatives, such as the Information Disorder Project at Harvard and Data & Society, have formed to build media literacy, disrupt fake news, and apply pressure on tech giants to support legitimate journalism and tighten their platform policies on disinformation and hate speech. Another important part of this corrective landscape is comprised of ethnic media outlets—media produced for a particular ethnic community—that continue to serve as bridges between mainstream society, and immigrants and communities of color. New America Media is the country's largest network of more than 3000 ethnic news organizations including TV, radio, online, and print publications. These outlets often have a closer relationship to their communities and tend to advocate for them. Nurses serving ethnically diverse populations can pitch story ideas or be available as health experts to journalists covering health and policy for these media outlets.

MEDIA TO PROMOTE HEALTH

There are a number of approaches to using media for health promotion. Media can help people change their health behaviors by equipping them with important information they lacked (public education) or through visual or verbal messaging that can shift a person's attitudes and beliefs (social marketing). Although these two approaches are used in political campaigns and to shape public policy, a third approach specifically targets policy: media advocacy. Read about Robin Cogan, a school nurse who has become a media maker on school nursing and health, in Box 12.1.

Media Advocacy

Media advocacy is the strategic use of media to apply pressure to advance a social or public policy initiative (Dorfman & Krasnow, 2014). This tool mobilizes constituencies and stakeholders to support or oppose specific policy changes as a means of political action. In contrast to social marketing and public education, media advocacy focuses on the individual as an advocate, not just an observer, and it aims to change the environment, not just the individual. It defines the primary problem as a *power* gap as opposed to an *information* gap, so stakeholder mobilization is necessary to influence the development of public policies.

Framing

Getting an issue on the agenda of the media, the public, and policymakers requires an understanding of *framing*. Framing "defines the boundaries of public discussion about an issue" (Wallack & Dorfman, 1996, p. 299). *Reframing* involves breaking out of the dominant perspective (or frame) on an issue to define a new way of thinking and potentially different, effective policy responses. Reframing requires working hard to understand the dominant frame, the values that underpin it, and its limitations; and then to

BOX 12.1   Robin Cogan: School Nurse and Media Maker

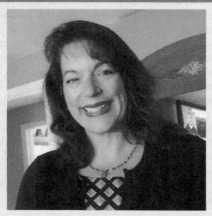

After 17 years as a practicing Nationally Certified School Nurse and educator of school nurses, I grew tired of the media's portrayal of school nursing: a retirement job for someone who puts Band-aids on the scraped knees of children. In this new digital age, I stepped up and became a media maker to counter this misinformation about school nursing.

In 2017, I launched *The Relentless School Nurse*, about school nursing that shifted to become a platform for social justice activism. This transformation moved quickly. It went from sharing stories from my school health office to highlighting the work of other school nurses. In February 2018, the focus of my work changed after the Parkland High School shooting, where my niece was a student. She survived, but 17 others did not. My family story is further complicated by an unimaginable tragedy my father experienced in 1949, when his parents and grandmother were murdered along with 10 other people in the first mass-murder in the country. Both my niece and my father survived by hiding in closets, 70 years apart.

To broaden my media outreach, I dipped my toe into the waters of Twitter and Facebook. In a short space of time I shifted to posting daily tweets, retweeting, following people who inspired and educated me, and forging relationships with other social activists. This all raised the visibility of my role as a school nurse activist and the role of school nurses in the health of children, families, and communities nationally.

My activism in addressing gun violence prevention since the Parkland shootings continues to grow. I have spoken at town hall meetings and professional conferences, and I have been a source for journalists on the issue. I have joined the ranks of health care professionals uniting to demand legislation to fund firearm prevention research. Following the mass shooting in 2018 at Southside Hospital in Chicago, where four people were killed, health care providers took to social media tweeting about their tragically frequent experiences treating patients in the aftermath of gun violence.

After the American College of Physicians called gun violence a "public health crisis," the National Rifle Association (NRA) mocked them with the tweet, "Someone should tell self-important anti-gun doctors to stay in their lane," which launched a massive Twitter response by the medical community using the hashtag #ThisIsOurLane.

For years, the NRA has lobbied to prevent the Centers for Disease Control (CDC) and the National Institutes of Health (NIH) from conducting research on gun violence prevention. We must change that. Dr. Joseph Sakran, a trauma surgeon and victim of gun violence, founded the not-for-profit ThisIsOurLane to organize health care professionals to find solutions to prevent firearm injury and death. I was invited to serve on the inaugural board of directors.

Speaking and writing about firearm violence prevention is not a topic that I would have chosen, but it seems to have chosen me. I have no choice but to use my family's story and my nursing lens to move this conversation forward. This engagement with digital media has moved me out of my comfort zone; but if that is what it takes to find solutions to preventing gun violence, I will stay uncomfortable until we make progress. I urge every nurse to add their voice and influence to address this public health crisis.

explore new frames. Chapter 62 provides an excellent example of reframing the issue of APRN scope of practice for West Virginia.

Framing for media coverage has two core dimensions. *Framing for access* to the media entails presenting the issue or a position on the issue in a way that will attract media attention. It helps to attach the issue to something already on the media's agenda or to a local concern, or you can make news by holding events that will attract the press.

Framing for content once you are in front of the media is more difficult. A compelling personal story may gain attention in some media, but there is no guarantee that the reporter or social media sharer will focus on the desired implications for policy change.

Reframing can be accomplished by (Wallack & Dorfman, 1996, p. 300):
- Emphasizing the social dimensions of the problem and translating an individual's personal story into a public issue

- Shifting the responsibility for the problem from the individual to the executive or public official whose decisions can address the problem
- Presenting solutions as policy alternatives
- Making a practical appeal to support the solution
- Using compelling images and symbols that resonate with the values of the audience
- Using the authentic voices of people who have experience with the problem
- Anticipating the opposition and knowing all sides of the issue.

EFFECTIVE USE OF MEDIA

Position Yourself as a Trusted Source

The 2017 *Woodhull Study Revisited* (Mason, Glickstein, & Westphaln, 2018b; www.go.gwu.edu/Woodhull) found that health journalists did not know how to find nurses as sources and could not rely on nurses to respond to their requests for interviews. The reporters noted that they would use nurses more often if they had easy access to them.

To become a trusted source journalists can rely on, it is critical that you attend to how you are (or are not) represented online. Decide where you want to be found (on your institution's website or on a professional networking site like LinkedIn.com) and craft a profile that spells out your expertise, including how your nursing education, credentials, research, and practice support your expertise. Consider your online profile as a pathway for journalists to know about you, your area of expertise, and the best means of contacting you.

Use social media to help build relationships with journalists in your local media outlets and nationally. Health reporters use social media platforms, particularly Twitter, and seek experts who can rapidly provide commentary on emerging issues (Mason et al., 2018a). The list-function within many social media platforms allows followers to group user profiles by interests such as "nurse scholars," "repro nurses," and "policy wonks." Be on top of the news cycle and comment on what a reporter is posting. Your research findings could be newsworthy on their own or you can make them applicable by hooking them to a current news story. Tweet about a story with a related #hashtag (searchable keywords on social media platforms; as in #HealthEquity) to make it searchable to the news being reported; or, when you know a major study in your field is about to be released, contact a journalist who reports on the topic and offer to comment.

Retweet a story that is important to you or on which you have special expertise and tag the journalists by including their Twitter handle (the "@name" users choose to identify themselves in Tweets). Thank them for covering the issue, suggest another angle they might consider, or offer assistance in covering the issue in future stories. When you repost or retweet messages, you are positioning yourself as a source. That means being careful about inadvertently amplifying "fake news" by sharing or responding to it. Nurses can be a resource for journalists, not just to be quoted but to help them understand an issue, interpret statistics and research, access hard-to-reach populations, or develop a frame for covering an issue that may be more aligned with your perspective.

Create Your Own Media Outlet

Whether through blogging, social media posting, or op-ed writing, you can create your own media outlet by consistently sharing your perspectives on policy matters and linking to reliable sources that enhance accurate news, fill knowledge gaps, and counter misinformation. A number of nurses provide models for accomplishing this media work. Rose Hoban is a nurse who became a journalist to improve health reporting (Box 12.2). Two of this chapter's authors (Mason and Glickstein) have produced and hosted radio programs on health for more than 35 years and view this work as their practice as public health nurses. Carole Myers, a professor of nursing at the University of Tennessee at Knoxville, produces podcasts on health policy that are shared through a local NPR radio station. She also blogs and writes op-eds, including for political and policy news outlets such as *The Hill*.

Writing op-eds can be a powerful way to get issues onto the public's agenda or reframe an issue that is already getting attention. As a professor of nursing at Rush University School of Nursing, Mona Shattell writes blogs for the *HuffPost* and other media outlets. She and her dean, Marquis Foreman, brought the Op-ed Project (www.opedproject.org) to the school to teach faculty how to write op-eds, commentaries, and blogs. As of 2018, participants had published 73 op-eds and other commentaries!

Know Your Medium and Your Message

Some approaches for framing and messaging work better for one medium and not another. Getting your message to the appropriate target audience requires careful analysis and planning of who the audience is, what media they use, and what form the messages take. For example, to get television coverage, a visual story works best. See Box 12.3 for guidelines for getting your message across in traditional media.

Debunking Falsehoods and Avoiding "Gotcha" Moments

If you are being interviewed for radio or television, look into the format of the program, approach of the host, and

BOX 12.2   Rose Hoban: The Nurse Is a Journalist

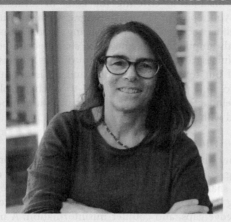

After a decade-plus of full-time nursing, I returned to school in 2000 to get a journalism degree. I was inspired by the bad information I was seeing in the media, and the time I had spent disabusing my patients of falsehoods they had heard on talk television. I got my first full-time job in broadcasting in 2005 as a health reporter for a North Carolina radio station. Informed by my nursing background, I quickly developed a reputation for seeing stories and developing angles other reporters missed.

The internet changed life as we know it, and it undermined the business model of traditional journalism. By 2010, most health reporters in North Carolina had been laid off or bought out or had quit in frustration. Consumers of news lost access to specialty reporting to help them understand complicated health care topics just as the system was undergoing massive change.

I took yet another leap of faith in 2012 (backed by a supportive spouse), launching NC Health News at www.northcarolinahealthnews.org. Our main focus is state health policy. Read by almost every politician and lobbyist in our capital, we have put them on notice that we are holding them accountable for their decisions! We also cover state government, environmental health, mental and rural health, and aging issues; we recently added a reporter to cover the Charlotte region.

As of 2018, we have 6 reporters, 100,000 readers monthly, and won multiple awards. We are launching a syndication service, realizing my initial vision of replacing some of the state's lost health reporting capacity.

---

audience served, and frame your discussion accordingly. During a time of "gotcha" media, be prepared for a host to make outrageous statements as a way of spicing up the interview. Simply bridge back to your key messages with statements such as, "What I know is . . . ." or "That's an interesting thought. What's important is . . . ." Restating an erroneous statement risks further embedding the thought in the minds of the audience. This is particularly important when someone is making claims without evidence to support them.

In some instances, providing an alternative causal account or story rather than refuting information with strong evidence has shown to be an effective way of changing people's opinions (Flynn, Nyhan, & Reifler, 2017). Directly offering corrections to misconceptions or providing a link to a credible third party can also be effective (Vraga & Bode, 2017).

ANALYZING MEDIA

To be credible sources of information, nurses must be skillful at analyzing media communications:

1. Check sources and facts.
   There are numerous online fact-checking sites that hold media producers and yourself accountable when sharing information. Examples include Snopes (www.snopes.com),

the oldest and largest fact checking site online that was launched in 1996; and PolitiFact (www.politifact.com/), a nonprofit that was awarded the Pulitzer Prize for National Reporting in 2009.

2. Consider the medium and who is creating and sending the message.
   Be alert for affiliations and websites that imitate names of recognized sources (mass media, academic, publishers, and so on). If in doubt, go to the website and click "About Us" to find out what the source is, who started it, the mission, and their funding.

3. What is the message and how is it communicated?
   Are certain emotions being provoked (anger, anxiety/fear) that influence interpretation of the information? Are "experts" quoted? One hallmark of a "fake news" story is the absence of quotes from known sources.

4. Is the information accurate? What is being omitted, and why?
   The 2018 Women's Media Center's "Media and #MeToo" report noted that, after October, 2017, the media wrote more news stories about sexual assault and harassment, as well as about reproductive health and the gender wage gap. In October 2017, *The New York Times* and *The New Yorker* published articles about decades of sexual assault allegations against movie producer

BOX 12.3   Guidelines for Getting Your Message Across

The following guidelines will help you to shape your message and get it delivered to the right media.

The Issue
- What is the nature of the issue?
- What is the context (e.g., timing, key stakeholders, history, current political environment)?

The Message
- Why is this relevant, or "so what"? Why does this matter?
- Be concise, focus on the news or novelty, and keep it simple. Is there a story or sound bite that represents the issue in a catchy, memorable or shareable way?
- How can you frame nursing's interests as the public's interests (e.g., as consumers, parents, women, taxpayers, and health professionals)?

The Target Audience
- Who is the target audience: the public, policymakers, or journalists? If the public, which segments?
- What medium is appropriate for the target audience? Does this audience rely on newspapers, TV, radio, or online media for their news?

Access to the Media
- Most journalists receive hundreds of pitches a day. Make your pitch worthwhile. Can you comment on what the reporter covers and pitch them your idea? Is this journalist the right fit? Do you know their format, style, (print, online, or broadcast), and their audience?
- Do you follow the journalist on Twitter? Have you responded directly to them about their recent news article and tagged them in your tweets?
- Research findings could be newsworthy and have significance to the public. It is your job to translate your research into a pitch to the journalist that helps them to sell the idea to their editor. Write in plain English, keep it short and impactful, hook it to a current news story, and include why it is important in the subject line and/or in the first line in your email. It is your job to make the reporter's job easy.

- If you get an interview request, then respond quickly if the answer is "yes." Journalists are often on hard deadlines and will move to the next potential source, so.

The Interview
- You are an expert on the issue, but always prepare up to three major points that you want to get across in the interview. Identify potential controversies, how you would respond to them, and rehearse the interview with a colleague.
- During the interview, be engaging and listening attentively. If on radio or TV, jump in and respond to statements made by the journalist or other guest. Get your primary points across more than once—repetition sticks. When asked questions that do not address your agenda, return the focus to your agenda with finesse and persistence (e.g., "That's an interesting question. What I can tell you is…").
- Come ready with rich, illustrative stories. Avoid yes or no answers.
- You do not have to answer all questions, and if you do not know the answer, say so and offer to get back to the interviewer with the information.
- Avoid being disrespectful or arguing with the interviewer.
- The more prepared you are for an interview, the less nervous you will be. Do not confuse being energized and excited for the media opportunity with being nervous. With the right preparation, you can secure a great piece of media coverage.
- After the interview, tell the journalist that you would be happy to be a source again and help to find other nurse experts for interviews. You can also share other story ideas you may have.

Follow-up
- Write a letter of thanks to the producer or journalist afterward, reinforcing other story ideas you have and your availability for identifying other nurse experts as sources.
- Provide feedback to the producer or journalist on any response you received to the interview, program, or coverage.

Harvey Weinstein. Actress Alyssa Milano encouraged women to share their stories using #MeToo *without* crediting Tarana Burke, an organizer and assault survivor who wanted to help survivors of sexual violence, particularly Black women and girls, and young women of color. Burke spoke out in solidarity with women with the words "Me Too." While Twitter was flooded with #MeToo stories in 2017 and 2018 that resulted in a global movement of women sharing their stories of sexual violence, women of color spoke out about the origins of #MeToo and Tarana Burke, and how once again Black women had been erased from the story.

CONCLUSION

Will another replication of the Woodhull Study in 20 years find changes in nursing's visibility in health news media? Here is our challenge: nurses can and should be leaders in the strategic use of media to shape health policy. As the professionals the public trusts most, nurses can demonstrate the ethical use of media to advance evidence-based policy.

DISCUSSION QUESTIONS

1. What are your main sources of health news? Do an analysis of each source and determine whether you are getting credible and accurate information.
2. What is your digital footprint? What steps can you take to make yourself more visible to journalists as an expert in nursing and health?
3. Evaluate your media skills. What knowledge and skills do you need to develop further to become an effective communicator with media?

REFERENCES

Allcott, H., & Gentzkow, M. (2017). Social media and fake news in the 2016 election. *Journal of Economic Perspectives, 31*(2), 211–236.

Berry, J.M., & Sobieraj, S. (2014). *The outrage industry: Political opinion media and the new incivility.* Oxford: Oxford University Press.

Brenan, M. (2018). *Nurses again outpace other professions for honesty, ethics.* Retrieved from https://news.gallup.com/poll/245597/nurses-again-outpace-professions-honesty-ethics.aspx.

Burton, C.W., McLemore, M.R., Perry, L., Carrick, J., & Shattell, M. (2017). Social media awareness and implications in nursing leadership: A pilot professional meeting campaign. *Policy, Politics and Nursing Practice, 17*(4), 187–197.

Dorfman, L., & Krasnow, I.D. (2014). Public health and media advocacy. *Annual Review of Public Health, 35,* 293–306.

Flynn, D.J., Nyhan, B., & Reifler, J. (2017). The nature and origins of misperceptions: Understanding false and unsupported beliefs about politics. *Political Psychology, 38*(S1), 127–150.

Fung, B. (2017). The FCC just repealed a 42-year-old rule blocking broadcast media mergers. *Washington Post.* Retrieved from www.washingtonpost.com/news/the-switch/wp/2017/11/16/the-fcc-just-repealed-decades-old-rules-blocking-broadcast-media-mergers/?utm_term=.1485351b8363.

Gabler, N. (2016, April 29). *Donald Trump, the emperor of social media.* Retrieved from http://billmoyers.com/story/donald-trump-the-emperor-of-social-media/.

Gennaro, S. (2015). Scientists and social media. *Journal of Nursing Scholarship, 475,* 377–378.

Gramlich, J. (2018). *Five facts about Americans and Facebook.* Retrieved from www.pewresearch.org/fact-tank/2018/04/10/5-facts-about-americans-and-facebook/.

Institute of Medicine. (2011). *The future of nursing: Leading change, advancing health.* Washington, DC: National Academies Press.

Jamieson, K.H. (2018). *Cyberwar: How Russian hackers and trolls helped elect a president— What we don't, can't, and do know.* Oxford, New York: Oxford University Press.

Kliff, S. (2016). *Why Obamacare enrollees voted for Trump.* Retrieved from www.vox.com/science-and-health/2016/12/13/13848794/kentucky-obamacare-trump.

Lazer, D.M.J., et al. (2018). The science of fake news. *Science, 359*(6380), 1094–1096.

Leonard, K. (2015). *Is the 'death panel' debate dead?* Retrieved from www.usnews.com/news/articles/2015/07/09/medicare-rule-revisits-death-panel-issue.

Mason, D.J., Glickstein, B., Nixon, L., Westphaln, K., Han, S., & Acquaviva, K. (2018a). *The Woodhull Study revisited: Nurses' representation in health news media.* Press conference, May 8, 2018, at the National Press Club, Retrieved from https://go.gwu.edu/Woodhull.

Mason, D.J., Glickstein, B., & Westphaln, K. (2018b). Journalists' experiences with using nurses as sources in health news stories. *American Journal of Nursing, 118*(10), 42-50. Retrieved from https://journals.lww.com/ajnonline/Fulltext/2018/10000/Original_Research___Journalists__Experiences_with.24.aspx.

Mason, D.J., Nixon, L., Glickstein, B. Han, S., Westphaln, K. & Carter, L. (2018c). The Woodhull Study revisited: Nurses' representation in health news media twenty years later. *Journal of Nursing Scholarship,50*(6), 695–704. Retrieved from https://sigmapubs.onlinelibrary.wiley.com/doi/full/10.1111/jnu.12429.

Meirick, P.C. (2013) Motivated misperception? Party, education, partisan news, and belief in 'death panels.' *Journalism & Mass Communication Quarterly, 90,* 39–57.

National Council of State Boards of Nursing (2011). *Nurses and social media: Regulatory concerns and guidelines.* Retrieved from www.ncsbn.org/4622.html.

Nyhan, B. (2010). Why the 'death panel' myth wouldn't die: Misinformation in the health care reform debate. *The Forum, 8*(1), 1–24.

Pew Research Center. (2017). *News use across social media platforms 2017.* http://www.journalism.org/2017/09/07/news-use-across-social-media-platforms-2017/.

Pew Research Center. (2018a). *News use across social media platforms 2018.* Retrieved from www.journalism.org/2018/09/10/news-use-across-social-media-platforms-2018/.

Pew Research Center. (2018b). *The public, the political system and American democracy.* Retrieved from www.people-press.org/2018/04/26/the-public-the-political-system-and-american-democracy/.

Pew Research Center. (2018c). *Social media use in 2018.* Retrieved from www.pewinternet.org/2018/03/01/social-media-use-in-2018/.

Polletta, F., & Callahan, J. (2017). Deep stories, nostalgia narratives, and fake news: Storytelling in the Trump era. *American Journal of Cultural Sociology, 5*(3), 392–408.

Polletta, F., Pang, C., Chen, B., Gardner, B.G., & Motes, A. (2011). The sociology of storytelling. *Annual Review of Sociology, 37,* 109–130.

Rapp, N., & Jenkins, A. (2018). Chart: These 6 companies control much of the U.S. media market. *Fortune.* Retrieved from http://fortune.com/longform/media-company-ownership-consolidation/.

Shattell, M., Burton, C.W., & McLemore, M. (2015a). Why nurses need Twitter. *Huffington Post Tech.* Retrieved from www.huffingtonpost.com/entry/why-nurses-need-twitter_b_7013762.html.

Shattell, M., McLemore, M., & Burton, C.W. (2015b). Scientist should contribute to, not shun, social media. *Huffington Post Tech.* Retrieved from www.huffingtonpost.com/entry/scientists-should-contrib_b_8164062.html.

Shattell, M., McLemore, M., & Burton, C.W. (2015c). What are the five best practices for Tweeting from conferences? *Huffington Post Tech.* Retrieved from www.huffingtonpost.com/entry/what-are-the-five-best-pr_b_7065090.html.

Shattell, M., Perry, L., Carrick, J., McLemore, M., & Burton, C.W. (2015d). How to infuse social media into a conference of tech-naive attendees. *Huffington Post Tech.* Retrieved from www.huffingtonpost.com/entry/how-to-infuse-social-media-into-a-conference-of-tech-naive-attendees_b_8712118.html.

Shearer, E. (2018). *Social media outpaces print newspapers in the U.S. as a news source.* Retrieved from www.pewresearch.org/fact-tank/2018/12/10/social-media-outpaces-print-newspapers-in-the-u-s-as-a-news-source/.

Silverman, C. (2016). *Here are 50 of the biggest fake news hits on Facebook from 2016.* Retrieved from www.buzzfeed.com/craigsilverman/top-fake-news-of-2016%3Futm_term%3D.vd7XmJPDq%23.wy0kgrobN?utm_term=.kdW4dPWjMw#.ncjvPKOB3j.

Silverman, C., Feder, J.L., Cvetkovska, S., & Belford, A. (2018, July 18). *Macedonia's pro-Trump fake news industry had American links, and is under investigation for possible Russia ties.* Retrieved from www.buzzfeednews.com/article/craigsilverman/american-conservatives-fake-news-macedonia-paris-wade-libert.

Silverman, C. & Singer-Vine, J. (2016). *Most Americans who see fake news believe it, new survey says.* Retrieved from www.buzzfeed.com/craigsilverman/fake-news-survey?utm_term=.dpVYQ5wGb1#.ki0dEQ51wW.

Statista, the Statistics Portal. (2018). *Most famous social network sites worldwide as of April 2018, ranked by number of active users.* Retrieved from www.statista.com/statistics/272014/global-social-networks-ranked-by-number-of-users/.

Sunstein, C.R. (2018). *# Republic: Divided democracy in the age of social media.* Princeton, NJ: Princeton University Press.

Vraga, E.K., & Bode, L. (2017). I do not believe you: How providing a source corrects health misperceptions across social media platforms. *Information, Communication & Society, 21*(10), 1337–1353.

Wallack, L., & Dorfman, L. (1996). Media advocacy: A strategy for advancing policy and promoting health. *Health Education Quarterly, 23*(3), 293–317.

Women's Media Center. (2018). *Media and #MeToo: How a movement affected press coverage of sexual assault.* Retrieved from www.womensmediacenter.com/reports/media-and-metoo-how-a-movement-affected-press-coverage-of-sexual-assault.

13

TAKING ACTION: Billboards and a Social Media Campaign

Monica R. McLemore

"The time is always right to do what is right."

Dr. Martin Luther King, Jr.

My nursing colleagues see it outside the abortion clinics where they work. My colleagues in reproductive health research see it in the ethically and scientifically questionable "reports" sent across their desks for comment. And as an educator, I see it infiltrating the very institution we rely on to provide continuing education to practicing nurses. The administration of progesterone to halt abortion after a patient has taken the first pill (mifepristone) in the medication abortion protocol is an untested and unproven practice that antiabortion extremists are calling "abortion reversal." Even Scott Lloyd, who served as Director of the Office of Refugee Resettlement in the Trump Administration, suggested that an undocumented pregnant teen in Texas could be made to "reverse" her much wanted and delayed medication abortion in this way (Sherman, 2018).

Despite the fact that this "reversal" procedure has not been proven to be effective—nor rigorously determined to be safe or harmful—antiabortion advocates stand outside abortion clinics evangelizing "reversal" to patients. They are also working to pass bills that would require providers to tell patients that it is a real option and have mounted a campaign to provide continuing education programs to teach "reversal" through the California Board of Registered Nursing (BRN). Crisis Pregnancy Centers (CPCs) have led the advocacy for medication abortion reversal, and the California BRN unknowingly legitimized this untested and unethical practice by certifying courses teaching this to nurses without considering that the content was not evidence based. Inadvertently, BRN officials did not realize that this approval has implications across the country, because 13 other state boards of nursing rely on the California BRN for the provision of continuing education credits.

CPCs, also known as "fake clinics," are mostly unlicensed (approximately 25% of CPCs in California are licensed as clinical facilities) and do not provide comprehensive, evidence-based reproductive health services. For example, despite pregnancy testing and ultrasound provision, prenatal care is not offered in most; nor are abortion or contraception services or referrals. They have been cited for using deceptive and coercive practices to delay or deny care to people seeking pregnancy-related care, including abortion and prenatal care (Wasko, 2018). A healthy dose of skepticism is warranted when it comes to whether they have women's best interest in mind.

CPCs assert that patients who seek abortion care have not arrived at a thoughtful decision, and that the physicians, nurses, and clinic staff who care for them have not fulfilled their legal obligation to provide fact-based information about and access to medication abortion reversal. However, the evidence base for medication abortion reversal is not strong; its efficacy and safety have not been established; and clear protocols have not been published. The decision-making process around whether to continue or end a pregnancy requires true *informed consent*. Building trusting and therapeutic relationships between patients and providers requires transparent discussions of factual information—not politically motivated, medically unproven claims.

In October of 2017, I shared a crazy idea I had with the board and staff of the Abortion Care Network (ACN) that has changed my life and my work. I had joined the ACN board and wanted to get right to work. I asked at a board meeting, "Could we use public service announcements, billboards, or some other type of traditional media to provide evidence-based information to the public?" The ACN is a membership organization of the independent clinics (both for-profit and not-for-profit) that provide the bulk of abortion care in the United States. At that time, we knew the Supreme Court was set to hear a case from California in Spring 2018 that would be argued by Attorney General Xavier Becerra regarding if CPCs could continue to lie to patients and communities about what services they offer or do not. The case, brought by the National Institute of Family and Life Advocates (NIFLA), made a first amendment free speech claim that their rights were violated by having to comply with the California Reproductive Freedom, Accountability, Comprehensive Care, and Transparency (FACT) Act (Chiu, 2015). According to their website, NIFLA "exists to protect life affirming pregnancy centers that empower abortion-vulnerable women and families to choose life for their unborn children" (NIFLA, 2018). The FACT Act requires licensed clinical facilities to provide the full range of pregnancy options to patients (i.e., abortion, adoption, contraception, and parenting) and to identify whether it is a licensed clinical facility.

In January 2018, we launched "Uniting Our Voices: Communications and Media Support for Independent Abortion Care Providers," a silent online and email campaign, asking the public to stand with us and patients for evidence-based care and to sign a petition on ending abortion deception. On February 5, 2018, six billboards went up around the Bay Area stating, "Patients need medically accurate information: Not politically motivated deception about abortion." And I was on the billboard as the expert! The press coverage was incredible, including Ms. Blog, Politico, Sacramento Bee, The Oakland Tribune/East Bay Examiner, and several others.

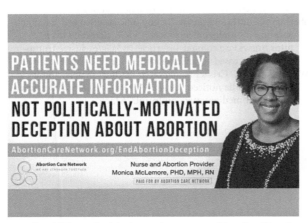

The first billboard with the author, created by the Abortion Care Network.

After hearing from advocates, activists, and clinicians, the California BRN proposed a change in language at its quarterly meeting on February 15, 2018, on criteria required for courses to meet approval for continuing

education credits. After a closed session, the California BRN decided to examine all criteria for continuing education and stated they would present new language at the end of 2018. Who knew when we started this campaign that we would have access to members of the public whom we could call upon to help us make change?

Coincidentally, at the end of this phase of the campaign, a landmark report was released from the National Academy of Science, Engineering, and Medicine (2018) on *The Safety and Quality of Abortion in the United States,* the first in 20 years to assess the current scientific findings and summarize the existing evidence on abortion using widely accepted standards of safety and quality. The study found that abortion is safe; quality services can be offered in a variety of settings; and current restrictions to abortion are not based in evidence, nor do they improve patient safety. Although CPCs are not specifically mentioned in the report, specific state regulations that target abortion providers and not CPCs are mentioned, as well as the importance of informed consent, patient access to care, and the time-sensitive nature of pregnancy decision making—the pinnacle of why access to fact-based information and identification of legitimate health clinics are important.

Fast forward to June 2018, when the decision in *NIFLA vs. Becerra* is released, written by Justice Clarence Thomas, in support of the NIFLA claims. The Supreme Court of the United States stated that it would constitute a violation of free speech rights for CPCs to have to provide a full range of options for pregnant people. In other words, CPCs would not have to abide by the same rules that licensed clinical facilities are held to unless the CPC is one of the 25% that are also a licensed facility. This decision, along with the 2019 changes to Title X (the federally funded family planning program) and the appointment of Brent Kavanaugh to the Supreme Court, inspired us to retool the campaign away from medication abortion reversal to a more general message that patients need care they can trust.

The purpose behind the new campaign, launched in August 2018, is to provide fact-based information to people seeking care. The ACN landing page provides geographic maps of independent abortion, family planning, and referrals for the full range of pregnancy options on their website, as well as links to report fake clinics. The new billboards were streamlined in messaging but retained the same graphics and were purposively placed in Sacramento and Fresno, California near CPCs where access to health centers for any abortion, adoption, or pregnancy-related care is limited. I hope that the people most impacted by both abortion restrictions and the closure of pregnancy services—low-income and Black women—will be able to use the billboards and the landing page of the ACN to get fact-based information to whatever pregnancy-related services they are seeking.

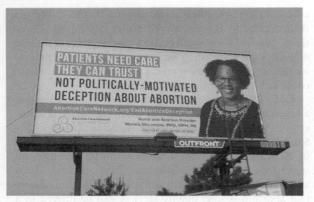

The second billboard created by the Abortion Care Network.

In February 2018, the California BRN voted to seek a regulatory change to modify the California Code of Regulations, Article 4, Section 1456 that governs continuing education courses under the California Nurse Practice Act. In December 2018 a draft of a comprehensive plan for overhauling the continuing education programs was discussed at the California BRN meeting and the approved plan is due to the legislature on January 1, 2019. I look forward to the California BRN open comment period in 2019 on their new requirements for courses that grant continuing education. I will work with ACN to ensure that those who signed on to the #EndAbortionDeception silent social media campaign will be notified so they can comment.

Nurses are extremely underrepresented in the media (Mason et al., 2018) and need to leverage the trust the public places in us and our profession to assist them to get the fact-based information they need to make the best decisions in their lives. People ask me all the time, "Have you had to deal with protesters?" "Have you been harassed?" I am proud to report that, to my knowledge, I have had no fallout from doing this. In fact, I have had an outpouring

of support and awe from nurses, other health professionals, and the public all over the country. There was a healthy debate both within the ACN board and with my academic and clinical employers about the positive and negative consequences for such a public campaign. More specifically, questions ranged from perceived bias in my scientific work, to fear for my physical safety in participating in such a public campaign. Ultimately, I landed on the principles from American Nurses Association Code of Ethics that inform my professional responsibilities—that patients have a right to self-determination and that part of self-determination is providing people with fact-based information then supporting them to make informed decisions about their health and their lives. Pregnant people and childbearing families are the experts in their own lives and deserve the full range of options and information to make those decisions. I hope you will join me in speaking out when we see injustices that fly in the face of safe and quality care.

REFERENCES

Chiu, D. (2015). *Reproductive Fact Act (AB775)*. Retrieved from https://leginfo.legislature.ca.gov/faces/billTextClient.xhtml?bill_id=201520160AB775.

National Academies of Sciences, Engineering, and Medicine. (2018). *The safety and quality of abortion care in the United States*. Washington, DC: The National Academies Press.

National Institute of Family and Life Advocates. (2018). *About NIFLA*. Retrieved from https://nifla.org/about-nifla/.

Sherman, C. (2018). Exclusive: Trump officials discussed "reversing abortion for undocumented teen." *VICE*. Retrieved from https://news.vice.com/en_us/article/yw5a5g/exclusive-trump-officials-discussed-reversing-abortion-for-undocumented-teen.

Wasko, S. (2018). Crisis Pregnancy center hurt people, and it's time the media noticed. *Media Matters for America*. Retrieved from www.mediamatters.org/print/763566.

14

Health Policy, Politics, and Professional Ethics

Carol R. Taylor and Susan I. Belanger

"To see what is right and not do it is want of courage."

Confucius

Writing in the *Encyclopedia of Bioethics,* Dan Callahan, one of the founders of U.S. bioethics, states that three paramount human questions lie at the heart of bioethics:

- What kind of person ought I be to live a moral life and make good ethical decisions?
- What are my duties and obligations to other individuals whose life and well-being may be affected by my actions?
- What do I owe the common good or the public interest in my life as a member of society?

The authors of this chapter believe that too few nurses take seriously their responsibilities as citizens, in spite of being frequently reminded that their sheer numbers as the largest group of health professionals (3.1 million) and as the public's most trusted professionals (Gallup, 2018), make us a formidable force. Ethics may be defined as the formal study of who we ought to be, how we should make decisions and behave, in light of our identity. This chapter centers around what it is reasonable to expect of professional nurses as citizens in regard to designing and delivering a just health system that meets the needs of all, with special concern for the most vulnerable.

Designing a system for delivering health care that adequately meets the needs of a diverse public is a complex challenge. Health care planners have always worried about access, quality, and cost. Who should get what quality of care and at what cost? What you think about health care in the United States largely depends on your past experiences. If you are well insured or independently wealthy, you can access the best health care in the world. If you lack insurance and have limited financial resources, you may die of a disease that might have been prevented or treated at an early stage if you had had access to quality care. The U.S. system has been criticized for providing too little care to some and too much of the wrong type of care to others. Many now believe that a moral society owes health care to its citizens. Health care is like clean water, sanitation, and basic education. Others believe that health care is a commodity, like automobiles, to be sold and purchased in the marketplace. If you lack the funds to buy a car, that may be unfortunate, but society has no obligation to purchase a car for you. As you read this chapter, ask yourself what you believe about health care. Is it simply unfortunate if people cannot afford the health care they and their families need?

People's health, well-being, and dying, as well as our daily nursing practice, are directly affected by decisions made by governments, insurers, and health care institutions. Nursing needs a seat at these decision-making tables, and nurses must be prepared and willing to take these seats. As the country's most trusted health care professionals, the nurses in these seats must be committed to ethical decision making. Drivers for much of human enterprise are power, position, prestige, profit, and politics (Barnet, n.d.). Strikingly absent from this list are people, patients, the public, and the poor! Nursing's challenge, as profits and politics increasingly dictate health priorities, is to keep health care strongly focused on the needs of patients, their families, and the public. Health care in the United States is a business, revenues need to be generated to make care possible, but health care can never be *only* a business. First and primarily, it is a service a moral society provides for its vulnerable members. Our relationships with patients are fiduciary, not merely contractual. Nurses play a critical role in keeping health care centered on the people it purports to serve.

This chapter opens with a description of the ethics of influencing policy and explores the professional ethics of nurses and their advocacy and health policy responsibilities. It offers a brief analysis of how nurses can use their voice to influence policy regarding scarce resource allocations and workplace issues. Throughout, short reflective practice vignettes invite readers to reflect on the adequacy of their moral agency in selecting and responding to advocacy challenges.

THE ETHICS OF INFLUENCING POLICY

An ethical critique of human behavior involves paying attention to the intention of the moral agent, the nature of the act performed, the consequences of the action, and the circumstances surrounding the act. Ethics has to do with right and wrong in this world, and policy and politics has everything to do with what happens to people in this world. Moreover, both ethics and politics have to do with making life better for oneself and others. Surely both deal with power and powerlessness, with human rights and balancing claims, with justice and fairness, and with good and evil. And good and evil are not the same as right and wrong. Right and wrong pertain to adherence to principles; good and evil pertain to the intent of the doer and the impact the deed has on other people. Surely policy and politics involves justice in the distribution of social goods; fairness and equity in relationships among and between people of different races, genders, and creeds; and access to education and assistance when one is in need. Although the goodness of an action lies in the intent and integrity of the human being who performs it, the rightness or wrongness of an action is judged by the difference it makes in the world. Therefore the principles applied in ethical analysis generally derive from a consideration of the duties one person owes another by virtue of commitments made and roles assumed, and/or a consideration of the effects that a choice of action could have on one's own life and the lives of others.

In a perfect world, legislators would all intend the good of the public they serve and use ethical means to achieve good outcomes. In the real world, legislators and lobbyists intend many things other than the good of the public and some use unethical means to achieve dubious ends. A democracy with an increasingly heterogeneous public necessarily involves compromise. Which strategies to influence policy can nurses use without sacrificing personal and professional integrity? Each advocacy strategy involves a variation of the same question—that is, what means can be legitimately used to achieve an end that someone (or a political party or the electorate) believes to be good? Should we assure the passage of health care insurance reform (a good end) by strong-arm tactics (an evil means)?

The price we pay for freedom and human rights is to grant them to all people, not just a favored few. And yes, it is risky and it may reduce our "efficiency," and in some cases it may even lead to loss of life, but the alternative is that no one has rights (i.e., just claims); rights become the privilege of a favored group, whereas all other individuals are utterly helpless before the power of the state.

Certainly the electorate does not consent to the corruption of the legislative process, and even if a majority did approve of bending the rules of fair engagement to ensure that a particular piece of legislation is passed, would that make it right? Would it not end up threatening the very foundations of a free society (because the foundation of a republic lies in the honesty of its processes)? What are the differences between normal legislative wrangling and abuse of power? What does it mean when political parties refuse to participate in the legislative process and/or use blatant scare tactics? What is legitimate dissent, and what is a refusal to accept democratic outcomes unless you happen to agree with them? Without civil disobedience, we would still have the Jim Crow laws. And without respect for the law, a society degenerates into either despotism or anarchy.

What is a true difference of judgment about what would benefit society versus knowingly lying to deceive the public to achieve a political end? Why do we now have numerous resources to uncover media bias and to fact check? When people ask whether it is wrong to lie about something (e.g., the number of people affected by a particular disease) to get funding for research and/or treatment of patients with a particular disease, in a word the answer is yes. It is wrong. Why is lying wrong? It's wrong because it undermines the foundation of any relationship: trust. Trust is the fabric that holds society together. In like manner, lying to further a political agenda is wrong not only because it undermines trust, but also because it fosters further dishonesty. Judging by the amount of political dishonesty reported in the media, one is led to the conclusion that there is a lot of lying going on! Adding to it, telling more lies to further our own agenda will only make matters worse.

Reflective Practice: Pants on Fire

Sarah Palin is famous for urging her supporters to oppose Democratic plans for health care using the scare tactic of death panels. She said the Democrats plan to reduce health care costs by simply refusing to pay for care:

> And who will suffer the most when they ration care? The sick, the elderly, and the disabled, of course. The America I know and love is not one in which my parents or my baby with Down Syndrome will have to stand in front of Obama's death panel so his bureaucrats can decide, based on a subjective judgment of their level of productivity in society, whether they are worthy of health care. Such a system is downright evil.

In fact, there was no panel in any version of the health care bills in Congress to judge a person's level of productivity in society to determine whether they are worthy of health care.

The truth is that the proposed health bill would have allowed Medicare, for the first time, to pay for optional doctors' appointments for patients to discuss living wills and other end-of-life issues with their physicians. Politi-Fact awarded Palin with the 2009 Lie of the Year for the death panel claim and it made the list of FactCheck's "whoppers," but the political impact of her statement is hard to overstate. In 2011, the Obama administration even deleted all references to end-of-life planning in a new Medicare regulation when opponents interpreted the move as a back-door effort to allow such planning. So even in the regulations, Palin achieved her goal (Holan, 2009).

1. How do you judge Palin's quote? Effective strategy to oppose Democrats' plans for health care reform or unethical scaremongering?
2. Reflect on what informs your judgment: commitment to advance care planning, analysis of facts, political party loyalties?
3. Is it right for nurses to endorse health reform legislation even if the legislation is not perfect? (The answer is yes; it may indeed be the right thing to do.)

Remember, politics is about relationships, and relationships cannot prosper when one party insists that the other party must agree with them on every (or even any) issue. It is not wrong to compromise; compromise is part of the give and take of relationships, and it is part of the give and take of politics. What is critical is knowing when it is possible to compromise without sacrificing personal integrity. This prompts the question of whether it can be acceptable to distort an issue to manipulate public opinion or to win the support of a particular piece of legislation. It is usually, however, possible to frame a discussion in a manner that is more acceptable to a certain constituency without lying in this manner. For example, in the health care arena, one can use words that appeal to known values, words such as tradition and legitimate authority (words that tend to appeal to conservatives), and words such as autonomous and experimental (words that tend to appeal to liberals). Knowing the target audience and framing the issue in words that will help them listen (or at least not harden their opposition) is smart, not unethical.

Any professional group has a duty to push forward laws and policies that protect or advance the best interests of those whom they serve. And any citizen, particularly a knowledgeable one, has a civic duty to speak out for the common good.

PROFESSIONAL ETHICS AND MORAL AGENCY

A professional ethic is built around three essential components: its purpose, the conduct expected of the professional, and the skills and outcomes expected in professional practice. Society demands that professionals be held to a separate moral standard of conduct because the choices professionals make affect other people's lives more than their own. Nursing's foundational documents make each nurse's advocacy and health policy responsibilities clear. Although some may think that advocacy and health policy are an ethical ideal, they are rather a nonnegotiable moral obligation embedded in the nursing role. The American Nurses Association (ANA) *Code of Ethics for Nurses* states: "The nurse promotes, advocates for, and protects the rights, health, and safety of the patient" (2015). Provision 8 of the code, reflecting the stronger emphasis of the 2015 edition on nursing's advocacy responsibilities, reads: "The nurse collaborates with other health professionals and the public to protect human rights, promote health diplomacy, and reduce health disparities." ANA's *Social Policy Statement: The Essence of the Profession* was published in 1980 and revised in 1995, 2003, and 2010. The introduction to the 2003 revision emphasizes nurses' central role in effecting health policy.

Nursing is the pivotal health care profession, highly valued for its specialized knowledge, skill, and caring in improving the health status of the public and ensuring safe, effective, quality care. The profession mirrors the diverse population it serves and provides leadership to create positive changes in health policy and delivery systems (p. 1).

The 2003 revision also included for the first time in its list of values and assumptions of nursing's social contract, "Public policy and the health care delivery system influence the health and well-being of society and professional nursing" (p. 4). This phrase appears again in the 2010 revision under the heading, "The elements of nursing's social contract" (p. 6). The 2010 revision also notes as a key social concern in health care and nursing "Expansion of health care resources and health policy" (p. 4).

Once professional nurses understand what is reasonable for the public to expect of them, the next step is to determine if one has the capacity to meet these expectations—that is, "Am I trustworthy?" Moral agency is quite simply the ability to be what is professed: a human, a parent, a professional nurse. Moral agency in any specific situation requires more than knowing what is the right thing to do; it also entails moral character, moral valuing, moral sensibility, moral responsiveness, ethical reasoning and discernment, moral accountability, and transformative moral leadership (Taylor, 2019).

Nurses who value their moral agency are familiar with the principles of bioethics which commit them, all things being equal, to (1) respect the autonomy of individuals, (2) act so as to benefit (beneficence), (3) not harm (non-maleficence), and (4) give individuals their due (justice). Other principles include keeping promises (fidelity) and responsiveness to vulnerability. A commitment to social justice and the common good has long characterized the profession of nursing. This commitment calls for the creation of a society in which all can flourish, not only the affluent, and the creation of a bottom floor, beneath which no one can fall regarding access to basic nutrition, safe housing, education, health care, and employment.

Reflective Practice: Negotiating Conflicts Between Personal Integrity and Professional Responsibilities

Shortly after the Department of Health and Human Services (HHS) announced the new federal rule that required all new private plans to cover prescribed Food and Drug Administration (FDA)–approved contraceptive methods without cost-sharing, a number of corporations sued, claiming that this new requirement violates their religious rights. These lawsuits have worked their way through the federal courts and on November 26, 2013, the Supreme Court agreed to hear two cases that involved for-profit corporations. The court agreed to hear a case from the Tenth Circuit Court of Appeals, which ruled in favor of Hobby Lobby, an Oklahoma-based chain of craft stores owned by a Christian family who claim that the contraceptive coverage requirement violates their company's religious freedom. The court also agreed to hear a case from the Third Circuit Court of Appeals, which ruled against the corporation and its owners, finding that Conestoga Wood Specialties, a cabinet manufacturer, does not have religious rights. The Supreme Court decided to take these cases to resolve the conflict between the two decisions along with other U.S. Courts of Appeals rulings (Sobel & Salganicoff, 2013).

1. You are a women's health nurse practitioner and are asked to collaborate on filing an amicus brief to the court supporting women's rights to free approved contraceptive methods. From your practice, you know how important women's accessibility to these methods are and have sat with many a tearful woman contemplating an unplanned pregnancy. You are Christian, however, and you support your church's stance on not using contraceptive methods. You feel torn between maintaining your personal integrity and fulfilling your nursing obligation to aid poor women without access to basic reproductive services. How will you reconcile your conflict?

2. Similarly, you believe that abortion is wrong, period. Life is a gift from God and not ours to initiate or terminate. That said, you understand that some women make tragic choices about ending a pregnancy and don't want to see them have to revert to back alley providers or coat hangers. You are torn about whether or not to vote for political candidates who are intent on eliminating funding for Planned Parenthood and passive restrictive legislation to drastically decrease access to safe abortion providers. You are actually surprised to see these efforts snowballing in your conservative state. You fully appreciate that the ANA Code of Ethics for nurses states that nurses have a duty to self-care that includes maintaining wholeness of character and integrity and your faith commitments are central to your identity as a Christian and integrity. As a nurse, you also understand your duties to patients. What will inform your vote?

3. If your state legalizes assisted suicide and authorizes nurse practitioners to write lethal prescriptions, should every qualified nurse practitioner be obligated to honor patient requests? What if the nurse for religious or other reasons believes that this is unethical? Should the ANA Code of Ethics for Nurses be changed to allow nurses to participate in assisted suicide? If you believe the answer is yes, how could you help to bring about this change?

Reflective Practice: Conscientious Objection

In January 2018, HHS announced the formation of a Conscience and Religious Freedom Division in its Office for Civil Rights with the goal to "protect the fundamental and unalienable rights of conscience and religious freedom" (HHS.gov). As nurses, we have long been aware of our right to opt out of processes or procedures that violate our conscience or religious values. These acts may include assisting in a surgical abortion, participating in assisted suicide, withdrawing life-sustaining treatments, deceiving patients, or administering blood products. The basis for this right of refusal is the protection of our moral integrity as health professionals and the preservation of our autonomy as individuals (Lewis-Newby et al., 2015). Moral integrity is a highly desirable professional trait and acting against our beliefs would constitute a form of self-betrayal or loss of self-respect (Magelssen, 2012). Provision 5.4 of the Code of Ethics for Nurses (2015) supports nursing's right to act with moral courage but likewise identifies corresponding obligations. As professional nurses, knowing our obligations to patients in the situation of conscientious objection (CO), will help ensure compliance with ethical standards.

An important deliberation in a claim of CO is the impact on those affected by our decision. Most significant is the question of harm. Magelssen (2012) points out four types of burdens to patients: (1) delay in care, (2) restricted access to treatment, (3) lack of information, and (4) a patient's sense of moral disapproval for hir or her choices. Will my decision harm my patient? If so, how can I mitigate or reduce the harm? The more life-threatening a situation, the less acceptable it is for a professional to refuse to treat, especially if the care can't be transferred to a competent colleague. We must also remember that under no circumstances should CO be based on medically irrelevant factors such as race, gender, religion, or sexual orientation. Doing so represents invidious discrimination, which is prohibited by law and discouraged by the *Code of Ethics for Nurses* (ANA, 2015; Lewis-Newby, 2015). As professionals, we are obligated to maintain patient safety, avoid patient abandonment, and ensure proper care is available.

1. Do health care settings where you work have policies on CO?
2. As the nurse leader of a mother-baby nursing unit, you receive a report that your newest employee is refusing to educate her patient on a new contraceptive medication. The nurse claims it's against her religious beliefs to do so. How would you address the situation? Which obligation should trump and why—the nurse's duty to provide a standard of care or the nurse's duty to protect her moral integrity?
3. Many ethicists believe protecting the moral integrity of clinicians may result in changes to professional norms and practices. What changes would you like to see?

U.S. HEALTH CARE REFORM

Put yourself in the shoes of a nurse working in a busy inner city emergency room. Every day he discharges patients with instructions for follow-up treatment that he knows will never happen because of a lack of financial or personal resources. His choices seem to be to stop caring in order not to experience frustration or distress, to show up for work like a robot and do his job, or to find meaning and purpose in working collaboratively to change the system.

A just and caring society provides for the health care needs of its people. Comparative studies of peer nations' health systems have documented that the United States is the most costly but consistently underperforms in most dimensions of a high-performance health system, including quality, access, equity, and healthy lives (Davis, Schoen, & Stremkis, 2010; Institute of Medicine, 2013). Included as factors linked to the U.S. disadvantage are inadequate health care, unhealthy behaviors, and adverse economic and social conditions. "The tragedy is not that the United States is losing a contest with other countries, but that

Americans are dying and suffering from illness and injury at rates that are demonstrably unnecessary" (Woolf & Aron, 2013).

Any discussion of health care access must include a review of human rights and a discussion of whether or not there is such a thing as a human right to health care services, and whether or not a just society would provide a legal right to such services. A human right is a justice claim to an essential, universal human need. The justice of the claim is affected by (1) the universality of the need, (2) the extent to which a person can meet his or her own needs, and (3) the extent to which others can help meet these needs without compromising their own fundamental needs. Some argue that health care services, or at least illness care services, are not a human right; however, a far larger number think that such needs can easily meet each of these criteria, at least under a variety of circumstances. For almost a century, presidents and members of Congress have tried and failed to provide universal health benefits to Americans. There are a few simple facts that are important: (1) the United States is the only developed country in the world that does not offer some type of universal health care; (2) each year tens of thousands of Americans lose their health care coverage caused by circumstances beyond their control; and (3) the main reason that Americans file bankruptcy is outstanding medical bills. The ANA website chronicles nurses' decades-long efforts to advocate for health care reforms that would guarantee access to high-quality health care for all.

Reflective Practice: Accepting the Challenge

The Affordable Care Act (ACA) has been challenged at every turn. In 2018, Congress and President Trump's administration remained focused on undoing benefits achieved by the ACA, including coverage of pre-existing conditions. Some Democrats talked about a single payer system—an option that President Obama couldn't even get the Senate to discuss in open floor dialogues.

1. You have mixed feelings about the ACA. You come from a family who greatly distrust big government and want the Act repealed. As a public health nurse you interact with families everyday who are complaining about difficulties enrolling in their state's online health insurance program. You've read about the successes some have had by contacting navigators in the governor's Office of Health Reform, but you know that many don't know how to initiate this contact. Are you obligated to do all you can to get coverage for the public you serve even if this means setting aside your political commitments?

Reflective Practice: Your State Turned Down Medicaid Expansion

As part of the ACA's broader effort to ensure health insurance coverage for all U.S. residents, the federal government from 2014 to 2017 has agreed to pay for 100% of the difference between a state's current Medicaid eligibility level and the ACA minimum. States that participate in the ACA expansion must provide Medicaid coverage to all state residents below a certain income level. As of January 2017, 33 states and the District of Columbia were expanding Medicaid (The Advisory Board Company, 2014). Dickman and colleagues (2014) reported that the Supreme Court's decision to allow states to opt out of Medicaid expansion would have adverse health and financial consequences. Based on recent data from the Oregon Health Insurance Experiment, they predicted that many low-income women would forego recommended breast and cervical cancer screening; people with diabetes would forego medications; and all low-income adults would face a greater likelihood of depression, catastrophic medical expenses, and death. Disparities in access to care based on state of residence will increase. Because the federal government will pay 100% of increased costs associated with Medicaid expansion for the first three years (and 90% thereafter), opt-out states are also turning down billions of dollars of potential revenue, which might strengthen their local economy.

1. You practice in a mobile van that serves poor children and families in the inner city. You have seen many media stories about families who are receiving badly needed health care for the first time in their lives because they now have coverage. You are exasperated with your state representatives who have repeatedly blocked efforts to expand Medicaid and worry about your state's ability to pay the costs of Medicaid in the future. You have personal knowledge of corruption within your state's current administration and are wondering if you should go public with your knowledge or feed it to the opposite party to ensure that current leaders will not be re-elected. What do you do?

ALLOCATING SCARCE RESOURCES

Health care resources are limited. No system has the financial resources to provide the best care to everyone in all situations (Hope, Reynolds, & Griffiths, 2002). Therefore, we look to the principles of distributive justice for answers.

Principles of Distributive Justice

Health care professionals, who are ideally situated to make microdistributive decisions and whose social role enables them to speak with authority to the general population about the impact of resource allocation decisions on the health and welfare of various segments of the population, must not allow social decisions to influence their clinical decisions. First, their ethical codes require, and for good reason, that health care professionals act in the best interests of the person on whom they are laying hands. Second, the will of the citizenry, as expressed through the votes of their elected representatives, should determine the distribution of the resources they have so diligently (if unwillingly) supplied to their governments. In general, the principles of distributive justice ought to be used to guide decision making at the sociopolitical levels. They are as follows:

1. *To each the same thing.* One of the simplest principles of distributive justice is that of strict or radical equality. The principle says that every person should have the same level of material goods and services.

2. *To each according to his need.* Rawls proposes the following two principles of justice: (1) each person has an equal claim to a fully adequate scheme of equal basic rights and liberties, and (2) social and economic inequalities are "to be to the greatest benefit of the least advantaged members of society" (Rawls, 1993, pp. 5–6). These principles give fairly clear guidance on what type of arguments will count as justifications for inequality. For example, the second principle would accept income disparities if these led to the greatest benefit to the least advantaged members of society (created job opportunities for the least well off) but would not support the rich getting richer at the expense of the poor.

3. *To each according to his ability to compete in the open marketplace.* Locke argued that people deserve to have those items produced by their toil and industry, the products (or the value thereof) being a fitting reward for their effort. His underlying idea was to guarantee to individuals the fruits of their own labor and abstinence. According to some contemporary theorists (Feinberg, 1970), people freely apply their abilities and talents, in varying degrees, to socially productive work. People come to deserve varying levels of income by providing goods and services desired by others (Feinberg, 1970). Distributive systems are just insofar as they distribute incomes according to the different levels earned or deserved by the individuals in the society for their productive labors, efforts, or contributions.

4. *To each according to his merits (desserts).* Merit-based principles of distribution differ primarily according to what they identify as the basis for deserving. Most contemporary proposals regarding merit fit into one of three broad categories (Miller, 1976, 1989):
   - *Contribution:* People should be rewarded for their work activity according to the value of their contribution to the social product.

- *Effort:* People should be rewarded according to the effort they expend in their work activity.
- *Compensation:* People should be rewarded according to the costs they incur in their work activity.

Reflective Practice: Barriers to the Treatment of Mental Illness

Austin Deeds, the son of Virginia State Senator Creigh Deeds, was discharged home in November 2013 from a Virginia hospital emergency room because there were no open psychiatric beds. He then stabbed his father and killed himself. The tragedy focused national attention on the need for a major investment in the nation's mental health system. In a 2008 report, Treatment Advocacy Center (TAC) found 17 public psychiatric beds per 100,000 U.S. citizens, down from 340 beds per 100,000 in 1955 (Torrey et al., n.d.). Although effective assisted outpatient treatment (AOT) programs are available in 45 states, TAC reports that implementation of AOT is often incomplete or inconsistent because of legal, clinical, official, or personal barriers to treatment. The center lists the following clinical barriers to treatment: (1) hospitals, physicians, and mental health professionals who are unaware of the laws and/or don't know how to use them and (2) identification mechanisms that would enable hospital emergency rooms, law enforcement, and others to immediately recognize individuals under court-ordered outpatient treatment. Official barriers include perceived or projected fiscal impacts on local government, shortage of public personnel with knowledge or training in implementing the laws, opposition by the mental health officials charged with implementing the laws and standards, and opposition from tax-funded protection and advocacy groups (TAC, 2014).

In 2018, the Centers for Disease Control and Prevention (CDC) reported that suicide rates in the United States have risen nearly 30% since 1999 and that underrecognized and untreated mental health conditions are one of several factors contributing to suicide. Unless states begin using a comprehensive evidence-based public health approach to prevent suicide risk before it occurs, identify and support persons at risk, prevent reattempts, and help friends and family members in the aftermath of a suicide, we can expect these numbers to increase (Stone, Simon, Fowler, et al. 2018).

Reflection Question

1. You chair a local chapter of the Emergency Nurses Association and practice in an inner city hospital serving a large number of individuals with mental health impairments in a state without an outpatient treatment program. You would like your chapter to address everyday challenges procuring mental health and psychiatric care in your state.

How can you leverage your health policy responsibilities for this population and bring about needed change?

HEALTH CARE DISPARITIES

Reverend Martin Luther King is often quoted as saying that of all the forms of inequality, injustice in health care is the most shocking and inhumane (1966). Some nurses can identify with Bill Gates when he noted during his 2007 commencement speech at Harvard:

> I left Harvard with no real awareness of the awful inequities in the world—the appalling disparities of health, and wealth, and opportunity that condemn millions of people to lives of despair. . . . But humanity's greatest advances are not in its discoveries—but in how those discoveries are applied to reduce inequity. Whether through democracy, strong public education, quality health care, or broad economic opportunity—reducing inequity is the highest human achievement.

Let's define a few terms:
- **Health equity:** This means efforts to ensure that all people have full and equal access to opportunities that enable them to lead healthy lives. No one should be denied this chance because of who they are or their socioeconomic opportunities (Health Equity Institute: http://healthequity.sfsu.edu/content/defining-health-equity).
- **Health inequities:** Differences in health that are avoidable, unfair, and unjust. Health inequities are affected by social, economic, and environmental conditions.
- **Health disparities:** Differences in health outcomes among groups of people.

Nurses can be on the frontlines of reducing inequities but many of us are affronted at the thought that we aren't treating everyone with the same degree of respect, compassion, and responsiveness. We are all too easily blind to implicit bias and institutional racism. When someone pointed out that the solution to the drug crisis when it mainly affected inner city Blacks was incarceration and compared this to the push to improve treatment options for Whites addicted to opioids in today's epidemic, many were stunned. Similarly, the disparity in research dollars to treat cystic fibrosis (predominantly a White disease) versus sickle cell disease—many fewer research dollars for a much larger Black population—becomes shocking when known.

Reflective Practice: Immigration

One of the divisive issues in the United States is what the United States owes immigrants in this country with undocumented status, whether they be dreamers (children brought here illegally with their parents) or others. At odds is whether health care professionals should report undocumented individuals or protect them and treat their health care needs. Suppose you work in a primary care practice that services a number of immigrant families. Recently you've noticed more fear in your local community as deportation efforts increase. This fear is resulting in fewer visits, including vaccination visits for children. You've read about sanctuary practices and talk with your colleagues about posting "The Sanctuary Providers' Pledge" in your waiting room (https://hsd.luc.edu/bioethics/content/sanctuary-doctor/). You believe that if someone's immigrant status is affecting his or her health, it should be a matter of concern for you. Other colleagues disagree and talk about practices who have been told by senior leadership to "cease and desist" aiding undocumented individuals.

- You believe that your sanctuary efforts are covered in the same way attorney-client privileges are addressed. How do you proceed?
- Review the Henry J. Kaiser Family Foundation Disparities in health and health care: five key questions and answers (https://www.kff.org/disparities-policy/issue-brief/disparities-in-health-and-health-care-five-key-questions-and-answers/).
- Do we each believe that health disparities exist in the United States, in each of our practice settings? That people like you and me experience indifference, disrespect, and worse every day, compromising their health and wellness? Are we part of the problem?
- How do we make sense of the disparities we encounter daily, and what are our obligations to hear a call to courage to advocate for those on the margins?

ETHICS AND WORK ENVIRONMENT POLICIES

Politics, defined as "any activity concerned with the acquisition of power, gaining one's own ends," is not just for elected officials (Politics, n.d.). Politics are alive and well in every aspect of health care, from the operating room of a small community hospital to the board room of a multibillion-dollar pharmaceutical company. Every day, health care administrators make decisions that impact both nurses and the populations of patients they serve. Nurses are in key positions to influence hospital decision makers and to share the realities of the day-to-day care of patients. Nurses have the greatest influence when they are well-informed, open-minded, collaborative, and willing to do what is right, even if there is a personal cost. Here we examine one workplace policy where nurses have the power to influence outcomes, the issue of mandatory flu vaccines.

Mandatory Flu Vaccination: The Good of the Patient Versus Personal Choice

A Pennsylvania nurse was 3 months' pregnant when she was fired from a home infusion company for refusing a mandatory flu vaccine. She was fearful that receiving the vaccine might cause her to miscarry her baby (Lowes, 2014). She had previously experienced two miscarriages before becoming pregnant again. When she presented the required documentation from a physician recommending she not be vaccinated, the note was rejected. Her agency noted the physician failed to cite a medical reason for the exemption. Fear and anxiety were not considered valid reasons. The agency was unwilling to grant the nurse the option of wearing a mask because, as a home care nurse, it would have been difficult to enforce and doing so also placed her immunocompromised patients at risk (Lowes, 2014).

Although we as individuals might make the same decision as our colleague from Pennsylvania, as a profession we also have the responsibility to serve the good of our patients. How do we maintain that balance? When considering mandatory flu vaccination policies, nurses must consider the interests of the individual with those of the population—in this case, the population of patients served. Ethical arguments in this situation weigh personal choice (autonomy) against the best interests of patients. Many argue that a nurse's duty not to harm patients outweighs any restriction on personal choice (Antommaria, 2013; Tilburt et al., 2008). Likewise, fairness and promoting the good of patients compels nurses to consider ways to provide protection for their vulnerable patients and to keep them safe (Steckel, 2007).

Working though challenging issues is not easy. Using the Ethics Inventory to evaluate our personal approach to ethical issues is a good step toward improving our moral sensibility and moral valuing. Asking ourselves the question "What counts as a good response?" can make us more aware of how we promote the common good and dignity of others. Do we maximize good and reduce harm for our patients? Do we act with virtue in difficult situations by speaking up when it may not be popular to do so? Do we act justly and/or advocate for justice in our work environments? Are we responsive to the vulnerabilities of others? Nurses are the most trusted of all professionals. Given our sheer numbers, think about the impact we could have if we shared one common voice to improve the care of the vulnerable.

CONCLUSION

Advocacy is the act or process of pleading for, supporting, or recommending a cause or course of action. Advocacy may be for persons (whether as an individual, group, population, or society) or for an issue such as potable water or global health (ANA Code of Ethics, 2015).

Denise Thornby, former president of the American Association of Critical Care Nurses, always charged nurses to make waves. She exhorted nurses to identify when health care was not working for people in need and to do whatever was necessary to address the need. She died in the summer of 2012. We cannot think of a better way to end this chapter than to repeat her charge to nurses everywhere:

Every day, every moment, you make choices on how to act or respond. Through these acts, you have the power to positively influence. As John Quincy Adams sagely said, "The influence of each human being on others in this life is a kind of immortality." So I ask you: What will be your act of courage? How will you influence your environment? What will be your legacy? (Thornby, 2001)

REFERENCES

Advisory Board Company. (2014, September 4). *Where states stand on Medicaid expansion.* Retrieved from www.advisory.com/daily-briefing/resources/primers/medicaidmap.

American Nurses Association. (2010). *Nursing's social policy statement* (2010 ed.). Silver Spring, MD: Author.

American Nurses Association. (2015). *Code of ethics for nurses with interpretive statements.* Silver Spring, MD: Author.

American Nurses Association. (2018). *Nurses role in addressing discrimination.* Retrieved from www.nursingworld.org.

Antommaria, A.H. (2013). An ethical analysis of mandatory influenza vaccination of health care personnel: Implementing fairly and balancing benefits and burdens. *American Journal of Bioethics, 13*(9), 30–37.

Barnet, R. (n.d.). Dr. Bob Barnet's human drivers: 5 P's. From Taylor, C.R. *Rethinking humane care for humans . . . trivial, superficial, unrealistic or essential?* Presented at the American University of Beirut. Retrieved from www.aub.edu.lb/fm/shbpp/ethics/public/Documents/Humane-care-presentation.pdf.

Davis, K., Schoen, C., & Stremkis, K. (2010). *Mirror, mirror on the wall: How the performance of the U.S. health care system compares internationally, 2010 update.* The Commonwealth Fund. Retrieved from www.commonwealthfund.org/publications/fund-reports/2014/jun/mirror-mirror-wall-2014-update-how-us-health-care-system.

Department of Health and Human Services. (2018, January 18). *HHS announces new conscience and religious freedom division.* Retrieved from www.hhs.gov/about/news/2018/01/18/hhs-ocr-announces-new-conscience-and-religious-freedom-division.html.

Dickman, S., Himmelstein, D., McCormick, D., & Woolhander, S. (2014). Opting out of Medicaid expansion: The health and financial impacts. *Health Affairs Blog.* Retrieved from healthaffairs.org/blog/2014/01/30/opting-out-of-medicaid-expansion-the-health-and-financial-impacts/.

Feinberg, J. (1970). *Justice and personal desert, doing and deserving.* Princeton, NJ: Princeton University Press.

Gallup. (2018). *Honesty/ethics in professions.* Retrieved from https://news.gallup.com/poll/245597/nurses-again-outpace-professions-honesty-ethics.aspx.

The Henry J. Kaiser Family Foundation. (2016, August 12). Disparities in health and health care: Five key questions and answers. Retrieved from www.kff.org/disparities-policy/issue-brief/disparities-in-healthand-health-care-five-key-questions-and-answers/.

Holan, A.D. (2009). Sarah Palin falsely claims Barack Obama runs a "death panel." *Politifact.com.* Retrieved from www.politifact.com/truth-o-meter/statements/2009/aug/10/sarah-palin/sarah-palin-barack-obama-death-panel/.

Hope, T., Reynolds, J., & Griffiths, S. (2002). Rationing decisions: Integrating cost-effectiveness with other values. In R. Rhodes, M. Battin, & A. Silvers (Eds.), *Medicine and social justice.* Oxford: University Press.

Kaiser Commission on Medicaid and the Uninsured. (2014, June). *Medicaid moving forward* [fact sheet]. The Henry J. Kaiser Family Foundation. Retrieved from www.kff.org/health-reform/issue-brief/medicaid-moving-forward/.

Lowes, R. (2014). *Pregnant RN fired for refusing flu vaccine: Not so simple? Medscape.* Retrieved from www.medscape.com/viewarticle/820234.

Magelssen, M. (2012). When should conscientious objection be accepted? *J Med Ethics, 38*, 18–21.

Miller, D. (1976). *Social justice.* Oxford: Clarendon Press.

Miller, D. (1989). *Market, state, and community.* Oxford: Clarendon Press.

Obama, B. (2014). *President Barack Obama's State of the Union address.* Retrieved from www.whitehouse.gov/the-press-office/2014/01/28/president-barack-obamas-state-union-address.

Politics. (n.d). *Collins English dictionary—Complete & unabridged* (10th ed.). Retrieved from dictionary.reference.com/browse/politics.

Rawls, J. (1971). *A theory of justice.* Harvard, MA: Harvard University Press.

Rawls, J. (1993). *Political liberalism.* New York: Columbia University Press.

The sanctuary providers' pledge. (2017). Retrieved from https://hsd.luc.edu/media/healthsciencesdivision/bioethics/documents/sanctuary-doctor-may2017.pdf.

Sobel, L., & Salganicoff, A. (2013). *A guide to the Supreme Court's review of the contraceptive coverage requirement* [Kaiser Family Foundation Women's Health policy]. Retrieved from kff.org/womens-health-policy/issue-brief/a-guide-to-the-supreme-courts-review-of-the-contraceptive-coverage-requirement/.

Steckel, C. M. (2007). Mandatory influenza immunizations for health care workers—An ethical discussion. *AAOHN Journal, 55*(1), 34–39.

Stone, D.M., Simon, T.R., Fowler, K.A., Kegler, S.R., Yuan, K., Holland, K.M., . . . & Crosby, A.E. (June 8, 2018). Vital signs: Trend in state suicide rates—United States, 1999-2016 and circumstances contributing to suicide—27 states, 2015. *CDC Weekly, 67*(22), 617–624.

Taylor, C. (2019). Values, ethics and advocacy. In C. Taylor, P. Lynn, & J. Bartlett. *Fundamentals of nursing: The art and science of person-centered care* (9th ed.). Philadelphia: Wolters Kluwer.

Thornby, D. (2001). *Make waves: The courage to influence practice.* Speech given at American Association of Critical-Care Nurses, National Teaching Institute and Critical Care Exposition. Anaheim, CA. Retrieved from www.aacn.org/wd/aacninfo/docs/board/pressspeech2001.pdf.

Tilburt, J.C., Mueller, P.S., Ottenberg, A.L., Poland, G.A., & Koenig, B.A. (2008). Facing the challenges of influenza in healthcare settings: The ethical rationale for mandatory seasonal influenza vaccination and its implications for future pandemics. *Vaccine, 26*(S4), D27–D30.

Torrey, E.F., Entsminger, K., Geller, J., Stanley, J., & Jaffe, D.J. (n.d). *The shortage of public hospital beds for mentally ill persons. A report of the Treatment Advocacy Center.* Retrieved from www.treatmentadvocacycenter.org/storage/documents/the_shortage_of_publichospitalbeds.pdf.

Treatment Advocacy Center. (2014). *Eliminating barriers to the treatment of mental illness.* Retrieved from www.treatmentadvocacycenter.org/problem/lack-of-implementation.

Woolf, S.H., & Aron, L. (Eds.), (2013). *U.S. Health in international perspective: Shorter lives, poorer health.* National Research Council and Institute of Medicine. Washington, DC: The National Academies Press.

15

The Changing United States Health Care System

Hillary Schneller and Barbara J. Safriet

"Of all the forms of inequality, injustice in health is the most shocking and inhumane."

Martin Luther King, Jr.

The U.S. health care system is complex and pluralistic. It is a mix of private and public initiatives and institutions that employ millions of workers in a myriad of settings to provide a wide range of health-related services to the diverse U.S. population across geopolitical environments that range from cities to rural areas. This chapter provides an overview of the current major components of the American health care system, which is in constant flux.

OVERVIEW OF THE U.S. HEALTH CARE SYSTEM

Public Insurance

The two principal public health insurance programs, Medicare and Medicaid, account for more than one-third of the nation's total health spending (Centers for Medicare and Medicaid Services [CMS], 2018).

Medicare. Title XVIII of the 1965 Social Security Act created Medicare as health coverage for individuals over age 65 and people with disabilities. It is financed through taxes, general revenues, and premiums paid by the enrollee (Klees, Wolfe, & Curtis, 2017). In 2017, Medicare covered care for nearly 60 million people at a cost of $702 billion (15% of federal spending in the United States) (Cubanski & Neuman, 2018). Medicare is divided

into four parts: A, B, C, and D (Klees et al., 2017). Part A pays for inpatient hospitalization, home health, hospice, and skilled nursing. Part B covers certain medical services and supplies such as outpatient health care, physician services, and services provided by Medicare-approved practitioners, including nurse practitioners, certified nurse anesthetists, clinical nurse specialists, and clinical psychologists working in collaboration with physicians. Part C, known as Medicare Advantage, expands beneficiaries' options for participation in private sector health care plans, which must cover the services covered by Parts A and B (except hospice services). Part D covers prescription drugs not otherwise covered by Parts A and B. Expenditures for the Medicare Drugs Program (Part D) was $99.5 billion in 2016 for over 43 million enrollees (Klees et al., 2017).

Medicaid. Title XIX of the Social Security Act created Medicaid in 1965 as a joint state-federal health coverage program for certain individuals and families with low incomes and low resources.

Medicaid is financed by the combination of state general funds and federal matching funds, and states must adhere to certain federal requirements to be eligible for federal funds. Within those broad federal requirements, and certain limitations, states develop and implement plans for their Medicaid programs.

A state's Medicaid program must cover certain basic services including, among others, inpatient and outpatient hospital services; family planning services and supplies; pregnancy-related care (except abortion care); vaccines for children; laboratory and x-ray services; pediatric and family nurse practitioner, nurse-midwife, and physician services; and rural health clinic and federally qualified health center (FQHC) services. States may also receive federal matching funds for certain optional services. In addition, most states have supplemental "state-only" programs that provide health coverage for individuals who do not otherwise qualify for Medicaid or that cover services for which the federal government does not provide matching funds (Klees et al., 2017).

Prior to 2014, federal law mandated state Medicaid programs to cover health services to certain federal minimum levels only low-income people who also met additional eligibility criteria. Thus, Medicaid coverage was required for pregnant women, children, parents of a dependent child, people with disabilities, and people 65 and older (Klees et al., 2017). Adults without dependent children were not included in these mandated categories for which states received federal matching funds, leaving millions without coverage (Henry J. Kaiser Family Foundation [KFF], 2013). The Patient Protection and Affordable Care Act (Affordable Care Act [ACA]) aimed to expand eligibility for Medicaid beginning in 2014 to all individuals under age 65 with incomes at or below 138% of the federal poverty level (see Table 15.1 for federal poverty levels; Klees et al., 2017). For this expanded group of eligible individuals, federal matching funds would be provided at 100% between 2014 and 2017 and then decrease incrementally 90% by 2020, with the states paying 10%. As with other

TABLE 15.1 Federal Poverty Guidelines		
Persons in Family/ Household	Poverty Guideline	138% of Federal Poverty Level
1	$12,140	$16,753
2	$16,460	$22,715
3	$20,780	$28,676
4	$25,100	$34,638
5	$29,420	$40,600
6	$33,740	$46,561
7	$38,060	$52,523
8	$42,380	$58,484

Federal poverty guidelines of the U.S. Department of Health and Human Services. (2018, January 18). Applicable to the 48 contiguous states and the District of Columbia. From the Federal Register. Retrieved from www.federalregister.gov/documents/2018/01/18/2018-00814/annual-update-of-the-hhs-poverty-guidelines.

federal rules governing the Medicaid program, states that do not comply with minimum federal guidelines face the loss of federal matching funds.

Shortly after the ACA was signed into law in March 2010, 26 states and others filed lawsuits arguing, among other things, it was unconstitutional to threaten states with loss of their existing federal matching funds if they declined to expand Medicaid. The Supreme Court agreed in a decision issued in 2012 (NFIB v. Sebelius, 2012). The Supreme Court's decision made the Medicaid expansion effectively optional for states. As of November 2018, 36 states and the District of Columbia had adopted the Medicaid expansion (KFF, 2018). In states that have not expanded Medicaid, many adults fall into a "coverage gap," without affordable health coverage options: based on their income, they are ineligible for both Medicaid and federal subsidies to help afford coverage in the ACA marketplaces. More than 2 million uninsured adults fall into this coverage gap (Garfield & Damico, 2017).

There is no deadline by which a state can expand Medicaid and receive federal matching funds. For instance, Virginia decided to expand Medicaid in 2018. In May, the Virginia legislature approved the expansion, although with a provision that newly eligible adults who do not have a disability volunteer or work as a condition of enrolling in Medicaid (Goodnough, 2018).

Private Health Insurance

The changes implemented by Medicare and Medicaid have always been made against the backdrop of a large private health insurance market in the United States. Most people in the United States continue to be insured through employer-sponsored health insurance, either as employees or dependents (KFF, 2016). The ACA implemented significant changes to the private health insurance market, many of which are covered in Chapter 18. In particular, the ACA aimed to increase coverage for individuals who do not obtain health coverage through their employers or public programs, as discussed in that chapter.

Veterans Administration Health Systems

The first federal Veterans hospital was authorized in 1811. Since that time, the U.S. Department of Veterans Affairs has expanded to become the largest integrated health care system in the United States, including 1240 health care facilities that serve over 9 million veterans with a $186.5 billion budget for FY18 (U.S. Department of Veterans Affairs, 2018b). A backlog of disability claims hit a recent peak in 2013, with over 600,000 claims pending for 125 days or longer. By the end of 2016, that number had dropped by 84%, to just under 100,000 claims, and has remained around that level (Veterans Benefit Administration, U.S.

Department of Veterans Affairs, 2017). The drop can be attributed in part to the agency's 2011 Transformation Plan, which aimed to modernize the agency, including moving its claims process from a paper-based system to an electronic one (U.S. Department of Veterans Affairs, 2016). A separate backlog for veterans who appeal the agency's initial benefits decision rose to over 470,000; legislation signed in 2017 aims to streamline the appeals process but applies primarily to newly filed appeals, not pending claims (Yen, 2018). Debate about privatizing veteran's health care intensified in 2017 and 2018, with a divide growing between Secretary David Shulkin and the White House, culminating in a reported attempt to remove Shulkin because he did not fully support privatization (Rein, 2018; Shulkin, 2018). In March 2018, President Trump announced Shulkin's firing via Twitter, and permanent leadership of the Veterans Administration was in limbo for several months after the president nominated his personal physician to the post; that nominee subsequently withdrew (Rein, Wax-Thibodeaux, & Dawsey, 2018). For a more detailed discussion of the U.S. Military and Veterans Health Administration System, see Chapter 37.

Indian Health Service

The U.S. Constitution recognizes a guardian or "trust relationship" between the United States and federally recognized Indian Tribes. In this role, as affirmed in treaties, executive orders, statutes, and Supreme Court cases, the federal government has a responsibility to provide health services to American Indians and Alaska Natives (National Indian Health Board, n.d.). It does so today through the Indian Health Service (IHS), an agency within the Department of Health and Human Services authorized by the Indian Health Care Improvement Act (IHCIA) of 1976. The ACA permanently reauthorized the IHCIA, meaning that it appropriates funds for fiscal year 2010 (the year the ACA was enacted) and each year thereafter (Heisler & Walke, 2010). In addition, as U.S. citizens and citizens of their states, American Indians and Alaska Natives are eligible to participate in all health programs available to the general population (IHS, 2015).

American Indians and Alaska Natives have long experienced poor health outcomes and lower life expectancies compared to other Americans (IHS, 2018). These health disparities are inseparable from poverty, social inequality, and discrimination experienced by American Indians and Alaska Natives, as well as inadequate health care services, housing, education, and other services (Belcourt, 2018). Access to culturally competent and quality health care is one critically important component of reducing these dramatic health disparities (Flowers, 2005).

In addition, workforce grants like the American Indians Into Nursing Program aims to increase the number of American Indian and Alaska Native nurses who provide health services to American Indian and Alaska Native communities (IHS, n.d.).

Infrastructure

Health services are delivered in a variety of settings, including community health clinics, clinicians' offices, nursing homes, and hospitals.

Hospitals. The American Hospital Association (2016) reports that in 2016, there were 5534 hospitals that meet the association's criteria for accreditation as a hospital by Joint Commission on Accreditation of Healthcare Organizations or are a certified provider of acute services under Title 18 of the Social Security Act. Approximately 51% of these hospitals are nonprofit community hospitals, 19% are for-profit/investor-owned hospitals, and 17% are state and local government hospitals.

Hospital mergers have substantially increased over the past several years: in 2012, 105 hospital mergers were reported, compared with between 50 and 60 annually between 2005 and 2007 (Dafny, 2014). Mergers have the potential to improve efficiency and lower costs for patients and providers. This trend, however, can also have negative consequences that result from reduced competition, such as higher costs and a reduction in access to care. Some of these consolidations—horizontal mergers of providers that supply similar services in the same geographic area, as well as vertical integration of services including urgent and long-term care—have received attention as potential violations of antitrust law (Dafny, 2014). The Federal Trade Commission (FTC), which enforces federal antitrust law to prevent anticompetitive activity that deprives consumers of the benefits of competition including in the health care market, has brought a number of challenges to hospital consolidations (Meier, Albert, & Brau, 2018). The share of religiously affiliated hospitals has grown as a result of mergers. By 2015, four of five of the largest health care systems were religiously affiliated, and Catholic hospitals account for one in six acute care hospital beds (Hill & Slusky, 2017). Such consolidations can decrease access to certain health services, including reproductive and end-of-life health care (Hill & Slusky, 2017; Khaikin, Uttley, & Winkler, 2016).

Community Health Centers. According to the National Association of Community Health Centers (NACHC), community health centers serve as the primary health care access point for more than 27 million people in over 10,000 rural and urban communities across the country

(NACHC, 2015). These "safety net" providers are also commonly referred to as FQHCs because they meet high quality of care, service, and cost standards and are thus qualified to receive enhanced Medicaid and Medicare reimbursement (NACHC, 2011). FQHCs provide primary and preventive health care along with health services not often offered in primary care settings, including dental care, behavior health, and pharmacy services. Yet in 2015, 95% of community health centers reported vacancies for clinical positions, including 50% vacancies for nurse practitioners and 41% vacancies for registered nurses (NACHC, 2016).

Nursing Homes. Nursing homes are the primary providers of long-term care in the United States. They provide inpatient medical services, skilled nursing and rehabilitative services, and assistance with the activities of daily living such as bathing and dressing (KFF, 2017a). As of 2015, there were just over 15,500 nursing homes certified to care for Medicare or Medicaid beneficiaries, and 92% of nursing homes are certified for both programs (Boccuti, Casillas, & Neuman, 2015). These nursing homes care for nearly 1.4 million residents (KFF, 2017a). Most nursing home residents are seniors, and one in three people turning 65 will need nursing home care at some point in their lives. Although most nursing home residents are Medicare beneficiaries, Medicaid is the primary payer for over 60% of nursing facility residents (KFF, 2017a).

Public Health. Public health is the promotion and protection of the health of people and communities where they live, at a population level, whether that be at the local, national, or regional level. Public health thus encompasses research and education on the conditions that allow people to live healthy lives; research about disease and injury prevention; and tracking, preventing, and responding to infectious diseases and other health care crises (Centers for Disease Control and Prevention [CDC] Foundation, n.d.). Public health programs include maintaining drinking water quality, immunizations, infectious disease monitoring, injury, asthma, and cancer prevention, among others (Office of Disease Prevention and Health Promotion [ODPHP], n.d.-a).

A variety of public and private agencies and organizations engage in public health work, but only approximately 3% of all health spending is directed to public health (Trust for America's Health, 2018). At the federal level, the CDC is the United States' primary public health agency and administers funding for many population-based prevention efforts. The CDC funds state and local health departments, although the allocation of the funding varies widely. More than half of states have a "decentralized" or largely decentralized public health governance, meaning that local health units are primarily led by local authorities and independent of state government (Association of State and Territorial Health Officials [ASTHO], 2014). The remaining states have either a centralized public health department or a shared structure (ASTHO, 2014). State public health agency leadership is closely tied to state government leadership: in the vast majority of states, the governor appoints the top state health official, and that person may also be subject to confirmation by another body such as a board or commission, or by the legislature (ASTHO, 2014). For that reason, among others, politicians can have a strong influence on state public health agencies (ASTHO & NORC, 2012).

Nurses are essential public health workers; indeed, public health nurses are the largest part of professional public health workforce (Boulton & Beck, 2013). Public health nursing aims to improve population health by focusing on prevention and addressing multiple determinants of health. It includes aspects advocacy, policy, development, and planning, as well as a social justice perspective to public health issues (American Public Health Association, 2013). Like other public health workers, public health nursing initiatives aim to leverage community participation. An early example is Lillian Wald's Henry Street Settlement in New York City, founded as the Nurses' Settlement in 1893 to provide care to the poor (Henry Street Settlement, n.d.). It evolved into an agency that not only provided services, but also advocated for and educated others about the population it served (Fee & Liping, 2010). And in Mississippi in 1921, Mary D. Osborne brought her expertise in maternity nursing to the position of Director of Public Health Nursing within the state Board of Health, where one of her primary focuses was maternal and child health care. The state had the highest maternal death rate and the highest infant mortality rate in the country. Osborne developed a collaboration between public health nurses and midwives: nurses spent at least 2 months in a county conducting classes for groups of midwives and hold prenatal and well-baby conferences and immunization clinics (Mississippi State Department of Health, 2014; American Nurses Association [ANA], 1996).

Public health officials continue to play a critical role in responding to crises through public education and preventive measures and by bringing together experts from a variety of fields to generate innovative responses on a population level. Although preventive health initiatives and disease outbreaks are typical examples of an issue demanding a public health response, other issues may similarly benefit from a public health approach. For example, the ANA has considered gun violence a public health issue since 1994 (ANA, 2018). In 2016, the American Medical Association [AMA] (2016), followed suit, officially declaring gun violence—which kills approximately 30,000 people per year in the United States—a public health crisis. In addition to gun violence, Kent State University recently identified three other emergencies that call for a public health response: toxic drinking water in Flint, Michigan; the abuse of opioids; and the deaths of immigrants at the U.S.-Mexican border (Kent State University, 2017).

TRANSFORMING HEALTH CARE THROUGH TECHNOLOGY

Two facets of health care technology include health information technology (health IT or HIT) and telehealth. Health IT involves the electronic transfer of health information (Office for Civil Rights, U.S. Department of Health and Human Services, 2017). Telehealth is the provision of remote or long-distance clinical health care, public health, and health education through the use of telecommunications technology (Center for Connected Health Policy [CCHPCA], n.d.). Advancements in health IT and telehealth hold the promise for improving quality of care, increasing efficiency, and reducing costs and other burdens for payers, providers, and patients. Health IT and telehealth programs also bring challenges and concerns.

Health Information Technology

Examples of health IT include electronic health records (EHRs) and electronic prescribing.

EHRs aim to enable health care providers to better management of patient care through the sharing of health information in a secure manner (Office of the National Coordinator for Health Information Technology [ONCHIT], n.d.). Ideally, EHRs enable a provider to (1) record accurate and complete information about a patient's health, (2) quickly provide care, (3) better coordinate the care that is given, and (4) better share information with patients and their caregivers (ONCHIT, n.d.).

EHRs date to 1971, when Lockheed engineers designed the first commercial EHR system for El Camino Hospital (Thede, 2012). This system was successful because it integrated physicians, nurses, and pharmacy processes, and a respect for the nursing workforce was apparent in the system design (Thede, 2012). The system freed nurses from established tasks, such as multiple documentation, enabling them to spend more time with patients. This system, however, has not necessarily been replicated in informatics design throughout the U.S. health care system. Concerns exist regarding the lack of consistent evidence for the effectiveness of EHRs (Balestra, 2017). In addition, despite

incentives, health care providers may not adopt EHRs for a variety of reasons—including challenges with implementing EHR systems, especially in a large health system (Congressional Budget Office [CBO], 2008).

Nonetheless, there are significant incentives to use health IT. For example, the 2009 Health Information Technology and Economic and Clinical Health Act appropriated billions of dollars to promote providers' adoption and use of federally certified EHRs, and as of 2014, the federal government had distributed $28.1 billion to eligible providers through the Medicare and Medicaid EHR program (Mennemeyer, 2015).

Often EHRs are discussed with physicians as the focus; however, the success of EHR systems has been found to correlate with designs that respect nursing practice. Several years ago, the American Association of Colleges of Nursing and the National League of Nursing, two nursing accrediting agencies, required that beginning informatics be added to the curriculum in all nursing schools (Thede, 2012). This requirement is consistent with that of the National Academies of Sciences, Engineering, and Medicine (NASEM), which requires that informatics education be provided for all health care professionals (Thede, 2012). Nursing schools now offer graduate degrees in informatics, which are largely focused on system design for hospitals, community health centers, and home care that are clinically directed (Moen & Knudsen, 2013).

Telehealth

As Americans continue to struggle with chronic disease and health care workforce shortages, access to health care providers is a challenge (Rutledge, 2017). Many Americans live in health professional shortage areas (HSPAs), meaning that they do not have adequate provider-to-population ratio in the areas of primary, dental, and/or mental health care (KFF, 2017b). Telehealth is becoming an essential means by which Americans can, at a minimum, access cost-effective quality health care.

"Telemedicine" is often used as synonymous with "telehealth," but the latter is a more universal term that covers an array of health care fields—including dentistry, counseling, and physical therapy, among others. Telehealth may encompass a variety of interactions. For instance, it may involve live videoconferencing between a patient and provider. This "real-time" interaction may substitute for an in-person visit to a clinician and can be used for consultations as well as diagnostic and treatment services. Telehealth may also include transmission of health history through an electronic communications system to the provider who uses the information to evaluate the patient or provide a service but not in a live interaction. In addition, it can include monitoring: electronic collection of personal health data that is transmitted to the provider for use in care and support. Mobile health is also a domain of telehealth and encompasses public health practice and education, like text message reminders to promote healthy behavior or to alert about disease outbreaks (CCHPCA, 2018).

Although telehealth has the power to improve access to care, many of the challenges for telehealth replicate the challenges in other areas of the health care system. For instance, although telehealth has the power to improve the health of individuals in rural communities, those very communities may lack the infrastructure—including a lack of access to high-speed internet—to access its benefits (Rural Health Information Hub, 2017).

HEALTH STATUS AND TRENDS

It is common to evaluate the health care system on three dimensions: quality, access, and cost. Health care systems can also be evaluated as the extent to which they secure justice.

Quality

Quality of care is the degree to which health services for individuals and populations increase the likelihood of desired outcomes and are consistent with current knowledge. A variety of quality measures exist, which generally fall into three broad categories: structure, process, and outcome (AHRQ, 2015). Patient experience is also a key quality measure (AHRQ, 2017).

Cross-nation comparisons help situate the United States' health system within a global context. The Commonwealth Fund reported on the findings of the Organization for Economic Cooperation and Development (OECD), which tracks and reports on more than 1200 health system measures across 35-member countries. Some of the highlights of the U.S. system, when compared with 12 other high-income nations, include that the United States has one of the lowest numbers of practicing physicians per 1000 population (2.6); the OECD mean was 3.2 per 1000. The United States also ranked at the top of the list of countries using medical technology, including diagnostic imaging and pharmaceuticals. In addition, adults in the United States regularly take more prescription medications (2.2 per adult) than adults in other countries (Squires, 2015).

Quality improvement in nursing was first introduced by Florence Nightingale during the Crimean War. Nurses remain involved in improving process but have evolved to emphasize patient care outcomes as a measurement of quality. In a landmark report entitled *The Future of Nursing*, NASEM (formerly the Institute of Medicine) identified

the nursing profession as crucial to improving quality in the changing health care system. That report presented four key messages (NASEM, 2010):
- Nurses should practice to the full extent of their education and training.
- Nurses should achieve higher levels of education and training through an improved education system that promotes seamless academic progression.
- Nurses should be full partners, with physicians and other health care professionals, in redesigning health care in the United States.
- Effective workforce planning and policymaking require better data collection and an improved information infrastructure.

Implementation of the four key messages of the NASEM can enable nursing to take a leading role in the ever-challenging endeavor to improve quality while being cost-effective.

Access

Access is the ability to obtain quality health care to achieve the best health outcomes in a timely way. According to the Department of Health and Human Services, access requires entry into the health care system, access to sites of care, and finding providers who meet the needs of individual patients (AHRQ, 2011). Despite many initiatives, access remains a serious challenge.

Discussions about health care often use "access" as a substitute for health coverage, but the two are not the same. In general, however, individuals with health coverage have better access to care (Giled, Ma, & Borja, 2017). An estimated 19.2 million non-elderly people gained health coverage between 2010 and 2015. In that same time, the number of uninsured adults ages 19 to 34 decreased by 42% and by 33% for adults 35 to 54 decreased (Garrett & Gangopadhyaya, 2016). (Despite these significant gains, as noted earlier in this chapter, many people remain without coverage in part due to the refusal of some states to expand Medicaid.) To return to "access": a Commonwealth Fund analysis demonstrated that the ACA's Medicaid expansion and implementation of state health insurance exchanges not only decreased the number of uninsured, but also improved access to care for those who obtained coverage (Giled et al., 2017).

Cost

The cost of health care can be considered from several perspectives. For patients or consumers, cost is the price of purchasing needed health care goods and services and includes insurance premiums, co-pays, and deductibles; out-of-pocket health expenditures not covered by insurance; taxes (Social Security, federal, and state) that support health programs; and in-kind services such as caring for aging parents or sick children. For health care providers, cost includes producing health care products and services and delivering them to patients. The cost of health care is also how much the state or nation spends on it, including as measured by the percentage of total domestic production health care consumes. Incentives and policy measures that address the cost of health may benefit one, some, or none of these groups.

Most developed countries have a health insurance system funded, subsidized, or managed by the national government and, with very few exceptions, the categorical delineation between countries with some type of national health system and those without is the country's economic development (Fisher, 2012). The great exception remains the United States. Nonetheless, the United States spends 17.2% of its gross domestic product (GDP) on health care expenditures—which is eight percentage points higher than the average of its peer countries, and higher than any peer countries, including those with national health systems (OECD, 2017).

Justice

Athough health care systems are typically measured on the three above measures—quality, access, and cost—another important measure is whether a health care system is just, fair, and equitable. As Georges C. Benjamin, MD, former executive director of the American Public Health Association, stated: "one of our biggest misconceptions—and perhaps, obstacles—is misconstruing access for equity" (Benjamin, 2015). This misconception can be seen in health disparities, including the racial disparities in maternal health outcomes that exist across income levels described above. Why, despite progressively accessible and affordable health care in the United States, do these disparities persist? Because health outcomes are linked to the quality, access, and cost of health care, along with social determinants like safe housing, a living wage, affordable health care, and other conditions that shape a person's ability to attain good health. In addition, health status is also linked to racism, discrimination, and bias (Benjamin, 2015; Daniels, 2017).

Health Status of the United States

Despite continuing to spend the most money on health care than any other country (Papanicolas, Woskie, & Jha, 2018), the United States ranks poorly on several important health indicators. *Healthy People 2020* reports leading health indicators are access to health services; clinical preventive services; environmental quality; injury and violence; maternal, infant, and child health; mental health; nutrition, physical activity, and obesity; oral health; reproductive and sexual health; social determinants; substance abuse; and tobacco (ODPHP, n.d.-b). The NASEM's Committee on the State of the USA Health Indicators identified a framework for health indicator development. Table 15.2 summarizes their findings.

The United States is ranked 28th for life expectancy at birth out of 35 peer countries determined by the OECD (2108). In addition, the United States has the highest maternal mortality ratio in the industrialized world: among OECD member countries with "advanced" and "emerging" economies, the United States has a higher maternal mortality ratio than any country except Mexico, which is considered an emerging economy (Kassebaum, 2016). Racial disparities in maternal health outcomes are stark: Black women who give birth in the United States are nearly four times more likely to die than White women are (Creanga, 2014). This disparity applies across all education levels and persists even after controlling for differences in socioeconomic status (Agrawal, 2014; Singh, 2010).

Health Reform

There have been many major milestones in health care policy over the last several decades in the United States. These include the Public Health Service Act of 1944, the Social Security Amendments of 1965, the Health Insurance Portability and Accountability Act of 1996, and the Patient Protection and ACA of 2010. Two of the major questions drive health care reform: the cost of health care and the right to health care.

The latest milestone in health care policy is the ACA. The ACA requires individuals to have health insurance and eliminated the power of insurance companies to deny or terminate coverage based on a person's preexisting condition. As explained above, the ACA also set out an expansion of Medicaid, and provided for health care exchanges or marketplaces through which individuals and small businesses could purchase health coverage with subsidies available based on income (KFF, 2013).

The most recent effort at health care reform is the ACA, which has been a political target even before it was enacted. As of 2017, Republicans had voted dozens of times to repeal the ACA (Cowan & Cornwell, 2017). President Trump's administration has weakened federal rules governing health care in an effort to undermine the ACA, even if they have been unable to repeal it (Luhby, 2018). On the other hand, many see the ACA as a starting point for further improvements (Obama, 2016); others see it as a foundation for more dramatic change in the health care system. For instance, since Medicare's inception, there have been advocates for a single-payer "Medicare for all" system, and today some Democrats have renewed that rallying cry (Scott, 2018).

TABLE 15.2 Framework for Health and Health Indicator Development

Social and Physical Environment		Health Outcomes
Socioeconomic status	→	Mortality
Race/ethnicity		Life expectancy at birth
Social support		Infant mortality
Health literacy		Life expectancy at age 65 years
Limited English proficiency		Injury-related mortality
Physical environments (where people live, learn, work, and play)		
Health-Related Behaviors		
Smoking	→	Health-related quality of life
Physical activity		(morbidity)
Excessive drinking		Self-reported health status
Nutrition		Unhealthy days
Obesity		
Condom use among youth		
Health Systems		
The health system is broadly defined as a set of institutions and	→	Condition specific outcomes
players whose purpose is to maintain or improve people's health.		Chronic disease prevalence
Cost		Serious psychological distress
Health care expenditures		
Access		
Insurance coverage		
Unmet medical, dental, and prescription drug needs		
Effectiveness of care		
Preventive services		
Childhood immunizations		
Preventable hospitalizations		

No single measure can capture the health of the nation. Indicators are needed that reflect a broad range of factors such as health, risk for illness, and health system performance. The set of indicators presented here should not be viewed as perfect or permanent; rather, the committee identified potential indicators that met the data constraints and then applied the framework to determine the final selection of indicators.

From the Committee on the State of the USA Health Indicators, Institute of Medicine of the National Academies. (2009). *State of the USA health indicators*. Washington, DC: The National Academies Press. Retrieved from www.nap.edu/download.php?record_id=12534#.

OPPORTUNITIES AND CHALLENGES FOR NURSING IN THE U.S. HEALTH CARE SYSTEM

Nurses are largest group of health professionals in the United States (Bureau of Labor Statistics, 2018). Most health care services involve some form of care by nurses, and nurses comprise the largest component of hospital staff, are the primary providers of hospital patient care, and deliver most of the country's long-term care (American Association of Colleges of Nursing, 2011). Nurses are well-positioned to contribute, lead, and improve efforts of the ever-changing U.S. health care system. Yet nurses and the nursing profession continue to face barriers that prevent them from fully

contributing their training, education, and perspective to those efforts.

One barrier is antiquated legal barriers that prevent nurses from practicing to the full extent of their license. In many states, there is a gap between the health services nurses are able, by means of their role, training, and education, to provide and the health services regulation allows nurses to provide (Safriet, 2002). And, despite substantial evidence and experience that advanced practice registered nurses (APRNs), such as nurse practitioners, are safe and effective independent health care providers of the many health services within the scope of their training, licensure, certification, and practice, APRN scope of practice varies widely across states, and many states require APRNs to practice pursuant to a written agreement with a physician.

In 2014, the Federal Trade Commission (FTC) surveyed APRN scope-of-practice laws and concluded that the wide variety in APRN scope of practice, the ability to practice independently, and requirements for physician supervision existed for reasons unrelated to their ability, education, training, or safety concerns. Instead, the report attributed the variations to "political decisions of the state in which they work." In particular, the FTC raised concerns about physician supervision requirements because "they effectively give one group of health care professionals the ability to restrict access to the market by another competing group of health care professionals, thereby denying health care consumers the benefits of greater competition." The FTC concluded: facts matter. It strongly urged that states not impose restrictions on APRN scope of practice unless those restrictions were based on "well-founded safety concerns" (Gilman & Koslov, 2014).

Health policy experts have concluded that eliminating unnecessary APRN scope of practice restrictions is a key component to better delivery of effective health care (NASEM, 2010). This is because nurses are quality health care providers and tend to make up a greater share of the primary care workforce in less densely populated areas, less urban areas, and lower income areas, as well as in health care provider shortage areas. And, compared to primary care physicians, APRNs are more likely to practice in underserved areas and care for large numbers of minority patients, Medicaid beneficiaries, and uninsured patients (Gilman & Koslov, 2014).

Another barrier stems from the fact that, despite being the largest part of the health care workforce and in particular in underserved areas, nurses remain underrepresented in arenas where policy, politics, economic, social, and professional decisions regarding the U.S. health care system are made.

One sign of this underrepresentation is nurses' low visibility in the media—a public representation of debate and discussion about the U.S. health care system. In 1998, the landmark Woodhull Study on Nursing and the Media: Health Care's Invisible Partner found that, in September 1997, nurses were identified as sources in only 4% of health-related stories in leading print national and regional newspapers and 1% of weeklies and industry media, and they were never cited in health news stories about policy (Woodhull Study Advisory Group, 1998). Twenty years later, preliminary findings from researchers revisiting nurses' representation in the media indicate that not much has changed. The updated study shows that in September 2017, nurses were identified as sources

in only 2% of health-related stories (Mason, Glickstein, Nixon, Westphaln, & Acquaviva, 2018). Nurses and the profession were mentioned in only 13% of articles about health care and were more likely to be mentioned in articles about labor, the profession, quality, and education but likely not to be included in articles about research, the ACA, and business. The study also examines health reporters' experiences using nurses as sources and why nurses are not better represented. Core themes that emerged included that "biases about women, nurses, and positions of power in the health care system can act as barriers to the use of diverse sources in health reporting," as well as a lack of understanding of what nurses do (Mason et al., 2018).

These two examples exemplify a broader challenge for nursing: how to recognize the contributions of the profession—not as separate accomplishments of individual nurses, selected nursing schools, or a particular hospital where nurses are making substantial contributions—but to let the public know that embedded in the fabric of nursing are the knowledge, skills, and desire to make significant contributions to transform health care and that nursing is essential to the challenges that come with that change.

DISCUSSION QUESTIONS

1. What change(s) in the U.S. health system do you think will provide an opportunity for nursing to improve health care?
2. What challenges do you think the profession of nursing faces as the U.S. health delivery system changes? Do you think these changes are going to improve patient care? Do you think they will improve the visibility and status of nursing?
3. What perspective does the nursing profession bring to the changing U.S. health care system?

REFERENCES

Agency for Healthcare Research and Quality, U.S. Department of Health and Human Services. (2011). *Access to health care: 2011 National healthcare disparities report.* Retrieved from https://archive.ahrq.gov/research/findings/nhqrdr/nhdr11/chap9.html.

Agency for Healthcare Research and Quality, U.S. Department of Health and Human Services. (2015, February). *Types of quality measures.* Retrieved from www.ahrq.gov/professionals/quality-patient-safety/talkingquality/create/types.html.

Agency for Healthcare Research and Quality, U.S. Department of Health and Human Services. (2017, March). *What is patient experience?* Retrieved from www.ahrq.gov/cahps/about-cahps/patient-experience/index.html.

Agrawal, P. (2014, September 12). Same care no matter where she gives birth: Addressing variation in obstetric care through standardization. *Health Affairs Blog*. Retrieved from www.healthaffairs.org/do/10.1377/hblog20140912.041347/full/.

American Association of Colleges of Nursing. (2011, April 1). *Nursing fact sheet*. Retrieved from www.aacnnursing.org/News-Information/Fact-Sheets/Nursing-Fact-Sheet.

American Hospital Association. (2018, February). *Fast facts on U.S. hospitals 2018*. Retrieved from www.aha.org/statistics/fast-facts-us-hospitals.

American Medical Association. (2016, June 14). *AMA calls gun violence "a public health crisis."* Retrieved from www.ama-assn.org/ama-calls-gun-violence-public-health-crisis.

American Nurses Association. (1996). *Mary D. Osborne (1875-1946)—Hall of fame 1996 inductee*. Retrieved from http://ojin.nursingworld.org/FunctionalMenuCategories/AboutANA/Honoring-Nurses/NationalAwardsProgram/HallofFame/19962000Inductees/osbomd5560.html.

American Nurses Association. (2018, June 15). *Stop the madness: End the violence!* Retrieved from www.nursingworld.org/news/news-releases/2018/stop-the-madness-end-the-violence/.

American Public Health Association. (2013). *The definition and practice of public health nursing*. Retrieved from www.apha.org/-/media/files/pdf/membergroups/phn/nursingdefinition.ashx.

Association of State and Territorial Health Officials. (2014). *ASTHO profile of state public health, volume three*. Retrieved from www.astho.org/Profile/Volume-Three/.

Association of State and Territorial Health Officials & NORC. (2012). *State public health agency classification: Understanding the relationship between state and local public health*. Retrieved from www.norc.org/PDFs/Projects/Classification%20of%20State%20Health%20Agencies/ASTHO%20NORC%20Governance%20Classification%20Report.pdf.

Balestra, M.L. (2017, February). Electronic health records: Patient care and ethical and legal implications for nurse practitioners. *Journal of Nurse Practitioners, 13*(2), 105–111. Retrieved from www.npjournal.org/article/S1555-4155(16)30510-4/pdf.

Belcourt, A. (2018, January 25). The hidden health inequalities that American Indians and Alaskan Natives face. *The Conversation*. Retrieved from http://theconversation.com/the-hidden-health-inequalities-that-american-indians-and-alaskan-natives-face-89905.

Benjamin, G.C. (2015, May 19). Health equity and social justice: A health improvement tool. *Grantmakers in Health: Views from the Field*. Retrieved from www.apha.org/~/media/files/pdf/topics/equity/health_equity_social_justice_apha_may_2015.ashx.

Boccuti, C., Casillas, G., & Neuman, T. (2015, May 14). *Reading the stars: Nursing home quality star ratings, nationally and by state*. Henry J. Kaiser Family Foundation. Retrieved from www.kff.org/report-section/reading-the-stars-nursing-home-quality-star-ratings-nationally-and-by-state-issue-brief/.

Boulton M.L., & Beck A.J. (2013, June 1). *Enumeration and characterization of the public health nurse workforce*. Robert Wood Johnson Foundation. Retrieved from www.rwjf.org/en/library/research/2013/06/enumeration-and-characterization-of-the-public-health-nurse-work.html.

Bureau of Labor Statistics, U.S. Department of Labor. (2018, March 30). *Occupational employment and wages—May 2017*. Retrieved from www.bls.gov/news.release/pdf/ocwage.pdf.

Center for Connected Health Policy. (2018, October). *Telehealth resource centers: A framework for defining telehealth*. Retrieved from www.cchpca.org/sites/default/files/2018-10/Telehealth%20Definintion%20Framework%20for%20TRCs_0.pdf.

Center for Connected Health Policy. (n.d.). *What is telehealth?* Retrieved from www.cchpca.org/about/about-telehealth.

Centers for Disease Control and Prevention Foundation. (n.d.) *What is public health?* Retrieved from www.cdcfoundation.org/what-public-health.

Centers for Medicare and Medicaid Services, U.S. Department of Health and Human Services. (2018). *National health expenditures 2016 highlights*. Retrieved from www.cms.gov/Research-Statistics-Data-and-Systems/Statistics-Trends-and-Reports/NationalHealthExpendData/downloads/highlights.pdf.

Congressional Budget Office. (2008, May 20). *Evidence on the costs and benefits of health information technology*. Retrieved from www.cbo.gov/publication/41690.

Cowan, R., & Cornwell, S. (2017, January 13). House votes to begin repealing Obamacare. *Reuters*. Retrieved from www.reuters.com/article/us-usa-obamacare-house-votes-to-begin-repealing-obamacare-idUSKBN14X1SK.

Creanga, A.A., Bateman B.T., Kuklina, E.V., & Callaghan W.M. (2014, May). Racial and ethnic disparities in severe maternal morbidity: A multistate analysis, 2008-2010, *American Journal of Obstetrics & Gynecology, 210*(5):435.e1–e8.

Cubanski, J., & Neuman, T. (2018, June 22). *The facts on Medicare spending and financing*. Henry J. Kaiser Family Foundation. Retrieved from www.kff.org/medicare/issue-brief/the-facts-on-medicare-spending-and-financing/.

Dafny, E. (2014, January 16). Hospital industry consolidation—Still more to come? *New England Journal of Medicine, 370*(3), 198-99.

Daniels, N. (2017, October 17). Justice and access to health care. In E.N. Zalta (Ed.), *The Stanford encyclopedia of philosophy* (Winter 2017 ed.). Retrieved from https://plato.stanford.edu/archives/win2017/entries/justice-healthcareaccess/.

Fee, E., & Liping, B. (2010, July). The origins of public health nursing: The Henry Street visiting nurse service. *American Journal of Public Health, 100*(7), 1206-1207.

Fisher, M. (2012). Here's a map of the countries that provide universal health care (America is still not on it). *The Atlantic*. Retrieved from www.theatlantic.com/international/print/2012/06/heres-a-map-of-the-countries-that-provide-universal-health-care-americas-still-not-on-it/259153/.

Flowers, D.L. (2005, February) Culturally competent nursing care for American Indian clients in a critical care setting. *Critical Care Nurse, 25*(1), 45–50. Retrieved from http://ccn.aacnjournals.org/content/25/1/45.full.pdf.

Garfield, R., Damico, A., & Orgera, K. (2018, June 18). *The coverage gap: Uninsured poor adults in states that do not expand Medicaid*. Henry J. Kaiser Family Foundation. Retrieved from www.kff.org/medicaid/issue-brief/the-coverage-gap-uninsured-poor-adults-in-states-that-do-not-expand-medicaid/.

Garrett, B., & Gangopadhyaya, A. (2016, December). *ACA implementation—Monitoring and tracking: Who gained health insurance coverage under the ACA, and where do they live?* The Urban Institute. Retrieved from www.urban.org/sites/default/files/publication/86761/2001041-who-gained-health-insurance-coverage-under-the-aca-and-where-do-they-live.pdf.

Giled, S.A., Ma S., & Borja A. (2017, May 8). *Effect of the Affordable Care Act on health care access.* The Commonwealth Fund. Retrieved from www.commonwealthfund.org/publications/issue-briefs/2017/may/effect-affordable-care-act-health-care-access.

Gilman, D.J., & Koslov, T.I. (2014, March) *Policy perspectives: Competition and the regulation of advanced practice nurses.* Office of Policy Planning, Federal Trade Commission. Retrieved from www.ftc.gov/system/files/documents/reports/policy-perspectives-competition-regulation-advanced-practice-nurses/140307aprnpolicypaper.pdf.

Goodnough, A. (2018, May 8). After years of trying, Virginia finally will expand Medicaid. *New York Times.* Retrieved from www.nytimes.com/2018/05/30/health/medicaid-expansion-virginia.html.

Heisler, E.J., & Walke, R. (2010, March 30). *Indian health care improvement act provisions in the Patient Protection and Affordable Care Act (P.L.111-148).* Congressional Research Service. Retrieved from www.ncsl.org/documents/health/indhlthcare.pdf.

Henry J. Kaiser Family Foundation. (2013, April 25). *Summary of the Affordable Care Act.* Retrieved from www.kff.org/health-reform/fact-sheet/summary-of-the-affordable-care-act/.

Henry J. Kaiser Family Foundation. (2016). *Health insurance coverage of the total population.* Retrieved from www.kff.org/other/state-indicator/total-population/.

Henry J. Kaiser Family Foundation. (2017a, June 20). *Medicaid's role in nursing home care.* Retrieved from www.kff.org/infographic/medicaids-role-in-nursing-home-care/.

Henry J. Kaiser Family Foundation. (2017b, December). *Primary care health professional shortage areas (HPSAs).* Retrieved from www.kff.org/other/state-indicator/primary-care-health-professional-shortage-areas-hpsas.

Henry J. Kaiser Family Foundation. (2018, November 7). *Status of state action on the Medicaid expansion decision.* Retrieved from www.kff.org/health-reform/state-indicator/state-activity-around-expanding-medicaid-under-the-affordable-care-act.

Henry Street Settlement. (n.d.). *About.* Retrieved from www.henrystreet.org/about/.

Hill, E.L., & Slusky, D.J.G. (2017, March 31). *Medically necessary but forbidden: Reproductive health care in Catholic-owned hospitals.* National Bureau of Economic Research working paper No. 23768. Retrieved from https://economics.ku.edu/sites/economics.ku.edu/files/files/Seminar/papers1617/april%2026.pdf.

Indian Health Service, U.S. Department of Health and Human Services. (2015, January). *Basics for health services.* Retrieved from www.ihs.gov/newsroom/factsheets/basisforhealthservices/.

Indian Health Service, U.S. Department of Health and Human Services. (2018, April). *Disparities.* Retrieved from www.ihs.gov/newsroom/factsheets/disparities/.

Indian Health Service, U.S. Department of Health and Human Services. (n.d.). *American Indians Into Nursing Program.* Retrieved from www.ihs.gov/dhps/dhpsgrants/americanindiansnursingprogram/.

Kassebaum, N.J., et al. (2016, October 8) Global, regional, and national levels of maternal mortality, 1990-2015: A systematic analysis for the Global Burden of Disease Study 2015. *The Lancet, 388,* 1775-1812. Retrieved from www.thelancet.com/pdfs/journals/lancet/PIIS0140-6736(16)31470-2.pdf.

Kent State University. (2017, April 25). *4 Devastating public health crises of the decade.* Retrieved from https://onlinedegrees.kent.edu/4-devastating-public-health-crises-decade/.

Khaikin, C., Uttley, L., & Winkler, A. (2016). *When hospitals merge: Updating state oversight to protect access to care.* The MergerWatch Project. Retrieved from https://static1.squarespace.com/static/568ad532cbced6b473f20732/t/57962bcc414fb5c7c3766775/1469459434906/MergerWatch_CON_report_June2016.pdf

Klees, B.S., Wolfe, C.J., & Curtis, C.A. (2017). *Brief summaries of Medicare and Medicaid, Title XVIII and Title XIX of the Social Security Act as of November 20, 2017.* Office of the Actuary, Centers for Medicare and Medicaid Services, Department of Health and Human Services. Retrieved from www.cms.gov/Research-Statistics-Data-and-Systems/Statistics-Trends-and-Reports/MedicareProgramRatesStats/Downloads/Medicare-MedicaidSummaries2017.pdf.

Luhby, T. (2018, October 22). Trump administration gives states new power to weaken Obamacare. *CNN.* Retrieved from www.cnn.com/2018/10/22/politics/obamacare-trump/index.html.

Mason, D.J., Glickstein, B., Nixon, L., Westphaln, K., & Acquaviva, K.D. (2018, May). The Woodhull Study revisited: Nurses' representation in health news, preliminary findings. Center for Health Policy and Management, George Washington University. Retrieved from https://nursing.gwu.edu/woodhull-study-revisited.

Meier, M.H., Albert, B.S., & Brau, S.C. (2018, August). *Overview of FTC actions in health care services and products.* U.S. Health Care Division, Bureau of Competition, Federal Trade Commission. Retrieved from www.ftc.gov/system/files/attachments/competition-policy-guidance/overview_health_care_april_2017.pdf.

Mennemeyer, S.T., Menachemi, N., Rahurkar, S., & Ford, E.W. (2016, March 1). Impact of the HITECH Act on physicians' adoption of electronic health records. *Journal of Informatics in Health and BioMedicine, 23*(2), 375–379.

Mississippi State Department of Health. (2014, November 4). *1920-1929: Beginnings and focus of public health nursing in Mississippi.* Retrieved from https://msdh.ms.gov/msdhsite/index.cfm/19,10786,378,html.

Moen, A., & Knudsen, L. (2013). Nursing informatics: Decades of contribution to health information. *Healthcare Informatics Research, 19*(2), 86-92. Retrieved from www.ncbi.nlm.nih.gov/pmc/articles/PMC3717442/.

National Academies of Sciences, Engineering, and Medicine. (2010, October 5). *The future of nursing: Leading change, advancing health.* Retrieved from www.nationalacademies.org/hmd/Reports/2010/The-Future-of-Nursing-Leading-Change-Advancing-Health.aspx.

National Association of Community Health Centers. (2011, July). *A practical guide for starting a federally qualified health center.* Retrieved from http://iweb.nachc.com/Downloads/Products/11_START_CHC.pdf.

National Association of Community Health Centers. (2015, June). *About our health centers.* Retrieved from www.nachc.org/about-our-health-centers/.

National Association of Community Health Centers. (2016, March). *Staffing the safety net: Building the primary care workforce at america's health centers.* Retrieved from www.nachc.org/wp-content/uploads/2015/10/NACHC_Workforce_Report_2016.pdf.

National Indian Health Board. (n.d.). *Indian health 101.* Retrieved from www.nihb.org/tribal_resources/indian_health_101.php.

NFIB v. Sebelius, 567 U.S. 519 (2012).

Obama, B. (2016, August 2). United States health care reform: Progress to date and next steps. *Journal of the American Medical Association, 316*(5), 525–532. Retrieved from https://jamanetwork.com/journals/jama/fullarticle/2533698.

Office for Civil Rights, U.S. Department of Health and Human Services. (2017, June). *Health information technology.* Retrieved from www.hhs.gov/hipaa/for-professionals/special-topics/health-information-technology/index.html.

Office of Disease Prevention and Health Promotion, U.S. Department of Health and Human Services. (n.d.-a). *Healthy People 2020: General health status.* Retrieved from www.healthypeople.gov/2020/about/genhealthabout.aspx.

Office of Disease Prevention and Health Promotion, U.S. Department of Health and Human Services. (n.d.-b). *Healthy People 2020: Public health infrastructure.* Retrieved from www.healthypeople.gov/2020/topics-objectives/topic/public-health-infrastructure.

Office of the National Coordinator for Health Information Technology, U.S. Department of Health and Human Services. (n.d). *Health IT and health information exchange basics.* Retrieved from www.healthit.gov/topic/health-it-and-health-information-exchange-basics/health-it-and-health-information-exchange.

Organization for Economic Cooperation and Development. (2017). *Health at a glance 2017: OECD indicators—How does the United States compare?* Retrieved from www.oecd.org/unitedstates/Health-at-a-Glance-2017-Key-Findings-UNITED-STATES.pdf.

Organization for Economic Cooperation and Development. (2018). *Life expectancy at birth indicator.* Retrieved from https://data.oecd.org/healthstat/life-expectancy-at-birth.htm.

Papanicolas, I., Woskie, L.R., & Jha, A.K. (2018, March 13). Health care spending in the United States and other high-income countries. *Journal of the American Medical Association 319*(10), 1024-1039. Retrieved from https://jamanetwork.com/journals/jama/article-abstract/2674671?resultClick=1.

Rein, L. (2018, March 9). "It's killing the agency": Ugly power struggle paralyzes Trump's plan to fix veterans' care. *Washington Post.* Retrieved from www.washingtonpost.com/politics/its-killing-the-agency-ugly-power-struggle-paralyzes-trumps-plan-to-fix-veterans-care/2018/03/08/1c33d6fe-2085-11e8-badd-7c9f29a55815_story.html.

Rein, L., Wax-Thibodeaux, E., & Dawsey, J. (2018, March 29). Trump taps his doctor to replace Shulkin at VA, choosing personal chemistry over traditional qualifications. *Washington Post.* Retrieved from www.washingtonpost.com/world/national-security/trump-ousts-veterans-affairs-chief-david-shulkin-in-administrations-latest-shake-up/2018/03/28/3c1da57e-2794-11e8-b79d-f3d931db7f68_story.html?

Rural Health Information Hub. (2017, August 2). *Telehealth use in rural healthcare.* Retrieved from www.ruralhealthinfo.org/topics/telehealth#improve-access.

Rutledge, C.M., Kott, K., Schweickert, P.A., Poston, R., Folwer, C., & Haney, T.S. (2017). Telehealth and eHealth in nurse practitioner training: Current perspectives. *Advances in Medical Education and Practice, 8,* 399–409. Retrieved from www.ncbi.nlm.nih.gov/pmc/articles/PMC5498674/.

Safriet, B.J. (2002). Closing the gap between can and may in health-care providers' scope of practice: A primer for policymakers, *Yale Journal on Regulation, 19,* 301–334.

Scott, D. (2018, July 2). The "pleasant ambiguity" of Medicare-for-all in 2018 explained. *Vox.* Retrieved from www.vox.com/policy-and-politics/2018/7/2/17468448/medicare-for-all-single-payer-health-care-2018-elections.

Shulkin, D.J. (2018, March 28). David J. Shulkin: Privatizing the V.A. will hurt veterans [op-ed]. *New York Times.* Retrieved from www.nytimes.com/2018/03/28/opinion/shulkin-veterans-affairs-privatization.html.

Singh, G.K. (2010). *Maternal mortality in the United States, 1935-2007: Substantial racial/ethnic, socioeconomic, and geographic disparities persist.* U.S. Department of Health and Human Services, Health Research and Services Administration, Maternal and Child Health Bureau. Retrieved from www.hrsa.gov/sites/default/files/ourstories/mchb75th/mchb75maternalmortality.pdf.

Squires, D. (2015, October 8). *U.S. health care from a global perspective: Spending, use of services, prices, and health in 13 countries.* The Commonwealth Fund. Retrieved from www.commonwealthfund.org/publications/issue-briefs/2015/oct/us-health-care-from-a-global-perspective.

Thede, L. (2012, January 23). Informatics: Where is it? *Online Journal of Issues in Nursing 17*(1). Retrieved from www.nursingworld.org/MainMenuCategories/ANAMarketplace/ANA-Periodicals/OJIN/TableofContents/Vol-17-2012/No1-Jan-2012/Informatics-Where-Is-It.html.

Trust for America's Health. (2018, March). *A funding crisis for public health and safety: State-by-state public health funding and key health facts.* Retrieved from www.tfah.org/wp-content/uploads/archive/assets/files/TFAH-2018-InvestInAmericaRpt-FINAL.pdf.

U.S. Department of Veterans Affairs. (2016, May). *My VA putting veterans first: Transformation update.* Retrieved from www.va.gov/opa/publications/docs/myva_transformation_update_8x10.pdf.

U.S. Department of Veterans Affairs. (2018a). *About VA.* Retrieved from www.va.gov/about_va/vahistory.asp.

U.S. Department of Veterans Affairs. (2018b). *2019 Congressional submission: Budget in brief.* Retrieved from www.va.gov/budget/docs/summary/fy2019VAbudgetInBrief.pdf.

Veterans Benefit Administration, U.S. Department of Veterans Affairs. (2018). *Veterans Benefits Administration reports: Claims backlog.* Retrieved from https://benefits.va.gov/reports/mmwr_va_claims_backlog.asp.

Woodhull Study Advisory Group. (1998). *The Woodhull Study on Nursing and the Media: Health care's invisible partner.* Center Nursing Press, Sigma Theta Tau International. Retrieved from www.nursingrepository.org/bitstream/handle/10755/624124/WoodhullReport1997.pdf?sequence=1&isAllowed=y.

Yen, H. (2018, January 6). AP fact check: Trump overstates progress in veterans' care. *Associated Press.* Retrieved from www.apnews.com/2ad7e0e3606043f9835140632deffbbc.

ONLINE RESOURCES

Agency for Healthcare Research and Quality
www.ahrq.gov
Henry J. Kaiser Family Foundation
www.kff.org
Organization for Economic Cooperation: Health
www.oecd.org/health

16

A Primer on Health Economics of Nursing and Health Policy

Len M. Nichols[a]

"The price of light is less than the cost of darkness."

Arthur Nielsen

Economics is the study of how resources are allocated by people operating in the real world, that is, with constraints on their time, their money, and their knowledge. It can be summarized as the study of choices people make under constraints. Because some constraints are operable on everyone, economists say the real world is a world of scarcity, by which they mean no one, and certainly not everyone, can have everything they might want. Sometimes choices today can relax constraints in the future (e.g., studying for an advanced degree can enable someone to earn higher wages and have more income to spend on goods and services in the future). Sometimes choices today are extremely limited by effective constraints (e.g., when the only jobs available pay the minimum wage; no matter how hard one works or how much one makes, there are only 24 hours in a day and every human must sleep).

ECONOMICS AS A DISCIPLINE

Choices under constraints produce trade-offs, which usually boil down to the fact that you can have more of one desirable thing only if you give up another. Time for money is the classic trade-off, and allocating a limited budget over competing priorities is something every manager (household or business) in the modern world is familiar with. This sets up the fundamental economic concept of opportunity cost, or what must be given up to get something else. This is a better definition of cost than price or out-of-pocket payment, both of which can be distorted by

insurance, taxes, or subsidies from the true total cost of acquiring any good or service.

Economics is a social science, which means it uses logic and analytic tools to develop models that attempt to characterize and explain the essence of a human choice situation. Models must omit some details to be manageable, and the art of creating models is deciding which details are essential (and measurable) and which can be omitted. The results of the models are predictions or hypotheses about how the real world works, how choices will be made, or what the implications of choices already made will be. These predictions and hypotheses can then be tested against real world observations or data.

When the models are confirmed as correct, then the results are added to the body of economic knowledge and passed on to others. When the models and predictions are shown to be inaccurate, then the models and thinking about the type of problem under study are revised. In that sense, economics is empirically driven or evidence based. Economics has evolved over time and continues to evolve, as new data emerge and new models, theories, and hypotheses are created; they compete with old models, theories, and hypotheses virtually all the time. This constant evolution is also partly why economists rarely reach unanimous consensus, but if a preponderance of evidence exists at a point in time, then a majority of economists will lean in a certain direction, just like health or other professionals do as evidence evolves in their fields.

Why Health Care Is a Hard Economic Case

Health care has some particular features that make it different from most markets, even though economic analysis can still be applied with appropriate attention to these

---

[a]This chapter is reprinted from the seventh edition of the book with minor revisions by Diana Mason.

details. Number one is unavoidable information asymmetry. This means either buyers or sellers have knowledge the other does not about a good or service. This asymmetry violates one of the key tenets of competitive markets and creates the opportunity for some market participants to take advantage of others without safeguards and institutions to protect them. Health professionals know more than most patients will ever fully understand about the patient's condition and treatment options. This information gap is why the Hippocratic Oath and the Nursing Code of Ethics came into being and use long ago. In the extreme case, malpractice law and the procedures that health care organizations undertake to protect themselves from liability claims also protect patients. Plans and employers and consumer-oriented organizations try to act as agents on the patient's behalf, but they are almost always working from an informational disadvantage that affects market outcomes. The current movement toward transparent quality metrics is helping, but informational asymmetry is present in almost every health care transaction.

The second big difference in health care is the importance of third party payers compared with most markets. Public and private insurers (and sometimes employers, as self-insured organizations) pay the bulk of the cost of health care, but decisions about what services to deliver are made by clinicians and patients, sometimes far removed from knowledge of total cost. Therefore direct market participants cannot weigh the true cost and benefit of choices, which again violates a key assumption of competitive markets.

Finally, the reality is that health care is sometimes a matter of life and death, and for humanitarian and professional ethics reasons, services are sometimes delivered regardless of a patient's ability to pay. This uncompensated care must be financed, and it is, by a combination of government subsidies, higher charges to private payers who can pay more, and some health care workers accepting little or no compensation for some of their efforts. Each of these three deviations from normal competitive conditions means that market signals from health care transactions can be distorted, which can in turn distort investment and resource allocation decisions across the board. Distortions from competitive market norms require that economic analysis takes these features into account when analyzing health care markets.

A FUNDAMENTAL ECONOMIC TOOL

Supply and Demand

The first tool in the economists' tool kit is supply and demand analysis, which we apply to registered nurses (RNs) in a hospital setting to illustrate its use. This tool can explain wage and employment trends and help to make predictions about the future.

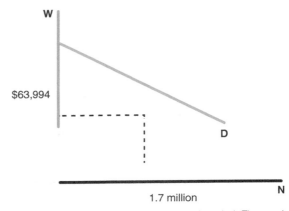

Fig. 16.1 Demand (D) for nurses in the hospital. The vertical axis is wage (W), which could be hourly, weekly, monthly, or annually, but must be specified to be precise. The horizontal axis is the number of nurses (N).

Let's start with the demand curve for nurses. Centuries of evidence suggest that almost all demand curves are downward sloping, that is, as the price of whatever falls, consumers will want more of it, and vice versa. The price of a nurse to a consumer is the wage or salary, plus the costs of necessary benefits that an employer, the hospital, and consumer in this case must pay. Thus economists postulate that the demand for nurses in the hospital setting looks something like what is shown in Fig. 16.1.

The U.S. Department of Health and Human Services (HHS) Health Resources and Services Administration (HRSA) (2010) provides the most recent estimates at the annual level, so we will use annual figures for this illustration. The average wage was $63,994 and 1.7 million were employed in hospitals (2.8 million were working nurses in all fields).

As wages fall, more nurses would be demanded by hospitals, and conversely, as wages rise, fewer nurses will be sought after. We will discuss cycles of nursing wages and employment trends in a bit, but for now, we want to make clear what might shift the entire curve or demand schedule and thus change the number of nurses that would be demanded at each wage. Graphically, we are asking what might shift the curve from D1 to D2, as in Fig. 16.2.

Factors that are assumed to be constant for each demand curve and, if they change, will shift the entire demand curve include:
- The size and health of the population that might need hospital care, inpatient or outpatient
- The percentage of that population that is well managed and coordinated by an independent primary care group that minimizes the need for hospital care

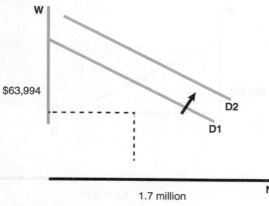

Fig. 16.2 Demand (D) for nurses in the hospital. The vertical axis is wage (W), which could be hourly, weekly, monthly, or annually but must be specified to be precise. The horizontal axis is the number of nurses (N).

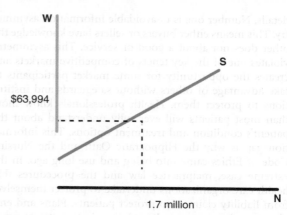

Fig. 16.3 The supply (S) of nurses in the hospital. The vertical axis is wage (W), which could be hourly, weekly, monthly, or annually but must be specified to be precise. The horizontal axis is the number of nurses (N).

- The number of hospitals, the number of beds in those hospitals
- The number of outpatient units
- The number of physicians and or advanced nursing practices, nursing homes, or home health agencies the hospitals own
- The production function of delivering care (substituting more or fewer other health professionals for RNs in the technology of care delivery)
- The prices/wages of potential substitutes or other complementary health professionals (e.g., licensed practical nurses, advanced practice nurses, or physicians)

Changes in any of these factors can shift the curve outward from D1 to D2, or inward (not shown). Changes in these factors help explain employment and wage trends for nurses over time.

The supply curve for hospital nurses is even more straightforward. The greater the wage, the more nurses are willing to work in the hospital setting or settings the hospital owns, as shown in Fig. 16.3.

The factors that would shift the entire supply curve for nurses include:

- Net growth in qualified nursing personnel willing to work in hospitals, such as new entrants from nursing schools and programs minus retirements
- Working conditions in hospitals versus other employment alternatives (e.g., nursing homes, skilled nursing facilities, assisted living facilities, independent physician's offices, home health agencies, other ambulatory clinics, ambulatory surgery centers, diagnostic laboratories)
- Wages in alternative employment

- Other household income (either from a spouse or invested wealth)

Note the first supply-shifting factor, net growth in qualified nursing personnel, reflects the impact of nursing faculty, federal support for nursing education, and preceptor shortage realities. Combing the pieces of the tool, Fig. 16.4 displays equilibrium in the market for hospital nurses. Fig. 16.4 depicts an equilibrium in the economist's sense that the wage has no tendency to rise or fall, because the quantity demanded equals the quantity supplied. A change in the number of hospitals or the wages of nurses in nursing homes, for example, would shift demand

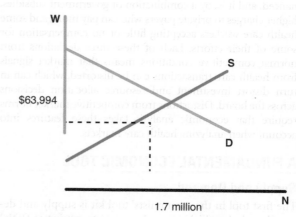

Fig. 16.4 The demand (D) and supply (S) of nurses in the hospital. The vertical axis is wage (W), which could be hourly, weekly, monthly, or annually but must be specified to be precise. The horizontal axis is the number of nurses (N).

or supply, respectively, and upset the equilibrium in this market over time. Demand and supply curves, once stable, do engender forces that tend to push prices/wages to the market clearing levels, which is when the market reaches equilibrium and the demand equals supply and there is then no tendency to change.

Vacancy Rates

The purpose of this primer is to use economics to explain key dimensions of the markets for nurses and their implications for health policy. All nurse managers know that hospitals usually face nursing vacancies, so they might be wondering, how can there be a positive vacancy rate in hospitals and also strong tendencies to equilibrium wages? Doesn't the persistence of vacancy rates that never go away render the traditional tools of economics inaccurate for nursing markets? No, and here's why.

A vacancy rate, the percentage of nursing positions that are unfilled, is a reflection of a shortage, where demand exceeds supply. Shortages should not persist if wages adjust upward to market (equilibrium) clearing levels. The actual history of vacancy rates and nursing wage adjustments suggests that the standard economic model works reasonably well to explain movements in wages and employment but with a lag for real world inertia. This inertia in raising wages is commonly caused by reluctance to raise nurses' pay until other options for recruitment are exhausted, as well as the time lag before information about higher wages and aggressive recruitment is well known enough to encourage more entry into nursing schools, reentry to work, or increasing hours of nursing work (Fig. 16.5) (Feldstein, 2011).

One technical note about Fig. 16.5; the darker line shows real wage growth, or wages adjusted for inflation. This is a relevant concept because, if wages do not rise as much as inflation, this amounts to a wage cut, because actual purchasing power of the wage level would have declined.

Two inferences should be drawn from Fig. 16.5: (1) Real wage growth can be negative if vacancy rates are low enough or falling long enough and (2) vacancy rates did not fall below 4% between 1979 and 2009. This suggests there is a natural floor in vacancy rates below which hospital administrators are not comfortable hiring; that is, they do not really want the market for nurses to clear completely, possibly because they fear how high equilibrium wages might actually be at that moment, and those high wages would significantly increase hospital costs, very possibly forever. Thus equilibrium in nursing markets is effectively reached when hospital vacancy rates are approximately 4%.

COST-EFFECTIVENESS OF NURSING SERVICES

In this era of hyper–cost consciousness, every part of the health care system is often required and wants to demonstrate its unique value. Cost-effectiveness is a technique that allows analysts to compare the costs and outcomes, in nonmonetary units such as body mass index reduction or quality-adjusted life years (QALYs) saved, across two or more possible strategies. It differs from cost-benefit analysis in that the outcomes are not measured in monetary terms but in health-related terms. Thus, if intervention A is more cost-effective than intervention B, either it yields the

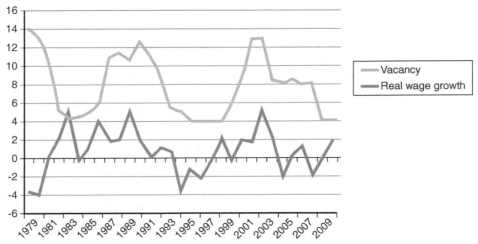

Fig. 16.5 Registered nurse (RN) vacancy rate and real wage growth.

same health benefit for a lower cost or it delivers more health benefit per dollar cost. The relevant metric is usually cost per QALY saved.

Cost-effectiveness studies are surprisingly rarely done on alternative nursing staffing patterns and care delivery modalities. The literature is much more likely to report analyses of a small number of advanced practice nurses partially or wholly replacing physicians or being added to a physician-led team. It is far simpler, frankly, to investigate the impact on cost and outcomes from a specific *marginal* intervention, for example, adding a care-coordination nurse to a primary care practice, than to compare the cost-effectiveness of 7:1 versus 5:1 hospital patient to nurse staffing ratios across hospitals in the United States. The former requires only an accounting of changes in costs and outcomes, and marginal costs are typically just the nurses' salaries, whereas the marginal outcome effect might be reduced admissions, reduced emergency room visits, better hypertension control, and so on. The latter requires complete transparency of different hospital accounting systems, congruence on allocation of fixed costs and variable costs, and so on. This is why the few studies of the effect of nurse staffing patterns on cost that have been done have typically focused on the impact on quality or patient outcomes, not overall hospital costs. It is simply too difficult to compare costs across hospitals because of variable accounting practices.

A notable exception is the paper by Rothberg and colleagues (2005) that estimated the cost-effectiveness of moving the patient/nurse ratio from 8:1 to 4:1, using total hospital costs as the cost metric. Those costs depend on nursing wages, and how much they would have to rise to call forth the proposed increase in staffing ratios (acknowledging the supply curve for nursing labor is upward sloping, as we postulated and drew previously); cost per hospital day; impact of more nursing hours on adverse events, mortality, and length of stay; and the risk of nurse dissatisfaction from high patient/nurse ratios and the cost of turnover. The most important feature of a good cost-effectiveness analysis is to do a complete inventory of existing and differential costs and impacts on outcomes. Rothberg and colleagues (2005) used estimates of the range of these costs and impacts from the published literature and did sensitivity analyses of the values of the key variables along with a Monte Carlo technique, which essentially runs the experimental calculation (or gamble, hence the name) repeatedly to yield the range of possible outcomes and the best possible estimate of the most likely outcome from lower patient-to-nurse ratios.

Rothberg and colleagues (2005) found that reducing patient/nurse ratios from 8:1 to 4:1 reduced mortality and increased costs, but that the incremental mortality gain per dollar fell as the ratio got closer to 4:1. In other words, cost per life saved rose as the ratio fell toward 4:1. Moving from 8:1 to 7:1 cost $24,900 per life saved (in 2005 dollars), whereas moving from 5:1 to 4:1 cost $136,300 per life saved, more than five times as much. The former would clearly be within the $50,000 per life saved threshold typically used by U.S. insurers and government agencies around the developed world to decide if a treatment is worth covering (Grosse, 2008; Neumann & Cohen, 2018; Weinstein, 2008). The latter incremental gain in mortality would not pass this threshold test. Still, most states leave staffing decisions to hospitals, and they are, predictably, all over the map in the absence of a definitive empirical study and national regulation. Thus the final decision is left to the market.

IMPACT OF HEALTH REFORM ON NURSING ECONOMICS

The Affordable Care Act (ACA) has many features which impact nursing and the entire health care system, but the most far reaching for nursing are those which relate to payment and delivery reforms. The increasingly explicit aim of the ACA is to catalyze, through public programs and multipayer incentives, a transformation across the health care system from fee-for-service medicine (which is basically pay-for-volume) to more accountable health care that will be closer to pay-for-value. This approach is reflected in the ACA's shared savings programs, especially Pioneer Accountable Care Organizations, the ACA Patient-Centered Medical Home (PCMH) experiment, and the Comprehensive Primary Care Initiative, as well as with bundled payments. The underlying assumption, widely shared, is that enabling most health delivery organizations to provide high-value care is the only way the health system as a whole is going to be financially sustainable, while serving all of us, as the ACA also envisions, rather than some of us, as the U.S. health care system currently does.

Although the new emerging models of care obviously differ in details, they share one common theme, which is to pay groups of providers for larger and larger units of service. For example, instead of paying physicians separately for each visit and associated tests with fee-for-service and then paying hospitals separately for each admission with a diagnosis-related group (DRG)–based payment, pay one lump sum to a team to take care of the patient for a given episode (bundled payment) or length of time (global capitation). The opportunity for nursing is that nurses' inherent skill set, patient-focused care, communication, and coordination across silos of care can help both physicians and hospitals to deliver higher-quality care more efficiently than today. The challenge for nursing is that the price is largely hidden, within the per visit charges of physicians and within the per diem charges of hospitals. This means that current data systems are unable to credibly estimate the value of nursing services and the optimal configuration of nurses within multidisciplinary clinical teams. Keeping a clear eye on nursing value to the team is essential for truly cost-effective and high-quality care to be priced and delivered, and not all managers are able to do this at the moment (Buerhaus, 2010).

These types of payment reforms are being adopted by private payers, in some cases faster than the government pilots can spread, such as with PCMHs. What they all have in common, for the first time in American health care (except for the closed staff model health maintenance organizations such as Kaiser Permanente and Group Health Cooperative), is that providers have powerful incentives to reorganize care delivery and coordination processes to seek the Triple Aim: cost-effective, timely, and efficacious care. Although this transformation is likely to be good for nurses at the RN level and above in the medium and long term, the transformation is not without risks and probably bodes some pain for some nurses in the short term.

The first-order effect of these incentive changes has been to modernize the nation's nurse practice acts to reflect current standards. The intense battles in many state houses over the scope of practice of advanced practice nurses have become relatively moot, because now health delivery organizations gain from using advanced practice nurses and others to practice at the top of their education and training. Too often, restrictive state nurse practice acts are still intent on protecting physicians' short-run economic interests at the expense of higher-cost care and limited access to qualified providers for all concerned. The ACA and the incentives it unleashed will eventually lead to full practice authority for these nurses.

This general incentive realignment is extending to reorganizing physician offices, starting with primary care because of the sheer number of PCMHs already in existence (attributable to public and private initiatives), but it will soon extend to specialists and hospitals also. Care-coordination nurses and nurses who function well within and even lead team-based delivery of care can earn premium wages, because communication across former silos of care will be paramount to reduce the avoidable hospital admissions and readmissions that have been huge cost drivers for patients with multiple chronic conditions. Systems which learn how to lower the costs on high-cost patients who account for most health care expenditures and attain satisfactory outcomes at the same time will be the systems that flourish. Nurses and social workers are becoming the backbone and sinew of care coordination and these new, more efficient systems of care.

A short-run cost could materialize for those nurses who work for hospitals and physician groups who deny, delay, or resist this incentive realignment and do not clearly see the value of nursing services, long past the point of being behind their peers. Top-level managers of these organizations may not be doing appropriate cost-effectiveness analyses of how best to reorganize care to align with new incentive structures but may rather be focused on preserving their top-level incomes even as overall revenue inevitably falls. The only solution they may see is to increase patient/nurse ratios by laying off relatively expensive RNs and either not replacing them or replacing them with lower-trained and less-expensive health professionals. And some small outlying hospitals will close owing to lack of demand for their services in a world focused on the ability of enhanced primary care to prevent hospitalizations and readmissions.

The marketplace will then have two strategies in competition: (1) a lower-cost and more team-based approach and (2) a higher-cost and more libertarian or traditional cowboy style go-it-alone health care. The lower-cost and team-based approach will surely win, but it may take a while before the evidence is clear to the common public, and the traditional providers will, in the meantime, claim loudly that they are the only high-quality alternative left. Credible quality measurement infrastructures, price, and quality transparency for consumers to make comparison shopping possible will hasten the demise of the old school strategy, but even so it may take 10 years at least before it disappears altogether.

The ACA will then ultimately create a more welcoming environment for nurses and their many talents, but some might have a more painful transition to this better world than others.

DISCUSSION QUESTIONS

1. Describe at least three issues that make the health care market behave differently from other markets.
2. According to economic principles, what forces go into play as demand for nursing goes up?
3. What role could nurses play, enlarge, or expand in value-driven care delivery models such as Primary Care Medical Homes and Accountable Care Organizations?

REFERENCES

Buerhaus, P.I. (2010). Health care payment reform: Implications for nurses. *Nursing Economics, 28*(1), 49-54. Retrieved from https://proxy.library.upenn.edu/login?url=https://search.proquest.com/docview/236936730?accountid=14707.

Feldstein, P.J. (2011). *Health policy issues: An economic perspective.* Chicago, IL: Health Administration Press.

Grosse, S. (2008). Assessing cost-effectiveness in healthcare: history of the $50,000 per QALY threshold. *Expert Review of Pharmacoeconomics & Outcomes Research*, 8(2), 165–178.

Neumann, P., & Cohen, J.T. (2018). QALYs in 2018—Advantages and concerns. *JAMA, 319*(24), 2473-2474.

Rothberg, M., Abraham, I., Lindenauer, P., & Rose, D. (2005). Improving nurse to patient staffing ratios as a cost-effective safety intervention. *Medical Care, 43*(8), 785–791.

U.S. Department of Health and Human Services, Health Resources and Services Administration, Bureau of Health Professions. (2010). *The registered nurse population: Initial findings from the 2008 National Sample Survey of Registered Nurses.* Retrieved from bhpr.hrsa.gov/healthworkforce/rnsurveys/rnsurveyinitial2008.pdf.

Weinstein, M. (2008). How much are Americans willing to pay for a quality-adjusted life year? *Medical Care, 46*(4), 343–344.

17

Financing Health Care in the United States

Joyce A. Pulcini and Betty Rambur

> *"What does U.S. health care have in common with an exotic international bazaar? The prices at one are almost never posted, whether for a heart bypass operation or antique rug. And the final price will almost certainly have little to do with the seller's opening bid."*
>
> **Susan Dentzer**

Health care financing in the United States is fragmented, complex, and fuels the most costly care in the world. Despite this expense, the United States consistently ranks low in quality and the last in health outcomes among 11 wealthy countries (Schneider et al., 2017). As designed, our system leaves many overtreated (Lyu et al., 2017)—and, paradoxically, underserved (Grady & Redberg, 2010)—others undertreated, and all riddled with unnecessary, inefficient, and harmful care (Berwick & Hackbarth, 2012). Representing roughly one-fifth of the U.S. economy, medical errors are recognized as the third leading cause of death in the country (Makary & Daniel, 2016).

The Affordable Care Act (ACA) of 2010 took steps to reshape how health care is paid for, enhance transparency, and test new payment and delivery models, but its primary purpose was to extend insurance coverage to the large number of uninsured Americans through private insurance regulation, expansion of public insurance programs, and creation of health insurance marketplaces to foster competition in the private health insurance market. Despite ACA implementation and revisions, health insurance affordability and cost containment are significant ongoing policy challenges (see Chapter 18 for more on the ACA). This chapter will provide an overview of U.S. health care financing, reimbursement and payment reform, including the impact of the ACA, the Tax Cuts and Jobs Act of 2017 (TCJA) (P.L. 115-97, Congress.gov, n.d.)—an amendment to the Internal Revenue Code with health care implications—and selected federal administrative rules changes and state-led initiatives.

HISTORICAL PERSPECTIVES ON HEALTH CARE FINANCING

Understanding today's complex and often confusing approaches to financing health care requires an examination of the nation's values and historical context. Some dominant values underpin the U.S. political and economic systems. The United States has a long history of individualism, an emphasis on freedom to choose alternatives, and an aversion to large-scale government intervention into the private realm. Compared with other industrialized nations, social programs have been the exception rather than the rule and have been adopted primarily during times of great need or social and political upheaval. Examples of these exceptions include the passage of the Social Security Act of 1935 and the passage of Medicare and Medicaid in 1965.

Health care in the United States had its origins in the private sector market with an aim of assuring reimbursement to physicians and hospitals (Starr, 1982), rather than providing care to consumers. The political power of physicians, hospitals, and the insurance industry has fueled a continuing debate about the degree to which government should be involved in health care. Other highly developed countries, such as Canada, the United Kingdom, France, Germany, and Switzerland, use a range of private and public financing mechanisms to provide health care for all their citizens. In contrast, the United States has viewed health care as a market-based commodity, readily available to those who can pay for it but not available universally to all people. The passage of the ACA was significant, though controversial, in its approach to expand access to affordable health insurance.

The debate over the role of government in social programs intensified in the decades after the Great Depression. The Social Security Act of 1935 brought sweeping social welfare legislation, providing Social Security payments, workman's compensation, welfare assistance for the poor, and certain public health, maternal, and child health services, but it did not provide health care insurance for all Americans. During the decade following the Great Depression, nonprofit Blue Cross and Blue Shield (BC/BS) emerged as a private insurance plan to cover hospital and physician care. The idea that people should pay for their medical care through insurance before they actually got sick ensured some level of security for both providers and consumers of medical services. The creation of insurance plans effectively defused a strong political movement toward legislating a broader, compulsory, government-run health insurance plan at the time (Starr, 1982). After a failed attempt by President Truman to legislate a national health plan in the late 1940s, no progress occurred on this issue until the 1960s, when Medicare and Medicaid were enacted as amendments to the original Social Security Act.

BC/BS dominated the health insurance industry until the 1950s, when for-profit commercial insurance companies entered the market and were able to compete with BC/BS by holding down costs through their practice of excluding sick people (those with preexisting conditions) from insurance coverage. Over time, the distinction between BC/BS and commercial insurance companies became increasingly blurred as BC/BS began to offer financially competitive for-profit plans (Knickman & Kovner, 2015). In the 1960s, the United States enjoyed relative prosperity, along with a burgeoning social conscience, and an appetite for change that led to a heightened concern for the poor and older adults and the impact of catastrophic illness. In response, Medicaid and Medicare, two separate but related programs, were created in 1965 as amendments to the Social Security Act. Medicare is a federal government-administered health insurance program for the disabled entitled to Social Security Disability Insurance (SSDI) benefits, those over 65 years, and those with end-stage renal disease (started in 1973) or amyotrophic lateral sclerosis (started in 2001) regardless of age. Medicaid is a federal program administrated by states but funded by both federal and state monies. It is subject to state rules within parameters required by the federal government. It was designed to serve low-income people who are in certain categories, such as pregnant women with children and elderly or disabled individuals who meet certain income limits.

GOVERNMENT PROGRAMS

Current Public/Federal Funding for Health Care in the United States

National health expenditures (NHE) are substantial in the United States, totaling $3.3 trillion in 2016 or $10,348 per person and accounting for 17.9% of the gross domestic product (GDP) (Centers for Medicare and Medicaid Services [CMS], 2018b). The proportion of health care spending by type of care in 2015 is presented in Fig. 17.1.

Medicare outlays were $672.1 billion in 2016 and accounted for 20% of all NHE. Medicaid outlays in 2016 were $565.5 billion and accounted for 17% of total NHE. In 2016, hospital and physician expenditures and clinical services expenditures had slower growth rates than in 2015 by 5.7% and 5.9%, respectively, and prescription drug spending was 8.9% slower than in 2015 (CMS, 2018b). The federal government's share of this health care spending was 28.3%; the proportion of Medicare spending as a share of total federal spending on health care as of 2017 is seen in Fig. 17.2. Why so expensive?

In the United States, no single public entity oversees or controls the entire health care system, making the payment for and delivery of health care complex, inefficient, and expensive. Instead, the system is composed of many public and private programs that form interrelated parts at the federal, state, and local levels. The public funding systems continue to represent a larger and larger proportion of health care spending and include Medicare, Medicaid, the Children's Health Insurance Program (CHIP), the U.S. Department of Veterans Affairs (VA), and the U.S. Department of Defense Military Health System program TRICARE for military personnel, military retirees, and their families. Other examples of federal programs are the Indian Health Service, which covers American Indians and Alaskan Natives, and the Federal Employees Health Benefits (FEHB) Program, which covers all federal employees unless excluded by law or regulation. The U.S. system is often perceived as a private or pluralistic system inclusive of both private and public payers; but, starting in 1965, the government was and continues to be deeply involved with U.S. health care. Himmelstein and Woolhandler (2016) reported that 64.3% of U.S. health care was financed through a governmental mechanism in 2014, and this is projected to rise to 67.1% by 2024, while Canada—a nation with single-payer financing offering universal coverage—is roughly 70% publicly funded. Notably, their study included all forms of public funding inclusive of direct governmental payments for Medicare, Medicaid and the other public programs described above, public employee's health insurance, and federal, state, and local tax subsidies to health care.

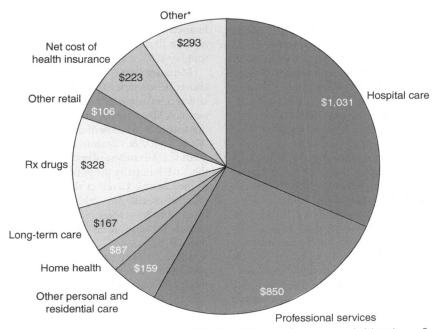

Fig. 17.1 National health expenditures by category, 2015 ($bn). *Other = Government administration + Government public health activities + Investment (noncommercial research, structures, and equipment). (Courtesy of Kaiser Family Foundation. National health expenditure projections. [2014–2024]. Spending growth faster than recent trends. *Health Affairs, 34*(8), 1407–1417. Centers for Medicare and Medicaid Services, Office of the Actuary, National Health Statistics Group.)

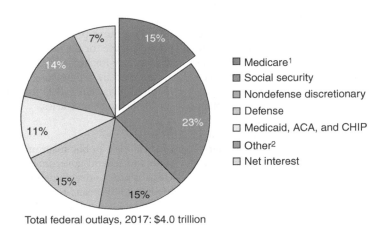

Total federal outlays, 2017: $4.0 trillion
Net federal medicare outlays, 2017: $591 billion

Note: All amounts are for federal fiscal year 2017. [1]Consists of mandatory medicare spending minus income from premiums and other offsetting receipts [2]Includes spending on other mandatory outlays minus income from offsetting receipts. ACA is Affordable Care Act. CHIP is Children's Health Insurance Program.

Fig. 17.2 Medicare as a share of the federal budget, 2017. (Courtesy of Kaiser Family Foundation. Retrieved from www.kff.org/medicare/issue-brief/the-facts-on-medicare-spending-and-financing/.)

Medicare

Before the enactment of Medicare in 1965, older adults were more likely to be impoverished by excessive health care costs. The proportion of elders covered with health insurance shifted from 56% prior to Medicare to 98% now. Roughly 17% of people with Medicare are younger than 65 and are disabled (National Committee to Preserve Medicare and Medicaid, 2018). Medicare provides access to care and medical technology, and, since 2006, prescription drug coverage.

But health coverage may not be enough to ensure that older adults are able to live healthy lives. The percentage of persons over age 65 years living below the poverty line decreased from 35% in 1959 (when older adults had the highest poverty rate of the population) to 9.3% in 2016 (U.S. Census Bureau, 2018); however, there is now evidence of increasing poverty among older population on fixed incomes. The National Council on Aging (NCOA, 2018b) reports that more than 25 million individuals over 60 are living at or below 250% of poverty. They also note that 21% of Social Security recipients who are married and 43% of single recipients aged 65+ depend on Social Security for 90% or more of their income.

Medicare and Social Security payments come in part from payroll deductions taken during working years and are not merely "government handouts" as some claim. At the same time, entitlement funding can fuel overtreatment. Disproportionate funding of the older population—particularly for care that is of low value, wasteful, or unnecessary—raises concerns about intergenerational injustice, because these public funds may not be available for other segments of society such as children (Newacheck & Benjamin, 2014). The Medicare trustees annual report regularly projects that the Medicare hospital insurance trust fund will be depleted by certain dates. For example, the 2018 report projects that the fund will be depleted in 2026, 3 years earlier than the projection in 2017 (Cubanski & Newman, 2018), and fiscal concerns are likely to accelerate as more baby boomers obtain Medicare eligibility.

Americans are eligible for Medicare Part A at age 65 years, the age for Social Security eligibility, or sooner if they are determined to be disabled. Medicare Part A accounted for $280.5 billion in benefit spending in 2016 and covered 56 million Americans. Medicare Part A covers hospital and related costs and is financed through payroll deduction to fund the hospital insurance trust fund at the payroll tax rate of 2.9% of earnings paid by employers and employees (1.45% each) (CMS, 2017a). Medicare Part B, which accounted for $289.5 billion in spending in 2016, covers 80% of the fees for physician services, outpatient medical services and supplies, home care, durable medical equipment, laboratory services, physical and occupational

therapy, and outpatient mental health services. Part B is financed through subscriber premiums and general revenue funding as well as cost-sharing with beneficiaries set at roughly 20% of costs of care used.

Medicare Part C, or the Medicare Advantage Program, allows beneficiaries to enroll in a private health plan and also receive some extra services such as vision or hearing services. Medicare Advantage enrollment has been increasing and covered 33% of all Medicare beneficiaries in 2017 (Cox, Levitt, & Claxton, 2017). In 2018, CMS provided Medicare Advantage plans with a 3.4% increase, well above the 1.84% initially proposed (Dickson, 2018). An element of the Chronic Care Act also expands Medicare Advantage reimbursement for telehealth provided outside rural areas and allows these plans to participate in new payment models for chronically ill patients (Veterans Administration, 2018).

Medicare Part D is a voluntary, subsidized outpatient prescription drug plan with additional subsidies for low- and modest-income individuals. It accounted for about $99 billion in benefit spending in 2016 and enrolled 43 million beneficiaries in 2016 (CMS, 2017a). Medicare Part D is financed through general revenues and beneficiary premiums, as well as state payments for "dual eligibles"—recipients who get both Medicare and Medicaid (Kaiser Family Foundation [KFF] 2014). The ACA will phase out by 2020 the Medicare Part D "donut hole" period of noncoverage for prescription drugs that left many seniors unable to pay out-of-pocket for their medications (CMS, 2017a).

The ACA authorized that certified nurse midwives (CNMs) be reimbursed at 100% of the physician payment rate. Other advanced practice registered nurses (APRNs), including nurse practitioners (NPs), are paid 85% of the physician rate for the same services. In addition, Medicare will not pay for home care or hospice services unless they are ordered by a physician. And, unfortunately, the ACA required physician orders for durable medical equipment for Medicare beneficiaries.

Medicaid

Medicaid is a public insurance program jointly funded by state and federal governments but administered by individual states under guidelines of the federal government. Medicaid is a means-tested program, as eligibility is determined by financial status. Before changes by the ACA, only low-income people within certain categories were eligible. These categories included recipients of Supplemental Security Income (SSI), families receiving Temporary Assistance to Needy Families (TANF), and children and pregnant women whose family income is at or below 133% of the poverty level. To qualify for federal Medicaid matching grants, a state must provide a minimum set of benefits, including hospitalization, physician care, laboratory services, radiology studies, prenatal care, and preventive services; nursing home and home health care; and medically necessary transportation. Some states opt to provide a greater set of services than the minimum and also allow eligibility at a higher percent of poverty. The proportion of residents on Medicaid also varies dramatically by state, with New Mexico the highest at 31% of its residents on Medicaid and CHIP, and Utah the lowest at 10%, with a nationwide average of 19% (KFF, 2018a) (Fig. 17.3). Medicaid programs are also required to pay the Medicare premiums, deductibles, and copayments for "dual eligible" persons who are often medically complex, frail, and thus expensive to insure.

Medicaid is increasingly becoming a long-term care financing program for older adults in nursing homes,

representing nearly two-thirds of total nursing home spending. Although roughly half of long-term care is delivered in nursing homes and half in community settings, nursing homes account for 70% of the cost (KFF, 2017a). Many older adults "spend down" their life savings to become low income and be eligible for Medicaid, an issue with ethical concerns on both sides of the argument. One view is that these funds should be a genuine safety net available only for those without the means to care for themselves. Others find it reasonable that people should be able to spend down—in essence giving their wealth to family or friends—and be cared for through public funds. Regardless of one's perspective, the overall impact of aging baby boomers on Medicaid funds is substantial, growing and directly competing with other state priorities such as public school funding.

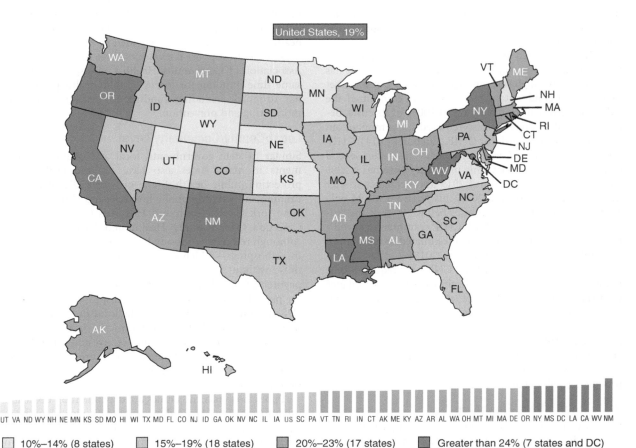

Fig. 17.3 Percentage of people on Medicaid or State Child Health Insurance Program (SCHIP) by state. (Courtesy of Kaiser Family Foundation. Further details available at Kaiser Family Foundation. [2018]. *Medicaid state facts*. Retrieved from www.kff.org/interactive/medicaid-state-fact-sheets/.)

In keeping with its goal to expand health insurance coverage to more Americans, the ACA expanded eligibility for the Medicaid program to any legal resident under the age of 65 years with an income up to 138% of the federal poverty level. One intent of the law was to have one eligibility standard across all states and eliminate eligibility by specific categories (Rosenbaum, 2011). The federal government agreed to pay for nearly all the expansion costs to insure more low-income people. The U.S. Supreme Court, however, struck down the mandate to expand Medicaid and ruled that states could decide whether or not to expand the program. As of May 13, 2019, 37 states and the District of Columbia had expanded Medicaid, and 14 have not (KFF, 2019). Some states are also seeking and receiving waivers to Medicaid requirements deemed restrictive. This option originated to allow states to try novel payment and delivery models, such as community-based approaches to long-term care. Starting in 2018, waivers were granted to states that intend to impose work or community engagement requirements or ongoing education as a condition of Medicaid eligibility.

CHIP was created in 1997 to help cover uninsured children whose families were not eligible for Medicaid. It has been funded through state and federal funds, but states set their own eligibility standards. The ACA committed the federal government to paying up to 100% of its costs, beginning in 2015. The ACA also required states to maintain their eligibility standards for CHIP (Emanuel, 2014). CHIP was reauthorized for 6 years in January 2018 after several delays and public outcry. This program continues a 23% enhanced federal match until 2019 and decreases it after that. Also, after October 1, 2019, this program would only apply to those with incomes at or below 300% of the federal poverty level (KFF, 2018b). CHIP continues to enroll a high number of children, with an estimated enrollment of 35.5 million in 2018 (Medicaid.gov, 2018).

Family and pediatric NPs and CNMs are required to be reimbursed under federal Medicaid rules if, in accordance with state regulations, they are legally authorized to provide Medicaid-covered services. Reimbursement varies by state from 75% to 100% of physician rates. However, restrictions still apply as Medicaid managed care programs are not all fully reimbursing NPs at the same rate as physicians or for all primary care services rendered by these providers (Bellot et al., 2017).

State Health Care Financing

State governments not only administer and partially fund some public insurance programs such as Medicaid and CHIP but they are also responsible for individual state public health programs. The mission of public health as defined by the Institute of Medicine (IOM), now called the National Academy of Medicine, is to ensure conditions in which people can be healthy (IOM, 1988). Whereas medicine focuses on the individual patient, public health focuses on whole populations even when serving individuals, for example, with immunizations. Medical care for the individual patient is associated with payment by health insurance. Public health programs are instead usually funded by local, county, and state revenues, often combined with grants from the federal government in areas such as maternal and child health, obesity prevention, human immunodeficiency virus/acquired immunodeficiency syndrome (HIV/AIDS), substance abuse, and environmental health. In addition to overseeing such public health initiatives, states will continue to have a major responsibility for the regulation of health insurance, health care providers and professionals.

Safety net health services such as those offered by community health centers, including federally qualified health centers (FQHCs), are funded primarily through the Community Health Centers Fund, which increased from $1 billion in 2011 to $3.6 billion in 2017. This community health center funding was extended in March of 2018 to $5.4 billion to support the work of these centers (National Association of Community Health Centers, 2018). At the same time, funding for foreign public health prevention has dropped, including funding for infectious disease monitoring and prevention.

Local/County/Community Level

Similar to state governments, local and county governments in many states also have the responsibility of protecting public health. Some provide indigent care by funding and running public hospitals and clinics, such as New York City's Health and Hospitals Corporation and Chicago's Cook County Health and Hospitals System. Although receiving a subsidy from their local government, these hospitals—which serve primarily poor patients and those without health insurance—also receive additional payments from Medicare and/or Medicaid. Such payments are provided hospitals that serve a disproportionate share (DSH, pronounced "dish") of Medicaid or Medicare patients and hospitals that meet the criteria for Medicare DSH, Medicaid DSH, or both and receive additional Medicare and/or Medicaid payments. The future status of DSH payments is in flux, creating uncertainty in those organizations that depend on them.

Public hospitals and clinics are dependent on taxes and other forms of public funding, and their budgets have been squeezed during times of fiscal restraint by local, state, and federal governments, putting in jeopardy their long-term sustainability. It was also anticipated that successful, full implementation of the ACA would remove the need for safety net public hospitals because all would be insured.

Paradoxically, Medicaid expansion states have improved financial outlooks in their safety net hospitals (Dobson et al., 2017), a phenomenon found across hospital sectors inclusive of rural hospitals (Lindrooth et al., 2018).

In addition, critical access hospitals and federally designated health centers (rural health clinics and community health centers) receive augmented reimbursement as an organization deemed essential to a community that would otherwise not be financially viable.

THE PRIVATE (COMMERCIAL) HEALTH INSURANCE

Although commercial health insurance has been the dominant nongovernmental payer, most Americans have little understanding of how insurance markets function, how insurance premiums are set, and the manner in which health care economics differs from classic free markets.

Pricing in Free Markets

The prime driver of the cost of health insurance is the price and volume of health services used. In general, Americans use more high-cost, low-value services than international counterparts. Although there may be an impression that "insurance is paying for it," these costs are collectively borne by those in an insurance pool. Therefore, high utilization in the form of a medical trend and pharmaceutical trend provides the basis for next year's premium increase. Insurance companies also must prepare for unexpected utilization—such as from an unexpected epidemic—through a contribution to reserves. The contribution to reserves (conceptually analogous to saving) supports the creation of financial resources sufficient for adherence within prescribed risk-based capital (RBC) ratios. The RBC ratio is a framework created by The National Association of Insurance Commissioners and widely adopted by state insurance regulators. It exists to assure that insurance companies have sufficient financial resources to meet their obligations (Liner, 2017). In other words, monitoring RBCs provides insurance regulators the data they need to be confident an insurance company remains "solvent", that is, able to reimburse providers for care given to patients as outlined in the terms of the insurance benefits package. Ponder the alternative: an insurance company becomes bankrupt and is not able to reimburse providers for services received, leaving it to the patient to pay out of pocket or to the provider to bear as uncompensated care. If the latter, uncompensated care is then built into the rate request for other commercial payer groups, again increasing the cost of insurance. Administrative costs including salaries for employees and leadership complete the cost structure for insurance companies.

Consumers, unaware of underlying cost structure, may be high utilizers of health care yet decry the very cost of increased insurance premiums they helped create. Although some insurance companies are profitable, others have experienced substantial financial strain. Still others have benefited from changes in tax law. The TCJA reduced the corporate tax rate from 35% to 21% and eliminated the minimum alternative tax, returning $2.3 billion to some BC/BS companies, despite them being "nonprofit" (Livingston, 2018). Some have suggested that health insurance is an inherently flawed design, given that insurance typically is for an unlikely event, such as a flood or car accident, not natural human phenomena such as health and illness.

In addition to the cost and high use of services, some unique aspects of health care markets create inefficiencies relative to classic free markets. In classic free markets, for example, consumers ration their own expenses based on the cost and perceived value of the purchase because they bear the financial consequences in an immediate way. Cost sharing in the form of deductibles, copayment, and coinsurance is one way to reflect these principles in health care. Yet classic free markets rely on a complementary principle: consumers are aware of the value and quality of items they might purchase and are in a powerful position to purchase or walk away. Health care is, instead, characterized by an "asymmetry of information" whereby the providers of health care largely drive the decision-making, the cost, and the cost consequences (see Chapter 16 on health economics).

Employer-Based Insurance

Most Americans' commercial health insurance is obtained as a benefit of employment in the form of group health insurance. It is important to note, however, that although it may appear that the employer is paying for the insurance, the cost is borne by the employee as part of their overall compensation package. Thus, some economists consider employer-based health insurance a hidden tax.

Cost-shifting also compounds the financial burden by increasing the cost of services paid for by commercial insurance to off-set lower payments by governmental payers. Medicare reimbursement is theoretically set at the cost of care but is less than the deemed actual cost, sometimes called "Medicare lite" reimbursement. Medicaid generally reimburses providers less than Medicare for the same services, and thus substantially less than the deemed actual cost. All of these "underpayments," including uncompensated care in the form of bad debt and charity care, are shifted to commercial insurance charges, meaning that those with commercial insurance pay more for the same service because they are compensating for underpayment by Medicare and Medicaid. Price variability and the lack of price transparency represent serious health financing problems in the United States (Potter, 2015).

Until the passage of the ACA, employers had no obligation to provide employee health insurance, leaving many Americans uninsured, especially those working in lower-wage jobs. Underinsurance was also common before the ACA and its "essential benefits package." Pre-ACA, one way for an insurance company to offer a less expensive insurance product was for it to cover fewer health services. Although enjoying a less expensive premium, the consumer was often unwittingly underinsured and obtained health services that the insurance company was not obligated to pay for. If, for example, a woman—either by intention or accident—chose a health insurance plan that did not include maternity benefits and became pregnant, costs related to prenatal, delivery and postpartum care would not be covered.

As this example illustrates, the "essential benefits" requirement of the ACA creates a social and financial safety net, but it does not create less expensive insurance premiums because, in general, the more services that are covered, the more expensive the premium. This issue has created ongoing political dialogue. A 2018 CMS administrative rule now allows states to determine which benefits are deemed "essential" in individual and small group health plans. Set to start in 2020, it is expected that more conservative states will not include some women's reproductive care as "essential," and some states will allow "skimpy" benefits packages that are less expense but leave insurance plan beneficiaries underinsured, creating more out-of-pocket expenses for consumers and greater potential for uncompensated care for providers. As private health insurance premiums have risen, employers have asked employees to pay for a greater percentage of their insurance premium and to enroll in plans that require more cost-sharing in the form of copayments, deductibles, and coinsurance.

Individual Insurance Market

Approximately 7% of insured Americans have purchased their health insurance from the nongroup individual insurance market (Cox, Levitt, & Claxton, 2017). Prior to the ACA, these plans typically were more expensive and insurers in all but a few states had been able to deny insurance to applicants with preexisting medical conditions and impose lifetime caps. The ACA outlawed these discriminatory practices based on medical history. Because private insurers are regulated by individual states, wide disparities exist in coverage from state to state, and there is a great deal of uncertainty in the individual insurance market, a particularly paradoxical circumstance given that one role of insurance is to minimize uncertainty.

Health insurance is generally regulated by a state agency or process. Some states now mandate that NPs be considered primary care providers and eligible for credentialing and payment by private insurers, but there is wide variation in the extent to which APRNs are included in insurers' provider panels. This variation can be seen among states, among insurers within a given state, and among the plans offered by an insurer (Brassard, 2014).

THE PROBLEM OF CONTINUALLY RISING HEALTH CARE COSTS

Many factors influence the growth in national health care expenditures, including

- *Weak price controls.* Unlike other industrialized countries, the U.S. federal and state governments do much less price setting and regulation of what can be charged for health care services and supplies.
- *Administrative burden.* There are complex, multipayer administrative systems of insurers and providers.
- *Care patterns.* The use, and often overuse, of expensive medical technology and medical specialists persists, in the face of a lack of focus on primary care and upstream social determinants of health.
- *Inflationary payment models.* The incentive in fee-for-service (FFS) reimbursement is for providers to increase their volume of services and provide unnecessary health care.
- *Consumer expectations.* Consumers have lacked knowledge of the actual cost and value of their care; furthermore, consumers perceive more expensive care to be better care, even if the evidence does not support this (Kliff, 2014).
- *Pharmaceutical costs.* Ongoing development of new medications heralds new forms of treatment. Americans uses many of these drugs, but also pay more for them than people in other countries.

Future costs will also be impacted by the aging of the population and increasing number of people with complex chronic illness who use a disproportionately high percentage of the health care dollars. Twenty-five percent of all of Medicare's expenses for those over 65 years of age are incurred in the last year of life (Cubanski et al., 2016). Chronic illness accounts for nearly two thirds of all health care expenditures; and, if you add mental health conditions, that number is 86% (National Center for Chronic Disease Prevention and Health Promotion, 2018). In 2015, about 1% of the population accounted for nearly a fifth (23%) of all out-of-pocket spending on health services, mostly because of chronic illnesses, whereas 50% of the population accounted for 3% of all out-of-pocket health spending (KFF, 2017b) (Fig. 17.4).

In summary, although medical *costs* are projected to continue flat growth, overall health care *expenditures*—driven by new services and pharmaceuticals as well as

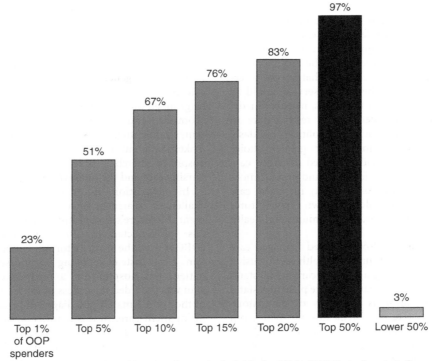

Fig. 17.4 Contribution to total health expenditures by individuals, 2016. *OOP,* Out of pocket. Source: Kaiser Family Foundation analysis of Medical Expenditure Panel Survey, Agency for Healthcare Research and Quality, U.S. Department of Health and Human Services. Courtesy of Kaiser Family Foundation. [2019]. *Peterson Kaiser Health System tracker: How do health expenditures vary across the population?* Retrieved from www. healthsystemtracker.org/chart-collection/health-expenditures-vary-across-population/?sf_data=results&_sft_category=spending&sf_paged=2%20]#item-discussion-of-health-spending-often-focus-on-averages-but-a-small-share-of-the-population-incurs-most-of-the-cost_2016.)

market consolidation resulting in higher prices—represent an increasingly unsustainable trend (PricewaterhouseCoopers, 2018). A 2018 poll found 65% of Americans "very concerned" about the cost of health care, inclusive of premiums and cost sharing such as deductibles and copayments. These concerns span demographics, including millennials and baby boomers, Democrats and Republicans, and diverse racial and ethnic groups (Reuters, 2018).

Cost-Containment Efforts

Over time, two approaches have been primarily used to contain costs.

Regulation Versus Competition. During the 1970s, modest government regulation attempted to contain health care costs through state rate-setting agencies and health planning mechanisms, such as certificate of need (CON) programs and regional health systems agencies (HSAs), which evaluated and approved applications for the construction of new facilities, beds, and new technology. During the 1980s and early 1990s, when proponents of competition and free market health care became politically more influential, rate setting and CON programs were weakened and HSAs were eliminated. Although free-market principles, as they apply to health care, have few similarities to a fully competitive market in economic terms, the rise of managed care programs and competition among health insurance plans in the 1980s may have temporarily slowed the growth of health costs before they began to rise again.

Managed Care. The origins of today's managed care plans were in early prepaid health plans of the 1920s, which evolved into health maintenance organizations (HMOs) in the 1970s, and into a variety of models in the subsequent 30 years, including preferred provider organizations (PPOs). A managed care system shifts health care delivery and payment from open-ended access to providers, paid for through FFS reimbursement, toward one in which the provider is a gatekeeper or manager of the patient's health care and assumes some degree of financial responsibility for the care that is given through a capitated budget. Originally, in managed care, the primary care provider was the gatekeeper, deciding what specialty services were appropriate and where these services could be obtained at the lowest cost. In the 1990s, negative media attention concerning the incentives to restrict care in the managed care model fueled a political backlash. Consumer and provider demands for greater choice in services and access to providers caused managed care plans to loosen gatekeeper requirements and provide more direct access to specialists. As a result, managed care became less effective in holding down expenditures and fueled a rise in health insurance premiums and health care costs.

Medicaid and Medicare also promoted managed care plans to control their expenditures for health care by using capitated payment and managing patient care. All 50 states offer some type of Medicaid-managed care plan, and states can decide if participation is voluntary or mandatory. Some states created state-run Medicaid-only plans, but others enroll Medicaid recipients in private managed care organizations. By 2010, when the ACA was passed, 70% of the Medicaid population received some or all of their services through Medicaid-managed care plans (Kaiser Health News, 2010). Medicaid-managed care spending for long-term care increased by $29 billion (284%). from FY 2012 through 2016 (Eiken et al., 2018),

REIMBURSEMENT MECHANISMS AND PAYMENT REFORM

The prior sections detail financing mechanisms. Governmental entities such as Medicare and Medicaid are not only financers—that is, sources of tax revenue for health care—but also serve as regulators and payers. The following section details payment mechanisms and the dramatic changes in health care delivery that are fueled by payment reform, but first, a bit of payment history.

Fee-for-Service Reimbursement

Until the 1980s, Medicare and private health insurers paid providers through retrospective FFS reimbursement. In FFS, providers charge a fee for each service, procedure, and supply, and then providers or patients submit claims to insurers for payment. FFS payment creates a strong incentive for providers to increase the volume of services and raise prices to increase their revenue. In addition, through the reimbursement mechanisms of their patients who are on Medicare, the federal government initially paid

hospitals (Medicare Part A) on a per diem basis according to the number of Medicare recipients hospitalized. Such retrospective per diem reimbursement created incentives for long hospital stays. Thus, hospital stays—particularly for high-intensity specialty care—and physician services were revenue generators, regardless of the value of that care. By contrast, nursing services in hospitals continued to be grouped into an aggregate hospital fee or as part of the room fee, rendering nursing care to be viewed as a cost center rather than a revenue generator. This mechanism makes it difficult to measure the value of nursing care in hospitals, whereby "value" is the product of the cost of nursing care and the quality/outcomes of that care.

In recognition of the inherent and exploding cost challenges created by retrospective per diem reimbursement, Medicare's prospective payment system for hospitals was enacted in 1983. Diagnosis-related groups (DRGs) were the strategy for implementation of this system. Now, instead of being reimbursed for each day a patient was hospitalized, a prospective, predetermined sum was provided regardless of the length of stay for each of the approximately 500 diagnostic groups typically used in inpatient care. In this manner, although Medicare retained financial risk for the overall number of hospitalizations, the hospital assumed financial risk for the length of stay. Thus, the DRG-based payment financially incentivizes short lengths of stay because hospitals receive the same payment regardless of length of stay. Nursing care remained bundled into the cost of the hospitalization, whereas some other "ancillary" services such as anesthesia remained FFS and generate additional revenue for the organization. Led by Medicare, Medicaid and commercial insurance quickly followed the move to prospective payments for hospitals.

The prospective payment approach helped to slow the rate of growth of payment for hospital care, shortening average length of stay, and increasing patient acuity in hospitals (Heffler et al., 2001), initially without demonstrable negative impacts on quality (Davis & Rhodes, 1988). Over time, however, premature hospital discharge was associated with readmissions and other complications, and these—initially—received additional reimbursement. As a result, poor quality care was actually reimbursed at a higher level than high quality care. Initial attempts to address this paradox included public reporting of hospital readmission rates. This, however, did not turn the tide on premature discharges; in 2012, Section 3025 of the ACA, The Hospital Readmission Reduction Program, resulted in hospitals receiving a financial penalty if the "same cause" readmission rate was above a defined level. This was just one element of the move from volume-based care toward value-based care, which is designed to create better alignment of the financial consequence and quality. Hospital-directed, value-based initiatives are critical to affordability, given that nearly one-third of total U.S. health care expenditures are hospital payments (Centers for Disease Control and Prevention [CDC], 2017). Hospitals traditionally have been the largest employer of nurses, and changes in reimbursement that lead to care redesign also shape needed nursing skills, such as with care transitions and enhanced primary care nursing (Bodenheimer & Mason, 2016).

Physician/Clinician Reimbursement Under Fee-for-Service. Payment for physician and clinical services encompasses approximately 20% of total NHEs (CMS, 2017b)—a significant driver of health care costs. FFS is still the predominant way of reimbursing for physician and clinician services. In this model, public and private health insurers pay physicians through a complicated formula related to medical coding and medical billing to determine the final payment (Emanuel, 2014).

The American Medical Association (AMA) created Current Procedural Terminology (CPT), a coding system for visits to physicians and other providers. There are codes for evaluation and management, office visits, emergency room visits, prevention services, anesthesia, radiology, pathology, laboratory codes, and medicine codes, such as for dialysis (Emanuel, 2014). These codes are then linked to a specific diagnosis, as outlined initially in the International Classification of Diseases ICD–9 and, now, ICD–10, and then assigned payment levels.

In the past, insurers paid what physicians billed. But in 1992, under Medicare Part B physician payment reform, payment was linked to a resource-based relative value scale (RBRVS), which was based on the degree of physician work (time, skill, training, intensity), practice expertise (non-physician labor and practice expenses), and the cost of malpractice for the specialty, as well as the geographic cost of living (Emanuel, 2014). Although the goal was to use relative value units (RVUs) not only to reduce expenses but also to redistribute physician services to increase primary care services and decrease the use of highly specialized physicians, this system still favored specialist care and hospital-based care. Still the Medicare RVUs per service ratings were adopted by private insurers, but they used different conversion factors, enabling them to pay more for each service.

In addition, the same procedure done in a hospital is reimbursed at a higher rate than if done in a physician's office. This "facility fee" has been one driver of physician market consolidation, that is, fewer independent physician/physician groups. Research has demonstrated that the incentive is to do more procedures in hospital-owned facilities and is a threat to the affordability of health care (Capps, Dranove, & Ody, 2017). One effort to correct this perverse incentive started in 2019, when CMS instituted "site neutral" payments for clinic visits or services provided in hospital outpatient departments. Site neutral payments simply means that reimbursement will be the same regardless of the setting in which the service is delivered. This policy shift is projected to save Medicare $380 million in 2019 (LaPointe, 2018). Nevertheless, site neutral payments are opposed by hospitals because they create a loss of valuable hospital revenue. In response, some hospitals have sued the Department of Health and Human Services (HHS) in an effort to stop site neutral payments (Bannow, 2019)

Since 1997, the Medicare program has also attempted to contain costs by limiting how much physician payments can increase through the sustainable growth rate (SGR), a target based on physician costs, Medicare enrollment, and the GDP (Emanuel, 2014). The intent of the original law was to reduce Medicare payments to physicians if the SGR was exceeded. There was, however, no incentive in the SGR for individual physicians to contain costs because the SGR is calculated for physician services for the entire country. Moreover, Congress regularly passed a so-called "doc-fix" bill to prevent SGR cuts from going into effect, enabling higher Medicare payment rates for physicians, APRNs, and other providers (Lowrey, 2014). By 2015, the SGR was considered unsustainable and ineffective in limiting physician spending growth or fostering better care (McClellan et al., 2015). It was replaced by the Medicare Access and CHIP Reauthorization Act of 2015 (MACRA). MACRA is bipartisan-supported legislation that amends section 1848(a)(8)(A) of the Social Security Act and, in addition to replacing the unpopular SGR, consolidates quality reporting programs and shifts Medicare payments toward value rather than volume. MACRA's quality component, the Merit-based Incentive Payment System (MIPS), replaced three legacy Medicare reporting programs: the Electronic Health Record (ERH) Incentive Program, also called "Meaningful Use"; the Physician Quality Reporting System; and the Value-Based Payment Modifier (CMS, n.d.). Clinicians reimbursed by Medicare, including NPs, who meet the minimum threshold of patients/services have the option of FFS reimbursement subject to a $+/-$ modification based on their performance on MIPS criteria or, alternatively, delivering care in a qualified advanced alternative payment model (APM) and receiving an additional 5% incentive payment. Although the administrative rules guiding this legislation continue to evolve, moving providers from traditional FFS to APM models remains a priority of CMS (Daly, 2018). Understanding APMs is thus essential for the contemporary clinician.

Value-Based Advanced Alternative Payment Models

An estimated 86% to 95% of payments to providers are still paid through the FFS payment system, creating an inherent incentive to increase volume and costs (Pearl, 2017). In response, value-based APMs are being tested throughout the United States. These new models are best understood when conceptualized as least-to-most-like FFS, within two broad categories: models in which reimbursement is linked to outcomes of care and those in which provider accountability includes not only outcomes but also cost.

Accountability for Outcomes—Pay for Performance and Patient-Centered Medical Homes.
Pay for performance (P4P) models complement FFS by providing additional reimbursement if performance outcomes are met. The patient-centered medical home (PCMH) can be construed as a particular form of P4P in which the model of primary care is team based, emphasizing care coordination and communication. Quality and outcomes are measured; settings that achieve defined targets receive additional reimbursement.

Although conceptually appealing, payment for outcomes in primary care has been somewhat mixed. It is possible that primary care practices have not been fully transformed to realize the potential in the PCMH model. Indeed, previous studies have found a "physician-centric mindset" and unimaginative use of NPs and physician assistants to be a barrier (Nutting, Crabtree, & McDaniel, 2012). In a similar vein, registered nurses have not yet realized their potential in primary care (Bodenheimer & Mason, 2016). New models are being developed that maximize use of all health care providers including registered nurses in primary care settings, but this innovation has yet to be fully implemented (Bodenheimer & Bauer, 2016). Taken as a whole, disappointing results in cost containment spur payers' interest in financial risk-sharing and risk-bearing models of reimbursement (see chapter 31 for more on the PCMH).

Accountability for Outcomes and Cost—Accountable Care Organizations.
Accountable care organizations (ACOs) are groups of providers who agree to take accountability for the cost and outcomes of care. The three iterations are pioneer ACOs, shared savings ACOs, and next generation ACOs. Both pioneer and next generation ACOs require substantial financial risk sharing. Shared savings ACOs have an option for *upside-only risk*, meaning if the cost of care for a population is less than expected, providers receive those savings and share them with the payer. If,

however, the cost of care is greater than projected for a population, they do not share that loss with the payer. In contrast, *two-sided risk* includes *downside risk*, whereby the cost of care that is above that projected creates a financial loss that is also shared between the providers and payer or, in the case of *full risk bearing*, borne by the provider group.

Some observers have proffered that upside-only shared savings offer "training wheels" or "on ramps" (Berenson et al., 2016, p. 5) to risk bearing for FFS provider groups that are not prepared or willing to assume financial risk for their clinical decision-making. Medicare upside-only ACOS may be eliminated through CMS administrative rule changes (Gregory, 2018), with Medicaid and commercial insurance likely to follow. Notably, only ACOs in which providers bear substantial financial risk for cost of care are recognized as advanced APMs, exempt from MIPS, and eligible for the 5% incentive payment under MACRA.

An "attributed provider" is the lead provider for a patient or panel of patients, accountable for the outcomes of care in upside-only ACOs, and outcomes *and* costs in two-sided risk models. One current limitation of ACOs is that NPs are not able to be an attributed provider under Medicare, while states determine if NPs can be attributed providers in Medicaid and commercial insurance, leading to dramatic variations by states. An additional serious limitation is the practice of "incident to billing" in which NPs can bill under a physician's national provider number (Buerhaus et al, 2018). These practices mask the contribution of NPs and undermine the goal of payment form directed at provider accountability for the cost and outcomes of their care.

Accountability for Outcomes and Cost—Bundled Payments.
Bundled payments offer a predetermined reimbursement for the cost of care for an episode of care and are sometimes called "episode-based payments." They are conceptually similar to DRGs, but the fixed payment is not just for the hospitalization, but for all pre- and posthospitalization care for an episode, including readmissions. Thus, providers bear financial risk for their decision-making, treatments, complications, etc., across care settings, not just in the hospital. Initially voluntary, the Obama administration moved to mandatory bundled payments for joint replacement in 75 randomly selected health services areas representing nearly 800 hospitals, with the intention of adding three new mandatory bundles. Thirty-two new voluntary bundled payments were announced in 2018. Although the required quality metrics associated with these 32 bundled payments vary somewhat by procedure/condition, all include two metrics that nurses can powerfully influence: (1) all-cause readmission rates and

(2) advanced care planning, predetermining the care an individual would want or decline if they could not speak for themselves, shared via advanced directives, medical proxies, or naming durable power of attorney for health care.

The administration of President Trump initially truncated the Obama administration's planned mandatory bundles and supported only those arrangements in which providers voluntarily choose to participate. Late in 2018, however, this stance was reversed, and administrative support for mandatory bundles was reinstated (Landi, 2018). Given that 17 conditions account for more than 50% of Medicare spending (Cutler & Ghosh, 2012), and that the first year of mandatory bundles resulted in half of the participating hospitals maintaining quality while creating substantial cost saving (Liao & Navathe, 2019), it is likely that more mandatory bundled payment initiatives will emerge.

Accountability for Outcomes and Cost—Global Budgets.
Global budgets take the concept of a bundled or risk-bearing ACO to a more comprehensive level. Statewide all-payer global budget approaches are being tested in the United States, and the approach varies by state. Maryland is focused on hospitals (CMS, 2018a), Vermont's approach is as part of an all-payer ACO, Pennsylvania focuses on rural hospitals, and Massachusetts has set an all-payer target (not a cap) to contain health care spending growth (Murphy, Hughes, & Conway, 2018; Murray, 2018; Zemel & Riley 2016).

WHAT IS NEXT?

The U.S. health care system continues to be undergoing a massive transition spurred in part by unsustainable costs, variable quality, and access barriers. There is, however, less agreement on what to do about it. The TCJA of 2017 removed the tax penalty the ACA placed on those who do not have health insurance. This effectively removed the individual mandate, despite that element of the ACA withstanding a Supreme Court challenge. The ACA required "essential benefits" remains in effect in the law; however, the CMS administrative rule change that allows states to determine their own essential benefits will likely create wide differences among basic health insurance plans. There is, however, support for continuance of the value-based payment initiatives started in the Obama administration. A dramatic explosion of new delivery models inclusive of telehealth, remote monitoring, and virtual care is also occurring. These innovations are driven, in part, by payment reform but also by technological innovations, increasing societal comfort with digital and virtual solutions, and innovative disruptors such as Amazon. Administrative rule changes such as those allowing VA physicians, nurses, and other providers to administer care to veterans using telehealth and virtual technology regardless of patient location (Office of Public and Intergovernmental Affairs, 2018) illustrate that innovation and care transformation is permeating the nation.

The complexity and magnitude of the changes in the U.S. health care system, as well as the economic and ethical imperatives for change, make it an ideal time for informed, bold action on the part of nurses and others toward a goal of a more equitable, sustainable, cost-effective, and safe system. The health of this nation depends on it.

DISCUSSION QUESTIONS

1. Which payment reform models have the greatest potential for enhancing nurses' potential to impact care, increase quality, and decrease costs? Why?
2. Imagine that you have just been named the U.S. health care czar. Your first assignment is to design a new health care system for the nation. How do you finance it? What do you measure? How do you determine what services should be covered, i.e., what constitutes "essential" care?

REFERENCES

Bannow, T. (2019). Dozens of hospitals sue to end site-neutral payment policy. *Modern Healthcare.* Retrieved from www.modernhealthcare.com/article/20190122/NEWS/190129991/dozens-of-hospitals-sue-to-end-site-neutral-payment-policy.

Bellot, J. et al. (2017). Does contracting with managed care organizations remain a barrier for nurse practitioners? *Nursing Economics, 35*(2), 57-63.

Berenson, R., Upadhyay, D., Delbanco, S, & Murray, R. (2016). *Payment method and benefits designs: How they work and how they work together to improve health care.* Washington DC; Urban Institute.

Berwick, D., & Hackbarth, G. (2012). Eliminating waste in U.S. health care. *JAMA, 307*(14), 1513-1516.

Bodenheimer, T., & Bauer, L. (2016). Rethinking primary care workforce: An expanded role for nurses. *New England Journal of Medicine, 375*(11), 1015-1017.

Bodenheimer, T. & Mason, D.J. (2016). *Registered nurses: Partners in transforming primary care.* New York: Josiah Macy Jr. Foundation.

Brassard, A. (2014). Making the case for NPs as primary care providers. *The American Nurse.* Retrieved from www.theamericannurse.org/index.php/2013/07/01/making-the-case-for-nps-as-primary-care-providers/.

Buerhaus, P., Skinner, J., McMichael, F., Auerbach, D., Perloff, J., Staiger, D., & Skinner, L. (2018). The integrity of MACRA may be undermined by "incident to billing" coding. *Health Affairs Blog.* Retrieved from www.healthaffairs.org/do/10.1377/hblog20180103.135358/full.

Capps, C., Dranove, D. & Ody, C. (2017). *The effect of hospital acquisitions of physician practices on prices and spending*. Retrieved from http://economics.mit.edu/files/12747.

Centers for Disease Control and Prevention. (2017). *National health expenditures, average annual percent change, and percent distribution, by type of expenditure: United States, selected years 1960–2016*. Retrieved from https://www.cdc.gov/nchs/data/hus/2017/094.pdf.

Centers for Medicare and Medicaid Services. (2017a). *Brief summary of Medicare and Medicaid*. Retrieved from www.cms.gov/Research-Statistics-Data-and-Systems/Statistics-Trends-and-Reports/MedicareProgramRatesStats/Downloads/MedicareMedicaidSummaries2017.pdf.

Centers for Medicare and Medicaid Services. (2017b). *National health expenditures: 2016*. Retrieved from www.cms.gov/Research-Statistics-Data-and-Systems/Statistics-Trends-and-Reports/NationalHealthExpendData/downloads/highlights.pdf.

Centers for Medicare and Medicaid Services. (2018a). *Maryland all-payer model*. Retrieved from https://innovation.cms.gov/initiatives/Maryland-All-Payer-Model/.

Centers for Medicare and Medicaid Services. (2018b). *NHE fact sheet*. Retrieved from www.cms.gov/Research-Statistics-Data-and-Systems/Statistics-Trends-and-Reports/NationalHealthExpendData/NHE-Fact-Sheet.html.

Centers for Medicare and Medicaid Services. (n.d.). *MIPS overview*. Retrieved from https://qpp.cms.gov/mips/overview Congress.gov.

Congress.gov. (n.d). Tax Cuts and Jobs Act. Retrieved from www.congress.gov/bill/115th-congress/house-bill/1.

Cox, C., Leavitt, L., & Claxton, G. (2017) *Insurer financial performance in the early years of the Affordable Care Act*. Kaiser Family Foundation. Retrieved from http://files.kff.org/attachment/Data-Note-Insurer-Financial-Performance-in-the-Early-Years-of-the-Affordable-Care-Act.

Cubanski, J., Neuman, T., Griffin, S., & Damico, A. (2016). *Medicare spending at the end of life: A snapshot of beneficiaries who died in 2014 and the cost of their care*. The Henry J. Kaiser Family Foundation. Retrieved from http://files.kff.org/attachment/Data-Note-Medicare-Spending-at-the-End-of-Life.

Cubanski, J. & Neuman, T. (2018). *The facts on Medicare spending and financing*. The Henry J. Kaiser Family Foundation. Retrieved from www.kff.org/medicare/issuebrief/the-facts-on-medicare-spending-and-financing.

Cutler, D. & Ghosh, K. (2012). The potential for cost savings through bundled payments. *New England Journal of Medicine, 366*, 1075-1077.

Daly, R. (2018) MACRA improvement coming, says top CMS official. *Healthcare Finance Management Association*. Retrieved from www.hfma.org/Content.aspx?id=60085.

Davis, C. & Rhodes, D. (1988). The impact of DRGs on the cost and quality of health care in the United States. *Health Policy, 9*(2), 117-131.

Dickson, V. (2018). CMS gives Medicare Advantage plans a raise. *Modern Healthcare*. Retrieved from www.modernhealthcare.com/article/20180402/NEWS/180409987.

Dobson, A., DaVanzo, J., Haught, R., & Luu, P. (2017). *Comparing the Affordable Care Act's financial impact on safety-net hospitals in states that expanded Medicaid and those that did not*. The Commonwealth Foundation. Retrieved from www.commonwealthfund.org/publications/issue-briefs/2017/nov/comparing-affordable-care-acts-financial-impact-safety-net.

Eiken, S, Sredl, K, Burwell, B., & Amos, A. (2018). *Medicaid expenditures for long-term care services and supports in FY 2016*. Retrieved from www.medicaid.gov/medicaid/ltss/downloads/reports-and-evaluations/ltssexpenditures2016.pdf.

Emanuel, E. (2014). *Reinventing American health care*. New York: Public Affairs.

Grady, D., & Redberg, RF. Less is more: How less health care can result in better health. *Archives of Internal Medicine, 170*, 749-750.

Gregory, J. (2018, May 8). CMS's Verma suggest upside-only ACOs are not producing results. *Health Exec*. Retrieved from www.healthexec.com/topics/leadership/cmss-verma-suggests-upside-only-acos-are-not-producing-results.

Heffler, S., Levit, K., Smith, S., Smith, C., Cowan, C., Lazenby, H., et al. (2001). Health care spending growth up in 1999: Faster growth expected in the future. *Health Affairs, 20*(2), 193–203.

Himmelstein, D. & Woolhandler, S. (2016). The current and projected share of US health costs. *American Journal of Public Health, 106*(3), 449-451.

Institute of Medicine. (1988). *The future of public health*. Washington, DC: National Academy Press.

Kaiser Family Foundation. (2014). *The Medicare prescription drug benefit fact sheet*. Retrieved from www.kff.org/medicare/fact-sheet/an-overview-of-the-medicare-part-d-prescription-drug-benefit/.

Kaiser Family Foundation. (2017a). *Medicaid's role in nursing home care*. Retrieved from www.kff.org/infographic/medicaids-role-in-nursing-home-care/.

Kaiser Family Foundation. (2017b). Peterson Kaiser Health System tracker. *Contribution to total health expenditures by individuals—2015*. Retrieved from https://www.healthsystemtracker.org/chart-collection/health-expenditures-vary-across-population/?sf_data=results&_sft_category=spending&sf_paged=2.

Kaiser Family Foundation. (2018a). *Medicaid state facts*. Retrieved from www.kff.org/interactive/medicaid-state-fact-sheets/.

Kaiser Family Foundation. (2018b). *Status of state action on the Medicaid expansion decision*. Retrieved from https://www.kff.org/health-reform/state-indicator/state-activity-around-expanding-medicaid-under-the-affordable-care-act/?activeTab=map&currentTimeframe=0&selectedDistributions=current-status-of-medicaid-expansion-decision&sortModel=%7B%22colId%22:%22Location%22,%22sort%22:%22asc%22%7D.

Kaiser Family Foundation. (2019). *Medicaid expansion decisions*. Retrieved from www.kff.org/medicaid/issue-brief/status-of-state-medicaid-expansion-decisions-interactive-map/.

Kaiser Health News. (2010). *Research roundup: Medicare spending, community health centers, children's dental services*. Retrieved from www.kaiserhealthnews.org/Daily-Reports/2010/February/05/Research-Roundup.aspx.

Kliff, S. (2014). *Half of Americans think expensive medical care is better—They're wrong*. Retrieved from www.vox.com/2014/7/21/5922835/half-of-americans-think-expensive-medical-care-is-better-theyre-wrong.

Knickman, J. & Kovner, A. (2015). *Jonas and Kovner's health care delivery in the United States* (11th ed.). New York: Springer.

Landi, H. (2018). *HHS Secretary Azar: HHS is planning new mandatory bundled payment models.* Patient-Centered Primary Care Collaborative. Retrieved from www.pcpcc.org/2018/11/09/hhs-secretary-azar-hhs-planning-new-mandatory-bundled-payment-models.

LaPointe, J. (2018). Site-neutral payment for hospital clinic visits starting in 2019. *Revcycle Intelligence: Policy and Regulation News.* Retrieved from https://revcycleintelligence.com/news/site-neutral-payments-for-hospital-clinic-visits-starting-in-2019.

Liao, J. & Navathe, A. (2019). Should Medicare's mandatory bundled-payment for U.S. hospitals be scaled up? *The Commonwealth Fund.* Retrieved from www.commonwealthfund.org/publications/journal-article/2019/jan/should-medicares-mandatory-bundled-payment-program-us.

Lindrooth, R., Perraillon, M., Hardy, R., & Tung G. (2018). Understanding the relationship between Medicaid expansion and hospital closures. *Health Affairs, 37*(1), 111-120,

Liner, D. (2017). Regulatory capital strategies in an evolving health insurance landscape. *Milliman White Paper.* Retrieved from http://us.milliman.com/uploadedFiles/insight/2017/regulatory-capital-strategieshealthcare.pdf.

Livingston, S. (2018). Blues reap billions from GOP tax cut. *Modern Healthcare.* Retrieved from www.modernhealthcare.com/article/20180615/NEWS/180619929?utm_source=modern healthcare&utm_medium=email&utm_content=20180615-NEWS-180619929&utm_campaign=dose.

Lowrey, W. (2014). For 17th time in 11 years, Congress delays Medicare reimbursement cuts as Senate passes "doc fix." *Washington Post.* Retrieved from www.washingtonpost.com/blogs/post-politics/wp/2014/03/31/for-17th-time-in-11-years-congress-delays-medicare-reimbursement-cuts-as-senate-passes-doc-fix/.

Lyu, H., Xu, T., Brotman, D., Mayer-Blackwell, B., Cooper, M., Daniel, M., et al. (2017). Overtreatment in the United States. *PLoS ONE, 12*(9), e0181970.

Makary, M., & Daniel, M. (2016). Medical error—The third leading cause of death in the US. *British Medical Journal, 353,* i2139.

McClellan, M., Berenson, R., Chernew, M., Kramer, W., Lanksy, D., & Milstein, A. (2015). *Medicare physician payment reform: Securing the connecting between value and payment. Brooking Institute.* Retrieved from www.brookings.edu/wp content/uploads/2016/06/012715-Medicare-Physician-Payment-Refom-WEB.pdf.

Medicaid.gov. (2018). *Medicaid & CHIP enrollment data highlights.* Retrieved from www.medicaid.gov/medicaid/program-information/medicaid-and-chip-enrollment-data/report-highlights/index.html.

Murphy, K., Hughes, L., & Conway, P. (2018). A path to sustain rural hospitals. *JAMA, 319*(12), 1193-1194.

Murray, R. (2018*). Toward hospital global budgeting: State considerations.* Global Health Payment, Inc. Retrieved from www.shvs.org/resource/toward-hospital-global-budgeting-state-considerations/.

National Association of Community Health Centers. (2018). *NACHC statement on the FY 2018 omnibus appropriations.* Retrieved from www.nachc.org/news/nachc-statement-on-the-2018-omnibus-legislation-passed-by-congress/.

National Center for Chronic Disease Prevention and Health Promotion. (2018). *Health and economic costs of chronic diseases.* Retrieved from www.cdc.gov/chronicdisease/about/costs/index.htm.

National Committee to Preserve Medicare and Medicaid. (2018). *Fact sheet.* Retrieved from www.ncpssm.org/our-issues/medicare/medicare-fast-facts/.

National Council on Aging. (2018a). *Chronic disease self-management facts.* Retrieved from www.ncoa.org/news/resources-for-reporters/get-the-facts/chronic-disease-facts/.

National Council on Aging. (2018b). *Fact sheet: Economic security.* Retrieved from www.ncoa.org/wp-content/uploads/NCOA-Economic-Security.pdf.

Newacheck, P., & Benjamin, A. (2004). Intergenerational equity and public spending. *Health Affairs, 23*(5), 142-146.

Nutting, P., Crabtree, B., & McDaniel, R. (2012). Small primary care practices face four hurdles—including a physician-centric mind-set—in becoming medical homes. *Health Affairs, 31*, 11:2417-2422.

Office of Public and Intergovernmental Affairs. (2018). *VA expands telehealth by allowing health care providers to treat patients across state lines.* Retrieved from www.va.gov/opa/pressrel/pressrelease.cfm?id=4054.

Pearl, R. (2017). Healthcare's dangerous fee-for-service addiction. *Forbes.* Retrieved from www.forbes.com/sites/robertpearl/2017/09/25/fee-for-service-addiction/#ea9130c8adbe.

Potter, W. (2015). *The enduring myth of cost shifting.* The Center for Public Integrity. Retrieved from www.publicintegrity.org/2015/03/30/17009/enduring-myth-cost-shifting

PricewaterhouseCoopers. (2018). *Medical cost trend: Behind the numbers 2019.* Retrieved from www.pwc.com/us/en/health-industries/health-research-institute/assets/pdf/hri-behind-the-numbers-2019.pdf

Reuters. (2018). *Soaring costs, loss of benefits top Americans' healthcare worries.* Retrieved from www.reuters.com/article/us-usa-healthcare-worries/soaring-costs-loss-of-benefits-top-americans-healthcare-worries-reuters-ipsos-poll-idUSKBN1JB1FD?feedType=RSS&feedName=healthNews&utm_source=feedburner&utm_medium=feed&utm_campaign=Feed%3A+reuters%2FhealthNews+%28Reuters+Health+News%29.

Rosenbaum, S. (2011). *The basic health program: Health reform GPS.* Retrieved from healthreformgps.org/wp-content/uploads/basic-health-plan.pdf.

Schneider, E.C., Sarnak, D.O., Squires, D., Shah, & Doty, M.M. (2017). *Mirror, mirror 2017: International comparison reflects flaws and opportunities for better U.S. health care.* New York: The Commonwealth Fund.

Starr, P. (1982). *The social transformation of American medicine.* New York: Basic Books.

U.S. Census Bureau. (2018). *People in poverty by selected characteristics: 2015-2016.* Retrieved from www.census.gov/library/publications/2017/demo/p60-.

Veterans Administration, Office of Public and Intergovernmental Affairs. (2018). *VA expands telehealth by allowing health care providers to treat patients across state lines.* Retrieved from www.va.gov/opa/pressrel/pressrelease.cfm?id=4054&utm_source=Telehealth+Enthusiasts&utm_campaign=3762ff526e-EMAIL_CAMPAIGN_2018_07_10_03_56&utm_medium=email&utm_term=0_ae00b0e89a-3762ff526e-353224725.

Zemel, S., & Riley, T. (2016). *Addressing and reducing health care costs in states: Global budgeting initiatives in Maryland, Massachusetts, and Vermont.* Retrieved from https://nashp.org/wp-content/uploads/2016/01/Global-Budgets1.pdf.

ONLINE RESOURCES

Agency for Health Care Research and Quality
www.ahrq.gov
Commonwealth Fund
www.commonwealthfund.org
Kaiser Family Foundation
www.kff.org

18

The Affordable Care Act: An Uncertain Future

Carole R. Myers

"By persisting in your path, though you forfeit the little, you gain the great."

Ralph Waldo Emerson

When President Barack Obama signed the Patient Protection and Affordable Care Act (PPACA), as amended by the Health Care and Education Reconciliation Act (HCERA), into law on March 30, 2010, it brought to fruition attempts at national health care reform spanning almost a century. The PPACA represented the most sweeping health care reform in the United States since the enactment of Medicare and Medicaid in 1965. The establishment of what is now commonly referred to as the Affordable Care Act (ACA) was contentious and reflects philosophical and political divisions that persist today and may be getting worse. The early fallout from the year of debate about the ACA included the ascendancy of the Tea Party, which now is represented in part by the House Freedom Caucus, and grassroots protests that continue today.

Despite a growing body of evidence about the positive impact of the ACA, favorable public opinion, and increasing stability of key provisions, the future of the ACA is uncertain. Naysayers contend the ACA is not working—and in some regards, the law is not working as originally enacted—and they do not concur with the design or the stated goals of the law. Support, or the lack of it, for the ACA is a metaphor for growing political divisions in the United States.

The ACA survived two early Supreme Court challenges, three major congressional repeal and replacement attempts in 2017, and the November 2018 midterm elections. However, actual and threatened reversals of key components of the law and cuts in funding and other support by the executive branch since 2017 are causing turmoil and confusion, as well as changes in how the law is implemented, that are eroding the ACA's potential positive impact. Despite gains by Democrats in the 2018 midterm elections, there is still uncertainty about the future of the ACA. Democrats gained 23 seats and control of the House of Representatives (235 Democrats and 199 Republicans in the 116th session of Congress) but lost two seats in the Senate (47 Democrats versus 53 Republicans). President Trump continued to consider opportunities to roll back or erode provisions of the ACA by executive order or regulatory action, and these executive actions prompted court challenges that are likely to continue into the foreseeable future.

AFFORDABLE CARE ACT DESIGN ELEMENTS

The problems that led to the passage of the ACA relate to access, costs, and quality. These problems are well documented (American Public Health Association, 2017). There has been progress in addressing some of the problems and little progress on other problems. Some of the initial gains associated with the ACA are now being lost.

- Evaluating ACA performance is predicated upon comparing intended outcomes with actual outcomes. An evidence-based evaluation aims to look at the adequacy of the provisions in the law designed to achieve intended outcomes and in what ways the implementation of the ACA has been true to original intentions. Therefore, to understand ACA performance, we must first understand the ACA provisions. The three main aims of the ACA were to reduce the number of uninsured Americans; improve fairness, quality, and affordability of health insurance coverage; and improve health care value by increasing quality and efficiency and decreasing wasteful spending (Rosenbaum, 2011). When enacted, the ACA (Kaiser Family Foundation [KFF], 2013)

- Included an individual mandate requiring Americans to have health insurance coverage that would provide minimum essential benefits;
- Established provisions for Medicaid expansion, a key component of ensuring coverage for many of the uninsured, and the Health Insurance Exchanges for providing free or low-cost insurance coverage;
- Provided subsidies to assist with purchase of coverage based on income eligibility;
- Prohibited denial, cancellation, or extra charges for insurance because of preexisting conditions;
- Added coverage for preventive care;
- Allowed young adults to remain on a parent's plan up to age 26 years;
- Removed lifetime limits on benefits of coverage;
- Limited insurance company profits.

The ACA benefitted nurses and the nursing profession in several ways. Specific provisions included support for the nursing workforce, expansion of the National Health Services Corps, and funding to support home visits by nurses to expectant mothers in high-risk communities and nurse-managed health centers (Wakefield, 2010). It also included support for expanding models that keep older adults in their homes instead of nursing homes, transitional care, and other ways to improve outcomes and decrease health care expenditures. In addition, it used the language of "providers" or "practitioners" in most places, which permits the inclusion of advanced practice registered nurses for reimbursement and rendering services.

Table 18.1 includes a high-level review of selected ACA provisions related to addressing access, cost, and quality problems.

TABLE 18.1   Major Affordable Care Act (ACA) Mechanisms for Addressing Problems Related to Health Care Costs, Access, and Quality

Increased Access

Medicaid expansion	National standard that allows anyone with incomes up to 138% of the federal poverty level to qualify for Medicaid; originally Medicaid expansion was mandatory for all states, but it was later ruled optional by the Supreme Court
Health Insurance Exchanges (Marketplaces)	State and federally run and regulated markets that facilitate purchase of individual health plans
Premium tax credits	Tax credit that can be used to lower premiums for Marketplace plans; based on income
Cost savings reductions[a]	Discount on deductibles, copayments, and coinsurance for Marketplace plans; based on income

Insurance/Market Reforms

Guaranteed issue and renewability	Opportunity for any eligible applicant to secure a health care plan regardless of health status
Individual mandate[a]	ACA requirement to have health plan coverage; noncompliance results in a penalty or fine; eliminated effective 2019
Employer requirement to offer coverage	Similar to individual mandate except applies to employers
Ban on preexisting conditions exclusions	A preexisting condition is a medical condition present prior to health plan enrollment; prior to the ACA, insurance companies frequently denied coverage to individuals with preexisting conditions and/or charged higher rates
Ban on annual and lifetime plan maximums	Eliminate practice of limiting health plan payments to a certain annual or lifetime dollar amount
Essential benefits package[a]	Items and services approved by states in 10 categories, including: ambulatory patient services, emergency services, hospitalization, maternity and newborn care, mental health and substance disorders services, prescription drugs, rehabilitative and habilitative services and devices, laboratory services, preventive and wellness services, chronic disease management, and pediatric services up to age 19, including oral and vison care
Expanded eligibility for young adults	Refers to provision that allows children up to 26 years old to remain on their parents' health plan

TABLE 18.1   Major Affordable Care Act (ACA) Mechanisms for Addressing Problems Related to Health Care Costs, Access, and Quality—cont'd

Coverage of preventive services	Three sets of free preventive services (for children, all adults, and women)
Elimination of Medicare prescription drug donut hole	Reduction of Medicare Part D (prescription drug coverage) beneficiary expenses in and eventual elimination of the donut hole, a coverage gap after plan expenses reach a certain limit
Medical loss ratios	Requirement that health plans spend at least 80% in the individual and small group markets and 85% in the large group market of premium income on health care and health care improvement
Premium rate reviews	Requirement that insurers planning significant rate plan premium increases submit their rates to either the state of federal government for review
Cost Reductions/Fees	
Medicare cost savings	Includes reduction excessive payments for Medicare Advantage plans, reduced provider payments, elimination of fraud and abuse, and lowered payments for hospital-acquired conditions, re-admissions, and adjustments to premium subsidies
Reimbursement reforms	Changes in the methods used to pay various providers
Accountable Care Organizations (ACOs)	Group of health care providers organized to provide coordinated care and chronic disease management with aim of improving quality of care and outcomes. Payment to ACOs is tied to meeting goals and outcomes while reducing costs.
Bundled payments	Strategy for reimbursing multiple care providers for a clinically based episode of care with a single preset payment
Pay for performance	Reimbursement strategies aimed at improving the value of health care, which includes maximizing quality and efficiency
Delivery reforms	Changes in the organization and delivery of health care services
Patient-centered medical homes (PCMHs)	Model for organizing and delivering care that achieves the core functions of primary care: Patient-centered, comprehensive, easily accessible, coordinated, high-quality and safe care
Health Insurance Exchanges (Marketplaces)	State and federally run and regulated markets that facilitate purchase of individual health plans
Reduce hospital errors and inefficiency	Reduced Medicare payments in the event of excess (preventable) hospital readmissions and hospital-acquired conditions
Independent Payment Advisory Board	Provision establishing 15-member independent board charged with submitting legislative proposals to manage Medicare costs; never implemented
Quality Improvements	
Reduce hospital errors and inefficiency	Reduced Medicare payments in the event of excess (preventable) hospital readmissions and hospital-acquired conditions
Comparative effectiveness research	Establish nonprofit Patient Centered Outcomes Research Institute

[a]Items that have been changed since President Trump was inaugurated.
Sources: Kaiser Family Foundation, 2013; Kaiser Permanente, n.d.; HealthCare.gov, n.d.

AFFORDABLE CARE ACT IMPLEMENTATION AND MANAGEMENT

Policymaking consists of two major steps: (1) establishment of broad parameters of government actions, such as the passage of the ACA in 2010 and (2) the translation of intentions into policy and programmatic results, including the establishment of rules and regulations and appropriation of the funds necessary to operate programs. It is not uncommon for there to be a discrepancy between what is implemented and what was originally envisioned, underscoring the importance of the regulatory process. Policies are dynamic and reflective of the sociopolitical milieu or context in which they exist. Policy implementation and operation is influenced by administrative agencies and program interpretation by the courts and regulatory bodies. As such, funding levels and other indicators of support, changes in leaders' perspectives and priorities, and other factors related to policy implementation, program operation, and interpretation must be considered when evaluating a policy.

The historic passage of the ACA was championed by Democratic congressional leaders and President Obama. The U.S. House of Representatives passed an ACA-like bill on November 7, 2009, with a vote of 220 in favor to 215 in opposition. One Republican voted in support and 39 Democrats in opposition. The Senate passed the ACA bill on December 24, 2009, with a vote of 60 to 39 (passage of the bill required a super-majority of 60; one lame duck Republican Senator did not vote). At the time of this vote, Senator Ted Kennedy, a staunch supporter of health care reform, had died and an interim Democratic Senator had been appointed. The dynamics changed unexpectedly when a Republican, Scott Brown, was elected to complete Senator Kennedy's term. The prevailing thought among Democrats had been that the Senate Christmas Eve bill would be reconciled to the November House bill. However, this was no longer possible since the Democrats no longer held a super-majority in the Senate. Instead, the House passed a bill identical to the Senate ACA bill by a vote of 219 to 212. No Republican Representatives voted for the ACA bill (Price & Norbeck, 2014; Washington Post Staff, 2010). In contrast, Medicare and Medicaid enjoyed bipartisan support when they were finally passed (Social Security Administration, n.d.). Just shy of seven years after the ACA became law, President Trump, who made a campaign promise to repeal the ACA, was inaugurated. Thus began a new phase of the ACA.

The implementation of various provisions of the ACA occurred in a staged fashion over several years. Some ACA provisions were never implemented. A multiyear timeline was employed for several reasons. Prominent among these reasons was the lead time needed to ready the necessary infrastructure to manage the provision. Table 18.2 provides an overview of the start date for key ACA provisions.

Court Challenges to the Affordable Care Act

There have been numerous challenges to the legality of the ACA. A Supreme Court decision, *NFIB v. Sebelius*, upheld the constitutionality of the individual mandate while ruling that the mandatory Medicaid expansion was unconstitutional. Consequently, Medicaid expansion became optional. Prior to the 2018 midterm elections, 34 states had opted in for the expansion of Medicaid eligibility, the cost of which would be borne mostly by the federal government (KFF, 2018a). During the 2018 elections, Idaho, Nebraska, and Utah passed ballot initiatives expanding

TABLE 18.2 Implementation Timeline for Select Affordable Care Act Provisions

Year	Provisions Implemented
2010	Coverage for dependent adult children up to age 26
	Prohibition lifetime benefits limit
	Allowable preventive services without cost-sharing in Qualified Health Plans
2011	No cost-sharing for allowable preventive services added for Medicare beneficiaries
2012	Accountable Care Organization (ACO) cost-savings
	Medicare payments reduced for preventable admissions
	Medicare value-based purchasing
	Reduction of rebates for Medicare Advantage plans
2014	Individual mandate implemented
	Guaranteed issue and renewability in effect
	Essential benefits package (EBP)
	Health Insurance Exchanges (Marketplaces)
	Premium subsidies
	Medicaid expansion
	Prohibition annual benefits limit

Source: Kaiser Family Foundation. (April 27, 2010). *Health reform implementation timeline.* Retrieved from http://leg.wa.gov/JointCommittees/Archive/HRI/Documents/May2010/HRITimeline.pdf.

Medicaid. A ballot initiative failed in Montana. The Governor-elect in Maine is on record in support of implementing a Medicaid expansion ballot initiative voted on previously and subsequently blocked by the prior Governor. The states of Kansas and Wisconsin elected pro–Medicaid expansion governors (KFF, 2018b).

Another Supreme Court case, *King v. Burwell*, upheld tax subsidies for both the federal and state insurance exchanges on June 25, 2015. Then, the Tax Cuts and Jobs Act of 2017 eliminated the ACA individual mandate penalty, the ACA requirement that everyone have health insurance or pay a tax penalty. Following this, a coalition of 20 Republican-led states filed a case in early February 2018 challenging the legality of the ACA in total. The plaintiffs assert that the elimination of the individual mandate as a result of the 2017 tax reform bill invalidates the entire bill. The case gained steam June 8, 2018, when the U.S. Justice Department took a different tack, arguing the individual mandate is unconstitutional and protections for people with preexisting conditions should be invalidated (Johnson, 2018; Luhby, 2018). The loss of protections for individuals with preexisting is predicted to adversely impact the

BOX 18.1 Trump Administration Erosion of the Affordable Care Act (ACA)

Actions	Dates
Executive Orders	
President Trump directs federal agencies to use administrative power to dismantle the ACA, within the bounds of law, to delay/avoid ACA taxes, fees, and payments	1/20/2017
President Trump instructs Internal Revenue Service (IRS) to not enforce the ACA individual mandate penalty	2/04/2017
President Trump directs relevant agencies to consider ways to allow people to buy plans exempt from ACA requirements, such as the essential benefits and community rating provisions. This action could pave way to deny insurance to individuals with preexisting conditions.	10/12/2017
Public Relations	
Department Health and Human Services (HHS) releases 23 videos and Tweets featuring individuals describing ACA ill-effects	2017
Content promoting ACA removed from HHS website	2017
Marketplace Support	
Navigator funding decreased by 84%	2017–2019
Decreased enrollment outreach, including enrollment ads	2017–2018
Elimination of federal payment to insurance companies for cost-sharing reductions	10/2017
Contracts with two private firms for in-person enrollment cancelled	7/20/2017
Medicaid Support	
President Trump sends letter to Governors indicating willingness to break precedent and permit Medicaid waivers that result in cuts to Medicaid eligibility and benefits	3/14/2017
Elimination Select ACA Provisions	
Trump administration allows employers to opt-out of covering contraception based on religious and moral objections	10/06/2017
Tax reform legislation eliminates the ACA individual mandate	2017
Trump administration proposes new rule to expand enrollment in association health plans; removes consumer protections and adversely impacts ACA plans by attracting younger, healthier enrollees	12/20/2017
Trump administration proposes rule to expand use of short-term plans that bypass ACA standards	1/04/2017

Source: Center on Budget and Policy Priorities. (2018). *Sabotage watch: Tracking efforts to undermine the ACA.* Retrieved from www.cbpp.org/sabotage-watch-tracking-efforts-to-undermine-the-aca.

availability of access to health care insurance for up to 52 million Americans or 27% of the population (Claxton, Cox, Damico, Levitt, & Pollitz, 2016). Public support for protections for people with preexisting conditions is strong. Overall, 52% of Americans rank continuing protections as very important with the following party splits: Democrats, 63%; Independents, 48%; and Republicans, 43% (Kirzinger, Wu, & Brodie, 2018). A third group comprised of attorneys general from 18 states argued that the individual mandate remains constitutional and the constitutionality of the rest of the law is not contingent upon the mandate (Kodjak & Davis, 2018; Levitt, 2018; Luhby, 2018). In December 2018, a federal judge in Texas ruled the ACA to be unconstitutional. The decision was appealed, and a ruling is expected in mid-2020 (National Public Radio, 2019).

Executive Branch Efforts to Weaken the Affordable Care Act

President Trump and key leaders in his administration serving in the executive branch have been unabashed in words and actions to undermine the ACA, consistent with long-standing conservative opposition to the health reform law. It must be remembered that the ACA passed with the slimmest majority and no Republican votes. In the ensuing time a Republican has been elected President and Republicans secured a majority in the U.S. House and Senate in 2016. The Trump administration has employed a broad complement of strategies and tactics to erode the ACA. Box 18.1 includes a summary of changes to the ACA, and the following discussion highlights key changes.

Of the individuals who enrolled in Marketplace (originally referred to as Health Insurance Exchanges) plans through February 2018, 87% qualified for premium tax credits to assist with the purchase of a health insurance plan. In addition, 53% of Marketplace enrollees are receiving cost-sharing reductions (CSRs). Whereas premium subsidies help with the purchase of a health insurance plan, CSRs reduce out-of-pocket expenses. Both benefits are based on income. Prior to October 2017, the federal government directly reimbursed insurance carriers to cover the costs of CSRs.

The Trump administration eliminated CSR payments to insurance companies in late 2017. Subsequently, the cost of CSRs was added to 2018 plan premiums (Luthi, 2018; Norris, 2018). It is important to note that even without federal reimbursement for CSRs, insurers are required to offer Silver plans, the most popular of the Marketplace plans, with cost-sharing to eligible individuals (Kamal, Semanskee, Long, Claxton, & Leavitt, 2017).

A provision of the ACA requires health insurance Marketplaces to establish a Navigator program. Navigator programs provide outreach, education, and enrollment assistance to individuals eligible for Marketplace plans or Medicaid. Navigators are required to provide fair and impartial information about ACA qualified health plans (QHPs) enrollment, available premium credits, and cost-saving reductions.

Since President Trump has been in office, federal Navigator funding has been reduced by 84%. For the 2017 enrollment, $63 million in federal funding was provided. This was reduced to $36 million for the 2018 enrollment and then $10 million for 2019 enrollment. The Trump administration contends that because the Marketplaces have evolved and public awareness is growing, labor-intensive, face-to-face enrollment is no longer needed (Pollitz, Tolbert, & Diaz, 2018). The annual enrollment period has also been reduced.

Enrollment for 2019 Marketplace plans dipped about 4%. Modest year-to-year increases are expected (Kodjak, 2018).

Legislative Efforts to Repeal and Replace the Affordable Care Act

During the summer and early fall of 2017, consistent with Republican philosophy, party positions, and campaign promises, the Republicans launched three major legislative efforts to repeal or replace the ACA. The efforts included the House American Health Care Act of 2017 (H.R. 1628), the Senate Better Care and Reconciliation Act of 2017, and the joint House and Senate Graham-Cassidy bill. Despite holding a sizable majority in the House of Representatives and a slim majority in the Senate, Republican efforts were

stymied. The divisions within the Republican Party were more significant than Republican and Democrat differences (Oberlander, 2017).

The 2018 midterm elections resulted in a divided Congress with a Democratic majority in the House and Republican majority in the Senate. Whether these changed dynamics will result in protections and even advancements of the ACA remains to be seen.

Public Opinion and Activism: An Unexpected Force

The debate about repeal and replacement of the ACA in 2017 was influenced by an unexpected, insurgent force—the American public. Public support for the ACA belied the strong Republican opposition and highlighted a growing gap between elected officials and their constituents fueled by hyperpartisanship (Edwards, 2011; Mann & Ornstein, 2012). The grassroots opposition to the threats associated with the repeal and replacement efforts, including threats to Medicaid projected to have a significant impact on funding, eligibility, and benefits; loss of consumer protections such as prohibition of coverage denials based on preexisting condition and basic benefits included in the essential benefits package; and rising premiums, costs, and numbers of uninsured Americans, resulted in a high level of activism and protest.

During the debates about ACA repeal and replacement, public support was strong for improving, not dismantling, the ACA. In August 2017, 60% of Americans polled were pleased that Congress failed to repeal or replace the ACA and 62% opposed President Trump's suggested approach that Congress persist with anti-ACA activities before taking on tax reform and other issues. In addition, a large public majority favored Republicans in Congress working with Democrats to improve the ACA (Kirzinger, DiJulio, Wu, & Brodie, 2017).

IMPACT OF THE AFFORDABLE CARE ACT

The ACA was enacted to address problems associated with health care costs, access, and quality. One measure of the success of the law is how well the problems have been addressed. The results are mixed eight years after the ACA was enacted, some owing to the previously discussed efforts to undermine the law.

Bending the Cost Curve

An important question is whether the ACA has contributed to reducing the rate of growth in health care spending, commonly referred to as "bending the cost curve." Major provisions of the ACA with the greatest potential for bending the cost curve include the Marketplaces; Medicare hospital payment adjustments; the Independent Payment Advisory Board (IPAB) authorized to slow the growth of Medicare spending by recommending payment reductions to Congress; a variety of strategies for reforming the organization of health care delivery, including Accountable Care Organizations (ACOs) and patient-centered medical homes (PCMHs); and various reimbursement approaches, including bundled payments, pay-for-performance, and value-based purchasing. The verdict on bending the cost curve is mixed and affordability expectations have not been met for many Americans.

Looking at health care costs in the ACA era is nuanced. National health care expenditures increased 5.3% in 2014 and 5.8% in 2015, following a low 2.9% increase in 2013. Major ACA coverage expansions were implemented in 2014. Between 2013 and 2015, the number of insured Americans increased 4.9% from 86.0% to 90.9% (Martin, Hartman, Washington, Catlin, & National Health Expenditures Account Team, 2017). ACA coverage expansion is primarily attributable to Medicaid expansion and, to a much lesser extent, the Marketplaces.

Per capita health care costs increased 5.0% in 2015. The breakdown for this increase is 0.6% attributed to changes in demographics (age and sex), 1.2% to price growth, and 3.2% to the mix of services provided (Martin et al., 2017). Medical prices are predicted to account for an increasing share of cost growth, as opposed to growth in use and intensity of services (Keehan et al., 2017). Underlying trends, irrespective of the ACA, need to be considered. These trends include aging of the population, changing economic conditions, and faster medical and pharmaceutical price growth (Martin et al., 2017).

Americans must face the reality that bending the cost curve will require focused strategies and a political will that has been absent to date. One example—albeit a relatively minor one—indicative of the unwillingness or inability to address costs directly is the ACA "Cadillac tax." This is a tax on expensive private insurance plans that was designed to save money by restraining excessive health care spending, in part fostered by the tax-favored status of employee health care benefits. The rationale for the plan is relatively sound, but the tax has been opposed by employers and generally wealthy individuals who participate in the plans (Oberlander, 2018). The Cadillac tax, a 40% excise tax, applies to employer-sponsored health benefits exceeding $10,200 per year for individuals and $27,500 for families. Included in what counts towards these thresholds are employer and employee premium contributions and most employer pretax contributions for health savings accounts (HSAs), medical savings accounts (MSAs), flexible spending accounts (FSAs), and health reimbursement accounts (HRAs). Criticisms of the Cadillac tax include the progressive

nature of the tax and the expected modest impact on total health care spending. The Cadillac tax is expected to disproportionately impact workers with high health care costs and those with generous benefits such as select union workers and highly paid employees (Gilead & Striar, 2016). The Trump administration delayed implementation of the Cadillac tax until 2022 (Japsen, January 23, 2018).

Similarly, the IPAB was never implemented and was eventually repealed on February 09, 2018. The IPAB, authorized by the ACA, was established to slow growth in Medicare spending (Cubanski & Neuman, 2017). Early on, the IPAB, given the moniker "Death Panel" by vice-presidential candidate Sarah Palin, was opposed by the health care industry and many others, including Democrats. Although an imperfect example of an attempt to cut costs, it nevertheless exemplifies the troubling dilemma commented on by Larry Leavitt of the Kaiser Family Foundation in a Tweet when he said, "Potential repeal of IPAB, along with continuing delays in the Cadillac plan tax, reveals a bipartisan consensus that health care cost containment generally seems better in theory than in practice" (Sanger-Katz, 2018).

When President Trump issued an anti-ACA executive order on January 20, 2017, he predicated his action upon the goal of encouraging the development of *free and open markets.* There are arguments against a pure market-based approach to health care. Shi and Singh (2019) contend health care in the United States is an *imperfect* market. Health care fails the test of a free market because: (1) buyers and sellers do not operate independently of one another and therefore supply and demand dynamics are atypical; (2) competition is thwarted in health care markets because of health care plans and provider consolidation; (3) patients do not have the information and often the time to make informed decisions; (4) patients do not directly bear the cost of services provided; and (5) comparable, comprehensive, easy-to-understand, and transparent price and quality data are not available to patients. The year 2017 saw the highest number of health care–related mergers and acquisitions in the recent past. This was followed by a record number of mergers in the first half of 2018, with acquisitions by American companies predominating (Grocer, 2018).

Access

One of the most noteworthy accomplishments associated with the ACA is the reduction in the number of uninsured Americans. In 2010, 18.2% of nonelderly adults were uninsured. By the end of 2016, this percentage decreased to 10.3% (KFF, 2017). However, the trend is reversing. Since 2014, four million working-age people have lost coverage, in part because of the federal government not acting to address ACA weaknesses and exacerbation of existing weaknesses by the Trump administration. Lower income adults are particularly hard hit—the uninsured rate for this group was 20.9% in 2016 and 25.7% in 2018 (Collins, Gunja, Doty, & Bhpal, 2018).

Quality

Has the ACA improved quality? The verdict is still out on this question, and much still needs to be done. However, a review of select studies on this question involving Medicaid expansion reveals some promising trends.

The fact that, as of 2019, 34 states have expanded Medicaid and 17 have not allows for important comparisons. Over 200 studies have examined differences between Medicaid expansion states and nonexpansion states. A select few of the studies are briefly summarized. Larger gains for individuals newly diagnosed with cancer (Jemal, Lin, Davidoff, & Han, 2017) and diabetes (Kaufman, Chen, Fonseca, & McPhaul, 2015) have been seen in expansion states. The rate of decline in infant mortality rates from 2010 to 2016 in Medicaid expansion states exceeded that of the national average more so than the rate in nonexpansion states (Bhatt & Beck-Sague, 2018). In another study, Medicaid expansion was shown to be associated with patients' obtaining care earlier in the disease course for five common surgical conditions (Loehrer et al., 2018).

CONCLUSION

Health care has been called "both the most personal and the most complex policy issue" (Washington Post, 2010). It is not surprising that the debate about health care reform exposes differences across the political spectrum at a time when political polarization is so dominant. Divisions between Republicans and Democrats reached a record high during the Obama administration and continued to grow after President Trump was elected (Pew Research Center, October 05, 2017), and the share of Americans holding a mix of liberal and conservative views declined from 1994 to 2015. This has resulted in a relative collapse of the political middle (Pew Research Center, 2017).

Although not specific to health care, one trend is telling and troubling. On the topic of government aid for the needy, the share of Democrat or Democrat-leaning Independents support has risen from 54% to 71% from 2011 to 2017. During the same time period, the Republican and Republican-leaning support changed from 25% to 24%. Of note is the precipitous decline of support for government assistance for needy people from 45% to 25% among Republican and Republican-leaning Independents from 2007 to 2011 (Pew Research Center, 2017).

However, in a political environment of divisions, public support for key components of the ACA is strong, adding a new layer of complexity. Public support was strong for the ACA during the 2017 deliberations about ACA repeal and replacement. When asked, 79% of respondents to a 2018 survey said it was most important or very important for 2018 candidates to talk about health care (Kirzinger, Wu, & Brodie, 2018). Furthermore, 76% of survey respondents supported continuing ACA provisions prohibiting insurance companies from denying coverage because of preexisting conditions, including 88% of Democrats, 77% of Independents, and 58% of Republicans. Similarly, 72% of respondents supported not charging sick people higher premiums, another ACA consumer protection currently in place; splits were 85%, 70%, and 58% for Democrats, Independents, and Republicans, respectively. These results likely reflect a more personal than policy perspective. While 50% of Americans held a favorable view of the ACA, 41% viewed the law unfavorably.

It is misdirected to say the ACA is not working when the implementation and management of the law has been so disrupted. It is also unrealistic to think that a law of the magnitude of the ACA would not require ongoing evaluation and improvement. Too little attention has been focused on making the ACA work better in reducing costs at all levels while improving access and quality of care. Americans are benefitting from increased access, consumer protections, and early improvements in outcomes. It is important to build upon these successes and as a nation come together to find common ground on how we build upon and extend early success and address those areas that are not yet meeting expectations. ACA repeal and replacement efforts should not be used as a political ploy or vehicle to reduce access and coverage and negate positive gains in the delivery of health care without having a real solution for addressing the underlying problems that led to the passage of the ACA. A commitment to a productive future of the ACA is far better.

DISCUSSION QUESTIONS

1. Which features of the ACA are essential for ensuring that the United States can reduce the number of people without health coverage?
2. Which features of the ACA are most troubling to you and why?
3. How has the ACA affected you, your family, or friends? Your patients?

REFERENCES

American Public Health Association [APHA] (2017). *Why do we need the Affordable Care Act?* Retrieved from www.apha. org/~/media/files/pdf/topics/aca/why_need_aca_2017.ashx.

Bhatt, C.B., & Beck-Sague, C.M. (2018). Medicaid expansion & infant mortality in the United States. *American Journal of Public Health, 108,* 565-567. Retrieved from www.ncbi.nlm. nih.gov/pubmed/29346003.

Center on Budget and Policy Priorities (2018). *Sabotage watch: Tracking efforts to undermine the ACA.* Retrieved from www.cbpp.org/sabotage-watch-tracking-efforts-to-undermine-the-aca.

Claxton, G., Cox, C., Damico, A., Levitt, L., & Pollitz, K. (2016). *Pre-existing conditions & medical underwriting in the individual insurance market prior to the ACA.* Kaiser Family Foundation. Retrieved from www.kff.org/health-reform/issue-brief/pre-existing-conditions-and-medical-underwriting-in-the-individual-insurance-market-prior-to-the-aca/.

Collins, S.R., Gunja, M.Z., Doty, M.M., & Bhupal, H.K. (2018). *First look at health insurance coverage in 2018 finds ACA gains beginning to reverse.* Retrieved from www.commonwealthfund. org/blog/2018/first-look-health-insurance-coverage-2018-finds-aca-gains-beginning-reverse.

Cubanski, J. & Neuman, T. (2017). *FAQs: What is the latest on the IPAB?* Kaiser Family Foundation. Retrieved from www. kff.org/medicare/issue-brief/faqs-whats-the-latest-on-ipab/.

Edwards, M. (2011). How to turn Republicans and Democrats into Americans. *The Atlantic.* Retrieved from www.theatlantic. com/magazine/archive/2011/07/how-to-turn-republicans-and-democrats-into-americans/308521/.

Gilead, S.A., & Striar, A. (2017). *Looking under the hood of the Cadillac tax.* The Commonwealth Fund. Retrieved from www.commonwealthfund.org/publications/issue-briefs/2016/jun/looking-under-hood-cadillac-tax.

Grocer, S. (2018). A record $2.5 trillion in mergers were announced in the first half of 2018. *New York Times: Business & Policy.* Retrieved from www.nytimes.com/2018/07/03/business/dealbook/mergers-record-levels.html.

HealthCare.gov. (n.d.). *Glossary.* Retrieved from www.healthcare. gov/glossary/.

Japsen, B. (2018). Big employers win delay for Obamacare's Cadillac tax once again. *Forbes.* Retrieved from www.forbes. com/sites/brucejapsen/2018/01/23/big-lobbies-and-employers-once-again-win-delay-for-obamacares-cadillac-tax/#f75c1323ed41.

Jemal, A., Lin, C.C., Davidoff, A.J., & Han, X. (2017). Changes in insurance coverage and stage at diagnosis among non-elderly patients with cancer after the Affordable Care Act. *Journal of Clinical Oncology, 35,* 3906-3915. Retrieved from http:// ascopubs.org/doi/abs/10.1200/jco.2017.73.7817.

Johnson, C.Y. (2018). ACA lawsuit could jeopardize 52 million Americans' access to health care. *Washington Posy Wonkblog.* Retrieved from www.washingtonpost.com/news/wonk/wp/2018/06/08/aca-lawsuit-could-jeopardize-52-million-americans-access-to-health-care/?utm_term=.8f2c0088a347.

Kaiser Family Foundation. (April 27, 2010). *Health reform implementation timeline.* Retrieved from http://leg.wa.gov/JointCommittees/Archive/HRI/Documents/May2010/HRITimeline.pdf.

Kaiser Family Foundation. (April 25, 2013). *Summary of the Affordable Care Act.* Retrieved from www.kff.org/health-reform/fact-sheet/summary-of-the-affordable-care-act/.

Kaiser Family Foundation. (2017). *Key facts about the uninsured.* Retrieved from www.kff.org/uninsured/fact-sheet/key-facts-about-the-uninsured-population/.

Kaiser Family Foundation. (September 11, 2018a). *Status of Medicaid expansion decisions.* Retrieved from www.kff.org/health-reform/slide/current-status-of-the-medicaid-expansion-decision/.

Kaiser Family Foundation. (November 7, 2018b). *What does the outcome of the midterm elections mean for Medicaid expansion?* Retrieved from www.kff.org/medicaid/fact-sheet/what-does-the-outcome-of-the-midterm-elections-mean-for-medicaid-expansion/.

Kamal, R., Semanskee, A., Long, M., Claxton, G, & Levitt, L. (2017). *How the loss of cost-sharing subsidy payments is affecting 2018 premiums.* Kaiser Family Foundation. Retrieved from www.kff.org/health-reform/issue-brief/how-the-loss-of-cost-sharing-subsidy-payments-is-affecting-2018-premiums/.

Kaufman, H.W., Chen, Z., Fonseca, V.A. & McPaul, M.J. (2015). Surge in newly identified diabetes among Medicaid patients in 2014 within Medicaid expansion states under the Affordable Care Act. *Diabetes Care, 38*(5), 833-837.

Keehan, S.P., Stone, D.A., Poisal, J.A., Cuckler, G.A., Sisko, A.M., Smith, S.D., ... & Lizonitz, J.M. (2017). National health expenditure projections, 2016-25: Price increases, aging push sector to 20 percent of economy. *Health Affairs, 36,* 553-563. Retrieved from www.healthaffairs.org/doi/10.1377/hlthaff.2016.1627.

Kirzinger, A., Wu, B., & Brodie, M. (2018). *Kaiser tracking poll— June 2018: Campaigns, pre-existing conditions, and prescription drug ads.* Kaiser Family Foundation. Retrieved from www.kff. org/health-costs/poll-finding/kaiser-health-tracking-poll-june-2018-campaigns-pre-existing-conditions-prescription-drug-ads/.

Kirzinger, A., DiJulio, B., Wu, B., & Brodie, M. (2017). *Kaiser tracking poll—August 2017: The politics of ACA repeal and replace efforts.* Kaiser Family Foundation. Retrieved from www.kff.org/health-reform/poll-finding/kaiser-health-tracking-`poll-august-2017-the-politics-of-aca-repeal-and-replace-efforts/.

Kodjak, A. (2018). Affordable Care Act insurance sign-ups fall slightly for 2019. *National Public Radio: Health, Inc.* Retrieved from www.npr.org/sections/health-shots/2018/12/14/676526601/aca-sign-ups-have-lagged-for-2019-but-what-does-that-mean.

Kodjak, A. & Davis, S. (2018). Trump administration move imperils pre-existing condition protections. *National Public Radio: Politics.* Retrieved from www.npr.org/2018/06/08/618263772/trump-administration-move-imperils-pre-existing-condition-protections.

Levitt, L. (2018). Legal & political fights over pre-existing condition protections. *JAMA News Forum.* Retrieved from https://newsatjama.jama.com/2018/06/25/jama-forum-the-looming-legal-and-political-fights-over-preexisting-condition-protections/.

Loehrer, A.P., Chang, D.C., Scott, J.W., Hutter, M.M., Patel, V.I., Lee, J.E., & Sommers, B.D. (2018). Association of the Affordable Care Act Medicaid expansion with access to and quality of care for surgical conditions. *JAMA, 153,* e175568. Retrieved from https://jamanetwork.com/journals/jamasurgery/fullarticle/2670459.

Luhby, T. (September 5, 2018). GOP lawsuit that could bring down Obamacare goes to court. *CNN Politics.* Retrieved from www.cnn.com/2018/09/05/politics/texas-affordable-care-act-obamacare-lawsuit/index.html.

Luthi, S. (2018). House drops CSRs, reinsurance from spending bill. *Modern Healthcare.* Retrieved from www.modernhealthcare.com/article/20180319/NEWS/180319894.

Mann, T.E. & Ornstein, N.J. (2012). *It's even worse than it looks: How the American Constitutional system collided with the politics of extremism.* New York: Basic Books.

Martin, A. B., Harman, M., Washington, B., Catlin, A., & National Health Expenditure Accounts Team. (2017). National health spending: Faster growth in 2015 as coverage expands and utilization increases. *Health Affairs (Millwood), 36*(1), 166-167.

National Public Radio. (July 9, 2019). *The Affordable Care Act is back in court: 5 facts you need to know.* Retrieved from www.npr.org/sections/health-shots/2019/07/09/739653482/the-affordable-care-act-is-back-in-court-5-facts-you-need-to-know.

Norris, L. (2018). *The ACA's cost-sharing subsidies.* Retrieved from www.healthinsurance.org/obamacare/the-acas-cost-sharing-subsidies/.

Oberlander, J. (2017). The art of repeal—Republicans health care reform muddle. *New England Journal of Medicine, 376,* 1497-1499. Retrieved from www.nejm.org/doi/full/10.1056/NEJMp1703980.

Oberlander, J. (2018). Hard promises: Has the ACA made health care more affordable? *North Carolina Medical Journal, 79,* 158-159. Retrieved from www.ncmedicaljournal.com/content/79/1/58.full.

Pew Research Center. (2017). *The partisan divide on political values grows even wider: Sharp shifts among Democrats on aid to needy, race, & immigration.* Retrieved from www.people-press.org/2017/10/05/the-partisan-divide-on-political-values-grows-even-wider/.

Pollitz, K., Tolbert, J., & Diaz, M. (2018). *Data note: Further reductions in Navigator funding for federal marketplace states.* Kaiser Family Foundation. Retrieved from www.kff.org/health-reform/issue-brief/data-note-further-reductions-in-navigator-funding-for-federal-marketplace-states/.

Price, G. & Norbeck, T. (2014). A look back at how the President was able to sign Obamacare into law four years ago today. *Forbes.* Retrieved from www.forbes.com/sites/physiciansfoundation/2014/03/26/a-look-back-at-how-the-president-was-able-to-sign-obamacare-into-law-four-years-ago/#61e98c18526b.

Rosenbaum, S. (2011). The Patient Protection and Affordable Care Act: Implications for public policy & practice. *Public Health Report, 126*(1), 130-135. Retrieved from www.ncbi.nlm.nih.gov/pmc/articles/PMC3001814/

Sanger-Katz, M. (2018). Another of Obamacare's unloved provisions is gone. *Upshot—New York Times.* Retrieved from www.nytimes.com/2018/02/09/upshot/obamacare-ipab-medicare-congress.html.

Shi, L. & Singh, D.A. (2019). *Delivering health care in America.* Burlington, MA: Jones & Bartlett.

Social Security Administration. (n.d.). *Vote tallies for passage of Medicare in 1965.* Retrieved from www.ssa.gov/history/tally65.html.

Wakefield, M.K. (2010). Nurses & the Affordable Care Act. *American Journal of Nursing, 110*(9), 9-11. Retrieved from https://journals.lww.com/ajnonline/Fulltext/2010/09000/Nurses_and_the_Affordable_Care_Act.2.aspx.

Washington Post Staff. (2010). *Landmark: The inside story of America's new health care law—The Affordable Care Act—and what it means for all of us.* New York: Perseus Books.

ONLINE RESOURCES

The Affordable Care Act
http://housedocs.house.gov/energycommerce/ppacacon.pdf
Center on Budget and Policy Priorities
www.cbpp.org
Kaiser Family Foundation
www.kff.org

19

The National Association of Hispanic Nurses Educating Multicultural Communities on the Patient Protection and Affordable Care Act

G. Adriana Perez

> "I first learned about the outreach and enrollment work of the Phoenix chapter through a fellow nurse. She said I needed to watch a news story that ran on NBC, which starred your Chapter President, Dr. Adriana Perez. Needless to say, I was mightily impressed with the great work that nurses were doing in Arizona to get people insured."
>
> *Mary K. Wakefield, RN, PhD*

When I graduated from my doctoral program at Arizona State University, in 2009, President Barack Obama was our commencement speaker. In his first commencement speech as President, he encouraged graduates to make a commitment to do what is meaningful to them, help others, and do what makes a difference in the world. I wanted to use my research and cultural knowledge to improve, inform, and implement policies that could advance the health of aging Latinos. In 2011, I was selected as one of the few nurses and the first Health and Aging Policy Fellow (HAPF) from Arizona to work on environmental health policy issues with funding from the Centers for Disease Control and Prevention and The Atlantic Philanthropies. This was a historic time in our nation, since President Obama had signed into law the Affordable Care Act (ACA) in 2010 and implementation efforts would require major outreach, education, resources, and support for populations who had never had health insurance coverage before.

LATINOS AND ACCESS TO HEALTH INSURANCE COVERAGE

There are many factors that contribute to Latinos' health disparities, including access to health care coverage and preventative care; language barriers; the lack of bilingual/bicultural health care providers; and health literacy. Latinos are concentrated in low-wage, service-industry jobs where employers are less likely to offer health insurance and other employee benefits. Latinos remain the highest uninsured population in the United States, particularly in states that did not expand access to Medicaid, such as Texas and Florida, where some of the largest Latino populations reside (Barnett & Vornovitsky, 2016).

Prior to the implementation of the ACA, most Latinos without dependent children would not qualify for Medicaid in most states, regardless of how low their income was. Despite their lawful presence, most Latino immigrants continue to be ineligible for Medicaid and health coverage under the ACA, due to a 5-year waiting period for Medicaid and the Children's Health Insurance Program (CHIP) in most states, and ineligibility in other states regardless of their length of time in the country.

Through my experience in the HAPF Program, I had the opportunity to make connections with key state and national organizations that saw the ACA as an opportunity to design strategies and initiatives aimed at reducing health disparities experienced by Latinos and other ethnic minorities, by increasing access to health insurance coverage. I knew that increasing access to health coverage would require thoughtful implementation that should combine health insurance literacy and enrollment for Latinos who had never been insured before and would benefit from bilingual assistance navigating our complex health care system.

While attending an AARP Arizona ACA workshop, I learned that Latinos 50 years and older were very interested in learning more about health care reform, since much of the information they were receiving was incorrect or politically motivated. A room of more than 200 older adults asked important questions, particularly regarding the Health Insurance Marketplace. Indeed, a survey by Doty, Blumenthal, and Collins (2014) found that Latinos were (1) interested in health insurance coverage but had a lower awareness of key aspects of the ACA; (2) more likely to report the enrollment as confusing; (3) more likely to prefer in-person assistance; (4) intended to sign up for health insurance coverage but were not able to; and (5) enrolled later in the period.

A CALL TO ACTION FOR THE NATIONAL ASSOCIATION OF HISPANIC NURSES

The Phoenix Chapter of the National Association of Hispanic Nurses (NAHN) seized health care reform as an opportunity to promote health and wellness among Latinos, using the ACA as a platform to teach multicultural communities about the protections, benefits and insurance options under the law. In partnership with AARP, we designed an education module developed specifically for bilingual, bicultural nurses. The Chapter received support from state and national offices of AARP, and the Future of Nursing: Campaign for Action at AARP's Center to Champion Nursing in America, to pilot the program in Arizona. In 1 year, NAHN members documented more than 50 community forums/education sessions throughout Maricopa, Pima, and Yuma Counties, reaching more than 1000 Latino families. Preliminary findings demonstrated the feasibility of this project and acceptability among Latinos. The success of the pilot project reached national attention, with stories featured on NBC Nightly News, *Modern Healthcare*, as well as in blogs and social media. As principal investigator, I was invited by U.S. Health and Human Services (HHS) Secretary Kathleen Sebelius to join a national call urging health care providers to embed ACA education and outreach in their practices.

PARTNERSHIPS TO INCREASE COVERAGE IN COMMUNITIES INITIATIVE

One year later, we used data from the pilot to expand ACA outreach and education through a unique grant opportunity. NAHN became one of 13 grantees—and the only professional nursing organization—to receive funding by the HHS Office of Minority Health for a project we called "Hispanic Nurses Educating Multicultural Communities

on the ACA." Its overarching purpose was to promote health insurance coverage, access to health care services, and health insurance literacy among multicultural communities, particularly Latinos, while conducting health screenings and bilingual health education on prevention and wellness. The key strategy to achieve this was the development and implementation of a bilingual, bicultural train-the-trainer nursing curriculum delivered to a network of Latinx nurse leaders and members of NAHN in 10 states with the highest Latino populations. Thirty-two nurses representing 15 NAHN chapters completed training and then took the lead on educating and training more than 100 other state and local NAHN members, nurses, students, new graduates, and affiliates.

This project also sought to broaden and strengthen nurses' knowledge related to health care reform, as well as hone their skills for teaching, communication, and leadership. Educating multicultural communities, particularly Latinos, about enrollment was only the first step in decreasing health disparities. Nurses used this platform to emphasize establishing primary care, prevention, describing the free preventive services through the ACA, as they tailored education to fit the needs of the audience (i.e. prevention for women and children; health and wellness visits for older adults on Medicare; and new incentives for small business owners to promote employee wellness programs).

Training Plan

The training plan included:
- A bilingual "train-the-trainer" manual with ACA resources and references
- Online practice sessions in which nurses were able to present and practice key communication strategies to assist with staying on message (considered a leadership competency)
- Program management and tracking tools that included community/town hall session flyer templates for marketing and event promotion, calendars to organize activities, attendance tracking records, and bilingual handouts
- Refreshers and updates conducted primarily via webinars on a monthly basis to review ACA updates, using national and state/chapter websites and social media to promote culturally and linguistically appropriate communication strategies

The trained nurses were expected to set a goal of providing a minimum of five community group or family education sessions with an average of 20 attendees per session. Some nurses used this training to educate individuals and families, one at a time if needed, especially in rural, hard-to-reach communities and border towns.

The train-the-trainer manual included content on

- Learning outcomes, such as (a) understanding best practices for targeting and educating hard to reach communities; (b) bilingual assistance for individuals and families with the enrollment process; and (c) connecting applicants to trained enrollment assisters for completion of application to determine eligibility and purchase of health insurance offered through the Marketplace. Training adhered to the National Standards for Culturally and Linguistically Appropriate Services in Health and Health Care (National CLAS Standards) and included "Coverage to Care" materials using multiple languages adapted from the Centers for Medicare and Medicaid Services (CMS) (https://go.cms.gov/c2c).
- An overview of the current "health status" of the designated state/community particularly focused on underserved, ethnic minority, vulnerable populations and how communities can benefit from the ACA.
- ACA fundamentals, including how to access its options for health coverage, creating a culture of health; prevention and health promotion as part of the solution to decrease health disparities.
- Health education relevant to specific populations focused on disease prevention and wellness; for example, free preventive health services specifically targeting adults, women, children (including oral health), older adults on Medicare, and employee wellness programs.
- Promoting community health centers, access to primary care to ensure a regular source of care and care coordination. Each NAHN chapter led a community referral process to help guide newly insured families to bilingual providers within their community and health insurance selection.
- Strategies for communicating public health policy in community settings.
- Strategies for training others on the ACA and how to effectively reach out to diverse populations and community groups.
- Development of a community resource guide, specific to targeted communities that can be used to help educate and support session attendees.

ACTION THAT IS RESULTS ORIENTED

Nationally, more than 100 bilingual, bicultural nurses participated in our virtual training, as well as in our national conference and monthly chapter meetings. Throughout the 2-year grant period, we reached our goal and educated 7068 individuals and families nationwide. Our main challenge was tracking and follow-up of families who actually obtained coverage. We relied on self-report to evaluate the obtaining health insurance component; however, some families provided minimal demographic or contact data.

In addition, we reached approximately 1680 individuals through traditional print media, including through our own NAHN newsletter, plus an additional 1000 through online broadcast of radio presentations. We reached more than 5000 through Facebook, Twitter, LinkedIn, and our dedicated ACA web page. A key to this success was our partnership and participation through the Latino ACA Coalition in Washington, DC, as well as state-based health insurance coverage coalitions.

We reached a diverse population: non-Hispanic Whites (12%), non-Hispanic Blacks/African Americans (12%), Latinos (66%), Asians (5%), American Indians/Alaska Natives (3%), and other (2%). Most participants were female (64%). We targeted pregnant women, new mothers, preschool sites, young parents, and grandparents caring for young families; thus, 2% of those we reached were newborns and infants; 3% were 1 to 5 years old; 5% were 6 to 12 years old; 5% were13 to 17 years old. We worked with partners such as The Young Invincibles, an organization that works to amplify the voices of young adults in entrepreneurship and the political process, to target our outreach efforts to young students attending all levels of college programs/trade schools, so 25% were18 to 24 years old. Adults (25 to 64 years old) were 40% of the population served; and 20% were older adults (65 years and older). At each site, education focused on serving the local community, including employees/staff, educators, other health care providers, school leaders, faith-based communities, nonprofits, and small businesses who would also help promote events and education offerings.

A major accomplishment of this grant included the growth of partnerships between NAHN and network/partner agencies—both in health care and nontraditional partners. We formed 145 partnerships nationwide! They included nursing schools, ranging from community colleges to universities, to educate and recruit nursing students interested in mentorship. NAHN educators shared how beneficial the "Coverage to Care" materials were in educating multicultural families. We leveraged existing resources and local community resources through a strong partnership with federally qualified community health centers in each state. Many of our partners have shared a commitment to continuing to provide support and resources, such as meeting/event space, logistical support, marketing and communication resources, building of coalitions, printing of education materials, audio-visual equipment for presentations, volunteer services to help organize and manage public events, and social media promotion efforts.

One of our most effective partnerships to improve consistency and coordination of access to health coverage was with Enroll America, since they had offices/teams in each state. We are also part of the Latino ACA Coalition, which

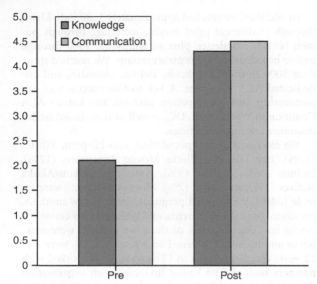

Fig. 19.1 Nursing outcomes for "Hispanic Nurses Educating Multicultural Communities on the Affordable Care Act."

includes other nonprofit organizations such as The Young Invincibles. Together, we developed and tested culturally tailored messages for health insurance enrollment through various social media platforms and we have presented our collaborative work at conferences and through live webinars. We worked with other nursing groups, including The Future of Nursing: Campaign for Action's state action coalitions, the Colorado Center for Nursing Excellence, and our sister ethnic minority nursing organizations.

Project outcomes included leadership development through knowledge of current health care reform, health insurance coverage, health insurance literacy, and health disparities in each state. This outcome is depicted as "knowledge" in Fig. 19.1. "Communication" measured nurse readiness and comfort with public presentations, especially as it relates to public policy. Both were measured on a Likert-type scale with 1 = Strongly Disagree and 5 = Strongly Agree. Overall, nurses benefited significantly from the training and improved on both outcome measures.

Based on feedback from those who attended the community forums, we found that nurses are uniquely positioned and qualified to educate the public on the fundamentals of the ACA and the importance of health insurance coverage. Moreover, Latinx nurses understand the health care challenges experienced by Latino communities. As Latinos gain health coverage for the first time, nurses are able to address their need for guidance on using the health care system and referrals to local community health centers for primary care services.

LESSONS LEARNED AND RECOMMENDATIONS FOR FUTURE EFFORTS

This project demonstrates that innovative, diverse nurse-led projects can make a positive impact in advancing health equity. In this case, professional nursing organizations, working in partnership with community nonprofits, faith-based leaders, small businesses, education/academic institutions, consumer groups, hospitals and other health care organizations, contributed significantly to educating and preparing individuals and families to navigate health insurance and health care systems.

It also serves as an example of how health professions can provide real-life, hands-on experiences to students and new graduate nurses. With the shortage of diverse students in science, technology, engineering, and math (STEM) careers, the activities that were part of this project were especially useful for bilingual, bicultural nurses who reported positive changes toward readiness/leadership to continue working in nontraditional community settings.

Overwhelmingly, data show that efforts that focus on educating the public about our health care system and health insurance literacy must continue and must include nurses, the most trusted profession in the United States. Both the trainers (91% nurses) and participants (96%) reported the need for continued education and resources in this area. Changes in the delivery of health care, both locally and nationally, must consider the inclusion of diverse outreach, especially to reach multicultural families.

REFERENCES

Barnett, J.C., & Vornovitsky, M.S. (2016). *Health insurance coverage in the United States: 2015*. Washington, DC: US Government Printing Office.

Doty, M.M., Blumenthal, D., & Collins, S.R. (2014). The Affordable Care Act and health insurance for Latinos. *JAMA, 312*(17), 1735-1736.

20

Patient Engagement and Public Policy: Emerging New Paradigms and Roles

Jane Clare Joyner and Mary Jo Kreitzer[a]

"Even in an age of hype, calling something 'the block-buster drug of the century' grabs our attention. In this case, the 'drug' is actually a concept—patient activation and engagement—that should have formed the heart of health care all along."

Susan Dentzer

Over the past 5 years, there has been a significant shift in the role and expectations of people seeking health care. Historically, the role of the patient was to be passive and do what they were told to do. Patients who did not follow orders were labeled as noncompliant. These roles were congruent with a hierarchical health care system in which the physician was most often perceived to be in charge. According to *Merriam-Webster Online Dictionary* (n.d.), the Latin word from which patient is derived literally means to suffer.

Although the language remains controversial, many people are more inclined to see themselves, along with their family members and caregivers, as consumers or clients of the health care system, and they seek relationships with health care providers that are on par with other purchasing arrangements of goods and services in their lives. As purchasers of a service or product, they want choice, transparency of information, and data about quality and outcomes. They are also concerned about value.

The landmark Institute of Medicine (now National Academy of Medicine) report *Crossing the Quality Chasm* (2001) was one of the first federal policy reports to describe the radical changes needed within the health care system to better meet the needs of patients. A set of new rules was identified that redefined the locus of control and relationships by emphasizing that care should be based on continuous healing relationships and be customized based on patient needs and values, that the patient should be in control of health care decisions, that patients should have unfettered access to clinical knowledge and their own medical information, and that the health care system should anticipate needs rather than react to events.

Recognizing the critical role of the consumer in determining health outcomes, the Center for Advancing Health (2010) defines engagement as "the actions we take to benefit from the health care available to us." Engagement behaviors range from accessing credible and easy to understand information, finding good care, communicating with health professionals, organizing health care, paying for care, and making good treatment decisions.

In exploring the idea of engagement in health care, Boissy (2017) observes that the phrase people engagement (rather than patient experience) may be more accurate, as navigating the health care system often involves the patient's family and caregivers, as well as health care providers and the community as a whole. Boissy also notes that while patient experience can be passive (i.e., what happens to the patient), the concept of an engaged patient suggests that the patient is actively interacting in some way with the health care system.

There is evidence that patient engagement, also called patient activation, can be measured (Hibbard et al., 2004). Although much of the impetus for engagement comes from people's changing expectations, there is also growing evidence (Hibbard & Greene, 2013; Hibbard et al., 2013; Katon et al.,1995; Robinson et al., 2008) that engagement is directly linked to health outcomes. In their work on

[a]The opinions expressed are those of the authors and do not necessarily reflect the views of the Department of Labor or the U.S. government.

conceptualizing patient activation, Hibbard et al. (2004) report that patients who are activated and engaged are more likely to seek health information, engage in disease prevention activities such as health screenings, and undertake self-management of their health through exercise, diet, or medication compliance.

A framework developed by Carman et al. (2013) describes patient engagement as taking place at three levels: the direct care level, including engagement with clinicians as well as health-related groups and resources; the design and governance level, where the patient perspective is considered and integrated into the organization; and the policymaking level, including development of programs and policies at the local, state, and national level. Nielsen et al. (2012) also describe patient engagement as taking place in distinct spheres: at the clinical encounter level, the practice or organizational level, the community level, and the policy level.

Current efforts to redesign the health care system are focused on achieving what is called the Triple Aim. The Institute for Healthcare Improvement (n.d.) defines the Triple Aim as:

- Improving the patient experience of care (including quality and satisfaction)
- Improving the health of populations
- Reducing the per capita cost of health care

To achieve the Triple Aim, changes are needed within health care environments, as well as in provider and consumer behavior. This chapter examines nursing and federal policy initiatives focused on patient engagement, highlights exemplary models of patient engagement, and identifies critical strategies for hearing and embracing the patient's voice.

INNOVATIVE EXEMPLARS OF PATIENT ENGAGEMENT

This section will highlight innovative initiatives designed to increase patient engagement through new models of care (the Veterans Health Administration [VHA] and Medical-Legal Partnerships [MLPs]) and tools and technologies designed to enable the public to access online credible health information (Choosing Wisely) and to assist patients with chronic disease manage their care (Healthy Interactions).

Veterans' Health Care

The VHA, part of the U.S. Department of Veterans Affairs (VA), is the largest integrated health care system in the United States, with 1240 health care facilities (VA, n.d.). A number of recent innovations at the VA have the potential to significantly impact patient engagement.

The VA is a leader in utilizing electronic tools to engage patients by giving them access to their health information. One such tool is the Blue Button initiative. The appearance

of the Blue Button icon signals that a patient is able to download his or her digital health record and share it with caregivers, family members, or other health care professionals. Such ready access to health information makes it easier for patients to monitor and engage in their health care. The VA was the first organization to utilize Blue Button. Since its launch in the VA in 2010, hundreds of organizations have joined the Blue Button Pledge Program, including Medicare and private health care insurers, as well as the Department of Defense (Ricciardi et al., 2013). In 2018, the VHA introduced a new online feature to allow veterans to view, download, and print many images and reports from their VA electronic health record (EHR), and to share them with other providers outside the VA system (VA, 2018).

The VA's implementation of patient-centered medical homes (PCMHs) in primary care clinics across the nation also has the potential to improve patient engagement. The PCMH has been described by Nielson et al. (2012) as "a model of primary care that is patient-centered, comprehensive, team-based, coordinated, accessible and focused on quality and safety." They describe the empirical support for the PCMH model and identify data showing how PCMHs improve care and outcomes while lowering costs. Within the VA, the aim of the PCMH initiative is to improve continuity of care and care management and coordination, improve patient access, and increase the use of preventative services (Kline 2011; Rosland et al., 2013). The VA utilizes patient-aligned care teams (PACTs) to provide integrated health care. Implementation of the program is monitored through various metrics, including measures of patient engagement and satisfaction (Kline, 2011). Metrics utilized to measure patient engagement include patient complaints and satisfaction survey results, enrollment in the VA's personal health record, My HealtheVet, and the number of patients who seek in-person authentication in order to utilize secure messaging (Kline, 2011).

The VA's Whole Health model was developed by VHA's Office of Patient-Centered Care and Cultural Transformation. The aim of this systemwide initiative is to activate and engage individual veterans in their health care. The Whole Health model moves away from episodic and disease-based care and combines personalized health planning with conventional medicine and preventive care (VA, VHA Directive, 2018).

The VA, like many health care facilities in the private sector, has begun to offer complementary and alternative medicine (CAM), now often called "integrative" health or medicine. According to a 2011 survey (Ezeji-Okoye et al., 2013) by the VA's Health Care Analysis and Information Group, the use of CAM has grown significantly over the past decade. According to the survey, about 9 in 10 VA facilities directly provide CAM therapies or refer patients to outside licensed practitioners. CAM is used in the VA most commonly to help veterans manage stress, promote general wellness, and to treat problems, including anxiety, post-traumatic stress disorder, depression, back pain, arthritis, fibromyalgia, and substance abuse. Offering integrative therapies is aligned with approaches in the VA to provide care that is personalized, proactive, and patient-centered. This is consistent with broader trends in health care that reflect the incorporation of integrative therapies and healing practices into care models.

Medical-Legal Partnerships

Social determinants of health (SDOH) impact patient engagement efforts and health outcomes. Fleming et al. (2017) report that conditions such as housing or food insecurity, homelessness, poverty, mental health, or substance use may impact the ability of patients to engage in their health care or comply with treatment recommendations. They suggest that access to such resources may be preconditions for effective engagement by marginalized patients.

MLPs have developed as a means to address social determinants that impact the ability of patients to fully engage in health care. MLPs integrate legal professionals into a health care organization to address unmet legal needs (including substandard housing, lack of insurance and poverty) that impact health care outcomes. The National Center for Medical-Legal Partnerships (NCMLP, 2018) describes MLPs as embedding legal professionals into health care organizations to address legal needs that are generally not addressed in a health care setting. NCMLP reports that bringing together health care and legal teams in MLPs may lower health care costs while improving patient engagement and health outcomes. Additional research is necessary to understand the full impact of MLPs on patient engagement and health outcomes. Martinez et al. (2017) reviewed published articles addressing the impact of MLPs. While they identified some research studies where MLP interventions resulted in improved well-being and health, most efforts to evaluate the effectiveness of MLPs focus on legal rather than health outcomes. They suggest that more vigorous research is essential to fully evaluate the impact of MLPs.

Tools and Technologies Designed to Increase Patient Engagement

Healthy Interactions, a company based in Chicago, has created innovative approaches to improving outcomes for patients with chronic conditions. Their programs focus on creating meaningful and ongoing dialogue between health care providers and health care consumers. Tools, including what are called Conversation Maps, create structured interactions that can be delivered in a one-on-one environment or in small groups. Digital tools support consumers in moving toward their goals with information, tracking, and ongoing peer and health professional interactions. Deployed in 120 countries and 38 languages and delivered through over 100,000 facilitators, these tools are achieving important patient outcomes including improved self-care, decision making, and adherence (Healthy Interactions, n.d.).

Accessible via the web or a phone application, Choosing Wisely helps patients choose health care that is supported by evidence, free from harm and truly necessary. Supported by the American Board of Internal Medicine (ABIM), this initiative helps patients engage in conversations with providers about their health care, including recommended tests and procedures that follow established guidelines. Participating clinician groups include specialty medical societies, nursing organizations, and organizations representing other clinician groups. The initiative's aim is to encourage patients to engage in conversations with their providers about the appropriate and necessary use of health care resources (Choosing Wisely, n.d.).

PATIENT ENGAGEMENT AND FEDERAL INITIATIVES

The federal government plays an important role in driving policy initiatives to foster patient engagement. Laws passed by Congress are implemented and clarified by regulations and policies issued by executive branch agencies. The federal government can also affect patient engagement policy through the awarding of research grants. This section highlights examples of federal policy initiatives impacting patient engagement.

The Affordable Care Act

Legislation can be a powerful driver of patient engagement policy. For example, the Affordable Care Act (ACA)[b] included a number of elements that sought to impact and advance patient engagement initiatives. While some provisions in the ACA were met with opposition (including the individual mandate/individual shared responsibility payment, which was reduced to zero by the Tax Cuts and Jobs Act of 2017 [Public Law 115-97]), other provisions currently remain in place.[c]

---

[b]The ACA refers to two laws passed in 2010: the Patient Protection and Affordable Care Act (Public Law 111-148) and the Health Care and Education Affordability Reconciliation Act (Public Law 111-152). [c]Following passage of Public Law 115-97 and the elimination of the tax penalty, Texas and a number of other states filed a complaint in federal court challenging the ACA's constitutionality. The District Court held that the entire ACA is unconstitutional. The decision was appealed to the U.S. Court of Appeals for the Fifth Circuit, which held oral arguments in the case in July 2019. Regardless of the ruling by the Fifth Circuit, it is likely that their decision will ultimately be appealed to the Supreme Court. The ongoing litigation concerning the ACA (commencing with its initial passage and continuing through this latest legal challenge) highlights one of the challenges of developing health care policy through legislation.

Accountable Care Organizations. Section 3022 of the ACA created a new Medicare shared savings program—Medicare Accountable Care Organizations (ACOs). A Medicare ACO consists of a group of providers (physicians, hospitals, and other health care providers) who are jointly responsible for the cost of care and the quality of care provided to their patient population. The law, which added a new section 1899 to the Social Security Act (42 U.S.C. 1395, et seq.), aims to incentivize providers to provide quality care at low cost and penalize those who provide high cost or low-quality care. The law requires groups of providers and suppliers to have a shared governance structure and stipulates a number of additional requirements to participate as a Medicare ACO. The statute requires ACOs to promote patient engagement and evidence-based medicine, coordinate care, and report cost and quality metrics.

Final regulations for the program were published in 2011 by the U.S. Department of Health and Human Services (HHS; HHS Federal Register Notice, November 2, 2011). The Federal Register notice emphasized that the new approach to delivering services to Medicare beneficiaries was designed to further a three-part aim to:

1. Provide better care for individuals.
2. Promote better health for populations.
3. Lower growth in expenditures for Medicare Parts A and B.

The rule explained that the goal of the value-based purchasing is to reward better outcomes, innovations, and values. It further articulated the statutory requirement for ACOs to have a governing body with a mechanism for shared decision-making and governance, including authority to define processes that promote patient engagement. It explained that patient engagement, defined as "the active participation of patients and their families in the process of making medical decisions," is a necessary part of patient-centered care. The final rule describes four patient-centeredness requirements that overlap with patient engagement:

1. Evaluation of the health needs of the population assigned to the ACO
2. Effective communication of clinical knowledge to beneficiaries
3. Recognizing the patient's unique needs, preferences, values, and priorities, while engaging in shared decision making
4. Having written standards for communicating with patients and allowing patient access to their medical record

The final rule also describes ways to promote patient engagement, including shared decision-making methods and tools, methods to promote health literacy, use of a beneficiary experience of care survey, and the involvement of patients in the governing processes of the ACO. The HHS Centers for Medicare and Medicaid Services (CMS) provides extensive resources describing the operation and requirements of ACOs (HHS, CMS, 2018).

The requirements for ACOs, including efforts to advance patient engagement, continue to evolve. The budget deal passed by Congress early in 2018 (Bipartisan Budget Act of 2018, Public Law 115-123) contained the ACO Beneficiary Incentive Program, which encourages patient engagement by authorizing ACOs to provide incentive payments to patients when they receive certain qualifying health care services.

Partnership for Patients. Another ACA innovation with a potential to impact patient engagement is the Center for Medicare and Medicaid Innovation (CMMI), which was established by section 3021 of the ACA. CMMI was created to reduce program expenditures and enhance quality of care for the Children's Health Insurance Program, Medicare, or Medicaid beneficiaries through testing of innovative payment and service delivery models. One initiative of CMMI is the *Partnership for Patients*, an organization consisting of more than 7500 partners, including organizations representing health care providers, consumers, and patients, as well as hospitals and health care systems and state and federal agencies (HHS, CMMI, 2012). Patient and family engagement is one focus of *Partnership for Patients*, which views the relationship between patients and families and health care providers as a key part of improving health care and reducing readmissions to hospitals (Partnership for Patients, 2013).

Patient-Centered Outcomes Research Institute. The Patient-Centered Outcomes Research Institute (PCORI), an independent, nonprofit health research organization, was created by section 6301 of the ACA. Washington and Lipstein (2011) explain that the organization, which focuses on patient-centered outcomes research, "will support many studies encompassing a broad range of study designs and outcomes that are relevant to patients, aiming to assist people in making choices that are consistent with their values, preferences, and goals." PCORI collaborates with federal agencies, such as the National Institutes of Health (NIH) and the Agency for Healthcare Research and Quality (AHRQ), to further patient-centered outcomes research, including patient engagement methods. PCORI seeks input on their work through a number of Advisory Panels, including a panel on patient engagement that includes representatives of patients as well as research and practicing clinicians (PCORI, n.d.).

Health Information Technology

There is evidence that providing online access to EHRs may empower patients to more fully contribute to their care (Woods et al., 2013), and that patients want to share access to their health information (Zulman et al., 2011). A section of the American Recovery and Reinvestment Act of 2009 (Public Law 111-5), the Health Information Technology for Economic and Clinical Health Act (HITECH Act) provisions, sought to stimulate the adoption of health information technology (Health IT or HIT) by authorizing financial incentives to providers for the adoption and meaningful use of EHRs.

Under this program, the federal government gives incentive payments to eligible professionals and hospitals that demonstrate efforts to implement certified EHR technology. While participation is voluntary, payment of Medicare and Medicaid fees will be negatively adjusted for those who do not participate. The program was implemented in three stages, with the final Stage 3 rule published in 2015 (HHS Federal Register Notice, October 15, 2015). The rule ties incentive payments to eight objectives and measures, which include a component on coordination of care through patient engagement.

A number of HIT policy initiatives at the federal level are driving patient engagement strategies. The HHS Office of the National Coordinator (ONC) for Health Information Technology has developed the Health IT Playbook, which provides strategies and best practices to support Health IT initiatives. The patient engagement portion of the playbook presents tips, guidance, and tools for using health IT, such as EHRs, to engage and activate patients (HHS, ONC, n.d.). While the Playbook provides resources for providers and hospital staff, ONC's Guide to Getting and Using Your Health Records, released by ONC in 2018, provides step-by-step guidance to patients and caregivers on how to access health records, check the accuracy of records, and effectively use the information (HHS, ONC, 2018).

Additional Federal Initiatives

Federal advisory committees can also further policy initiatives such as patient engagement. These entities, authorized by the Federal Advisory Committee Act of 1972 (Public Law 92-463), provide advice to the executive branch of the federal government (General Services Administration [GSA], n.d.). For example, one of the purposes of the U.S. Food and Drug Administration's (FDA) Patient Engagement Advisory Committee is to "increase the integration of patient perspectives into the regulatory process for medical devices" (HHS, FDA Federal Register Notice, September 9, 2015). In the same Federal Register announcement FDA opened docket to allow the public to provide input on a range of topics to help inform agency policy concerning patient engagement.

Other federal entities have also developed patient engagement policy initiatives. AHRQ developed an extensive policy document entitled Guide to Patient and Family Engagement in Hospital Quality and Safety (AHRQ, 2013). The AHRQ publication is an evidence-based resource for hospitals that identifies strategies to promote patient and family engagement in the quality and safety of hospital care. AHRQ has also developed an online resource center on PCMH, which includes resources to engage patients, families, and caregivers (AHRQ, 2011).

A new initiative from the NIH, called *All of Us*, seeks to engage a million people in a research effort to share their unique health data in a database. Approved researchers will have access to the data to research how health can be impacted by things such as genetics, lifestyle, and the environment. *All of Us* is a part of NIH's precision medicine program, which explores how a patient's unique genetics and other factors can impact how disease or illness is treated (HHS, NIH, n.d.). This type of initiative moves engagement efforts from the individual to the broader community level.

THE ROLE OF NURSING IN ADVANCING PATIENT ENGAGEMENT

A core theme from the Institute of Medicine report titled *The Future of Nursing: Leading Change, Advancing Health* (2011) is that nurses should be leaders in redesigning health care in the United States, and be full partners in developing and shaping health policy and in implementing health care reform. A follow-up report, *Assessing Progress on the Institute of Medicine Report The Future of Nursing* (2016), reemphasized the important role of nurses as leaders in care delivery and the redesign of health care. Patient engagement initiatives, likened to the "block-buster drug of the century" (Dentzer, 2013), offer nurses the opportunity to advance health policy and reform the health care system.

By definition, patient engagement involves individuals taking action to benefit from health care. Advancing patient engagement requires that nurses identify what will encourage patients (or others acting on a patient's behalf) to take action to benefit from available health care. Much of what is called "patient engagement" has been within the domain of nursing for decades. For example, in her *Notes on Nursing* published in 1860, Florence Nightingale advocated that the role of the nurse was to help the patient attain the best possible condition so that nature could act and self-healing could occur (Dossey, 2000). The American Nurses Association's Code of Ethics for Nurses With Interpretive Statements (2015) highlights the nurse's commitment to the unique needs of the individual patient and the importance of engaging patients in planning their care.

Nurses are on the front lines of delivering health care. They provide patient care across the health care spectrum and in more settings than any other health care profession. Also, for many patients, nurses hold a position of trust. Nurses have consistently been ranked as the most trusted profession (Gallup, 2017). As health reform advances, the health care environment is moving from a system where the patient is passive to a system in which health care consumers are engaged and share accountability for health outcomes with health providers and the system as a whole. As the largest segment of the health care workforce, nursing is well positioned to promote this transition. Nursing competencies, such as fostering behavior changes through the use of patient education, case management, and aligning patient needs to the health care system, are assets to making this transition (O'Neil, 2009).

In 2013, the Nursing Alliance for Quality Care, a group composed of leading nursing organizations and consumer advocacy groups, published a paper addressing the role of the nurse in advancing patient and family engagement (Sofaer & Schumann, 2013). The paper identifies opportunities and strategies to further nursing's role in patient engagement. Several strategies, including aligning incentives to encourage patient engagement and enforcing regulatory expectations and standards that support patient engagement principles in practice, would require nurses to engage with other stake-holders to advance these public policy initiatives. As trusted providers of health care, nurses are in an optimal position to advance patient engagement through policy initiatives.

Hassmiller and Bilazarian (2018) conducted a literature search and key informant interviews to identify the leadership strategies and practices of nurse leaders that advance consumer engagement. They found links between patient and family engagement and improved organizational outcomes measured by decreased length of stay and medication errors, and increased patient experience scores. Through this process they identified barriers and challenges to engagement, as well as a range of promising practices from key informant interviews that support both family and patient engagement as well as nurses. Promising practices included the use of patient activation measure tools, rounding by clinical nurse leaders, bedside charting to allow patients to more easily view their charts, and the use of shared decision-making tools.

FROM PATIENT ENGAGEMENT TO CITIZEN HEALTH

Twenty-five years ago, in the book *Through the Patient's Eyes: Understanding and Promoting Patient-Centered Care,*

Margaret Gerteis and her colleagues broke new ground in summarizing data obtained from thousands of patients through surveys and focus groups that advanced the perspective that "institutional" does not need to be synonymous with "impersonal." Seven areas were identified as important to improving the patient experience: respecting patients' values and preferences, coordinating care, providing information and education, attending to physical comfort, providing emotional support, involving family and friends in care, and ensuring continuity among providers and treatment settings (Gerteis, 1993). As fundamental and basic as these core tenets of patient-centered care are, they have been largely ignored until recently with the re-emergence of patient-centered care as an imperative, not an option.

Applying design-thinking to the process of care redesign is a very helpful strategy to ensure that the consumer's voice is heard. As described by Tim Brown (2009) in *Change by Design*, design thinking is a human-centered planning process that includes three overlapping steps:
1. Inspiration (the search for solutions)
2. Ideation (the process of generating developing and testing ideas)
3. Implementation (the path leading from project room to market)

It is an iterative, nonlinear process that involves continuously testing and revisiting assumptions and adhering to a philosophy of fail earlier to succeed sooner. The foundation of design thinking is planning around three overlapping criteria:
1. Desirability—What makes sense to people, and what is needed or desired?
2. Feasibility—What is functionally possible?
3. Viability—What is likely to be sustainable?

Engaging people at the beginning of a planning process, whether the process focuses on care, education, or public policy, increases the likelihood that their voices and perspectives will be heard and the outcome desirable, or even optimal.

Citizen health care is a bold vision proposed by Doherty and Mendenhall (2006) that goes beyond the activated patient to the activated community. They argue that patients, families, and communities should be co-producers of health and health care with professionals acquiring community organizing skills to enable them to effectively work with people who see themselves as citizens of health care, as builders of health in clinics and communities, rather than merely as consumers of medical services.

CONCLUSION

Although this chapter highlights governmental, professional (nursing), and organizational strategies aimed at shifting behavior to achieve patient engagement through policy initiatives, perhaps more thought and focus needs to be centered on what people can do for themselves and for each other to advance health and well-being. Determinants of well-being (Kreitzer, Delagran, & Uptmor, 2014) include health (physical, mental, emotional, and spiritual) as well as purpose, relationships, community, safety and security, and the environment.

In considering broader societal aspirations of human flourishing and economic sustainability, it is critical to consider ways to harness our cultural and democratic roots in service of advancing wellbeing and the common good. In *Healing the Heart of Democracy*, Parker Palmer (2011) notes that "when all of our talk about politics is either technical or strategic, to say nothing of partisan and polarizing, we loosen or sever the human connections on which empathy, accountability, and democracy itself reside." His central point is that we need to create a politics worthy of the human spirit, one that has a chance to serve the common good. This requires more than an engaged patient; it requires an engaged and informed citizenry.

DISCUSSION QUESTIONS

1. What is the role of the profession of nursing in creating an informed citizenry that is empowered to advance wellbeing within individuals, families, and communities?
2. What can you do in your practice to engage and empower patients and families?
3. What governmental, institutional, or private sector policies could enhance patient engagement and activation?

REFERENCES

Agency for Healthcare Research and Quality. (2011). *The patient-centered medical home: Strategies to put patients at the center of primary care*. Retrieved from www.pcmh.ahrq.gov/page/patient-centered-medical-home-strategies-put-patients-center-primary-care.

Agency for Healthcare Research and Quality. (2013). *Guide to patient and family engagement in hospital quality and safety*. Retrieved from www.ahrq.gov/professionals/systems/hospital/engagingfamilies/guide.html.

American Nurses Association. (2015). *Code of ethics for nurses with interpretive statements*. Silver Spring, MD: Nursebooks.org. Retrieved from www.nursingworld.org/practice-policy/nursing-excellence/ethics/code-of-ethics-for-nurses/coe-view-only/.

American Recovery and Reinvestment Act of 2009, Public Law 111–5. (2009). Retrieved from www.gpo.gov/fdsys/pkg/PLAW-111publ5/pdf/PLAW-111publ5.pdf.

Bipartisan Budget Act of 2018, Public Law 115-123. (2018). Retrieved from www.congress.gov/bill/115th-congress/house-bill/1892.

Boissy, A. (2017). Patient engagement versus patient experience. *New England Journal of Medicine Catalyst*. Retrieved from https://catalyst.nejm.org/patient-engagement-vs-patient-experience/.

Brown, D. (2009). *Change by design: How design thinking transforms organizations and inspires innovation*. New York: Harper Business.

Carman, K., Dardess, P., Maurer, M., Sofaer, S., Adams, K., Bechtel, C., et al. (2013). Patient and family engagement: A framework for understanding the elements and developing interventions and policies. *Health Affairs, 32*(2), 223-231.

Center for Advancing Health. (2010). *A new definition of patient engagement: What is engagement and why is it important*. Retrieved from Document9 www.cfah.org/pdfs/CFAH_Engagement_Behavior_Framework_current.pdf.

Choosing Wisely. (n.d.). Retrieved from www.choosingwisely.org.

Dentzer, S. (2013). Rx for the "blockbuster drug" of patient engagement. *Health Affairs, 32*(2), 202.

Doherty, W.J., & Mendenhall, T. (2006). Citizen health care: A model for engaging patients, families and communities as coproducers of health. *Family, Systems and Health, 24*, 251-263.

Dossey, B. M. (2000). *Florence Nightingale: Mystic, visionary, healer*. Springhouse, PA: Springhouse Corp.

Ezeji-Okoye, S., Kotar, T., Smeeding, S., & Dufree, J. (2013). State of care: Complementary and alternative medicine in Veterans Health Administration—2011 survey results. *Federal Practitioner, 30*(11), 15-20.

Fleming, M.D., Shim, J.K., Yen, I.H, Thompson-Lastad, A., Rubin, S., Van Natta, M., & Burke, N.J. (2017). Patient engagement at the margins: Health care providers' assessments of engagement and the structural determinants of health in the safety net. *Social Science & Medicine, 183*, 11-18.

Gallup. (2017). *Nurses keep healthy lead as most honest, ethical profession*. Retrieved from http://news.gallup.com/poll/224639/nurses-keep-healthy-lead-honest-ethical-profession.aspx.

Gerteis, M., Edgeman-Levitan, S., Daley, J., & Delbanco, T.L. (Eds.), (1993). *Through the patient's eyes: Understanding and promoting patient-centered care*. San Francisco: John Wiley & Sons, Inc.

Hassmiller, S. & Bilazrian, A. (2018). The business, ethics, and quality cases for consumer engagement in nursing. *Journal of Nursing Administration, 48*(4), 184-190. Retrieved from https://journals.lww.com/jonajournal/Fulltext/2018/04000/The_Business,_Ethics,_and_Quality_Cases_for.5.aspx.

Healthy Interactions. (n.d.). Retrieved from http://healthyinteractions.com/.

Hibbard, J., & Greene, J. (2013). What evidence shows about patient activation: Better health outcomes and care experiences; fewer data on costs. *Health Affairs, 32*(2), 207-214.

Hibbard, J., Greene, J., & Overton, V. (2013). Patients with lower activation associated with higher costs; delivery systems should know their patients' scores. *Health Affairs, 32*(2), 216-222.

Hibbard, J., Stockard, J., Mahoney, E., & Tusler, M. (2004). Development of the patient activation measure (PAM): Conceptualizing and measuring activation in patients and consumers. *Health Services Research, 39*(4/1), 1005-1026.

Institute for Healthcare Improvement. (n.d.). The Triple Aim. Retrieved from www.ihi.org/offerings/Initiatives/TripleAim/Pages/default.aspx.

Institute of Medicine. (2001). *Crossing the quality chasm: A new health system for the 21st century.* Washington, DC: National Academies Press.

Institute of Medicine. (2011). *The future of nursing: Leading change, advancing health.* Washington, DC: National Academies Press.

Institute of Medicine. (2016). *Assessing progress on the Institute of Medicine report The Future of Nursing.* Washington, DC: National Academies Press.

Katon, W., Von Korff, M., Lin, E., Walker, E., Simon, G. E., et al. (1995). Collaborative management to achieve treatment guidelines: Impact on depression in primary care. *Journal of the American Medical Association, 273*(13), 1026-1031.

Kline, S. (2011). *The Veterans Health Administration: Implementing patient-centered medical homes in the nation's largest integrated delivery system.* Commonwealth Fund. Retrieved from www.commonwealthfund.org/~/media/Files/Publications/Case%20Study/2011/Sep/1537_Klein_veterans_hlt_admin_case%20study.pdf.

Kreitzer M.J., Delagran, L. & Uptmor, A. (2014). Advancing wellbeing in people, organizations and communities. In M.J. Kreitzer & M. Koithan (Eds.), *Integrative nursing.* New York: Oxford University Press.

Martinez, O., Boles, J., Muñoz-Laboy, M., Levine, E.C., Ayamele, C., Eisenberg, R., Manusov, J., & Draine, J. (2017). Bridging health disparity gaps through the use of medical legal partnerships in patient care: A systematic review. *Journal of Law, Medicine & Ethics, 45,* 260-273.

National Center for Medical-Legal Partnerships. (2018). *Medical-legal partnerships: Where they are, how they work, and how they are funded.* Retrieved from http://medical-legalpartnership.org/wp-content/uploads/2017/12/Health-Center-based-Medical-Legal-Partnerships.pdf.

Nielsen, M., Langner, B., Zema, C., Hacker, T., & Grundy, P. (2012). *Benefits of implementing the primary care patient-centered medical home: A review of cost and quality results.* Patient-Centered Primary Care Collaborative. Retrieved from www.pcpcc.org/sites/default/files/media/benefits_of_implementing_the_primary_care_pcmh.pdf.

O'Neil, E. (2009). Four factors that guarantee health care change. *Journal of Professional Nursing, 25*(6), 317-321

Palmer, P. J. (2011). *Healing the heart of democracy.* New York: Jossey-Bass.

Partnership for Patients. (2013). *Welcome to the Partnership for Patients.* Retrieved from http://partnershipforpatients.cms.gov/about-the-partnership/patient-and-family-engagement/the-patient-and-family-engagement.html.

Patient. (n.d.). In *MerriamWebster Online.* Retrieved from www.merriam-webster.com/dictionary/patient.

Patient Centered Outcomes Research Institute. (n.d.). Retrieved from www.pcori.org/engagement/engage-us/join-advisory-panel/advisory-panel-patient-engagement.

Patient Protection and Affordable Care Act (Public Law 111-148) and the Health Care and Education Affordability Reconciliation Act (Public Law 111-152).

Ricciardi, L., Mostashari, F., Murphy, J., Daniel, J., & Siminerio, E. (2013). A national action plan to support consumer engagement via e-health. *Health Affairs, 32*(2), 376-384. Retrieved from www.healthaffairs.org/doi/abs/10.1377/hlthaff.2012.1216.

Robinson, J. H., Callister, L. C., Berry, J. A., & Dearing, K. A. (2008). Patient‚Äêcentered care and adherence: Definitions and applications to improve outcomes. *Journal of the American Academy of Nurse Practitioners, 20*(12), 600-607.

Rosland, A., Nelson, K., Sun, H., Dolan, E., Maynard, C., et al. (2013). The patient-centered medical home in the Veterans Health Administration. *American Journal of Managed Care, 19*(7), e263-e272. Retrieved from www.ajmc.com/publications/issue/2013/2013-1-vol19-n7/The-Patient-Centered-Medical-Home-in-the-Veterans-Health-Administration.

Sofaer, S. & Schumann, M.J. (2013). Fostering successful patient and family engagement: Nursing's critical role. Washington, DC: Nursing Alliance for Quality Care. Retrieved from www.naqc.org/WhitePaper-Patient Engagement.

Tax Cuts and Jobs Act of 2017 (Public Law 115-97). Retrieved from www.congress.gov/bill/115th-congress/house-bill/1/text.

U.S. Department of Health and Human Services, Center for Medicare and Medicaid Innovation. (2012). *Report to Congress.* Retrieved from http://innovation.cms.gov/Files/reports/RTC-12-2012.pdf.

U.S. Department of Health and Human Services, Centers for Medicare and Medicaid Services, (2011). *Accountable care organizations.* Federal Register, 76 Fed. Reg. 67802. Retrieved from www.gpo.gov/fdsys/pkg/FR-2011-11-02/pdf/2011-27461.pdf.

U.S. Department of Health and Human Services, Centers for Medicare and Medicaid Services. (2018). *Shared savings program.* Retrieved from www.cms.gov/Medicare/Medicare-Fee-for-Service-Payment/sharedsavingsprogram/index.html.

U.S. Department of Health and Human Services, Centers for Medicare and Medicaid Services. (2015). *Electronic health record incentive program—Stage 3 and modifications to meaningful use in 2015 through 2017.* Federal Register, 80 Fed. Reg. 62762. Retrieved from www.gpo.gov/fdsys/pkg/FR-2015-10-16/pdf/2015-25595.pdf.

U.S. Department of Health and Human Services, Food and Drug Administration. (2015). *Establishment of a patient advisory committee; establishment of a public docket.* Federal Register, 80 Fed. Reg. 57007. Retrieved from www.gpo.gov/fdsys/granule/FR-2015-09-21/2015-23521.

U.S. Department of Health and Human Services, National Institutes of Health. (n.d.). *About the All of Us research program.* Retrieved from https://allofus.nih.gov/about/about-all-us-research-program.

U.S. Department of Health and Human Services, Office of the National Coordinator for Health Information Technology. (2018). *The guide to getting and using your health records.* Retrieved from www.healthit.gov/how-to-get-your-health-record/.

U.S. Department of Health and Human Services, Office of the National Coordinator for Health Information Technology.

(n.d.). *Patient engagement playbook*. Retrieved from www.healthit.gov/playbook/pe/.

U.S. Department of Veterans Affairs. (2018). VA medical images and reports user guide. Retrieved from www.myhealth.va.gov/documents/25286/25831/VA_Medical_Images_and_Reports_User_Guide.pdf.

U.S. Department of Veterans Affairs. (n.d.). Retrieved from www.va.gov/health/.

U.S. Department of Veterans Affairs, Veterans Health Administration. (2018). VHA Directive 1120.02, Health promotion and disease prevention core program requirements. Retrieved from www.prevention.va.gov/Publications/VHA_Prevention_Policies_and_Guidelines.asp.

U.S. General Services Administration. (n.d.) *FACA 101*. Retrieved from www.gsa.gov/policy-regulations/policy/federal-advisory-committee-management/finding-information-on-faca-committees/faca-101.

Washington, A., & Lipstein, S. (2011). The Patient-Centered Outcomes Research Institute—Promoting better information, decisions, and health. *New England Journal of Medicine, 365*, e31. Retrieved from www.nejm.org/doi/full/10.1056/NEJMp1109407.

Woods, W., Schwartz, E., Tuepker, A., Press, N., Nazi, K., et al. (2013). Patient experiences with full electronic access to health records and clinical notes through the My HealtheVET Personal Health Record Pilot: Qualitative study. *Journal of Medical Internet Research,15*(3), e65. Retrieved from www.jmir.org/2013/3/e65/.

Zulman, D., Nazi, K., Turvey, C., Wagner, T., Woods, S., & An L. (2011). Patient interest in sharing personal health record information: A web-based survey. *Annals of Internal Medicine, 155*(12), 805-810.

ONLINE RESOURCES

Agency for Healthcare Research and Quality: Guide to Patient and Family Engagement in Hospital Quality and Safety
www.ahrq.gov/professionals/systems/hospital/engagingfamilies
Center for Spirituality and Healing: Taking Charge of Your Health and Wellbeing
www.takingcharge.csh.umn.edu

21

The Marinated Mind: Why Overuse Is an Epidemic and How to Reduce It

Rosemary Gibson

"Our minds have been marinated to believe more is better."

Rosemary Gibson

The Institute of Medicine (now the National Academy of Medicine) identified three health care quality challenges in the United States: underuse, misuse, and overuse. Overuse is when the potential for harm of a health care service exceeds the possible benefit. Dedicated clinicians, journalists, and public interest advocates are creating the urgency for policymakers to reduce it.

COMMONLY OVERUSED INTERVENTIONS

Commonly overused health care interventions in the United States were first identified in 2008 by the National Priorities Partnership, which was convened by the National Quality Forum. The interventions include prescription drugs, laboratory tests, diagnostic imaging, procedures such as back surgery and prostatectomy, and treatments at the end of life. A frequent example of overuse is antibiotic treatment of a cold virus. It confers no benefit and reduces the effectiveness of antibiotics because bacteria mutate and develop resistance. The surge of antibiotic-resistant bacteria is a testament to the misuse of antibiotics, and the public health impact is rightly worrisome.

Other forms of overuse put patients at immediate risk of harm, disability, and death. Research on back surgery published in the Journal of the American Medical Association identified overuse of complex fusion procedures for spinal stenosis. Patients suffered more major complications and higher mortality compared with evidence-based, less-intensive surgical interventions (Deyo et al., 2010). A study of implanted cardiac defibrillators reported that 23% of patients who had surgery to implant the device did not meet evidence-based guidelines (Al-Khatib et al., 2011). The risk of in-hospital death was significantly higher in patients who received a nonevidence-based device than in patients who received an evidence-based device. Certain hospitals had especially high rates, 40% or more, of inappropriate use of defibrillators.

Studies such as these do not report the names of the hospitals performing unnecessary surgeries. The defibrillator study was funded by the National Institutes of Health and paid for by taxpayers, but the public is precluded from knowing the hospitals that are putting patients in harm's way. In addition to the human cost, overuse has a high financial cost. More than $210 billion is wasted every year on unnecessary treatments and tests (Institute of Medicine, 2012). The cost of overuse draws resources away from care that underserved populations desperately require. It contributes to the unsustainably high levels of health care spending that are a growing burden on families, employers, and federal and state governments.

REASONS FOR OVERUSE

Multiple reasons explain overuse. Uncertainty is a fundamental challenge in health care. In the face of uncertainty, a clinician may try to address a patient's concern. A provider's belief, rather than knowledge, may guide practice.

Physicians, nurses, and patients have different beliefs about the role of medical care. Some believe that medical interventions are risky and a "less is more" approach is desirable. Others believe in the possibilities of medicine and that they should be explored in a context of uncertainty. Beliefs may evolve and become dogma, which is authoritative and reinforced by habit rather than evidence. Clinicians and patients can become enthusiastic about a treatment even when evidence unequivocally points to its folly.

Fear of missing a diagnosis drives overuse. A physician or nurse practitioner does not want to miss a diagnosis of cancer or other serious disease. The risk of medical liability can propel overuse.

Providers' expectations of each other can prompt overuse. When a primary care physician refers a patient for a diagnostic imaging test, a radiologist may not believe the test is warranted but performs it anyway because a colleague requested it. A specialist may not want to jeopardize future referrals. In addition, it can be time consuming to contact the referring physician and explain why the test is not needed.

Patient expectations drive overuse. When a patient requests an inappropriate antibiotic or screening test, busy primary care providers may comply to save time or placate a patient, even though they know they should not.

A clinician's competence and diagnostic skills affect whether patients receive appropriate care. Young physicians in training, who have yet to hone their diagnostic skills, may order more tests than are necessary.

Financial Incentives as the Major Cause of Overuse

Fee-for-service payment for health care services has been the main driver of overuse. With virtually no limit on the volume of services that providers can bill, the design of the payment system has propelled overuse to epidemic proportions and launched a highly lucrative business model.

When Medicare was established, no health care companies were on the Fortune 100 list. Currently, there are 15. Publicly traded health care companies have a fiduciary duty to shareholders to increase revenue and profitability. Shareholder expectations can be met in a limited number of ways: raise prices, increase sales volume, and reduce expenses. Not-for-profit organizations are not immune from the incentive structure and are also at risk of overtreating patients.

Higher volume of prescription drugs, diagnostic imaging, hospital admissions, and surgery strengthens the financial bottom line. Manufacturers that sell products, equipment, and supplies to hospitals have the incentive to sell more, not to choose wisely. This is the reason why overuse remains the most neglected quality challenge in the United States. Fixing it will cause revenue reductions for providers and manufacturers. Not fixing it means that the health care enterprise is propped up by putting patients in harm's way.

Through this lens, overuse causes two additional harms. First, physicians, nurses, and pharmacists are required by their organizations to accommodate a faster workflow. They do more procedures, administer more medications, and fill more prescriptions in the same amount of time. Demands for higher productivity in a health care system that is yet to be free from faulty design and defects inevitably cause more patients to be harmed. When a clinician makes a mistake, his or her confidence can be shaken, creating a risk for more mistakes.

Even the most competent clinician is at risk of harming a patient when forced to work at a pace faster than human factors engineering suggests is feasible. Moral distress is heightened. Highly skilled clinicians desire to meet their professional duty to the patient while their employer's requirements preclude them from doing so. A clinician cannot serve two masters whose interests are diametrically opposed.

This profound and disturbing conflict can drive out highly skilled, caring professionals from patient care as they seek other ways to use their skills. Health care delivery systems are at risk of being caught in a downward spiral whose logical conclusion is not a safer system for patients and caregivers.

The Marinated Mind

The business model of health care requires consumers and patients to be high users of health care services. A steady stream of advertisements for drugs, medical devices, tests, and procedures creates public expectations for medical care that may be unrealistic, unnecessary, and harmful. Television medical dramas portray testing and surgery as the norm to an unsuspecting public whose mind has been marinated to believe that more treatment is better (Gibson & Singh, 2010). The benefits of treatment are extolled while risks are underplayed.

A subset of the public is becoming more aware of overuse. An analysis of cardiac bypass surgery trends in a California hospital conducted by Dartmouth Atlas researchers shone a light on communities where patients were at risk of overuse of unnecessary bypass surgery. The analysis identified a hospital in Redding, California as having the highest rate of cardiac bypass surgery in the country in 2001 and 2002 (Dartmouth Atlas of Health Care, 2005). The rate had nearly doubled during the preceding decade. A sudden outbreak of serious heart disease warranting the increase in surgery volume was unlikely to be the underlying cause of the upward trend. Although this information was publicly available, Medicare officials did not intervene.

The overuse trend was interrupted only when a patient who was diagnosed as having blockages that required bypass surgery obtained a second opinion elsewhere and was given a clean bill of health. After he contacted the Federal Bureau of Investigation, it was determined that more than 700 patients had unnecessary heart procedures.

The hospital and doctors paid nearly $500 million in fines and penalties (Lucas, 2005).

Large-scale overuse of cardiac procedures occurred at a Maryland hospital. A U.S. Senate investigation that was widely reported in the media found that approximately 600 patients had been given unnecessary cardiac stents (U.S. Senate Committee on Finance, 2010). A patient complaint launched the initial inquiry, which resulted in the doctor losing his medical license and the hospital paying fines.

Five years later, the federal Department of Justice fined 457 hospitals more than $250 million for inappropriate use of implantable cardioverter defibrillators in people covered by Medicare (U.S. Department of Justice, 2015b). Over a period of 7 years, the defibrillators were implanted contrary to evidence-based guidelines. In another case a Michigan doctor administered unnecessary chemotherapy to 553 patients who were given a false diagnosis of cancer (U.S. Department of Justice, 2015a). Eliminating overuse can be one of the most effective ways to keep patients safe and to reduce costs. Relying on patients to pull the emergency brake when overuse is evident is not an effective strategy. Public policies that enable public reporting of providers who are performing unnecessary tests and procedures are needed.

PHYSICIAN AND NURSE ACKNOWLEDGMENT OF OVERUSE

A breakthrough in the recognition of overuse as a widespread patient safety concern occurred with the launching of the Choosing Wisely campaign by the American Board of Internal Medicine Foundation. The aim of the campaign has been to encourage physicians, other health care providers, and patients to engage in conversations to reduce overuse of tests and procedures (American Board of Internal Medicine Foundation, 2014). Approximately 50 medical specialty societies and other organizations have identified top-five lists of tests or procedures commonly used whose necessity should be questioned and discussed. For example, the American Geriatrics Society recommends that antipsychotics should not be used as a first choice to treat behavioral and psychological symptoms of dementia (American Geriatrics Society, 2014). The American College of Radiology recommends that patients do not have imaging tests when they have a common headache without risk factors (American College of Radiology, 2014).

The American Academy of Nursing participated in Choosing Wisely and identified 25 things that nurses and patients should question (American Academy of Nursing, 2014). They include not placing or maintaining an indwelling urinary catheter in a patient unless there is a specific indication. The aim is to prevent catheter-associated urinary tract infections.

Consumer Reports joined the Choosing Wisely campaign to translate the information on overused tests and procedures for consumers to help them talk with their doctors so they can get the care they need, not the care they do not need (Consumer Reports Health, 2014). Consumer Reports distributed information to the public through employer organizations, such as the National Business Coalition on Health and the Pacific Business Group on Health.

PUBLIC REPORTING TO REDUCE OVERUSE

Public reporting of hospital-specific information is a strategy to reduce overuse. As an example, the Leapfrog Group, an employer-driven hospital quality watchdog group, asked hospitals to voluntarily report their rate of elective deliveries before 39 completed weeks of pregnancy. Babies have a higher risk of morbidity and mortality and mothers have a higher risk of postpartum complications when delivery occurs before a full 39 weeks' gestation.

The Leapfrog Group publicly reported these rates, and they generated substantial media attention (Leapfrog Group, 2013). By highlighting hospitals' overuse of early elective deliveries, public awareness created urgency for reform and improvement. Since the first hospital rates were publicly reported, the rate of early deliveries without medical necessity has been declining significantly. Many organizations are working to reduce these high-risk births, including the American College of Obstetrics and Gynecology and the American College of Nurse-Midwives.

Public reporting of overuse of diagnostic imaging has also helped to reduce unnecessary testing. Medicare's Hospital Compare website reports the hospitals that perform double chest computed tomography (CT) scans. These double scans occur when patients receive two imaging tests consecutively, one without contrast and a second with contrast. Experts say that patients should receive one or the other, not both, to avoid excess exposure to radiation.

Radiation exposure has risks. Researchers at the National Cancer Institute estimated that approximately 29,000 future cancers and 14,500 deaths could be related to CT scans performed in the United States in 2007. Chest CT scans are among the contributors to the increase risk (Berrington de González et al., 2009).

The New York Times and the Washington Post published the first round of data from Medicare's website using interactive maps that allowed readers to identify hospitals that performed high rates of double chest CT scans (Appleby & Rau, 2011; Bogdanich & McGinty, 2011).

More than 75,000 Medicare patients had double scans. Because Medicare data exclude patients with private and other insurance, the number of people having unnecessary scans is likely to be higher.

Members of the public are consumers of these data, as are hospital leaders and board members whose hospitals are overusing these scans. A hospital's visibility in the mainstream media can be a powerful stimulus for improvement. The reporting of overuse has encouraged some hospitals to reduce double chest CT scans (Chedekel, 2013).

JOURNALISTS ADVOCATE FOR MORE TRANSPARENCY ABOUT OVERUSE

Enterprising journalists have provided the public with valuable information about overtreatment. In addition, they have helped to change public policy to enable more data transparency on overuse.

The Wall Street Journal published a series of articles in 2010 that used Medicare claims data to identify billing patterns of individual doctors who participate in the program. The claims data are a computerized record of the bills Medicare pays. The journalists' analysis revealed clear cases of overtreatment. However, the journalists could not use the Medicare data to publish details of individual doctors' billings because of a 1979 court order barring disclosure of that information. Using additional sources, journalists pieced together profiles of physicians who were putting their patients at risk. For example, they identified a neurosurgeon who had the highest rate of multiple spinal-fusion surgeries among his peers and operated on some of his patients' spines as many as seven times (Carreyrou & McGinty, 2011).

The newspaper's parent company, Dow Jones, filed a lawsuit in 2011 to overturn a long-standing prohibition against the release of information on individual doctors' Medicare billing practices. In a major step toward transparency, a Florida judge ruled in May 2013 that the federal government should make the information available. In 2014 the Centers for Medicare and Medicaid Services (CMS) made Medicare data on physician payment information more transparent and accessible, while maintaining the privacy of beneficiaries (Blum, 2014). Journalists and researchers, along with the public, currently have greater access to data to shine a light on overuse.

INCREASE IN THE PEER-REVIEWED LITERATURE ON OVERUSE

The literature documenting overuse is expanding, which reflects growing interest in the topic. In 2016, more than 1200 articles were identified compared with 821 in 2015 and 440 in 2014 (Morgan et al., 2016). A study of emergency department visits for upper respiratory tract symptoms (sore throats and nasal congestion) and lower respiratory tract symptoms (cough and shortness of breath), found that CT use increased 400% from 2001 and 2002 to 2009 and 2010 (Drescher et al., 2016). The largest increase was for patients with nonacute upper respiratory tract symptoms who were less likely to benefit. No change in hospital admissions and antibiotic prescriptions were found during these time periods. The findings suggest that the increase in use of CT and consequent patient exposure to ionizing radiation did not change treatment decisions.

Overuse occurs not because of a lack of evidence for what to do. A randomized trial of 47 practices found that inappropriate antibiotic prescribing for acute respiratory tract infections was reduced from 24% to 13% after automated interventions provided feedback to the prescriber (Meeker et al., 2016). The three interventions were: suggestions for alternative treatment options, required written justification, and emails that allowed the prescribing clinicians the opportunity to compare their prescribing practices with peers who prescribed antibiotics more appropriately.

Shared decision-making can help to reduce unnecessary cardiac imaging in low-risk patients, according to a study of 898 patients with chest pain who went to one of six emergency departments (Hess et al., 2016). They were randomized into two groups. One group received usual care, and the other group received a decision aid that explained the interventions and the risks and benefits. Patients who received usual care were more likely to choose advanced cardiac testing. Those who received decision aids were less likely to choose cardiac testing. They also had more knowledge of their risk for acute heart conditions and were more involved in the decision process. No major adverse cardiac events occurred.

Public policies to prevent overtreatment need to be strengthened. The most effective actions required are stronger enforcement of unlawful billing and payment for unnecessary medical services, as well as stepped-up prosecution of individuals engaged in medically inappropriate treatment that harms patients. These efforts will serve as a deterrent to others and help to assure the public that they are protected from treatment traps that undermine confidence in the nation's health care system. The wise use of health care resources is imperative. The amount of money available for health care services is not unlimited. With proper stewardship, the nation can ensure that all Americans will receive the care they need, not the care they do not.

DISCUSSION QUESTIONS

1. Have you had medical care that you thought was unnecessary?
2. What are your top five most overused interventions in medicine and nursing?
3. What public policies can reduce overuse?

REFERENCES

Al-Khatib, S. M., Hellkamp, A., Curtis, J., Mark, D., Peterson, E., Sanders, G.D., et al. (2011). Non-evidence-based ICD implantations in the United States. *JAMA, 305*(1), 43–49.

American Academy of Nursing. (2014). *Twenty-five things nurses and patients should question.* Retrieved from www.aannet.org/initiatives/choosing-wisely.

American Board of Internal Medicine Foundation. (2014). *Choosing Wisely.* Retrieved from www.choosingwisely.org/about-us/.

American College of Radiology. (2014). *Choosing Wisely.* Retrieved from www.choosingwisely.org/doctor-patient-lists/american-college-of-radiology/.

American Geriatrics Society. (2014). *Choosing Wisely.* Retrieved from www.choosingwisely.org/doctor-patient-lists/american-geriatrics-society/.

Appleby, J., & Rau, J. (2011). Many hospitals overuse double CT scans, data show. *Washington Post.* Retrieved from www.washingtonpost.com/national/health-science/many-hospitals-overuse-double-ct-scans-data-shows/2011/06/16/AGvpTAaH_story.html.

Berrington de González, A., Mahesh, M., Kim, K., Bhargavan, M., Lewis, R., Mettler, H.F., et al. (2009). Projected cancer risks from computed tomographic scans performed in the United States in 2007. *JAMA Internal Medicine, 169*(22), 2071–2077.

Blum, J. (2014). CMS modifies policy on disclosure of physician payment information. *CMS Blog.* Retrieved from www.healthdata.gov/blog/cms-modifies-policy-disclosure-physician-payment-information.

Bogdanich, W., & McGinty, J.C. (2011). Medicare claims show overuse for CT scanning. *New York Times.* Retrieved from www.nytimes.com/2011/06/18/health/18radiation.html?pagewanted=all&_r=0.

Carreyrou, J., & McGinty, T. (2011). Medicare records reveal troubling trail of surgeries. *Wall Street Journal.* Retrieved from www.wsj.com/articles/SB10001424052748703858404576214642193925996.

Chedekel, L. (2013). *Dempsey Hospital makes progress reducing double CT scans.* Connecticut Health I-Team. Retrieved from http://c-hit.org/2013/04/04/dempsey-hospital-makes-progress-reducing-double-ct-scans-2/.

Consumer Reports Health. (2014). *The Choosing Wisely campaign.* Retrieved from www.consumerreports.org/video/view/healthy-living/drugs-medication/2142290539001/choosing-wisely-for-better-healthcare/.

Dartmouth Atlas of Health Care: Studies of Surgical Variation. (2005). *Cardiac surgery report.* Retrieved from http://archive.dartmouthatlas.org/downloads/reports/Cardiac_report_2005.pdf.

Deyo, R.A., Mirza, S.K., Martin, B.I., Kreuter, W., Goodman, D.C., & Jarvik, J.G. (2010). Trends, major medical complications and charges associated with surgery for lumbar spinal stenosis in older adults. *JAMA, 303*(13), 1259–1265.

Drescher, F.A., & Sirovich, B.E. (2016). Use of computed tomography in emergency departments in the United States: A decade of coughs and colds. *Journal of the American Medical Association Internal Medicine, 176*(2), 273-275.

Gibson, R., & Singh, J.P. (2010). *The treatment trap.* Chicago: Ivan R. Dee.

Hess, E.P., Hollander, J.E., Schaffer, J.T., et al. (2016). Shared decision making in patients with low risk chest pain: prospective randomized pragmatic trial. *BMJ, 355*, i6165.

Institute of Medicine. (2012). *Better care at lower cost: The path to continuously learning health care in the United States.* Retrieved from www.nationalacademies.org/hmd/~/media/Files/Report%20Files/2012/Best-Care/BestCareReport Brief.pdf.

Leapfrog Group. (2013). *New data: Early elective deliveries decline at hospitals as health leaders caution against unnecessary deliveries.* Retrieved from www.leapfroggroup.org/news-events/new-data-early-elective-deliveries-decline-hospitals-health-leaders-caution-against.

Lucas, A. (2005). *Redding settlement in heart surgery fraud case: Victims could get $32.5 million from doctors, insurers.* Retrieved from www.sfgate.com/health/article/REDDING-Settlement-in-heart-surgery-fraud-case-2594884.php.

Meeker, D., Linder J.A., Fox, C.R., et al. (2016). Effect of behavioral interventions on inappropriate antibiotic prescribing among primary care practices: A randomized clinical trial. *JAMA, 315*(6), 562-570.

Morgan, D., Dhruva, S., Coon, E., Wright, S., & Korenstein, D. (2018). 2017 update on medical overuse: A systematic review. *Journal of the American Medical Association Internal Medicine, 178*(1), 110-115.

U.S. Department of Justice. (2015a). *Detroit area doctor sentenced to 45 years in prison for providing medically unnecessary chemotherapy to patients.* Retrieved from www.justice.gov/opa/pr/detroit-area-doctor-sentenced-45-years-prison-providing-medically-unnecessary-chemotherapy.

U.S. Department of Justice. (2015b). *Nearly 500 hospitals pay United States more than $250 million to resolve False Claims Act allegations related to implantation of cardiac devices.*

Retrieved from www.justice.gov/opa/pr/nearly-500-hospitals-pay-united-states-more-250-million-resolve-false-claims-act-allegations.

U.S. Senate Committee on Finance. (2010). *Staff report on cardiac stent usage at St. Joseph Medical Center*. S. PRT. 111–157. Retrieved from www.finance.senate.gov/imo/media/doc/12062010%20Finance%20Committee%20Staff%20Report%20on%20Cardiac%20Stent%20Usage%20at%20St%20Joseph%20Medical%20Center.pdf.

ONLINE RESOURCES

Leapfrog Group
www.leapfroggroup.org
Medicare Hospital Compare
www.medicare.gov/hospitalcompare/search.html
ProPublica (a public interest investigative journalism group)
www.propublica.org

22

Policy Approaches to Address Health Disparities

Nadia Campos de Andrade and Carmen Alvarez

"The call to the nurse is not only for the bedside care of the sick, but to help in seeking out the deep-lying basic cause of illness and misery."

Lillian Wald

ORIGINS OF HEALTH EQUITY POLICIES

In 1984, former U.S. Department of Health and Human Services (HHS) Secretary Margaret Heckler presented to Congress a report outlining health trends among the American people in 1983. Despite demonstrating significant improvements in most health measures, that year's report also—as stated by Secretary Heckler—"signaled a sad and significant fact; there was continuing disparity in the burden of death and illness experienced by Blacks and other minority Americans as compared with our nation's population as whole," (Heckler, 1985, ix). Accordingly, Secretary Heckler called a panel of experts to conduct a comprehensive study of the health of minorities, which resulted in the publication of the landmark 1985 HHS Report of the Secretary's Task Force on Black and Minority Health (Heckler Report). This report marks the beginning of important changes in research, policy, and legislations that have fueled national, state, and local efforts to end health disparities. The creation of the Health and Human Services Office of Minority Health (OMH) in 1986 is one of the most significant changes following the report.

In September 1990, HHS released Healthy People 2000: National Health Promotion and Disease Prevention Objectives, which included reducing health disparities. Healthy People 2010 added the objective to eliminate, not just reduce, health disparities. The latest initiative, Healthy People 2020, expands the objectives even further, to include achieving health equity. But what actually are health disparities? Or health equity? Or social determinants of health (SDOH)? Over the past 20 years, much literature has been published on the topic and many terms have emerged to describe the troubling findings outlined in the Heckler Report.

HEALTH DISPARITIES AND SOCIAL DETERMINANTS OF HEALTH

Health disparities are "a particular type of *health difference* that is closely linked with social, economic, and/or environmental disadvantage" (OMH, 2018). These differences are often related to unequal distribution of power, money, and resources, which more often impact the most vulnerable populations. In recognizing the importance of accounting for the impact of social and environmental factors on health, the World Health Organization (WHO) established the Commission on Social Determinants of Health and published the report *Closing the gap in a generation: Health equity through action on the social determinants of health* (Marmot, Bell, Houweling, Taylor & Commission on Social Determinants of Health, 2008). In October 2011, WHO hosted the first World Conference on Social Determinants of Health in Rio de Janeiro, Brazil. The SDOH are "the conditions in which people are born, grow, work, live, and age, and the wider set of forces and systems shaping the conditions of daily life" (WHO, 2017). Healthy People 2020 has developed a framework that groups SDOH into five key areas (Table 22.1): (1) Economic Stability; (2) Education; (3) Social and Community Context; (4) Health and Health Care; and (5) Neighborhood and Built Environment.

The goal of addressing SDOH is to ultimately achieve health equity. Health equity is the "attainment of the highest level of health for all people" (OMH, 2018). If equity is described as fairness and opportunity, health equity refers to the principle of eliminating health disparities and the barriers inhibiting opportunity to obtain optimal

TABLE 22.1	Social Determinants of Health
Economic Stability	Employment; Food Insecurity; Housing Instability; Poverty
Education	Early Childhood Education and Development; Enrollment in Higher Education; High School Graduation; Language and Literacy
Social and Community Context	Civic Participation; Discrimination; Incarceration; Social Cohesion
Health and Health Care	Access to Health Care; Access to Primary Care; Health Literacy
Neighborhood and Built Environment	Access to Foods that Support Healthy Eating Patterns; Crime and Violence; Environmental Conditions; Quality of Housing

health (Braveman, 2014). The National Partnership for Action to End Health Disparities (NPA) draft document states that "achieving health equity requires valuing everyone equally with focused and ongoing societal efforts to address avoidable inequalities, historical and contemporary injustices, and the elimination of health and health care disparities" (Beadle & Graham, 2011 p. 9).

In summary, in order to eliminate *health disparities*, we must investigate and act upon the *social determinants of health* to ultimately achieve *health equity*. Health inequities in the United States remain a problem for, among others, racial and ethnic minorities as well as low-income populations. An established contributor to poor health outcomes is a lack of access to health care. Increased access to health care services has been an anticipated result of the implementation of Patient Protection and Affordable Care Act (ACA).

FROM THE HECKLER REPORT TO THE AFFORDABLE CARE ACT: ONGOING CHANGES

The past 30 years have seen great advancements in policies aimed at addressing health disparities. One of the most significant has been the enactment of the ACA in March 2010. The ACA offers the potential to reduce health disparities through increasing access to coverage and more efficient/cost-effective health care delivery models for preventive services and wellness (ACA, 2010). One of the initial provisions of ACA aimed at addressing health disparities was requiring the establishment of Offices of Minority Health within all HHS agencies (Box 22.1). These offices, along with the NIH National Institute on Minority Health and Health Disparities (NIMHD), have since become the main players in developing policies and procedures aimed at improving the health of U.S. minorities. In 2011, the HHS Action Plan to Reduce Racial and Ethnic Health Disparities was launched, which outlined five goals (Table 22.2). Additionally, the ACA permanently reauthorizes the Indian Health Care Improvement Reauthorization Extension Act of 2009.

BOX 22.1 Federal Agencies With Established Office of Minority Health

- Center for Medicare & Medicaid Services (CMS) Office of Minority Health
- Health and Human Services (HHS) Office of Minority Health
- Agency for Healthcare Research and Quality (AHRQ), Office of Minority Health
- Food and Drug Administration, Office of Minority Health (OMH)
- Health Resources and Services Administration, Office of Health Equity (OHE)
- National Institute on Minority Health and Health Disparities (NIMHD)
- Substance Abuse and Mental Health Services Administration (SAMHSA) Office of Behavioral Health Equity
- Department of Veterans Affairs Center for Health Equity Research and Promotion

---

As we quickly approach the 10th anniversary of ACA's enactment, its impact on health disparities have become more evident through the publication of numerous studies tracking changes in health care access and utilization after 2013. Between 2013 and 2015, the first 2 years of ACA coverage expansion, the uninsured rate dropped 9% for Black adults ages 19 to 64, and by 12% for Latino adults (Hayes, Riley, Radley, & McCarthy, 2017). Similarly, non-Latino Whites, despite already having much lower uninsured rates, saw a 5% decline in the uninsured rate (Hayes et al., 2017). In absolute population numbers, this drop means that an estimated 2 million more Black adults, 3.5 million more Latino adults, and 6.7 million more White adults had health insurance in 2015 compared to 2013 (Hayes et al., 2017). In that same 2-year period, the number of U.S. adults without a usual source of care (e.g., access to a personal health care provider) dropped 4% for Blacks and Latinos, while Whites had a smaller 1% decrease (Haynes et al., 2017).

Population mean out-of-pocket expenses decreased by 11.9% in the first 2 years after expansion, with mean

TABLE 22.2   **Health and Human Services Action Plan to Reduce Racial and Ethnic Health Disparities**

Goals	Efforts (2011–2014 Report)
Goal I: Transform Health Care	• Expansion of Medicaid and Introduction of the Health Insurance Marketplace. • From Coverage to Care (C2C) Initiative. • The Health Resources and Services Administration's (HRSA) National Health Service Corps (NHSC).
Goal II: Strengthen the Nation's Health and Human Services Infrastructure and Workforce Care (National CLAS Standards).	• National Standards for Culturally and Linguistically Appropriate Services in Health and Health
Goal III: Advance the Health, Safety, and Well-Being of the American People	• Health Profession Opportunity Grants (HPOG). • Public-Private Partnerships to Improve Vaccination Rates. • Community Transformation Grants (CTG) Program
Goal IV: Advance Scientific Knowledge and Innovation	• Native Hawaiian/Pacific Islander National Health Interview Survey. • Community Networks Program Centers (CNPCs)
Goal V: Increase Efficiency, Transparency, and Accountability of HHS Programs	• Health System Measurement Project

HHS, Health and Human Services.

spending by Medicaid-eligible households (lowest-income ≤138% Federal Poverty Level [FPL]) decreasing by 21% (Goldman, Woolhandler, & Himmelstein, 2018). As for cost concerns, the percentage of Black adults who skipped a doctor's visit because of cost decreased from 21% in 2013 to 17% in 2015 (Hayes et al., 2017). For Latinos, the number of adults skipping needed care because of costs decreased from 27% in 2013 to 22% in 2015, while their non-Latino White counterparts saw a 2% decrease, from 12% (2013) to 10% (2015) (Hayes et al., 2017).

Additionally, socioeconomic disparities in health coverage significantly narrowed between 2011 and 2015. The absolute gap in insurance coverage between people in households with annual incomes below $25,000 and those in households with incomes above $75,000 fell from 31% to 17% (46% relative reduction) in expansion states, and from 36% to 28% in non-expansion states (23% reduction), (Griffith, Evans, & Bor, 2017). Among sexual minorities, the percentage of uninsured lesbian, gay, and bisexual (LGB) individuals decreased from 19% in 2013 to 10% in 2016. As for Medicaid utilization, LGB individuals had an 8% increase in coverage, going from 7% in 2013 to 15% in 2016 (Dawson, Kates, & Damico, 2018).

ACA AND DISPARITIES IN MEDICAID COVERAGE

A provision central to ACA is the expansion of Medicaid, which intends to reduce the percentage of uninsured adults

with family income at or below 138% of the FPL, or approximately $33,000 for a family of four in 2014. As of 2018, 34 states plus the District of Columbia have adopted the expansion (Box 22.2) (Kaiser Family Foundation, 2018). States adopting the expansion saw Medicaid coverage increased from 18.1% (2011–2013) to 23.6% (2014) and 28.1% in 2015. Those same states saw the uninsured rate declined from 32.4% in 2011 to 2013, to 24.4% in 2014, and 18.8% in 2015 (Wehby & Lyu, 2017). Non-expanding states saw a small increase in Medicaid coverage in 2014 to 2015 (1.5%) and uninsured rates decline of nearly half of those observed in expanding states (Wehby & Lyu, 2017). Latinos saw the largest effects of expansion with a 6.9% take-up increase and a 5% decline in the uninsured rate as compared to a 6.6% increase in take-up and a 4.5% decrease in uninsured rate among non-Latino Blacks (Wehby & Lyu, 2017).

Medicare and Health Equity

In September 2015, the Centers for Medicare and Medicaid Services (CMS) Office of Minority Health, to address one of ACA's key provisions for reducing disparities, released the *CMS Equity Plan for Improving Quality in Medicare* (CMS Equity Plan for Medicare). The plan outlines six priority areas (Table 22.3) (CMS, 2016) aimed at advancing health equity by improving the quality of care provided to minority and other underserved Medicare beneficiaries. In October 2016, the first report on the actions and results related to each of the six priority was published.

BOX 22.2 Current Status of Medicaid Expansion Decision by States (as of July 2018)

Alabama	Not Adopted	Montana	Adopted
Alaska	Adopted	Nebraska	Considering Expansion
Arizona	Adopted	Nevada	Adopted
Arkansas	Adopted	New Hampshire	Adopted
California	Adopted	New Jersey	Adopted
Colorado	Adopted	New Mexico	Adopted
Connecticut	Adopted	New York	Adopted
Delaware	Adopted	North Carolina	Not Adopted
District of Columbia	Adopted	North Dakota	Adopted
Florida	Not Adopted	Ohio	Adopted
Georgia	Not Adopted	Oklahoma	Not Adopted
Hawaii	Adopted	Oregon	Adopted
Idaho	Considering Expansion	Pennsylvania	Adopted
Illinois	Adopted	Rhode Island	Adopted
Indiana	Adopted	South Carolina	Not Adopted
Iowa	Adopted	South Dakota	Not Adopted
Kansas	Not Adopted	Tennessee	Not Adopted
Kentucky	Adopted	Texas	Not Adopted
Louisiana	Adopted	Utah	Considering Expansion
Maine	Adopted	Vermont	Adopted
Maryland	Adopted	Virginia	Adopted
Massachusetts	Adopted	Washington	Adopted
Michigan	Adopted	West Virginia	Adopted
Minnesota	Adopted	Wisconsin	Not Adopted
Mississippi	Not Adopted	Wyoming	Not Adopted
Missouri	Not Adopted		

Adapted from www.kff.org/health-reform/state-indicator/state-activity-around-expanding-medicaid-under-the-affordable-care-act/?currentTimeframe=0&sortModel=%7B%22colId%22:%22Location%22,%22sort%22:%22asc%22%7D#note-1.

TABLE 22.3 Centers for Medicare and Medicaid Services (CMS) Equity Plan for Improving Quality in Medicare

	Priority Areas	Actions (2016 Report)
Priority 1	Expand the Collection, Reporting, and Analysis of Standardized Data	Making Medicare disparities data more accessible and easier to use. The *Mapping Medicare Disparities (MMD)* interactive tool uses Medicare fee-for-service data to show the prevalence of 18 chronic conditions, health care utilization, and costs by race, ethnicity, sex, disability, and age.
Priority 2	Evaluate Disparities' Impacts and Integrate Equity Solutions Across CMS Programs	Developed and piloted *the Disparities Action Statement (DAS)*—a tool that enables CMS and CMS stakeholders to evaluate the impact of a policy or program on health disparities. Developed a Health Equity Technical Assistance team to provide solutions through coaching for organizations working on health disparities.
Priority 3	Develop and Disseminate Promising Approaches to Reduce Health Disparities	Launched the *Building an Organizational Response to Health Disparities—Resource Guide* developed the *Guide to Preventing Readmissions among Racially and Ethnically Diverse Medicare Beneficiaries*

Continued

TABLE 22.3   Centers for Medicare and Medicaid Services (CMS) Equity Plan for Improving Quality in Medicare—cont'd

	Priority Areas	Actions (2016 Report)
Priority 4	Increase the Ability of the Health Care Workforce to Meet the Needs of Vulnerable Populations	Created a *Medicare Learning Network (MLN) training module* to raise awareness of the importance of collecting Sexual Orientation and Gender Identity data for health care providers and developed a set of standards for collecting Sexual Orientation and Gender Identity status in clinical settings.
Priority 5	Improve Communication and Language Access for Individuals with Limited English Proficiency and Persons with Disabilities	Estimated language and communication needs at national, state, and local levels. Data brief on these geographic profiles is being developed highlighting how providers can use data to determine and meet the needs of their limited English-proficient and vision- and hearing-impaired patients.
Priority 6	Increase Physical Accessibility of Health Care Facilities	Proposed a change to the Medicare Physician Fee Schedule (PFS) for Calendar Year 2017, in order to improve quality and access to care for individuals with mobility-related disabilities. The proposed rule included a new payment code to recognize the increased resource costs associated with the medically necessary use of specialized mobility-assistive technology, such as adjustable height chairs or tables, patient lifts, and adjustable padded leg supports, during an office visit.

Adapted from Centers for Medicare and Medicaid Services, Office of Minority Health. (2016). The CMS equity plan for improving quality in Medicare. Retrieved from www.cms.gov/About-CMS/Agency-Information/OMH/OMH_Dwnld-CMS_EquityPlanforMedicare_090615.pdf.

HEALTH DISPARITIES REMAIN AFTER ACA

It is undeniable that in the past 30 years, the United States has seen progress toward becoming a country with a more equitable health system. Nonetheless, many disparities affecting the health of the most vulnerable populations remain. Evidence shows that the ACA has contributed to improvements in gaps related to access and utilization, but many challenges remain. The 2016 National Healthcare Quality and Disparities Report (QDR) showed that only 20% of its 250 disparity measures saw improvement from 2014 to 2015, with Blacks and Latinos seeing gains greater than other racial and ethnic groups (AHRQ, 2017). Additionally, more than 50% of measures show that poor and low-income households have worse care than high-income households; for middle-income households, more than 40% of measures show worse care than high-income households. For insurance type, nearly 66% of measures show that uninsured people had worse care than privately insured people (AHRQ, 2017).

The ACA has focused on policies that improve quality and increase access. Quality health care is as critical as access to health care. Research has established that low-income and minority groups often receive lower quality care than their wealthier White counterparts (AHRQ, 2013). The ACA calls

for elevating quality of primary care for patients and funding the testing of models of care, such as the Patient-Centered Medical Home (PCMH). There are several provisions in the ACA directed at the establishment and promotion of the PCMH.

The PCMH has been the model of care with the most promise to improve receipt of quality care and health outcomes. PCMH membership has been associated with a lower probability of inpatient hospitalization from the emergency department (ED) among behavioral health patients (Adaji, Melin, Campbell, Lohse, Westphal, & Katzelnick, 2018), lower ED, hospital, and ambulatory care utilization, including among individuals with disabilities, chronic illnesses and veterans (Cuellar, Helmchen, Gimm, Want, Burla, Kells, & Nichols, 2016; Green, Chang, Markovitz, & Paustian, 2018; Chu, Sood, Tu, Miller, Ray, & Sayles, 2017; Hearld, Hearld, & Guerrazzi, 2017; Randall, Maynard, Chan, Devine, & Johnson, 2017; Neal, Chawla, Colombo, Snyder, & Nigam, 2015), reduction in pharmacy spending among those 65 and older (Salzberg, Bitton, Lipsitz, Franz, Shaykevich, Newmark, Kwatra, & Bates, 2017), and an increase in use of advanced practice staff (nurse practitioners [NPs] and physician assistants) (Park, Wu, Frogner, & Pittman, 2018). Although PCMH holds promise in reducing health disparities, findings from studies suggest that low-income and minority groups are less likely to have access to a PCMH (Strickland et al., 2011).

DISPARITIES IN HEALTH CARE ACCESS AND THE NEED FOR NURSES

Affording health insurance is an essential step in attempting to achieve health equity. Throughout the United States, there is still lack of access to the health care infrastructure and health care providers for primary care and wellness services. Over 58 million Americans live in areas known as Health Professional Shortage Areas (HPSAs), a number that varies greatly by state—specifically, 1.4% in Nebraska to 57.3% in Mississippi (Van Vleet & Paradise, 2015).

To address work force development in areas with limited access to primary care, ACA dedicated $1.5 billion dollars toward HRSA's National Health Service Corps (NHSC) program, which provides loan repayment and scholarships to NPs and other clinicians who commit to work in underserved areas, and has since 2010 added 1900 NPs to fill care access gaps (Erickson, 2016). Nurse-managed health clinics and federally qualified health centers (FQHCs), which serve low-income minorities and are largely staffed by NPs, were authorized $11.5 billion under ACA, placing an additional 94,000 patients under the care of NPs (Erickson, 2016). According to the American Association of Nurse Practitioners (AANP, 2018), 86.6% of NPs are certified in an area of primary care, 77.8% of all NPs deliver primary care, 84.9% of NPs are accepting Medicare patients, and 82.9% are accepting Medicaid patients. Also, the evidence consistently demonstrates that NPs deliver high-quality care (DesRoches, Clarke, Perloff, et al., 2017; Buerhaus, Perloff, Clarke, et al., 2018).

Expanding the role of registered nurses (RNs) in primary care settings provides another opportunity for enhancing access to primary care services, particularly in underserved areas. The growing shortage of the primary care workforce (Department of Health and Human Services, 2013) could potentially worsen access to primary care services in already disparate communities. Smolowitz and others (2015) outline multiple ways in which RNs can contribute to primary care services and increase access to care. The RN-provided services include medication reconciliation, health coaching, case management, and all critical services for improving chronic disease management. Support for the RN role in primary care exists in part in the shift from fee-for-service to value-based care. As part of team-based care, RN services are valuable for enhancing patient-centered care and improving health behavior, particularly for chronic disease management (Bauer &

Bodenheimer, 2017). These services are paramount in health centers serving ethnic minority and low-income patients, as they are more likely to be disproportionately affected by uncontrolled chronic diseases.

SUMMARY

This is an opportune time for NPs and nurse researchers to highlight the unique contributions of nursing to health promotion, particularly for low-income populations. Nursing expertise will be critical to implement the needed health system reforms, and our continued professional involvement with research, advocacy, community outreach, and policy will help ensure that underserved populations' health challenges are addressed. However, to successfully eliminate health disparities, a broad range of policy solutions must be developed. Nurses should continue their advocacy for eliminating scope-of-practice restrictions that prohibit nurses from practicing to the extent of their education and consequently decreasing access to care.

REFERENCES

Adaji, A., Melin, G.J., Campbell, R.L., Lohse, C.M., Westphal, J.J., & Katzelnick, D.J. (2018). Patient-centered medical home membership is associated with decreased hospital admissions for emergency department behavioral health patients. *Population health management, 21*(3), 172-179.

Agency for Healthcare Research and Quality. (2013). *2012 National healthcare disparities report.* Retrieved from www.ahrq.gov/research/findings/nhqrdr/nhdr12/2012nhdr.pdf.

Agency for Healthcare Research and Quality. (July, 2017). *2016 National healthcare quality and disparities report.* AHRQ Pub. No. 17-0001. Rockville, MD: Agency for Healthcare Research and Quality.

American Association of Nurse Practitioners. (2018). *AANP—NP fact sheet.* Retrieved from www.aanp.org/all-about-nps/np-fact-sheet.

Bauer, L., & Bodenheimer, T. (2017). Expanded roles of registered nurses in primary care delivery of the future. *Nursing Outlook, 65*(5), 624-632.

Beadle, M.R., & Graham, G.N. (2011). *National stakeholder strategy for achieving health equity.* Retrieved from https://drum.lib.umd.edu/handle/1903/23622.

Bitton, A., Martin, C., & Landon, B.E. (2010). A nationwide survey of patient centered medical home demonstration projects. *Journal of General Internal Medicine, 25*(6), 584-592.

Braveman, P.A. (2011). Monitoring equity in health and healthcare: A conceptual framework. *Journal of Health, Population, and Nutrition, 21*(3), 181-192.

Buerhaus, P., Perloff, J., Clarke, S., O'Reilly-Jacob, M., Zolotusky, G., & DesRoches, C.M. (2018). Quality of primary care provided to medicare beneficiaries by nurse practitioners and physicians. *Medical Care, 56*(6), 484-490.

Chu, L., Sood, N., Tu, M., Miller, K., Ray, L., & Sayles, J.N. (2017). Reduction of emergency department use in people with disabilities. *American Journal of Managed Care, 23*(12), e409-e415.

Centers for Medicare and Medicaid Services & Office of Minority Health. (2015). The CMS equity plan for improving quality in Medicare. Retrieved from www.cms.gov/About-CMS/Agency-Information/OMH/OMH_Dwnld-CMS_EquityPlan-forMedicare_090615.pdf.

Cuellar, A., Helmchen, L.A., Gimm, G., Want, J., Burla, S., Kells, B.J., ... & Nichols, L.M. (2016). The CareFirst patient-centered medical home program: Cost and utilization effects in its first three years. *Journal of General Internal Medicine, 31*(11), 1382-1388.

Dawson, L., Kates, J., & Damico, A. (2018). *The Affordable Care Act and insurance coverage changes by sexual orientation.* The Henry J. Kaiser Family Foundation. Retrieved from www.kff.org/disparities-policy/issue-brief/the-affordable-care-act-and-insurance-coverage-changes-by-sexual-orientation/.

DesRoches, C.M., Clarke, S., Perloff, J., O'Reilly-Jacob, M., & Buerhaus, P. (2017). The quality of primary care provided by nurse practitioners to vulnerable Medicare beneficiaries. *Nursing Outlook, 65*(6), 679-688.

Erickson, F. (2016). *The role of nurse practitioners in health care reform* [blog]. Online.nursing.georgetown.edu. Retrieved from https://online.nursing.georgetown.edu/blog/ACA-and-NPs/.

Esperat, M. C.R., Hanson-Turton, T., Richardson, M., Tyree Debisette, A., & Rupinta, C. (2012). Nurse-managed health centers: Safety-net care through advanced nursing practice. *Journal of the American Academy of Nurse Practitioners, 24*(1), 24–31.

Goldman, A.L., Woolhandler, S., Himmelstein, D.U., Bor, D.H., & McCormick, D. (2018). Out-of-pocket spending and premium contributions after implementation of the Affordable Care Act. *JAMA Internal Medicine, 178*(3), 347-355.

Green, L.A., Chang, H.C., Markovitz, A.R., & Paustian, M.L. (2018). The reduction in ED and hospital admissions in medical home practices is specific to primary care–sensitive chronic conditions. *Health Services Research,* 53(2), 1163-1179.

Griffith, K., Evans, L., & Bor, J. (2017). The Affordable Care Act reduced socioeconomic disparities in health care access. *Health Affairs, 36*(8), 1503-1510.

Hayes, S.L., Collins, S.R., Radley, D.C., & McCarthy, D. (2017). *What's at stake: States' progress on health coverage and access to care, 2013–2016.* Issue brief (Commonwealth Fund), 2017, 1-20.

Hearld, L.R., Hearld, K.R., & Guerrazzi, C. (2017). Patient-centered medical home capacity and ambulatory care utilization. *American Journal of Medical Quality, 32*(5), 508-517.

Heckler, M. (1985). *Report of the Secretary's task force on Black and minority health.* U.S. Department of Health and Human Services.

Kaiser Family Foundation (2018). *Current status of state Medicaid expansion decisions.* The Henry J. Kaiser Family Foundation. Retrieved from www.kff.org/health-reform/slide/current-status-of-the-medicaid-expansion-decision/.

Ku, L., Shin, P., Jones, E., & Bruen, B. (2011). Transforming community health centers into patient-centered medical homes: The role of payment reform. The Commonwealth Fund. Retrieved from www.commonwealthfund.org/publications/fund-reports/2011/sep/transforming-community-health-centers.

Marmot, M., Friel, S., Bell, R., Houweling, T.A., Taylor, S., & Commission on Social Determinants of Health. (2008). Closing the gap in a generation: Health equity through action on the social determinants of health. *The Lancet, 372*(9650), 1661-1669.

Neal, J., Chawla, R., Colombo, C.M., Snyder, R.L., & Nigam, S. (2015). Medical homes: Cost effects of utilization by chronically ill patients. *American Journal of Managed Care, 21*(1), e51-e61.

Nichols, M., Stein, A.D., & Wold, J.L. (2014). Health status of children of migrant farm workers: Farm worker family health program, Moultrie, Georgia. *American Journal of Public Health, 104*(2), 365-370.

Office Of Minority Health. (February 22, 2018). *Glossary of terms.* Retrieved from https://minorityhealth.hhs.gov/npa/templates/browse.aspx?lvl=1&lvlid=34.

Park, J., Wu, X., Frogner, B.K., & Pittman, P. (2018). Does the patient-centered medical home model change staffing and utilization in the community health centers? *Medical Care, 56*(9), 784-790.

Patient Protection and Affordable Care Act, 42 U.S.C. § 18001 (2010).

Randall, I., Maynard, C., Chan, G., Devine, B., & Johnson, C. (2017). Assessing the effect of the VHA PCMH model on utilization patterns among veterans with PTSD. *American Journal of Managed Care, 23*(5), 291-296.

Salzberg, C.A., Bitton, A., Lipsitz, S.R., Franz, C., Shaykevich, S., Newmark, L.P., ... & Bates, D.W. (2017). The impact of alternative payment in chronically Ill and older patients in the patient-centered medical home. *Medical Care, 55*(5), 483-492.

Shin, P., Sharac, J., Alvarez, C., & Rosenbaum, S. (2013). *Community health centers in an era of health reform: An overview and key challenges to health center growth.* Kaiser Commission on Medicaid and the Uninsured, Kaiser Family Foundation. Retrieved from kff.org/health-reform/issue-brief/community-health-centers-in-an-era-of-health-reform-overview/.

Shin, P., Sharac, J., Zur, J., Alvarez, C., & Rosenbaum, S. (2014). *Assessing the potential impact of state policies on community health centers' outreach and enrollment activities.* RCHN Community Health Foundation. Retrieved from www.rchn-foundation.org/wp-content/uploads/2014/01/GG-policy-brief-CHC-OE-FINAL-unembargoed.pdf.

Smolowitz, J., Speakman, E., Wojnar, D., Whelan, E. M., Ulrich, S., Hayes, C., & Wood, L. (2015). Role of the registered nurse in primary health care: meeting health care needs in the 21st century. *Nursing Outlook, 63*(2), 130-136.

Strickland, B.B., Jones, J.R., Ghandour, R.M., Kogan, M.D., & Newacheck, P.W. (2011). The medical home: Health care access and impact for children and youth in the United States. *Pediatrics, 127*(4), 604–611.

U.S. Department of Health and Human Services, Health Resources and Services Administration, National Center for Health Workforce Analysis. (2013). *Projecting the supply and demand for primary care practitioners through 2020.* Rockville, MD: U.S. Department of Health and Human Services.

Van Vieet, A., & Paradise, J. (2015). Tapping nurse practitioners to meet rising demand for primary care. The Henry J. Kaiser Family Foundation. Retrieved from www.kff.org/medicaid/issue-brief/tapping-nurse-practitioners-to-meet-rising-demand-for-primary-care/.

Wehby, G.L., & Lyu, W. (2018). The impact of the ACA Medicaid expansions on health insurance coverage through 2015 and coverage disparities by age, race/ethnicity, and gender. *Health Services Research*, 53(2), 1248-1271.

World Health Organization. (September 25, 2017). *Social determinants of health.* Retrieved from www.who.int/social_determinants/sdh_definition/en/.

23

TAKING ACTION: Policy Advocacy for American Indian/Alaska Native Children: School Nutrition and Indigenous Food Sovereignty

Regina S. Eddie (Dine') and Dorinda L. Welle

"I must go and do more."

Annie Dodge Wauneka (1918–1997), first woman elected to the Navajo Nation Tribal Council and lifelong activist for community health

AMERICAN INDIAN/ALASKA NATIVE HEALTH CHALLENGES

Across the nation, there are 573 federally recognized American Indian/Alaska Native (AI/AN) tribes (U.S. Department of Interior, n.d.) accounting for 2% of the U.S. population or 5.2 million people (U.S. Census Bureau, 2014). Whether living in reservation or urban communities, AI/ANs experience widespread disparities in health compared to the general population, including higher rates of heart disease, cancer, diabetes, and shorter life expectancies (Indian Health Service [IHS], 2018).

AI/AN children face alarming health disparities. Childhood obesity affects all U.S. children but is a greater concern for AI/AN children. While 17% of U.S. children aged 2 to 19 years are obese (Ogden, Carroll, Kit, & Flegal, 2014), the IHS estimates 25% of AI/AN children ages 2 to 5 and 31% of youth ages 12 to 19 are obese (IHS, 2011). Given the serious health risks associated with childhood obesity, including (adult obesity, diabetes, heart disease, asthma, and low self-esteem (Centers for Disease Control and Prevention [CDC], 2016), the need for immediate solutions is elevated (Box 23.1).

HISTORICAL INFLUENCES ON CHILDHOOD OBESITY

Childhood obesity is a complex health problem with no single cause, and is attributed to factors beyond individual genetic predisposition, behaviors, or choices (Gates, Skinner, & Gates, 2014; Ohri-Vachaspati et al., 2014). In the colonial context of AI/AN communities, childhood obesity is connected to more deeply rooted causes associated with multiple social, historical, political, and economic disparities (Mitchell, 2012). European contact and subsequent Federal policies forced AI/ANs from their sacred lands. Families were involuntarily relocated to newly established reservations or cities, children were forcibly separated from their families, homes, and food traditions, and sent to boarding schools or adoptive families hundreds of miles away (Deloria & Lytle, 1983).

A SHIFT IN NUTRITIONAL HEALTH

After forced relocations or displacement from AI/AN sacred lands, traditional subsistence activities such as farming, hunting, gathering, and herding gradually diminished or were banned by federal and state policies. This

BOX 23.1 Food Enterprise

Strategic approaches to nutrition and food policy advocacy include food enterprise, food security, food justice, and food sovereignty (Holt-Giménez, 2010). Food enterprise projects can revitalize food production, cultural practices, and economic development (Feldman, 2017). In New Mexico, where less than 1% of agricultural land "is devoted to growing fruit, nuts, and vegetables" (Feldman, 2017, p. 22), food enterprise can help fill this gap, but may place different priority on the process and sustainability of producing food versus the opportunity to sell to consumers (Cadieux & Slokum, 2015).

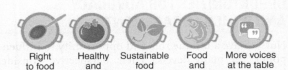

| Right to food | Healthy and sustainable | Sustainable food systems | Food and reconciliation | More voices at the table |

Five big ideas for a better food system. (Courtesy Food Secure Canada, 2017.)

BOX 23.2 Food Security

Food security promotes family and community access to adequate amounts of nutritious food for the healthy development of children and activities to sustain livelihood. Food security scholars challenge advocates to re-think "food security governance," noting that national-level governance is not always "a problem-solving mechanism" (Candel, 2014, p. 585). Rather, advocacy for food security is needed at "sub-national" levels of governance—such as city, county, state, tribal, and chapter house levels.

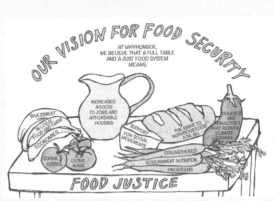

Source: *Hunger: Just the facts.* (May 20, 2015). Retrieved from https://whyhunger.org/category/uncategorised/just-the-facts/.

removed a primary supply of natural foods high in protein and low in fat, sugar, and carbohydrates, arguably a dietary pattern that protected against nutrition-related diseases (Styne, 2010). Traditional foods were replaced by processed, Western foods with minimal or no nutritional value, instead high in fat, sugar, sodium, and chemical content (Frisbie, 2018) (Box 23.2).

ROLE OF SCHOOLS IN NUTRITIONAL HEALTH OF AI/AN CHILDREN

Schools are a crucial setting for providing and modeling quality, healthy nutrition in AI/AN communities. Historically, obesity prevention studies conducted in or near reservation schools have shown school meal programs to be only partially successful in meeting recommended dietary needs for AI/AN children. The Pathways study documented baseline high fat content of school meals: children drinking high fat whole milk, not consuming recommended intake of fruits or vegetables, and having second servings of meals (Synder et al., 1999). These earlier findings are consistent with national studies identifying widespread availability of low-quality foods and beverages laden with fat, sugar, and calories in schools (Burghardt, Devaney, & Gordon, 1995; Fox, Crepinsek, Connor, & Battaglia, 2001). Several studies have called for continued improvement (Fox & Condon, 2012; Turner, Chaloupka, & Sandoval, 2012) (Box 23.3).

BOX 23.3 Food Justice

Food justice addresses structural aspects of inequality by: "(1) confronting historical, collective social trauma and persistent race, gender, and class inequalities; (2) designing exchange mechanisms that build communal reliance and control; (3) creating innovative ways to control, use, share, own, manage, and conceive of land...that place them outside the speculative market and the rationale of extraction; and (4) pursuing labor relations that guarantee a minimum income and are neither alienating nor dependent on (unpaid) social reproduction by women" (Cadieux & Slokum, 2015, p. 13).

In the United States, which has no city or state agencies specifically tasked to address food, Food Policy Councils involve stakeholders representing five sectors of the food system: production, consumption, processing, distribution, and waste recycling (Harper et al., 2009). See the many Food Policy Council Achievements at their website: Foodpolicynetworks.org.

MY ROLE IN ADVOCACY FOR SCHOOL NUTRITION

Advocacy can take many forms and occur in a myriad of ways. As a Dine' (Navajo) nurse, this begins with my own commitment to Dine' traditional perspective, embracing my cultural identity and roots, and weaving these into my nursing practice. I also bring a profound understanding of many issues and disparities that affect my own Dine' communities. The poor quality of food sources and limited access to healthy, affordable foods in many AI/AN communities is alarming. The term "food desert" accurately characterizes conditions on rural, isolated reservations devoid of large supermarket chains or other sources of healthy food (Walker, Keane, & Burke, 2010). Instead, many communities have only gas stations or convenience stores offering inexpensive, energy-dense, empty-calorie foods. Food deserts are further complicated by poor economic conditions where job opportunities are scant. Many AI/AN households struggle for economic and social survival because of lower education and income levels and higher unemployment rates (Office of Minority Health, n.d.).

The challenges in addressing AI/AN children's nutritional health have served as a tremendous inspiration to my nursing work and pursuit of graduate education. A Navajo elder once asked me, "If you don't do this work, who else is going to do it?" Through a PhD nursing program with a health policy concentration, I was introduced to new and unfamiliar roles for nurses, engaging as health policy leaders, researchers, and advocates. For a health policy field placement course, my role was to assess the impact of a state bill on AI/AN children's health and nutrition and provide recommendations to tribal communities.

I completed my dissertation research in the Navajo Nation that examined school nutrition policies and practices. Every step of the dissertation journey offered chances to take action in my communities. I engaged in policy research and analysis to understand relevant tribal, state, and federal policies pertinent to school health, nutrition, and wellness. It was also important to understand how the state administered the federal National School Lunch Program (NSLP) to school entities on the Navajo Nation and the role of tribal policy in child health and nutrition in schools.

My engagement with communities to gain access for conducting research was a process of educating school officials, school board members, and local community officials about the concerns with the school food environment and the need to use research to understand in greater depth how schools were contributing to the health of Navajo children. I heard many concerns and comments that supported the project, suggestions for ways to improve the school food environment, and expressions of appreciation for my presence and intention to take action. These interactions validated and strengthened my commitment to bring a unique nursing and cultural perspective to the research process.

OPPORTUNITIES FOR ADVOCACY AND POLICY ENGAGEMENT

Nurses have a unique role and opportunity to influence policy on many levels. Their perspective considers health and wellness for patients, families, and communities in a holistic way, which better equips them to address and shape policy issues. Advocacy and activism can span a wide range of activities, including research and scholarship, community dissemination, promotion of indigenous rights on the global stage, and advocating for specific policy change by tribal, federal, state, county, and local governments and school boards (Box 23.4).

Nurses can engage with organizations and grassroots projects to revitalize local food systems, including clinic-based and school-based projects. School nurses can leverage the support of state-wide nursing organizations and state and local organizations of AI/AN nurses to advocate for policy reform. Research studies are needed to document how indigenous communities pursue policy change and food sovereignty through reviving "country food traditions, individual and community gardens, agriculture, [and] better quality imported foods" (Rudolph & McLachlan, 2013, p. 1079). Culture-centered schools, classrooms, and families and communities that teach traditional philosophy and immerse students in indigenous approaches to living can enable AI/AN students to experience the deep nourishment that is their right and their heritage. Such efforts develop policy knowledge "from the ground up" (Dumas & Anderson, 2014, p. 1), using indigenous knowledge as a guide to address the food crisis and develop sustainable food systems.

BOX 23.4   Indigenous Food Sovereignty

La Vía Campesina, an organization of "peasants, small-scale farmers, farm workers, and indigenous communities," introduced food sovereignty in 1993, advocating for "the right of nations and peoples to control their own food systems, including their own markets, production modes, food cultures and environments" (Wittman, Desmarais, & Wiebe, 2014, p. 2). Internationally, indigenous activists have promoted efforts to protect or restore land, water quality, and water rights, increasing access to healthy food through policies that honor indigenous communities' traditional knowledge and self-governance (Working Group on Indigenous Food Sovereignty, n.d.).

Indigenous food sovereignty may bring educational and school nutrition goals into a comprehensive approach. Culture-centered curricula and resources, such as Frisbie's (2018) *Food Sovereignty the Navajo Way: Cooking with Tall Woman*, can instill indigenous perspectives on land, food systems, traditional foods, and food as medicine.

The STAR (Service To All Relations) School in Arizona represents indigenous food sovereignty at work. The first "off-the-grid" solar and wind-powered charter school in the United States, STAR School considers its Farm to School project as integral to "place-based" education, treating "the natural environment, the people, and the culture of the area in which students' families live" as students' educational context (Newell, 2013).

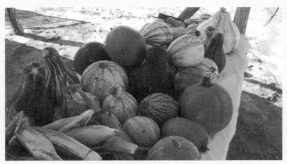

Image courtesy of Leupp Family Farms and the STAR School.

DISCUSSION QUESTIONS

1. What food policy opportunities exist in your communities to advance children's nutritional health?
2. What federal, state, and local policies have negatively or positively impacted the food system in your region?

REFERENCES

Burghardt, J., Devaney, B., & Gordon, A. (1995). The school nutrition dietary assessment study: Summary and discussion. *American Journal of Clinical Nutrition, 61*(1), 252S-257S.

Cadieux, K.V., & Slokum, R. (2015). What does it mean to *do* food justice? *Journal of Political Ecology, 22*, 1-26.

Candel, J.J.L. (2014). Food security governance: a systematic literature review. *Food Security, 6*(4), 585-601.

Centers for Disease Control and Prevention. (2016). *Overweight and obesity*. Retrieved from www.cdc.gov/obesity/childhood/causes.html.

Deloria, V., & Lytle, C. (1983). *American Indians, American justice*. Austin, TX: University of Texas Press.

Dumas, M.J., & Anderson, G. (2014). Qualitative research as policy knowledge: Framing policy problems and transforming education from the ground up. *Education Policy Analysis Archives, 22*(11), 1-24.

Feldman, D. (2017). *Another way forward: Grassroots solutions from New Mexico*. Albuquerque, NM: Dede Feldman Company.

Food Secure Canada. (2017). *Five big ideas for a better food system: A proposal from Food Secure Canada on national food policy*. Retrieved from https://foodsecurecanada.org/five-big-ideas.

FoodPolicyNetworks.org. (2016). *Food policy council achievements*. Retrieved from http://222.foodpolicynetworks.org/directory/online.

Fox, M., & Condon, E. (2012). *USDA food and nutrition service: School nutrition dietary assessment study–IV: Summary of findings*. Retrieved from www.fns.usda.gov/sites/default/files/SNDA-IV_Findings_0.pdf.

Fox, M., Crepinsek, M., Connor, P., & Battaglia, M. (2001). *School nutrition dietary assessment study–II: Summary of findings*. Retrieved from https://fns-prod.azureedge.net/sites/default/files/SNDAIIfind.pdf.

Frisbie, C. (2018). *Food sovereignty the Navajo way: Cooking with Tall Woman*. University of New Mexico Press: Albuquerque, NM.

Gates, A., Skinner, K., & Gates, M. (2014). The diets of school-aged Aboriginal youths in Canada: A systematic review of the literature. *Journal of Human Nutrition and Dietetics, 28*, 246-261.

Harper, A., Shattuck, A., Holt- Giménez, E., Alkon, A., & Lambrick, F. (2009). *Food policy councils: Lessons learned*. Washington, DC: Institute for Food and Development Policy.

Holt-Giménez, E. (2010). Food security, food justice, or food sovereignty? *Food First Backgrounder, 16*(4): 1-4.

Indian Health Service. (2011). *Healthy weight for life: A vision for health weight across the lifespan of American Indians and Alaska Native*. Retrieved from www.ihs.gov/healthyweight/includes/themes/newihstheme/display_objects/documents/HW4L_TeamsLeaders.pdf.

Indian Health Service. (2018). *Disparities*. Retrieved from www.ihs.gov/newsroom/factsheets/disparities/.

Mitchell, F. (2012). Reframing diabetes in American Indian communities: A social determinants of health perspective. *Health & Social Work, 37*(2), 71-90.

National Congress for American Indians (2017). *Fiscal year 2017 Indian Country budget request.* Retrieved from www.ncai.org/resources/ncai-publications/08_FY2017_health_care.pdf.

Newell, S. (2013). *Healthy foods for Navajo schools: Discoveries from the first year of a Navajo farm to school program.* Flagstaff, AZ: Native American Development Associates.

Office of Minority Health. (n.d.). *Profile: American Indian/Alaska Native.* Retrieved from https://minorityhealth.hhs.gov/omh/browse.aspx?lvl=3&lvlid=62.

Ogden, C., Carroll, M., Kit, B., & Flegal, K. (2014). Prevalence of childhood and adult obesity in the United States, 2011-2012. *JAMA, 311*(8), 806-814.

Ohri-Vachaspati, P., DeLia, D., DeWeese, R., Crespo, N., Todd, M., & Yedida, M. (2014). The relative contribution of layers of the social ecological model to childhood obesity. *Public Health Nutrition, 11*, 1-12.

Rudolph, K.R. & McLachlan, S.M. (2013). Seeking Indigenous food sovereignty: Origins of and responses to the food crisis in northern Manitoba, Canada. *Local Environment: The International Journal of Justice and Sustainability, 18*(9), 1079-1098.

Styne, D. (2010). Childhood obesity in American Indians. *Journal of Public Health Management & Practice, 16*(5), 381-387.

Synder, P., Anliker, J., Cunninham-Sabo, L., Dixon, L., Altaha, J., Chamberlain, A., … & Weber, J. (1999). The Pathways study: A model for lowering the fat in school meals. *American Journal of Clinical Nutrition, 69*(4), 810S-815S.

Turner, L., Chaloupka, F., & Sandoval, A. (2012). *School policies and practices for improving children's health: National elementary school survey results: School years 2006-07 through 2009-10* (vol. 2). Retrieved from www.bridgingthegapresearch.org/_asset/3t94yf/ES_2012_execsumm.pdf.

U.S. Census Bureau. (2014). *Facts for features: American Indian and Alaska Native Heritage: November 2015.* Retrieved from www.census.gov/newsroom/facts-for-features/2015/cb15-ff22.html.

U.S. Department of Interior Indian Affairs. (n.d.). *About us.* Retrieved from www.bia.gov/about-us.

Walker, R., Keane, C., & Burke, J. (2010). Disparities and access to healthy food in the United States: A review of food deserts literature. *Health & Place, 16*(5), 876-884.

Whittman, H., Desmarais, A., & Wiebe, N. (Eds.) (2014). *Food sovereignty: Reconnecting food, nature and community.* Oakland, CA: Food First Books.

Whyhunger.org. (May 20, 2015). *Hunger: Just the facts.* Retrieved from https://whyhunger.org/category/uncategorised/just-the-facts/

Working Group on Indigenous Food Sovereignty. (n.d.). *Indigenous food sovereignty.* Retrieved from www.indigenousfoodsystems.org/food-sovereignty.

ONLINE RESOURCES

National Congress of American Indians: Consultation with USDA to Address School Lunch Funding for Tribal Schools
www.ncai.org/resources/resolutions/consultation-with-usda-to-address-school-lunch-program-funding-for-tribal-schools
Native American Food Sovereignty Alliance
https://nativefoodalliance.org

24

TAKING ACTION: Addressing the Health Needs of Immigrant/Migrant Farmworkers

Maria Elena Ruiz

> *"It's ironic that those who till the soil, cultivate and harvest the fruits, vegetables, and other foods that fill your tables with abundance have nothing left for themselves."*
>
> Cesar Chavez

Over 55 million Americans (20%), many of lower socioeconomic status, are living in rural areas with limited access to health care and at greater risk for poor health (Institute of Medicine, 2005). These include almost 4 million farmworkers who harvest our crops and contribute to our bountiful food supply, yet they are at greater risk for poverty and occupational dangers with little to no access for nutritional, housing, health, and basic environmental safety.

HISTORICAL CONTEXT OF MIGRATION: FARMWORKERS

Despite recent media attention, the migration of foreign-born workers to the United States is not a new phenomenon. Instead, the in-migration of migrant workers to the United States has occurred over many decades with peaks and flows dependent on economic and sociopolitical factors from the sending (primarily Mexico) and receiving country (United States). However, not all Mexican-origin workers have had to cross borders "sin papeles" (without documentation). For many older generations, no legal documents were required, as U.S. boundaries encroached south into Mexican territory several times. As the U.S. border shifted south, families living in the annexed territory became U.S. residents, while others left in the constricted Mexican regions remained Mexican citizens. This pattern divided some families between two countries; some became U.S. citizens, while others had to request permits in order to visit relatives in "el norte" (the United States).

At other times, some Mexican residents were invited to migrate north when young male workers were recruited to support the U.S. economy. During the first wave of 1910 to 1921, as the United States entered World War I, over 700,000 Mexican workers were brought into the United States as agricultural workers (National Farm Worker Ministry, n.d). These workers were systematically excluded from receiving labor benefits, including the right to unionize, receive overtime pay, worker protection, and other benefits. This exclusionary pattern of selective labor restriction set the stage for the exploitation of farmworkers and ill will that persists among some generations.

As a result, many generations of Mexican workers in the United States and Mexico have a long history with the guest worker and Bracero Program of the 1940s, with conflicting views on whether the programs offered positive opportunities or exploited immigrant workers. For older generations, such programs "had a jaded history with regard to worker treatment and implications for their health status, but on the other hand, afforded them the opportunity for U.S. citizenship" (Ruiz, Phillips, Kim & Woods, 2016, p. 11).

THE BRACERO PROGRAM (1942–1964)

During World War II, the United States initiated a binational Farm Labor Agreement with Mexico (Bracero Program), formally enticing thousands of men with promises of visas and agricultural jobs. Drawn by the prospects for work and residency, thousands of Mexican nationals crossed into the United States, leading to massive exploitation and abuse by agricultural owners and immigration and law enforcement officials. By 1954, the Operation Wetback (anti-Mexican), backed by agricultural growers, businesses, and the U.S. Border Patrol, gained prominence. This led to thousands to millions of arrests, including deportation of some U.S. citizens (Blakemore, 2018). By 1964, when the Bracero Program ended, over 4.5 million agricultural workers had arrived in the United States. Multiple factors led to the demise of the program, including the anti-immigrant climate, complaints of human rights abuses, poor housing and work conditions, unpaid salaries, and high fees for unsanitary housing and food (UNCO.edu, n.d).

THE RISE OF THE UNITED FARMWORKERS UNION

During the Bracero Program, Cesar Chavez and Dolores Huerta advocated for reforms and joined Filipinos in their organizing efforts, founding the National Farm Workers Association, later changed to the United Farm Workers (UFW) of California. Supported by faith organizations, college students, and key politicians (including Senator Robert Kennedy), the UFW went on to become not only a California-based powerful force for farmworkers, but also a national cause for Latino immigrants. Fueled by the civil rights era of the 1960s and the "La Causa" movement of the UFW, it became a major driving force, advocating for class, economic, gender, indigenous and migrant social justice issues.

Chavez is also recognized for various accomplishments that improved the living and working conditions for farmworkers, including demands for basic human rights such as housing, potable water and toilets in the fields, rest periods, and higher salaries for men as well as for the growing number of women and children who toiled in the fields along with their parents. An experienced farmworker, Chavez also brought attention to the backbreaking trauma inflicted by the bending movement associated with the short-handle hoe. Through his sociopolitical efforts, the short hoe was declared unsafe in 1975, a major landmark for fieldworkers. Chavez' charismatic non-violent approach and ability to link faith, civil rights, and social justice contributed to his status as a civil rights icon. Later, Dolores Huerta gained recognition as co-founder of the UFW.

Today, agricultural workers continue to be imported under an expanded temporary guest worker program, with over 200,000 workers approved last year alone (Gutierrez, Wallace, & Castañeda, 2004).

MIGRANT FARMWORKERS: DEMOGRAPHIC PROFILE

Unlike earlier generations of Latinos who tended to migrate to well-established communities supportive by large ethnic enclaves, newer subgroups are diversifying non-traditional states and migrating to regions throughout the United States, including the Midwest and the northeastern coast. Most farmworkers are from Mexico (76%) and are Spanish-speaking males (70%), with increasing numbers of indigenous workers with unique cultural, language, social, and diverse health needs (Association of Farmworker Programs 2017). Despite some prevailing stereotypes, 27% of farmworkers are U.S. born, up to one-third are U.S. citizens, and over half (59%) have lived in the United States over 10 years (National Center for Farmworker Health [NCFH], 2014). Average individual incomes range from $15,000 to $19,000 annually, with family income ranging from $17,000 to almost $20,000. Overall, the majority are subsisting at high poverty levels, with limited access to food, housing, and health care, with a life expectancy of 49, or 30 to 40 years below the national average (Hansen & Donohoe, 2003).

MIGRANT FARMWORKERS: OCCUPATIONAL HEALTH

Despite the accomplishments of the UFW, the conditions under which farmworkers live and work continue to be a major source of shame in this country. Over 30 years ago, the landmark report *The Occupational Health Risks of Migrant and Seasonal Farmworkers* (Farmworker Justice Fund, 1986) documented the health risks and paucity of research on the health of farmworkers. The report not only noted the multiple health risks of agricultural workers; including skin, eye, respiratory and musculoskeletal conditions, gastrointestinal and renal problems, and infectious disorders, but also traumatic equipment-related injuries. The report highlighted the third-world living conditions that farmworkers toil under in a first-world country as the United States. Violations included the lack of sanitation facilities and potable water, pesticide exposures, equipment hazards, crowded unsanitary housing conditions often without indoor plumbing, child labor abuses, plus other environmental and access barriers that exacerbated chronic conditions made worse by the inhumane housing and work conditions and lack of health access.

Cesar Chaves, Dolores Huerta, and the UFW may have brought attention to the plight of immigrant farmworkers as early as the 1960s. Over 50 years later, research continues to document the numerous health risks and abuses faced by the largely invisible and impoverished farmworkers.

EPIDEMIOLOGICAL STUDIES: UPDATE

Agricultural work is one of the most dangerous occupations in the United States, yet gaps in research persist, as limited attention has been given to the association between rural living, farmworking, and migration. For limited English-speaking migrant workers, the occupational risks are even higher, due to the nature of seasonal work, language and cultural differences, inadequate training, and protective equipment as well as lack of protective measures (Ramos, Fuentes, & Trinidad, 2016). Even when eligible for governmental support, workers may not report unsafe working conditions or may postpone health care due to fear or threats of deportation (Perez-Escamilla, Garcia, & Song, 2010).

Despite the comprehensive landmark report published in 1986, updated epidemiological studies continue to document the long-term health risks by not only individuals who toil in the fields, but also their families and surrounding communities. Newer research also documents the long-term damage related to pesticide exposure, including reproductive organ damage to women, as well as congenital birth disorders in children and various types of cancers (McCauley et al., 2006). Migrant Health Centers also report a greater need for family-focused care for women and children, along with greater needs for dental care, hearing, and vision care due to equipment noise and traumatic injuries (NCFH, 2014).

Emerging issues also call attention to rising mental health needs due to stress and loss of family and social support networks, as well as sexual harassment and violence against women in the fields (Galvez, Mankowski, McGlade, Ruiz, & Glass, 2011).

A CALL FOR SOCIAL JUSTICE AND SOCIAL DETERMINANTS OF HEALTH APPROACH

Farmworkers have been economically exploited and politically excluded from basic human rights protection and public services. The gaps in research call for an integrative approach that encompasses not only a rural versus urban examination of disparities, but for a social justice approach that incorporates race/ethnicity, migration, and culture.

Medical care alone cannot close the inequality gap or improve the living and sociopolitical environment that farmworkers toil under (Castaneda et al., 2014). Instead of relying on a downstream systematic approach where we seem to be applying temporary band aids to major ills and superficial fixes, nurses and other health providers may find an upstream approach more effective for attacking the roots of the problem in order to address the racism, inequities, and the multiple social factors confronting farmworking communities (Braverman, Egerter, & Williams, 2011). Nurses are the foremost trusted health workforce in the nation; the public depends on nurses to advocate and bring about public policy changes.

TAKING ACTION: HEALTH CARE IN THE FIELDS

Almost 15 years ago, I volunteered with a mobile van program, providing health care to agricultural workers in the fields. Through an arrangement with agricultural owners, the van would roll into the beautiful fields where crop workers were tilling the crops, and we would park off to the side, away from the public's view. I always wondered why we needed to park a distance away from the entrance to the buildings. Were the health workers, like the field workers, to remain invisible?

At first, I was impressed with the beauty of the fields, and the support from the growers that welcomed our health services. I quickly began to question if the farmworkers were using their breaks or lunchtimes or perhaps losing invaluable time allotted for picking crops, thus losing some of their salary.

An eye-opening experience arose when I requested to use the bathroom and I was directed to the "honey buckets" (portable toilets). A fieldworker suggested I might not want to visit these. At some sites, the portable toilets were nearby; at others, they were a good distance away from our view. Some had soap and water, many were malodorous. Some health staff used these "facilities" (same ones used by the field workers). A few times, the growers (company owners) would invite us to use the indoor, clean facilities inside the building (facilities provided for the business company staff).

As I spent more time in the fields, my sorrowful and ethical concern rose as I witnessed the separate and unequal facilities for the migrant workers: no visible drinking water, limited breaks, no visible shade nor sitting areas for the workers who toil, 6 to 7 days per week for minimum pay. Some colleagues expressed that these were great improvements from what was previously available. I thank the health staff for their passion and patience, but these continue to be inhumane third-world conditions in a first-world country.

I first became involved with the UFW and "La Causa" in California as a teenager, drawn by the civil rights movement many years ago, collecting supplies while caravanning Delano in central California. Viewed through my lenses, not much has changed in more than 40 years. Some colleagues may see these improvements as the glass half full and rising. I see the glass as half empty and in urgent need of repair.

As an immigrant, Latina, university professor, Advanced Practice Nurse, researcher, and social justice leader and advocate, I would hope nurses and all health workers would dig deeper for a more just society and advocate for more than a Band-aid approach in our system of health care.

DISCUSSION QUESTIONS

1. Discuss a downstream approach that nurses may rely on to decrease pesticide-related health risks. What upstream approach may be more constructive?
2. Some individuals may express concern that immigrants are taking jobs away from American citizens. Provide an example of one occupation where this has occurred.
3. List a local or national labor and health care policy that nurses can develop to improve the health of farmworker rural communities?

REFERENCES

Association of Farm Worker Programs. (2017). *Where are they now: Migrant farm workers*. Retrieved from https://afophs.wordpress.com/2017/01/24/where-are-they-now-migrant-farm-workers.

Blakemore, E. (2018). The largest mass deportation in American history. Retrieved from www.history.com/news/operation-wetback-eisenhower-1954-deportation.

Braverman, P., Egerter, S., & Williams, D.R. (2011). The social determinants of health: Coming of age. *Annual Review of Public Health, 32,* 381-98.

Castaneda, H., Holmes, S.M., Madrigal, D.S., de Trinidad Young, M., Beyler, N., & Quesada, J. (2015). Immigration as a social determinant of health. *Annual Review of Public Health, 36,* 375-92.

Farmworker Justice Fund. (1986). *The occupational health risks of migrant and seasonal farmworkers*. Washington, DC: National Rural Health Association.

Galvez, G., Mankowski, E.S., McGlade, M., Ruiz, M.E., & Glass, N. (2011). Work-related intimate partner violence among immigrants from Mexico. *Psychology of Men & Masculinity, 12*(3), 230-246.

Gutiérrez, V.F., Wallace, S.P., & Castañeda, X. (2004). Demographic profile of Mexican immigrants in the United States. *Health Policy Fact Sheet*. Retrieved from www.researchgate.net/publication/242491308_Demographic_Profile_of_Mexican_Immigrants_in_the_United_States.

Hansen, E, & Donohoe, M. (2003). Health issues of migrant and seasonal farmworkers, *Journal of Health Care for the Poor and Underserved, 14*(2), 153-163.

Institute of Medicine (2005). *Quality though collaboration: The future of rural health*. National Academies Press. Washington DC.

McCauley, L., Anger, W., Keifer, M., Langley, R., Robson, M., & Rohlman, D. (2006). Studying health outcomes in farmworker populations exposed to pesticides. *Environmental Health Perspectives, 114*(6), 953-960.

National Center for Farmworker Health. (2014). *A profile of migrant health: An analysis of the uniform data system 2010*. Retrieved from www.NCFH.org?fact-sheets–research.html.

Perez-Escamilla, R., Garcia, J., & Song, D. (2010). Health care access among Hispanic immigrants: ¿Alguien esta escuchando? *American Anthropological Association, 34*(1), 47-67.

Ramos, A., Fuentes, A., & Trinidad, N. ((2016). Perception of job-related risk, training, and use of personal protective equipment among Latino immigrant hoc CAFO workers in Missouri. *Safety, 2*(25), 3-11.

Ruiz, M., Phillips, L, Kim, H., & Woods, D. (2016). Older Latinos: Applying the ethnocultural gerontological nursing model. *Journal of Transcultural Nursing, 27*(1), 8-17.

UNCO.edu. (n.d.). The Bracero Program. Retrieved from www.unco.edu/colorado-oral-history-migratory-labor-project/pdf/Bracero_Program_PowerPoint.pdf.

25

The Unfulfilled Promise of Mental Health and Addiction Parity

Freida H. Outlaw, Jake Coffey, Sita M. Diehl, and Patricia K. Bradley

"We are concerned about the constant use of federal funds to support this most notorious expression of segregation. Of all the forms of inequality, injustice in health is the most shocking and the most inhuman because it often results in physical death…I see no alternative to direct action and creative nonviolence to raise the conscience of the nation."

Dr. Martin Luther King, Jr., at the Second National Convention of the Medical Community for Human Rights, Chicago, March 25, 1966

"The Mental Health Parity and Addiction Equity Act of 2008, which required insurers to provide mental health services that were on par with physical health services, and the Affordable Care Act, which built on the Parity Act, laid some critical groundwork. However, mental health care is still separate and unequal due to unchecked practices occurring in payment and reimbursement. The only way we're going to change this is by requiring health insurance companies to be more transparent so that they can be held accountable under federal law. [As advocates we need to] find our voice. That means turning your thoughts and feelings into action."

Patrick Joseph Kennedy II, at the College of Charleston, October 11, 2017

Throughout decades of struggle for U.S. health reform, demands for the recognition and protection of mental health have encountered many challenges, disappointments, and victories. Health insurance, as it is generally understood today, began post-World War II. Since its inception, coverage of mental health services has been more limited and restrictive than other types of medical care (Peterson & Busch, 2018; Rochefort, 1989). Deinstitutionalization, and the attendant reduction of federal and state funding for community mental health centers, led to greater reliance on private insurance strategies. In the ensuing years, although there was a marked increase in the proportion of insurance plans with mental health and substance abuse benefits, limitations and restrictions on that coverage became more stringent (Barry, 2006; Barry, Goldman, & Huskamp, 2016; Peterson & Busch, 2018).

Over the past 20 years, federal parity legislation, culminating in the passage of The Paul Wellstone and Pete Domenici Mental Health Parity and Addiction Equity Act of 2008 (MHPAEA), has contributed to improvements in disparities between behavioral health (mental health and substance use conditions) and medical health insurance benefits. While evidence suggests that the MHPAEA has contributed to improvements in financial protections for people with behavioral health conditions, increased the utilization of services, and reduced quantitative treatment limits (QTLs) (e.g., number of covered treatment visits or inpatient days) (Busch et al., 2013; Grazier, Eisenberg, Jedele, & Smiley, 2015; Horgan et al., 2015; Thalmayer, Friedman, Azocar, Harwood, & Ettner, 2016), a number of national studies have documented significant violations and noncompliance with federal parity law, meaning that individuals with mental illness and addictive disorders continue to be routinely denied the care to which they are entitled (Bendat, 2014; Dixon, 2009; Frank, 2017; Heller, 2016; Melek, Perlman, & Davenport, 2017; National Alliance on Mental Illness [NAMI], 2017).

Behavioral health conditions are extremely common, with millions of Americans affected every year. Approximately 1 in 5 adults in the United States experiences mental illness in a given year (Substance Abuse and Mental Health Services Administration [SAMHSA] Center for Behavioral Health Statistics and Quality, 2017), and approximately 1 in 25 or 9.8 million adults experience a serious mental illness that substantially interferes with or limits one or more major life activities. Additionally, among the 20.2 million adults with a substance use disorder, over half had a co-occurring mental illness (SAMHSA, 2017). Discriminatory health insurance practices that lead to barriers in care place insurance beneficiaries at greater risk of unemployment and homelessness, and people may turn to substance abuse to self-medicate, which makes their symptoms worse. Risk of suicide and incarceration are exacerbated by lack of access to care. Marginalized populations with poor access to mental health services are made more vulnerable when those services are denied. The social costs of lack of or underinsurance are well documented (Institute of Medicine, 2003).

This chapter describes the recent history of behavioral health advocacy and the adoption of a national parity-focused legislative strategy to address discriminatory mental health substance abuse insurance practices, detailing legislative milestones, beginning with the Mental Health Parity Act (MHPA) of 1996, moving through the far more comprehensive MHPAEA of 2008, the expansion and strengthening of parity protections under the Patient Protection and Affordable Care Act (or ACA) of 2010, and the Mental Health Parity provisions contained within the 21st Century Cures Act of 2016. The chapter describes the gaps in mental health and substance abuse coverage and the ongoing challenges of implementing and enforcing parity laws at both state and national levels. Recommendations are offered for all nurses with specific attention to Advanced Practice Psychiatric Nurses.

In 1966, Martin Luther King Jr. joined with the Medical Committee for Human Rights in opposing the persistent denial of care and substandard treatment faced by African Americans in Southern and Northern hospitals, in violation of the Civil Rights Act of 1964 and the recently passed 1965 Medicaid and Medicare legislation (Galarneau, 2018). Theoretically, the passage of federal and state parity laws would have brought an end to a system in which it is legal for health insurers to limit coverage for mental health and substance abuse conditions and to require patients to pay more out-of-pocket costs than are required for other

medical conditions. The reality, however, is that today—just as was the case with racially segregated hospitals in 1966—passing laws is one thing and enforcing them quite another. Absent the full implementation and enforcement of parity law, discriminatory health insurance coverage will continue to place a disproportionate financial burden on people with mental health and substance use disorders and lead to barriers to accessing care.

FEDERAL LEGISLATIVE MILESTONES TOWARD ACHIEVING BEHAVIORAL HEALTH PARITY

Mental Health Parity Act (1996)

Although the first national attempt to regulate mental health parity in private insurance plans began in 1963 when President John F. Kennedy directed the Civil Service Commission to offer equal insurance coverage for mental health, federal legislation was not introduced until 1992 by Senators Pete Domenici (R-NM) and John Danforth (R-MO) (Barry, 2006; Barry, Huskamp, & Goldman, 2010; Peterson & Busch, 2018). During the debates over national health reform (1993–1994), the issue of mental health and substance use disorder parity again gained some national attention. Although national health reform failed, the push for parity contained within it led to the passage of the MHPA of 1996, which went into effect in 1998. Co-sponsored by Senators Domenici (R-NM) and Paul Wellstone (D-MN), the bill represented a compromise approach to parity that even at that time was recognized as largely symbolic rather than substantive. Although the MHPA did not require full parity, it took the initial steps of removing annual or lifetime dollar limits on mental health care that were more restrictive than those required for other types of medical care. However, it did not require insurers to provide mental health services as part of their plans and it did not apply to other benefit-design features such as higher cost sharing or annual limits on inpatient days or outpatient visits. Small companies (<50 employees) were exempt from the law, and employers could also apply for exemptions if compliance led to cost increases. Furthermore, MHPA standards did not apply to the individual (nongroup) health insurance market and did not cover substance use disorder treatment services (Barry, 2006; Barry et al., 2010).

Mental Health Parity and Addiction Equity Act (2008)

Twelve years later, the passage of The Paul Wellstone and Pete Domenici MHPAEA of 2008 significantly expanded upon the MHPA. The MHPAEA required that all standards limiting the type or duration of benefits involving a number of visits, days, or costs for mental health or substance use disorders be comparable with those applied to other types of medical care in employment-based plans (Barry et al., 2016; Frank, 2017). These types of limits are called QTLs. In the final rules and regulations that came out of the MHPAEA, parity requirements were also extended to non-quantitative treatment limits (NQTLs), those non-numerical limits on the scope or duration of treatment or management techniques that may be used to curb the use of behavioral health treatments. The MHPAEA required the processes by which these standards are determined for mental health and substance use disorders be comparable and no more restrictive than processes used to determine medical care management. Examples of NQTLs include provisions related to management techniques used to affect treatment patterns, such as utilization review, standards for provider admission to plan networks, and prior authorization and step therapy strategies. The MHPAEA's final rules also provided six classifications by which plans could determine if benefits were equivalent to medical/surgical care: in-network inpatient, out-of-network inpatient, in-network outpatient, out-of-network outpatient, emergency care, and prescription drugs (see Box 25.1 for a summary of federal parity law protections).

Patient Protection and Affordable Care Act (2010)

Congress enacted the ACA in 2010, representing perhaps the most significant health care bill passed in U.S. history. The law extended the impact of parity in several important ways. This law set consumer protection standards. For example, under this law, health plans could no longer reject applicants or charge more for having a long-term or pre-existing health condition such as mental illness. The law also barred health plans from having lifetime or annual limits for addiction treatment or mental health care. The ACA allowed states to expand Medicaid to cover low-income Americans (at or below 138% of the federal poverty level), who tend to have a higher concentration of mental health and substance use disorders (Beronio, Po, Skopec, & Gilead, 2013; Frank, Beronio, & Glied, 2014; Noonan & Boraske, 2015). Since its passage, over half of the states have expanded Medicaid, representing an additional 15 million new enrollees who could potentially have access to needed behavioral health services (Kaiser Family Foundation [KFF], 2017). This law extended parity requirements to all individual and small group health plans, whether they are sold through the health insurance exchange or not. It also required parity in private health

---

BOX 25.1   Parity Protections

Types of Care
- Hospital or residential treatment
- Outpatient visits
- Emergency or crisis care
- Prescription drugs
- Both in-network and out-of-network

Out-of-Pocket Costs
Costs for mental health or addiction treatment must not be greater than costs for most other medical care
- Co-pays: Flat fee per visit or service
- Co-insurance: Percentage of total service cost
- Maximum out-of-pocket costs: What you pay before the plan pays 100%
- Deductibles: What you pay before the plan begins to pay
- Annual or lifetime dollar limits: The most a plan will pay in a year or lifetime

Treatment Limits
The number of visits or days for mental health or addiction treatment must be no less than limits for most other medical care
- Number of outpatient visits
- Number of days in hospital or residential care
- Limits on prescription medications
- Excluded types of treatment or situations

Other Limits
Other types of limits must not be more restrictive for mental health or addiction treatment than for other types of medical care
- Prescription drug costs or requirements
- Prior-approval requirements
- Clinical standards used to approve or deny care
- + Availability of providers

Source: National Alliance on Mental Illness. Retrieved from www.nami.org/Find-Support/Living-with-a-Mental-Health-Condition/Understanding-Health-Insurance/What-is-Mental-Health-Parity.

---

plans used in Medicaid expansion and the Children's Health Insurance Program (CHIP). The ACA set up health insurance exchanges in every state to offer health plans that meet quality standards. The law provided for tax credits in advance to make the plans affordable. The ACA also required all individual and small group plans to cover ten categories of Essential Health Benefits (EHB), of which behavioral health is one. Benefits in all EHB categories must meet MHPAEA standards, not only within the behavioral health category, but also in other categories such as emergency care (Beronio et al., 2013; Frank et al., 2014; Noonan & Boraske, 2015).

The ACA *required* insurers to cover mental health and substance use care for individual and small group plans. This mandate is stronger than the *if/then* standard of the MHPAEA, which applies to large employer-sponsored plans. Finally, the ACA made care more affordable for members by setting limits on annual out-of-pocket costs. The ACA substantially broadened insurance benefits for mental health and substance use disorder services. Combined, the MHPAEA and the ACA expanded health insurance access for more than 170 million people (Frank, 2017).

21st Century Cures Act (2016)

Despite the expanded parity protections and increased health insurance access afforded under both the MHPAEA and ACA, there remained a lack of guidance or measurable standards to identify payer and provider compliance with the enacted parity coverage requirements, particularly related to NQTLs. Title XII of the 21st Century Cures Act—the mental health parity provisions contained within the Cures Act—was an attempt to do just that. The provisions clarified that Medicaid is to permit same-day billing for the provision of both primary care and mental health services. It also clarified the application of parity law to eating disorder benefits. Additionally, the Cures Act required new federal guidance on parity compliance and required a public meeting of stakeholders to create an action plan to improve federal and state coordination on parity requirements. Finally, these provisions required the U.S. Government Accountability Office to conduct a study on parity enforcement and provide recommendations for increasing enforcement results (American Psychiatric Association, 2018). The Cures Act is another step forward for parity, but real-time progress in changes to federal and state regulatory enforcement and health plans' compliance with parity requirements is still ongoing.

GAPS, CHALLENGES, AND THREATS TO PARITY LAW

Some types of health plans are not required to follow federal parity law (Table 25.1). Medicare, which provides health insurance for over 55 million—46 million people age 65 and older and 9 million younger people—is not subject to the MHPAEA, although the 2008 Medicare Improvements for Patients and Providers Act (MIPPA) phased out a statutory provision requiring a higher co-pay for outpatient mental health services. Still at issue is the fact that Medicare continues to impose a 190-day lifetime limit for psychiatric inpatient care, unlike other types of inpatient care.

Medicaid fee-for-service programs are also not subject to parity law, though most state Medicaid programs use managed care organizations, which must comply. TRICARE, the federal health care program for uniformed military service members and their families, is also excluded from parity law, although parity issues are

Type of Plan	Parity?	Notes
Employer Sponsored		
Large employer (>50 employees)	Yes	Not required to provide mental health or addiction benefits, but if they do, coverage must be on par with other medical benefits.
Small employer (2–50 employees)	Depends	*If created after March 23, 2010*, must provide mental health benefits. Required to follow federal parity law.
Federal Employee Health Benefits Plan (FEHBP)	Yes	Must provide mental health benefits; required to follow federal parity law.[a]
Non-federal government	No	Some health plans for state or local government workers can opt out of federal parity law.
Faith-based organizations	No	Plans for employees of faith-based organizations can opt out of federal parity law.
Retiree only	No	Plans that only cover retirees can opt out of federal parity law.

TABLE 25.1   **Health Plans and Federal Parity**

TABLE 25.1 Health Plans and Federal Parity—cont'd		
Type of Plan	**Parity?**	**Notes**
Government Programs		
Medicare	No	Federal health plan for people who are age 65 or older and people with disabilities. Federal parity law does not apply.
Children's Health Insurance Program (CHIP)	Yes	Government health plan for low-to-middle income children. Federal parity law applies.
Medicaid	Depends	Government health plan for certain low-income children and adults.[b] Federal parity law applies to Medicaid managed care plans, but not Medicaid Fee-for-Service (FFS) plans.
TRICARE	No	Federal health care program for uniformed military service members and their families
Individual Plans		
Individual health plans (you buy for self or family)	Depends	*If created after March 23, 2010, or changed since,* must provide mental health benefits; required to follow federal parity law.

[a]U.S. Office of Personnel Management, FEHB Program Carrier Letter, No. 2008-17. (November 10, 2008). Retrieved from www.opm.gov/healthcare-insurance/healthcare/carriers/2008/2008-17.pdf.
[b]Federal law restricts the use of Medicaid dollars for service to adults between the ages of 21 and 64 in certain types of free-standing psychiatric hospitals and residential facilities. 42 U.S.C. 1369(d).
Source: National Alliance on Mental Illness. Retrieved from www.nami.org/Find-Support/Living-with-a-Mental-Health-Condition/Understanding-Health-Insurance/What-is-Mental-Health-Parity.

uncommon within the program. Small state and local government health plans with 50 or fewer employees and health plans for employees of faith organizations can opt out of federal parity requirements. Finally, grandfathered plans, small group and individual plans purchased before 2010, are not subject to parity requirements if the plan is unchanged since the ACA was enacted. Despite these exclusions, most Americans are covered by health plans subject to one or more federal parity laws.

Ten years after the passage of the MHPAEA, the promise of parity has not been realized, and large gaps still exist between behavioral health and general medical care among health plans that are required to follow federal parity requirements. This unfulfilled promise is largely due to enforcement issues. Recent studies indicate that insurers continue to deny mental health and substance use claims twice as often as they do other medical benefits (NAMI, 2017). According to a report published by Milliman, a management consulting company, out-of-network service use remains significantly higher for mental health care than other types of medical care, forcing individuals to pay much higher out-of-pocket costs for mental health care than other medical conditions (Melek et al., 2017). The study found that psychiatrists are paid more than 20 percent lower on average than medical and surgical physicians for the same or similar service codes, reducing incentives

for psychiatrists to participate in insurance networks. In fact, participation would likely result in large financial losses (Melek et al., 2017).

Reduction of regulatory burdens undermine the ACA parity protections. The expansion of Short-Term Limited Duration Plans and Association Health Plans, for example, could negatively impact access to behavioral health care because these types of plans are not subject to EHB requirements. The sale of these plans can result in adverse selection against the ACA individual market, as younger, healthier people opt for less robust coverage, leaving those with significant health care needs in the individual market with elevated premiums.

STATE-LEVEL IMPLEMENTATION

Before federal parity legislation, beginning in the 1970s, states led efforts to regulate insurance coverage for behavioral health services (Barry, 2006; Barry et al., 2016, 2010). In the intervening years between the enactment of the MHPA and the passage of the MHPAEA, most states passed their own parity laws, although these state-based laws varied considerably in scope. Insurance regulation, in fact, is largely understood to be a state, not a federal function. However, federal policy is recognized as essential to require self-insured companies otherwise exempt from state regulation under the Employee Retirement Income Security Act (ERISA) of 1974 to comply with a parity mandate (Peterson & Busch, 2018). Today, in the wake of the MHPAEA, many of the implementation and enforcement challenges have returned to the states.

A number of strategies should be deployed to address the MHPAEA's implementation and enforcement issues at the state level. These include supporting interagency collaboration between state insurance agencies and state mental health agencies; the adoption of workbooks and templates that provide standard formats for state insurance agencies to assess parity compliance; deploying market conduct examinations and network adequacy assessments with an explicit focus on the MHPAEA; and strengthening and expanding public education campaigns to increase awareness about the MHPAEA rules among the public and providers (Purtle, Borchers, Clement, & Mauri, 2018).

IMPLICATIONS FOR MENTAL HEALTH NURSES: ISSUES AND STRATEGIES

Nurses and other allied professions provide the bulk of mental health and substance abuse services in the U.S. All nurses, and especially psychiatric mental health nurses at the general and advanced practice levels who work closest to and have everyday contact with patients receiving mental health and substance abuse services, can play a critical role in the movement toward mental health parity (Pearson et al., 2014).

Issue: While the MHPAEA and the ACA strengthen protections for mental health and substance abuse benefits, there remains a critical nationwide shortage of mental health care providers. This provider shortage can be partly attributed to reimbursement inequity and treatment limitations out of compliance with federal parity law.

Strategy: **Legislative Advocacy**—Psychiatric mental health nurses can impact parity policy through advocacy from a unique vantage point. Their clinical experience directly serving patients with mental health and addiction care needs positions them to be effective advocates. Psychiatric mental health nurses can draw upon their experiences with patients, and navigating the health care system themselves as providers, in order to advocate for the full implementation and greater enforcement of the MHPAEA (see the resources section for information about access to current advocacy efforts in your state). Advocacy efforts around state implementation and enforcement of federal parity law might include:

• Join local and national advocates to pursue full enforcement of the federal parity law

• Get to know state insurance department regulators and ensure their familiarity with federal and state statutes.
• Assess the power of the state insurance department to enforce federal regulations both statutorily and with resources such as enough personnel and adequate training
• Advocate with state policymakers to address deficits

Issue: Consumers, family members, employers, purchasers, clinicians, policymakers, and the general public all require greater education regarding the scope of federal parity law. There is a general lack of awareness among consumers and providers about how federal parity law can address barriers to care, and how consumers can exercise their parity rights and identify common violations. Public education is needed to raise awareness among consumers of mental health and substance abuse services and their families.

Strategy: **Promoting Consumer Education and Leadership**—Nurses need be knowledgeable about parity law to help patients and their families understand their parity rights and identify potential parity violations. Psychiatric mental health nurses can play an important role in facilitating and supporting mental health consumers in leadership roles as advocates and educators. Nurses must also be familiar with patient advocacy groups such as the NAMI, Mental Health America (MHA), and the Depression Bipolar Support Alliance (DBSA) and their consumer education efforts.

Issue: Psychiatric mental health nurses can play an important role in developing and forwarding a research agenda to inform practice and policy about the effects of parity.

Strategy: **Developing a Research Agenda**—There are many avenues for future research, including the impact of NQTL noncompliance, effects of parity on individuals with serious mental illness or substance use disorders, and a better understanding of the relationship between parity and mental health and substance abuse workforce shortages, to name a few. These research opportunities are ripe for collaborative research endeavors between and among psychiatric mental health nurses interested in the intersectionality of knowledge generation, evidence-based clinical practice, and quality improvement and policy.

DISCUSSION QUESTIONS

1. Are mental health parity laws in your state more comprehensive or less comprehensive than the federal laws and in what ways?
2. How are consumers in your workplace (hospital, community mental health center, etc.) educated about the benefits that they are entitled to as a result of the MHPAEA and the ACA?

3. What educational program for consumers and/or advocacy resources would you suggest to your patients and their families to help them learn more about the benefits of the MHPAEA?

REFERENCES

American Psychiatric Association. (2018). Mental Health reform provisions in H.R. 34, the 21st Century Cures Act. Retrieved from www.psychiatry.org/File%20Library/Psychiatrists/Advocacy/Federal/Comprehensive-Mental-Health-Reform/APA-Summary-Mental-Health-Reform-Provisions-21st-Century-Cures-Act.pdf.

Barry, C.L., Goldman, H.H., & Huskamp, H.A. (2016). Federal parity in the evolving mental health and addiction care landscape. *Health Affairs, 35*(6), 1009–1016.

Barry, C.L., Huskamp, H.A., & Goldman, H.H. (2010). A political history of federal mental health and addiction insurance parity. *The Milbank Quarterly, 88*(3), 404–433.

Bendat, M. (2014). In name only? Mental health parity or illusory reform. *Psychodynamic Psychiatry, 42*(3), 353–375.

Beronio, K., Po, R., Skopec, L., & Gilead, S. (2013). *Affordable Care Act expands mental health and substance use disorder benefits and federal parity protections for 62 million Americans* (ASPE issue brief) (p. 3). Washington, DC: U.S. Department of Health & Human Services. Retrieved from http://aspe.hhs.gov/health/reports/2013/mental/rb_mental.cfm.

Busch, A.B., Yoon, F., Barry, C.L., Azzone, V., Normand, S.-L.T., Goldman, H.H., & Huskamp, H.A. (2013). The effects of mental health parity on spending and utilization for bipolar, major depression, and adjustment disorders. *American Journal of Psychiatry, 170*(2), 180–187.

Dixon, K. (2009). Implementing Mental Health Parity: The challenge for health plans. *Health Affairs, 28*(3), 663–665.

Frank, R.G. (2017). Realizing the promise of parity legislation for mental health. *JAMA Psychiatry, 74*(2), 117–118.

Frank, R.G., Beronio, K., & Glied, S.A. (2014). Behavioral health parity and the Affordable Care Act. *Journal of Social Work in Disability & Rehabilitation, 13*(1–2), 31–43.

Galarneau, C. (2018). Getting King's words right. *Journal of Health Care for the Poor and Underserved, 29*(1), 5–8.

Grazier, K.L., Eisenberg, D., Jedele, J.M., & Smiley, M.L. (2015). Effects of mental health parity on high utilizers of services: Pre-post evidence from a large, self-insured employer. *Psychiatric Services, 67*(4), 448–451.

Heller, B.D., (2016). Revolutionizing the Mental Health Parity and Addiction Equity Act of 2008: Comments. *Seton Hall Law Review, 47*, 569–602.

Horgan, C.M., Hodgkin, D., Stewart, M.T., Quinn, A., Merrick, E.L., Reif, S., … & Creedon, T.B. (2015). Health plans' early response to federal parity legislation for mental health and addiction services. *Psychiatric Services, 67*(2), 162–168.

Institute of Medicine. (2003). Economic and social implications of uninsurance within communities. In *A shared destiny: Community effects of uninsurance* (pp. 120-137). Washington, DC: The National Academies Press.

Kaiser Family Foundation. (2017). *Analysis of Medicaid enrollment data collected from the Centers for Medicare and Medicaid Services (CMS) Medicaid Budget and Expenditure System (MBES)*. Retrieved from www.kff.org/health-reform/state-indicator/medicaid-expansion-enrollment/.

Melek, S., Perlman, D., & Davenport, S. (2017). *Addiction and mental health vs. physical health: Analyzing disparities in network use and provider reimbursement rates*. Milliman. Retrieved from www.milliman.com/uploadedFiles/insight/2017/NQTLDisparityAnalysis.pdf.

National Alliance on Mental Illness. (2017). *The doctor is out—Continuing disparities in access to mental and physical health care*. Retrieved from www.nami.org/About-NAMI/Publications-Reports/Public-Policy-Reports/The-Doctor-is-Out.

Noonan, K.G., & Boraske, S.J. (2015). Enforcing mental health parity through the Affordable Care Act's essential health benefit mandate. *Annals of Health Law, 24*, 252–285.

Pearson, G.S., Evans, L.K., Hines-Martin, V.P., Yearwood, E.L., York, J.A., & Kane, C.F. (2014). Promoting the mental health of families. *Nursing Outlook, 62*(3), 225–227.

Peterson, E., & Busch, S. (2018). Achieving mental health and substance use disorder treatment parity: A quarter century of policy making and research. *Annual Review of Public Health, 39*(1), 421–435.

Purtle, J., Borchers, B., Clement, T., & Mauri, A. (2018). Interagency strategies used by state mental health agencies to assist with federal behavioral health parity implementation. *Journal of Behavioral Health Services & Research, 45*(3), 516–526.

Rochefort, D.A. (Ed.). (1989). *Handbook on mental health policy in the United States*. New York: Greenwood Press.

Substance Abuse and Mental Health Services Administration Center for Behavioral Health Statistics and Quality. (2017). *Results from the 2016 National Survey on Drug Use and Health: Detailed tables*. Retrieved from www.samhsa.gov/data/sites/default/files/NSDUH-DetTabs-2016/NSDUH-DetTabs-2016.pdf.

Thalmayer, A.G., Friedman, S.A., Azocar, F., Harwood, J.M., & Ettner, S.L. (2016). The Mental Health Parity and Addiction Equity Act (MHPAEA) Evaluation Study: Impact on quantitative treatment limits. *Psychiatric Services, 68*(5), 435–442.

ONLINE RESOURCES

Federal Enforcement Agencies

Department of Labor (DOL) Employee Benefits Security Administration (EBSA) (handles parity complaints involving self-insured private employer health plans; for assistance, call [866] 444-3272)
www.askebsa.dol.gov

Department of Health and Human Services (HHS), Centers for Medicare and Medicaid Services (CMS) (handles parity complaints involving state and local government employer plans that are self-insured; complaints can be filed through the HHS parity complaint portal [www.parity.hhs.gov]; by phone with the CMS Health Insurance Helpline at [877] 267-2323, extension 6-1565; or by email to phig@cms)
www.hhs.gov or *www.cms.gov*

Advocacy Resources

Depression Bipolar Support Alliance (DBSA)
www.dbsalliance.org
The Kennedy Forum
www.thekennedyforum.org

Mental Health America
www.mentalhealthamerica.net
National Alliance on Mental Illness (NAMI)
www.NAMI.org/parity
Parity Registry (an online tool that allows consumers to file an appeal with their health plan, send a complaint directly to state enforcement officials, and access step-by-step appeals guidance; the data shared will help shape public policy and future legislation)
www.parityregistry.org
Parity Track (provides a comprehensive listing of legislative, regulatory, and legal parity activities in all 50 states and at the Federal level to monitor implementation and best practices)
www.paritytrack.org

26

Improving LGBTQ+ Health: Nursing Policy Can Make a Difference

Sarah Stover Filer Zollweg, Valerie Tobin, Zil Garner Goldstein,
David M. Keepnews, and Peggy L. Chinn

"ANA is committed to the elimination of health disparities and discrimination based on sexual orientation, gender identity, and/or expression within health care. LGBTQ+ populations face significant obstacles accessing care such as stigma, discrimination, inequity in health insurance, and denial of care because of an individual's sexual orientation or gender identity."

American Nurses Association position statement, June 2018
(ANA Center for Ethics and Human Rights, 2018)

The nursing profession has made significant strides over the last several years in contributing to efforts to achieve health equity for lesbian, gay, bisexual, transgender, and queer (LGBTQ+)[a] communities. (For more information on definitions and terminology, see Table 26.1.) As the American Nurses Association (ANA) recently recognized formally (above), LGBTQ+ individuals face numerous health disparities, many of which stem from stigma and discrimination and are further exacerbated by structural and institutional-level inequities. Despite being uniquely positioned to address these inequities, the nursing profession has been slow to recognize LGBTQ+ health disparities and slow to take action (Eliason, Dibble, & DeJoseph, 2010; Harrell & Sasser, 2018). Keepnews (2011), while recognizing the deficit in nursing literature, also noted a foundation of nursing activism. Advocacy by LGBTQ+ nurses led to support by the ANA for antidiscrimination legislation. In the early days of the human immunodeficiency virus/acquired immunodeficiency virus (HIV/AIDS) epidemic, when homophobia often led to discrimination and/or poor care (despite the fact that HIV/AIDS—while affecting large numbers of gay men—was never a "gay disease"), the ANA and other nursing organizations strongly opposed discrimination and advocated for access to quality HIV/AIDS care. But then nursing remained largely quiet on LGBTQ+ issues for many years.

In recent years, nursing organizations have increased their support of LGBTQ+ people and made up some lost ground. The ANA, American Academy of Nursing (AAN), International Society for Psychiatric-Mental Health Nurses, National Association of School Nurses, National Student Nurses' Association, American College of Nurse Midwives, and others have all contributed to the recognition and prioritization of LGBTQ+ health inequities (see a summary of actions taken by nursing organizations in Table 26.2). This chapter is not an exhaustive review of LGBTQ+ health issues and health policy, rather it provides an overview of principles to guide policy and to outline nursing actions that contribute to achieving health equity for LGBTQ+ communities.

RECOGNIZING AND ADDRESSING LGBTQ+ ISSUES

In order to address LGBTQ+ health inequities, it is first necessary to recognize that they exist and to identify them. There was little recognition and knowledge of these inequities until recently, with many major social and political developments in the last few years. In December 2010 the

---

[a]The acronym LGBTQ+ is used throughout this chapter to indicate lesbian, gay, bisexual, transgender, queer, plus the many additional identities within the community beyond those who identify as LGBT or Q.

TABLE 26.1   Definitions and Terminology

Term	Definition
Sexual orientation	This term is used to describe to whom a person is or is not attracted. Examples of sexual orientation include lesbian, gay, bisexual, pansexual, etc.
Gender identity	This term is used to describe which gender(s) a person may identify with, such as man, woman, genderqueer, etc.
Lesbian	A woman who is primarily attracted to other women and identifies as a lesbian.
Gay	An adjective used to describe an individual who is primarily attracted to people of the same sex or gender and identifies as gay.
Bisexual	An individual who is attracted to both men and women and identifies as bisexual.
Pansexual	An individual whose romantic and sexual attraction are not dependent primarily on the sex or gender of their partners and identifies as pansexual.
Transgender or trans	Individuals whose gender identification and/or expression differs from the sex assigned at birth. Trans men were assigned female at birth; trans women were assigned male at birth. Some have surgeries or use hormones to alter their bodies and some do not. Identifying as trans does not necessarily mean that an individual identifies with being a man or a woman; a transgender individual may identify with neither gender, both genders, or all genders. Note that the term transsexual may be seen as derogatory.
Queer	Some people do not identify their sexual orientation with terms like lesbian, gay, or bisexual, but consider themselves to be outside of the mainstream heterosexual identity. Many people use the term "genderqueer" to indicate that they do not fit gender norms. Queer is a derogatory term that has often been used as a slur against the LGBTQ+ community and has been reclaimed.
Nonbinary or gender nonconforming	An individual who does not necessarily identify with being either male or female or may identify with being both male and female, or who does not feel that they conform to gender norms.
Agender	An individual who does not identify with any gender and may identify with being genderless.
Questioning	Some individuals are not sure what sexual or gender identification best fits them and are in the process of exploring identities. This can happen at any age.
Intersex	A small subset of the population is born with genetic, endocrine, and/or anatomical differences that place their bodies somewhere on the spectrum between male and female. Because of the stigma often associated with a body that does not conform to societal norms, many people with intersex conditions have similar experiences of hiding their condition or experiencing shame and guilt about it as do LGBT people. Some people who are intersex identify as LGBTQ.
Two-Spirit	Two-Spirit is a term used by many American Indian, Native, First Nations, and Indigenous people to describe diversity in gender, gender expression, and/or sexual orientation. This term is reflective of an expansive understanding of gender in many Native cultures that predates colonialism. It is not interchangeable with LGBTQIA or other western terms or concepts for gender or sexual orientation and is a community organizing tool rather than an identity.
Same Gender Loving	Same Gender Loving is a culturally affirming term used by many African Americans to describe attraction to the same gender.
Allies	Many people who do not identify as LGBTQ are strong and active supporters of the struggle for LGBTQ equality.
LGBT, LGBTQ, LGBTQ+, LGBTQI, LGBTQIA, and so on	Organizations vary in how inclusive they are regarding the varieties of sexual and gender identifications. The most common acronym is LGBT, but if the organization serves many people with other identities, they may choose to include them all in their written materials. Every agency must make decisions about whom to include (and whom to exclude) when they issue policies or statements about cultural sensitivity.
Behavioral terms	Men who have sex with men (MSM) and women who have sex with women (WSW) are terms often used by public health professionals to encompass individuals who have sex with others of the same sex or gender but who may not identify as lesbian, gay, or bisexual.

TABLE 26.1	Definitions and Terminology—cont'd
Term	**Definition**
Pronouns	The pronouns that an individual identifies with. Examples include she/her/hers, he/him/his, they/them/theirs, ze/hir/hirs*, and ze/zir/zirs.* Please note that there are many other terms beyond the ones in this table; please make sure to check that they are appropriate and not derogatory before using them. Many terms may be reclaimed by the LGBTQ+ community and used by members of the community that may be offensive when used by people who do not identify as LGBTQ+.

*These are gender-neutral pronouns that someone may use if that individual does not identify with male or female pronouns.
Source: Retrieved from https://lavenderhealth.org/lgbtqpolicy-chapter-8th-edition/.

TABLE 26.2	LGBTQ+ Supportive Actions by Nursing Organizations
Nursing Organization	**Supportive Statements and Actions**
American Nurses Association (ANA)	ANA Center for Ethics and Human Rights. (2018). *Policy statement: Nursing advocacy for LGBTQ+ populations.* American Nurses Association. Retrieved from www.nursingworld.org/~49866e/globalassets/practiceandpolicy/ethics/nursing-advocacy-for-lgbtq-populations.pdf. American Nurses Association. (July 28, 2017). *Statement in support of equality and human rights for the LGBTQ community.* (Press release). Retrieved from www.nursingworld.org/news/news-releases/2017-news-releases/statement-insupport-of-equality-and-human-rights-for-the-lgbtq-community. American Nurses Association. (2015a). *Code of ethics for nurses with interpretive statements.* Silver Spring, MD: Author. Retrieved from http://nursingworld.org/Code-of-ethics. American Nurses Association. (2010). *ANA applauds house action to repeal "don't ask, don't tell."* (Press release). Retrieved from http://ojin.nursingworld.org/MainMenuCategories/ANAMarketplace/ANAPeriodicals/OJIN/Columns/ANA-Position-Statements/ANA-Position-Statement-Advocacy-for-LGBTQ.html. American Nurses Association. (1992a). *Compendium of HIV/AIDS position statements, policies, and documents.* Washington, DC: Author. American Nurses Association. (1992b). *Discrimination against gays and lesbians by military.* Washington, DC: Author. American Nurses Association. (1988). *Personal heroism, professional activism: Nursing and the battle against AIDS.* Kansas City, MO: Author. American Nurses Association Convention '80. (1980). ANA position statement: Nursing advocacy for LGBTQ+ population. *American Journal of Nursing, 80*(7), 1317–1332. American Nurses Association Convention '78. (1978). ANA position statement: Nursing advocacy for LGBTQ+ population. *American Journal of Nursing, 78*(7), 1231–1246.
American Academy of Nursing (AAN)	American Academy of Nursing. (n.d.). *Expert panel on LGBTQ health.* Retrieved from www.aannet.org/expertpanels/ep-lgbtq-health. Expert Panel on LGBTQ Health. (2015a). American Academy of Nursing: Position statement: Employment discrimination based on sexual orientation and gender identity. *Nursing Outlook, 63*(3), 366. Expert Panel on LGBTQ Health. (2015b). American Academy of Nursing position statement on reparative therapy. *Nursing Outlook, 63*(3), 368. Expert Panel on LGBTQ Health. (2015c). American Academy of Nursing: Same-sex partnership rights: Health care decision making and hospital visitation. *Nursing Outlook, 63*(1), 95.

Continued

TABLE 26.2 LGBTQ+ Supportive Actions by Nursing Organizations—cont'd	
Nursing Organization	**Supportive Statements and Actions**
International Society for Psychiatric-Mental Health Nurses	International Society of Psychiatric-Mental Health Nurses. (2010). *Position statement on reparative therapy.* Retrieved from www.ispn-psych.org/assets/docs/ps-reparativetherapy.pdf.
National Association of School Nurses	National Association of School Nurses. (2017). *LGBTQ students: The role of the school nurse.* Retrieved from www.nasn.org/advocacy/professional-practice-documents/position-statements/ps-lgbtq.
National Student Nurse Association	National Student Nurses Association. (2016). *Improving professional support and advocacy for lesbian, gay, bisexual, transgender, questioning, intersex, and asexual (LGBTQIA) nurses.* Retrieved from https://lavenderhealth.files.wordpress.com/2016/04/2016-nsna-resolution-lgbtqia.pdf.
American College of Nurse Midwives	American College of Nurse Midwives. (2012). *Transgender/transsexual/gender variant health care.* Retrieved from www.midwife.org/ACNM/files/ACNMLibraryData/UPLOADFILENAME/000000000278/Transgender%20Gender%20Variant%20Position%20Statement%20December%202012.pdf.

U.S. Department of Health and Human Services newly included LGBTQ+ health as a topic area in Healthy People 2020. In 2011 the Institute of Medicine (IOM) issued a landmark report that described the state of LGBTQ+ health, identified research gaps, and provided recommendations for a research agenda to address disparities (IOM, 2011). Also in 2011, the Joint Commission created a field guide for improving LGBTQ+ care and began to require hospitals to prohibit discrimination based on sexual orientation and gender identity (SOGI) (The Joint Commission, 2011). The National Institutes of Health (NIH) established the Sexual and Gender Minority Research office in 2015 in order to augment research efforts on LGBTQ people (https://dpcpsi.nih.gov/sgmro). In 2016 the NIH formally designated sexual and gender minorities as a health disparity population for research purposes (Pérez-Stable, 2016). These actions have increased the visibility of LGBTQ+ health inequities and paved a way forward to address disparities.

IMPORTANCE OF SEXUAL ORIENTATION AND GENDER IDENTITY DATA COLLECTION

In order to adequately address LGBTQ+ health disparities, it is necessary to understand what disparities exist and how different LGBTQ+ individuals are affected, and how LGBTQ+ disparities overlap and interact with racial/ethnic and other disparities (Cahill & Makadon, 2017). One important way to gather this information is through national surveys. The Trump administration will not include questions about gender identity in the 2020 U.S. Census, and will only capture data on same-sex couples if

they are living together (Necati, 2018). While it is a huge step forward to ask about same sex relationships, it ignores large portions of LGBTQ+ communities. The Trump administration has also removed questions on SOGI from the National Survey of Older Americans Act Participants (NSOAAP) and from the Annual Program Performance Report for Centers for Independent Living (Singh, Durso, & Tax, 2017). A question about sexual orientation has been added back to the NSOAAP after backlash from Congress, LGBTQ+ advocacy groups, and the general public, but at this time there are still no questions on gender identity (Maril, 2017).

LGBTQ+ ACROSS THE LIFESPAN

LGBTQ+ seniors and minors require particular policy protections. Needs may differ for those who are cisgender LGBQ+ and those who are transgender and gender nonbinary.

Youth

Health disparities among LGBTQ+ adolescents include higher rates of suicide, suicidal ideation, depression, anxiety, and sexually transmitted infections (STIs) (Hafeez, Zeshan, Tahir, Jahan, & Naveed, 2017). They also experience high rates of psychosocial risk for poor health, including bullying (Earnshaw, Bogart, Poteat, Reisner, & Schuster, 2016), multiple forms of victimization such as dating violence and abuse (Sterzing, Ratliff, Gartner, McGeough, & Johnson, 2017), placement in child welfare systems (McCormick, Schmidt, & Terrazas, 2016), and homelessness ("Missed Opportunities: Youth Homelessness in America," 2018).

Trauma in early life may lead to poorer health throughout the lifespan (Felitti et al., 1998).

Children who do not conform to gender norms are more likely to face abuse in the home than their peers, regardless of actual gender or sexual identity (Roberts, Rosario, Corliss, Koenen, & Austin, 2012). As adolescents, they are more likely to be evicted from their homes (Choi, Wilson, Shelton, & Gates, 2015). In the foster care system, LGBTQ+ young people report more frequent placements, more psychiatric hospitalizations, and more likelihood of placement in a group home rather than a family home (Wilson, Cooper, Kastanis, & Nezhad, 2014).

According to recent estimates, LGBTQ+ youth are *120%* more likely to be homeless than their peers (Missed Opportunities: Youth Homelessness in America, 2018). Recent estimates are over 30% of homeless youth are LGBTQ+ (Choi et al., 2015). It is incumbent on homeless agencies to be aware of the needs of LGBTQ+ youth and to have well-prepared staff to meet their needs. Safety in the setting is vital, particularly for gender unique youth, since sleeping arrangements are often determined by gender.

Schools are often not a safe place for LGBTQ+ young people. Over 80% of LGBTQ students reported verbal harassment at school and 13% report being physically assaulted (Kosciw, Greytak, Giga, Villenas, & Danischewski, 2015). Retrospectively, 54% of transgender and nonbinary persons who were out or perceived as transgender or nonbinary in grades K-12 report verbal harassment and almost one-quarter report being physically assaulted (James et al., 2016). As of January 15, 2019, only 17 states and Washington, DC states protect public elementary and high school students from discrimination based on sexual orientation and only 15 from discrimination based on gender identity (Human Rights Campaign, 2019b). Gay-straight alliances (or gender-sexuality alliances as some schools now name these groups, i.e. GSAs) in schools decrease victimization of LGBTQ adolescents (Kosciw, Greytak, Giga, Villenas, & Danischewski, 2015).

Family therapists who are prepared and experienced in work with LGBTQ+ young people and their parents are vital. The most protective factor for the mental health of LGBTQ+ youth is a supportive parental relationship (McConnell, Birkett, & Mustanski, 2015; Ryan, Russell, Huebner, Diaz, & Sanchez, 2010). Mental health care, in the form of family therapy, must be accessible and available for these young people and their families.

It is vital for nurses who come into contact with children, adolescents, and families to be prepared to respond to the needs of SOGI diverse children and their parents. Gender expansive children may benefit from suppression and delay of puberty, which can vastly improve a transgender person's mental health and quality of life (McNeil, Bailey, Ellis, Morton, & Regan, 2012). Treatment needs for

transgender and nonbinary children and adolescents include access to nursing, mental health, and medical providers who are prepared to address their unique developmental needs (Hembree et al., 2017).

School district policies that support LGBTQ+ young people include: support of GSAs; LGBTQ+-inclusive curriculum; preparing teachers and counselors about creating an affirming environment for LGBTQ+ adolescents, parents, and staff. Children and youth have urgent needs for well-designed, sensitive, and accurate sex education, including information about LGBTQ+ experience, healthy sexuality, and how to protect themselves from STIs and pregnancy. Transgender and nonbinary children and adolescents benefit from gender inclusive policies that include consistent instructions for supporting students who are transitioning or have a unique gender expression, including use of correct pronouns, names, and facilities (Gender Spectrum: Education, n.d.).

Elders

LGBTQ+ elders face considerable health disparities, particularly those who are transgender, bisexual, living with HIV, African American, Latino, poor, and those who are in advanced old age. Elders who are LGBTQ+ often have poorer health and health behavior such as drinking and smoking, and more functional limitations than peers (Emlet & Fredriksen-Goldsen, 2017). They have higher rates of disability and poor physical and mental health. Over 71% of transgender older adults have considered suicide (Fredriksen-Goldsen et al., 2017).

They are also more likely to face health risks. Over 80% of LGBTQ+ elders report victimization at some point in their lives (Fredriksen-Goldsen et al., 2017). Many of the disparities that elders in general face are also true for those who are LGBTQ+. There is a lack of affordable housing for elders, and this is made worse for LGBTQ+ elders living in states without protection in housing for LGBTQ+ people (Movement Advancement Project & Sage, 2017).

Important policy changes include protections to assure availability of housing for LGBTQ+ elders, workforce development programs for elders that are LGBTQ+ inclusive, and LGBTQ+ education for all staff in agencies that serve older people, including senior housing, assisted living, and nursing homes. Nondiscrimination policies are also important for all organizations that may provide services to the older population. Adding the LGBTQ+ population to the Older Americans Act as a "population of greatest need" would make more funding available to support needed services to protect LGBTQ+ elders. Some LGBTQ+ people who were discharged from the U.S. military under the "Don't ask, don't tell" law lost their veteran's benefits (Movement Advancement Project & Sage, 2017). This can be remedied with the "Restore Honor to Service Members Act" (Schatz, 2017) and by guarding against future discharges of transgender service members. Additionally, transgender elders are now able to receive gender confirmation care under Medicaid, but may not know that this is the case and they may be unable to find or afford appropriate health care (Fredriksen-Goldsen et al., 2017).

RECENT POLICY ISSUES

Internationally there have been important strides toward equity for LGBTQ+ communities as well as steps back. Increasing numbers of countries have legalized marriage equality and created policies protecting LGBTQ+ rights, whereas state-sponsored violence toward LGBTQ+ communities remains common in other countries (Reid, 2018). However, LGBTQ+ Americans continue to face discrimination in housing, employment, health care, and the military as well as in many other aspects of public life. In 2017 President Trump signed an executive order on "religious liberty" that potentially opens the door for discrimination against LGBTQ+ individuals based on religious beliefs (Gruberg, Bewkes Frank, Franke, & Markham, 2018). In 2019, the Trump Administration issued the Conscience Rule, making it legal to deny care on religious grounds, including denial of care to LGBTQ+ people based on SOGI (Fenway Health, 2019). Additionally, only 20 states and Washington, DC prohibit discrimination in public accommodations based on SOGI, with 1 additional state prohibiting public accommodation discrimination by sexual orientation but not gender identity (Human Rights Campaign, 2018c). Discrimination by organizations and businesses, whether someone is refused service by a store or restaurant or does not have access to an appropriate restroom, limits individuals' ability to participate in public life. The sections that follow present important issues that illustrate progress to protect the health and wellbeing of LGBTQ+ people and explain the challenges that still remain.

Marriage Equality

On June 26, 2015, the U.S. Supreme Court recognized the rights of individuals to marry, regardless of sex (U.S. Supreme Court, 2015). This means, among other things, that all rights given to married male/female couples in the hospital setting can and should be extended to married same-sex couples as well. This includes visitation rights for partners and children, as well as inclusion of same-sex partners in medical decision making.

Adoption, Surrogacy, and Reproductive Care and Access

Many of the options LGBTQ+ people have for becoming parents are not guaranteed on the federal level. LGBTQ+ people considering surrogacy and assisted reproductive

technologies are subject to a wide variety of legal protections and prohibitions on a state-by-state basis and individual agencies or states may exercise bias against LGBTQ+ people. The legality of surrogacy, or the use of a third party to carry a pregnancy to term, varies highly on a state-to-state basis, from outright bans to no regulation to explicit protections through both legislative and court rulings ("U.S. Surrogacy Law by State," n.d.). It is important for providers to be familiar with state regulations as well as those of nearby states. Access to reproductive technologies is subject to both individual providers' biases as well as insurance coverage.

Provider bias is often expressed through lack of education in working with LGBTQ+ people and the special needs that may arise when, for example, discussing fertility options with a transgender man taking testosterone. Health insurance also often excludes or limits coverage for reproductive technologies, and LGBTQ+ people are often excluded from definitions of infertility required to qualify for coverage (Bowerman, May, & Rossma, 2017).

Bathroom Access

Access to the bathroom consistent with gender identity is an important issue for transgender people. It is an issue of basic dignity as well as a safety issue, as transgender people are at risk for being assaulted or physically removed from bathrooms. Transgender people's access to appropriate bathrooms may vary by state and locality. In 2016, North Carolina enacted House Bill (HB) 2, requiring people using a public or school bathroom to use the bathroom consistent with the sex stated on their birth certificate which, under another North Carolina law, cannot be amended without documentation of what the law calls "sex reassignment surgery." After widespread national outrage, which also led to significant consequences to the state's economy, the state legislature repealed HB 2 in 2017 via compromise legislation that also placed a moratorium on local antidiscrimination laws for the following three years (Berman & Phillips, 2017).

Insurance Coverage

More and more states are mandating insurance coverage for transition-related health care for transgender patients. Coverage for transition-related services should be seen as an essential right that nurse advocates can promote. Access to the wide spectrum of health care, including transition-related health care, is crucial for quality of life and well-being. Transgender people currently suffer a 41% suicide attempt rate, and health interventions can help improve quality-of-life outcomes (Agarwal, Scheefer, Wright, Walzer, & Rivera, 2018; Hess et al., 2018; James et al., 2016). Along with advocacy for transition-related coverage, it is important for nurses to advocate for health care facilities to offer transition-related services, such as mental health care, hormone therapy, and surgery, so that people have appropriate places to obtain care.

Military Service

The ban on U.S. military service by LGB and Q people was lifted in 2010. Toward the end of the Obama Administration, a longtime ban on transgender service members was to be ended, allowing transgender persons to serve openly. In 2017, the Trump administration sought to reinstate the ban, but multiple court challenges halted its implementation. As of January 22, 2019, the Supreme Court lifted injunctions on implementing the ban on transgender military service, and the Department of Defense began to implement the ban on April 12, 2019, though litigation is still underway (Human Rights Campaign, 2018c). The ANA opposed the ban on lesbian, gay, and bisexual service members in 1992 and supported repeal of "Don't ask, don't tell" in 2010 (ANA Center for Ethics and Human Rights, 2018). The AAN also supported the repeal of "Don't ask, don't tell" and issued a letter to the U.S. Secretary of Defense opposing a return to the ban on transgender service members (Berkowitz, 2017). These are examples of how nursing organizations can leverage their power and visibility to support and advocate for LGBTQ+ communities.

Housing and Employment

Housing and job insecurity remain major issues within LGBTQ+ communities and have profound impacts on health. Only 22 states and the District of Columbia (DC) protect from housing discrimination based on sexual orientation, with only 21 of those also protecting against gender identity discrimination (Human Rights Campaign, 2018b). LGBTQ+ people experience significant housing discrimination; rates are higher still for LGBTQ+ people of color and transgender people of any race due to multiple overlapping systems of oppression ("Facing Barriers: Experiences of LGBT People of Color in Colorado," n.d.; Kattari, Whitfield, Eugene Walls, Langenderfer-Magruder, & Ramos, 2016).

Only 33 states and DC have employment protections based on sexual orientation, 11 of which only apply to public employees; only 28 states and Washington, DC protect based on gender identity, 7 of which only protect public employees (Human Rights Campaign, 2018a). Kattari et al. (2016) found that 25.1% of cisgender LGBQ participants and 50% of transgender participants reported workplace discrimination based on SOGI and that these numbers increase the longer an individual has been out of the closet. One Colorado study found that nearly 43% of LGBTQ+ people of color and nearly 38% of LGBTQ+ Whites reported employment discrimination based on SOGI ("Facing Barriers: Experiences of LGBT People of Color in Colorado," n.d.). In 2015 the AAN issued a position statement opposing employment discrimination against LGBTQ+ people and acknowledging the many ways employment discrimination contributes to LGBTQ+ health disparities (AAN, 2015b). This is an example of how nursing organizations can use their power and influence to help achieve health equity.

"Conversion Therapy"

Despite multiple United States health organizations stating that it lacks scientific evidence and is harmful (Flentje, Heck, & Cochran, 2014), only 17 states and Washington, DC have regulations in place to prohibit licensed mental health professionals from administering so-called conversion therapy to individuals under 18 (Human Rights Campaign, 2019a). This practice may also be called sexual reorientation therapy, reorientation therapy, or reparative therapy. Both the International Society of Psychiatric-Mental Health Nurses (ISPN) and the AAN have come out with position statements opposing conversion therapy, stating that it is a harmful and ineffective practice and affirming the fact that homosexuality is not a disorder (AAN, 2015a; ISPN Diversity and Equity Committee, 2008).

NURSING EDUCATION POLICY

Policy that drives the quality of nursing education is established by accreditation standards, notably the standards developed by the Commission on Collegiate Nursing Education (which provides baccalaureate and higher degree accreditation), the Accreditation Commission for Education in Nursing, and the National League for Nursing (which provides accreditation across the academic spectrum including Licensed Practical Nurse/Licensed Vocational Nurse, diploma, associate, bachelor's, master's, and clinical doctorate degree programs). These groups have taken stands promoting diversity in nursing education, but only recently have they begun to include gender and sexual diversity as crucial dimensions of diversity. However, nursing education at all levels, including continuing education, is widely regarded as lacking in LGBTQ+ content (Lim, Johnson, & Eliason, 2015). Faculty may hold persistent anti-LGBTQ+ prejudices, or be uninformed of the importance of LGBTQ+ health issues. But even when faculty are interested in including LGBTQ+ content, many lack the knowledge and skills required to address gender and sexual diversity (Bosse, Nesteby, & Randall, 2015).

A first step to remedy the neglect of LGBTQ+ curriculum content is faculty education and discussion to overcome prevailing attitudes and stereotypes toward LGBTQ+ people and families, to learn ways to address the needs of LGBTQ+ people and families skillfully, and to acquire accurate knowledge related to LGBTQ+ experience. Additionally, even as nurses begin to incorporate LGBTQ+ content into curricula, previous generations of nurses as well as some non-nursing members of the health care team will still lack the education unless this material is incorporated into health care organizations' continuing education and required competencies (Bonvicini, 2017). LGBTQ+ concerns need to be included throughout nursing curricula at every level (see Table 26.3 for LGBTQ+ education guidelines and Table 26.4 for continuing education resources for LGBTQ+ competent care).

TABLE 26.3   Guidelines for LGBTQ+ Education

LGBTQ+ Inclusive Factors	Why	How

Inclusive language in syllabi, lectures, exams	Noninclusive language contributes to enforced closeting and stigma	• Eliminate pronouns or use plural forms.
		• Use "they/them" as both singular and plural.
		• Avoid binary language
		  • "people" instead of "men" or "women"
		  • "trans" instead of "trans man/woman"
		• Beware of language that assumes legal or casual heterosexual relationships—wife, husband, girl-/boyfriend. Use significant other, partner, spouse instead

Create welcoming climates	There are likely to be a wide diversity of gender and sexual identities in the classroom; you cannot assume they are all "not gay"	• Display rainbow symbols throughout in offices, classrooms, hallways. • Use posters that reflect diversity in family structures, relationships. • Create and maintain space for LGBTQ+ students and faculty to be open about their identities.
Clear and accessible antidiscrimination policies and actions	Prevailing cultures sustain tolerance of discrimination toward LGBTQ+ people	• Emphasize no-tolerance policies for LGBTQ+ discrimination in writing and frequent verbal affirmation. • Follow through on even the slightest discriminatory words or actions. • Include antidiscrimination language in course syllabi, and in discussions of all elements of each course. • Address ethical issues related to inclusion and acceptance of diversity to promote wellness for all. • Provide frequent forums for discussion of inclusive practices.
Integrated LGBTQ+ issues in each and every element of the curriculum.	LGBTQ+ people and families are found in each and every population, and as part of every other "minority" group.	• Mention LGBTQ+ people in each and every lecture, class, or clinical experience. • Include case studies featuring LGBTQ+ people and families—at least 3 in every course—to emphasize the particular challenges of gender and sexual diversity in the contexts of common health challenges. • Revise tools used to teach interviewing skills to assure that students learn appropriate language for gender and sexual identities and histories.

TABLE 26.4   Continuing Education Resources for LGBTQ+ Competent Care

Provider education	Association of American Medical Colleges (AAMC): Videos and resources on diversity and inclusion: www.aamc.org/initiatives/diversity/431388/videos.html
	The Joint Commission Field Guide: www.jointcommission.org/-/media/enterprise/tjc/imported-resource-assets/documents/lgbtfieldguide_web_linked_verpdf.pdf?db=web&hash=1EC363A65C710BCD1D4E14ED120CB23
	National LGBT Health Education Center, Fenway Institute: www.lgbthealtheducation.org/
	Re-Examining LGBT Healthcare, National LGBT Cancer Network: www.LGBTcultcomp.org
	Lavender Health (2012) educational materials for nurse educators, including a syllabus, media references, and learning activities: https://lavenderhealth.org
	National Coalition for LGBT Health general health information, fact sheets, and annual meeting focused on LGBT health: https://healthlgbt.org

TABLE 26.4	Continuing Education Resources for LGBTQ+ Competent Care—cont'd
	Substance Abuse and Mental Health Services Administration (SAMHSA) (2012) top health issues for LGBT populations information and resource kit: https://store.samhsa.gov/system/files/sma12-4684.pdf *LGBTQ Cultures: What Health Care Professionals Need to Know About Sexual and Gender Diversity* (Eliason & Chinn, 2015)
Transgender care	World Professional Association for Transgender Health (WPATH): www.wpath.org UCSF Center of Excellence for Transgender Health: www.transhealth.ucsf.edu *Endocrine Treatment of Gender-Dysphoric/Gender-Incongruent Persons: An Endocrine Society, Clinical Practice Guideline* (Hembree et al., 2017)
LGBT advocacy	GLMA: Health Professionals Advancing LGBTQ Equality: www.glma.org National Gay and Lesbian Task Force: www.thetaskforce.org National Resource Center on LGBT Aging: www.lgbtagingcenter.org Services and advocacy for LGBT elders: www.sageusa.org Human Rights Campaign—includes Healthcare Equality Index (HEI) with guidelines and hospital rankings: www.hrc.org

References: Radix, A., & Maingi, S. (2018). LGBT cultural competence and interventions to help oncology nurses and other health care providers. *Seminars in Oncology Nursing, 34*(1), 80-89; Bosse, J.D., Nesteby, J.A., & Randall, C.E. (2015). Integrating sexual minority health issues into a health assessment class. *Journal of Professional Nursing, 31*(6), 498-507.

HEALTH CARE ORGANIZATIONS AND POLICY

In the absence of comprehensive state and federal nondiscrimination laws for LGBTQ+ people, hospitals, health systems, and other health care organizations can take the initiative to protect their employees, patients, and visitors with policies prohibiting discrimination based on SOGI. These policies establish an organizational culture and commitment to promote inclusion and a safe environment for LGBTQ+ communities. Many LGBTQ+ individuals, and especially transgender people, report experiencing a hostile health care environment due to discrimination and lack of respect by providers, contributing to avoidance of care and inadequate care (Grant et al., 2010; Radix & Maingi, 2018).

Notably, nurses have stepped up to address the harmful effects of discrimination that has pervaded many workplaces where nurses are employed (see Table 26.5 showing a LGBTQ+ Welcoming and Inclusive Services Checklist developed by nurses for nurses). For further recommendations, refer to the Healthcare Equality Index Scoring Criteria, Fenway Health "Ten Things: Creating Inclusive Environments for LGBT People," and the GLMA Nursing Section Workplace Climate Scale (www.hrc.org/hei/hei-scoring-criteria).

TABLE 26.5	LGBTQ+ Welcoming and Inclusive Services Checklist (Amended From Chapter 78 in 7th edition)	
Yes	**No**	**Institution or Agency Policies and Procedures**
☐	☐	We have a nondiscrimination policy for staff members that includes sexual orientation and gender identity
☐	☐	We have a nondiscrimination policy for patients that includes sexual orientation and gender identity
☐	☐	Our mission statement is inclusive; it names LGBTQ+ people
☐	☐	We offer domestic partner benefits to LGBTQ+ employees
☐	☐	Patient confidentiality policies include how to deal with patients who do not want information about sexuality or gender on their records
☐	☐	Our sexual harassment policy includes LGBTQ+ issues
☐	☐	We have a procedure for staff or patients to grieve issues of discrimination based on sexuality and/or gender

Continued

TABLE 26.5   LGBTQ+ Welcoming and Inclusive Services Checklist (Amended From Chapter 78 in 7th edition)—cont'd

Yes	No	Institution or Agency Policies and Procedures
☐	☐	Written notice is given to patients about when and for what reason information about them may be disclosed to a third party
		Staff Training/Conduct
☐	☐	All staff get basic training on LGBTQ+ people and issues at least once, and ideally ongoing
☐	☐	Some staff get advanced training
☐	☐	At least one staff member has expertise in working with LGBTQ+ patients
☐	☐	The board and senior management are actively engaged. This may take the shape of an LGBTQ+ task force or advisory group that works with the board and senior management as a "champion."
☐	☐	All staff treat LGBTQ+ patients with respect and honor confidentiality
☐	☐	Staff members know how to intervene when patients act in a discriminatory manner to LGBTQ+ patients or their families
		Inclusive Language: Forms/Assessments/Treatment
☐	☐	Written forms have inclusive language and encourage disclosure
☐	☐	Assessments are inclusive and encourage discussion of whether gender or sexuality issues need to be addressed in treatment
☐	☐	Case management, treatment, and aftercare plans include issues related to sexuality and gender if appropriate
☐	☐	Staff members are prepared to obtain an inclusive sexual history from all patients
☐	☐	Treatment groups, social activities, and all aspects of the institution are safe for LGBTQ+ patients (receptionists, laboratory technicians, housekeepers, ward clerks, kitchen staff, clergy)
		Visibility of LGBTQ+ People and Issues
☐	☐	We advertise employment opportunities in LGBTQ+ publications
☐	☐	The workplace has a defined and visible interest/support group that provides a safe space for LGBTQ+ nurses and allies to gather, network, and socialize.
☐	☐	We have openly LGBTQ+ people on staff
☐	☐	We have openly LGBTQ+ people on the board of directors, community advisory panels, agency task forces, and so on
☐	☐	We have openly LGBTQ+ people as volunteers, sponsors, mentors
☐	☐	Our nondiscrimination policy that includes LGBTQ+ is prominently displayed
☐	☐	Families of LGBTQ+ patients are included in visitation policies and decision making
☐	☐	LGBTQ+ issues are discussed in treatment groups, health education sessions, case management sessions, and other group settings when appropriate
☐	☐	Posters, pamphlets, magazines, and other materials reflect our LGBTQ+ patients
☐	☐	We do outreach/market our services to local LGBTQ+ communities
		Resources and Linkages
☐	☐	We have checked our referral sources to make sure that they are LGBTQ+-sensitive (home care, clinics for follow-up care, community agencies, and so on)
☐	☐	We have linkages to our local LGBTQ+ community
☐	☐	We screen clergy, guest speakers, volunteers, mentors, sponsors, and so on to make sure they know that we are welcoming and inclusive of LGBTQ+ people

RECOMMENDATIONS

Nurses are well situated to advocate for LGBTQ+ rights within communities and at state and national levels worldwide. The following are key recommendations that provide a focus for nursing policy related to LGBTQ+ populations.

Research

- Create a strong LGBTQ+ research agenda.
- Continually work to identify current gaps in knowledge and to determine areas of need and take action to fill these gaps.

- Advocate within nursing research organizations to increase emphasis on LGBTQ+ health disparities.
- Actively recruit faculty, researchers, and students who will pursue LGBTQ+ research topics.
- Advocate for SOGI data collection in electronic health records, research, and in local and national surveys.

Public and Organizational Policy

- Take a lead in nursing organizations to take strong actions and develop strong statements in support of LGBTQ+ communities.
- Pressure health care organizations and institutions of higher learning to create policies that foster environments that are safe and affirming for LGBTQ+ individuals.
- Hold organizations accountable for following protective and affirming LGBTQ+ policies.
- Advocate for nondiscrimination policies (local, state, national) on housing, employment, K-12 education, military, health care organizations, businesses, nursing homes, assisted living.
- Advocate for a ban on any practice that harms LGBTQ+ people, such as conversion therapy or limiting access to bathrooms based on gender identity.
- Call for insurance coverage that is inclusive of LGBTQ+ needs, particularly transition/gender-affirming treatment and reproductive technology access.
- Advocate for all agencies that provide services to children, youth, and the older population to recognize and provide services appropriate for LGBTQ+ people.

Nursing Education

- Develop accreditation standards and take leadership to assure that LGBTQ+ health issues and care are incorporated in all educational programs at all levels.
- Develop standards that require LGBTQ+ content in continuing education offered through health care organizations.
- Create policies that foster a safe and affirming environment for LGBTQ+ students, faculty, and staff.
- Include questions that test for competency and knowledge of LGBTQ+ care and disparities in all licensing examinations.
- Recruit and retain LGBTQ+ faculty, staff, and students in nursing schools.

Nursing Practice and the Care Environment

- Develop policies that require adequate LGBTQ+ competencies for all nurses and others providing direct health care services.
- Develop organizational policies that support open and welcoming environments for LGBTQ+ people and families.

- Develop data collection forms that are LGBTQ+ inclusive.
- Create all-gender and/or single stall restrooms that are safe for all regardless of gender identity or expression.
- Develop policies to enforce nondiscrimination and anti-bullying that include safe reporting avenues and outline clear consequences when discrimination occurs.
- Recruit and retain LGBTQ+ staff.

CONCLUSION

Nurses are in an exciting yet precarious moment in time. There has been a huge increase in LGBTQ+ research, affirming national policy, and nursing literature. On the other hand, negative attitudes about LGBTQ+ communities persist, especially toward transgender individuals (Brown, 2017; Norton & Herek, 2013). Nursing has a great opportunity as well as a great responsibility to build on positive momentum and make change in research, education, policy, and practice to take us down a road toward equity.

DISCUSSION QUESTIONS

- Identify and discuss resources available in your community to serve LGBTQ+ people.
- Discuss ways your work setting can be more supportive of LGBTQ+ people.
- Discuss the reasons for LGBTQ+ health disparities and ways to address them. How might you contribute?
- Discuss how you can make your institution friendlier to LGBTQ+ patients and staff.

REFERENCES

Agarwal, C.A., Scheefer, M.F., Wright, L.N., Walzer, N.K., & Rivera, A. (2018). Quality of life improvement after chest wall masculinization in female-to-male transgender patients: A prospective study using the BREAST-Q and Body Uneasiness Test. *Journal of plastic, reconstructive & aesthetic surgery: JPRAS, 71*(5), 651–657.

American Academy of Nursing. (2015a). American Academy of Nursing position statement on reparative therapy. *Nursing Outlook, 63*(3), 368–369.

American Academy of Nursing. (2015b). Position statement: Employment discrimination based on sexual orientation and gender identity. *Nursing Outlook, 63*(3), 366–367.

American Nurses Association Center for Ethics and Human Rights. (2018). *Policy statement: Nursing advocacy for LGBTQ+ populations.* American Nurses Association. Retrieved from www.nursingworld.org/~49866e/globalassets/practiceandpolicy/ethics/nursing-advocacy-for-lgbtq-populations.pdf.

Berkowitz, B. (August 8, 2017). *Letter to Secretary Mathis.* Retrieved from https://higherlogicdownload.s3.amazonaws.com/AANNET/c8a8da9e-918c-4dae-b0c6-6d630c46007f/UploadedImages/docs/Policy%20Resources/Cosigned%20Letters/2017_Ltr_DoD_Secy_Trans_8_8_17.pdf.

Berman, M., & Phillips, A. (March 30, 2017). North Carolina governor signs bill repealing and replacing transgender bathroom law amid criticism. *The Washington Post.* Retrieved from www.washingtonpost.com/news/post-nation/wp/2017/03/30/north-carolina-lawmakers-say-theyve-agreed-on-a-deal-to-repeal-the-bathroom-bill/.

Bonvicini, K.A. (2017). LGBT healthcare disparities: What progress have we made? *Patient Education and Counseling, 100*(12), 2357–2361.

Bosse, J.D., Nesteby, J.A., & Randall, C.E. (2015). Integrating sexual minority health issues into a health assessment class. *Journal of Professional Nursing: Official Journal of the American Association of Colleges of Nursing, 31*(6), 498–507.

Bowerman, M., May, A., & Rossma, S. (April 22, 2017). Should the definition of infertility be more inclusive? *USA Today.* Retrieved from www.usatoday.com/story/news/nation-now/2017/04/22/same-sex-couples-covered-infertility-insurance/100644092/.

Brown, A. (June 13, 2017). *5 Key findings about LGBT Americans.* Pew Research Center. Retrieved from www.pewresearch.org/fact-tank/2017/06/13/5-key-findings-about-lgbt-americans/.

Cahill, S.R., & Makadon, H.J. (2017). If they don't count us, we don't count: Trump administration rolls back sexual orientation and gender identity data collection. *LGBT Health, 4*(3), 171–173.

Carabez, R., Eliason, M.J., & Martinson, M. (2016). Nurses' knowledge about transgender patient care: A qualitative study. *ANS: Advances in Nursing Science, 39*(3), 257–271.

Choi, S.K., Wilson, B.D.M., Shelton, J., & Gates, G.J. (2015). *Serving our youth 2015: The needs and experiences of lesbian, gay, bisexual, transgender, and questioning youth experiencing homelessness.* The Williams Institute with True Colors Fund. Retrieved from https://williamsinstitute.law.ucla.edu/wp-content/uploads/Serving-Our-Youth-June-2015.pdf.

Earnshaw, V.A., Bogart, L.M., Poteat, V.P., Reisner, S.L., & Schuster, M.A. (2016). Bullying among lesbian, gay, bisexual, and transgender youth. *Pediatric Clinics of North America, 63*(6), 999–1010.

Eliason, M.J., Dibble, S.L., & DeJoseph, J. (2010). Nursing's silence on lesbian, gay, bisexual, and transgender issues. *ANS: Advances in Nursing Science, 33*(3), 206–218.

Emlet, C.A., & Fredriksen-Goldsen, K.I. (2017). Green light given to more research on health disparities in LGBT elders. *Aging Today: The Bimonthly Newspaper of the American Society on Aging, 38*(1), 13.

Facing barriers: Experiences of LGBT people of color in Colorado. (n.d.). One Colorado. Retrieved from www.one-colorado.org/wp-content/uploads/2013/10/LGBT_POC_SurveyResults2mb.pdf.

Felitti, V. J., Anda, R. F., Nordenberg, D., Williamson, D. F., Spitz, A. M., Edwards, V., ... & Marks, J.S. (1998). Relationship of childhood abuse and household dysfunction to many of the leading causes of death in adults: The Adverse Childhood Experiences (ACE) Study. *American Journal of Preventive Medicine, 14*(4), 245–258. Retrieved from www.ajpmonline.org/article/S0749-3797(98)00017-8/fulltext.

Fenway Health. (May 2, 2019). *Trump Administration finalizes rule that will make it harder for LGBT people to access health care.* Retrieved from https://fenwayhealth.org/trump-administration-finalizes-rule-that-will-make-it-harder-for-lgbt-people-to-access-health-care/.

Flentje, A., Heck, N.C., & Cochran, B.N. (2014). Experiences of ex-ex-gay individuals in sexual reorientation therapy: reasons for seeking treatment, perceived helpfulness and harmfulness of treatment, and post-treatment identification. *Journal of homosexuality, 61*(9), 1242–1268.

Fredriksen-Goldsen, K.I., Kim, H., Emlet, C.A., Muraco, A., Erosheva, E.A., Hoy-Ellis, C.P., Goldsen, J., et al. (2017). *The aging and health report: Disparities and resilience among lesbian, gay, bisexual, and transgender older adults.* Retrieved from www.age-pride.org/wordpress/wp-content/uploads/2011/05/Full-Report-FINAL-11-16-11.pdf.

Gender Spectrum: Education. (n.d.). Gender Spectrum. Retrieved from www.genderspectrum.org/resources/education-2/.

Grant, J.M., Mottet, L.A., Tanis, J., Herman, J.L., Harrison, J., Keisling, M., et al. (2010). *National Transgender Discrimination Survey report on health and health care.* National Center for Transgender Equality and the National Gay and Lesbian Task Force. Retrieved from www.kwncbxw.thetaskforce.org/downloads/resources_and_tools/ntds_report_on_health.pdf.

Gruberg, S., Bewkes Frank J., Franke, K., & Markham, C. (April 3, 2018). *Religious liberty for a select few—Center for American Progress.* Center for American Progress. Retrieved from www.americanprogress.org/issues/lgbt/reports/2018/04/03/448773/religious-liberty-select/.

Hafeez, H., Zeshan, M., Tahir, M.A., Jahan, N., & Naveed, S. (2017). Health care disparities among lesbian, gay, bisexual, and transgender youth: A literature review. *Cureus, 9*(4), e1184.

Harrell, B.R., & Sasser, J.T. (2018). Sexual and gender minority health: Nursing's overdue coming out. *International Journal of Nursing Studies, 79*, A1–A4.

Hembree, W. C., Cohen-Kettenis, P. T., Gooren, L., Hannema, S. E., Meyer, W. J., Murad, M. H., Rosenthal, S. M., ... & T'Sjoen, G.G. (2017). Endocrine treatment of gender-dysphoric/gender-incongruent persons: An Endocrine Society clinical practice guideline. *Journal of Clinical Endocrinology & Metabolism, 102*(11). 3869 -3903.

Hess, J., Breidenstein, A., Henkel, A., Tschirdewahn, S., Rehme, C., Teufel, M., ... & Hadaschik, B. (2018). Satisfaction, quality of life and psychosocial resources of male to female transgender after gender reassignment surgery. *European Urology Supplements, 17*(2), e1748.

House Bill 2. (2016). Retrieved from www.ncleg.net/Sessions/2015E2/Bills/House/PDF/H2v4.pdf.

Human Rights Campaign. (June 7, 2018a). *State maps of laws and policies: Employment.* Retrieved from www.hrc.org/state-maps/employment.

Human Rights Campaign. (June 11, 2018b). *State maps of laws and policies: Housing.* Retrieved from www.hrc.org/state-maps/housing.

Human Rights Campaign. (June 11, 2018c). *State maps of laws and policies: Public accommodations.* Retrieved from www.hrc.org/state-maps/public-accommodations.

Human Rights Campaign. (July 25, 2019a). *State maps of laws and policies: Conversion therapy.* Retrieved from www.hrc.org/state-maps/conversion therapy/.

Human Rights Campaign. (January 15, 2019b). *State maps of laws and policies: Education.* Retrieved from www.hrc.org/statemaps/education.

Human Rights Campaign. (October 1, 2019c). *Transgender military service.* Retrieved from www.hrc.org/resources/transgender-military-service/.

Institute of Medicine. (2011). *The health of lesbian, gay, bisexual, and transgender people: Building a foundation for better understanding.* [Report brief.] Retrieved from www.nationalacademies.org/hmd/~/media/Files/Report%20Files/2011/The-Health-of-Lesbian-Gay-Bisexual-and-Transgender-People/LGBT%20Health%202011%20Report%20Brief.pdf.

International Society of Psychiatric-Mental Health Nurses Diversity and Equity Committee. (2008). *International Society of Psychiatric-Mental Health Nurses (ISPN) position statement on reparative therapy.* Retrieved from www.ispn-psych.org/assets/docs/ps-reparativetherapy.pdf.

James, S.E., Herman, J.L., Rankin, S., Keisling, M., Mottet, L., & Anafi, M. (2016). *The report of the 2015 US Transgender Survey: Executive summary.* National Center for Transgender Equality. Retrieved from www.transequality.org/sites/default/files/docs/USTS-Full-Report-FINAL.PDF.

The Joint Commission. (November 8, 2011). *Advancing effective communication, cultural competence, and patient- and family-centered care for the lesbian, gay, bisexual and transgender (LGBT) community: A field guide.* Retrieved from www.jointcommission.org/assets/1/18/LGBTFieldGuide.pdf.

Kattari, S.K., Whitfield, D.L., Eugene Walls, N., Langenderfer-Magruder, L., & Ramos, D. (2016). Policing gender through housing and employment discrimination: Comparison of discrimination experiences of transgender and cisgender LGBQ individuals. *Journal of the Society for Social Work and Research.* Chicago: University of Chicago Press. Retrieved from www.journals.uchicago.edu/doi/10.1086/686920.

Keepnews, D.M. (2011). Lesbian, gay, bisexual and transgender (LGBT) health issues and nursing: Moving toward an agenda. *ANS: Advances in Nursing Science, 34,* 163–170.

Kosciw, J.G., Greytak, E.A., Giga, N.M., Villenas, C., & Danischewski, D.J. (2015). *GLSEN 2015 National School Climate Survey (NSCS) executive summary: The experiences of lesbian, gay, bisexual, transgender, and queer youth in our nation's schools.* GLSEN. Retrieved from www.glsen.org/sites/default/files/GLSEN%202015%20National%20School%20Climate%20Survey%20%28NSCS%29%20-%20Executive%20Summary.pdf.

Lim, F., Johnson, M., & Eliason, M.J. (2015). A national survey of faculty knowledge, experience, and readiness for teaching lesbian, gay, bisexual, and transgender health in baccalaureate nursing programs. *Nursing Education Perspectives, 36*(3), 144–152.

Maril, R. (June 22, 2017). *HRC marks victory for older LGB Americans.* Human Rights Campaign. Retrieved from www.hrc.org/blog/hrc-marks-victory-for-older-lgb-americans-hhs-to-restore-sexual-orientation/.

McConnell, E.A., Birkett, M.A., & Mustanski, B. (2015). Typologies of social support and associations with mental health outcomes among LGBT youth. *LGBT Health, 2*(1), 55–61.

McCormick, A., Schmidt, K., & Terrazas, S.R. (2016). Foster family acceptance: Understanding the role of foster family acceptance in the lives of LGBTQ youth. *Children and Youth Services Review, 61,* 69–74. Retrieved from www.sciencedirect.com/science/article/pii/S0190740915301195.

McNeil, J., Bailey, L., Ellis, S., Morton, J., & Regan, M. (2012). *Trans Mental Health Study 2012.* UK Equality Network. Retrieved from www.gires.org.uk/wp-content/uploads/2014/08/trans_mh_study.pdf.

Missed opportunities: Youth homelessness in America. (2018). Voices of Youth Count. Retrieved from http://voicesofyouthcount.org/brief/national-estimates-of-youth-homelessness/.

Movement Advancement Project, & Sage. (2017). *Understanding issues facing LGBT older adults.* MAP: Movement Advancement Project. Retrieved from www.lgbtmap.org/policy-and-issue-analysis/understanding-issues-facing-lgbt-older-adults.

Necati, Y. (April 6, 2018). The 2020 US census will fail to recognise all LGBT+ people who aren't currently in a same sex relationship. *The Independent.* Retrieved from www.independent.co.uk/news/world/americas/us-census-lgbt-same-sex-relationship-recognise-donald-trump-a8292561.html.

Norton, A.T., & Herek, G.M. (2013). Heterosexuals' attitudes toward transgender people: Findings from a national probability sample of U.S. adults. *Sex Roles, 68*(11), 738–753.

Pérez-Stable, E.J. (October 6, 2016). *Director's message: Sexual and gender minorities formally designated as a health disparity population for research purposes.* NIH National Institute on Minority Health and Health Disparities. Retrieved from www.nimhd.nih.gov/about/directors-corner/message.html.

Pruden, H. (October 26, 2016). *UBC TEFA talks Two Spirit with Harlan Pruden.* [Video]. Retrieved from https://twospirit-journal.com/?p=659.

Radix, A., & Maingi, S. (2018). LGBT cultural competence and interventions to help oncology nurses and other health care providers. *Seminars in Oncology Nursing, 34*(1), 80-89.

Reid, G. (April 16, 2018). *After a grim year for LGBT rights, the way forward.* Human Rights Watch. Retrieved from www.hrw.org/news/2018/04/16/after-grim-year-lgbt-rights-way-forward.

Roberts, A.L., Rosario, M., Corliss, H.L., Koenen, K.C., & Austin, S.B. (2012). Childhood gender nonconformity: A risk indicator for childhood abuse and posttraumatic stress in youth. *Pediatrics, 129*(3), 410-417.

Ryan, C., Russell, S.T., Huebner, D., Diaz, R., & Sanchez, J. (2010). Family acceptance in adolescence and the health of LGBT young adults. *Journal of Child and Adolescent Psychiatric Nursing: Official Publication of the Association of Child and Adolescent Psychiatric Nurses, Inc, 23*(4), 205-213.

Schatz, B. (2017). *Restore Honor to Service Members Act.* Retrieved from www.congress.gov/bill/115th-congress/senate-bill/1366.

Singh, S., Durso, L.E., & Tax, A. (March 20, 2017). The Trump administration is rolling back data collection on LGBT older adults. Center for American Progress. Retrieved from www.americanprogress.org/issues/lgbt/news/2017/03/20/428623/trump-administration-rolling-back-data-collection-lgbt-older-adults/.

Sterzing, P.R., Ratliff, G.A., Gartner, R.E., McGeough, B.L., & Johnson, K.C. (2017). Social ecological correlates of polyvictimization among a national sample of transgender, genderqueer, and cisgender sexual minority adolescents. *Child Abuse & Neglect, 67,* 1-12.

U.S. Supreme Court. (June 26, 2015). *Obergefell v. Hodges,* 576 U.S. ____ (2015). *Justia Law.* Retrieved from https://supreme.justia.com/cases/federal/us/576/14-556/opinion3.html.

U.S. Surrogacy Law by State. (n.d.). *The surrogacy experience.* Retrieved from www.thesurrogacyexperience.com/u-s-surrogacy-law-by-state.html.

Wilson, B.D.M., Cooper, K., Kastanis, A., & Nezhad, S. (2014). *Sexual and gender minority youth in foster care: Assessing disproportionality and disparities in Los Angeles.* Retrieved from https://escholarship.org/uc/item/6mg3n153.

ONLINE RESOURCES

Fenway Health Institute
http://fenwayhealth.org/the-fenway-institute/
GLMA: Health Professionals Advancing LGBT Health Equality
http://glma.org
Human Rights Campaign
www.hrc.org
Lavender Health
https://lavenderhealth.org

27

Reproductive Health Policy

Carol F. Roye and Monica R. McLemore

"You cannot have maternal health without reproductive health."

Hillary Clinton

Reproductive health is a foundation of public health. Since 2002, the countries of the United Nations (UN) sought to determine the highest priorities for promoting health and reducing poverty globally. In 2015 the UN member states adopted the 2030 Agenda for Sustainable Development that includes 17 Sustainable Development Goals (UN, 2015). Several are specific to the health and well-being of people with capacity for reproduction, including gender equality, good health and well-being, and reduced inequalities. These goals are essential to improving maternal and child health and to ensure reproductive well-being for people of all ages.

When viewed as a human rights framework, reproductive justice posits that individuals have a human right to have children and to determine the conditions under which they birth (Ross & Solinger, 2017). Individuals have a human right to decide if they will become pregnant or not, have a baby, and have the full range of options for preventing or ending pregnancies. In addition, individuals have a right to parent the children they already have with dignity, free from violence from other individuals and the government. Finally, individuals have the human right to disassociate sex from reproduction. Using this framework, it is easier to understand that reproductive health serves as a barometer for the health of a nation.

HISTORICAL PERSPECTIVES ON WOMEN'S HEALTH AND U.S. POLICY

In the second half of the 20th century, women's health[a]—defined here as access to the full range of reproductive health services, including abortion, adoption, contraception, and infertility treatment—became a controversial topic that was viewed through a religious lens. However, this had not been the case earlier in American history. Until the middle of the 19th century, legal abortion, like so much else in this country, was governed by British common law. This held that abortion was criminal only if performed without due cause after the woman felt fetal movement, which usually occurs at about the 16th week of pregnancy. This was known as the "quickening doctrine" after the medical term for the mother's perception of fetal movement. It is not even clear that late abortions were prosecuted. In fact, in 1800 there was no American legislation at all on the subject of abortion.

Similarly, there was no legislation on contraception, because there were no medically recognized means of preventing conception (Mohr, 1979). In the early 19th century, there were no laboratory tests to reliably diagnose pregnancy. Common signs and symptoms of early pregnancy, such as absence of menstruation and nausea, can be caused by other factors. Thus a physician, or a woman herself, could take steps to correct her blocked menstrual flow. There were widely advertised products and medicines to help women restore menstruation or cure blocked or delayed menstruation. The fine print stated that the products should not be used by married women because they could cause miscarriages; this served as a signpost to women who wanted to end a pregnancy. Such was the nonchalant view of abortion that these ads could be found

---

[a]A note on language: This chapter is edited from previous versions that did not include gender-neutral language. Despite the fact that the authors recognize that gendered language is inconsistent with reproductive justice principles, we are retaining the use of *women* and *women's health* to align with past versions of this chapter.

not only in newspapers but also in the religious press (Brodie, 1994).

Many of those drugs and practices were unscientific and ineffective. Some, such as douching with carbolic acid, were downright dangerous. It was actually the concern about the danger of these methods that led to the first antiabortion laws in some states in the 1820s. Given that many of the early providers of abortion were nurses, lay midwives, and granny midwives who were committed to caring for individuals across the reproductive spectrum, the Flexner Report and the professionalism of medicine, combined with perceived danger of abortion, criminalized termination of pregnancy (Ehrenreich & English, 2010).

It also should be noted that abortion is safer than carrying a pregnancy to term (Raymond & Grimes, 2012). Furthermore, some women have always been so distressed by an unwanted, unintended, or mistimed pregnancy that they have knowingly risked their lives to end the pregnancy. Not surprisingly, then, women were accessing illegal abortions before it was decriminalized in the United States and were dying from infections from unhygienic abortions. Survivors of these procedures often became so scarred that they lost their fertility.

The story of abortion policy in the United States is long and tangled (Roye, 2014). By 1880 most states had antiabortion laws, and by 1910 every state had them except Kentucky, where the courts had outlawed the practice. Some of the laws enacted in the late 1800s remain on the books and 23 of 50 states will revert back to abortion being illegal if the 1973 *Roe v. Wade* decision is overturned (Center for Reproductive Rights, 2018).

In the mid-20th century, physicians began to agitate to legalize abortion, this time out of concern for their patients' health. Religious bodies, such as the Southern Baptist Convention, advocated for the legalization of abortion to help women who were at risk of being maimed and killed by illegal, unsafe procedures. Indeed, members of the clergy banded together and formed networks to help women access safe abortions. The best known of these, the Clergy Consultation Service on Abortion, was formed by Reverend Howard Moody, a Texas-born Baptist minister (Moody, 1971). For complex reasons, having primarily to do with politics, power, and money rather than women's health or public health, abortion became a hot button political issue after *Roe v. Wade*. Currently the introduction of laws limiting women's access to reproductive health care, and the fate of those laws, depend on who is in power in a given state and in the federal government.

Roe v. Wade has been attacked by state and federal legislators who want to overturn the law. For example, in 2000, in the case of *Stenberg v. Carhart,* a sharply divided Supreme Court struck down a Nebraska statute banning so-called partial birth abortion because the law placed an undue burden on a woman's right to have an abortion because it did not allow for an exception when the mother's health is threatened by continuing the pregnancy. Yet an almost identical federal law, the Partial-Birth Abortion Ban Act of 2003, was upheld by the Supreme Court in 2007 (Mears, 2007). A partial-birth abortion, correctly called intact dilation and evacuation, is a rare procedure typically performed to protect the mother's health or when a fetus is found to have a severe, often life-limiting congenital defect.

Despite this legal success, abortion opponents realized that it would be very difficult to have *Roe v. Wade* struck down, so they turned their efforts to the states. In some states, abortion is very difficult to access, especially for poor women, because of multiple reasons, including but not limited to distance traveled to abortion clinics, mandated waiting period between a required visit to the abortion facility and the procedure, and other Targeted Restrictions of Abortion Providers (TRAP) laws (Guttmacher, 2018b). These regulations can entail days off from work and finding transportation and childcare on multiple occasions. Other states are likely to have no abortion providers in the near future because of onerous and medically unnecessary requirements being placed on these facilities, such as a requirement that the physical building where abortions are performed meet the same standards as an ambulatory surgery center and a requirement that the abortion doctor have admitting privileges at a local hospital. Currently, women's access to abortion varies widely by the state in which they reside and remains contentious.

WHEN WOMEN'S REPRODUCTIVE HEALTH NEEDS ARE NOT MET

Infant Mortality

The infant mortality rate (IMR) in the United States is much lower than it is in the world's poorest countries; however, in 2017, the rate in the United States was higher than the rate in Saint Kitts and Nevis and other resource-poor nations (Central Intelligence Agency [CIA], 2017). Three critical factors influencing pregnancy outcomes are:

1. *Age at which women conceive.* For biological reasons, teenage mothers and mothers in their 40s are more likely than women in their 20s and 30s to have infants who do not survive.
2. *Spacing of pregnancies.* The chance of dying in infancy increases by 60% to 70% for a child born less than 2 years after an older sibling.
3. *Having too many children.* Children born fourth or higher in birth order have a threefold greater risk of dying than those lower in birth order.

In the United States, access to birth control (defined as whether or not a state pays for comprehensive contraceptive services for poor women through Medicaid) influences the IMR. A state's failure to allow Medicaid to pay for comprehensive contraceptive services is a statistically significant predictor of a higher IMR (Roye, 2014). In addition, large family size and unplanned pregnancies and births place children at risk for physical abuse and neglect (Aztlan-James, et al., 2017; Guterman, 2015). Even when you consider socioeconomic status (SES), Black women are more likely to have low birth-weight babies and preterm births (Centers for Disease Control and Prevention [CDC], 2016), which can lead to infant mortality. In states that expanded Medicaid, in response to the Patient Protection and Affordable Care Act (ACA), infant mortality decreased more than it did in nonexpansion states (Bhatt & Beck-Sagué, 2018). Clearly, one easily implemented solution to these problems is to provide women with access to the full range of contraception and safe abortions.

Maternal Mortality

Although the United States saw a sevenfold reduction in maternal mortality in the 20th century (Loudon, 2000), deaths related to pregnancy and childbirth persist even though most are preventable. Evidence shows that maternal mortality is greatly underestimated. As with infant mortality, the global ranking of the United States on maternal mortality is dismal, worse than a number of lower-resource Eastern European nations; moreover, unlike most nations, the rate in the United States has increased since 1990, whereas it has decreased in most other nations (World Bank, 2018).

Predictors of maternal mortality are similar to those for infant mortality. Recent data have shown that the Black-White disparity gap—where Black women are three to four times more likely to die from a pregnancy-related complication (CDC, 2018)—is preventable when health care professionals and teams are able to recognize signs and symptoms of deterioration (Main et al., 2017; Macdorman et al., 2016). Several efforts have been focused on raising awareness of the epidemic of maternal morbidity among Black women, including the fact that a little more than half of pregnancies in the United States are unintended (Finer et al., 2016). New data highlight an urgent need to reduce so called "mother blame" (McLemore, 2019; Scott, Britton, & McLemore, 2019; McLemore, 2018) to begin to reduce maternal morbidity and mortality. Clearly, access to comprehensive reproductive health care for all people with the capacity for pregnancy would have a significant effect on public health by improving health outcomes for mothers and children.

WHAT IS EQUITABLE REPRODUCTIVE HEALTH POLICY?

One might wonder why reproductive health deserves special attention from policy experts. First, women's unique reproductive health needs have been targeted by politicians because of the potential for pregnancy. Over the years, as reproductive health care has advanced (including contraception and abortion techniques), it has become a focus of political rhetoric and a hot-button issue. This has extended to political battles over who has control over the pregnant body, including, the criminalization of pregnancy (Paltrow & Flavin, 2013).

Second, women's reproductive health needs are a nexus where health and sex (thus sexual taboos) meet. With our history of Puritanism, sex has always been a particularly sensitive topic in the United States. Moreover, there is a misguided concern that any discussion of sex will lead to promiscuity. The context of the issue of women's health is the resurgence of orthodox religion, particularly the Religious Right, in the 1970s. Indeed, Randall Balmer, an evangelical Christian and religious historian, said that after holding a 2-year seminar on fundamentalist religions, an Ivy League university determined that: "the defining feature of fundamentalism, across religions, is an attempt to control women and their sexual behavior" (Roye, 2014). This religious influence has increased over the years, making it more difficult for women to access needed health care. It has, in many ways, overtaken the discussion of women's health and affected policymakers who now may feel that by preventing access to reproductive health care, they are taking a moral stand.

However, as we have seen, there are serious public health consequences for everyone when women are not able to access comprehensive reproductive health care. As a result of this religious influence over legislators in some states, there were more abortion restrictions enacted by states that have not been shown to improve reproductive health. As of June 1, 2018, in the United States, 1327 state level sexual and reproductive health policies had been introduced; 21 were abortion restrictions and only 75 provisions that improve access to health care were enacted (Guttmacher, 2018a). In addition, two recent reports (National Academies of Science, Engineering, and Medicine [NASEM], 2018; Ravi, 2018) have shown that limiting abortion access contributes to poor maternal health outcomes.

ABORTION POLICY AND CONTRACEPTION

There are thoughtful people on both sides of the abortion debate nowadays. Many of those who oppose legal abortion earnestly believe that abortions are tantamount to infanticide, and therefore abortions should be outlawed. However, among those who hold this view, there remains debate about whether abortion should be allowed in cases of incest, rape, or threat to the life of the mother. This is a key point because if women in need of an abortion were not able to get that care and were thus fated to die as a result of a severe complication of pregnancy, then there is room for legitimate discussion among them about whether policies banning or allowing abortion are also tantamount to killing women. Indeed, as noted previously, access to safe abortions reduces maternal and infant mortality significantly.

The ACA mandates comprehensive preventive health care for women, including contraceptive services without copays and access to contraception, particularly for poor women. Women who can afford to get health care and pay for contraception have always been able to purchase it. However, for poor women who rely on public insurance (i.e., Medicaid), access may again depend on the state in which they reside. Some states allow full access to contraception (and abortion) for poor women, although other states do not.

In 2018, several changes were enacted at the Department of Health and Human Services (DHHS) under the Trump Administration that included the installation of administrators who worked throughout their careers to restrict access to contraception and to promote abstinence-only education (Byrd, 2018). In addition, the 2019 rules for grants supported by the Title X program, which provides contraception and family planning services to low-income people who do not qualify for Medicaid, changed the eligibility for funding from programs that offer comprehensive contraception services to those offering the rhythm method of contraception and abstinence, despite their lower rates of efficacy. These funds currently support clinical providers including Planned Parenthood, some federally qualified health centers, and other public health–run clinics; however, under the new proposed rules, organizations that do not provide clinical services such as crisis pregnancy centers (also known as "fake clinics") could be eligible for funding. In 2019, states filed multiple challenges to the rule change, and its impact is under consideration in the House of Representatives. One of the authors of this chapter (MM) provided written and oral testimony to the 116th Congress in support of Title X in 2019.

Another public health issue related to contraception that became a political football is approval of over-the-counter (OTC) access to emergency contraception (EC): the morning-after pill. EC had been used successfully for years overseas before it became available in the United States. It is a very safe medication (usually 1 or 2 doses of a common birth control pill formulation), which may prevent pregnancy if taken within 3 to 5 days of unprotected intercourse. Commercial preparations include Plan B and Ella. Despite the U.S. Food and Drug Administration's scientific panel overwhelmingly agreeing that EC should be available to women OTC, it took years to receive approval

because of political opposition. The objection stemmed, in part, from the erroneous belief by some that EC causes an abortion by preventing implantation of a fertilized ovum. EC first became available OTC for women aged 18 and older, despite the evidence demonstrating that it is a safe medication for all women. In 2013 a judicial ruling finally made it legally available for adolescent and adult women of all ages.

Affordable Care Act

The ACA could dramatically improve the reproductive health landscape for women who have insurance. As noted, it mandates comprehensive preventive health care for women, including contraceptive services, without copays (White House Blog, 2013). This care was included in the ACA because of a recommendation in the Institute of Medicine's (IOM's) 2011 report *Clinical Preventative Services for Women: Closing the Gaps*, calling for women's health services be covered without copays when a network provider delivers them. It should be noted that religious organizations, with a specific religious mission, are exempt from this regulation (Liptak, 2013). However, other employers, who have for-profit, nonreligious businesses, such as Hobby Lobby, a chain of craft shops with stores across the country, sued to exempt themselves from this regulation because the employers have personal objections to contraception. In 2014 the Supreme Court ruled that the owners of "closely-held" profit-making corporations (with company shares held by one person or a small group of people) cannot be forced by the ACA to provide their employees with contraceptives that offend their religious beliefs.

In 2018, these rules were further codified within the DHHS to widen the number of employers who could claim religious exemption (National Women's Law Center [NWLC], 2018). The proposed rules were meant to protect the "conscience" of physicians and other health care providers to refuse to provide services such as care to transgender individuals or people seeking infertility treatment for same sex couples.

Reproductive Justice-Informed Policies

In 2018, more than 80 pieces of legislation were introduced to address maternal morbidity and mortality in the United States and only one was signed into law by President Trump (Mahone, 2019; Congress.gov, 2018). Many of the proposed bills addressed different aspects of factors known to be associated with poor reproductive health outcomes, including implicit bias, education and training for the health care workforce; greater access to midwives, doulas, and other health professionals; and the establishment of maternal morbidity and mortality review committees.

These policies are important and crucial to improve reproductive health outcomes but are not sufficient. Policies that support a reproductive agenda where all individuals are able to become pregnant, prevent or end pregnancies, and have supports to parent with dignity free from violence from individuals or the state are important to achieve reproductive health equity.

DISCUSSION QUESTIONS

1. Thinking about the national conversation about women's reproductive health policies nowadays, how would you respond to those who wish to limit women's access to contraception or abortion?
2. Investigate your state's policies on access to contraception and abortion for women with insurance and those without. What are your state's infant and maternal mortality rates? Discuss the possible relationship between these factors.

REFERENCES

Aztlan-James, E., McLemore, M.R., & Taylor, D. (2017). Multiple unintended pregnancies in U.S. women: A systematic review. *Women's Health Issues, 27*(4), 407-413.

Bhatt, C.B., & Beck-Saque, C.M. (2018). Medicaid expansion and infant mortality in the United States. *American Journal of Public Health, 108*(4), 565-567.

Brodie, J.F. (1994). *Contraception and abortion in nineteenth-century America.* Ithaca, NY: Cornell University Press.

Byrd, A. (2018). Trump's choice to run family planning program is staunchly anti-choice. *Colorlines.* Retrieved from www.colorlines.com/articles/trumps-appointee-run-family-planning-program-staunchly-anti-choice.

Center for Reproductive Rights. (2018). *What if Roe fell—A state-by-state alert system if Roe fell.* Retrieved from www.reproductiverights.org/what-if-roe-fell.

Centers for Disease Control and Prevention. (2016). *Infant mortality.* Retrieved from www.cdc.gov/reproductivehealth/maternalinfanthealth/infantmortality.htm.

Central Intelligence Agency. (2017). *The world factbook—Infant mortality rates, 2017.* Retrieved from www.cia.gov/library/publications/the-world-factbook/rankorder/2091rank.html.

Congress.gov. (2018). *H.R. 1318, Preventing Maternal Death Act of 2018.* Retrieved from www.congress.gov/bill/115th-congress/house-bill/1318.

Ehrenreich, B. & English, D. (2010). *Witches, midwives, & nurses* (2nd ed.). New York: Feminist Press.

Finer, L.B. & Zolna, M.R. (2016). Declines in unintended pregnancy in the United States, 2008–2011, *New England Journal of Medicine, 374*(9), 843-852.

Guterman, K. (2015). Unintended pregnancy as a predictor of child mistreatment. *Child Abuse & Neglect, 48*, 160-169.

Guttmacher Institute. (2018a). *State policy updates: Major developments in sexual and reproductive health.* Retrieved from www.guttmacher.org/state-policy.

Guttmacher Institute. (2018b). *Targeted regulation of abortion providers.* Retrieved from www.guttmacher.org/state-policy/explore/targeted-regulation-abortion-providers.

Institute of Medicine. (2011). *Clinical preventive services for women: Closing the gaps.* Washington, DC: National Academy of Sciences.

Liptak, A. (2013). Court confronts religious rights of corporations. *New York Times.* Retrieved from www.nytimes.com/2013/11/25/us/court-confronts-religious-rights-of-corporations.html.

Loudon, I. (2000). Maternal mortality in the past and its relevance to developing countries today. *American Journal of Clinical Nutrition, 72*(1), 241S.

Macdorman, M.F., Declercq, E., Cabral, H., & Morton, C. (2016). Recent increases in the U.S. maternal mortality rate: Disentangling trends from measurement issues. *Obstetrics & Gynecology, 128*(3), 447-455.

Mahone, R. (2019, April 12). State legislators are finally doing something about the Black maternal health crisis. *Rewire. News.* Retrieved from https://rewire.news/article/2019/04/12/black-maternal-health-is-still-in-crisis-legislators-are-finally-taking-notice/.

Main, E.K., Cape, V., Abreo, A., Vasher, J., Woods, A., Carpenter, A., & Gould, J.B. (2017). Reduction of severe maternal morbidity from hemorrhage using a state perinatal quality collaborative. *American Journal of Obstetrics and Gynecology, 216*(3), 298.e1-298.e11.

McLemore, M.R. (2018). *What blame the mother stories get wrong about birth outcomes among Black women.* Retrieved from www.centerforhealthjournalism.org/2018/02/18/what-blame-mother-stories-get-wrong-about-birth-outcomes-among-black-moms.

McLemore, M.R. (2019). To prevent women from dying in childbirth, first stop blaming them. *Scientific American, 5*(320), 48-51.

Mears, B. (2007). Justices uphold ban on abortion procedure. *CNN.com.* Retrieved from www.cnn.com/2007/LAW/04/18/scotus.abortion/.

Mohr, J. (1979). *Abortion in America: The origins and evolution of national policy.* New York: Oxford University Press.

Moody, H. (1971). Abortion: Woman's right and legal problem. *Theology Today, 28*(3), 337-346.

National Academies of Science, Engineering, and Medicine. (2018). *The quality and safety of abortion care in the United States.* Washington, DC: National Academies Press. Retrieved from http://nationalacademies.org/hmd/Reports/2018/the-safety-and-quality-of-abortion-care-in-the-united-states.aspx

National Women's Law Center. (2018). *Trump administration proposes sweeping rule to permit personal beliefs to dictate health care.* Retrieved from https://nwlc.org/resources/trump-administration-proposes-sweeping-rule-to-permit-personal-beliefs-to-dictate-health-care/.

Paltrow, L. & Flavin, J. (2013). Arrests of and forced interventions on pregnant women in the United States, 1973-2005: Implications for women's legal status and public health. *Journal of Health, Politics, Policy, and Law, 38*(2), 299-343.

Ravi, A. (2018). *Limiting abortion access contributes to poor maternal health outcomes.* Center for American Progress. Retrieved from www.americanprogress.org/issues/women/reports/2018/06/13/451891/limiting-abortion-access-contributes-poor-maternal-health-outcomes/

Raymond, E.G., & Grimes, D.A. (2012). The comparative safety of legal induced abortion and childbirth in the United States. *Obstetrics and Gynecology, 119*(2/1), 215-219.

Ross, L., & Solinger, R. (2017). *Reproductive justice: A new vision for the 21st century.* Oakland, CA: University of California Press.

Roye, C. (2014*). A woman's right to know.* Pleasantville, NY: Frances Price Enterprises.

Scott, K.A., Britton, L., & McLemore, M.R. (2019). The ethics of perinatal care for Black women: dismantling the structural racism in "mother blame" narratives. *Journal of Perinatal and Neonatal Nursing, 33*(2),108-115.

United Nations. (2015). *The 2030 agenda for sustainable development.* Retrieved from https://sustainabledevelopment.un.org/?menu=1300.

White House Blog. (2013). *How the Affordable Care Act improves the lives of American women.* Retrieved from www.whitehouse.gov/blog/2013/10/24/how-affordable-care-act-improves-lives-american-women.

World Bank. (2018). *Databank: World development indicators.* Retrieved from http://databank.worldbank.org/data/reports.aspx?source=2&series=SH.STA.MMRT&country=.

ONLINE RESOURCES

Advancing New Standards in Reproductive Health
www.ansirh.org
Alan Guttmacher Institute
www.guttmacher.org
Gynuity
www.gynuity.org
The Henry J. Kaiser Family Foundation
www.kff.org
Ibis Reproductive Health
www.ibisreproductivehealth.org
SisterSong Reproductive Justice Collective
www.sistersong.net
United States Health Resources and Services Administration
www.hrsa.gov/womensguidelines

28

Public and Population Health: Promoting the Health of the Public

Susan Swider and Heide Cygan[a]

> *"What public health really is is a trust....It's a trust between the government and the people."*
>
> **Laurie Garrett**

PUBLIC HEALTH, POLICY, AND NURSING

Public health is the science of protecting the health of populations and improving the conditions of the communities in which they work, play, and live (CDC Foundation, 2018). The seminal report *The Future of Public Health* defined public health as "What we as a society do collectively to assure the conditions in which people can be healthy" (Institute of Medicine [IOM], 1988). By its very nature, public health addresses health for all people and includes services and policies designed to meet the IOM definition.

Nurses play a crucial role in the robust, interdisciplinary, public health workforce charged with assuring the health of the public. In fact, nurses make up the largest segment of the public health workforce (American Public Health Association [APHA], 2013), with approximately 41,000 public health nurses working in state and local health departments, making up 18% of the workforce (Beck, Boulton, & Coronado, 2014). Public health nurses possess a wide range of skills, working with populations and communities through disease surveillance, epidemiology, health promotion and education, community- and individual-level diagnostics and treatment, and policy development. They provide direct patient care to underserved populations, and engage in population-level health promotion and prevention activities. However, while nurses are in an ideal position to influence public health practice and policy, less than 6% hold leadership positions in state and local health departments, such as director or administrator (Beck & Boulton, 2016).

Historically, nurses naturally fulfilled the role of public health worker and policy influencer. Florence Nightingale may be best known as the founder of modern nursing; she also served as a public health activist, epidemiologist and statistician, and social reformer (Monteiro, 1985). Nightingale stressed health promotion and disease prevention, developing the well-known Environment Theory, which focuses on caring for the patient's environment as a means to improve health outcomes (Nightingale, 1860). She understood that health was impacted by factors such as decent housing and quality childcare, and used statistics to guide decision makers and influence policy. Nightingale applied her nursing knowledge to treat her patient population and improve the condition of the communities in which they lived—one of public health's primary missions (Monteiro, 1985).

Lilian Wald created the term "public health nurse" to describe nurses who worked outside of the hospital, in poor communities (Jewish Women's Archive, n.d.). As a public health nurse and social activist, she developed the Henry Street Settlement House in New York to address the health needs of women and children. Wald supported nurses in schools, insurance coverage for public health nursing services, and restrictions on child labor (Visiting Nurse Service of New York, 2018). As an advocate for immigrants' rights, her efforts to improve working conditions for immigrant laborers led to the creation of the New York State Bureau of Industries (Jewish Women's Archive, n.d.).

Like Nightingale and Wald, nurses must understand the role policy plays in the health of individuals and populations and in our health care system. Armed with this knowledge,

---

[a]This chapter builds on a previous chapter originally developed by Mary Mincer Hansen, PhD, RN.

nurses can advocate for evidence-based, public health policies that improve population health outcomes.

THE STATE OF PUBLIC HEALTH AND THE PUBLIC'S HEALTH

The U.S. public health system, designed to ensure conditions in which people can be healthy, has been credited with much of the improvement in life expectancy and improved health outcomes during the past 40 years (Box 28.1) (University of Pennsylvania, 2016). Key U.S. public health accomplishments include:

- Vaccine preventable diseases
- Prevention and control of infectious disease
- Tobacco control
- Maternal and infant health
- Motor vehicle safety
- Cardiovascular disease prevention
- Occupational safety
- Cancer prevention
- Childhood lead poisoning prevention
- Public health preparedness and response (Centers for Disease Control and Prevention [CDC], 2011)

Despite dramatic successes, the share of the U.S. health care budget spent on prevention and public health remains low. This is due in part to high costs of pharmaceutical and technological innovations in health care and a national focus on medical treatment rather than prevention. Whereas one-third of health care spending is attributed to hospital care, less than 3% is used for public health efforts. Total public health expenditures rose from 1.36% in 1960 to a high of 3.18% in 2002. By 2014, they had fallen to 2.65%—a decline of 17% (Himmelstein & Woolhandler, 2016). This funding disparity occurred despite data indicating that traditional

BOX 28.1 U.S. Health Outcome Improvements, 1975–2015

Between 1975 and 2015, the following improvements in U.S. health outcomes occurred:

- Life expectancy increased from 72.6 to 78.8 years
- Infant mortality rate decreased 63%, from 16.07 to 5.90 deaths per 1000 live births
- Death rates for heart disease decreased from 431.2 to 168.5 deaths per 100,000 people
- Death rates for cancer decreased from 200.1 to 158.5 deaths per 100,000 people.

Source: National Center for Health Statistics. (2017). *Health, United States, 2016: With chartbook on long-term trends in health*. Hyattsville, MD. Retrieved from www.cdc.gov/nchs/data/hus/hus16.pdf.

clinical services are responsible for roughly only 20% of health outcomes (County Health Rankings, 2016).

Although U.S. public health policies and practices have influenced improvements in population health outcomes, these outcomes are still abysmal when compared to those in peer countries (Organisation for Economic and Co-operative Development, 2018). The United States spends more money on health care ($9892 per capita in 2016) than any other nation, and compared to other high-income countries, more than double the average of $4006. This high level of spending has not resulted in better population health outcomes. Among high-income countries, the U.S. infant mortality rate is the highest at 5.8 deaths per 1000 live births (mean = 3.6 deaths/1000 live births), and the overweight and obesity rate of 70.1% is the highest (mean = 55.6%). Further, U.S. life expectancy is the lowest at 78.8 years (mean = 81.7 years). Increased spending without improved population health outcomes has precipitated a call for health care reform.

The current leading causes of death in the United States are heart disease, cancer, lower respiratory infection, accidents, and cerebrovascular diseases (Murphy, Xu, Kochanek, Curtin, & Arias, 2017). While 630,000 deaths in 2015 were attributed to heart disease, almost all of those deaths can more accurately be attributed to a combination of tobacco use, poor diet, and physical inactivity (Mokdad, Marks, Stroup, & Gerberding, 2004). Cigarette smoking is the leading, preventable cause of death, leading to 480,000 deaths per year (U.S. Department of Health and Human Services [DHHS], 2014). It is estimated that nearly half of deaths from cardiometabolic diseases are a result of dietary factors (Micha et al., 2017), and replacing sedentary time with just 10 minutes of physical activity decreases cardiovascular mortality risk (Dohm, Kwak, Oja, Sjostrom, & Hagstromer, 2018). Based on these facts, an increase in public health programs that address underlying causes of death, and not simply provide clinical services to treat the health condition, should be a practice and policy priority. Our current national health care landscape is one in which curative services are often prioritized over preventative practices. Despite the health benefits and cost-effectiveness of prevention, Americans use preventative services at merely half the recommended rate; those who are economically or socially disadvantaged seek preventative care even less (CDC, 2017). When we invest in prevention, the impact is beyond dollars saved and disease rates lessened: children grow up in families and communities that foster healthy living, adults are productive at home and at work, and businesses profit from increased community stability.

Whereas data and science provide the underpinnings for public health services, social and political values shape policies and programs. A focus of public health is achieving health equity in which all people have the opportunity to attain their highest level of health. This calls for addressing the social determinants of health (SDOH), focusing efforts on vulnerable populations, and addressing social conditions such as racism, which negatively impact health (APHA, 2015). Public health nurses are equipped with the knowledge and skills to assess and address the SDOH that contribute to underlying causes of many chronic diseases and disparities in related health outcomes for individuals and populations.

THE PUBLIC HEALTH SYSTEM

The U.S. public health system is a complex web of organizations that work together to ensure the health of the public. Public health systems are defined as "all public, private, and voluntary entities that contribute to the delivery of essential public health services within a jurisdiction" (CDC, 2018b). The public health system is a wide-ranging system of connections across organizations, including private organizations and all levels of government (local, state, and national) (Fig. 28.1).

Professional nursing organizations are a part of this complex web, and provide resources through research and practice. The Association of Public Health Nurses, the Association of Community Health Nursing Educators, and the Public Health Nursing section of the APHA all provide input into public health debates and policy development. Supported in part by the CDC, the American Association of Colleges of Nursing (AACN) provides public and population health resources as part of an effort to enhance nursing competency in public and population health (AACN, 2018a).

Local Public Health

There are over 2500 U.S. local health departments, including city, county, and tribal health departments (National Association of County & City Health Officials, 2016). Local health departments are on the front lines of public health, acting as the eyes and ears of the system. Because they derive their authority from the state, the roles and responsibilities of local health departments differ based on state policy and governing relationships. Considering that public needs vary widely across jurisdictions, local systems and

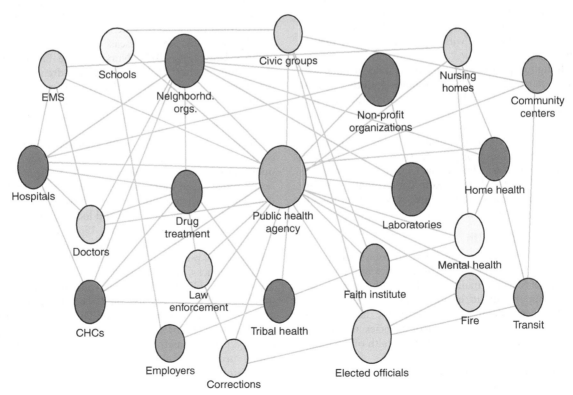

Fig. 28.1 The public health system (CDC, 2018b). *CHCs,* Community health centers; *EMS,* emergency medical services.

services are unique and diverse to meet these needs. For example, a local health department in a large, metropolitan area may offer a wide variety of services through a sophisticated system of agencies and partners. In contrast, a smaller health department is likely to provide fewer services. Local health department roles include: immunization provision, communicable disease surveillance, tuberculosis screening, food service inspection, environmental health surveillance, and school/daycare inspections (APHA, 1974). Not only do they gather and share local public health data, they also receive and analyze shared data. This reciprocal relationship is particularly evident between local and state health departments.

State/Territorial Public Health

There are 59 state/territorial health departments (Association of State & Territory Health Officials, 2017). State health departments maintain the primary responsibility for the health of the public within their geopolitical region (Public Health Law Center, 2015). At the state level, the health department is greatly influenced by elected officials as state legislatures set public health policies and appropriate funding for public health efforts. Based on policies and funding, state health departments delegate authority and resources to local health departments. In addition, the state serves as the conduit between local and federal governments and collaborates with other state health departments.

Although responsibilities vary from state-to-state, state health departments fulfill the following duties: disease surveillance and data collection, state laboratory services, disaster preparedness and response, primary prevention for populations, health care services, regulation of licensed professionals, environmental health services, and technical assistance and training for partners (including local health departments) (Public Health Law Center, 2015). Whereas the duties of local and state health departments may vary and overlap in some instances, both serve critical roles in protecting the health of the public.

Federal Public Health

Federal public health agencies serve to coordinate public health policy and response across all states and localities. They also serve as the main repository and creator of science to support public health knowledge and actions. While the key federal agency for public health is the DHHS, there are a large number of agencies and departments that work together to assure the health of the public (Table 28.1).

Public health nurses hold various positions within federal agencies. For example, within the CDC, nurses work with the Emergency Operations Center to monitor and

TABLE 28.1 DHHS Federal Public Health Agencies	
Agency/Department	Website
Centers for Disease Control and Prevention (CDC)	www.cdc.gov
Environmental Protection Agency (EPA)	www.epa.gov
Health Resource and Service Administration (HRSA)	www.hrsa.gov
Indian Health Service (IHS)	www.ihs.gov
National Vital Statistics System	www.cdc.gov/nchs/nvss/index.htm
National Institutes of Health (NIH)	www.nih.gov
Public Health Service	www.usphs.gov
United States Department of Agricultural (USDA)	www.usda.gov
United States Food and Drug Administration (FDA)	www.fda.gov

respond to national and global outbreaks such as influenza, and nurses collect and analyze data that answer questions brought forward by state health departments within the Division for Heart Disease and Stroke Prevention (Emory University, 2013). Nurses at the Environmental Protection Agency (EPA) protect children from lead exposure by developing, implementing, and evaluating community-based health promotion programs (http://whsc.emory.edu/home/publications/nursing/emory-nursing/fall2013/the-cdc-nurse.html).

Together, federal public health agencies ensure all levels of government have the capabilities to provide essential public health services. They coordinate a response when health threats span more than one state, region, or the nation. They act when solutions may be beyond state jurisdiction by collaborating with state and local governments and other relevant stakeholders (IOM, 1988). Federal agencies assist states when they lack expertise or resources to respond effectively in a public health emergency (e.g., disasters, bioterrorism attacks, or emerging diseases).

Federal public health agencies and private organizations provide resources for public health improvement across the country. For example, CDC (2018a) publishes the *Morbidity and Mortality Weekly Report (MMWR)*, the agency's primary method of sharing accurate and timely public health information and recommendations. The Community Preventive Services Task Force publishes the *Guide to Community Preventive Services*, a collection of evidence-based findings supporting community-level, public health interventions (The Community Guide, n.d.). The *Practical Playbook*, published by the de Beaumont Foundation in partnership with Duke University, CDC, and Health Resources and Services Administration (HRSA), is a web-based tool designed to facilitate public health and primary care integration through a wide variety of resources (Michener, Koo, Castrucci, & Sprague, 2016).

PUBLIC HEALTH CORE FUNCTIONS

In order to ensure conditions in which people can be healthy, public health has three core functions: assessment, policy development, and assurance (Fig. 28.2).

Assessment involves ongoing monitoring of the public's health, diagnosing and investigating health problems. *Policy development* is defined as creating and advocating for policies and interventions to improve population health outcomes, including education about public health concerns, and developing partnerships to sustain these interventions. *Assurance* is the function of ensuring that such policies are implemented and evaluated, via enforcing laws and codes, educating a competent workforce, connecting people to needed health services, conducting research into new solutions for health concerns, and providing data that feeds back into the assessment function in a quality improvement loop (CDC, 2018b).

To address all of the factors that impact health outcomes, the public health system needs to include a diverse set of stakeholders who are concerned with clinical care, innovative clinical prevention, and population or community-wide prevention. This includes understanding and addressing the SDOH, the non-clinical, social, and environmental factors known to impact health and shown to be largely responsible for poor health outcomes (Fig. 28.3). In order to increase impact on the health of the public, the public health system is moving away from episodic care toward a system that serves the public outside of traditional care settings and addresses the SDOH through implementation of interventions that reach entire populations. The public health system can then serve as coordinator for health improvement efforts across all populations (DiSalvo et al., 2017).

Policy Exemplars for Public Health

The Patient Protection and Affordable Care Act (ACA) (2010) was enacted in 2010 with a primary focus on expanding access to care as a means to improve the health of the public (see Chapter 18). Two additional aspects of the ACA critical to public health include: (1) the National Prevention Strategy (NPS), and (2) the move to a system of value-based payments.

The NPS was designed to direct the country to focus on prevention as one way of improving health, controlling costs, and enhancing client satisfaction. The strategy of the initiative "envisions a prevention-oriented society where all sectors recognize the value of health for individuals, families, and society and work together to achieve better health for Americans" (DHHS, n.d.). The NPS includes four strategic directions and seven strategic priorities to address the principle causes of early death and disability (Fig. 28.4). By encouraging all stakeholders to be involved in promoting health, the NPS engages many types of community partners such as individuals and families, businesses, churches, health care systems, and all levels of government. The strategy also addresses the SDOH, and promotes collaboration across all sectors of society to improve health for all (DHHS, n.d.).

Examples of how the NPS has been used across the nation include in Chicago, where the Chicago Department of Public Health (CDPH) developed the citywide strategic plan modeled on the NPS, called *Healthy Chicago 2.0* (Dircksen et al., 2016). This plan prioritizes health equity, collaboration, meaningful use of statistics, and addressing the SDOH. *Healthy Chicago 2.0* is a plan that involves citywide goals and concrete, actionable strategies to reach these goals through the collaboration of city agencies, businesses, community organizations, faith groups, and individuals (Dircksen et al., 2016). An example of a nurse-led, academic-practice partnership designed to reach *Healthy Chicago 2.0* goals is found in the Box 28.2.

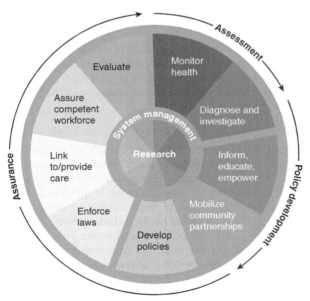

Fig. 28.2 Public health: 3 core functions and 10 essential services (CDC, 2018b).

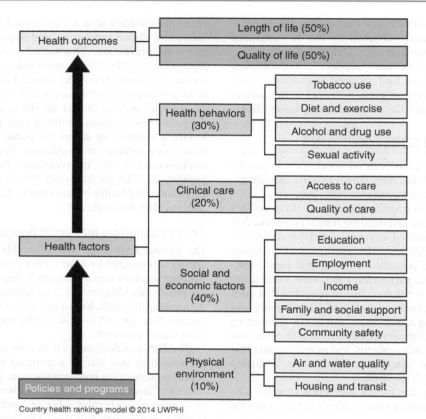

Fig. 28.3 County health rankings model (County Health Rankings, 2016).

Moving to a value-based payment system was another important aspect of the ACA. Value-based payment systems are designed to hold providers accountable for the quality and cost of services by encouraging health care providers to focus more on quality of care, rather than the quantity. The relevant ACA provisions addressing value-based payments focus on three broad areas: testing new delivery models and disseminating successful ones; encouraging the shift toward payment based on the value/outcomes of care provided; and developing resources for system-wide improvement (Centers for Medicare and Medicaid Services, 2018).

A variety of demonstration efforts for value-based payment systems funded under the ACA remain in place, as data on their impact is collected, analyzed, and disseminated (The Commonwealth Fund, 2015). These include primary care transformation initiatives, state-level demonstration projects, model Accountable Care Organizations, and bundled payment for care improvement initiatives. Studies have also demonstrated the contributions of nurses

to a value-based payment system (Koshinsky et al., 2018). Preliminary results are positive and much of the payment reforms remain intact, even as the overall ACA has been debated for its expansion of coverage initiatives (The Commonwealth Fund, 2015).

The Shift to Population Health and the Triple Aim

Early in the 21st century, the concept of "public health" began to shift to "population health." Kindig and Stoddart (2003) offered one of the earliest definitions of *population health*: "the health outcomes of a group of individuals, including the distribution of such outcomes within the group" (p. 381). Population health includes patterns in the SDOH and health outcomes, as well as the policies and programs that link the two. This definition differs from that of public health, in that it addresses health outcomes for *groups* of individuals (whether by location, demographics, or diagnoses), and examines a wide variety of factors impacting outcomes, such as the SDOH, across the continuum of care. The concept of population health is not

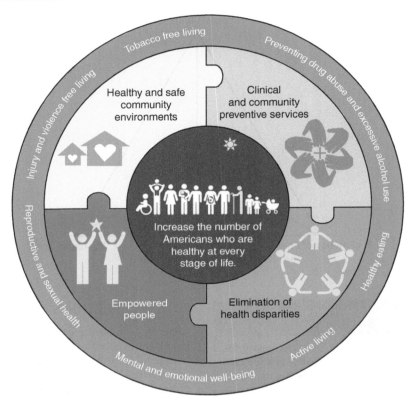

Fig. 28.4 The National Prevention Strategy (DHHS, n.d.).

BOX 28.2 Public Health Nurses and Health Chicago 2.0: Healthy Students Are Better Learners

Public health nurses at an academic institution in Chicago developed a partnership with Chicago Public Schools (CPS) to address goals set forth by *Healthy Chicago 2.0* (Dircksen et al., 2016) through increased access to sexual health education for Chicago youth. This partnership aims to address several priorities of *Healthy Chicago 2.0*, including education as a social determinant of health (SDOH), and the health outcome areas of "Strengthening Adolescent and Child Health" and "Preventing the Burden of Infectious Disease." Since 2014, graduate nursing students have taught comprehensive, medically accurate sexual health education to over 2500 CPS students across grades 4–12. As a result, CPS student knowledge has increased, and they report increased comfort in talking about sexual health with peers and parents. Through this partnership, the city moves closer to *Healthy Chicago 2.0* goals and alignment with the National Prevention Strategy (Cygan et al., 2018).

new to nurses. Public health nurses working with individuals, families, and communities identify patterns across populations, and develop, implement, and evaluate broadbased interventions (Storfjell et al., 2017). As the largest, and most trusted, profession in the nation (Gallup, 2017), it is the nursing profession's duty to promote population health.

The shift to using the term population health is related to the development and promotion of the Triple Aim framework (Institute for Healthcare Improvement [IHI], 2018). In 2007, IHI developed the Triple Aim framework to address the performance of the U.S. health care system in three dimensions: improving the health of populations, improving the patient experience and quality of health care, and decreasing the per capita cost of health care (Fig. 28.5).

Nurses work across these components to develop and implement policies and programs to create the conditions in which people can be healthy (Storfjell et al., 2017) (Box 28.3). Using this framework, organizations and health care professionals can better understand the populations they serve, empower populations to take actions that

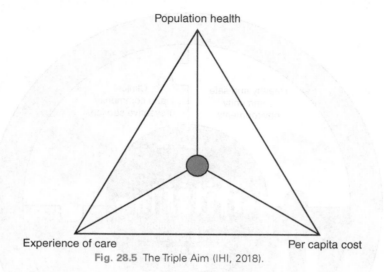

Fig. 28.5 The Triple Aim (IHI, 2018).

BOX 28.3   The Triple Aim in Action: The Role of the Nurse

Researchers from the University of Texas are making the case for Doctor of Nursing Practice (DNP)–directed care as the preferred method to reach the Triple Aim for breast cancer survivorship care. Breast cancer survivor care delivered by nurse practitioners has been shown to improve the quality of care and patient satisfaction scores. DNP-prepared nurse practitioners have the skills to collaborate with stakeholders and develop care plans that are shown to improve population health outcomes (Pandey & Nguyen, 2017). Additionally, nurse practitioners deliver "equal or better" care than physician peers at a lower cost (Pandey & Nguyen, 2017).

---

improve their health, and leverage community assets to achieve the Triple Aim.

The goals of the Triple Aim are in alignment with the definitions of public and population health and are impacted by the 10 essential public health services. Answering the call for a health care system that spends less and produces better outcomes, the Triple Aim framework has improved patient outcomes and experiences and decreased costs. As positive outcomes continue to be documented, health care leaders are calling for more policies that support Triple Aim expansion and innovation (Verma & Bhatia, 2016). It is critical that nurses understand the approach and have a voice in national advocacy efforts to promote the Triple Aim.

FUTURE DIRECTIONS

Given the complexity of the changes in health care, it is important to consider the most effective role for nurses in both public health practice and policy. Nurses can leverage their patient care expertise, reputation as the most trusted profession, and presence across all health care settings to be instrumental in developing and implementing interventions to address the SDOH and initiate upstream prevention initiatives. Encouraging nursing education, practice, and research into public and population health will have the benefits of highlighting nursing's contribution to public health outcomes and supporting those populations in achieving improved health.

DISCUSSION QUESTIONS

1. How does public health nursing practice contribute to a value-based health care reimbursement system?
2. What core nursing competencies, across all areas of practice, will help nurses improve population health outcomes?

REFERENCES

American Association of Colleges of Nursing. (2017). *Academic partnerships to improve health.* Retrieved from www.cdc.gov/ophss/csels/dsepd/academic- partnerships/index.html.

American Association of Colleges of Nursing. (2018a). *Population health nursing.* Retrieved from www.aacnnursing.org/Population-Health-Nursing.

American Association of Colleges of Nursing. (2018b). *Public/population health learning hubs.* Retrieved from www.aacnnursing.org/Population-Health-Nursing/Public Health-Learning-Hubs.

American Public Health Association. (1968). *The state health department: Policy 6812.* Retrieved from www.apha.org/policies-and-advocacy/public-health-policy- statements/policy-database/2014/07/21/09/50/the-state-health-department.

American Public Health Association. (1974). *The role of official local health agencies: Policy 7434.* Retrieved from www.apha.org/policies-and-advocacy/public-health-policy-statements/policy-database/2014/07/15/14/41/the-role-of-official-local-health-agencies.

American Public Health Association. (2013). *Strengthening public health nursing in the United States: Policy 201316.* Retrieved from www.apha.org/policies-and-advocacy/public-health-policy-statements/policydatabase/2014/07/23/11/02/strengthening-public-health-nursing-in-the-united-states.

American Public Health Association. (2015). *Better health through equity.* Retrieved from www.apha.org/-/media/files/pdf/topics/equity/equity_stories.ashx?la=en&hash=DB7341 D9CA82547EAFD8DF9DCAE718A0CD6B92DC .

Association of State and Territory Health Organizations. (2017). *ASTHO profile of state and territorial public health.* Retrieved from www.astho.org/Profile/Volume-Four/2016-ASTHO-Profile-of-State-and-Territorial-Public-Health/.

Beck A.J., & Boulton, M.J. (2016). The public health nurse workforce in U.S. state and local health departments, 2012. *Public Health Reports, 131*(1), 145-142.

Beck A.J., Boulton, M.L., & Coronado, F. (2014). Enumeration of the governmental public health workforce. *American Journal of Preventative Medicine, 47*(5 Suppl 3), S306-S313.

CDC Foundation. (2018). *What is public health?* Retrieved from www.cdcfoundation.org/what-public-health.

Centers for Disease Control and Prevention. (2011). *Ten great public health achievements—United States, 2001-2010.* Retrieved from www.cdc.gov/mmwr/preview/mmwrhtml/mm6019a5.htm.

Centers for Disease Control and Prevention. (2017). *Preventative health care.* Retrieved from www.cdc.gov/healthcommunication/toolstemplates/entertainmented/tips/Preventiv eHealth.html.

Centers for Disease Control and Prevention. (2018a). *The public health system and the ten essential public health services.* Retrieved from www.cdc.gov/stltpublichealth/publichealthservices/essentialhealthservices.html.

Centers for Disease Control and Prevention. (2018b). *Morbidity and Mortality Weekly Report.* Retrieved from www.cdc.gov/mmwr/index.html.

Centers for Medicare and Medicaid Services. (2018). *Value based programs.* Retrieved from www.cms.gov/Medicare/Quality-Initiatives-Patient-Assessment-Instruments/Value-Based-Programs/Value-Based-Programs.html.

The Commonwealth Fund. (2015). *The Affordable Care Act's payment and delivery system reforms: A progress report at five years.* Retrieved from www.commonwealthfund.org/publications/issue-briefs/2015/may/affordable-care-acts-payment-and-delivery-system-reforms.

The Community Guide. (2012). *Tobacco use and secondhand smoke exposure: Smoke-free policies.* Retrieved from www.thecommunityguide.org/findings/tobacco-use-and-secondhand-smoke-exposure-smoke-free-policies.

The Community Guide. (n.d.). *The community guide.* Retrieved from www.thecommunityguide.org/.

County Health Rankings. (2016). *County health rankings model.* Retrieved from www.countyhealthrankings.org/county-health-rankings-model.

Cygan, H., McNaughton, D., Reising, V., & Reid, B. (2018). An academic practice partnership: Building capacity to meet sexual health education policy requirements of a public school system. *Public Health Nursing, 35*(5), 414-419.

DeSalvo K.B., Wang Y.C., Harris A., Auerbach J., Koo D., & O'Carroll P. (2017). Public health 3.0: A call to action for public health to meet the challenges of the 21st century. *Preventing Chronic Disease, 14,* 170017.

Dircksen, J.C., Prachand, N.G., Adams, D., Bockskay, K., Brown, J., Cibulskis, A., … & White, M. (2016). *Healthy Chicago 2.0: Partnering to improve health equity.* Retrieved from www.cityofchicago.org/content/dam/city/depts/cdph/CDPH/Healthy%20Chicago/HC2.0Upd4152016.pdf.

Dohm, I., Kwak, L., Oja, P., Sjostrom, M., & Hagstromer, M. (2018). Replacing sedentary time with physical activity: A 15-year follow-up of mortality in a national cohort. *Clinical Epidemiology, 10,* 179-186.

Emory University. (2013). *The CDC nurse.* Retrieved from http://whsc.emory.edu/home/publications/nursing/emory-nursing/fall2013/the-cdc- nurse.html.

Gallup. (2017). *Nurses keep healthy lead as most honest, ethical profession.* Retrieved from https://news.gallup.com/poll/224639/nurses-keep-healthy-lead-honest-ethical-profession.aspx?g_source=Economy&g_medium=newsfeed&g_campaign=tiles.

Gross, W.L., Cooper, L., Boggs, S., & Gold, B. (2017). Value based care and strategic priorities. *Anesthesiology Clinics, 35*(4), 725-731.

Himmelstein, D.U., & Woolhandler, S. (2016). The current and projected taxpayer shares of U.S. health costs. *American Journal of Public Health, 106*(3), 449-452.

Institute for Healthcare Improvement. (2018). *Triple Aim.* Retrieved from www.ihi.org/Engage/Initiatives/TripleAim/Pages/default.aspx.

Institute of Medicine. (1988). *The future of public health.* Washington, DC: The National Academies Press.

Jewish Women's Archive. (n.d.). *Lilian Wald.* Retrieved from https://jwa.org/womenofvalor/wald.

Kindig, D., & Stoddart, G. (2003). What is population health? *American Journal of Public Health, 93*(3), 380-383.

Koshinsky, J.L., Krall, J., Ruppert, K., Kantner, J. Solano, F.X. & Siminerio, L.M. (2018). Diabetes educator impact in value based care models. *Diabetes, 67*(Suppl 1). Retrieved from https://diabetes.diabetesjournals.org/content/67/Supplement_1/253-OR.

Micha, R., Peñalvo, J.L., Cudhea, F., Imamura, F., Rehm, C.D., & Mozaffarian, D. (2017). Association between dietary factors and mortality from heart disease, stroke, and type 2 diabetes in the United States. *JAMA, 317*(9), 912-924.

Michener, J.L., Koo, D., Castrucci, B.C., & Sprague, J.B. (2016). *The practical playbook: Public health and primary care together.* New York: Oxford University Press.

Mokdad, A.H., Marks, J.S., Stroup, D.F., & Gerberding, J.L. (2004). Actual causes of death in the United States, 2000. *JAMA, 291*(10), 1238-1245.

Monteiro, L. (1985). Florence Nightingale on public health nursing. *American Journal of Public Health, 75*(2), 181-186.

Murphy, S.L., Xu, J., Kochanek, K, Curtin, S.C., & Arias, E. (2017). *Deaths: Final data for 2015.* Retrieved from www.cdc.gov/nchs/data/nvsr/nvsr66/nvsr66_06.pdf.

National Association of County & City Health Organizations. (2016). *2016 National profile of local health departments.* Retrieved from www.nacchoprofilestudy.org/.

National Center for Health Statistics. (2017). *Health, United States, 2016: With chartbook on long-term trends in health.* Hyattsville, MD. Retrieved from www.cdc.gov/nchs/data/hus/hus16.pdf.

Nightingale, F. (1860). *Notes on nursing: What it is, and what it is not.* London: Harrison

Organisation for Economic and Co-operative Development. (2018). *Health data.* Retrieved from www.oecd.org/els/health-systems/health-data.htm.

Pandey, P., & Nguyen, V. (2017). Achieving the Triple Aim through doctor of nursing practice directed breast cancer survivorship care. *The Journal for Nurse Practitioners, 13*(4), 277-283.

Patient Protection and Affordable Care Act, 42 U.S.C. § 18001 et seq. (2010).

Public Health Law Center (2015). State and local public health: An overview of regulatory authority. Retrieved from http://publichealthlawcenter.org/sites/default/files/resources/phlc-fs-state-local-reg-authority-publichealth-2015_0.pdf.

U.S. Department of Health and Human Services. (2014). *The health consequences of smoking: 50 years of progress: A report of the Surgeon General.* Atlanta: U.S. Department Health and Human Services, Centers for Disease Control and Prevention, National Center for Chronic Disease Prevention and Health Promotion, Office on Smoking and Health.

U.S. Department of Health and Human Services. (2015). *HHS agencies and offices.* Retrieved from www.hhs.gov/about/agencies/hhs-agencies-and-offices/index.html.

U.S. Department of Health and Human Services. (n.d.). *National prevention strategy.* Retrieved from www.surgeongeneral.gov/priorities/prevention/strategy/index.html.

University of Pennsylvania. (2016). *Mortality in the United States: Past, present, and future.* Retrieved from http://budgetmodel.wharton.upenn.edu/issues/2016/1/25/mortality-in-the-united-states-past-present-and-future.

Verma, A., & Bhatia, S. (2016). A policy framework for health systems to promote Triple Aim innovation. *Healthcare Papers, 15*(3), 9-23.

Visiting Nurse Service of New York. (2018). *Lillian Wald.* Retrieved from www.vnsny.org/who-we-are/about-us/history/lillian-wald/.

ONLINE RESOURCES

AACN Population Health Nursing
www.aacnnursing.org/Population-Health-Nursing
The Community Guide
www.thecommunityguide.org
The County Health Rankings
www.countyhealthrankings.org
Healthy People 2020
www.healthypeople.gov
The Practical Playbook
www.practicalplaybook.org

29

TAKING ACTION: Influencing Public Health in a Politically Charged Environment

Gina Miranda-Diaz

"Be the change you want to see in the world."

Mahatma Gandhi

The New Jersey State Department of Health (NJSDOH) defines a health officer as:

> the public health chief executive officer of a municipal, regional, county, or contractual health agency. This individual is responsible for evaluating health problems, planning appropriate activities to address these health problems, developing necessary budget procedures to finance these activities and directing staff to carry out these activities efficiently and economically. (NJSDOH, n.d.)

On October 27, 2015, I was appointed to be the first Latina in New Jersey's history to hold both titles of Health Officer for West New York (WNY), New Jersey, and Advanced Public Health Nurse. Feeling a little daunted and out of my comfort zone, I nonetheless believed what I lacked in experience as a Health Officer, I had in abundance as a passionate, public health nurse and advocate.

NOT A POLITICIAN

I am not a politician. Working in a politically charged environment is demanding. The learning curve was steep, but it soon became apparent that everyone, from the commissioners and mayor to the director of public affairs, wanted to place their imprimatur on every project. Determined to move full steam ahead, I dove right in, ready to steer the health department in a new direction. Soon, I would arrive at the sad realization that municipal government is laden with multiple layers of red tape, with each of the key players at town hall having their ideas about how things are done.

Although the health officer is defined as a nonpolitical, statutory appointee, it is difficult not to become engulfed in the political quagmire in a municipality. My loyalty to

the mayor—a physician and my friend—thrust me into the center of a political war. Politics in Hudson County, New Jersey takes no prisoners. You can only hope that you end up on the right side of history. From the inside, one truly values a politician whose focus is the community and well-being of all its citizens. However, in this town, the government became fractured between the mayor and three commissioners on his team who wanted to "run" the town without him….and me. My department was dismantled and I was forced out of my role, the first of many casualties of this political war. However, during my 5-year tenure as the health officer, I was able to accomplish a great deal.

A TALE OF TWO CITIES IN WEST NEW YORK

On the second day as health officer, I put on my public health nurse hat and assessed the community. What I discovered was astounding. There were million-dollar homes along an 18.5 linear/nautical mile area on the Hudson River that was described as the "Gold Coast," with a breathtaking view of the New York City skyline. This exclusive area is less than a mile from the predominantly immigrant neighborhoods of WNY. It is a tale of two cities: waterfront properties, high-end restaurants, and supermarkets are juxtaposed with a blue-collar community filled with tenements, bodegas, and food vendors lining the streets. And there were stark differences in environmental and social justice issues.

Residents who live on the Gold Coast do not interact with their neighbors across town. A majority work in New York City and commute to work via ferry or bus. A large marble stone with a cascading water facade and lighting at the ferry station marks the entry point into this community. Carved into the stone is "Port Imperial" and, below in smaller lettering, "West New York." Developers of this community have adorned all the lamp posts with flags that establish the area as Port Imperial. Noteworthy is the absence of the town's name on the lamp post flags as if to distinguish themselves from their neighbors atop the hill. Interactions between myself and this wealthy part of WNY are limited to annual inspections of the annual "food truck" festival, upscale restaurants, spas, ice cream shops, and supermarkets.

Although WNY is among the smallest cities in New Jersey, it is among the top 10 cities in the state with the most significant numbers of Spanish-speaking residents. More than 83% of the population older than 5 years of age speaks a language other than English (NJ.com, 2017). Spanish is the native language for 68% of residents (DataUS, 2018). Being bilingual (English/Spanish) is indispensable for assisting residents in this community. Now everyone in town had access to a public health official who was linguistically and culturally competent. Communication is a barrier for one out of four Latinos, which can have a lasting impact on access to care, public health, and well-being.

The health goals for WNY are aligned with *Healthy New Jersey 2020* (NJSDOH, n.d.), which details health goals for New Jersey residents modeled on the federal government's *Healthy People 2020*. Consistent with established public health priorities, efforts have been implemented at the WNY health department to improve access to public health providers and create organizational partnerships for improving health for all the citizens. Collaboration with community-based and national organizations, houses of worship, and health care partners has improved access to health care resources. One such partnership was Safe Kids Day (SKD).

SAFE KIDS DAY

On May 18, 2013, WNY launched its first SKD, an event observed around the globe. Introducing an evidence-based safety fair to the community provided both parents and children with information about the importance of safety on and off wheels (e.g., bikes or skateboards). Head trauma for children younger than 18 years of age not wearing a protective helmet when cycling is an important issue. Bicycle safety laws are often ignored by more than 50% of cyclists. New Jersey had established its own bicycle and pedestrian safety law in 2005 mandating that "all children under the age of 17 must wear a helmet while riding a bicycle, skateboarding, roller skating, and inline skating" (New Jersey Division of Highway and Traffic Safety, n.d.). Opportunities to highlight many safety issues are the core of its success: donning bicycle helmets, pedestrian, fire, medication, and driving safety.

August 7, 2018, marked the sixth anniversary since our inaugural SKD event. For the past 3 years, "Safe Kids Day" and "National Night Out," a community-building campaign that promotes police-community partnerships for safer communities, have merged to provide opportunities for the public to interact with the health department and law enforcement. Other community partners, such as the National Association of Hispanic Nurses New Jersey Chapter, donated bicycles. Hospitals, clinics, AARP, and the Supplemental Nutrition Assistance Program educated attendees and offer food samples. Linking these events drew hundreds of residents and provided an opportunity for neighbors to socialize. As of 2018, 626 helmets had been distributed to children accompanied by a parent/guardian.

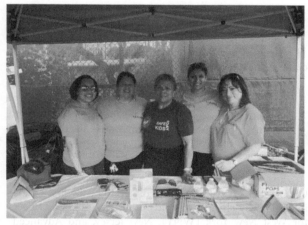

Author Gina Miranda-Diaz (middle) with members of the National Association of Hispanic Nurses on Safe Kids Day 2017.

FLU FIGHTERS

The Centers for Disease Control and Prevention (CDC) (2018) predicted that 2017–2018 would surpass 2009 as the deadliest flu season—a wake-up call to the world to get vaccinated. Even more devastating was the record number of pediatric deaths from the flu-related illness. Sadly, one of our smallest neighbors became one of these statistics. Overwhelmed with sadness and determined to prevent this from happening to another child, the health department held its first Emergency Flu Clinic.

Hackensack-Meridian Hospital, located in the neighboring town, contributed 150 vaccines to the WNY Health Department. Joining forces with the local hospital, nurses from neighboring Union City, health department staff, and student interns became "Flu Fighters."

On February 21, 2018, the Flu Fighters sprang into action, and the response was unprecedented and overwhelming. Approximately 350 parents and children arrived at our doorstep with children in tow to receive their "free vaccine." During the 5-hour clinic, the Flu Fighters administered 136 vaccines to neighborhood children younger than the age of 17. This was bittersweet, yet a heartwarming moment, as we were able to shield 136 children from the flu and perhaps from a flu-related death.

INFLUENCING POLICY AND REVISING ORDINANCES

After my first winter at the Health Department, I recognized an environmental injustice unique to the working poor of the community—lack of heat during the winter. Unfortunately, daily heat complaints are not uncommon among individuals who reside in tenement housing. A majority of building owners live outside of town and are unavailable to address the needs of the tenants. If the landlord answers the telephone, oftentimes concerns about heating are met with indifference, excuses, and delays in addressing the tenants' grievances.

For the period extending from October 1 through May 1, the "Heating Ordinance" is in effect. When the outdoor temperature dips to less than 55°F anytime for 24 hours, the landlord is responsible for providing heat until the temperature at the residence reaches 68°F. A survey of the "heat complaints" during the 2015–2016 winter season revealed more than 1500 calls from tenants who were supplied little or no heat. Heat is not a luxury; it is the right of all individuals to live in a warm home.

One winter season proved to be a rude awakening for the "slumlords" who were surprised by a revised ordinance and my relentless efforts to enforce it. A review of the town ordinance revealed that the fines associated with these violations were minimal and did not serve as a deterrent. The fines ranged from $50 to $200 per incident, depending on how often the violations occurred during the season. The landlord of a multidwelling building would pay the fines as though it was the cost of doing business. I immediately worked with the town attorney to ensure that the ordinance was revised to impose harsher fines to deter this behavior. Revisions to the ordinance included a $500/unit fine per day without heat. In addition, there was a fine for failure to notify the health department within 4 hours of malfunction of the heating unit/system. In the event the living conditions were deemed hazardous, an additional $500 fine could be imposed. The revised "Heating" ordinance was approved by the mayor and commissioners in July 2017. Enforcement action would be taken immediately against violators of the law.

One bitterly cold night during the 2017 holiday season, residents of a seven-unit building called the health department to report the absence of heat since October 1. Unfortunately, the residents did not complain until December 28. Delays in tenants' reporting heat complaints are typical because of fear of retribution by the landlord. In this case, many tenants claimed the landlord acted violently, kicked their front door, left vulgar voicemail messages, and imposed arbitrary fines if the rent was not paid on the due date (violation of rent control ordinance).

On the night of December 30, 2017, the inspector "on call" notified me that the heating situation had grown dire. After entering the tenement, I was horrified at the condition of the tenement apartments. Tenants ranged in age from 6 months to 93 years of age, and apartment temperatures were 38.5°F to 55°F on the ambient thermometer. The shared hallway registered 32°F. Even my snow boots were no match for the freezing temperature of the floor tiles. Residents had to send their children to live with relatives during the holiday season. Exasperated with the landlord's feeble attempt at convincing the health department that he was addressing the situation, I condemned the building because I deemed it hazardous. Everyone in the apartment building was relocated to a nearby hotel, where they remained for 3 weeks until the boiler was repaired.

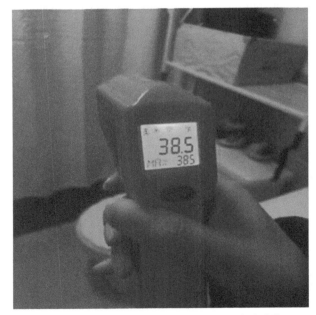

Bathroom temperature of the "condemned" building on December 30, 2017.

Summonses for violating the ordinance were issued to the landlord and required him to reimburse the town $12,000 for the 3-week hotel expense required to house the displaced tenants. In addition to the hotel expenses, $165,500 in summonses were issued to the landlord for multiple heating ordinance violations.

Social justice prevailed when I discovered the tenants were overcharged up to three times the rent allowed by Rent Control laws. All of the residents did not pay rent during the time that they were deprived of heat. In a final ruling, all of the tenants under the rent control contract received credit for overpayment of rent.

Engaging in advocacy is a critical component of environmental and social justice. Merging the health officer and advanced public health nurse roles was effective in changing the lives of seven families.

ADVOCATING FOR SOCIAL JUSTICE

During my tenure as health officer, I influenced policies in sanitary and environmental health despite the bureaucracy of local government. Challenges may have discouraged me at times, but I learned to become flexible and adapt to the workings of local government. Each obstacle became a teachable moment, and that afforded me the opportunity to grow into my role.

Forging alliances with local organizations, public health nurses, and local town hall employees benefited the health of the community. Although the New Jersey Association of City and County Health Officials is not a nursing organization, membership afforded me the opportunity to discuss issues through the lens of an advanced public health nurse. As the former President of the New Jersey chapter of the National Association of Hispanic Nurses, I was able to engage its members in community events and expand our network within WNY and other communities in the state. These and other nursing and health-related organizations are involved in activism and use their political know-how and strength in numbers to influence policy. Partner with others, but do not leave advocacy for someone else.

REFERENCES

Centers for Disease Control and Prevention. (2018). *Influenza (flu)*. Retrieved from www.cdc.gov/flu/.

Document18DataUSA. (n.d.). *West New York*. Retrieved from https://datausa.io/profile/geo/west-new-york-nj/#category_heritage.

New Jersey Division of Highway and Traffic Safety. (n.d.). *Safe passage: Moving to zero fatalities*. Retrieved from www.nj.gov/oag/hts/index.html.

New Jersey State Department of Health. (n.d.). *Licensure for health officers*. Retrieved from https://nj.gov/health/lh/professionals/licensing/.

NJ.Com. (2017). *About 2.6M people in N.J. don't speak English at home, new census data shows*. Retrieved from www.nj.com/data/2017/12/new_jersey_now_has_more_non-english_speakers_censu.html.

30

Disaster Response and Public Health Emergency Preparedness

Tener Goodwin Veenema, Roberta Proffitt Lavin, and Clifton P. Thornton

> *"By failing to prepare, you are preparing to fail."*
>
> *Benjamin Franklin*

PURPOSE STATEMENT

Disasters and public health emergencies of international concern (PHEICs) are heralded as "breaking news" and garner aggressive and sustained media coverage regardless of their scope and impact. This coverage often results in a mandate for a political response, which may drive the creation of disaster health policies by Congress. These policies, although well-intentioned but frequently politically motivated, address the public outcry for action from the most recent disaster but may have unexpected short- and long-term consequences, both positive and negative. This chapter focuses on the challenges the United States and its communities face in disaster and public health emergency preparedness and the policy responses to these challenges.

BACKGROUND AND SIGNIFICANCE

According to the National Centers for Environmental Information (NCEI), the United States continues to experience a dramatic increase in the frequency and intensity of natural and manmade disasters and acts of terrorism. During 2017–18, the United States experienced two historic years of weather and climate disasters. In 2017 alone, the United States was impacted by 16 separate billion-dollar disaster events, tying 2011 for the record number of billion-dollar disasters for an entire calendar year (National Oceanic and Atmospheric Administration [NOAA], 2018). More notable than the high frequency of these events was the cumulative cost, which exceeded $300 billion in 2017, a new U.S. annual record (Fig. 30.1). The cumulative damage of the 16 U.S. events during 2017 is $309.5 billion (consumer price index [CPI]-adjusted to present), which shattered the previous U.S. annual record cost of $219.2 billion (also CPI-adjusted) that occurred in 2005 from the impacts of Hurricanes Dennis, Katrina, Rita, and Wilma (NOAA, 2018).

Disaster health policies are established and evolve in response to the events of our times. These policies affect all of those impacted by a disaster, including public and private health and human service responders, hospital-based receivers, suppliers, and community members. The passage of federal, state, and local policies that alter scope of practice and standards of care can ensure greater access to care or can create barriers to care. Disasters and PHEICs often result in a sudden unanticipated demand for care or "patient surge." This surge creates a significant burden for health care systems, and the providers who work within them, to rapidly adapt and expand capacity in order to create or sustain a unique environment that allows nurses and physicians to care for people and save lives. Because of their intimate involvement in responding to all types and levels of disasters, health care providers should be involved in the planning and policymaking phase of disaster and PHEIC response to avoid unintended consequences and ensure effective policy and planning that maintains human dignity and is guided by social justice (American Medical Association [AMA], 2018; American Nurses Association [ANA], 2017). Awareness of current and proposed disaster health policies as well as the agencies charged with executing them is critical to both planning and response initiatives.

PRESIDENTIAL DECLARATIONS OF DISASTER AND THE STAFFORD ACT

Recognizing that disasters have the potential to cause loss of life, property damage, human suffering, income loss,

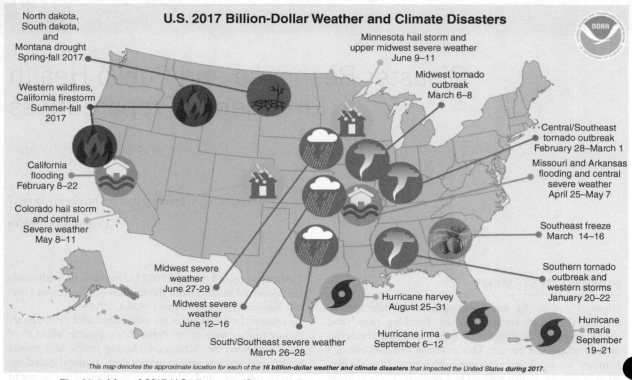

Fig. 30.1 Map of 2017 U.S. disasters. (Courtesy of National Oceanic and Atmospheric Administration.)

and great financial burdens to all levels of government, the United States enacted the Robert T. Stafford Disaster Relief and Emergency Assistance Act (Public Law 100-707) on November 23, 1988. Amended in 2016, the Act constitutes the statutory authority for most federal disaster response activities and charges the Federal Emergency Management Agency (FEMA) with the responsibility to coordinate and conduct relief efforts through coordination of 28 federal agencies and nongovernmental agencies. The cornerstone of disaster preparedness lies in planning to ensure that local and state organizations are prepared for the event. As "all disasters are local," it is these local groups that are ultimately responsible for dealing with the immediate consequences of the disaster. The Stafford Act outlines how the *federal* government will assist local, state, and tribal organizations in disaster response by coordinating with them and facilitating a unified command (Stafford Act, 2016). Congress has passed additional disaster legislation in the Post-Katrina Emergency Management Reform Act (PKEMRA), enacted after Hurricane Katrina (2006), and in response to Hurricane Sandy, Congress enacted the Sandy Recovery Improvement Act (SRIA, 2013) in an effort to reduce costs and improve effectiveness of several disaster assistance programs authorized by the Stafford Act (House Report 1678, 2017).

POST-KATRINA EMERGENCY MANAGEMENT REFORM ACT (2006)

Gaps that became apparent in the response to Hurricane Katrina in 2005 led to the PKEMRA (2006), which significantly reorganized FEMA, provided it substantial new authority to remedy gaps in response, and included a more robust preparedness mission for FEMA (FEMA, 2018). This act:

- Establishes a Disability Coordinator and develops guidelines to accommodate individuals with disabilities.
- Establishes the National Emergency Family Registry and Locator System to reunify separated family members.
- Coordinates and supports precautionary evacuations and recovery efforts.
- Provides transportation assistance for relocating and returning individuals displaced from their residences in a major disaster.
- Provides case management assistance to identify and address unmet needs of survivors of major disasters.

SEPTEMBER 11, 2001: A SENTINEL EVENT

The extended media coverage of the terrorist attacks of September 11, 2001, contributed to congressional policy changes that significantly increased presidential authoritative power to (Sylves, 2008) declare a state of emergency. The Homeland Security Act was signed into law on November 25, 2002. It created the U.S. Department of Homeland Security (DHS), headed by the Secretary of Homeland Security; established the Cyber Security Enhancement Act; and moved many programs involved in disaster response to new leadership under DHS (Homeland Security Act, 2002, Section 102).

THE POLITICS UNDERLYING DISASTER AND PUBLIC HEALTH EMERGENCY POLICY

Disaster policy in the United States has been performed in a predominately retrospective manner. The government develops policies and procedures for handling disasters after one has occurred. For instance, the formation of the DHS followed the 9/11 terrorist attacks, Project BioShield was introduced after the anthrax attacks, and the PKEMRA resulted from Hurricane Katrina. Disaster plans were created in response to those policies and/or disasters. For a more comprehensive list of disaster policies that followed national disasters and large-scale public health emergencies, see Fig. 30.2 and

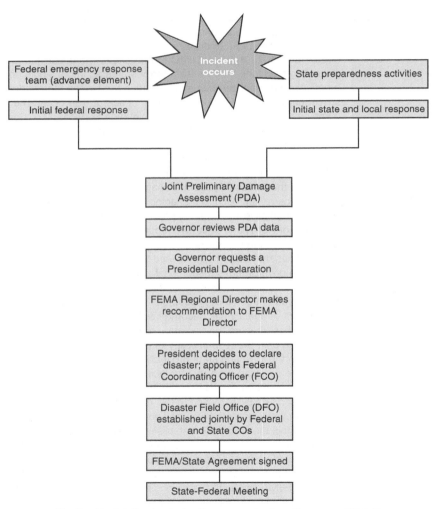

The Presidential disaster declaration process begins with a request from the Governor of the affected State; the response is ultimately determined by the President.

Fig. 30.2 Flowchart of a disaster declaration and the provisions of the Stafford Act. *FEMA,* Federal Emergency Management Agency.

Table 30.1. The implementation of disaster health policies created in direct response to a previous disaster often results in a knee-jerk response characterized by shining a laser, focused on correcting one glaring deficit while frequently overlooking another.

PROJECT BIOSHIELD (2004)

In reaction to the 2001 anthrax attacks, President George W. Bush introduced Project BioShield to prepare for

future bioterrorism attacks, signing it into law on July 21, 2004 (Cohen, 2011; Gottron & Shea, 2011; U.S. Department of Health and Human Services [HHS], 2016). Protection of the general population was thought to be best achieved by obtaining medical countermeasures (MCMs) against chemical, biologic, radiologic, and nuclear (CBRN) threats (Gottron & Shea, 2011). A sum of $5.6 billion was initially approved for 10 years to be used for the development and purchase of MCMs (DHS, 2013a). Evaluation of the progress of BioShield, however, revealed excessive

TABLE 30.1 U.S. Disaster Policies Enacted Since 9/11

Policy	Date Enacted	Description
Homeland Security Act (HSA)	November 2002	Created the U.S. Department of Homeland Security (DHS); this is the first new federal executive department since 1989 in response to the terrorist attacks of September 11, 2001. The act aims to restructure the departments responsible for protecting the United States from terrorist attacks into a single department. It functions to prevent terrorist attacks within the United States, decrease the susceptibility to attacks, and respond to attacks if they occur. The department combines the U.S. Citizenship and Immigration Services, U.S. Coast Guard, U.S. Customs and Border Protection, Federal Emergency Management Agency, U.S. Immigration and Customs Enforcement, and the Transportation Security Administration together to integrate their individual regulatory responsibilities into carrying out the provisions outlined by the DHS (HSA, 2002, Section 102).
Homeland Security Presidential Directive-5 (HSPD5)	February 2003	Established the National Incident Management System (NIMS) to fill the need for a comprehensive approach to managing crises and their consequences as a single entity through all levels of government across the nation. Under this act, the Secretary of Homeland Security is responsible for preventing, preparing for, responding to, and recovering from terrorist attacks, major disasters, and other emergencies that occur in the United States. The secretary will initiate coordination of the government's resources if a federal department or agency requests the assistance of the secretary; federal assistance has been requested by state and local authorities whose resources have been depleted; more than one federal department or agency has become involved in response to an event; or the President has directed the secretary to begin management. The directive is not designed to shift the responsibility of planning for and responding to disasters away from the local and state organizations to the federal government but rather provide the secretary as a tool for local and state organizations to use if they become overwhelmed by an event (DHS, 2003).
Post-Katrina Emergency Management Reform Act (PKEMRA)	July 2006	This act began as a bill proposed to the 109th Congress to amend the Homeland Security Act and aimed to keep the Federal Emergency Management Agency (FEMA) within the DHS while establishing new provisions to plan, respond, and recover from disasters. It also implemented an all-hazards strategy for preparedness and promoted planning for the protection and postdisaster restoration of necessary infrastructures and resources. Most notably, the act redefined the role of the administrator of FEMA and added provisions ranging from outlining the presidential roles and responsibilities in disasters to providing counseling for victims. PKEMRA also addressed staffing issues; education regarding planning, preparedness, and training; and fraud, waste, and abuse within the system (S.3721, 2006).

TABLE 30.1 U.S. Disaster Policies Enacted Since 9/11—cont'd

Policy	Date Enacted	Description
Pandemic and All-Hazards Preparedness Act (PAHPA)	December 2006	Amended the Public Health Service Act within the U.S. Department of Health and Human Services (HHS) with the goal to improve upon the public health and medical preparedness and response capabilities of the United States for all disasters and emergencies. The act also established a new Assistant Secretary for Preparedness and Response (ASPR) as well as new authorities for other programs. The act established new construction and acquisition of medical countermeasures and strives to develop a quadrennial National Health Security Act. The secretary is responsible for organizing a nationwide public health situational awareness communication network that will allow the rapid detection and response to public health issues. The legislation also required the HHS and ASPR to disseminate novel and best practices of outreach to and care of at-risk individuals before, during, and following public health emergencies (Public Law 109-417).
National Response Framework (NRF)	January 2008 May 2013	Replacing the older National Response Plan, the NRF serves as the nation's all-hazards response guide to handling natural and manmade disasters. Its guidelines detail how leaders at all levels of government along with private sector partners and health care providers must prepare for and provide a unified domestic response through enhanced coordination and integration. The Framework is scalable and adaptable to a variety of different events and works to align key roles and responsibilities across the United States. The priorities of response are to save lives, protect property and the environment, stabilize the incident, and provide for basic human needs. The Framework is always in effect, and elements of the plan can be implemented at any time as they are needed. Besides the main body of the document, the NRF also comprises Emergency Support Function (ESF) Annexes, Support Annexes, and Incident Annexes. ESF Annexes assign resources and capabilities that are most frequently needed in a national response into functional areas. Support Annexes detail the essential supporting processes and considerations that are most common to the majority of incidents. Lastly, Incident Annexes describe the unique response aspects of incident categories. The second edition of the framework was released in May 2013 (DHS, 2008; DHS, 2013b).
National Health Security Strategy (NHSS); National Health Security Strategy Implementation Plan 2015–2018	December 2009; 2015	A society that is able to manage and function well during large-scale incidents that affect the health of workers who are responsible to provide food, water, and health care to the greater population helps strengthen security and stability for the United States. The NHSS was designed to minimize the consequences from these incidents by coordinating the stakeholders responsible for providing these important resources. The strategy offers a framework in which to improve relevant portions of the Pandemic and All-Hazards Preparedness Act, legislation meant to improve the preparedness and response of the country to emergencies. Developed by the HHS, the two stated goals of the NHSS are to build community resilience and to strengthen and maintain health and emergency response systems (HHS, 2009).
Homeland Security Presidential Directive-8 (HSPD8)	March 2011	In recognition that emergency preparedness is an effort that requires input from multiple sectors of government as well as input from civilians, President Barack Obama drafted PPD-8 in 2011. This directive aims to strengthen the security and resilience of the United States through preparation for acts of terrorism, cyber-attacks, pandemics, and natural disasters. It views preparation for these events as a shared responsibility among the private and nonprofit sector, government, and individuals.

Continued

TABLE 30.1	U.S. Disaster Policies Enacted Since 9/11—cont'd	
Policy	**Date Enacted**	**Description**
		The directive itself is aimed at the responsibilities of the government in establishing safeguards against the aforementioned threats, but it also addresses the fact that complete preparedness is an all-of-nation effort. This directive serves as a call to action to prepare the nation to establish an effective national preparedness system. Once this system is established, it will allow evaluation and tracking of the efforts made to prevent, protect against, dampen the effects of, or respond to and recover from, threats to the nation's security. Coordinating this preparedness system is the responsibility of the Assistant to the President for Homeland Security and Counterterrorism, while the Secretary of Homeland Security is responsible for developing the preparedness goal (DHS, 2011c).
National Preparedness Goal	September 2011	Outlines the approach of the United States to preparation for all types of disasters through a shared-responsibility model. The directive describes the responsibilities of the population and emphasizes that the individual, community, private and non-profit sectors, faith-based organizations, and federal, state, and local governments should be involved in national security. The focus of the directive is to use individual and community preparedness to contribute to national security to provide benefit to all. The National Preparedness Goal aspires to involve all of these individuals and groups in the five mission areas of prevention, protection, mitigation, response, and recovery with regard to disasters. The directive outlines specific core capabilities for each of these mission areas that must be achieved to meet the goal (DHS, 2011a).
National Preparedness System	November 2011	The National Preparedness System holds the same view of an all-of-nation approach to preparing for and managing disasters. The system outlines an organizational process for all community members to use while moving forward in preparing to achieve the National Preparedness Goal. The National Preparedness System is composed of six parts. These include identifying and assessing risk, estimating capability requirements, building and sustaining capabilities, planning to deliver capabilities, validating capabilities, and reviewing and updating the plans developed through these processes (Federal Emergency Management Agency, 2014).
Homeland Security Presidential Directive-21 (HSPD21)	February 2013	This directive addresses the need for a critical infrastructure of security and resilience that aims to advance a national unity of effort in strengthening and maintaining a secure, functioning, and resilient critical infrastructure. The directive recognizes the importance of infrastructure that is essential to the nation's safety, prosperity, and well-being. The directive also recognizes the vast complexity of this infrastructure, noting that it includes both physical and cyber space that is controlled by government, business, private, and individual owners. All components of this infrastructure must be secure and be able to withstand or recover from threats to safety. Because these components of the infrastructure share ownership among federal, state, local, tribal, territorial, public, and private owners, a team effort must be used to establish security. An all-hazards approach to identifying possible threats and planning for these events is taken to begin preparation for security. The federal government functions to help direct and guide planning for the remaining sectors and owners, with a particularly large role to be performed by the Secretary of Homeland Security (U.S. Office of the Press Secretary, 2013).

TABLE 30.1	U.S. Disaster Policies Enacted Since 9/11—cont'd	
Policy	**Date Enacted**	**Description**
Pandemic and All-Hazards Preparedness Reauthorization Act (PAH-PRA)	March 2013	The law builds on work the HHS has undertaken to advance national health security. These include authorizing funding for public health and medical preparedness programs, such as the Hospital Preparedness Program and the Public Health Emergency Preparedness Cooperative Agreement, amending the Public Health Service Act to grant state health departments greatly needed flexibility in dedicating staff resources to meeting critical community needs in a disaster, authorizing funding through 2018 for buying medical countermeasures under the Project BioShield Act, and increasing the flexibility of BioShield to support advanced research and development of potential medical countermeasures. PAHPRA also enhances the authority of the U.S. Food and Drug Administration to support rapid responses to public health emergencies.
Public Health Emergency Preparedness Act	Pending 2018 legislation	To make a supplemental appropriation for the Public Health Emergency Fund and for other purposes including support for the Strategic National Stockpile.

spending for a vaccine that had limited commercial value and unintended consequences (Sell & Watson, 2013).

Through BioShield, the federal government had the authority to create a market and enter into contracts with companies promising the purchase of certain products if developed (Gottron & Shea, 2011; Kadlec, 2013). The first BioShield contract was with VaxGen and cost $877.5 million for the acquisition of 75 million doses of a new anthrax vaccine (Kadlec, 2013). VaxGen had never produced a vaccine licensed with the U.S. Food and Drug Administration (FDA), and 2 years later, VaxGen still had no vaccine. The government terminated the contract despite already paying $1.5 million to the company (Cohen, 2011; Kadlec, 2013). As of 2018, Project BioShield has been involved in procurement of 27 MCMs against 6 identified threats (anthrax, botulism, smallpox, nerve agents, radiation, and Ebola [Daschle & Gregg, 2018]). However, it should be noted that of the 27 agents the program has procured, only 6 have been approved by the FDA and several are agents already approved to treat side effects caused by CBRN agents.

PUBLIC READINESS AND EMERGENCY PREPAREDNESS ACT 2005

The Public Readiness and Emergency Preparedness (PREP) Act authorized the Secretary of HHS to issue a PREP Act Declaration ("Declaration") that provides immunity from liability for any loss caused, arising out of, relating to, or resulting from administration or use of countermeasures to diseases, threats, and conditions determined in the Declaration to constitute a present or credible risk of a future public health emergency. In general, the liability immunity applies to entities and individuals involved in the development, manufacture, testing, distribution, administration, and use of MCMs described in a Declaration. The only statutory exception to this immunity is for actions or failures to act that constitute willful misconduct. A PREP Act Declaration is specifically for the purpose of providing immunity from liability and is different from, and not dependent on, other emergency declarations issued by HHS or other government agencies.

NATIONAL COMMISSION ON CHILDREN AND DISASTERS 2009, 2013

Every major disaster event has had a significant impact on our nation's children, and yet little attention was given to them in the legislation until the National Commission on Children and Disasters (NCCD) was established pursuant to the Kids in Disasters Well-being, Safety, and Health Act of 2007, as provided in Division G, Title VI of the Consolidated Appropriations Act of 2008. The objective of the NCCD was to examine and assess the needs of children in all phases of a disaster and to make policy recommendations at the local, state, and federal levels. The intended consequence was to be the most comprehensive review of the impact of disaster on children that had been undertaken to date and the recommendation of policies to address the gaps. The NCCD concluded in 2010 with the issuance of their final report.

Sadly, the recommendations published in the 2010 NCCD final report quickly lost traction, and little was accomplished to advance the care of children following disasters. Distressed by the lack of progress, former Commission members advocated for and were successful in launching a second Commission to continue their work. The National Advisory Committee on Children and Disasters (NACCD) was established in 2014 with the stated purpose to: provide advice and consultation with respect to the activities carried out pursuant to section 2814 of the PHS Act as applicable and appropriate (42 U.S.C. § 300hh-16); evaluate and provide input with respect to the medical and public health needs of children as they relate to preparation for, response to, and recovery from all-hazards emergencies; and provide advice and consultation with respect to state emergency preparedness and response activities for children, including related drills and exercises pursuant to the preparedness goals under section 2802(b) of the PHS Act (42 U.S.C. § 300hh-1). The NCAAD report can be found at www.phe.gov/Preparedness/legal/boards/naccd/meetings/Documents/naccd-hs-wg-rpt082017.pdf, (NACCD, 2017b) and much work remains to be done for this group of vulnerable individuals who cannot advocate for themselves.

NATIONAL TERRORISM ADVISORY SYSTEM (2011)

The signing of Homeland Security Presidential Directive-3 in 2002 established the Homeland Security Advisory System (HSAS) to communicate information concerning the threat of terrorist attacks to the federal, state, and local organizers (Homeland Security Presidential Directive-3, 2002; Sharp, 2013). At the time, the system was composed of five levels of perceived threat and a color to accompany each: green (low), blue (guarded), yellow (elevated), orange (high), and red (severe) (Homeland Security Presidential Directive-3, 2002). By assigning a color to each level, the federal government was aiming to quickly and clearly communicate the threat level to the general population and key organizations involved in protecting the United States from terrorist attacks (DHS, 2011b), however the information communicated was greatly misunderstood. It contained little record as to what caused the change in threat level and what people should do in response (Sharp, 2013). As a result, very few states incorporated HSAS threat level information into their disaster plans or even addressed the topic (Shapiro & Cohen, 2007; Sharp, 2013). In 2011, the DHS replaced the poorly adopted color-coded alerts of the HSAS with the National Terrorism Advisory System (NTAS), designed to more effectively communicate information about terrorist threats by providing timely, detailed information to the American

public. Since 2015, the DHS has used the NTAS bulletins to highlight the continuing terror threat to the U.S. homeland. In May of 2018, DHS issued a bulletin stating that "the United States is engaged in a generational fight against terrorists who seek to attack the American people, our country, and our way of life. An informed, vigilant and engaged public remains one of our greatest assets to identify potential terrorists and prevent attacks" (DHS, 2018).

NATIONAL HEALTH SECURITY STRATEGY AND IMPLEMENTATION PLAN (2015–18)

The National Health Security Strategy 2015–18 (NHSS) provides strategic direction to ensure that efforts to improve health security nationwide over the 4 years of the plan are guided by a common vision; based on sound evidence; and carried out in an efficient, collaborative manner. ASPR led the development of the NHSS in collaboration with a broad range of stakeholders, including representatives from local, state, territorial, tribal, and federal governments; community-based organizations; private-sector firms; and academia. The strategy is one of the most important documents for the public health, health care, and emergency management communities, providing a framework to build community resilience, strengthen and sustain health emergency response systems, improve capabilities, and prioritize resources on current and future budgets. The NHSS describes a vision ("a nation that is secure and resilient in the face of diverse incidents with health consequences, with people in all communities enjoying a high level of security against threats to their health and well-being") and goal (sustain communities' abilities to prevent, protect against, mitigate the effects of, respond to, and recover from incidents with negative health consequences) for national health security and identifies five strategic objectives (Table 30.2).

PANDEMIC AND ALL-HAZARDS PREPAREDNESS REAUTHORIZATION ACT (2013)

In March 2013 Congress passed and the President signed the Pandemic and All-Hazards Preparedness Reauthorization Act (PAHPRA), Public Law No. 113-5. The 2013 law builds on work of the HHS to advance national health security. These include authorizing funding for public health and medical preparedness programs, such as the Hospital Preparedness Program and the Public Health Emergency Preparedness Cooperative Agreement, amending the Public Health Service Act to grant state health departments greatly needed flexibility in dedicating staff resources to meeting critical community needs in a disaster, authorizing funding

TABLE 30.2 National Health Security Strategy (NHSS) Strategic Objectives

Strategic Objective 1: Build and sustain healthy, resilient communities	The NHSS aims to improve community health resilience—a community's ability to use its assets to strengthen public health and health care systems and to improve the community's physical, behavioral, and social health in order to withstand, adapt to, and recover from adversity. This objective focuses on encouraging social connectedness, enhancing coordination of health and human services through partnerships, and building a culture of resilience.
Strategic Objective 2: Enhance the national capability to produce and effectively use both medical countermeasures and nonpharmaceutical interventions	Countermeasures are used to protect communities from and limit the adverse health impacts of chemical, biological, radiological, and nuclear (CBRN) attacks, outbreaks of infectious diseases, and other incidents. This objective aims to make available a range of medical countermeasures and nonpharmaceutical interventions to protect health during incidents; expand non-federal stakeholder involvement in the Public Health Emergency Medical Countermeasures Enterprise (PHEMCE) process; focus research and translation of findings on nonpharmaceutical interventions (NPIs); and improve distribution and dispensing of medical countermeasures.
Strategic Objective 3: Ensure comprehensive health situational awareness to support decision-making before incidents and during response and recovery operations	Active and timely situational awareness provides the foundation for decisions and actions that may result in better resource utilization, successful prevention and mitigation of emerging threats, and improved health security for the nation. This objective focuses on improving data-sharing, using innovative systems and tools for health situational awareness (HSA), improving operational capabilities to meet the full range of HSA needs across stakeholders, developing a collaborative oversight body for HSA, and addressing technological and policy barriers to HSA.
Strategic Objective 4: Enhance the integration and effectiveness of the public health, health care, and emergency management systems	The integration of public health, health care, and emergency management systems means that they are able to work together effectively and efficiently routinely, mutually supporting one another so that they can seamlessly scale up to handle increased requirements or demands during the mitigation, response, and recovery phases of an incident. This objective seeks to strengthen health care coalitions and regional planning alliances, build on and improve routine services and systems, ensure that the integrated systems can scale to meet the access and functional needs of at-risk individuals, strengthen health security workforce education, increase the number of trained workers and volunteers, and effectively manage and use that workforce.
Strategic Objective 5: Strengthen global health security	Global health security refers to preparedness for, response to, and recovery from incidents that adversely affect health and that also could pose a risk to security, destabilize economies, disrupt social cohesion, and affect the critical business of government. This objective seeks to improve global health security by supporting the implementation of the World Health Organization (WHO) International Health Regulations.

Source: U.S. Department of Health and Human Services, Office of the Assistant Secretary for Preparedness and Response. Retrieved from www.phe.gov/Preparedness/planning/authority/nhss/Pages/strategy.aspx.

through 2018 for buying MCMs under the Project BioShield Act, and increasing the flexibility of BioShield to support advanced research and development of potential MCMs. PAHPRA enhanced the authority of the FDA to support rapid responses to public health emergencies. The purpose of the PAHPRA is "to reauthorize certain programs under the Public Health Service Act and the Federal Food, Drug, and Cosmetic Act with respect to public health security and all-hazards preparedness."

OFFICE OF THE ASSISTANT SECRETARY FOR PREPAREDNESS AND RESPONSE (2018)

In January 2018, the Director of the Assistant Secretary for Preparedness and Response (ASPR) testified before Congress as to ASPR's four key priority areas for the future described in *Facing 21st Century Public Health Threats: Our Nation's Preparedness and Response Capabilities, Part 1* (Statement of Robert Kadlec, MD, MTM&H,

MS, ASPR, January 17, 2018). Dr. Kadlec's testimony stated the following:

> First, provide strong leadership, including clear policy direction, improved threat awareness, and secure adequate resources. Second, seek the creation of a "national disaster healthcare system" by better leveraging and enhancing existing programs—such as the Hospital Preparedness Program (HPP) and the National Disaster Medical System (NDMS)—to create a more coherent, comprehensive, and capable regional system integrated into daily care delivery. Third, advocate for the sustainment of robust and reliable public health security capabilities, primarily through the Centers for Disease Control and Prevention (CDC), but also through other components of HHS, including an improved ability to detect and diagnose infectious diseases and other threats, as well as the capability to rapidly dispense medical countermeasures in an emergency. Fourth, advance an innovative medical countermeasures enterprise by capitalizing on additional authorities provided in the 21st Century Cures Act, as well as advances in biotechnology and science, in order to develop and maintain a robust stockpile of safe and efficacious vaccines, medicines, and supplies to respond to emerging disease outbreaks, pandemics, and chemical, biological, radiological, and nuclear incidents and attacks. (ASPR, 2018)

PUBLIC HEALTH EMERGENCY PREPAREDNESS ACT (2018)

In May 2018, a Senate committee approved the Public Health Emergency Preparedness Act (HR 3579) to reauthorize federal programs for health emergencies like large-scale disease outbreaks or major catastrophes. The pandemic-related bill would primarily renew and set funding levels for several HHS programs that support research into treatments or vaccines for emergency uses and purchase those and other medical supplies needed to respond to health emergencies. The programs are due to expire, and the bill would give them authority to operate through fiscal 2023. Although appropriations legislation would ultimately need to fund these programs for fiscal 2019 and beyond, the bill would allow for increased spending on them. The Biomedical Advanced Research and Development Authority (BARDA), which funds early-stage private sector research into new medical products, would be authorized at approximately $612 million per year. It received nearly $537 million in the fiscal 2018 omnibus (PL 115-141). The BioShield Special Reserve Fund, which is used to invest in products that are closer to being ready and to purchase some of them, would be authorized at $3.5 billion for the entire fiscal 2019–23 period, with the money available until it is spent. At this time, it is unclear whether the Appropriations Committee will accept that kind of advanced appropriation.

STRATEGIC NATIONAL STOCKPILE

The Public Health Service Act authorizes the secretary of HHS, in coordination with the secretary of Homeland Security, to maintain a stockpile of drugs, vaccines, and other medical products and supplies, known as the Strategic National Stockpile (SNS), to provide for the emergency health security of the United States and its territories (Public Health Service Act §319F-2; 42 U.S.C. § 247d-6b). The current SNS program has its origin in the National Pharmaceutical Stockpile (NPS), which Congress required the HHS and the CDC to create in 1999. The mission of the NPS was to assemble large quantities of essential medical supplies to provide to states and communities during an emergency within 12 hours of a federal decision to deploy the stockpile. In 2003, the NPS was renamed the SNS (CDC, 2018). The SNS according to the Health Emergency Preparedness bill described above, would be authorized at $610 million, the same amount it received in fiscal 2018. Oversight and control of the SNS has engendered political controversy. Previously administered by the CDC, the current administration has shifted authority over the stockpile to the HHS ASPR. ASPR also oversees the funds for BARDA and Project BioShield.

CONCLUSION

Disaster health policies should be thoughtfully designed and drafted in anticipation of the next disaster or public health emergency event. Policies and the resultant plans they inspire should be constructed through collaboration and in coordination with the planned stakeholders of the policy, community, and organizational members and the health care personnel responding to the event. Nurses and other health care providers are in a unique position to contribute to these policy discussions. To fulfill this role, nurses must be aware of challenges faced in disaster planning and to previous policy successes and failures.

DISCUSSION QUESTIONS

1. How can the evaluation of policies be better incorporated into the planning phase of policy? Consider which aspects of policymaking, funding requirements, personnel needs, and timing for evaluation of programs would be involved.
2. What can be done to direct the planning of disaster policy to be more proactive instead of retroactive?
3. How can the involvement of a community of interest be used to avoid the unintended consequences?

REFERENCES

American Medical Association. (2018). *AMA code of medical ethics.* Retrieved from www.ama-assn.org/delivering-care/physicians-responsibilities-disaster-response-preparedness.

American Nurses Association. (2017). *Who will be there? Ethics, the law, and a nurse's duty to respond in a disaster.* Retrieved from www.nursingworld.org/MainMenuCategories/WorkplaceSafety/Healthy-Work-Environment/DPR/Disaster-Preparedness.pdf.

Centers for Disease Control and Prevention. (2019, September 24). *Strategic national stockpile.* Retrieved from www.cdc.gov/phpr/stockpile/stockpile.htm.

Cohen, J. (2011). Biodefense: 10 years after: Reinventing project BioShield. *Science, 333*(6047), 1216–1218.

Daschle, T., & Gregg, J. (2018). *Budgeting for medical countermeasures: An ongoing need for preparedness.* Bipartisan Policy Center. Retrieved from https://bipartisanpolicy.org/wp-content/uploads/2018/02/BPC-Health-Budgeting-For-Medical-Countermeasures-An-Ongoing-Need-For-Preparedness.pdf.

Federal Emergency Management Agency. (2018). *Post-Katrina Emergency Management Reform Act of 2006.* Retrieved from https://emilms.fema.gov/is230c/fem0101200.htm.

Gottron, F., & Shea, D.A. (2011). *Federal efforts to address the threat of bioterrorism: Selected issues and options for Congress.* Congressional Research Service. Retrieved from digital.library.unt.edu/ark:/67531/metadc103084/m1/1/high_res_d/R41123_2011Feb08.pdf.

Homeland Security Act. (2002). Public Law No. 107-296, S. 102, 107th Congress.

Homeland Security Presidential Directive-3. (2002). Retrieved from georgewbush-whitehouse.archives.gov/news/releases/2002/03/20020312-5.html.

House Report 1678. (2017). *To amend the Robert T. Stafford Disaster Relief and Emergency Assistance Act concerning the statute of limitations for actions to recover disaster or emergency assistance payments, and for other purposes.* Retrieved from www.congress.gov/bill/115th-congress/house-bill/1678/actions?r=40&pageSort=asc.

Kadlec, R. (2013). *Renewing the project BioShield Act: What has it brought and wrought?* Center for a New American Security. Retrieved from www.cnas.org/files/documents/publications/CNAS_RenewingTheProjectBioShieldAct_Kadlec.pdf.

Kean, T.H., & Hamilton, L.H. (2004). *The 9/11 Commission report.* Retrieved from www.9-11commission.gov/report/911Report.pdf.

Leonard, B. (Ed.). (2009). *Decline of the National Disaster Medical System: Report by the Committee on Government Reform, Minority Staff, US House of Representatives.* Darby, PA: Diane Publishing.

McCarthy, F. (2011). *Federal Stafford Act disaster assistance: Presidential declarations, eligible activities, and funding.* Congressional Research Service. Retrieved from https://fas.org/sgp/crs/homesec/RL33053.pdf

National Advisory Committee on Children and Disasters. (2017a). *Charter on the National Advisory Committee on Children and Disasters.* Retrieved from www.phe.gov/Preparedness/legal/boards/naccd/Documents/naccd-charter.pdf.

National Advisory Committee on Children and Disasters. (2017b). *Exploring approaches and strategies for human services and child-serving institutions to promote resiliency and recovery for children and youth affected by natural disasters.* Retrieved from www.phe.gov/Preparedness/legal/boards/naccd/meetings/Documents/naccd-hs-wg-rpt082017.pdf.

National Oceanic and Atmospheric Administration, National Centers for Environmental Information. (2018). *Billion dollar weather and climate disasters overview.* Retrieved from www.ncdc.noaa.gov/billions.

Pandemic All-Hazards Preparedness Act. (2006). Public Law 109-417. 109th Congress.

Pandemic and All-Hazards Preparedness Reauthorization Act. (2013). Public Law No. 113-5. 113th Congress.

Post-Katrina Emergency Management Reform Act of 2006. (2006). Public Law 109-295. 109th Congress. Retrieved from www.doi.gov/sites/doi.gov/files/uploads/Post_Katrina_Emergency_Management_Reform_Act_pdf.pdf.

Public Readiness and Emergency Preparedness Act. (2005). Retrieved from www.phe.gov/Preparedness/legal/prepact/Pages/default.aspx.

Robert T. Stafford Disaster Relief and Emergency Assistance Act. (2016). Public Law 93-288, as amended, 42 U.S.C. 5121 et seq., and Related Authorities. S.3721, 109th Congress. Retrieved from www.fema.gov/media-library/assets/documents/15271.

Sell, T.K., & Watson, M. (2013). Federal agency biodefense funding, FY2013-FY2014. *Biosecurity and Bioterrorism: Biodefense Strategy, Practice, and Science, 1*(3), 196–216.

Shapiro, J.N., & Cohen, D.K. (2007). Color bind: Lessons from the failed Homeland Security Advisory System. *International Security, 32*(2), 121–154.

Sharp, V.H. (2013). *Faded colors: From the Homeland Security Advisory System (HSAS) to the National Terrorism Advisory System (NTAS)* (Master's thesis). Monterey, CA: Naval Postgraduate School.

Sylves, R. (2008). *Disaster policy and politics: Emergency management and homeland security.* Washington, DC: CQ Press.

U.S. Department of Health and Human Services. (2009). *National Health Security strategy of the United States of America.* Retrieved from www.phe.gov/Preparedness/planning/authority/nhss/Pages/default.aspx.

U.S. Department of Health and Human Services. (2013). *Project BioShield acquisitions: Public health emergency: Public health and medical emergency support for a nation prepared.* Retrieved from www.phe.gov/about/amcg/Pages/projectBioShield.aspx.

U.S. Department of Health and Human Services. (2016). *Medical countermeasures.* Retrieved from www.medicalcountermeasures.gov/barda/cbrn/project-bioshield-overview.aspx.

U.S. Department of Homeland Security. (2003). *Homeland Security Presidential Directive-5.* Retrieved from www.dhs.gov/publication/homeland-security-presidential-directive-5.

U.S. Department of Homeland Security. (2008). *National Response Framework.* Retrieved from www.fema.gov/pdf/emergency/nrf/nrf-core.pdf.

U.S. Department of Homeland Security. (2011a). *National preparedness goal*. Retrieved from www.fema.gov/media-library-data/20130726-1828-25045-9470/national_preparedness_goal_2011.pdf.

U.S. Department of Homeland Security. (2011b). *National Terrorism Advisory System public guide*. Retrieved from www.dhs.gov/xlibrary/assets/ntas/ntas-public-guide.pdf.

U.S. Department of Homeland Security. (2011c). *Presidential Policy Directive/PPD 8: National preparedness*. Retrieved from www.dhs.gov/presidential-policy-directive-8-national-preparedness.

U.S. Department of Homeland Security. (2013a). *Chronology of changes to the Homeland Security Advisory System*. Retrieved from www.dhs.gov/homeland-security-advisory-system.

U.S. Department of Homeland Security. (2013b). *National Response Framework* (2nd ed.). Retrieved from www.fema.gov/media-library-data/20130726-1914-25045-1246/final_national_response_framework_20130501.pdf.

U.S. Department of Homeland Security. (2018, May 9). *National Terrorism Advisory System: Bulletin*. Retrieved from www.dhs.gov/sites/default/files/ntas/alerts/18_0509_NTAS-Bulletin_0.pdf.

U.S. Federal Emergency Management Agency. (2014). *National Preparedness System*. Retrieved from www.fema.gov/national-preparedness-system.

U.S. Office of the Press Secretary. (2013). *Presidential policy directive—Critical infrastructure security and resilience*. Retrieved from www.whitehouse.gov/the-press-office/2013/02/12/presidential-policy-directive-critical-infrastructure-security-and-resil.

ONLINE RESOURCES

Centers for Disease Control and Prevention: Emergency Preparedness and Response
https://emergency.cdc.gov
Federal Emergency Management Agency
www.fema.gov
Overview of the National Response Framework through the Federal Emergency Management Agency
www.fema.gov/national-response-framework
The Robert T. Stafford Disaster Relief and Emergency Assistance Act, as amended, and Regulated Authorities as of August 2016
www.fema.gov/media-library/assets/documents/15271
U.S. Department of Labor, Office of the Assistant Secretary for Policy
www.dol.gov/dol/aboutdol/history/carter-asper.htm

31

Advancing New Models of Primary Care

Margaret Mary Flinter and Mary Blankson

"Change will not come if we wait for some other person or some other time. We are the ones we've been waiting for. We are the change that we seek."

Barack Obama

Primary care is not a new concept, but a new vision of primary care is emerging. Forty years ago, the World Health Organization (WHO, 1978) released the Declaration at Alma-Ata affirming attainment of optimum health as a human right and a social goal. The promise of the Declaration may not have been fully realized globally, but much progress has been made in the areas of health professions training, the organization and delivery of health care, and changes in policy, payment, and insurance coverage. The most significant legislative development of a generation, the Patient Protection and Affordable Care Act (ACA) of 2010 has had a significant impact on primary care, including making it more accessible to millions of people who gained health coverage.

The foundational principles of primary care as detailed by Starfield (1998)—accessibility, affordability, first contact, proximity to where people live and work, providing both preventative and curative services, and engaging the community—remain core to our understanding of primary care, even if we fall short. With its emphasis on first contact and care coordination, primary care has consistently been associated with fewer health disparities across subpopulations (Starfield, Shi, & Macinko, 2005). In addition, WHO emphasizes the importance of addressing social determinants of health (Van Lerberghe, 2008). Worries about the sustainability, affordability, and political will to achieve this vision of universal access to primary care remain; but nurses, particularly nurse practitioners (NPs), have shown a robust commitment to primary care, helping to ease these concerns (Bodenheimer, 2006).

In this chapter, we look back at the traditionally accepted definitions of primary care with a forward view of broad scientific and societal changes, along with health care workforce trends and emerging health threats and opportunities, and their policy implications. We consider primary care in the context of multiple settings that are the source of care in America today. These include federally qualified health centers (FQHCs), the nation's largest system of primary care, born of the civil rights movement and with a statutory mandate to care for the poor, the uninsured, special populations, and to deliver a comprehensive set of prevention and treatment services—all in a unique governance structure that requires a consumer-majority. In a time of significant debate and question about the concept of health care as a right, not a privilege, the bipartisan congressional support that has allowed FQHCs to grow, innovate, and test new models of primary care stands as a beacon of hope. No one system holds all the answers to health care, however. We consider multiple settings and systems, and the impact that broad changes are having on primary care today and into the future.

PRIMARY CARE AND SOCIAL DETERMINANTS OF HEALTH

The greatest influences on overall health outcomes are not derived from health care services, but from the social determinants of health (adequate income, housing, education, employment, safety, and social environment), genetic predisposition, and lifestyle, all of which have led to increased focus on health promotion and prevention (McGinnis, Williams-Russo, & Knickman, 2002). In 2008, WHO published *Closing the Gap in a Generation: Health Equity Through Action on the Social Determinants of Health* that identifies "the conditions in which people are born, grow, live, work, and age...shaped by the distribution of money, power, and resources at global, national, and local levels are mostly responsible for health inequities—the unfair and avoidable differences in health status seen within and between countries" (WHO, Commission on Social Determinants of Health, 2008).

Primary care must address these factors. This is not to say that investing more in health care alone will resolve social determinants inequities—far from it. The National Academy of Medicine provided a framework for primary care action that includes: (1) strengthen assessment and action on health-impacting social policies, (2) expand policies that increase resources and environments fostering healthy behaviors, and (3) transform the financing of health care services (Adler et al., 2016). Over the past decade, primary care has addressed upstream interventions—policies that can affect large populations through regulation, increased access, or economic incentives—such as school-based health centers (SBHCs), early childhood and parenting supports, and more widespread access to behavioral health services (Magnan, 2017). We have decades of evidence in support of home visiting programs for new mothers and young families, perhaps the best known of which is the Nurse Family Partnership (Magnan, 2017). We can reduce the negative impact of adverse conditions by assessing families who access primary care for eligibility for and awareness of the earned income tax credit, supplemental nutrition services, housing, energy, and childcare support services; acquiring insurance coverage through Medicaid and the health insurance exchange; and increasing the minimum wage (Magnan, 2017). In the United States, there has been renewed emphasis on screening for social determinants of health using tools that identify those who are "positive" or "at risk" by virtue of those factors, then adjusting care delivery, improving coordination of care, referring to community resources, and even reforming the primary care payment model (Chung et al., 2016; Gottlieb et al., 2016). There is interest in using this screening data to predict the need for social services and other interventions to reduce health risks, including risks of admission and readmission to acute care settings (Kasthurirathne et al., 2017). Providers can now code specifically for social determinants using standard International Classification of Diseases (ICD-10) definitions. The potential power of electronic health records to link these factors to health status and individual health risk, coupled with available public health data, bode well for the future of value-based, population-health management (Gottlieb et al., 2016).

Screening alone, of course, is insufficient, and a referral is ineffective if there are no available resources. Nursing has, at its core, a commitment to advocacy and thus must work to ensure that communities have the resources to address the social determinants that pose a threat to health, safety, and well-being.

ACCESS AND THE ACA

Access and first contact care remains the essential first pillar of primary care. The ACA has contributed significantly toward improving access to highly effective primary care by reducing the number of people without health coverage, particularly in states that expanded Medicaid. In the first 5 years following signing of the ACA, the proportion of residents with insurance increased by 5.9% in states that elected to expand their Medicaid programs, compared to 2.8 percentage points in states that did not (Courtemanche et al., 2017). Medicaid expansion has reduced the percentage of uninsured receiving care in community health centers (Huguet et al., 2018).

The ACA mandated that public and private insurance provide full coverage—without restriction or out-of-pocket payment—for essential primary care services, including high-cost preventive tests and services (such as colonoscopy, mammograms, and prenatal care) while preventing denial of coverage or higher premiums for pre-existing conditions. By 2018, Congress was proposing to change the mandate for coverage of pre-existing conditions and roll back essential benefits. However, by the time of the midterm elections, pre-existing conditions and the need to protect and preserve this very popular element of the ACA had become a talking point throughout the election season for both of the major parties.

Although the ACA is most closely associated with the expanded coverage (Title 1), it also addresses issues of core concern to nursing and primary care including the role of public programs (Title 2), the quality and efficiency of health care (including the development of new patient care models) (Title 3), prevention of chronic disease and improvement of public health, including creating healthier communities (Title 4), and health care workforce (Title 5). Despite the legal and political challenges to the legislation, it has increased the percentage of Americans with coverage and access to health care and, particularly, to primary care that includes greater access to preventive, chronic illness care. (For more on the ACA, see Chapter 18.)

TEAM-BASED CARE

In addition to addressing social determinants of health in primary care, there is renewed emphasis on screening for behavioral health disorders, substance use, trauma, intimate partner violence, and other problems associated with health risks. This has been the responsibility of the

BOX 3.1 Patient-Centered Medical Home Core Concepts

- **Team-Based Care and Practice Organization:** Helps structure a practice's leadership, care team responsibilities, and how the practice partners with patients, families, and caregivers.
- **Knowing and Managing Your Patients:** Sets standards for data collection, medication reconciliation, evidence-based clinical decision support, and other activities.
- **Patient-Centered Access and Continuity:** Guides practices to provide patients with convenient access to clinical advice and helps ensure continuity of care.
- **Care Management and Support:** Helps clinicians set up care management protocols to identify patients who need more closely managed care.
- **Care Coordination and Care Transitions:** Ensures that primary and specialty care clinicians are effectively sharing information and managing patient referrals to minimize cost, confusion, and inappropriate care.
- **Performance Measurement and Quality Improvement:** Improvement helps practices develop ways to measure performance, set goals, and develop activities that will improve performance.

Source: National Commission on Quality Assurance. Retrieved from www.ncqa.org/programs/health-care-providers-practices/patient-centered-medical-home-pcmh/pcmh-concepts/.

primary care practitioner (PCP), who is already overwhelmed with providing, improving, and reporting patient outcomes. One analysis estimates that a PCP with a 2500 person panel of medium-risk patients would have to spend 7.4 hours per day to perform all the recommended preventive screenings (Yarnall et al., 2003). This is a formidable challenge and better use of health information technology (HIT), as well as a team-based approach to care, a key component of the patient-centered medical home (PCMH) (Box 31.1).

Teamlets

As primary care embraces and further develops the fundamentals of the PCMH, teams will have to execute on processes such as care coordination that emphasize patient engagement (McDonald et al., 2007). Team composition varies based on issues such as workforce availability, regulatory guidelines and state scope of practice, and reimbursement models. The core team or "teamlet" is typically made up of the PCP—physician, doctor of osteopathy, advanced practice registered nurse (APRN), or physician assistant (PA)—a medical assistant (MA), and, at times, a primary care nurse (RN, LPN/LVN) (Bodenheimer, Thomas & Willard-Grace, 2016). Teamlets can vary in terms of ratios of support staff to PCP, such as 1:1 MA-to-provider ratio to 3:1 RN-to-provider ratio, largely depending on what kind of care is provided, how it is organized, and job descriptions (Sinsky et al., 2013; Mason, 2016). The move toward value-based care requires team roles to evolve to ensure implementation of all relevant screens, chronic illness care, and care coordination, as well as quality outcomes and payment.

Primary Care Providers. PCPs are required to perfect skills such as care coordination and delegation of team-based roles and tasks. However, these may not be well developed within the context of clinical rotations or even in the organizations where they ultimately enter the workforce. Focusing on these competencies within PCP education will become more mainstream as a team-based approach becomes fully realized, with providers functioning as team leaders, effectively delegating appropriate responsibilities to the extent they are able under legal scope of practice guidelines and leveraging the skills of all team members (both clinical and non-clinical). This is essential for delivering high-quality, high-value care that enhances the patient experience and reduces PCP and, hopefully, team member burnout (Bodenheimer et al., 2014).

NPs and PAs are projected to represent the majority of new health care providers joining the workforce by 2030, particularly in primary care (Auerbach, Staiger, & Buerhaus, 2018). The impact of NPs is increasingly felt everywhere in primary care. NPs constitute about 25% of providers in rural and 23% of providers in non-rural practices, up from 17% and 15%, respectively, in 2008 (Barnes, Richards, McHugh, & Martsolf, 2018). Naylor and Kurtzman (2010) emphasize that NP readiness and willingness to work in primary care plays a pivotal role in reinvesting in that care, calling for appropriate changes to state practice acts, reimbursement rules, and public reporting on quality to support this. Evidence suggests that full practice authority—practicing without legally mandated supervision or direction by physicians—is associated with a higher supply of NPs in areas with primary care health professional shortages (Xue et al., 2018).

Medical Assistants. The role of the MA has continued to advance to include functions including care coordination, patient navigation, health coaching, population health, and more (Ladden et al., 2013). The bureau of labor statistics predicts that the job growth for this role will increase by approximately 29% from 2016 to 2026, with the growth to be mainly in preventive and direct patient care services, including primary care (U.S. Department of

Labor, 2018a). Clinical organizations and leaders and individual provider groups will need to partner with academic programs to advocate for advances and clarifications in MA scope of practice (which varies by state), as well as to forge academic partnerships to offer valuable externship experiences that can contribute to proper training and competency (Bodenheimer et al., 2014). Scope of practice issues that should be addressed range from clarifying that all PCP groups and primary care registered nurses (PC RNs) can delegate tasks to MAs, to expansions of scope to improve their use in care coordination and other roles.

Registered Nurses. The role of the PC RN is one that also is coming to greater prominence. Not all team-based care models include a PC RN. At times, organizations may utilize LPNs/LVNs, which limits the full actualization of the nursing model because of their more limited scope of practice (Wagner et al., 2017). The 2017 Josiah Macy Foundation report, *Registered Nurses: Partners in Transforming Primary Care*, recommended that primary care use RNs to build capacity and enhance care quality, and highlighted several successful models currently implemented across the country as demonstrations of role development and actualization (Bodenheimer & Mason, 2017). The role of the PC RN should change from primarily a triage function to one that is responsible for complex care management, chronic disease management (including medication titration), primary and secondary prevention, and health promotion (Flinter et al., 2017). Payment reform is creating many new avenues to further legitimize and build the business case for PC RNs through current fee-for-service (FFS) payments, additional value-based payments, and global payments where these services are more specifically built into the overall cost and reimbursement of care (Needleman, 2017).

As the business case builds for this role, national accrediting bodies and professional associations should advocate for a more in-depth focus on primary care across all RN curriculums. A survey conducted to identify both facilitators and barriers to the addition of primary care to the nursing curriculum outlined barriers including lack of financial resources, experienced faculty, faculty buy-in, and a lack of RN role models in clinical settings (Wojnar & Whelan, 2017). These barriers will be addressed as strong academic and clinical partnerships are forged with high-functioning organizations, both dedicated to training the next generation and embracing new models such as the dedicated education unit (Edgecombe, Wotton, Gonda, & Mason, 1999). Federal funding opportunities have already begun to support this transformation, including the 2018 Health Resources and Services Administration's (HRSA's) grants program to develop academic-clinical partnerships, develop PC RN role models, and advance the team-based care implementation at rural organizations (U.S. HRSA, 2018b). Despite current challenges, the Bureau of Labor Statistics predicts job growth for the RN on the scale of about 15% from 2016 to 2026, with this growth solely in roles focused on chronic disease management, such as the PC RN (U.S. Department of Labor, 2018b).

Pharmacists. Pharmacists can also play key roles. A 2014 systematic review reported that pharmacists who are co-located with primary care delivered a variety of interventions that promoted favorable results with respect to chronic disease management and evidence-based use of medication in about 50% of studies reviewed, mixed results in another roughly 16%, and no effect in the final 34% (Tan, Stewart, Elliott, & George, 2014).

Behavioral Health Clinicians. Nearly one in five Americans struggles with mental health issues, including substance use disorders (Center for Behavioral Health Statistics and Quality, 2016). Many challenges exist to integrating behavioral health into primary care, such as staffing to care for the full range of behavioral health conditions. The Learning from Effective Ambulatory Practices (LEAP) project was funded in 2012 by Robert Wood Johnson Foundation as a national project to study 30 high-performing primary care practices across the country (Ladden et al., 2013). These exemplar practices focused most of their integration efforts in areas such as universal behavioral health screening, integration of behavioral health services into chronic disease management, collaboration in delivering full-spectrum care, and new models to enhance access (Blasi et al., 2018). This project has identified additional areas that need to be addressed to embrace behavioral health integration, such as enhanced HIT tools, overall staffing, funding, and the need for strategies to mitigate coding challenges, many of which are underway already.

Other Team Members. Social workers, community health workers, and legal experts are increasingly key members of primary care staff who assist patients with addressing social needs related to the social determinants of health. In addition, nutritionists, chiropractors, and complementary and alternative health care workers are playing key roles in primary care.

There are many ways to configure teams. Research on different staffing models and their effect on clinical and financial outcomes can help to ensure maximal impact and analyze the business case for each, given real and potential barriers in payment models.

THE VIRTUALIZATION OF PRIMARY CARE

Historically, primary care has been highly personal, delivered in the context of a continuous healing relationship (Dorsey & Topol, 2016). Of the many innovations that challenge this notion of primary care, virtualization of primary care appears to be one of the most disruptive. Virtual primary care is just one point on the telehealth continuum, a continuum which includes face-to-face, real-time communication via video, email, or phone in the context of an established or random relationship, asynchronous consultations between patients and providers (again both established and random), and asynchronous consultations between primary care providers and specialists initiated by the PCP in support of clinical care and decision making for a particular patient.

Is virtual primary care inherently contradictory to the traditional definition of primary care, or does it just require us to reframe our lens? Is it the case that only primary care *services* can be delivered virtually, or can an ongoing primary care *relationship* be developed in which those services can be delivered? Change is afoot in both the public and private sectors. Centers for Medicare and Medicaid Services (CMS) has issued a change to the physician payment schedule that reflects these developments. Under a 2018 rule (CMS-1693-P), Medicare has authorized adding brief virtual check-in visits, remote evaluation of prestored patient information, and interprofessional consultation between providers as covered services. This represents a dramatic advance in CMS policy and will likely accelerate the pace of change throughout the entire health care system.

In the private sector, non-physical contact primary care has been advancing for years. Jay Parkinson, MD, co-founder of Sherpaa Health, asserts that virtual primary care maintains the relationship between patient and provider over time and is personal, coordinated, and highly effective (Sherpaa Health Inc., 2017). In the non-profit sectors, Planned Parenthood (2018) provides online virtual services to residents of several states. The benefits for rural, underserved individuals, as well as the tech-savvy urban dweller who is accustomed to immediate response to requests for services of virtually all kinds, are obvious. Along with the development of the virtual care provider (VCP) (to which we would add virtual care nurse practitioner [VCNP]), we have the direct-to-consumer (DTC) health care movement, defined as "on-demand access to health care providers through personal devices" (Ashwood, Mehrotra, Cowling, & Uscher-Pines, 2017). It is suggested that virtual care increases access, particularly for those without a pre-existing source of care (Chen et al., 2014), but does not decrease costs and may increase utilization. Finally, even "traditional" primary care is moving toward offering virtual visits to their established patients, with commercial plans offering this service to their patients. This move to virtual care has in fact been underway for over a decade in self-funded, health maintenance organization (HMO) model plans such as the former Group Health, Inc. (GHI), now part of the Kaiser Permanente system (Pearl, 2014). GHI pioneered virtual visits via telephone encounters as part of a primary care system redesign in accord with the principles of the PCMH and traditional primary care. Its reported outcomes include decreased provider burnout, decreased overall costs, high patient satisfaction, and uptake of non-face-to-face care (Reid et al., 2010).

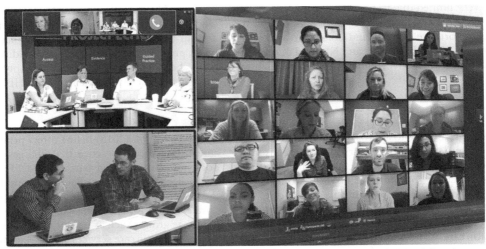

Community Health Centers of Connecticut's Weitzman Project ECHO is a case-based, didactic learning strategy that brings together expert clinical faculty with primary care teams from around the country (using videoconferencing) to address high-complexity issues like HIV, chronic pain, and opioid use disorder.

The Veterans Health Affairs (VHA) is also an innovator in this space, and provides over 2 million virtual visits a year, with a large portion of these visits focused on mental health concerns, with documented efficiencies in time and travel, and significant increases in efficacy of treatment of posttraumatic stress disorder (PTSD) for veterans in rural areas (U.S. Department of Veterans Affairs [VA], 2014). FQHCs are just beginning to report their telehealth services, with 44% of health centers providing care via telehealth in recent years (HRSA, 2017b). The majority of FQHCs reporting that they provide telehealth services are using telehealth to provide mental health services (52%), 20% use it for primary care, and 24% for chronic illness care (HRSA, 2017b). A study of 5441 patients and 144 physicians on their use and satisfaction with virtual visit encounters concluded that younger patients (and physicians) were more likely to use and provide virtual visits; patients liked the virtual visit format; and older and sicker patients were more likely to see a known provider, whereas the lowest socioeconomic groups were the least likely to see a known provider (McGrail, Ahuja, & Leaver, 2017).

For NPs and RNs in primary care, this has implications for education, training, and skill development in becoming effective telehealth providers. Rutledge et al. (2014) advocate for a multimodal training approach for NPs on the skills and knowledge needed to effectively utilize telehealth. One telehealth tool that is increasingly available to today's primary care provider is eConsults, through which PCPs pose a consult question with supporting detail to a designated specialist and receive an answer or guidance within a very short period of time (usually no more than 48 hours). It is a particularly important tool for PCPs practicing in safety net settings where access to specialists has been historically very limited due to financial, linguistic, transportation, specialist availability, and other reasons, but it has obvious importance for rural and isolated areas as well (Olayiwola et al., 2016). Both MDs and NPs find eConsults highly valuable to themselves and their patients (Liddy et al., 2018).

PRIMARY CARE SETTINGS

Today, consumers are able to approach primary care on an "à la carte" or on-demand basis. A survey of 1000 consumers reported 36% had visited a retail clinic in the past year, with 95% satisfaction; 75% of those surveyed would see a NP or PA for care; and 60% are open to a virtual doctor's visit (Health Research Institute, 2015). We posit that the ability for consumers to find, use, and pay out of pocket for virtual health care services may adversely affect current tracking and reporting systems for usual sources of care. One traditionally respected source of data on where care is

delivered is that of the National Medical Expenditure Panel Survey (MEPS) that includes nationally representative data on ambulatory care visits to physician offices in the United States. Stagnitti and colleagues (2017) used the 2015 MEPS Supplemental Medical Organizations Survey to include information on characteristics of practices of office-based providers who were identified by respondents as their usual source of care: 80% of the civilian, non-institutionalized population—about 249.6 million people—had a usual source of care, and, of these, 44.1% saw their usual source of care at least once during the year.

We urge constant vigilance on the central but unrealized tenet of equity—in access, quality, and care—as innovations in primary care evolve. In this section we look at some specific major contributors to ensuring access and quality in primary care in the United States, particularly but not exclusively for low-income and vulnerable populations. If we can achieve great outcomes with patients who are adversely affected by the social determinants of health such as poverty and low educational attainment, we should be able to do this everywhere.

Primary Care at Home

We have seen the value of home-based primary care (HBPC) for homebound, isolated, frail older population, and those for whom leaving the house is physically or emotionally impossible or costly. Innovation is called for as both public and private payers strive to meet the numbers of homebound patient populations. The Veterans Affairs has been a leader in this area, documenting increased satisfaction and decreased costs in veterans receiving primary care at home (Edes et al., 2014). Norman et al. (2018) studied six practices that included HBPC and noted that all were provider-led (physician or NP), with smaller practices tending to be provider-centered and larger practices having a team-based approach. Challenges include reimbursement, provider burnout and retention, difficulty with electronic health record linkages, and simply getting around. All practices noted the demand for HBPC far exceeded their practice's ability to meet it.

Direct Primary Care

Eskew and Klink (2015) define direct primary care (DPC) as a primary care practice that charges a periodic FFS, does not bill any third parties on a FFS basis, and any per-visit charges are less than the monthly equivalent of the periodic fee. Perhaps the best known of these is a corporate entity, Iora Health, which works with employers and large groups such as unions to provide their members with all primary care services at a set fee and with no direct patient billing. The model's mission is to restore humanity to health care and is based on a team concept with a provider, nurse, and health coach assigned to every patient (Howe, 2017).

Intensive Primary Care for the High-Need/High-Cost Patient

In response to the need for new models to provide appropriate and effective primary care to particularly challenging patients, a new focus on high-need/high-cost patients has emerged to address the need for complex care management within the context of effective primary care while reducing overall health care costs (Hochman & Asch, 2017). These include well-established, decades-old programs like PACE (Program of All-inclusive Care for the Elderly) and new models of high-intensity, multidisciplinary team-based care with dramatically smaller panels of patients (CMS, 2018c; Hochman & Asch, 2017; Powers, 2018). The challenge, as usual, is reimbursement, and these clinics are generally found within fully self-insured or fully at-risk plans since neither FFS Medicaid, Medicare, nor commercial insurers generally differentiate between reimbursements for primary care visits based on patient complexity. However, these are the type of patients seen in most safety net settings, further amplifying the challenges faced in systems where patients are disproportionately burdened by chronic illness, as well as challenged by adverse social determinants of health.

Retail Clinics

We recall the "dawn" of the retail clinics as a disruptive innovation whose time had come, coupling the corner pharmacy with the services of a NP who could educate, counsel, diagnose, and treat the most common episodic and acute illnesses. In the nearly two decades since the first clinics appeared, that premise has expanded to encompass thousands of stores owned by various major national corporations along with smaller alternatives. These national corporations have plans to significantly expand the offerings of clinical services and to engage more substantially in chronic illness management (Cassel, 2018; Frakt & Garthwaite, 2018).

Retail clinics are now part of the mainstream and expanding. The larger question for primary care is whether, as with virtual care, they might suffice as the source of "in-person" primary care—whether the "neighborhood retail clinic" might become the primary care provider, including redirection to urgent care when needed or other more specialized care. One criticism is that retail clinics may increase costs because of the ease of seeking out care for minor complaints that might have resolved with watchful waiting, or increased urgent care referrals due to the relatively limited scope of care at retail clinics (Cassel, 2018). Parents report high satisfaction with care received for their children, with parents reporting convenience, hours, difficulty getting an office appointment, and not wanting to "bother the pediatrician" for a minor problem as reasons for seeking care for a child at the retail clinic.

Federally Qualified Health Centers

Also referred to as health centers, community health centers, and FQHCs, these primary care organizations have a dramatic 50-year history of steady growth as a movement to address the primary health care needs of underserved populations and communities. They trace their historical roots to the work of Sydney and Emily Kark in South Africa in the 1940s in developing a new model of population-focused, data-driven, community-oriented health care that engaged local community members in organizing and delivering care (Kark, Kark, & Jack, 1999). The model was introduced to the United States by Jack Geiger, MD, who studied with the Karks. He returned to the United States, later proposing and securing federal funding that led to the development of the first U.S. health centers in Mound Bayou, Mississippi (Geiger, 2002; 2005).

From early on, health centers were defined by a set of core characteristics and values: private, independent non-profit organizations with consumer-controlled boards of directors, sliding scale fees for low-income persons, a comprehensive set of primary care services, and a focus on underserved geographic areas and populations. Community health centers have their own distinct enabling legislation, Section 330 of the Public Health Service Act (Title 42 U.S.C. s254b), which defines them in statute as an entity that serves a population that is medically underserved, or a special medically underserved population comprised of migratory and seasonal agricultural workers, the homeless, and residents of public housing. Organizations that meet all of the requirements of an FQHC but have not received funding under the health center program may apply to be designated FQHC Look-Alikes, which entitles them to many, though not all, of the benefits of being an FQHC (U.S. Department of Health and Human Services, 2018).

Health centers are subject to annual rigorous public reporting through a system known as the Uniform Data System (UDS). Health centers report on an extensive set of quality of care measures, health outcomes, population and patient demographic data, service utilization, workforce, and cost measures. This data is published annually for each individual health center, as well as in aggregate by state and nationally. The 2017 UDS data reported that 1373 FQHC organizations cared for 27,174,372 individuals. Health centers are leaders in providing substance abuse services in primary care, including medication-assisted treatment for opioid use disorder (HRSA, 2018b). They also achieve superior chronic illness management in hypertension and diabetes control compared to the national averages, despite the fact that their patients are overwhelmingly low income, publicly- or uninsured, and members of racial or ethnic minority groups.

NPs are a major component of the primary care workforce in this setting with 8851 FTE (full-time equivalent) NPs, compared with 12,893 FTE physicians and 3076 PAs (HRSA, 2017b). Nurses other than NPs are a strong element of the health care team in FQHCs, perhaps more so than in most primary care systems, with 17,663 FTE nurses (other than NPs) reported in 2017, along with 691 nurse midwives (HRSA, 2018a). Health centers have become leaders in training the next generation of primary care providers through physician, dentist, psychologist, and NP/PA residency and fellowship programs (Chen et al., 2012; Flinter, 2012). The broad distribution of health centers in both rural and urban areas has positioned them as first responders when threats like the opioid epidemic arise. As such, they have continued to secure bipartisan funding support.

Nurse-Managed Health Centers

Nurse-managed health centers (NMHCs) are nurse-led, primary care delivery sites located in the communities they serve and traditionally focused on vulnerable populations that lack access to care, such as homeless shelters, rural areas, or public housing communities (Vece, Sutter, Sutter, & Toulouse, 2016). NMHCs are often associated with academic institutions and provide clinically-based educational settings for undergraduates and graduate students across disciplines (National Nursing Center Consortium, 2018). In these diverse practices, NPs provide team-based care in collaboration with other providers and incorporate social needs care into their focus. The ability of these centers to grow and expand, despite evidence of effectiveness, is hampered by many challenges, including inconsistent recognition by both commercial insurers and Medicaid managed care organizations of their providers as primary care providers, and the lack of a consistent, ongoing, reliable source of federal funding unless they become FQHCs.

School-Based Health Centers

SBHCs are an often unrecognized but very important contributor to the primary care landscape, particularly for vulnerable children, families, and communities. They are operated by FQHCs, health departments, and private non-profit organizations in a collaborative, but generally independent, relationship. Although they have been around for decades and do not have any permanent legislative "home" in terms of funding and regulation, SBHCs

were included in the ACA as the recipients of funding, and legislation was introduced in 2018 to reauthorize that funding, which expired in 2014. There were 2315 SBHCs operating in 49 of 50 states and the District of Columbia in 2014 (School-Based Health Alliance, 2014); 800,000 students received care in an SBHC operated under the authority of a FQHC in 2018, and about 20% of SBHCs receive HRSA funding (HRSA, 2017a).

Although the model may vary from program to program, the trend is toward comprehensive care including primary medical care, behavioral health services, and oral health services. A systematic review confirmed that SBHCs improve health and advance health equity, particularly for low-income and racial/ethnic minority groups (Knopf et al., 2016). SBHCs are important as part of the whole-child/whole-school approach to education, with health improvements reported across multiple domains from management of chronic illness like asthma to decreased emergency department (ED) utilization and increased use of contraception among adolescents (Lewallen & Hunt, 2015). Those that are stand-alone clinics without FQHC designation or other HRSA or state funding struggle with financial sustainability in the absence of a consistent state or federal funding stream. Despite this, many states have embraced funding for SBHCs because of their ability to increase access to both primary care and behavioral health services, particularly in schools serving low-income populations.

Veterans Affairs

The VHA is America's largest integrated health care system, providing care at 1240 health care facilities, including 170 medical centers and 1061 outpatient sites of care of varying complexity (VHA outpatient clinics), and serving 9 million enrolled veterans each year (U.S. Department of Veteran Affairs, 2018). The VHA system has invested in primary care for all of its diverse and challenging populations, from homeless veterans to those with complex chronic illnesses. They do so through patient-aligned care teams (PACTs) as a way of meeting the needs of its patients and the standards of the PCMH (Kearney, Post, Pomerantz, & Zeiss, 2014; Hobson & Curtis, 2017). NPs have full practice authority in the VHA and play a key role on these teams. PACTs have been found to increase continuity and decrease ED visits (Chaiyachati et al., 2014). See Chapter 16 for more on the VHA.

TRANSITIONING FROM FEE-FOR-SERVICE TO VALUE-BASED PAYMENTS

A 2018 analysis of payment models and their influence on primary care concluded that no one payment model demonstrates consistent benefits across the quadruple aim of better quality, reduced cost, increased satisfaction with care, and increased provider satisfaction (Park, Gold, Bazemore, & Liaw, 2018). These models include traditional FFS, full risk capitation usually on a per-member per-month (PMPM) payment, pay for performance (PfP), bundled payment (episode of care, shared savings, blended FFS and capitation), comprehensive primary care payment, and finally, DPC. Implementing PMPM-based models, validating risk-adjustment tools, increasing investments in integrated behavioral health and social services, and connecting payments to patient-oriented and primary care–oriented metrics are all strategies to improve care and control costs.

In the years since the ACA was signed into law, there has been substantial change in the way health care is paid for, with a significant impact on primary care. However, these changes to date fall far short of what could be called a full transformation. The dominant payment model for primary care remains FFS—75% of all physician office visits in 2013 (Zuvekas & Cohen, 2016). On the federal level, the U.S. CMS (2018a), as well as its Center for Medicare and Medicaid Innovation (CMMI) that was authorized under the ACA, has been a leader in driving change since the ACA was implemented. On the state level, CMMI has funded the state innovation models (SIMS) to give states the funding to experiment with state-based redesign of primary care and to advance models of payment and delivery reform that lead to better quality, lower costs, and improved health for the population of the state (CMS, 2018d). Of note, CMS has authority to move innovations from pilot tests to covered benefit if found to reduce costs while improving care or outcomes. The Diabetes Prevention Program model is a prominent primary care example of a community-based intervention through YMCAs that had a positive impact on Medicare beneficiaries at high risk of developing type 2 diabetes (CMS, 2018b).

With two major initiatives launching in 2020, CMMI is continuing its commitment to innovations that improve outcomes, reduce costs, and satisfy patients and providers with a particular focus on higher complexity, need, cost, or utilization patients. First, the Emergency Triage, Treat, and Transport (ET3) Model (CMS, 2019a) provides an option for selected ambulance suppliers and providers to respond to an emergency call with options to (1) assess and treat on the scene, directly or by telehealth with a qualified health care practitioner, (2) transport the patient to a destination other than a hospital emergency room, such as a patient's primary care provider's office or an urgent care clinic, or (3) transport to an emergency room, including in situations when that is simply the patient's preference.

CMMI will also provide funding to the local or regional entities that oversee the 911 emergency response system in these selected areas to establish a medical triage line to screen for eligibility for medical triage services prior to ambulance initiation.

Second, the Primary Care First Model Options is designed to support the delivery of advanced primary care (CMS, 2019b). This initiative includes many elements of a high-performing primary care system that have already been addressed in this chapter. It goes further to encourage and incentivize primary care practices by giving participating providers more freedom to innovate in their care delivery model, reducing administrative burden and creating a simple payment structure that incorporates elements of population-based payments, flat primary care visit fees, shared savings, and performance transparency on their own performance and that of other participants. It also allows these advanced primary care practices to accept patients identified as Seriously Ill Population (SIP), including hospice and palliative care patients who lack a primary care provider. Payment amounts for these patients reflect the acuity and high need of these patients.

Both the ET3 and the Primary Care First Model Options point to a future for primary care as the bedrock of the health care system, embedded in community and responsive to the highly varied health care needs of individuals across the lifespan.

LOOKING TO THE FUTURE: WHERE WILL SCIENCE TAKE US?

The present and future hold enormous potential for radical and positive change based on the explosion of knowledge in basic science, engineering, and artificial intelligence, and the application of these to the human condition. One of the most exciting advances in primary care in recent years is the incorporation of the uniqueness of the individual patient's genomic constitution into decision making regarding both screening and treatment at the individual level, and the historic launch of a national effort, now known as the "All of Us" initiative to engage everyone in a far-reaching research initiative to advance our knowledge of health through understanding the influence and interplay of genetics and environment (Collins & Varmus, 2015). Advances in our understanding of the human genome and its application to detection, treatment, and even prevention is being felt in primary care as evidence-based screening guidelines have been put into place for common cancers, as systems to check pharmaceutical choice against genome become possible on a routine basis, and as patients ask us to help them understand what their family history means. Genetic screening in the presence of an identifiable risk became covered under the essential benefits of the ACA and made screening available to individuals who (1) had an identifiable risk and (2) had a provider who had incorporated routine screening of family history for identified risk into their practice (Fox & Shaw, 2015).

Finally, any discussion of primary care would be incomplete at a time when the death toll from drug overdose continues to rise and exceeded 66,000 deaths in 2016, with the majority coming from prescription opioids and illicit opioids, including powerful manufactured synthetics in recent years (Centers for Disease Control and Prevention, 2018). The epidemic speaks to the most urgent need for primary care to step up and respond with significantly increased capacity, competency, commitment, and service integration in the areas of behavioral health, substance abuse, addictions, and primary care prevention and treatment. There is no room for passive bystanders in the face of this epidemic among our national community of health care providers and organizations committed to primary care as a force for a healthy and just society.

CONCLUSION

We are at the dawn of yet another new era in primary care. We have the knowledge and basic elements in place for a just, equitable, effective primary care system. We have made significant progress in access to primary care, the way we deliver it, and how we pay for it. In this new era, nursing must be at the forefront of driving and shaping policy changes that support better health for all through a focus on primary care in its broadest sense: the promotion of health, the prevention of disease, and the management of chronic and acute illness in the context of the individual, the family, community, and society. Finding common ground in our highly polarized political system will continue to be a challenge. As individual nurses in service, education, public health, and policy and as nurse leaders across all domains, we will continue to innovate, transform, and advance models of primary care that build upon and reimagine a new era of primary care as defined by WHO 50 years ago.

DISCUSSION QUESTIONS

1. What is your source of primary care? To what extent does it deliver the kind of care defined by WHO, Starfield, and the authors?
2. What are the barriers to providing high-quality primary care?
3. What policies at the state and national level could strengthen primary care?

REFERENCES

Adler, N.E., Cutler, D.M., Jonathan, J.E., Galea, S., Glymour, M., Koh, H.K., & Satcher, D. (2016). *Addressing social determinants of health and health disparities.* Washington, DC: National Academy of Medicine. Retrieved from https://nam.edu/wp-content/uploads/2016/09/Addressing-Social-Determinants-of-Health-and-Health-Disparities.pdf.

Ashwood, J.S., Mehrotra, A., Cowling, D., & Uscher-Pines, L. (2017). Direct-to-consumer telehealth may increase access to care but does not decrease spending. *Health Affairs, 36*(3), 485-491.

Auerbach, D., Staiger, D.O., & Buerhaus, P. (2018). Growing ranks of advanced practice clinicians—Implications for the physician workforce. *New England Journal of Medicine, 378*(25), 2358-2360.

Barnes, H., Richards, M.R., McHugh, M.D., & Martsolf, G. (2018). Rural and nonrural primary care physician practices increasingly rely on nurse practitioners. *Health Affairs, 37*(6), 908-914.

Barnett, M.L., Yee Jr, H.F., Mehrotra, A., & Giboney, P. (2017). Los Angeles safety-net program eConsult system was rapidly adopted and decreased wait times to see specialists. *Health Affairs, 36*(3), 492-499.

Blasi, P.R., Cromp, D., McDonald, S., Hsu, C., Coleman, K., Flinter, M., & Wagner, E.H. (2018). Approaches to behavioral health integration at high performing primary care practices. *Journal of the American Board of Family Medicine, 31*(5), 691-701.

Bodenheimer, T. (2006). Primary care—Will it survive? *New England Journal of Medicine, 355*(9), 861-864.

Bodenheimer, T., Ghorob, A., Willard-Grace, R., & Grumbach, K. (2014). The 10 building blocks of high-performing primary care. *Annals of Family Medicine, 12*(2), 166-171.

Bodenheimer, T., & Mason, D. (2016). *Registered nurses: Partners in transforming primary care.* New York: The Josiah Macy Jr. Foundation. Retrieved from http://macyfoundation.org/docs/macy_pubs/Macy_Monograph_Nurses_2016_webPDF.pdf.

Bodenheimer, T., & Willard-Grace, R. (2016). Teamlets in primary care: Enhancing the patient and clinician experience. *Journal of the American Board of Family Medicine, 29*(1), 135-138.

Cassel, C.K. (2018). Can retail clinics transform health care? *JAMA, 319*(18), 1855-1856.

Center for Behavioral Health Statistics and Quality. (2016). *Key substance use and mental health indicators in the United States: Results from the 2015 national survey on drug use and health.* Retrieved from https://www.samhsa.gov/data/sites/default/files/NSDUH-FFR1-2015/NSDUH-FFR1-2015/NSDUH-FFR1-2015.pdf

Centers for Medicare and Medicaid Services. (2018a). *CMS Innovation Center.* Retrieved from https://innovation.cms.gov/.

Centers for Medicare and Medicaid Services. (2018b). *Medicare diabetes prevention program (MDFF) expanded model.* Retrieved from https://innovation.cms.gov/initiatives/medicare-diabetes-prevention-program/

Centers for Medicare and Medicaid Services. (2018c). *Programs of all-inclusive care for the elderly benefits.* Retrieved from www.medicaid.gov/medicaid/ltss/pace/index.html.

Centers for Medicare and Medicaid Services. (2018d). *State innovation models initiative.* Retrieved from https://innovation.cms.gov/initiatives/state-innovations/.

Centers for Medicare and Medicaid Services. (2019a). *Emergency triage, treat and transport (ET3) model.* Retrieved from https://innovation.cms.gov/initiatives/et3/.

Centers for Medicare and Medicaid Services. (2019b). *Primary care first model options.* Retrieved from https://innovation.cms.gov/initiatives/primary-care-first-model-options/.

Chaiyachati, K.H., Gordon, K., Long, T., Levin, W., Khan, A., Meyer, E., & Brienza, R. (2014). Continuity in a VA patient-centered medical home reduces emergency department visits. *PLoS One, 9*(5), e96356.

Chen, P.G., Mehrotra, A., & Auerbach, D.I. (2014). Do we really need more physicians? Responses to predicted primary care physician shortages. *Medical Care, 52*(2), 95-96.

Chung, E.K., Siegel, B.S., Garg, A., Conroy, K., Gross, R.S., Long, D.A., & Wade Jr, R. (2016). Screening for social determinants of health among children and families living in poverty: A guide for clinicians. *Current Problems in Pediatric and Adolescent Health Care, 46*(5), 135-153.

Collins, F.S., & Varmus, H. (2015). A new initiative on precision medicine. *New England Journal of Medicine, 372*(9), 793-795.

Courtemanche, C., Marton, J., Ukert, B., Yelowitz, A., & Zapata, D. (2017). Early impacts of the affordable care act on health insurance coverage in Medicaid expansion and non-expansion states. *Journal of Policy Analysis and Management, 36*(1), 178-210.

Dorsey, E.R., & Topol, E.J. (2016). State of telehealth. *New England Journal of Medicine, 375*(14), 1399-1400.

Edes, T., Kinosian, B., Vuckovic, N.H., Olivia Nichols, L., Mary Becker, M., & Hossain, M. (2014). Better access, quality, and cost for clinically complex veterans with home-based primary care. *Journal of the American Geriatrics Society, 62*(10), 1954-1961.

Edgecombe, K., Wotton, K., Gonda, J., & Mason, P. (1999). Dedicated education units: A new concept for clinical teaching and learning. *Contemporary Nurse, 8*(4), 166-171.

Eskew, P.M., & Klink, K. (2015). Direct primary care: Practice distribution and cost across the nation. *Journal of the American Board of Family Medicine, 28*(6), 793-801.

Flinter, M. (2012). From new nurse practitioner to primary care provider: Bridging the transition through FQHC-based residency training. *OJIN: The Online Journal of Issues in Nursing, 17*(1), 6.

Flinter, M., Hsu, C., Cromp, D., Ladden, M.D., & Wagner, E.H. (2017). Registered nurses in primary care: Emerging new roles and contributions to team-based care in high-performing practices. *Journal of Ambulatory Care Management, 40*(4), 287.

Fox, J.B., & Shaw, F.E. (2015). Clinical preventive services coverage and the affordable care act. *American Journal of Public Health, 105*(1), e10.

Frakt, A.B., & Garthwaite, C. (2018). The CVS–Aetna merger: Another large bet on the changing US health care landscape. *Annals of Internal Medicine, 168*(7), 511-512

Geiger, H.J. (2002). Community-oriented primary care: A path to community development. *American Journal of Public Health, 92*(11), 1713-1716.

Geiger, H.J. (2005). The first community health centers: A model of enduring value. *Journal of Ambulatory Care Management, 28*(4), 313-320.

Gottlieb, L., Tobey, R., Cantor, J., Hessler, D., & Adler, N.E. (2016). Integrating social and medical data to improve population health: Opportunities and barriers. *Health Affairs, 35*(11), 2116-2123.

Health Research Institute. (2015). *Primary care in the new health economy: Time for a makeover.* Retrieved from www.pwc.com/us/en/health-industries/our-perspective/assets/pwc-hri-primary-care-new-economy-2016.pdf

Hobson, A., & Curtis, A. (2017). Improving the care of veterans: The role of nurse practitioners in team-based population health management. *Journal of the American Association of Nurse Practitioners, 29*(11), 644-650.

Hochman, M., & Asch, S.M. (2017). Disruptive models in primary care: Caring for high-needs, high-cost populations. *Journal of General Internal Medicine, 32*(4), 392-397.

Howe, M. (2017). Profile: Iora Health transactional vs. relationship-based care. *Nursing Management, 48*(5):26-31.

Huguet, N., Springer, R., Marino, M., Angier, H., Hoopes, M., Holderness, H., & DeVoe, J.E. (2018). The impact of the Affordable Care Act (ACA) Medicaid expansion on visit rates for diabetes in safety net health centers. *Journal of the American Board of Family Medicine, 31*(6), 905-916.

Kark, S., Kark, E., & Jack, W. (1999). Promoting community health: From Pholela to Jerusalem. *Development, 20*, 305.

Kasthurirathne, S.N., Vest, J.R., Menachemi, N., Halverson, P.K., & Grannis, S.J. (2017). Assessing the capacity of social determinants of health data to augment predictive models identifying patients in need of wraparound social services. *Journal of the American Medical Informatics Association, 25*(1), 47-53.

Kearney, L.K., Post, E.P., Pomerantz, A.S., & Zeiss, A.M. (2014). Applying the interprofessional patient aligned care team in the Department of Veterans Affairs: Transforming primary care. *American Psychologist, 69*(4), 399.

Knopf, J.A., Finnie, R.K., Peng, Y., Hahn, R.A., Truman, B.I., Vernon-Smiley, M., … & Community Preventive Services Task Force. (2016). School-based health centers to advance health equity: A community guide systematic review. *Journal of Preventive Medicine, 51*(1), 114-126.

Ladden, M.D., Bodenheimer, T., Fishman, N.W., Flinter, M., Hsu, C., Parchman, M., & Wagner, E.H. (2013). The emerging primary care workforce: Preliminary observations from the primary care team learning from effective ambulatory practices project. *Academic Medicine, 88*(12), 1830-1834.

Lathrop, B. (2013). Nursing leadership in addressing the social determinants of health. *Policy, Politics, & Nursing Practice, 14*(1), 41-47.

Lewallen, T.C., Hunt, H., Potts-Datema, W., Zaza, S., & Giles, W. (2015). The whole school, whole community, whole child model: A new approach for improving educational attainment and healthy development for students. *Journal of School Health, 85*(11), 729-739.

Liddy, C., Moroz, I., Mihan, A., Nawar, N., & Keely, E. (2018). A systematic review of asynchronous, provider-to-provider, electronic consultation services to improve access to specialty care available worldwide. *Telemedicine and E-Health.* doi: 10.1089/tmj.2018.0005. [Epub ahead of print].

Magnan, S. (2017). *Social determinants of health 101 for health care: Five plus five.* National Academy of Medicine discussion paper. Retrieved from https://nam.edu/social-determinants-of-health-101-for-health-care-five-plus-five/.

Mason, D.J. (2016). Partnering with nurses to transform primary care. *JAMA, 316*(23), 2471-2472.

McDonald, K.M., Sundaram, V., Bravata, D.M., Lewis, R., Lin, N., Kraft, S.A., & Owens, D.K. (2007). *Closing the quality gap: A critical analysis of quality improvement strategies.* Rockville, MD: Agency for Health Research and Quality. Retrieved from www.ncbi.nlm.nih.gov/books/NBK44015/.

McDonough, J.E. (2018). The health reformers' dilemma. *The Milbank Quarterly, 96*(4), 631-634.

McGinnis, J.M., Williams-Russo, P., & Knickman, J. R. (2002). The case for more active policy attention to health promotion. *Health Affairs, 21*(2), 78-93.

McGrail, K.M., Ahuja, M.A., & Leaver, C.A. (2017). Virtual visits and patient-centered care: Results of a patient survey and observational study. *Journal of Medical Internet Research, 19*(5), e177.

National Nursing Center Consortium. (2018). About us: The National Nurse-Led Care Consortium (NNCC). Retrieved from www.nurseledcare.org/.

Naylor, M.D., & Kurtzman, E.T. (2010). The role of nurse practitioners in reinventing primary care. *Health Affairs, 29*(5), 893-899.

Needleman, J. (2017). Expanding the role of registered nurses in primary care: A business case analysis. *Journal of Medical Practice Management, 32*(5), 343-351.

Norman, G.J., Orton, K., Wade, A., Morris, A.M., & Slaboda, J.C. (2018). Operation and challenges of home-based medical practices in the US: Findings from six aggregated case studies. *BMC Health Services Research,*18(1), 45. Retrieved from https://bmchealthservres.biomedcentral.com/articles/10.1186/s12913-018-2855-x.

Olayiwola, J.N., Anderson, D., Jepeal, N., Aseltine, R., Pickett, C., Yan, J., & Zlateva, I. (2016). Electronic consultations to improve the primary care-specialty care interface for cardiology in the medically underserved: A cluster-randomized controlled trial. *Annals of Family Medicine, 14*(2), 133-140.

Park, B., Gold, S.B., Bazemore, A., & Liaw, W. (2018). How evolving United States payment models influence primary care and its impact on the Quadruple Aim. *Journal of the American Board of Family Medicine, 31*(4), 588-604.

Pearl, R. (2014). Kaiser Permanente Northern California: Current experiences with internet, mobile, and video technologies. *Health Affairs, 33*(2), 251-257.

Planned Parenthood Federation. (2018). *Planned Parenthood at a glance.* Retrieved from www.plannedparenthood.org/about-us/who-we-are/planned-parenthood-at-a-glance.

Powers, J.S. (2018). *Value driven healthcare and geriatric medicine.* New York: Springer.

Reid, R.J., Coleman, K., Johnson, E.A., Fishman, P.A., Hsu, C., Soman, M.P., ... & Larson, E.B. (2010). The group health medical home at year two: Cost savings, higher patient satisfaction, and less burnout for providers. *Health Affairs, 29*(5), 835-843.

Rutledge, C.M., Haney, T., Bordelon, M., Renaud, M., & Fowler, C. (2014). Telehealth: Preparing advanced practice nurses to address healthcare needs in rural and underserved populations. *International Journal of Nursing Education Scholarship, 11*(1), 1-9.

School-Based Health Alliance. (2014). *2013-14 Digital census report.* Retrieved from https://censusreport.sbh4all.org/.

Sherpaa Health, Inc. (2017). *What is virtual primary care (VPC)?* Retrieved from http://scope.sherpaa.com/virtual-primary-care-vpc/.

Sinsky, C.A., Willard-Grace, R., Schutzbank, A.M., Sinsky, T.A., Margolius, D., & Bodenheimer, T. (2013). In search of joy in practice: A report of 23 high-functioning primary care practices. *Annals of Family Medicine, 11*(3), 272-278.

Stagnitti, M.N., Soni, A., & Zodet, M.W. (2017). *Characteristics of practices used as usual source of care providers during 2015—Results from the MEPS medical organizations survey* [statistical brief #502]. Medical Expenditure Panel Survey (US). Rockville, MD: Agency for Healthcare Research and Quality (US). Retrieved from www.ncbi.nlm.nih.gov/books/NBK447181/.

Starfield, B. (1998). *Primary care: Balancing health needs, services, and technology.* New York: Oxford University Press.

Starfield, B., Shi, L., & Macinko, J. (2005). Contribution of primary care to health systems and health. *The Milbank Quarterly, 83*(3), 457-502.

Tan, E.C., Stewart, K., Elliott, R.A., & George, J. (2014). Pharmacist services provided in general practice clinics: A systematic review and meta-analysis. *Research in Social and Administrative Pharmacy, 10*(4), 608-622.

U.S. Department of Health and Human Services. (2018). *Health center program look-alikes.* Retrieved from https://bphc.hrsa.gov/programopportunities/lookalike/index.html.

U. S. Department of Labor, Bureau of Labor Statistics. (2018a). *Occupational outlook handbook: Medical assistants.* Retrieved from www.bls.gov/ooh/healthcare/medical-assistants.htm.

U.S. Department of Labor, Bureau of Labor Statistics. (2018b). *Occupational outlook handbook: Registered nurses.* Retrieved from www.bls.gov/ooh/healthcare/registered-nurses.htm.

U.S. Department of Veterans Affairs. (2014). *VA telehealth services served over 690,000 veterans in fiscal year 2014.* Retrieved from www.va.gov/opa/pressrel/pressrelease.cfm?id=2646.

U.S. Department of Veteran Affairs. (2018). *About Veterans Health Administration.* Retrieved from www.va.gov/health/aboutvha.asp.

U.S. Health Resources and Services Administration. (2017a). *School-based health centers.* Retrieved from www.hrsa.gov/our-stories/school-health-centers/index.html.

U.S. Health Resources and Services Administration. (2017b). *Uniform Data System (UDS).* Retrieved from https://bphc.hrsa.gov/datareporting/reporting/index.html.

U.S. Health Resources and Services Administration. (2018a). *Nurse Education, Practice, Quality and Retention (NEPQR)— Registered Nurses in Primary Care (RNPC) training program.* Retrieved from https://bhw.hrsa.gov/fundingopportunities/?id=f5ad18f6-eafc-4c72-baf1-5ad606a354c3.

U.S. Health Resources and Services Administration. (2018b). *FY18 HRSA opioids fundings.* Retrieved from www.hrsa.gov/opioids/HRSA-fy18-awards.html.

Van Lerberghe, W. (2008). *The world health report 2008: Primary health care: Now more than ever.* World Health Organization. Retrieved from www.who.int/whr/2008/en/.

Vece, L., Sutter, R., Sutter, C., & Toulouse, C. (2016). Impacting vulnerable populations through integrating oral health care into nurse-managed health centers. *Journal for Nurse Practitioners, 12*(9), 629-634.

Wagner, E.H., Flinter, M., Hsu, C., Cromp, D., Austin, B.T., Etz, R., & Ladden, M.D. (2017). Effective team-based primary care: Observations from innovative practices. *BMC Family Practice, 18*(1), 13.

Wojnar, D.M., & Whelan, E.M. (2017). Preparing nursing students for enhanced roles in primary care: The current state of prelicensure and RN-to-BSN education. *Nursing Outlook, 65*(2), 222-232.

World Health Organization. (1978). *Primary health care.* Geneva, Switzerland. Retrieved from http://apps.who.int/iris/handle/10665/39228.

World Health Organization, Commission on Social Determinants of Health. (2008). *Closing the gap in a generation: Health equity through action on the social determinants of health: Final report: Executive summary.* Retrieved from www.who.int/social_determinants/thecommission/finalreport/en/.

Xue, Y., Kannan, V., Greener, E., Smith, J.A., Brasch, J., Johnson, B.A., & Spetz, J. (2018). Full scope-of-practice regulation is associated with higher supply of nurse practitioners in rural and primary care health professional shortage counties. *Journal of Nursing Regulation, 8*(4), 5-13.

Yarnall, K.S., Pollak, K.I., Østbye, T., Krause, K.M., & Michener, J.L. (2003). Primary care: Is there enough time for prevention? *American Journal of Public Health, 93*(4), 635-641.

Zuvekas, S.H., & Cohen, J.W. (2016). Fee-for-service, while much maligned, remains the dominant payment method for physician visits. *Health Affairs, 35*(3), 411-414.

ONLINE RESOURCES

National Association of Community Health Centers
www.nachc.org
Primary Care Development Corporation
www.pcdc.org
Primary Care Progress
www.primarycareprogress.org

32

Family Caregiving and Social Policy

Susan C. Reinhard and Heather M. Young

"There are four kinds of caregivers in this world: Those who have been caregivers, those who currently are caregivers, those who will be caregivers, and those who will need caregivers."

Rosalynn Carter

The number of older adults over age 85 in the United States is increasing dramatically, from approximately 6 million today to around 20 million by 2060 (Mather, Jacobsen, & Pollard, 2015). With advanced age comes a higher prevalence of chronic conditions and functional limitations. Over half of older adults between 80 and 85 years of age and 75% of those over 90 years of age require help due to health or functional decline (Freedman & Spillman, 2014). Family caregivers (broadly defined to include relatives and friends) provide the majority of long-term services and support (LTSS) for older adults.

The demand for care is increasing while the availability of caregivers is decreasing. The current ratio of more than seven potential caregivers for every person age 80 and over will fall to 4 to 1 by 2030 and less than 3 to 1 by 2050 (Redfoot, Feinberg, & Houser, 2013). This decline stems from changes in family size and composition, notably in fertility rates of successive cohorts of baby boomers. Only 11.6% of women in their 80s in 2010 were childless compared with a projected 16.0% of women in their 80s in 2030 (Kirmeyer & Hamilton, 2011). The rising demand for caregivers with projected shrinking supply creates urgency to improve social policy to better serve the needs of older persons and those with disabilities. Family caregivers play a valuable, irreplaceable role in our society by supporting people who have LTSS needs.

WHO ARE THE FAMILY CAREGIVERS?

Approximately 39.8 million Americans over the age of 18 years provide unpaid care to adult relatives or friends (National Alliance for Caregiving [NAC] & AARP, 2015).

Caregivers include both women (60%) and men, the majority provide care for a relative (85%) and the average age is 49 years, with 7% over age 75. Millennials (born between 1980 and 1996) constitute about one-quarter of all caregivers (Flinn, 2018). The prevalence of caregiving is 21% among Latinx families, 20% among African-American and Asian-American families, and 17% among White, non-Hispanics. Nine percent of caregivers identify as lesbian, gay, bisexual, or transgender (LGBT). The average age of Latinx caregivers is younger (42.7 years) than African American caregivers (average age 44.2), Asian-American caregivers (46.6 years), and Whites (52.5 years). African American caregivers are more likely to be providing care for both an older person and a child under 18, are more likely to live with the older adult, and with Latinx caregivers, provide the most hours of care (average 30 hours/week). Veterans constitute another large group of individuals relying on family caregivers. Among veterans receiving care, 19% are over 75 years in age and the vast majority of caregivers for veterans (96%) are women, predominately spouses (70%) (National Alliance for Caregiving, 2010). Millennials are the most diverse group of caregivers, with 47% men, 54% from underrepresented minority groups, and 12% identifying as LGBT. While in the overall caregiving population about 60% work, 73% of millennial caregivers are employed. Most care recipients live in their own home (58%) with another 20% living in the home of their caregiver.

WHAT DO CAREGIVERS DO?

Caregiving is a long-term commitment, with an average duration of 4 years and an average intensity of 24 hours per week. Those receiving care most commonly have a long-term physical condition that necessitates assistance (59%), with a quarter (26%) having a memory problem. About one-third have multiple conditions (37%). Caregivers provide a range of supports, from personal care to physical assistance, to help managing the household and providing emotional and social support. Most commonly, caregivers help with mobility (43%), transportation (78%), shopping (76%), and housework (72%) (NAC and AARP, 2015).

Increasingly, caregivers are performing medical and nursing tasks as people of all ages are living with chronic conditions at home and are discharged with complex needs from hospitals. The Home Alone Revisited study revealed that 50% of caregivers are performing medical/nursing tasks, with 96% of these also assisting with activities of daily living (Reinhard, Young, Levine, Kelly, Choula, & Accius, 2019). These tasks include managing medications (82%), including complex medication schedules, injections, and intravenous therapy; helping with assistive mobility devices (51%); preparing special diets (48%); performing wound care (37%); using meters and monitors (34%); and using incontinence supplies (25%). Many find the tasks difficult to do because of the time and effort, fear of making a mistake, or resistance from the older adult. Importantly, over half (54%) of caregivers helping with medications never received instruction and support in learning this skill. Family caregivers are now performing tasks at home that previously occurred only in hospitals and were performed nurses and other health care professionals. More than half of family caregivers providing this care reported they had no other choice because there was no one else to do it or insurance would not cover professional help.

Finally, family caregivers play a critical role in advocacy and surrogacy for older adults (National Academies of Sciences, Engineering, and Medicine [NASEM], 2015). Care coordination is particularly vital with complex multiple conditions and an array of providers and treatment recommendations, along with health care decision making, managing insurance, services, and supplies. Family caregivers also often assume responsibility for legal and financial matters, including personal property and advance planning.

UNPAID VALUE OF FAMILY CAREGIVING

Family caregivers' contributions have enormous value to those in their care and to the nation. Caregivers provide high-quality care at low cost that is consistent with consumer preferences. In 2013, the economic value of family caregiving reached $470 billion, more than the total national spending for Medicaid, including federal and state contributions and

medical and long-term care, which totaled $449 billion in 2013 (Reinhard, Feinberg, Choula, & Houser, 2015).

Among noninstitutionalized persons needing assistance with activities of daily living, families remain the most important source of help. An estimated 78% of Americans expect that at some point they will be responsible for caring for an aging parent or relative (Parker & Patten, 2013). The work of family caregivers is irreplaceable, mainly because alternatives are difficult and costly. The value of this unpaid care is stunning, but it exacts a high, often hidden cost on the quality of life for family caregivers.

PERSONAL COSTS OF CAREGIVING

As a human experience, caregiving is deeply personal. Each caregiver has individual motivations and rewards for engaging in this important role and experiences particular strains over the course of the commitment. Caregivers make great sacrifices to provide care, enduring negative effects on their physical and mental health, as well as burnout and depletion of financial resources.

There is a well-established relationship between caregiving and health, due to both the chronic stress of caregiving and the tendency of caregivers to neglect their own health as they prioritize giving care to another person. Caregivers report greater anxiety, stress, emotional difficulty, and depressive symptoms and experience more chronic conditions (NASEM, 2015). Many factors place caregivers at higher risk for negative sequelae. These include baseline caregiver physical and mental health, having a choice to assume the role of caregiving, perceptions of the degree of suffering of the person in their care, the intensity of caring, the complexity of care (e.g., dementia), available supports, and the resources of the home environment. Stigma can prevent many caregivers from getting support. For example, more than eight million Americans are providing care to an adult with an emotional or mental health issue, with almost three in four reporting high emotional stress (NAC, Mental Health America [MHA], & National Alliance on Mental Illness [NAMI], 2016). Caregiving has all the features of a chronic stress experience as it creates physical and psychological strain over an extended period. Among family caregivers of persons with dementia, more than four out of five reported at least one chronic illness, and nearly two out of three reported multiple chronic illnesses (Wang, Robinson, & Carter-Harris, 2013).

Family caregivers often become secondary patients because they do not adhere to their own medication schedules or keep their own health appointments. The physical demands of caregiving, including lifting and positioning, pose risk for musculoskeletal injury such as back or muscle strain (NASEM, 2015). The strain of caring for family members with dementia results in their family caregivers using 25% more health care services compared with non-caregivers of the same age (NAC, 2011).

High levels of unpredictability and uncontrollability accompany family caregiving situations. Thus, caregiving can create secondary stress in multiple domains of life, such as work and family relationships. Caregivers often experience the demands of both caring for an older adult and caring for a younger family and balancing work demands. More than one in six employees who work full or part time care for a family member (Cynkar & Mendes, 2011). Given trends for late life employment for older women in particular, the percent of working family caregivers will increase (Feinberg, 2018).

Almost half of employed caregivers who were engaged in intensive caregiving (>20 hours/week) experience negative impacts on their ability to remain fully employed, having to quit their jobs, reduce work hours, or take a less demanding position (NAC & AARP, 2015). These reductions in full employment and salary have long-term financial consequences by reducing income, retirement savings, accrual of Social Security and benefits, limiting career opportunities, and threatening overall financial well-being (Feinberg, 2018). The estimated loss of income and benefits for family caregivers over 50 averages $303,880 over a lifetime (MetLife Mature Market Institute, 2011). In addition to loss of income, 78% of family caregivers incur out-of-pocket costs for household and medical needs, averaging $7000 per year (Rainville, Skufca, & Mehegan, 2016). These costs are highest for Latinx family caregivers, at over $9000 per year, and an even higher percentage of family income, at 44% versus 34% for African American caregivers and 14% for White caregivers. For millennial caregivers, of whom one-third earn less than $30,000 per year, the long-term financial implications are a serious concern.

SUPPORTING FAMILY CAREGIVERS

In the foreseeable future, we will never have as many caregivers per person for those who need care at 80 years and older than we have today and families are already beyond their capacity to serve (Redfoot et al., 2013). Family caregivers juggle their jobs and their complex caregiving responsibilities. They prevent hospitalizations and nursing home admissions. And as value-based purchasing models take hold, they also take their hospitalized family member straight home to avoid even a short-term rehabilitation stay (Reinhard, 2018).

Unpaid caregivers are looking for help from public policymakers, health care professionals, social networks, and employers (NAC & AARP, 2015):

- Two-thirds of caregivers support policy banning workplace discrimination against workers with caregiving responsibilities.
- Thirty percent would like financial help through income tax credits or payment for the care they provide. Lower-income caregivers are more interested in payment to provide care, while higher-income caregivers show greater interest in a tax credit. Those who give 20 or more hours a week are more likely to prefer some reimbursement for the hours of care they provide, while lower-hour caregivers are more likely to prefer the tax credit or a partially paid leave of absence.
- Nearly half (49%) of caregivers feel a policy to have their own name on the recipient's health care record would be helpful. Approximately 4 in 10 feel it would be helpful to require hospitals to demonstrate medical/nursing tasks or inform them about major decisions. As caregivers' age, education, and income rises, so too does the perceived helpfulness of including their names on medical chart, receiving instruction on medical/nursing tasks, and being informed of major decisions about the recipient's care.
- Getting a breakthrough respite services is important, particularly for higher-hour caregivers who live with their care recipient (44%). Respite is also appealing to high-burden caregivers (42%), co-resident caregivers (39%), those caring for someone with dementia (46%), and those caring for someone with a mental health issue (39%).

Public policymakers are beginning to pay more attention to the needs of family caregivers, perhaps because many of them are already caregivers themselves. Federal action has been slow, but there are some recent advances. More action is occurring at the state level. In addition, employers are starting to pay more attention.

FAMILY CAREGIVING POLICY

Federal Policy

The Family and Medical Leave Act (FMLA) of 1993 was an important step in helping working caregivers, providing up to 12 weeks of unpaid, job-protected leave to care for oneself, a new child, or certain ill family members (child, spouse, and parent) or military service member. The Department of Labor now includes workers in legal same-sex marriages under the FMLA. However, there are major limitations. First, it only applies to public sector entities and private employers with 50 or more employees; 60% of workers are not protected (Feinberg, 2018). Second, it is unpaid. Third, it does not cover the care of all family members, such as a sibling or grandparent. Thus far, federal attempts to address these limitations have failed. Nevertheless, some states are stepping in as described below.

The National Family Caregiver Support Program, established in 2000, provides grants to states to fund information and referral, individual counseling, caregiver training, and respite care. Limited funding and restriction to caregivers of people 60 years of age and older are ongoing advocacy issues. More recently, the NASEM report on Families Caring for an Aging America (NASEM, 2015) is raising more interest in family caregiving issues. In 2015, the U.S. Congress formed a bipartisan Assisting Caregivers Today (ACT) Caucus. This leadership group successfully promoted the 2018 enactment of the Recognize, Assist, Include, Support, and Engage (RAISE) Family Caregivers Act (AARP, 2018). This law requires the development of a national strategy to recognize and bolster family caregivers. It calls upon the Secretary of Health and Human Services to bring together the public and private sectors, including health care professionals, state and federal policymakers, employers, consumers, and advocates to recommend actions that providers, communities, government, and others can take to better support family caregivers. For example, the strategy may include ways that all providers can make person- and family-centered care a reality and improve methods and financing for information, education, training supports, referrals, and care coordination.

One of the major policy wishes of family caregivers is financial help (NAC & AARP, 2015). About 8 out of 10 family caregivers spend their own money to help with home modifications, medications, transportation, assistive devices, incontinence products, and other things needed to help their family member. They spend an average of 20% of their income (approximately $7,000 in 2016 dollars) on these caregiving expenses (Rainville et al., 2016). A proposed federal law would help respond to that need. The Credit for Caring Act would create a non-refundable tax credit of up to $3,000 for employed family caregivers (AARP, 2017).

Federal policy is also starting to include family caregivers in the management of chronic conditions. Since 2015, Medicare will pay primary care clinicians, including nurse practitioners, for non-face-to-face care management activities. This fee includes communication with family caregivers during transitions from acute care settings to home (Centers for Medicare and Medicaid Services, 2018). Medicare will also pay for telehealth services for Medicare beneficiaries and their family caregivers in rural areas, permitting licensed social workers and other mental health professionals to provide counseling services even

when the Medicare beneficiary is not included (Reinhard et al., 2015).

State Policy

States have become very active in addressing policies that can support family caregivers. State by state advocacy has resulted in over 300 new state laws—at least one in every state—since 2014 (Ryan, 2018, personal communication). These include funding for respite care, guardianship laws, telehealth funding, and more.

A major area of state legislative advocacy and activity followed the publication of the Home Alone research that identified the major gap between what family caregivers are expected to do and the support they receive (Reinhard & Ryan, 2017). Now enacted in 43 states and territories (Fig. 32.1), the Caregiver Advise, Record and Enable (CARE) Act requires hospitals to ask all who are admitted if they have someone who helps with their care (a family caregiver), and if so, whether they want that person(s) to be included in the health record. This routine admission procedure encourages the inclusion of the family caregiver into the hospital care team. If the family caregiver is expected to perform medical/nursing tasks after discharge, s/he must be offered instruction and informed of the discharge date as soon as possible.

A CARE Act National Scan is underway to uncover promising practices to quickly spread innovation. Nursing leaders are spotlighting this practice-changing policy (Mason, 2017), and the Home Alone Alliance (Box 32.1) is spearheading the development of evidence-based instructional videos to teach family caregivers how to perform specific medical/nursing tasks, such as injections, wound care, mobility support, specialized equipment, incontinence interventions, and more. The *American Journal of Nursing* (Fig. 32.2) disseminated this "No Longer Alone" series of videos, tip sheets, and peer-reviewed articles on the evidence underlying the instructions (Harvath, Lindauer, & Sexson, 2016; Kirkland-Kyhn, Generao, Teleten, & Young, 2018; Powell-Cope, Pippins, & Young, 2017; Reinhard & Young, 2016). The video and other resources can be found at www.aarp.org/nolongeralone.

The LTSS State Scorecard tracks many policies that are crucial in a high-performing LTSS system (Reinhard, Accius, Houser, Ujvari, & Fox-Grage, 2017). The passage of the CARE Act is one of several indicators. Examples of others include the following, with details provided at www.longtermscorecard.org:

- Thirteen states and the District of Columbia exceed the federal floor of protections provided in the FMLA. Some states cover family members who fall outside the federal definition of family, such as in-laws, step-parents, and grandparents. Others extend the length of leave or apply

The CARE Act is a commonsense solution that supports family caregivers when their loved ones go into the hospital, and provides for instruction on the medical tasks they will need to perform when their loved one returns home.

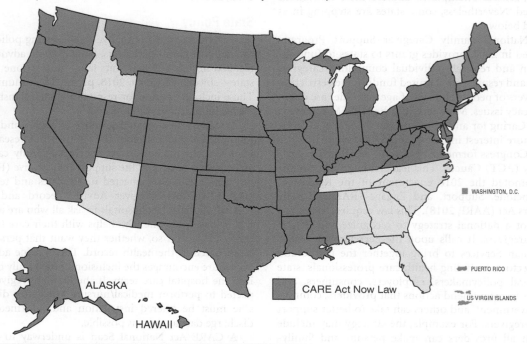

ALASKA

HAWAII

WASHINGTON, D.C.

PUERTO RICO

US VIRGIN ISLANDS

CARE Act Now Law

CARE Act goes into effect:
Alaska, 1/1/17; Arkansas, 7/2215; California. 1/1/16; Colorado, 5/8/15; Connecticut. 10/1/15; Delaware, 1/1/17; Hawaii, 7/1/17, Illinois, 1/27/16; Indiana, 1/1/16; Kansas, 7/1/18; Kentucky, 6/29/17; Louisana. 8/1/16; Maine, 10/15/15; Maryland, 10/1/16; Massachusetts, 11/8/17; Michigan, 7/12/16; Minnesota, 1/1/16; Mississippi. 7/1/15; Missouri, 8/28/18; Montana, 10/1/17; Nebraska, 3/30/16; Nevada, 10/1/15; New Hampshire, 1/1/16; New Jersey, 5/12/15; New Mexico, 6/17/15; New York, 4/23/16; North Dakota, 8/1/19; Ohio, 3/21/17; Oklahoma, 11/5/14; Oregon, 1/1/16; Pennsylvania, 4/20/17; Puerto Rico, 12/31/15; Rhode Island, 3/14/17; Texas, 5/26/17; Utah, 2/10/16; Virgin Islands, 3/30/16; Virginia, 7/1/15; Washington,7/6/16; Washington, DC, 7/6/16; West Virginia, 6/8/15; Wyoming, 7/1/16

**Updated on 4/10/2019

I♥Caregivers AARP Real Possibilities

Fig. 32.1 Enactment of the Caregiver Advise, Record, Enable (CARE) Act.

the provisions to smaller employers. In addition, 10 states and the District of Columbia have enacted state-wide or local ordinances to mandate paid sick days, an important step in helping employed caregivers take time off from work to provide care to a family member.
• Four states have made family caregivers a protected class under anti-discrimination laws.
• Seven states have laws to protect spouses from becoming impoverished due to a nursing home admission under Medicaid.
• Thirty-three states include family caregiver assessments when their family members are assessed for LTSS.

• Sixteen states permit nurses to delegate a full range of tasks, helping family caregivers who would otherwise need to leave work to perform these routine tasks.

In addition, six states and the District of Columbia have enacted laws to establish paid family leave (Feinberg, 2018). And states are beginning to pay for home telehealth services under Medicaid.

Employer Policies

As employers experience family caregiving responsibilities themselves and realize that one in six employees is a

BOX 32.1 Home Alone Alliance Resources

Videos and Written Resource Guides (Organized by Series)[a]

Medication Managements Series
- Beyond Pills: Eye Drops, Patches and Suppositories
- Dealing With Dementia-Related Resistance
- Giving Insulin Injections
- Hospital Discharge Planning[b]
- Organizing and Administering Pills

Mobility Series
- Preparing Your Home for Safe Mobility[b]
- Getting From a Car to a Wheelchair[b]
- What to Do When Someone Falls[b]
- Using a Walker or Cane and Navigating Stairs[b]
- Moving From a Walker to Shower or Bed[b]

Wound Care Series
- Treatment of Skin Tears
- Pressure Ulcers: Prevention and Skin Care
- Caring for and Maintaining Ostomy Bags
- Diabetic Foot Care: Treatment and Prevention[b]
- General Principles of Wound Care[b]
- Caring for Lower Extremity Wounds and Cellulitis

***American Journal of Nursing* Articles (in Reverse Chronological Order)[c]**
- Ostomy Care at Home (April 2018)
- Teaching Wound Care to Family Caregivers (March 2018)
- Caring for Aging Skin (February 2018)
- Preventing Falls and Fall-Related Injuries at Home (January 2018)
- Teaching Family Caregivers to Assist Safely With Mobility (December 2017)
- Nurses Supporting Family Caregivers (May 2017)[d]
- Discharge Planning and Teaching (May 2017)[d]
- Medication Management for People With Dementia (February 2017)[d]
- Teaching Caregivers to Administer Eye Drops, Transdermal Patches, and Suppositories (January 2017)[d]
- Administration of Subcutaneous Injections (December 2016)[d]
- Managing Complex Medication Regimens (November 2016)[d]

[a]All resources are available for free public access on the Home Alone Alliance's website: www.aarp.org/nolongeralone.
[b]Denotes videos also available in Spanish.
[c]All articles are available for free public access on the *American Journal of Nursing's* website: https://journals.lww.com/ajnonline/pages/default.aspx.
[d]Denotes an article included in a May 2017 supplement issue.

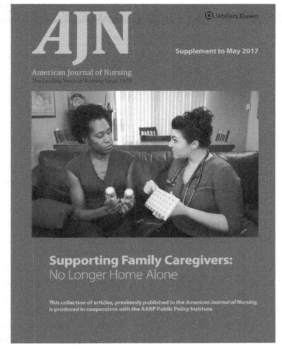

Fig. 32.2 *American Journal of Nursing,* May 2017 Supplement cover. (Retrieved from https://journals.lww.com/ajnonline/toc/2017/05001.)

caregiver (Cynkar & Mendes, 2011), they are becoming more interested in how they might help their employees (Table 32.1). Recent research by the Northeast Business Group on Health (NEBGH; Nobel, Weiss, Sasser, Sherman, & Pickering, 2017) highlights approaches taken to support employees:

- Leave policies that permit employees to use sick days to care for someone else or actually provide designated paid caregiver leave. It should be noted that although some employers offer paid leave, only 15% of private sector workers are affected (U.S. Bureau of Labor Statistics, 2017). This is an area that warrants advocacy in the private sector.
- Direct support to caregivers, such as in-person and telephonic counseling and support to help navigate the complexities of caregiving responsibilities.
- Facilitate access to outside caregiving services, such as back-up care at discounted rates.

AARP and the NEBGH are broadly disseminating a new Practical Guide for Employers, which includes a Helpful Tips resource (Nobel, Weiss, Sherman, Wilson-Meyers, & Pickering, 2017).

TABLE 32.1	Helpful Tips to Support Family Caregivers at Work
Tip	**Strategies**
Optimize Flex Time	• Encourage project teams to work with managers to achieve flexibility and predictability • Build out schedules that work for everyone on the team
Extend Telehealth Benefits	• Allow family members to use employee telehealth benefits to reduce transportation hassles and enable employees to spend more time at work • Telehealth conferences are a good way to involve employees and families in a family member's care
Provide Useful Tips to Ease the Burden	• For example, compile a directory of food delivery services on an employee portal • Make suggestions about how to automate bill paying • Little things can make a big difference
Connect Employees With Specialist Guidance	• Consultants can help employees develop a caregiving plan tailored to specific caregiving circumstances • Elder law and financial planning specialists exist in most communities • Caregivers should not have to do it all alone
Recognize Diversity	• Employees' family members may not speak English, so providing information in multiple languages can help • Consider content that's culturally appropriate
Be Sensitive to Privacy Needs	• Dedicate a huddle room or private area for phone calls or handling difficult emotions • Open plan offices lack privacy—and that can add to an employee-caregiver's stress level
Tailor Communications to Increase Engagement	• Have communications team members develop fact sheets on specific scenarios (e.g., "What do I need to know about being a caregiver?" or "My family member has dementia.") • Assemble publicly available background information and lists of resources, along with any employer-sponsored benefits and services • Get creative

Note: These tips and strategies are sourced from benefit managers, employers, and other experts, and were first published in a joint publication from AARP and the Northeast Business Group on Health.
Source: Nobel, J, et al. (2017). *Supporting caregivers in the workplace: A practical guide for employers.* Retrieved from https://nebgh.org/wp-content/uploads/2017/11/NEBGH-Caregiving_Practical-Guide-FINAL.pdf.

THE FUTURE

Caregiving is a global issue, and the United States is not an international leader in addressing the needs of family caregivers. Countries around the globe are grappling with the increasing demands placed on families to care for older and disabled members of society and testing approaches to support employed caregivers and increase national capacity for high-quality home-based care (Dossa & Coe, 2017; Ireson, Sethi, & Williams, 2018; Kodate & Timonen, 2017). There are positive trends that can help us pick up the pace in supporting family caregivers. As is true in other public policy areas, the states are leading the way. Some are leaders in helping employed caregivers, while others are promoting respite care. Most are mandating that caregivers of hospitalized patients be included in important decisions (with agreement from the individual) and given instruction in how to perform complex medical/nursing tasks. These policies are consistent with national payment penalties for unnecessary hospital readmissions and the research literature that shows family caregiver engagement is linked to substantial reductions in readmissions (Rodakowski et al., 2017).

We will all be or need caregivers one day. It is a personal, private sector, and public policy issue. We can all reach out to those who are caregiving now and offer whatever support we can. As health care professionals, we can recognize and actively include family caregivers in the care circle. And we can advocate to employers and policymakers that they can do more to help. This is a global issue that calls for creativity and action.

DISCUSSION QUESTIONS

1. What can you do in your current role to better support family caregivers?
2. What promising practices would you advocate to health care systems to successfully implement the CARE Act and/or support family caregivers?

REFERENCES

AARP. (2017). *The Credit for Caring Act*. Retrieved from www.aarp.org/caregiving/financial-legal/info-2017/credit-for-caring-act.html.

AARP. (2018). *Recognize, Assist, Include, Support, and Engage (RAISE) Family Caregivers Act Now Law*. Retrieved from www.aarp.org/politics-society/advocacy/caregiving-advocacy/info-2015/raise-family-caregivers-act.html.

Centers for Medicare and Medicaid Services. (2018). Connected care: The chronic care management resource. Retrieved from www.cms.gov/About-CMS/Agency-Information/OMH/equity-initiatives/chronic-care-management.html.

Cynkar, P., & Mendes, E. (2011). *More than one in six American workers also act as caregivers*. Retrieved from www.gallup.com/poll/148640/one-six-american-workers-act-caregivers.aspx.

Dossa, P., & Coe, C. (2017). *Transnational aging and reconfigurations of kin work*. New Brunswick, NJ: Rutgers University Press.

Feinberg, L. (2018). *Breaking new ground: Supporting employed family caregivers with workplace leave policies*. Retrieved from www.aarp.org/content/dam/aarp/ppi/2018/08/breaking-new-ground-supporting-employed-family-caregivers-with-workplace-leave-policies.pdf.

Flinn, B. (2018). *Millennials: The emerging generation of family caregivers*. Retrieved from www.aarp.org/ppi/info-2018/millennial-family-caregiving.html.

Freedman, V., & Spillman, B. (2014). Disability and care needs among older Americans. *Milbank Q, 92*(3), 509-541.

Harvath, T., Lindauer, A., & Sexson, K. (2016). Managing complex medication regimens. *American Journal of Nursing, 116*(11), 43-46.

Ireson, R., Sethi, B., & Williams, A. (2018). Availability of caregiver-friendly workplace policies (CFWPs): An international scoping review. *Health & Social Care in the Community, 26*(1), e1-e14.

Kirkland-Kyhn, H., Generao, S., Teleten, O., & Young, H. (2018). Teaching wound care to family caregivers. *American Journal of Nursing, 118*(3), 63-67.

Kirmeyer, S., & Hamilton, B. (2011). *Childbearing differences between three generations of U.S. women* (NHCS Brief No. 68). Retrieved from www.cdc.gov/nchs/data/databriefs/db68.pdf.

Kodate, N., & Timonen, V. (2017). Bringing the family in through the back door: The stealthy expansion of family care in Asian and European long-term care policy. *Journal of Cross-Cultural Gerontology, 32*(3), 291-301.

Mason, D. (2017). Supporting family caregivers, one state at a time: The CARE Act. *news@JAMA*. Retrieved from https://newsatjama.jama.com/2017/12/13/jama-forum-supporting-family-caregivers-one-state-at-a-time-the-care-act/

Mather, M., Jacobsen, L., & Pollard, K. (2015). Aging in the United States. *Population Bulletin, 70*(2).

MetLife Mature Market Institute. (2011). *The MetLife study of caregiving costs to working caregivers: Double jeopardy for Baby Boomers caring for their parents*. Retrieved from: https://www.caregiving.org/wp-content/uploads/2011/06/mmi-caregiving-costs-workingcaregivers.pdf.

National Academies of Sciences, Engineering and Medicine. (2015). *Families caring for an aging America*. Retrieved from www.nap.edu/catalog/23606/families-caring-for-an-aging-america.

National Alliance for Caregiving. (2010). *Caregivers of veterans—Serving on the homefront*. Retrieved from www.caregiving.org/data/2010_Caregivers_of_Veterans_FULLREPORT_WEB_FINAL.pdf.

National Alliance for Caregiving. (2011). *Caregiving costs: Declining health in the Alzheimer's caregiver as dementia increases in the care recipient*. Retrieved from www.caregiving.org/pdf/research/Alzheimers_Caregiving_Costs_Study_FINAL.pdf.

National Alliance for Caregiving, & AARP. (2015). *Caregiving in the U.S.* Retrieved from www.caregiving.org/wp-content/uploads/2015/05/2015_CaregivingintheUS_Final-Report-June-4_WEB.pdf.

National Alliance for Caregiving, Mental Health America, & National Alliance on Mental Illness. (2016). *On Pins & Needles: Caregivers of adults with mental illness*. Retrieved from www.caregiving.org/wp-content/uploads/2016/02/NAC_Mental_Illness_Study_2016_FINAL_WEB.pdf.

Nobel, J., Weiss, J., Sasser, E., Sherman, C., & Pickering, L. (2017). *The caregiving landscape: Challenges and opportunities for employers*. Retrieved from www.nebgh.org.

Nobel, J., Weiss, J., Sherman, C., Wilson-Meyers, C., & Pickering, L. (2017). *Supporting caregivers in the workplace: A practical guide for employers*. Retrieved from https://nebgh.org/wp-content/uploads/2017/11/NEBGH-Caregiving_Practical-Guide-FINAL.pdf.

Parker, A., & Patten, E. (2013). *Caregiving for older family members*. Retrieved from www.pewsocialtrends.org/2013/01/30/caregiving-for-older-family-members/.

Powell-Cope, G., Pippins, K., & Young, H. (2017). Teaching family caregivers to assist safely with mobility. *American Journal of Nursing, 117*(12), 49-53.

Rainville, C., Skufca, L., & Mehegan, L. (2016). *Family caregiving and out-of-pocket costs: 2016 report*. Retrieved from www.aarp.org/research/topics/care/info-2016/family-caregivers-cost-survey.html.

Redfoot, D., Feinberg, L., & Houser, A. (2013). *The aging of the baby boom and the growing care gap: A look at future declines in the availability of family caregivers*. Retrieved from www.aarp.org/home-family/caregiving/info-08-2013/the-aging-of-the-baby-boom-and-the-growing-care-gap-AARP-ppi-ltc.html.

Reinhard, S. (2018). The family context. In B.T. Fulmer (Ed.), *Handbook of geriatric assessment* (5th ed.). Burlington, Massachusetts: Jones & Bartlett Learning.

Reinhard, S., Accius, J., Houser, A., Ujvari, K., & Fox-Grage, W. (2017). *Picking up the pace of change, 2017: A state scorecard on long-term services and supports for older adults, people with physical disabilities, and family caregivers*. Retrieved from http://longtermscorecard.org/2017-scorecard.

Reinhard, S., Feinberg, L., Choula, R., & Houser, A. (2015). *Valuing the invaluable: 2015 update: Undeniable progress, but big gaps remain*. Retrieved from www.aarp.org/content/dam/aarp/ppi/2015/valuing-the-invaluable-2015-update-new.pdf.

Reinhard, S.C., Young, H.M., Levine, C., Kelly, K., Choula, R., & Accius, J. (2019). *Home Alone revisited: Family caregivers providing complex care*. Washington, DC: AARP Public Policy Institute. Retrieved from www.aarp.org/content/dam/aarp/ppi/2019/04/home-alone-revisited-family-caregivers-providing-complex-care.pdf.

Reinhard, S., & Ryan, E. (2017). *From Home Alone to the CARE Act: Collaboration for family caregivers*. Retrieved from www.aarp. org/ppi/info-2017/from-home-alone-to-the-care-act.html.

Reinhard, S., & Young, H. (2016). Nurses supporting family caregivers. *American Journal of Nursing, 116*(11), 7.

Rodakowski, J., Rocco, P., Ortiz, M., Folb, B., Schulz, R., Morton, S., & James, A. (2017). Caregiver integration during discharge planning for older adults to reduce resource use: A metaanalysis. *Journal of the American Geriatrics Society, 65*(8), 1748-1755.

U.S. Bureau of Labor Statistics. (2017). *Employee benefits survey, table 32—Leave benefits: Access, private industry workers*. Retrieved from www.bls.gov/ncs/ebs/benefits/2017/ownership/private/table32a.htm.

Wang, X., Robinson, K., & Carter-Harris, L. (2013). Prevalence of chronic illnesses and characteristics of chronically ill informal caregivers of persons with dementia. *Age and Ageing, 43*(1), 137–141.

ONLINE RESOURCES

Family Caregiving Alliance
www.caregiver.org
Family Caregiving Site at AARP
www.aarp.org/home-family/caregiving
National Alliance for Caregiving
www.caregiving.org
Prepare to Care: A Planning Guide for Families
www.aarp.org/content/dam/aarp/home-and-family/caregiving/ 2012-10/PrepareToCare-Guide-FINAL.pdf
Top 20+ Websites for Caregivers-Caregiving Café
www.caregivingcafe.com

33

Dual Eligibles: Challenges and Innovations in Care

Pamela Z. Cacchione

> *"The critical first step in integrating care for dual eligibles is designing a practical, achievable, and reasonable health care delivery system that can meet their individual needs and preferences."*
>
> **Community Catalyst**

People enrolled in both Medicare and Medicaid are known as "dual eligible." Persons who are dual eligible are receiving significant attention from state and national policymakers. These dual-eligible beneficiaries—also known simply as the "duals"—experience high rates of chronic illness, often due to multiple chronic conditions, and may have long-term care needs (Medicare-Medicaid Coordination Office [MMCO], 2018). Medicare is the main payer for the acute and post-acute care services. Medicaid coverage varies by state, levels of assistance with Medicare premiums, and cost sharing. For many Medicaid beneficiaries, Medicaid covers services not covered by Medicare, such as long-term services and supports (LTSS) (MedPAC & MACPAC, 2018).

This variation in coverage is due to the payment streams for Medicare and Medicaid. Medicare, a federal program, has uniform eligibility rules and a standard benefit package. Medicaid, a joint federal-state program, has eligibility rules and benefits that differ state by state (MedPAC & MACPAC, 2018). Duals make up a disproportionately large share of the cost of both Medicare and Medicaid programs (MMCO, 2018). Reducing the cost of the duals is a major driver of the attention from policymakers, but so too is the growing recognition that the duals need care coordination. Innovative nurses are in a position to shape new initiatives and models of care for dual-eligible beneficiaries.

In order to innovate for this population or provide coordinated care it is essential to gain an understanding of Medicare and Medicaid as well as the beneficiaries they serve. Because Medicare and Medicaid are separate payment streams for health care, duals must navigate two separate programs. The Patient Protection and Affordable Care Act established the Federal Coordinated Health Care Office known as the MMCO as part of the Centers for Medicare and Medicaid Services (CMS) to improve coordination of care for the duals (Feng, 2018). The MMCO's role is to improve the quality of services for dual individuals by: (1) implementing delivery system reform to eliminate cost shifting between the two programs; (2) investing in new methods to support duals in accessing care and understanding their benefits; (3) supporting states to develop new models to address regulatory conflicts between Medicare and Medicaid; (4) supporting providers and health plans to engage in new models to promote access to care, continuity of care, and safe transitions; (5) increasing accessibility to data to improve care; and (6) improving methodology to hold providers accountable for quality (MMCO, 2018).

WHO ARE THE DUALS?

In 2016, there were 11.7 million people who were enrolled in both Medicare and Medicaid (MMCO, 2017). These dual-eligibles typically have very low incomes, multiple complex chronic conditions and disabilities, multiple medical providers, and they account for a disproportionate share of spending in both programs (Feng, 2018; Samson, Chen, Epstein & Maddox, 2018). There is also significant diversity among the duals. In 2016, 40.6% of duals were under age 65, 37.5% were from minority race or ethnicity populations, 61% were women, and 68% had three or more chronic conditions (MedPAC & MACPAC, 2018). In addition, duals younger than 65 years old were more likely to have a mental health disorder or intellectual disability versus those 65 years and older who were more likely to have dementia and the following medical conditions: diabetes, heart failure, hypertension, and ischemic heart disease (MedPAC & MACPAC, 2018).

The journey to becoming dual eligible or a dual varies, primarily due to variation in Medicaid coverage by state. Medicare coverage is a little more straight forward. One becomes eligible for Medicare by age (65 years old and older) or for those under age 65, they become eligible for Medicare by having a permanent disability and are receiving Social Security Disability Insurance, or by having end-stage renal disease (Feng, 2018). Medicare beneficiaries qualify for Medicaid through several pathways. All states generally must provide Medicaid to Supplemental Security Income (SSI) beneficiaries, and states can extend Medicaid eligibility for other older adults and people with disabilities up to 100% of the federal poverty level ($12,060 for an individual in 2017) (Musumeci, 2017), thus providing a security net for those in poverty. States can also expand eligibility for Medicaid to Medicare recipients who need long-term care services in nursing homes or the community up to three times the SSI benefit rate (219% of the federal poverty level or $26,460 per year for an individual in 2017) with asset limits at the SSI level of $2000 (Musumeci, 2017). The majority of duals receive full Medicaid and Medicare

benefits. However, 25% of Medicare beneficiaries only receive partial Medicaid benefits to assist with Medicare deductibles for hospital stays, outpatient services, and/or Medicare monthly premiums (Feng, 2018; Musumeci, 2017).

Duals, by virtue of being impoverished with multiple chronic conditions and/or disabled, are a vulnerable population who would benefit by nursing innovation in the community along with care coordination. Over 20% of duals lived in an institution in 2013; this percentage increased to 27% when looking at duals over age 65 (Feng, 2018). Only 5% of older adults with only Medicare live in an institution (Feng, 2018). Most older adults in nursing homes have spent down to Medicaid. This is a very common route to becoming a dual. Based on the above statistics over 90% of all Medicare beneficiaries living in long-term care facilities are duals.

While older frail adults comprise 58% of the duals population, people with a disability under the age of 65 years comprise the other 42% (MedPAC & MACPAC, 2018). These individuals younger than age 65 may have a physical disability, end-stage renal disease, a behavioral or substance use disorder, or some combination of these conditions. Compared to duals older than age 65, those beneficiaries under age 65 are more likely to be male, White, or Black (Table 33.1) (MedPAC & MACPAC, 2018). Dual-eligibles younger than 65 were more likely to have a behavioral health diagnosis as compared to those older than 65 who were more likely to have a Alzheimer disease or related dementia diagnosis (23% vs. 4%) (MedPAC & MACPAC, 2018).

TABLE 33.1 Characteristics of Dual-Eligible Beneficiaries Calendar Year (CY) 2013				
	DUAL-ELIGIBLE BENEFICIARIES			
Demographic Characteristics	All (%)	Under Age 65 (%)	Ages 65 and Older (%)	Non-Dual Medicare Beneficiaries (%)
Gender				
Male	39	48	33	47
Female	61	52	67	60
Race/Ethnicity				
White/Non-Hispanic	57	61	53	84
African American/ Non-Hispanic	21	25	18	8
Hispanic	16	11	19	5
Other	7	3	10	3
Limitations in ADL				
None	44	45	44	74
1–2 ADL limitations	26	33	21	17
3–6 ADL limitations	30	22	36	9

TABLE 33.1 Characteristics of Dual-Eligible Beneficiaries Calendar Year (CY) 2013—cont'd				
	DUAL-ELIGIBLE BENEFICIARIES			
Demographic Characteristics	All (%)	Under Age 65 (%)	Ages 65 and Older (%)	Non-Dual Medicare Beneficiaries (%)
Self-Reported Health Status				
Excellent or very good	22	17	26	51
Good or fair	59	60	58	43
Poor	18	22	15	6
Unknown	1	1	15	<1
Living Arrangement				
Institution	21	11	27	5
Alone	28	27	28	24
Spouse	15	14	16	55
Children, non-relative, others	36	48	29	16

ADL, Activities of daily living.
Source: Medicare Payment Advisory Commission & Medicaid and CHIP Payment and Access Commission. (2018, January). *Data book: Beneficiaries dually eligible for Medicare and Medicaid.* Retrieved from https://www.macpac.gov/wp-content/uploads/2017/Jan18_MedPAC_MACPAC_DualsDataBook.pdf.

However, age differences are not the only reason this is a heterogeneous group (Musumeci, 2017). About 21% lived in a nursing homes in 2013 (Feng, 2018), another one out of five uses community-based LTSS, and one out of four has multiple chronic conditions, but no need for LTSS. Surprisingly, two out of five have one or no chronic conditions or LTSS, but as extremely low-income people, they face a host of social and environmental challenges. Their health and social needs vary substantially.

Despite their heterogeneity, compared with people who only receive Medicare (the nonduals), the duals are more vulnerable. Fig. 33.1 provides important comparisons. They are more than twice as likely to be in fair or poor health, and more likely to require help with activities of daily living (ADL), such as bathing, dressing, and eating (MedPAC & MACPAC, 2018; Musuceni, 2017). In addition, more than half of duals have a cognitive or mental impairment, compared with 29% of nonduals (MedPAC & MACPAC, 2018).

The complexity of coordinating the payments and services for this group of high-need, high-cost beneficiaries led to the development of the MMCO through the Affordable Care Act. The role of the MMCO is to integrate benefits and improve the coordination between state and federal governments to improve access to high-quality coordinated services to dual-eligible beneficiaries (MMCO, 2018). However there are still challenges to meeting these ideals for this vulnerable group of beneficiaries.

WHAT ARE THE CHALLENGES?

From a care perspective, the greatest challenge is delivering and coordinating services and supports to these vulnerable groups within the duals population. Many need complex health care, but many also need long-term supportive services such as housing and transportation. Furthermore, most desperately need help coordinating all of these services, some of which are covered by Medicare, some covered by Medicaid, and some offered through other public and private sources. Most existing delivery models for Medicare and Medicaid do not coordinate services. These individuals live in an unmanaged care world:

- If they are getting LTSS, their LTSS provider (paid by Medicaid) gets little information about the inpatient, clinician, and prescription services paid by Medicare.
- Data linking Medicare and Medicaid service use and expenditures at the individual level are lacking.
- Services that both Medicare and Medicaid cover, such as home health, hospice, and durable medical equipment, intersect in complex ways that few understand.
- If a person wants to appeal a denial for services, there are different appeal processes.

In a series of focus groups with older adults who are duals, most expressed interest in having care coordination (Reinhard, 2013). They felt supported when a case manager or others called to see how they were doing and if they got what they needed to take care of their condition, for example, checking their blood sugar. Family caregivers, the

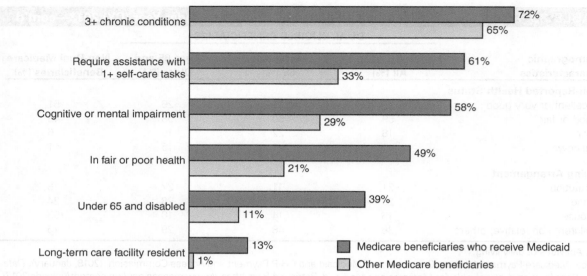

Fig. 33.1 Health and functioning of Medicare beneficiaries who receive Medicaid compared to other Medicare beneficiaries. (Source: Musumeci, M. [2017]. *Medicaid's role for Medicare beneficiaries* (issue brief). The Henry J. Kaiser Family Foundation. Retrieved from www.kff.org/medicaid/issue-brief/medicaids-role-formedi-care-beneficiaries/.)

primary coordinators of care, want to be included in care planning and execution, especially when they have a regular role in that execution. Also, consumers really want their clinicians and providers to communicate with one another so everyone is on the same page (Reinhard, 2013).

From a cost perspective, this uncoordinated care situation is untenable. The dual-eligible population represents a relatively small proportion of those covered by either Medicare or Medicaid (nonduals), while accounting for a higher part of total system costs. Of the separate programs (Medicare and Medicaid), the duals represent 20% of all Medicare recipients but account for 34% of Medicare expenditures. Of those on Medicaid only 15% of the beneficiaries are dual eligible and account for 32% of all of Medicaid expenditures (MMCO, 2018). Even within the duals population, two cost facts stand out. First, 20% of fee-for-service duals used Medicaid institutional LTSS but accounted for more than 34% of Medicare spending and more than 53% of total Medicaid spending in 2013 (MedPAC & MACPAC, 2018). High-cost duals tend to live in institutions, have three or more ADL limitations, and are substantially more likely to have diabetes or Alzheimer disease. Second, 49% of Medicaid spending on duals goes to institutional LTSS (MedPAC & MACPAC, 2018).

Given the heterogeneity of this relatively small group of people spread across the United States it is very important to develop financing and care models that target expert care and coordination for people and their families dealing with multiple physical conditions, serious behavioral health conditions, and LTSS needs that include crucial social aspects of care, such as housing and transportation. People cannot choose home and community care options for LTSS unless they have a place to live and can access health care.

HEALTH CARE DELIVERY REFORMS THAT HOLD PROMISE

After decades of trying to get federal and state policymakers to pay attention to this high-cost, vulnerable population, advocates are hopeful that change is possible. There is growing consensus that providing quality care for duals needs to be more efficient in terms of both the cost and delivery of care. Duals require better care coordination, particularly for high-cost individuals who receive many services without sufficient attention to the coordination or quality of those services. We need to measure quality of life as well as quality of care. Many duals need access to more integrated primary, acute, behavioral health, and LTSS, with a particular focus on blending health and social services. Families should be engaged and supported whenever possible, and people who are on both Medicare and Medicaid need harmony between the two sets of programs in terms of rules and procedures. The creation of the Medicare and Medicaid Coordination Office was a major step forward in this effort (Feng, 2018).

One of the most significant demonstration projects emerging from the new center is known as the Financial Alignment Initiative Demonstration in 13 states, although Virginia and Colorado ended their demonstrations in 2017 (Feng, 2018; Musumeci, 2013). This is a federal-state partnership to develop service and payment models that will better integrate care and align financial incentives across the Medicare and Medicaid programs. Currently, if a state invests resources to improve care of people who are on Medicaid but also on Medicare, the state may incur Medicaid costs while the federal government saves money. These new models offer a pathway to focus resources across the two programs in a way that may improve the quality and coordination of care, while reducing costs for both.

In most cases, demonstration states ($n = 10$) are experimenting with managed care plans to accomplish these goals (Feng, 2018). The plans receive a prospective blended rate for all primary, acute, behavioral health, and LTSS. Under this capitated approach, states and the CMS can share savings. A few states are exploring a managed fee-for-service financial alignment model that does not involve capitation. In the fee-for-service model the state is responsible for care coordination and the delivery of fully integrated Medicare and Medicaid benefits. The state receives a retrospective performance payment if a target level of Medicare savings is achieved (Walls et al., 2013). It takes time to build capacity for this multipronged approach to serve these populations and an infrastructure to integrate both Medicare and Medicaid services and financing with the intention to better align Medicare and Medicaid financing to integrate primary, acute, behavioral health, and LTSS for the duals (Feng, 2018). Preliminary research suggests they are effective at protecting consumer choices and continuity of care (Saucier, Burwell, & Halperin, 2013).

The number of people who need LTSS is expected to increase as the aging population grows. With this increased need for LTSS looming, states are again looking for opportunities to rebalance Medicaid LTSS toward less-restrictive, lower-cost, community-based care (Archibald, Kruse, Sommers, 2018). State movement toward managed LTSS (MLTSS) is accelerating, from 8 states in 2004 to 24 states in September of 2018 (MACPAC, 2018) (Fig. 33.2) with

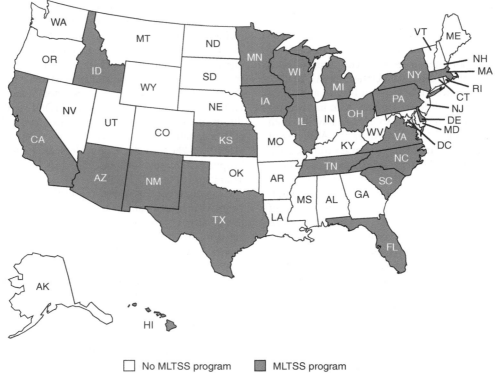

☐ No MLTSS program   ■ MLTSS program

Fig. 33.2 Managed long-term services and supports (MLTSS). (Source: Medicaid and CHIP Payment and Access Commission. [2018]. *Managed long-term services and supports: Status of state adoption and areas of program evolution.* Report to Congress on Medicaid & CHIP. Retrieved from www.macpac.gov/wp-content/uploads/2018/06/Managed-Long-Term-Services-and-Supports-Status-of-State-Adoption-and-Areas-of-Program-Evolution.pdf.)

roughly 1 million people enrolled (Archibald et al., 2018). States can use several Medicaid authorities to implement MLTSS: either section 115 waivers or combining 1912 home and community-based services waiver authority with section 1915(a), Section 1915(b), or Section 1932 managed care authorities (MACPAC, 2018). Managed LTSS is not integrated care in that it does not integrate primary, acute, and LTSS services, and it does not integrate Medicaid and Medicare. Yet, it is worth including here because many LTSS users are duals, and managed LTSS can be a step toward more fully integrated care models.

IMPLICATION FOR NURSES

Nurses and other advocates need to monitor the state and federal shift from fee-for-service models to managed care for duals. One should not be deluded into thinking that the fee-for-service world was wonderful and the managed care world will be dreadful. In fact, there are some success stories.

The Program for All-Inclusive Care of the Elderly (PACE), a capitated managed care program, was started by the On Lok Senior Health Services in 1973 as a way to provide comprehensive culturally appropriate care to older adults in the Chinatown-North Beach community of San Francisco. This community responded to the pressing LTSS needs of their elders. On Lok Senior Health Services was created to provide an interprofessional community-based system of LTSS (National PACE Association [NPA], 2018b). PACE has integrated health, behavioral health, and social services for frail, older adults to support them in the community as long as it is safe to do so. Nurses have been an integral part of this model. In fact, American Academy of Nursing Edge Runner Jennie Chinn Hansen founded On Lok and the University of Pennsylvania's School of Nursing had a nurse-run PACE program for duals known as the Living Independently for Elders (LIFE). LIFE UPenn was sold to Trinity Health PACE and has expanded the number of their participants to over 500. There are now 123 PACE sponsoring organizations with 250 centers in 31 states. The majority of these centers have fewer than 500 duals in each capitated program (NPA, 2018a). As of 2018, 90% of all PACE enrollees were dual eligible. Initially started as not-for-profit organizations, this restriction was removed in 2015 allowing for-profit organizations to enter the market (U.S. Department of Health and Human Services (HHS), 2015). Currently 8% of PACE organizations are for-profit (NPA, 2018a). Evaluations have shown that PACE successfully integrates acute and long-term care and reduces hospitalizations.

The Evercare model was founded in 1987 by two geriatric advanced practice nurses who had a vision for how better care might be delivered to frail older adults in nursing homes as part of United Healthcare (now known as Optum CarePlus) (Lipton, 2012). The target population was Medicare beneficiaries in nursing homes, who, as noted earlier, quickly spend down their resources paying for their nursing home stay and become dually eligible for Medicaid. Nurse practitioners were placed in the nursing homes to provide preventive care, monitor changes in health, make early diagnoses and interventions, and coordinate better communication including advanced care planning (Lipton, 2012). Eight years later, Evercare became a federal demonstration project that was evaluated by the University of Minnesota with excellent results, including a 50% reduction in emergency room visits and a 40% reduction in hospitalizations without changes in mortality (Kane et al., 2004). With these findings, federal policy moved this program into permanent status, converting them to special needs plans offered throughout the United States.

The Missouri Quality Initiative (MOQI) was spearheaded by Dr. Marilyn Rantz and other nursing leaders in Missouri. Dr. Rantz was funded by the CMS Innovations Center and the MMCO. These two offices sponsored an initiative to reduce avoidable hospitalizations among nursing facility residents (Rantz et al., 2017). The Missouri Quality Initiative was a 4-year project that assigned advanced practice registered nurses (APRNs) into 16 nursing facilities (Rantz et al., 2017). The APRNs were supported by an interprofessional team including a Project Medical Director, a Social Service Care Transitions Coach, Health Information Coordinator, and a Registered Nurse skilled in the Quality Improvement Program for Missouri Nursing Homes (QIPMO). Within 3 years, MOQI significantly reduced all-cause hospitalizations by 40%, potentially avoidable hospitalizations by 58%, emergency department (ED) visits by 54%, and decreased Medicare expenditures for hospitalizations by 34% and ED visits by 50% (Research Triangle Institute [RTI], 2017).

Nursing literature is growing in this area; there is evidence that nurses can make a significant contribution to the quality of care provided to older adults in plans targeted to duals. For example, using a nurse care manager model in a community-based dual-eligible special needs plan can improve patient outcomes (Roth et al., 2012). These nurse care managers are skilled at complex psychosocial assessments and behavior interventions that can address the social determinants so often neglected in traditional medical practices.

Evidence suggests some common features of successful care coordination programs (Brown & Mann, 2012): regular (monthly) face-to-face contact between the care coordinator and the consumer; strong rapport with the patient's primary clinician; an effective communication hub for providers and patients with the ability to know when patients are hospitalized so transition support can be provided; access to reliable information about prescriptions, with access to prescribers and pharmacists; and use of behavior change techniques to help people create and adhere to self-care plans, including medication adherence.

POLICY IMPLICATIONS

Care coordination is in the limelight, and nurses are in a position to make a critical contribution. As PACE, Evercare, and MOQI have demonstrated, interprofessional team-based care is essential in addressing the needs of the dual eligibles. Nurses are skilled at care coordination and person-centered care leading to decreased costs and better outcomes. It is essential that nurses fully engage in MLTSS and other demonstration projects to bring patient advocacy and strong care coordination to the team.

State experimentation is proceeding with more than 1.8 million people enrolled in MLTSS—primarily older adults and adults with physical disabilities (Lewis et al., 2018). Preliminary outcomes from the early adopters of MLTSS have found enrollees reported improved quality of life and a greater sense of independence (Archibald, et al., 2018). More evidence will emerge from the demonstrations as the programs mature. In the meantime, states are advancing certain elements of care coordination: use of care assessments, person-centered focus, comprehensive care plans, inclusion of the patient and family in care decisions, and the use of interdisciplinary teams. Some states are more prescriptive than others in how care coordination is to be defined and delivered and what entity should be designated the primary care coordinator, whereas others provide flexibility to managed care plans. Thus, there is a great deal of flux. However, the best advice for policymakers at this time, as it has been in the past, is to target high-risk cases and pay attention to subgroup differences. Everyone does not need, nor can we afford, one-to-one close care coordination, and one size will not fit all. A critical element to these demonstrations is the ability of a dual participant in the program to have the right to challenge decisions made effecting their MLTSS. Organizations have addressed this issue in a variety of ways from enrollment counselors to ombudsman programs. Nurses are in a key position to advocate on behalf of dual-eligible beneficiaries.

As we design new systems of care and people move from one program to another, we need to provide sufficient transition periods to avoid abrupt changes to the consumer's provider network, care manager, and other key aspects of care (Saucier, Burwell, & Halperin, 2013). Advocates also need to keep the attention on the adoption of clear, transparent public goals for what the new programs are designed to do, particularly in relation to the consumer's

experience, population health, and cost-reduction expectations (Burwell & Saucier, 2013). We need to build sufficient state and federal capacity to oversee the programs being created, especially to monitor quality and areas that might need improvement.

This continues to be a period of substantial change that brings opportunities for improved care, better use of resources, and important roles for nurses and other members of the team, but it also brings a clarion call for research and advocacy. We need more evidence to help us move in the right direction, and we need advocacy to keep a watchful eye on what is happening to those who most need the right changes: the people called duals, the people we know, the people we care for.

DISCUSSION QUESTIONS

1. What is the role of the Medicare Medicaid Coordination Office?
2. What are some current efforts to develop more coherent policies and programs to support people who have both Medicare and Medicaid coverage?
3. What are some key areas to monitor as new policies and programs are developed for the duals?

REFERENCES

Archibald, N.D., Kruse, A.M., & Somers, S.A. (2018). The emerging role of managed care in long-term services and supports. *Public Policy & Aging Report, 28*(2), 64-70

Brown, R., & Mann, D. (2012). *Best bets for reducing Medicare costs for dual eligible beneficiaries: Assessing the evidence.* Menlo Park, CA: The Henry J. Kaiser Family Foundation. Retrieved from kaiserfamilyfoundation.files.wordpress.com/2013/01/8353.pdf.

Burwell, B., & Saucier, P. (2013). Managed long-term services and supports programs are a cornerstone for fully integrated care. *Generations: Journal of the American Society on Aging, 37*(2), 33–38.

Feng, Z. (2018). Dual eligibles: Who are they and why are they important? *Public Policy & Aging Report, 28*(2), 56-63.

Kane, R.L., Flood, S., Bershadsky, B., & Keckhafer, G., (2004). The effect of an innovative Medicare Managed Care Program on the quality of care for nursing home residents. *The Gerontologist, 44*(1), 95-103.

Lewis, E., Eiken, S., Amos, A., & Saucier, P. (2018). *The growth of managed long-term services and supports programs: 2017 update.* Turven Health Analytics. Retrieved from www.medicaid.gov/medicaid/managed-care/downloads/ltss/mltssp-inventory-update-2017.pdf

Lipton, C. (2012). *UnitedHealthcare Nursing Home Plan Evercare Clinical Model telemedicine initiatives.* Retrieved from www.slideshare.net/gatelehealth/cathy-lipton-31512.

Medicaid and CHIP Payment and Access Commission. (2018). *Managed long-term services and supports: Status of state adoption and areas of program evolution* (Report to Congress on Medicaid and CHIP). Retrieved from www.macpac.gov/wp-content/uploads/2018/06/Managed-Long-Term-Services-and-Supports-Status-of-State-Adoption-and-Areas-of-Program-Evolution.pdf.

Medicare-Medicaid Coordination Office. (2017). *Medicare-Medicaid dual enrollment from 2006-2016.* Retrieved from www.cms.gov/Medicare-Medicaid-Coordination/Medicare-and-Medicaid-Coordination/Medicare-Medicaid-Coordination-Office/DataStatisticalResources/Downloads/Eleven-YearEver-EnrolledTrendsReport_2006-2016.pdf.

Medicare-Medicaid Coordination Office. (2018). *Fact sheet—February 2018.* Retrieved from www.cms.gov/Medicare-Medicaid-Coordination/Medicare-and-Medicaid-Coordination/Medicare-Medicaid-Coordination-Office/Downloads/MMCO_Factsheet.pdf.

Medicare Payment Advisory Commission & Medicaid and CHIP Payment and Access Commission. (2018, January). *Data book: Beneficiaries dually eligible for Medicare and Medicaid.* Retrieved from www.macpac.gov/wp-content/uploads/2017/Jan18_MedPAC_MACPAC_DualsDataBook.pdf.

Musumeci, M. (2013). *Long-term services and supports in the financial alignment demonstrations for dual eligible beneficiaries.* Washington, DC: The Henry J. Kaiser Family Foundation. Retrieved from kaiserfamilyfoundation.files.wordpress.com/2013/11/8519-long-term-services-and-supports-in-the-financial-alignment-demonstrations.pdf.

Musumeci, M. (2017). *Medicaid's role for Medicare beneficiaries* (issue brief). The Henry J. Kaiser Family Foundation. Retrieved from www.kff.org/medicaid/issue-brief/medicaids-role-formedicare-beneficiaries/.) Retrieved from www.kff.org/medicaid/issue-brief/medicaids-role-for-medicare-beneficiaries/.

National PACE Association. (2018a). *PACE by the numbers.* Retrieved from www.npaonline.org/sites/default/files/PACE%20Infographic%20Feb%202018.pdf.

National PACE Association. (2018b). *Understanding PACE.* Retrieved from www.npaonline.org/sites/default/files/Profile%20of%20PACE_December%202016.pdf.

Rantz, M.J., Popejoy, L., Vogelsmeier, A., Galambos, C., Alexander, G., Flesner, M., ... & Petroski, G. (2017). Successfully reducing hospitalizations of nursing home residents: Results of the Missouri Quality Initiative. *Journal of the American Medical Directors Association, 18*(11), 960-966.

Reinhard, S.C. (2013). What do older adults want from integrated care? *Generations: Journal of the American Society on Aging, 37*(2), 68–71.

Research Triangle Institute International. (2017). *Evaluation of the initiative to reduce avoidable hospitalizations among nursing home facility residents: Final annual report project year 3.* Retrieved from https://innovation.cms.gov/Files/reports/irahnfr-finalyrthreeevalrpt.pdf.

Roth, C.P., Ganz, D.A., Nickels, L., Martin, D., Beckman, R., & Wenger, N.S. (2012). Nurse care manager contribution to quality of care in dual-eligible Special Needs Plan. *Journal of Gerontological Nursing, 38*(7), 44–54.

Samson, L.W., Chen, L.M., Epstein, A.M., & Joynt Maddox, K.E. (2018). Dually enrolled beneficiaries have higher episode costs on the Medicare spending per beneficiary measure. *Health Affiaris, 37*(1), 86-94.

Saucier, P., Burwell, B., & Halperin, A. (2013). *Consumer choices and continuity of care in managed long-term services and support: Emerging practices and lessons.* Washington, DC: AARP Public Policy Institute. Retrieved from www.aarp.org/content/dam/aarp/research/public_policy_institute/ltc/2013/consumer-choices-report-full-AARP-ppi-ltc.pdf.

U.S. Department of Health and Human Services. (2015). Report to Congress: The Centers for Medicare & Medicaid Services evaluation of for-profit PACE programs under section 4804(b) of the Balanced Budget Act of 1997.

Walls, J., Scully, D., Fox-Grage, W., Ujvari, K., Cho, E., & Hall, J. (2013). *Two-thirds of states integrating Medicare and Medicaid services for dual eligibles.* Washington, DC: AARP Public Policy Institute. Retrieved from www.aarp.org/content/dam/aarp/research/public_policy_institute/health/2013/states-integrating-medicare-and-medicaid-AARP-ppi-health.pdf.

Walsh, E., Freiman, M., Haber, S., Bragg, A., Ouslander, J., & Wiener, J. (2010). *Cost drivers for dually eligible beneficiaries: Potentially avoidable hospitalizations from nursing facility, skilled nursing facility, and home and community based services waiver programs.* Washington, DC: Centers for Medicare and Medicaid Services. Retrieved from www.cms.gov/Research-Statistics-Data-and-Systems/Statistics-Trends-and-Reports/Reports/downloads/costdriverstask2.pdf.

ONLINE RESOURCES

AARP
www.aarp.org/research/ppi
Center for Health Care Strategies: Medicare-Medicaid Integration: An Online Toolkit
www.chcs.org/resource/medicare-medicaid-integration-online-toolkit/
The Henry J. Kaiser Family Foundation
www.kff.org/tag/dual-eligible
Medicare-Medicaid Coordination Office
www.cms.gov/Medicare-Medicaid-Coordination/Medicare-and-Medicaid-Coordination/Medicare-Medicaid-Coordination-Office/index.html
The Scan Foundation
www.thescanfoundation.org/categories/dual-eligibles-1

34

Home Care, Hospice, and Community-Based Care: Evolving Policy

Mary Ann Christopher, Sherl Brand, Florence Kariuki, and Maria LoGrippo

> *"Reform can only be accomplished when attitudes are changed."*
>
> **Lillian Wald**

Nurses are pivotal to the promotion of efforts that can and will build a "culture of health" that puts "well-being at the center of every aspect of our lives. Everyone has access to the care they need and all families have the opportunity to make healthier choices" (Robert Wood Johnson Foundation, 2018). This chapter focuses on the role of home care, hospice, and community-based care in meeting the Triple Aim to help individuals, families, and the nation live healthier lives.

FUNDAMENTAL UNDERPINNINGS

The value-based reimbursement framework, catalyzed by the Institute for Healthcare Improvement's Triple Aim (Berwick, Nolan, & Whittington, 2008) and the enactment of the Patient Protection and Affordable Care Act, highlights home health and community-based services as fundamental underpinnings of the achievement of better care and health at lower costs. Value-based reimbursement is the payment model by which purchasers of health care (government, employers, and consumers) and payers (public and private) hold the health care delivery system (physicians and other providers, hospitals, and so on) accountable for both quality and cost of care (American Academy of Family Physicians, 2018). Home and community-based services are consumer-centric, value-based alternatives to more costly, less appropriate settings of care. Policy mandates and practice initiatives set forth by the Centers for Medicare and Medicaid Services (CMS) (2018a) position home and community-based services at the forefront of strategies around securing a culture of health for our nation.

The home and community-based setting is where patient satisfaction is notably higher, health care spending is lower, and nurses can favorably impact outcomes. However, it is also the site that poses the greatest challenges. In facility-based settings, the health care system controls the level of care including treatments, administration of medications, meals, and even visitation for multiple patients in one location. An individual's home is just the opposite. In a patient's home, the patient is in control and the care is one-to-one. In the home, nurses must effectively support the patient's progress and/or maintenance as well as promote self-care management with a "visitor" mindset. Similarly, providers of community-based services must work collaboratively with and within communities and view them as partners. In order to preserve the right for people to receive care in their homes and communities, it is imperative for nurses to be leaders in advocacy, innovation, and the development of new payment and care models.

INNOVATIVE MODELS IN THE HOME AND IN THE COMMUNITY

Bundled Payment for Care Improvement

The Centers for Medicare and Medicaid Services Innovation's (CMMI, 2018d) Bundled Payment for Care Improvement (BPCI) program evolved from evidence that the post-acute transition of patients was unnecessarily directed to sub-acute facilities. CMMI proposed a demonstration project that based the transition to next site of care on evidence that factored in patients' functional status, support system, and preference. The results for Medicare patients with diagnoses that include orthopedic and cardiac surgeries and congestive heart failure overwhelmingly demonstrate that patient outcomes and consumer satisfaction are enhanced when the discharge is facilitated directly from hospital to homecare, skipping sub-acute facilities altogether whenever possible. Related impacts were the notable avoidance of unnecessary hospitalizations, lower rates of postoperative infections, earlier achievement of optimal functional ability, and enhanced patient satisfaction (The Lewin Group, 2017).

Transitional Care Model

Mary Naylor, PhD, RN, FAAN, Marian S. Ware Professor in Gerontology and Director of the New Courtland Center for Transitions and Health at the University of Pennsylvania, recognized that the rate of readmissions to hospital within 30 days of discharge was excessive and costly for Medicare recipients. She designed the Transitional Care Model that promotes the role of the advanced practice registered nurse (APRN) to deliver and coordinate care in collaboration with the interprofessional team for at-risk patients while in the hospital and then continuing that care in the home. Research on transition care models shows a reduction in the burden of costly readmissions by early detection and screening for at-risk patients, engaging family and caregivers early in the plans of care, and the prevention of breakdowns in care (Hirschman et al., 2015). Emerging from this work, other models of care have used registered nurses (RNs), coaches, and other trained individuals to support and coordinate care for at-risk patients. With the Coleman Care Transitions Intervention, for example, a trained individual follows a patient who is being discharged from acute care and offers support for self-management and functional recovery (Coleman, n.d.). With Medicare transitioning to value-based programs, these models offer hospital systems ways to improve performance, efficiency, and quality of care most associated with complex care of the older adult.

Hospital at Home

Hospital-level care at home continues to offer another innovative model of care for individuals living in the community. The Johns Hopkins Hospital at Home model allows eligible patients who present with an acute diagnosis usually predictive of hospital inpatient admission to receive the care alternatively in the home. Principal diagnoses for which the Hospital at Home program might be an alternative include congestive heart failure, chronic obstructive pulmonary disease (COPD), dehydration, and cellulitis. The patient might receive continuous in-home monitoring, hydration, and other supportive interventions through an interprofessional team that includes a physician, nurse practitioner, and nurse. While nurses are available 24 hours a day/7 days a week and prepared for urgent or emergency situations, they are essential members of the team providing the initial extended nursing care upon admission to home and then daily nursing visits when appropriate. Researchers have demonstrated

considerable cost savings, increased opportunities for patient teaching, and communication with caregivers while maintaining high-quality acute care in the home (Cryer et al., 2012; Marsteller et al., 2009).

Collaborative Partnerships

An essential component in achieving successful models of care in the community is the engagement of key partners. Home care organizations will have increased relevance to the health care system if they can convey to payers and to health systems who aggregate payment that they are valuable, high-performing organizations, as defined by top decile with patient satisfaction, process measures (including 24-hour admission turnaround times), electronic health record (EHR) connectivity, availability of high-tech infusion capabilities, and top decile performance on Home Care Compare (www.medicare.gov/homehealthcompare/) and other critical indicators.

Although payers and health systems are collaborating with home care providers that will deliver on expected performance, there are challenges from a patient perspective. The June 2018 report of the Medicare Payment Advisory Commission (MedPAC, 2018) noted that about 40% of Medicare acute inpatient hospital discharges result in use of post-acute care (PAC), which includes home health agencies. Ensuring that the patient is served by the appropriate type of PAC provider is critical, but the selection of a provider within a PAC category is a challenge. Home Health Compare (CMS, 2018c), a publicly available resource developed by CMS to provide insight into key quality indicators, indicated that the market share of high-quality providers has increased less than 1% during the period of 2001 to 2006 (Jung et al., 2016). There are notable reasons, including consumers' lack of understanding of information or access to available post-acute services, regulatory protection of patient choice, legislation that prevents hospital discharge planners from making recommendations, and limitations within the hospital discharge planning conditions of participation (CoPs). Medicare CoPs are federal regulations with which particular health care organizations must comply in order to participate and receive funding from the Medicare and Medicaid programs. They include CoPs for home health care and are published in the Code of Federal Regulations (CMS, 2018b).

Because Medicare discharge planning regulations place responsibility with hospitals and more specifically nurse discharge planners and case managers for connecting inpatient acute care hospital patients with their options for PAC, nurses must be knowledgeable about best practices to educate beneficiaries about their choices and to optimize access to PAC when necessary. Nurses in these roles must also recognize policy implications and develop strategic initiatives that can support patient preferences and guarantee beneficiary freedom of choice in selecting PAC providers.

The Balanced Budget Act of 1997 (BBA) required hospitals to provide lists of skilled nursing facilities (SNFs) and home health agencies to patients but not any quality information. To address this, the Improving Medicare Post-Acute Care Transformation Act of 2014 (IMPACT) required changes to the discharge planning CoPs to mandate that hospitals "take into account quality, resource use, and other measures . . . in the discharge planning process" (MedPAC, 2018). CMS proposed regulations in 2015 to put this mandate into effect but never finalized the regulation. To make the necessary changes to support informed decisions with a lens on quality, nurses in critical roles such as discharge planning and case management must advocate for updates to and clarity around existing regulations, specifically around having the flexibility to use data-driven resources to educate patients and caregivers for informed decision making.

Interdisciplinary Teams to Address Social Determinants of Health

Increasingly, engaging members of the interdisciplinary team to address the social determinants of health is being recognized as crucial to achieving the Triple Aim—factors such as housing, transportation, food, and safe environments. Increasingly, successful organizations across the country are testing models of care that integrate ways of addressing social determinants of health. The Mercy Health System, a Southeastern-based hospital system, created a team of a social workers, nurses, and community health workers (CHWs) working across the acute care, physician practice, and home care settings. The organization's leaders valued the role of CHWs by integrating them within home health care. The impact of the team within Mercy contributed to a 31.25% reduction in avoidable emergency department (ED) visits (Tyrrell & Sullivan, 2017).

Like Mercy, the University of Maryland St. Joseph Medical Center (a 232-bed hospital in Towson) and Maxim Healthcare (a home health company) partnered in 2015 to address their 25% readmission rate within 30 days of discharge by high-risk patients by using a CHW model. When in 2014 the Maryland Commission and CMS required Maryland hospitals to reduce the readmission gap by 2018 (Whitman, 2016), they turned to CHWs to address patients' urgent nonclinical factors related to social health determinants. As representatives of the community, CHWs hold an integral, respected place on interdisciplinary teams and can offer a bi-directional referral pathway. Cutting-edge research from the Penn Center for Community Health Workers (2018) provides substantial evidence to support the use of CHWs for Triple-Aim improvements through a standardized, exportable CHW model called Individualized

Management for Patient-Centered Targets (IMPaCT). Randomized controlled studies demonstrated the effectiveness of the CHW model in reducing hospital readmissions, supporting chronic disease management, and improving access to primary care and mental health services (Kangovi et al., 2017).

Home care organizations are testing various models of care and mechanisms that support a team approach for in-home visits for mothers and children and new roles for CHWs and home health aides (HHAs). Nurse leaders within policy think tanks, academic environments, and even the United Nations (UN) are crafting solutions around this work. The UN sponsored a steering committee to promote the adoption of CHWs within community-based interprofessional teams with the goal of drawing upon sustainable community models of care internationally (Arnhold Institute for Global Health, 2016). Nurses and health leaders within Horizon Blue Cross Blue Shield New Jersey participated in that workgroup and formed a partnership to test the model within the city of Newark. Focusing on four zip codes within the city, nurses and other health care leaders created a clinically integrated team comprised of a hospital-based APRN, a care coordinator, two CHWs, and a nursing care coordinator within the health plan. Social determinants most frequently identified included transportation, undiagnosed mental health issues, housing costs, food insecurity, and medication adherence related to lack of ability to make copayments. Payers and providers alike have demonstrated the impact of CHWs in the mitigation of social determinants for patients with Medicaid, Medicare, and commercial insurance plans. For example, a CHW worked with a 46-year-old patient with a diagnosis of hypertension who was discharged from the hospital but couldn't afford the drug copays, creating a risk for poor health outcomes and rehospitalization. The CHW worked with the hospitalist to change the prescriptions to less costly generic options and secured pharmaceutical assistance to promote medication compliance. In another example, a 42-year-old patient with heart failure could not afford transportation to attend regular primary care provider (PCP) visits, and instead would wait until he was unwell and call an ambulance. The CHW helped the patient apply for van services, which allowed him to attend all his PCP visits. Ultimately, examples like these show evidence to support how the CHW model can reduce unnecessary ED visits and hospitalizations, reduce health disparities, and improve health and health equity.

With the growing interest in CHW programs comes some challenges. Although the evidence clearly suggests that these programs can reduce health disparities and target social determinants, there continue to be challenges related to sustainability, payment and reimbursement, certification/training of CHWs, and the allocation of resources to address social concerns for the communities most in need (Nkouaga et al., 2017). To address these challenges, stakeholders from the payer, provider, government, employer, and community groups must collaborate to develop policies that promote and expand the role of the CHW.

FROM GRASSROOTS TO NATIONAL POLICY

It is critically imperative for nurses to implement and define home and community-based care services both at the grassroots and national level to address the tsunami of future workforce demands, the aging population, and increasingly more complex care needs of patients. The shift to provide care in the home increased significantly with the Olmstead Decision by the U.S. Supreme Court affirming that public entities must provide community-based services to individuals with disabilities (Olmstead v. L.C., 1999). The level and need for care at home continues to grow with the overall aging of the population, longer life expectancy, and overall redirection of care from facilities to home along with the prevalence of chronic care disease. By 2050, the proportion of the population aged 65 and older (15.6%) will be more than double that of children under age 5 (7.2%). This is unprecedented and will lead to a crisis in care delivery (He, Goodkind, & Kowal, 2015).

With the looming nursing workforce shortage, high numbers of consumers of care, and challenges facing disability advocates and Medicaid programs, health care professionals must seek evidence-based solutions. Nurse delegation to HHAs has become one such solution and a priority in many states, strongly aligning with one of the recommendations from the Institute of Medicine's report on *The Future of Nursing* that stresses the need for nurses to work at their highest level of training and education (Institute of Medicine [IOM], 2011).

Nurse Delegation

Key challenges to nurse delegation to HHAs has focused largely on scope of practice and nurse delegation regulations. Patients often require nursing care at home which may include tasks such as medication administration, wound care, and other medical treatments. These interventions fall under the nursing scope of practice clearly defined in Nurse Practice Acts in every state. In 2005, the American Nurses Association (ANA) and the National Council of State Boards of Nursing (NCSBN) in a joint statement defined delegation as the "the process for a nurse to direct another person to perform nursing tasks and activities." Additional barriers have included nurses' skill in delegation of tasks (Box 34.1), training of HHAs, liability

---

BOX 34.1   New Jersey Administrative Code 13.37-6.2 Delegation of Selected Nursing Tasks

(a) The registered professional nurse is responsible for the nature and quality of all nursing care including the assessment of the nursing needs, the plan of nursing care, the implementation, and the monitoring and evaluation of the plan. The registered professional nurse may delegate selected nursing tasks in the implementation of the nursing regimen to licensed practical nurses and ancillary nursing personnel. Ancillary nursing personnel shall include but not be limited to: aides, assistants, attendants, and technicians.

(d) In delegating selected nursing tasks to licensed practical nurses or ancillary nursing personnel, the registered professional nurse shall be responsible for exercising that degree of judgment and knowledge reasonably expected to assure that a proper delegation has been made. A registered professional nurse may not delegate the performance of a nursing task to persons who have not been adequately prepared by verifiable training and education. No task may be delegated which is within the scope of nursing practice and requires:

  1. The substantial knowledge and skill derived from completion of a nursing education program and the

specialized skill, judgment, and knowledge of a registered nurse;

  2. An understanding of nursing principles necessary to recognize and manage complications which may result in harm to the health and safety of the patient.

(c) The registered professional nurse shall be responsible for the proper supervision of licensed practical nurses and ancillary nursing personnel to whom such delegation is made. The degree of supervision exercised over licensed practical nurses and ancillary nursing personnel shall be determined by the registered professional nurse based on an evaluation of all factors including:

  1. The condition of the patient;

  2. The education, skill, and training of the licensed practical nurse and ancillary nursing personnel to whom delegation is being made;

  3. The nature of the tasks and the activities being delegated;

  4. Supervision may require the direct continuing presence or the intermittent observation, direction, and occasional physical presence of a registered professional nurse. In all cases, the registered professional nurse shall be available for on-site supervision.

concerns, and willingness of aides to take on delegated tasks in addition to their existing responsibilities. Nurses in New Jersey addressed these barriers by driving changes to the New Jersey Nurse Practice Act back in the early 1990s. Original language in the amendments allowed RNs to use judgment in delegating tasks to unlicensed assistive personnel without defining tasks or limits by setting, but later amendments were made to prohibit certified HHAs from administering medications, yet allowed delegation of other tasks under the RN's discretion (Young, Farnham, & Reinhard, 2016). The New Jersey Board of Nursing (NJBON) brought together key stakeholders from across the state, including the New Jersey Division of Disability Services of the New Jersey Department of Human Services, New Jersey Department of Health and Senior Services (HSS), and groups representing RNs, HHAs, and consumers, to provide the necessary evidence to support best practices and a clearer understanding of nurse delegation. A pilot study with 19 participating home care agencies in 2007 provided the evidence demonstrating higher patient, family, and HHA satisfaction with no adverse outcome and lower costs (Young, Farnham, & Reinhard, 2016). In 2018, NJBON rules were promulgated to reflect years of advocacy and evidence to support delegation of nursing tasks to HHAs. The decision remains solely with the RN and the approach is at a nurse by nurse, HHA by HHA, patient by patient level, meaning that all three aspects are considered in the determination of whether to delegate or not.

Driving Change and Impacting Health: Telehealth

With the public and payer shift to home and community-based care and a shrinking work force, telehealth can and will play an important role in allowing patients to heal and age at home and remain in their communities. The Public Health Institute Center for Connected Health Policy (2018) defines *telehealth* as a "a collection of means or methods for enhancing health care, public health and health education delivery and support using telecommunications technologies" and categorizes four telehealth modalities: live video, store-and-forward (recorded health history such as transmission of x-rays), remote patient monitoring (RPM), and mobile health (mHealth).

In 2010, the Department of Health in New York State funded a project involving telehealth services to provide effective and efficient monitoring of individuals' symptoms who were receiving health care from home care agencies. Other objectives of the project included improved communication with PCPs and the delivery of evidence-based treatments (Gellis et al., 2014). This randomized controlled trial involved a 3-month integrated telehealth depression intervention for older adults receiving home care, compared with usual care with in-home nursing and psychoeducation. Results of the Integrated Telehealth Education and Activation of Mood (I-TEAM) study revealed a 50% reduction in depression scores, improved problem-solving, and self-efficacy among those receiving the telehealth intervention. In addition, analysis of health care–related data collected 12 months before and after initiation of treatment revealed fewer ED visits among the intervention. In 2018, NY State Governor Cuomo announced innovative state regulatory measures including the provision of telehealth to patients through home care services.

Today telehealth is being utilized in all sectors of the health care continuum. In the home and community-based setting, the most common modality is RPM with some larger and more progressive agencies, like Trinity at Home, expanding into the mHealth space. In 2017, Erin Denholm, RN, MSN, led Trinity Health at Home to partner with Vivify Health, a remote care technology company, to launch Home Care Connect, an integrated virtual care program with a goal of reducing ED utilization and preventing avoidable hospital admissions. It provides patients with wireless peripheral devices including an easy-to-use tablet, a blood pressure cuff, a scale, and pulse oximeter. These devices provide health and medication information to the patient, monitor important vital statistics and patient health status to enable early intervention, and allow the patient to access clinicians 24/7 (Trinity Health at Home, 2017).

In densely populated urban communities like those found in New York City, home care agencies are tasked with caring for some of the nation's sickest children and can support a decrease in hospitalizations and readmissions utilizing technology like the RPM program. The use of telehealth is saving a considerable amount of money, time, and resources simply by checking in by phone with patients and their families on a regular basis. Elvira Fardella-Roveto, RN, administrator of patient services for St. Mary's Healthcare System for Children, said the RPM program saved the program roughly $2.17 million by eliminating some 77 hospitalizations in a 1-year span. When asked if the agency saw an improvement in clinical outcomes, Fardella-Roveto responded "anecdotal information indicates that we were successful" in improving the overall health of the children in their care. She also noted improved satisfaction rates for the families and caregivers, many of whom deal with a lot of stress in caring for the children. The program also revealed some unexpected results. With better communication between the agency and the patients/families, the agency was able to identify other issues, like caregiver stress, language barriers, and even home safety problems. In at least one case, Fardella-Roveto felt that the agency was able to help a family make needed home improvements to improve the care environment for a child (Wicklund, 2016).

Although the uptake of telehealth has been limited in the past, nursing leaders and other stakeholders have played a key role in influencing policy and reformation of payment to expand the access and utilization of telehealth. From a regulatory perspective, the way the government views telehealth is changing as exemplified by the recent enactment of the Creating High-Quality Results and Outcomes Necessary to Improve Chronic (CHRONIC) Care Act (Public Health Institute Center for Connected Health Policy, 2018). The Act expands the use of telehealth in Medicare Advantage plans and Accountable Care Organizations. It also allows telehealth access for patients on dialysis and expands telestroke services for Medicare beneficiaries. It specifically recognizes the patient's home as an originating site for telehealth services. Telehealth-related legislation at the federal and state levels continues to expand further, supporting the recognition of its value in care delivery for the future. The use of telehealth by nurses and other members of the health care team is transforming how care is being delivered, therefore nurses are expected to know, understand, and articulate the potential impact that telehealth has on improving access and quality and reducing costs. Such growth and expansion support new roles for nurses in business development around innovative home care business ventures and entrepreneurship.

Project Extension for Community Health Care Outcomes

There are additional examples of technologies that bring clinicians together to promote best practices, improve communication and collaboration, and ultimately drive for better care and outcomes. Starting in 2003, Project Extension for Community Healthcare Outcomes (ECHO) was a grassroots project that became a movement to inform and provide best practices for underserved people globally. When Sanjeev Arora, M.D., a liver disease physician in Albuquerque, became frustrated that many New Mexicans with Hepatitis C could not get care because there was no access to specialists, he found a way for local providers to team with specialists at academic medical centers in weekly virtual clinics or teleECHO clinics (Project ECHO, 2018).

A home and community-based provider that opted to utilize this solution was Visiting Nurse Association Health Group in NJ. The organization deployed the Project ECHO model to support its Central New Jersey Community-Based Care Transition Program, a CMS demonstration project. Under the leadership of Marie Perillo, RN, MSN, and Kimberly Mora, DNP, RN, the care transitions project engaged nurses and social workers from multiple hospitals, home health agencies, and community-based agencies to work together to drive improvements with all-cause readmissions. These individuals were geographically dispersed across multiple counties and embedded in the communities

they served. Using Project ECHO, Perillo and Mora were able to connect the remote team to enhance individual development, promote collaboration and consistency, and meet program goals. The outcomes included improved satisfaction among nurse and social worker participants, improved collaboration and improvements in practice based on lessons learned from case reviews, and a decrease in readmissions.

COMMUNITY-BASED PALLIATIVE CARE

As the U.S. population continues to age and the health industry moves further into risk-based contracting, health providers are turning to palliative care as a winning strategy for cutting costs and improving quality. In adopting community-based, consumer-centric care, progressive organizations are making strides toward providing palliative care beyond the traditional settings, with expanding focus on outpatient and home-based settings.

Fundamental understanding of the difference between "hospice" and" palliative care" is critical to the articulate formulation and implementation of laws, policies, and programs. The goal of *palliative care* is to provide quality care for patients experiencing life-limiting diseases or the severe symptom burden of acute or chronic illnesses. *Hospice care* includes palliative care and addresses the patient's physical, emotional, and spiritual needs as well. It is set aside for terminally ill patients during the last 6 months of life, when treatment is no longer curative and with the assumption that the disease will take its normal course. Although palliative care has historically faced significant political challenges, there continues to be significant advocacy and headway in formation of policies that increase access to these services. In July 2018, the Palliative Care and Hospice Education Training Act (PCHETA) was passed, making palliative care and end-of-life care more accessible to patients and families by supporting outreach and enhanced education for health care professionals (California State University Institute for Palliative Care, 2018). In addition, California and several other states have enacted policies that require provision of palliative care services for their Medicaid population. CMS is also actively reviewing proposals to develop Alternative Payment Models (APMs) that reimburse for palliative care.

At Horizon Blue Cross Blue Shield NJ, nurse leaders developed a program to offer health plan members access to palliative care services, using a team of highly-trained nurses with previous hospice experience. The program was branded the "Supportive Care Program (SCP)," to reduce barriers associated with patients' perceptions of the word "palliative." Through a predictive algorithm and referrals from case management and other providers, Horizon's members who could potentially benefit from palliative care

are identified, and then nurses conduct telephonic outreach to them, complete a comprehensive assessment, and facilitate interventions. The nurses help members to address symptoms such as pain and anxiety by referring them to appropriate providers and engaging the providers to ensure that needs are optimally addressed. They also connect members to other resources such as durable medical equipment that could improve the member's quality of life and outcomes. In a community-based approach, the SCP nurses refer members to community-based palliative care providers for additional community-based support. Since its' inception in April 2017, the SCP continues to show success, with a high engagement rate and total cost reduction.

Horizon's SCP nurses also make referrals to community-based palliative providers (CBPP), where an interdisciplinary team delivers a comprehensive set of palliative care services in the home. In each of the community-based palliative care settings, the team works under the leadership of a palliative-certified physician or NP to deliver care to the patient in their home. Teams consist of physicians, NPs, nurses, social workers, dietitians, chaplains, and nonclinical staff. Upon referral into the CBPP, the team begins with a comprehensive assessment that facilitates the development of an appropriate plan of care, leveraging the appropriate team member to provide care in the home. The CBPP programs encourage the delivery of a comprehensive set of services under a single case-rate payment per month for each engaged member. This is an important step in the evolution of the health industry from a fee-for-service model to a value-based reimbursement model, where providers are reimbursed for the quality of care provided, rather than the quantity.

Policies supporting the advancement of palliative care continue to make headway. In July 2018, the House of Representatives passed the groundbreaking PCHETA with bipartisan support. The Act would increase access to palliative and end-of-life care by supporting outreach and enhanced education for health care professionals (California State University-Institute for Palliative Care, 2018). Moving forward, policy initiatives that address workforce needs, research, and payment models linked to quality measures will further bring palliative care to scale in the country.

MEDICARE ADVANTAGE EXPANSION OF SUPPLEMENTAL BENEFITS

Just as nurses address the gaps in palliative care, they must also address the challenges in accessing non-traditional care and support for the frail and older population patients that exist with both government and private payers. Almost half of Medicare beneficiaries struggle with activities of daily living (ADLs), yet Medicare has not covered services in the home unless they are related to an acute care episode or support the improvement of a health condition (Willink & DuGoff, 2018). Often the services most needed are considered custodial and/or "unskilled" services and have long been deemed outside of the Medicare benefit. Supplemental benefits are included in Medicaid plans across the country to meet the needs of the aged and those with disabilities. Medicare Advantage plans often offer some relief; however, the traditional Medicare fee-for-service plan does not. Nursing as well as other advocacy groups can and must influence policymakers on efforts to expand services that can render the greatest benefit and equity.

ACCOUNTABLE HEALTH COMMUNITIES

Supported by federal demonstration project dollars, the accountable health communities (AHC) model is based on the premise that by systematically addressing social determinants of health, health outcomes are improved while costs go down. The model demands collaborations of clinical and social support systems within identified communities. Thirty-one programs were funded by CMS (CMS, 2018d). One such program was developed and led by Billie Lynn Allard MS, RN, at Southwestern Vermont Health Care. Within this ACH, Billie integrated the learnings of nurse leaders before her with a Transitional Care Nursing (TCN) program, a Community Care Team (CCT), an Interventions to Reduce Acute Care Transfers (INTERACT) program, a Diabetes Care and Prevention program, an integrated social worker, a Home Safety Initiative program, a Medication Management and Education program, an Emergency Department Imbedded Physical Therapists program, a Maternal Transitions of Care program, and a Communitive Collaborative program. This comprehensive AHC demonstrated a 56.1% reduction in hospital admissions and observation status visits among high-risk patients participating in the TCN program over 180 days, with a sustained decrease of 46.8% over a 1-year period. The CCT demonstrated a 34.7% reduction in ED visits among patients with addiction and mental illness who frequented the ED when comparing 6 months before intervention and 6 months after. A 12.4% reduction in hemoglobin A1c was achieved by patients working with a certified diabetes educator within primary care practices. After the implementation of a pulmonary rehabilitation program, the 30-day readmission rate decreased from 17.26% to 2.56% (American Academy of Nursing, n.d.).

CONCLUSION

With increasingly more vulnerable patients being cared for at home and in community-based settings, it becomes critical to educate all nurses to be leaders in developing policies that will support innovation and growth in community-based health and social services. Nurse leaders have the responsibility to translate results from innovative models of care into payment policy in both the public and private sectors. This activism will ensure that care becomes increasingly consumer centric and community centered, principles upon which meaningful health reform is predicated.

DISCUSSION QUESTIONS

1. What are the major factors nurses should consider in launching social determinant intervention strategies?
2. Consider one of the innovative models of care discussed in this chapter and describe the role of the nurse as an innovator and designer to impact the health policy discussion.
3. Review community-based palliative models of care and determine the key influencers on decision making that reduce costs while providing access to high-quality care.
4. Reflecting on home and community-based services, what are some of the ways nurses can be leaders and change agents in actualizing the Triple Aim?

REFERENCES

American Academy of Family Physicians. (2018). *Value-based payment*. Retrieved from www.aafp.org/about/policies/all/value-based-payment.html.

American Academy of Nursing. (n.d.). *Raise the voice edge runner: Accountable community of health*. Retrieved at www.aannet.org/initiatives/edge-runners/profiles/edge-runners—accountablecommunity.

Arnhold Institute for Global Health (2016). *Closing the gap: Applying global lessons toward sustainable community health models in the U.S.* Retrieved from www.healthenvoy.org/wp-content/uploads/2014/05/Closing-the-Gap-Applying-Global-Lessons-Toward-Sustainable-Community-Health-Models-in-the-U.S..pdf.

Berwick, D., Nolan, T., & Whittington, J. (2008). The Triple Aim: Care, health, and cost. *Health Affairs, 27*(3), 759-69.

California State University Institute for Palliative Care. (2018). *Palliative care education—Anytime, anywhere*. Retrieved from https://csupalliativecare.org/pcheta-2018/.

Centers for Medicare and Medicaid Services. (2018a). *Community-based care transitions program*. Retrieved from https://innovation.cms.gov/initiatives/CCTP/

Centers for Medicare and Medicaid Services. (2018b). *Home health agency (HHA) interpretive guideline*. Retrieved from www.cms.gov/Medicare/Provider-Enrollment-and-Certification/Survey CertificationGenInfo/Downloads/QSO18-25-HHA.pdf

Centers for Medicare and Medicaid Services. (2018c). *Home health compare*. Retrieved from www.medicare.gov/homehealthcompare/search.html.

Centers for Medicare and Medicaid Services. (2018d). *The CMS Innovation Center*. Retrieved from https://innovation.cms.gov/.

Coleman, E. (n.d.). *Care transitions program*. Retrieved from https://caretransitions.org/.

Cryer, L., Shannon, S., Van Amsterdam, M., & Leff, B. (2012). Innovation profile: Costs for "Hospital at Home" patients were 19 percent lower, with equal or better outcomes compared to similar inpatients. *Health Affairs, 31*(6), 1237–1243.

Gellis, Z., Kenaley, B., & Have, T. (2014). Integrated telehealth care for chronic illness and depression in geriatric home care patients: The Integrated Telehealth Education and Activation of Mood (I-TEAM) Study. *Journal of the American Geriatrics Society, 62*(5), 889-895.

He, W., Goodkind, D. & Kowal, P. (2016). *An aging world 2015: International population reports*. Washington, DC: U.S. Department of Commerce, Economics and Statistics Administration, U.S. Census Bureau.

Hirschman, K., Shaid, E., McCauley, K., Pauly, M., & Naylor, M. (2015). Continuity of care: The transitional care model. *OJIN: The Online Journal of Issues in Nursing, 20*(3).

Institute of Medicine. (2011). *The future of nursing: Leading change, advancing health*. Washington, DC: National Academies Press.

Jung, J.K., Wu, B., Kim, H., & Polsky, D. (2015). The effect of publicized quality information on home health agency choice. *Medical Care Research and Review. 73*(6), 703-723.

Kangovi, S., Mitra, N., Grande, D., Hairong, H., Smith, R.A., & Long, J.A. (2017). Community health workers support for disadvantaged patients with multiple chronic diseases: A randomized clinical trial. *American Journal of Public Health, 107*(10), 1660-1667.

The Lewin Group. (2017). *CMS bundled payments for care improvement initiative models 2-4: Year 3 evaluation and monitoring annual report*. Retrieved from https://downloads.cms.gov/files/cmmi/bpci-models2-4yr3evalrpt.pdf

Marsteller, A., Burton, L., Mader, B., Naughton, B., Burl, B., Guido, B., ... & Leff, B. (2009). Health care provider evaluation of a substitutive model of Hospital at Home. *Medical Care, 47*(9), 979–985.

Medicare Payment Advisory Commission. (2018). *Report to the Congress: Medicare and the health care delivery system*. Retrieved from www.medpac.gov/docs/default-source/reports/jun18_medpacreporttocongress_sec.pdf?sfvrsn=0.

Nkouaga, C., Kaufman, A., Alfero, C., & Medina, C. (2017). Diffusion of community health workers within Medicaid managed care: A strategy to address social determinants of health. *Health Affairs*. Retrieved from www.healthaffairs.org/do/10.1377/hblog20170725.061194/full/.

Olmstead v. L.C., 527 U.S. 581 (1999).

Project ECHO. (2018). *Project ECHO: A revolution in medical education and care delivery*. Retrieved from https://echo.unm.edu/.

Public Health Institute Center for Connected Health Policy. (2018). *National Telehealth Policy Resource Center*. Retrieved from www.cchpca.org/.

Robert Wood Johnson Foundation. (2018). *About a culture of health*. Retrieved from www.rwjf.org/en/cultureofhealth/about.html.

Trinity Health at Home. (2017). *Home care connect*. Retrieved from www.trinityhomehealth.org/home-care-connect.

Tyrrell, R. & Sullivan, D. (2017). *How Mercy Health overhauled its approach to care transitions—and cut ED visits by 30%*. Care Transformation Center Blog, The Advisory Board. Retrieved from www.advisory.com/research/care-transformation-center/care-transformation-center-blog/2017/06/mercy-care-transitions.

Whitman, E. (2016). Deploying community health workers to reduce readmission rates. *Modern Healthcare, 46*(43), 0032.

Wicklund, E. (2016). Remote monitoring platform is an mHealth lifeline for New York's sickest children. *mHealth Intelligence*. Retrieved from https://mhealthintelligence.com/news/remote-monitoring-platform-is-an-mhealth-lifeline-for-new-yorks-sickest-chi.

Willink, A., & DuGoff, E.H. (2018). Integrating medical and nonmedical services: The promise and pitfalls of the CHRONIC Care Act. *New England Journal of Medicine, 378*(23), 2153-2155.

Young, H.M., Farnham, J., & Reinhard, S.C. (2016). Nurse delegation in home care. *Journal of Gerontological Nursing, 42*(9), 7-15.

ONLINE RESOURCES

Accountable Health Communities Model
https://innovation.cms.gov/initiatives/ahcm/
National Association for Home Care and Hospice
www.nahc.org
National Hospice and Palliative Care Organization
www.nhpco.org
Visiting Nurse Associations of America
www.VNAA.org

35

Long-Term Services and Supports Policy Issues

Caroline Stephens, Michele Diaz, and Laura M. Wagner

"A policy is a temporary creed liable to be changed, but while it holds good it has got to be pursued with apostolic zeal."

Mahatma Gandhi

The U.S. population is aging, with the number of adults aged 65 and older projected to almost double between 2014 and 2060 from 43.1 million to 98 million (Mather, Jacobsen, & Pollard, 2015). By 2030, approximately one in five Americans will be 65 years or older (Colby & Ortman, 2015). Moreover, the number of the oldest old (aged 85 years and older) is projected to triple from 5.9 million in 2012 to 18.2 million in 2050, accounting for 4.5% of the total population (Ortman, Velkoff, & Hogan, 2014; U.S. Census Bureau, 2012). The demand for long-term services and supports (LTSS) and the need for nurses and other personnel to provide those services is growing rapidly. According to the Bureau of Labor Statistics, between 2016 and 2026, personal care aides and home health aides are projected to be the leading occupations with the most job growth. However, the Institute of Medicine (IOM, 2008) predicts a major shortage of health workers with geriatric training to address the growing needs of the aging population. In 2013, total LTSS spending was $305.4 billion, which constitutes 10.6% of the total U.S. personal health care expenditures. Although Medicaid is the largest payer of total LTSS expenditures (48% of total expenditures), Medicare is a significant source of spending with more than a 15-fold growth increase between 1988 and 2013 (Wiener, Knowles, & White, 2017).

This policy chapter focuses on some of the policy and political issues facing nursing in long-term care. First, it reviews the problems of poor quality of nursing home care, weak enforcement of federal quality regulations, and profit-making nursing homes. Second, it examines nursing home staffing and reimbursement policies. Third, it discusses the need for expanding home and community-based

service (HCBS) programs. Finally, nurses are urged to become advocates for older and disabled people who need long-term care services.

POOR QUALITY OF CARE

Poor nursing home quality has been documented since the early 1970s and culminated in the passage of the Omnibus Budget Reconciliation Act (OBRA) of 1987 to reform nursing home regulation. The federal law requires comprehensive assessments of all nursing home residents and assurance that residents maintain the highest possible mental and physical health. Although the federal government sets the standards, state survey and certification agencies conduct annual surveys and complaint investigations to verify compliance for a nursing home to be certified to receive federal funds.

Although the federal regulations are clear, many nursing homes provide poor quality of care. Nursing facilities are cited with deficiencies when they fail to meet requirements or regulations. Between 2009 and 2013, the average citation per facility declined from 9.33 to 7.28, and increased to 8.6 between 2013 and 2016. The number of nursing home deficiencies vary state by state. Some states have higher rates of citations across all deficiency categories. The percentage of facilitates *without* deficiencies decreased from 8.07% in 2013 to 6.5% in 2016 (Harrington et al., 2018). 1n 2016, many formal complaints were made to state regulatory agencies about poor nursing home quality, and one in five facilities received a citation for actual harm or immediate jeopardy to nursing home residents. Many nursing homes failed to provide adequate infection control, a safe environment, adequate food sanitation, optimal quality standards, and pharmacy consultation (Harrington et al., 2018).

WEAK ENFORCEMENT

Many studies have documented that the federal and state survey and enforcement system as well as the complaint investigation processes are weak (U.S. Government Accounting Office [GAO], 1999, 2011). State surveyors are often unable to detect serious problems with the quality of care. Some state survey agencies improperly downgrade the scope and severity of the deficiencies observed and do not refer nursing homes for intermediate sanctions. The timing of state surveys continues to be predictable and consumer complaint investigations are not timely (U.S. GAO, 2011). Poor state investigations and documentation of deficiencies, large numbers of inexperienced state surveyors, and weak federal oversight of state activities continue.

When violations are detected, few facilities have follow-up enforcement actions or sanctions taken against them (Harrington et al., 2008). The continued widespread variation in the number and type of deficiencies issued by states shows that states are not using the regulatory process consistently and are not following federal guidelines (U.S. GAO, 2011). More importantly, state enforcement problems are related to inadequate federal and state resources for regulatory activities, which have not kept pace with inflation.

One study documented the benefits of strong regulation in those states that more rigorously implemented federal regulations (Mukamel et al., 2012). Regulatory stringency was significantly associated with better quality for four of the seven measures studied and the regulations were found to be cost effective. To ensure the safety of residents, strong enforcement and increased funding for the survey and certification program are needed and poorly performing facilities need to be cut from the Medicare and Medicaid programs.

INADEQUATE NURSING STAFFING LEVELS

Low nurse staffing levels are the single most important contributing factor to poor quality of nursing home care in the United States. Over the past 25 years, numerous research studies have documented the important relationship between nurse staffing levels, in particular registered nurse (RN) staffing, and the outcomes of care (Bostick et al., 2006; Castle, 2008; CMS, 2001; Schnelle et al., 2004; Spilsbury et al., 2011). The benefits of higher staffing levels, especially RN staffing, can include lower mortality rates; improved physical functioning; and reduced antibiotic use,

pressure ulcers, catheterized residents, urinary tract infections, hospitalization rates, physical restraint and side-rail use, weight loss, and dehydration. States that have introduced higher minimum staffing standards for nursing homes have higher nurse staffing levels, lower deficiency citations, and improved quality of outcomes (Harrington, Swan, & Carrillo, 2007; Mukamel et al., 2012; Wagner, McDonald, & Castle, 2013a, 2013b).

In 2016, the average U.S. nursing home provided a total of 4.1 hours per resident day (HPRD) of total RN, licensed vocational nurse or licensed practical nurse (LVN/LPN), and nursing assistant (NA) time (Harrington et al., 2018). Of the total time, most HPRD is provided by NAs, who care for an average of 11 residents and are only required to have 2 weeks of training. RNs provide only 42 minutes (0.7 hour) of time per patient day (Harrington, Carrillo, Dowdell, Tang, & Blank, 2011). Although the average staffing hours have increased over time, there are wide variations, and some facilities have dangerously low staffing.

A Centers for Medicare and Medicaid Services (CMS) (2001) report found that staffing levels for long-stay residents that are below 4.1 HPRD result in harm or jeopardy for residents. (The total should consist of at least 1.3 HPRD for licensed nurses and 2.8 HPRD of NA time.) NA time should range from 2.8 to 3.2 HPRD depending on the care residents need, and this is just to carry out basic care activities (CMS, 2001; Harrington, Schnelle, McGregor, & Simmons, 2016). This amounts to 1 NA per 7 residents on both the day and evening shifts and 1 NA per 12 residents at night. On average, nonprofit and government nursing homes are more likely to meet the recommended standards than for-profit homes (Harrington et al., 2012). Establishing higher staffing levels should have the highest policy priority at both the state and federal levels.

CORPORATE OWNERSHIP

Many studies have shown that for-profit nursing homes operate with lower costs and staffing compared with nonprofit facilities, which provide higher staffing and higher quality of care and have more trustworthy governance (Comondore et al., 2009). Nevertheless, for-profit companies owned 69% of the nation's nursing homes, compared with nonprofit (24%) and government-owned facilities (7%) in 2016 (Harrington et al., 2018). For-profit corporate chains emerged as a dominant organizational form in the nursing home field during the 1990s, and they increased from 39% in the 1990s to 55% of all nursing homes in 2010 (Harrington, Carrillo, Dowdell, Tang, & Blank, 2011). The largest nursing home chains are publicly traded companies with billions of dollars in revenues. Many large nursing home chains own a number of related companies including residential care/assisted living facilities, home health agencies, hospices, pharmacies, therapy organizations, and staffing organizations. These related companies refer patients to each other and use their corporate interrelationships to maximize revenues.

Private equity companies have purchased many of the largest nursing home chains and these companies have few reporting requirements. Many large chains have multiple investors, holding companies, and multiple levels of companies involved such that property companies are separated from the management of facilities largely to avoid litigation (Wells & Harrington, 2013). The lack of transparency in the ownership responsibilities has made regulation and oversight by state survey and certification agencies problematic. To address these issues, the Patient Protection and Affordable Care Act included provisions for reporting corporate ownership information on the Medicare Nursing Home Compare website along with information regarding expenditures on staffing and direct care (Wells & Harrington, 2013). These changes arose from advocacy by consumer organizations and unions.

The 10 largest for-profit chains had residents with the highest acuity and the lowest nurse staffing hours compared with nonprofit and government nursing homes between 2003 and 2008 (Harrington et al., 2012). The study also showed that the 10 largest for-profit chains had the highest numbers of violations of federal quality regulations and the most serious deficiencies that caused harm or jeopardy compared with nonprofit and government nursing homes (Harrington et al., 2012). In addition, the four largest for-profit nursing home chains purchased by private equity companies between 2003 and 2008 had more deficiencies after being acquired.

Regulators need to undertake stronger enforcement actions when chains fail to meet the nursing home staffing requirements and quality regulations. Chains should be targeted for regulatory oversight by state survey agencies rather than the current procedure of focusing on individual facilities. Greater financial accountability for chains and private equity companies would address the quality problems.

FINANCIAL ACCOUNTABILITY

U.S. nursing home expenditures increased from $140.5 billion in 2010 to $162.7 billion in 2016 (CMS, 2017). Medicare covers up to 100 days of nursing home care after a medically necessary hospital stay of at least three days and Medicaid generally pays for those with low incomes who need long-term nursing home care. The estimated median annual cost of nursing home care (semi-private room) is $80,300 nationally, although these costs vary greatly by state (Genworth, 2015).

Nursing home reimbursement methods and per diem reimbursement rates are of great importance because they influence the costs and quality of care. State Medicaid reimbursement policies have primarily focused on cost containment at the expense of quality and have established very low payment rates. Facilities tend to respond by cutting nurse staffing levels and quality of care (Grabowski, Angelelli, & Mor, 2004). Nursing homes also keep wages and benefits low, which results in high employee turnover rates (Castle, Engberg, & Men, 2007; CMS 2001). Nursing home wages and benefits are substantially lower than those of comparable hospital workers and lower than many of those with jobs in the fast food industry and other unskilled jobs and are generally well below the level of a living wage (CMS, 2001).

Congress passed the Prospective Payment System (PPS) for Medicare reimbursement that was implemented in 1998 to control overall payment rates to skilled nursing homes (Medicare Payment Advisory Commission [MedPAC], 2012). Under the PPS, Medicare rates are based in part on the resident case mix (acuity) in each facility to take into account the amount of staffing and therapy services that residents require. Skilled nursing homes however do not need to demonstrate that the actual amount of staff and therapy time provided is related to the payments allocated under the PPS rates. Funds can be shifted from staffing into profits.

Excess profits have grown dramatically over time because Medicare does not limit the profit margins of nursing homes. In 2010, the profit margins on Medicare payments in for-profit nursing homes were 21%, while profit margins in nonprofit nursing homes were 9.5% (MedPAC, 2012). A study of total revenues and expenditures for all payers in California nursing homes found that administrative expenses grew only slightly, although profits grew by 80% of total revenues from 2007 to 2010. It also found that direct care expenditures have been steadily declining, and for-profit nursing homes had substantially higher administrative costs and profit levels three times greater than nonprofit facilities (Harrington et al., 2013).

One policy option is to revise the Medicaid and Medicare payment systems to specify the minimum proportion of the payments that must be used for nurse staffing and therapy services and the maximum payments for profits and administration costs. If the minimum amount of payments were regulated, nursing homes would be prevented from cutting nurse staffing and using the funds for profit making. If profits and administrative costs were capped at 20% for all payers (Medicare, Medicaid, private insurance, and self-pay), there could be a large savings in the United States (Harrington et al., 2013). Thus, quality could be improved and costs reduced by increasing nursing home financial accountability.

OTHER ISSUES

A large and growing percentage of older people are admitted and often readmitted to hospitals and emergency departments (EDs). Estimates suggest nursing home residents have more than 2.2 million ED visits annually, half of which result in a hospital admission (Wang et al., 2011). In addition, studies indicate that 24% to 67% of nursing home resident ED visits and 47% of hospitalizations are potentially preventable, resulting in more than $2.6 billion in unnecessary health care spending (Grabowski, O'Malley, & Barhydt, 2007; Stephens et al., 2012; Walsh, Wiener, Haber, Bragg, Freiman, & Ouslander, 2012). Unfortunately, these potentially preventable ED visits and hospitalizations unnecessarily expose individuals to the risks and complications associated with care transitions, such as higher morbidity and mortality, delirium, and functional decline, among others (Creditor, 1993; Ouslander et al., 2010).

Many of these often burdensome care transitions could be avoided with increased care capacity in the nursing home (Stephens, Hunt, Bui, Halifax, Ritchie, & Lee, 2018; Trahan, Spiers, & Cummings, 2016). For example, many of these transfers are caused by inadequate assistance with activities of daily living and instrumental activities of daily living, deficient monitoring and treatment of chronic conditions, and inadequate responses to acute conditions that could, at least under optimal conditions, be addressed within the facility (Ouslander et al., 2010). Moreover, a recent study found that nearly 70% of residents are eligible for palliative care services and supports, yet none receive it (Stephens et al, 2018). Increasing access to palliative care in the nursing home setting improves care quality and satisfaction, enhances symptom management, and reduces ED visits, particularly when such care is initiated earlier in the disease course (Hall, Kolliakou, Petkova, Froggatt, & Higginson, 2011; Miller, Lima, Intrator, Martin, Bull, & Hanson, 2016). Thus, lack of access to timely and appropriate primary and palliative care, appropriate RN care, and adequately trained staff and clinical resources appear to significantly contribute to inappropriate ED use.

Historically, the structure of Medicare and Medicaid's coverage of acute and long-term care created conflicting incentives regarding dually eligible beneficiaries, leading to increased rates of hospitalizations without accountability for care coordination (Grabowski, 2007). Since 2012, however, the CMS has monitored and imposed financial penalties to hospitals for excessive 30-day readmission rates. As a result of these penalties brought about by the ACA, many hospitals and health systems have developed "preferred" networks of closely aligned and/or higher-quality contract skilled nursing facility (SNF) providers to address the higher risk of patients discharged to the

SNF setting (Lage et al., 2015; Maly et al., 2012). Until recently, however, SNFs themselves have not been directly accountable for this readmission monitoring and financial penalty process.

In 2014, Congress passed the Protecting Access to Medicare Act (PAMA), which includes provisions for hospital readmission penalties for SNFs under the Skilled Nursing Facility Value Based Purchasing Program. As of 2018, facilities are now required to measure their potentially preventable 30-day post-discharge readmissions and will be subject to incentivized payments based on performance beginning in January 2019 (CMS, 2016). Identifying high-performing SNFs with low readmission rates may be a powerful strategy to improve patient outcomes and reduce the likelihood of rehospitalization and Medicare penalties (Rahman, McHugh, Gozalo, Ackerly, & Mor, 2017).

HOME AND COMMUNITY-BASED SERVICES

LTSS services that are needed for more than 90 days are focused on providing assistance with limitations in activities of daily living and supporting those with cognitive limitations and mental illness. About 11 million people living in the community receive assistance with activities of daily living; 92% of those individuals received informal help from family and friends, and only 13% received paid help (Kaye, Harrington, & LaPlante, 2010).

There are increased pressures to expand HCBS, especially in the Medicaid program which pays for most LTSS. The public increasingly reports a preference for LTSS provided at home over services in institutions. The 1990 Americans with Disabilities Act (ADA) and the subsequent legal judgment in the 1999 Olmstead Supreme Court decision require that states must not discriminate against persons with disabilities by refusing to provide community services when these are available and appropriate (Kaye, Harrington, & LaPlante, 2010).

In response to the increased demand, Medicaid HCBS programs grew by 52% (from 2.1 million to 3.2 million) and expenditures increased by 170% (from $19.5 to $52.7 billion) between 2000 and 2010 (Ng, Harrington, & Musumeci, 2013). In spite of the growth in HCBS, there are wide variations in access to services and expenditures across states. Moreover, states do not provide equitable access to groups such as those with developmental disabilities, the aged and disabled, individuals with mental health problems, children, and other groups (Ng, Harrington, & Musumeci, 2013). In 2012, only 32 states had Medicaid personal care attendant programs, and many states have limited services under their HCBS waiver programs. States have begun to shift individuals in HCBS programs to Medicaid managed care programs, even though most managed care programs have little or no experience providing LTSS.

Some states have rapidly expanded their HCBS programs, whereas others still lag behind, relying heavily on institutional services. The percentage of LTSS participants receiving HCBS increased from 56% in 2005 to 65% in 2010, and the percentage of LTSS expenditures for HCBS increased from 30% to 45% in the same period. Although progress has been made, the increased adoption of state cost control policies has led to large increases in persons on waiver wait lists. The waiting lists for Medicaid HCBS have increased from 192,000 reported in 2002 to more than 524,000 in 39 states in 2012, with waiting periods averaging 27 months for services across the country (Ng, Harrington, & Musumeci, 2013). Access could be improved by standardizing and liberalizing state HCBS policies, but state fiscal concerns are barriers to rebalancing between HCBS and institutional services.

The ACA included important new provisions to expand HCBS through a Medicaid state plan rather than a waiver. It also established the Community First Choice Option in Medicaid to provide personal care services to individuals, created the State Balancing Incentive Program to provide enhanced federal matching payments to eligible states, and extended the Medicaid Money Follows the Person Rebalancing Demonstration program. It also continued the Aging and Disability Resource Center initiatives. All these provisions to expand HCBS under Medicaid were advocated by ADAPT (www.adapt.org), an advocacy organization for individuals with disabilities, along with a coalition of consumer advocacy groups. It will be important to determine whether states take advantage of the new options to expand HCBS.

Although the cost of nursing home care is almost six times as much as HCBS (Harrington, Ng, & Kitchener, 2011), the main opposition to expanding Medicaid HCBS has been the potential for increased costs to states if additional Medicaid participants request new LTSS services. However, studies show that states offering extensive HCBS had spending growth comparable to those states with low HCBS spending (Kaye, 2012). States that had well-established HCBS programs had much less overall LTSS spending growth compared with those with low HCBS spending because these states were able to reduce institutional spending.

PUBLIC FINANCING

In the long run, the United States needs a comprehensive mandatory public long-term care insurance system for everyone. Currently, the only segment of the U.S. population whose cost of LTSS is covered is individuals who live below the poverty threshold enrolled in Medicaid. Except for short-term post-acute care, the rest of the U.S. population must either pay for care out-of-pocket or resort to privately purchased long-term care insurance. The financially crippling cost of nursing home care (as much as $90,000 per year) is one of the great fears confronting persons who are otherwise self-supporting. Yet relatively few individuals have either the means or motivation to insure themselves privately. Only about 7 million private long-term care policies were in force covering 3% of the population aged 20 and over in 2005 (Feder, Komisar, & Friedland, 2007). Few older adults can afford to purchase private long-term care insurance, so this does not appear to be a viable financing mechanism for the future (Wiener, 2009).

A mandatory social insurance program for LTSS offers distinct advantages over the current means-tested system. If everyone paid into the system, individuals would have access to coverage when they are chronically ill or disabled without the humiliation of having to become poor to receive services. By expanding the Medicare program to include LTSS, the payment of LTSS contributions early in a worker's life could prefund LTSS services that generally are required late in life, spreading the risk across the entire population. Germany, Japan, and countries in Scandinavia have adopted mandatory public long-term insurance systems that can serve as models for the United States. These countries generally provide protection and coverage for persons who need LTSS (Wiener, 2009). The nation should focus on public financing of LTSS insurance that would ensure that all citizens have access to high-quality LTSS.

CONCLUSION

We need a vision for advocacy in LTSS that is multidimensional and long range. Political efforts are needed at the local, state, and national levels. Community mobilization, public education, legislative reform, and legal actions are all needed to bring about policy changes to ensure access to high-quality LTSS services. Consumer advocates and organizations such as The Consumer Voice, ADAPT, and AARP have taken a lead in reform efforts, but they need help to make progress. Nurses and nursing organizations should form joint alliances with consumer organizations to advocate for needed changes in the long-term care system.

Organized nursing needs to place its considerable political influence into LTSS reform, including improving the quality of nursing home care and expanding HCBS. These efforts could improve the lives of residents in nursing homes as well as those who need HCBS. Nurses should act not only because of a concern for all those individuals who need LTSS, but also to ensure that they, their families, and their friends will have access to high-quality, appropriate LTSS in the future.

DISCUSSION QUESTIONS

1. What are the most important steps needed to improve the poor quality of nursing home care in the United States and the inadequate nurse staffing levels (RNs, LVNs, and NAs)?

2. Because consumers prefer HCBS, what policy changes are needed to ensure an adequate supply of services and a high-quality labor force?

3. What strategies can nurses use to effectively advocate for a higher quality of care, greater access to LTSS services, and adequate public funds to pay for LTSS?

REFERENCES

Bostick, J.E., Rantz, M.J., Flesner, M.K., & Riggs, C.J. (2006). Systematic review of studies of staffing and quality in nursing homes. *Journal of the American Medical Directors Association, 7*(6), 366–376.

Castle, N. (2008). Nursing home care giver staffing levels and quality of care: A literature review. *Journal of Applied Gerontology, 27*(4), 375–405.

Castle, N.G., Engberg, J., & Men, A. (2007). Nursing home staff turnover: Impact on Nursing Home Compare quality measures. *The Gerontologist, 47*(5), 650–661.

Centers for Medicare and Medicaid Services. (2001). Appropriateness of minimum nurse staffing ratios in nursing homes. In *Report to Congress: Phase II final* (vol. I to III). Baltimore: Author.

Centers for Medicare and Medicaid Services, Office of the Actuary, National Health Statistics Group, & U.S. Department of Commerce, Bureau of Economic Analysis, and the U.S. Census Bureau. (2016). *National health expenditures account: Methodology paper, 2016: Definitions, sources, and methods.* Retrieved from www.cms.gov/Research-Statistics-Data-and-Systems/Statistics-Trends-and-Reports/NationalHealthExpendData/Downloads/dsm-16.pdf.

Centers for Medicare and Medicaid Services, & U.S. Department of Health and Human Services. (2016). Medicare program: Prospective payment system and consolidated billing for skilled nursing facilities for FY 2017, SNF value-based purchasing program, SNF quality reporting program, and SNF payment models research: Final rule. *Federal Register, 81*(151), 51969-52053.

Colby, S.L., & Ortman, J.M. (2014). Projections of the size and composition of the U.S. population: 2014 to 2060. *Current Population Reports*, P25-1143. Retrieved from https://census.gov/content/dam/Census/library/publications/2015/demo/p25-1143.pdf.

Comondore, V.R., Devereaux, P.J., Zhou, Q., Stone, S.B., Bussey, J.W., Ravindran, N.C., ... & Guyatt, G.H. (2009). Quality of care in for-profit and not-for-profit nursing homes: Systematic review and meta-analysis. *British Medical Journal, 339,* b2732.

Creditor, M.C. (1993). Hazards of hospitalization of the elderly. *Annals of Internal Medicine, 118*(3), 219–223.

Feder, J., Komisar, H.L., & Friedland, R.B. (2007). *Long-term care financing: Policy options for the future.* Washington, DC: Georgetown University. Retrieved from ltcfinalpaper061107.pdf.

Genworth. (2015). *Genworth 2015 cost of care survey: Home care providers, adult day health care facilities, assisted living facilities and nursing homes.* Retrieved from www.genworth.com/dam/ Americas/US/PDFs/Consumer/corporate/130568_040115_gnw.pdf.

Grabowski, D.C. (2007). Medicare and Medicaid: Conflicting incentives for long term care. *Millbank Quarterly, 85*(4), 579–610.

Grabowski, D.C., Angelelli, J.J., & Mor, V. (2004). Medicaid payment and risk-adjusted nursing home quality measures. *Health Affairs, 23*(5), 243–252.

Grabowski, D.C., O'Malley, A.J., & Barhydt, N.R. (2007). The costs and potential savings associated with nursing home hospitalizations. *Health Affairs, 26*(6), 1753–1761.

Hall, S., Kolliakou, A. Petkova, H., Froggatt, K., & Higginson, I.J. (2011). Interventions for improving palliative care for older people living in nursing care homes. *Cochrane Database of Systematic Reviews, 16*(3), CD007132.

Harrington, C., Carrillo, H., Garfield, R., (2018). *Nursing facilities, staffing, residents and facility deficiencies, 2009 through 2016.* Retrieved from http://files.kff.org/attachment/REPORT-Nursing-Facilities-Staffing-Residents-and-Facility-Deficiencies-2009-2015.

Harrington, C., Carrillo, H., Dowdell, M., Tang, P.P., & Blank, B.W. (2011). *Nursing facilities, staffing, residents and facility deficiencies, 2005 through 2010.* San Francisco, CA: University of California, Department of Social and Behavioral Sciences. Retrieved from ualr.edu/seniorjustice/uploads/2011/11/FACILITY%20DEFICIENCIES.pdf.

Harrington, C., Ng, T., & Kitchener, M. (2011). Do Medicaid home and community based services save money? *Home Health Care Services Quarterly, 30*(4), 198–213.

Harrington, C., Olney, B., Carrillo, H., & Kang, T. (2012). Nurse staffing and deficiencies in the largest for-profit chains and chains owned by private equity companies. *Health Services Research, 47*(1, Pt. I), 106–128.

Harrington, C., Ross, L., Mukamel, D., & Rosenau, P. (2013). *Improving the financial accountability of nursing facilities.* Washington, DC: Kaiser Commission on Medicaid and the Uninsured, June. Retrieved from kaiserfamilyfoundation.files.wordpress.com/2013/06/8455-improving-the-financial-accountability-of-nursing-facilities.pdf.

Harrington, C., Schnelle, J.F., McGregor, M., Simmons, S. (2016) The need for higher minimum staffing standards in U.S. nursing homes. *Health Services Insights;* 9 ,13h Services Insights; J.F., McHarrington, C., Swan, J. H., & Carrillo, H. (2007). Nurse staffing levels and Medicaid reimbursement rates in nursing facilities. *Health Services Research, 42*(3, Pt. I), 1105–1129.

Harrington, C., Tsoukalas, T., Rudder, C., Mollot, R.J., & Carrillo, H. (2008). Study of federal and state civil money penalties and fines. *The Gerontologist, 48*(5), 679–691.

Institute of Medicine, Committee on the Future Health Care Workforce for Older Americans. (2008). *Retooling for an aging America: Building the health care workforce.* Washington, DC: National Academy of Science Press.

Kaye, H.S. (2012). Gradual rebalancing of Medicaid long-term services and supports saves money and serves more people, statistical model shows. *Health Affairs, 31*(6), 1195–1203.

Kaye, H.S., Harrington, C., & LaPlante, M.P. (2010). Long-term care in the United States: Who gets it, who provides it, who pays, and how much does it cost? *Health Affairs, 29*(1, special issue), 11–21.

Keehan, S.P., Cuckler, G.A., Sisko, A.M., Madison, A.J., Smith, S.D., Lizonitz, J.M., ... & Wolfe, C.J. (2015). National health projections: Modest annual growth until coverage expands and economic growth accelerates. *Health Affairs, 34*(8).

Lage, D.E., Rusinak, D., Carr, D., Grabowski, D.C., & Ackerly, D.C. (2015). Creating a network of high-quality skilled nursing facilities: Preliminary data on the postacute care quality improvement experiences of an accountable care organization. *Journal of the American Geriatrics Society, 63*(4), 804–808.

Maly, M.B., Lawrence, S., Jordan, M.K., Davies, W.J., Weiss, M.J., Deitrick, L., & Salas-Lopez, D. (2012). Prioritizing partners across the continuum. *Journal of the American Medical Directors Association, 13*(9), 811–816.

Mather, M., Jacobsen, L.A., & Pollard, K.M. (2015) Aging in the United States, *Population Bulletin, 70,* 2.

Medicare Payment Advisory Commission. (March, 2012). Report to Congress: Medicare payment policy. In *Skilled nursing facility services* (pp. 171–208). Washington, DC: MedPac. Retrieved from www.medpac.gov/documents/Mar12_EntireReport.pdf.

Miller, S.C., Lima, J.C., Intrator, O., Martin, E., Bull, J., & Hanson, L.C. (2016). Palliative care consultations in nursing homes and reductions in acute care use and potentially burdensome end-of-life transitions. *Journal of the American Geriatrics Society, 64*(11), 2280-2287.

Mukamel, D.B., Weimer, D.L., Harrington, C., Spector, W.D., Ladd, H., & Li, Y. (2012). The effect of state regulatory stringency on nursing home quality. *Health Services Research, 47*(5), 1791–1813.

Ng, T., Harrington, C., & Musumeci, M. (2013). *Medicaid home and community based service programs: 2010 data update.* Washington, DC: Kaiser Commission on Medicaid and the Uninsured.

Ortman, J.M., Velkoff, V.A., Hogan, H. (2014). An aging nation: The older population in the United States. Population estimates and projections. *Current Population Reports,* P25-1140. Retrieved from www.census.gov/prod/2014pubs/p25-1140.pdf.

Ouslander, J.G., Lamb, G., Perloe, M., Givens, J.H., Kluge, L., Rutland, T., & Saliba, D. (2010). Potentially avoidable hospitalizations of nursing home residents: Frequency, causes, and costs. *Journal of the American Geriatrics Society, 58*(4), 627–635.

Rahman, M., McHugh, J., Gozalo, P.L., Ackerly, D.C., & Mor, V. (2017). The contribution of skilled nursing facilities to hospitals' readmission rate. *Health Services Research, 52*(2), 656-675.

Schnelle, J.F., Simmons, S.F., Harrington, C., Cadogan, M., Garcia, E., & Bates-Jensen, B. (2004). Relationship of nursing home staffing to quality of care. *Health Services Research, 39*(2), 225–250.

Spilsbury, K., Hewitt, C., Stirk, L., & Bowman, C. (2011). The relationship between nurse staffing and quality of care in nursing homes: A systematic review. *International Journal of Nursing Studies, 48*(6), 732–750.

Stephens, C., Blegen, M., Newcomer, R., Miller, B., & Harrington, C. (2012). Emergency department use by nursing home residents: Effect of severity of cognitive impairment. *The Gerontologist, 52*(3), 383–393.

Stephens, C.E., Hunt, L.J., Bui, N., Halifax, E., Ritchie, C.S., & Lee, S.J. (2017). Palliative care eligibility, symptom burden, and quality of life ratings in nursing home residents. *Journal of the American Medical Association Internal Medicine, 178*(1), 141–142.

Trahan, L.M., Spiers, J.A. & Cummings, G.G. (2016). Decisions to transfer nursing home residents to emergency departments: A scoping review of contributing factors and staff perspectives. *Journal of the American Medical Directors Association, 18*(5), 445.

U.S. Bureau of Labor Statistics. (2018). *Employment projections: Occupations with the most job growth 2016 and projected 2026.* Washington, DC. Retrieved from www.bls.gov/emp/ep_table_104.htm.

U.S. Census Bureau. (December 12, 2012). U.S. Census Bureau projections show a slower growing, older, more diverse nation a half century from now. *News Room.* Washington, DC. Retrieved from www.census.gov/newsroom/releases/archives/population/cb12-243.html.

U.S. General Accounting Office. (1999). *Nursing homes: Additional steps needed to strengthen enforcement of federal quality standards.* Report to the Special Committee on Aging, U.S. Senate. GAO/HEHS-99-46. Washington, DC: Author.

U.S. Government Accountability Office. (April 7, 2011). *More reliable data and consistent guidance would improve CMS oversight of state complaint investigations.* GAO-11-280. Washington, DC: Author.

Wagner, L.M., McDonald, S.M., & Castle, N.G. (2013a). Staffing-related deficiency citations in nursing homes. *Journal of Aging and Social Policy, 25*(1), 83–97.

Wagner, L. M., McDonald, S. M., & Castle, N. G. (2013b). Nursing home deficiency citations for physical restraints and side rails. *Western Journal of Nursing Research, 35*(5), 546–565.

Walsh, E.G., Wiener, J.M., Haber, S., Bragg, A., Freiman, M., & Ouslander, J.G. (2012). Potentially avoidable hospitalizations of dually eligible Medicare and Medicaid beneficiaries from nursing facility and home- and community-based services waiver programs. *Journal of the American Geriatrics Society, 60,* 821-829.

Wang, H.E., Shah, M.N., Allman, R.M., & Kilgore, M. (2011). Emergency department visits by nursing home residents in the United States. *Journal of the American Geriatrics Society,* 59(10), 1864–1872.

Wells, J., & Harrington, C. (2013). *Implementation of Affordable Care Act provisions to improve nursing home transparency, care quality, and abuse prevention.* Washington, DC: Kaiser Commission on Medicaid and the Uninsured. Retrieved from www.kff.org/medicare/upload/8406.pdf.

Wiener, J.M. (2009). *Long-term care: Options in an era of health reform.* Washington, DC: RTI International.

Wiener, J.M., Knowles, M.E., & White, E.E. (2017). *Financing long-term services and supports: Continuity and change.* RTI Press Publication No. OP-0042-1709. Research Triangle Park, NC: RTI Press.

ONLINE RESOURCES

The Henry J. Kaiser Family Foundation
www.kff.org
Medicare Home Health Compare
www.medicare.gov/homehealthcompare/search.html
Medicare Nursing Home Compare
www.medicare.gov/nursinghomecompare/search.html

36

The United States Military and Veterans Administration Health Systems: Contemporary Overview and Policy Challenges

Jennifer Hatzfeld and Sheila Cox Sullivan[a]

"To care for him who shall have borne the battle and for his widow, and his orphan."

Abraham Lincoln

The health systems for military personnel and veterans are among the world's largest. Military health care plays a vital role in the security of the nation, ensuring that military personnel are ready for whatever duty calls and are provided the best of care when in need. Military service is accompanied by unique exposures, whether from the trauma of battle or toxic chemicals from the burning of oil fields in the Middle East. As such, the Veterans Health Administration (VHA) provides expert care to those who suffer the consequences of such exposures and provides routine health care for all veterans who qualify for services.

STRUCTURE OF MILITARY AND VETERANS HEALTH CARE

Military medicine in the United States was established during the Revolutionary War, although most physicians operated independently until 1818, when an Army Medical Department was established (U.S. Army Medical Department, 2018). This began a more coordinated effort to provide medical care to military members (Box 36.1). Toward the end of the Civil War in 1865, President Abraham Lincoln authorized the National Asylum for

---

[a]This chapter updates a previous edition chapter originally developed by John S. Murray, PhD, RN, CPNP-PC, CS, FAAN and draws upon his excellent work.

Disabled Volunteer Soldiers. This facility targeted Civil War veterans and was the first government-sponsored institution worldwide designated to provide health care to military personnel after their service. The Eastern Branch of the National Asylum for Disabled Volunteer Soldiers was built in Augusta, Maine and opened in 1866.

Today, the U.S. Military Health System (MHS) directly supports the operational mission of the Department of Defense (DoD) through "fostering, protecting, sustaining, and restoring health" (DoD, 2017, p. I-1). The MHS consists of an integrated network of military and civilian health care providers and facilities located around the world providing care to military members, military retirees, and family members. Within the MHS, the TRICARE program facilitates connection between the military and civilian parts and provides many of the functions of a medical insurance program. In fiscal year 2017, the 9.42 million eligible beneficiaries received care within the MHS including active duty military members, their families, retirees and their families, as well as other uniformed members, including the U.S. Coast Guard and the U.S. Public Health Service Commissioned Corps (Defense Health Agency [DHA] Decision Support Division, 2018) (Table 36.1).

There are 54 military hospitals and 377 military medical clinics serving MHS beneficiaries around the world, staffed by 147,165 personnel, a majority (57%) of whom are active duty members (DHA Decision Support Division, 2018; MHS, 2018). Historically, these medical facilities and personnel

BOX 36.1 Timeline of Key Events Within the Military and Veterans Health Services

Year	Event
1818	Army Medical Department established
1842	Navy Bureau of Medicine and Surgery established
1865	President Abraham Lincoln authorized the National Asylum for Disabled Volunteer Soldiers
1866	The first veteran health facility, Eastern Branch of the National Asylum for Disabled Volunteer Soldiers, opened in Augusta, Maine
1927	Congress created new benefits for veterans, such as disability compensation and rehabilitation programs
1930	President Hoover created the Veterans Administration (VA) by Executive Order 5398
1942	Department of Defense (DoD) establishes a ban on lesbian, gay, bisexual, and transgender (LGBT) service members
1945	VA established as a major research and education entity, as part of Public Law 293
1949	Air Force Medical Service established
1951	Defense Advisory Committee on Women in the Services (DACOWITS) established as an external advisor to the Secretary of Defense
1970	Senate Committee on Veterans' Affairs established
1988	Secretary of Veterans Affairs established as Cabinet position (previously part of DoD)
1991	Veterans Health Services and Research Administration became the Veterans Health Administration
1995	DoD and VA signed a Memorandum of Understanding making U.S. Military Health System (MHS) health care beneficiaries eligible to receive care at VA facilities
2011	DoD repealed ban on LGBT service members
2014	Defense Health Agency (DHA) established
2016	All career fields in the military opened to women
2017	Public Law 114-328, Section 702, introduced a new requirement that DHA, not the individual branch of the military, will be responsible for the administration of each military medical treatment facility

TABLE 36.1 Health System Overview

	Military Health System[a]	Department of Veterans Affairs
Enrolled Patient Population	9.42 Million	9.7 Million
Active Duty/Guard/Reserve	5.42 Million	
Active Duty/Guard/Reserve Family Members	2.46 Million	
Retired and Family Members	1.54 Million	
Hospitals (Inpatient Facilities)	54 (41 in U.S.)	171 in U.S., Puerto Rico, the Philippines, and Guam
Clinics (Outpatient Facilities)	377 (312 in U.S.)	1062
Personnel	147,165 (Military: 84,167; civilian: 62,998)	25,884 physicians 98,000+ nurses

[a]DHA Decision Support Division, 2018.

have been overseen separately by individual branches of the military (Army, Navy, and Air Force) with further oversight and management from the DHA (Fig. 36.1) (Smith, Bono, & Slinger, 2017).

The U.S. Department of Veterans Affairs is currently made up of three major departments (Fig. 36.2). The Veterans Benefits Administration (VBA) oversees approval and distribution of benefits such as health care, education, and housing. The Veterans Cemetery Association manages the 136 national cemeteries where veterans are interred. The VHA has 172 medical centers, over 1000 outpatient clinics, and nearly 140 long-term care facilities to provide care to the 9.7 million veterans of the U.S. Armed

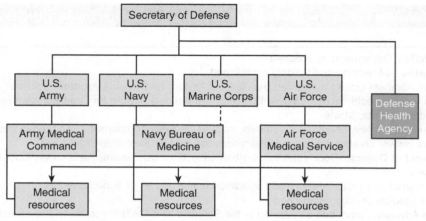

Fig. 36.1 Department of Defense oversight of medical resources. (Source: Smith, D.J., Bono, R.C., & Slinger, B.J. [2017]. Transforming the military health system. *JAMA, 318*[24], 2427–2428.)

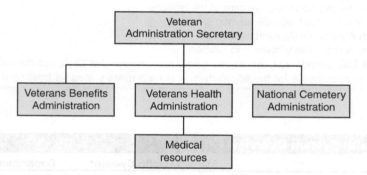

Fig. 36.2 Veteran Administration oversight of medical resources.

Forces. It is the largest health care system in the United States, employing nearly 100,000 nurses. Despite the three major administrations making up the larger Department of Veterans Affairs, most Americans still refer to the Department and its components as "the VA."

Because both the MHS and VHA are funded through the federal budgeting process, Congress can establish specific requirements as a condition of funding (Saturno, Heniff, Lynch, & Tollestrup, 2012). Additionally, specific laws can be created that direct the care provided through the MHS or VHA, but require an "act of congress," as a subsequent law must be passed to change these requirements. Congress can request or conduct inquiry into the management of these organizations, such as a Congressional Budget Office (CBO)

report, evaluating options to save MHS funds (CBO, 2017), or through inquiries raised by individuals receiving care within the system. Although this oversight can be burdensome, this process allows the government to ensure federal funds support the health of our nation's military and veterans. Congress maintains oversight of the MHS through separate "Committees on Armed Services" in the U.S. House of Representatives and Senate; oversight of the VHA occurs through separate "Committees on Veterans' Affairs."

Organization of Care

A key mission of the MHS is to maintain optimum health of military members so they are ready to deploy (DoD, 2017). As such, primary care and preventive services are a critical element of the MHS, and rely on a patient-centered medical home (PCMH) model for primary care. Military primary care facilities rely on a single, civilian organization to certify all MHS PCMH locations, using the same standard (DHA, 2017). The MHS has a maximum number of patients assigned to primary care managers, applied equally across physicians, nurse practitioners, and physician assistants. Inpatient care is provided primarily through one of the 54 military hospitals located within the United States, and in countries with permanently assigned military members. These hospitals are categorized into one of three types of facilities: small bedded, residency program, or a medical center. For any medical care that cannot be provided within a military facility, each military facility has a designated Referral Management Office that assists individuals to find appropriate specialty care (DHA, 2018).

During 2018, the VA modernized its structure. The VHA identified specific health care services (primary care, urgent care, mental health, geriatric and extended care, post-deployment health, war-related injury and illness study centers, and pain management/opioid safety) deemed to be those most attributable to military service, and areas for which the VHA seeks to excel. This care will be available at all VHA medical centers. For patients requiring other services, recent legislation known as the MISSION Act provides for these services to be covered at non-VA medical centers (U.S. Department of Veterans Affairs, 2018b).

MHS support of military operations during combat, deployments, or disasters is governed by Joint Publication 4-02 that outlines a formal process to combine resources and personnel from the individual armed services that provide medical services (only the Army, Navy, and Air Force) to meet a defined mission or requirement (DoD, 2017). In general, when medical support is needed for an operational mission, a "Joint Force Surgeon" or Task Force, is designated for the mission with four primary lines of effort: Plans and Operations, Medical Logistics, Force Health Protection, and Liaison Officers. Military members assigned as the Joint Force Surgeon or to any of the other lines of effort may be physicians, nurses, or another medical profession, depending on the nature of the mission. The intent is that the basic "Joint Force Surgeon" organizational structure remains consistent and can expand to meet the unique requirements for each mission (DoD, 2017).

UNIQUE CARE TOPICS ACROSS THE CONTINUUM

Traumatic Brain Injury

Military service is associated with unique exposures that can create health problems seldom seen in the private sector. Traumatic brain injury (TBI) has been identified as a "signature injury" of the conflicts in Iraq and Afghanistan. These combat operations have resulted in over 350,000 TBI diagnoses among military members between 2000 and 2016, or approximately 20% of those deployed to Iraq or Afghanistan during that time (Swanson et al., 2017). Since 2009, all military members suspected of a TBI follow a standardized assessment and treatment guideline (Management of Concussion/mTBI Working Group, 2016), one that helped standardize the initial evaluation and treatment. Since objective measures to validate mild TBI do not currently exist (it relies on self-reported symptoms), the lack of diagnostic tools has led to concerns of over-reporting, and a perception of secondary gain from the diagnosis (Soble, Cooper, Lu, Eapen, & Kennedy, 2018).

Since monitoring began in 2000, nearly 400,000 veterans have been diagnosed with TBI (Defense and Veterans Brain Injury Center, 2018). Mild TBI is often concurrent with post-traumatic stress disorder (PTSD) (88%), major depressive disorder (44%), and alcohol (43%) and substance (22%) abuse (Wojtowicz et al., 2017). These increases in comorbid diagnoses for patients with TBI have enhanced the synergetic provision of the medical and mental health management of patients. For those with more serious TBI, VHA developed a poly-trauma system for treatment of concurrent injuries and TBI at several VA medical centers nationwide. The VA is also working with the families of veterans with TBI to improve their ability to manage the needs of the injured veteran. One innovative strategy is multi-family group support (Straits-Troster et al., 2013). By allowing multiple families with a common, isolating condition to engage in a shared medical appointment, families were able to acknowledge their challenges while finding new ways to cope, and develop a support system.

Musculoskeletal Injuries

Compared with previous conflicts, musculoskeletal injuries were a significant proportion of combat-related injury in Iraq and Afghanistan (Belmont, Owens, & Schoenfeld, 2016). This has been attributed to the widespread use of body armor protecting the head and vital organs and the use of unconventional weapons such as improvised explosive devices. Extremity injuries, including soft-tissue injuries, fractures, and amputations, were found to require a higher proportion of MHS resources and were the most common reason for medical discharge compared with other combat injuries (Masini et al., 2009). Non-battle injuries are also a significant cause of orthopedic injuries, requiring continued treatment and management (Le et al., 2018). Chronic pain affected 80% of Iraq or Afghanistan veterans and was associated with psychological, functional, and family issues (Lew et al., 2009). Given these lessons learned and the likelihood that future conflicts will see similar injury patterns, the MHS must ensure that appropriate care and resources are available to stabilize and treat orthopedic injuries.

Amputation is the most challenging orthopedic issue. The VA Amputation System of Care manages care for the veteran from the time of amputation throughout their life. There are seven Regional Amputation Centers (Level 1) and 18 Polytrauma/Amputation Network Sites (Level 2) nationwide to assist with prosthetic fitting, veteran adaptation, and rehabilitation. A VA Peer Visitation Program was identified by participants as a key component of their successful recovery (U.S. Department of Veterans Affairs, 2015).

Mental/Behavioral Health

Compared with civilian populations, military members experience relatively high rates of mental and behavioral disorders, including PTSD, depression, and panic or anxiety disorders, with the highest incidence of PTSD and panic/anxiety disorders among combat deployers (Crum-Cianflone, Powell, LeardMann, Russell, & Boyko, 2016; Millennium Cohort Study, n.d.). Although there is no evidence that deployment increases the risk, suicides are almost twice as high since the start of conflict in Iraq and Afghanistan (Reger, 2015). A comprehensive review of the care provided by the MHS for PTSD and depression found they were successfully screening patients for suicide and substance use but needed to improve follow-up and evidence-based psychotherapy once patients were diagnosed (Hepner et al., 2018). Program reviews such as these identify the complexity of tracking these important mental health needs within a large and mobile population and highlight the need to strengthen the quality of mental health care provided within the MHS.

Psychological resilience has been found to be higher among military veterans compared to the general population (Isaacs et al., 2017), and suicide ideation rates for younger veterans (under the age of 35) are comparable to civilians (Logan, Bohnert, Spies, & Jannausch, 2016). However, data estimated 20 veterans a day completed suicide, making suicide prevention a top priority for the VA (VA Suicide Prevention Program, 2016). In response, the VA has developed an integrated care strategy where mental health services are available at the same location as primary care services, and worked to improve access to mental health services, including hiring additional mental health providers (Knopf, 2017). The Veterans Crisis Line (1-800-273-8255) provides 24/7 access to mental health counseling assistance. The VA has expanded mental health care to all service veterans, added telephone applications for management of PTSD, sleep disorders, depression, and learning mindfulness, and provided support groups for veterans and their family members (VA Suicide Prevention Program, 2016).

Military-Related Sexual Trauma

Military-related sexual trauma (MST) is a high-priority issue. In an effort to eliminate sexual assault within the military, the number of sexual assaults from every branch of the military has been reported annually to Congress since 2011 (DoD, 2018). There were 6769 reported sexual assaults in 2017, up nearly 10% compared to 2016, which the reports suggest could be due to an increased willingness to report (DoD, 2018). While the rates of sexual crimes against women by military members is similar to civilian rates, the rates of all other crimes are significantly lower than their civilian counterparts (Wood & Toppelberg, 2017). The reasons for the higher rate of sexual crimes against women is complex, but theorized to reflect a culture of hyper-masculinity and clear, hierarchical (rank) structures (Wood & Toppelberg, 2017), as well as the value of performance, frequent moves to new assignments, team allegiance, and an emphasis on problem resolution at the lowest level (Castro, Kintzel, Schuyler, Lucas, & Warner, 2015). The military has established several new policies and campaigns to address this issue, through prevention training programs and outreach to leadership (DoD, 2018b).

MST continues to haunt military service members long after discharge. One study of over 6 million veterans found that 1.1% of men and over 20% of women reported MST during their period of service. The study further noted that the hazard ratio of suicide among those reporting MST was 1.69 (95% confidence interval [CI] 1.45, 1.97) among men, but 2.27 (95% CI 1.70, 2.24) for women (Kimerling, Makin-Byrd, Louzin, Ignacio, & McCarthy, 2016). Primary care providers in the VHA receive clinical reminders in the electronic health record (EHR) to screen for MST in order to intervene once the service member is ready to report an incident.

POLICY CHALLENGES

U.S. Military Health System Policies

LGBTQ Service Members. In 2011, the military repealed the ban of lesbian, gay, bisexual, transgender, and queer (LGBTQ) service members, which had been in place since 1942 (Golbach & Castro, 2016). Since the end of the second World War, homosexual military members were prohibited due to the belief that homosexuality would negatively impact national security (Sinclair, 2009). The 1993 "Don't Ask, Don't Tell" policy was a compromise that left the ban in place, but allowed homosexual members to serve honorably in the military unless their status was revealed. It was because of this potential for exposure that many medical personnel did not routinely assess health risk factors for the LGBTQ population (particularly for men who have sex with men) nor was open dialogue about sexual orientation encouraged within the medical community (Campbell, Jahan, Bavaro, & Carpenter, 2017). More recently, the uncertainty about the status of transgender military members has become a similar topic that is difficult for patients to navigate within the context of medical care (Goldbach & Castro, 2016). Because of this history of secrecy and uncertainty, there remain continued policy challenges to ensure the LGBTQ population does not continue to experience disparities in access to appropriate health services (Campbell, Jahan, Bavaro, & Carpenter, 2017).

Women in Combat Roles. In January 2016, all military career fields were opened to women, including combat-specific roles that had been limited to men. This policy change required training, staffing models, promotion rates, and other factors be addressed to ensure women were seamlessly integrated into the combat training environments, particularly with physical standards and living arrangements (Committee on Armed Services, 2016). Established in 1951 as an external advisor to the Secretary of Defense, the Defense Advisory Committee on Women in the Services (DACOWITS, 2017) has carefully tracked the progress and challenges encountered during gender integration in the military. Their 2017 report recommended further strategic communication about the status of incorporating women into combat positions, sharing "lessons learned" among the different branches of the military. A key recommendation was to ensure that physical training methods for advanced combat training incorporate evidence-based, physiologic differences for women when compared with men. While there is evidence to guide policy decisions, the differences of physiologic response to traumatic injuries and impact of more frequent combat deployments for women is not yet well known (Rank & Heroux, 2018).

Health Care Management Consolidation. The 2017 National Defense Authorization Act (Public Law 114-328) introduced a new requirement: the DHA, and not the individual branch of the military, would be responsible for the management and administration of military medical treatment facilities (U.S. Congress, 2016). This consolidation is challenging as each facility located on military bases has traditionally "belonged" to an individual branch of service. While this may represent the largest consolidation of a health care organization, lessons learned from private sector mergers and acquisitions may provide a roadmap for the services (Robbins, 2018). While the review and integration of the cultural differences between different branches of service are currently not part of the implementation plan, identifying and integrating shared assumptions, beliefs, and values is particularly important within a health care team to ensure positive patient outcomes, staff retention, and overall satisfaction of care.

Veteran Health System Policies

Contrary to popular belief, not all veterans qualify for completely free health care. For example, members of the military reserves or National Guard who served as active duty personnel only when training do not meet basic eligibility requirements. Although the VA determines who qualifies for care based in part on how their health care issues are related to their service, the process to determine eligibility is sometimes challenging.

Currently the VA provides 4.9 million veterans with $76.52 billion in compensation, inclusive of death and service-connected disabilities (U.S. Department of Veterans Affairs, 2018c). Although the VA goal for processing claims is 120 days, there is substantial evidence that these goals are unmet, with claims processing often taking over a year (Nuss, n.d.). The VA has opened a variety of enrollment options for new claims including by phone, completing online applications, or applying in person and the newer process promises a decision within 30 days. Despite improvements, there are still significant process delays. President Donald Trump signed the Veterans Appeals Improvement and Modernization Act in August of 2017 to (1) decrease time to decision, (2) improve notification of VA decisions, and (3) provide earlier claim resolution and enhance timeliness of an effective date (U.S. Department of Veterans Affairs, 2018d). Outcomes of these changes are not currently available at the time of this writing.

In 2014, wait times at various VA medical centers nationwide commanded the nation's attention. Although to date no government investigation has supported the claim of harm or death related to delays, these allegations were sufficiently disturbing to cause congressional and public concern. To increase access to VHA services in a timely fashion, the VA Office of Nursing Services proposed the exertion of Federal Supremacy to allow advanced practice registered nurses (APRNs) full practice authority at VHA facilities. This clause of the U.S. Constitution (Article VI, Clause 2, establishing precedence of federal law over state or local laws) allows the VHA to establish full scope of practice for APRNs working for the VA that may exceed the authority provided by state law, including those states where APRN practice is limited. The intended outcome was to increase access to primary and specialty care services in all clinics. In December of 2016, the acting VA Secretary implemented the change, but limited the policy change to nurse practitioners, clinical nurse specialists, and nurse midwives (excluding certified registered nurse anesthetists) and determined the transition would be implemented at individual medical centers rather than as a national mandate (U.S. Department of Veterans Affairs, 2016). The VHA Office of Nursing Services was responsible for the implementation of this directive and, as of this writing, about

50% of 172 individual medical centers have implemented APRN full practice authority. A rigorous evaluation process will provide outcomes from this effort.

In addition, there have been efforts to privatize more of veterans care through the VA Choice Program developed in 2014 to allow veterans to get care in the private sector if they are long distances from a VA health center or face excessive wait times. The VA then pays for that private care. Initially lauded as a way to expedite access to care for veterans, a June 2018 report by the U.S. Government Accountability Office found that many veterans still faced months of delays in getting appointments for care; and a December 2018 report by ProPublica confirmed that wait times were excessive, some appointments were inappropriate (an appointment with a neurologist instead of a urologist), and excessive amounts of overhead being paid to the two private companies hired to manage the program (Arnsdorf & Greenberg, 2018). The privatization of veterans' health care is likely to be a contentious issue for years to come.

Intersection of Military and Veteran Health System Policies

Service-Related Injuries. As mentioned previously, the primary reason for VHA eligibility is based on a disability as a result of a service-related event. Therefore, military health policies that address prevention activities, initial medical response, and availability of early rehabilitation resources have a direct impact on the long-term health needs of the veteran following discharge or retirement from military service. While this continuum is well documented and accepted for physical injuries, mental health is less clear for individual patients and the health systems. In some cases, mental health injuries may not be evident or well-measured prior to leaving the military. Navigating the review and approval process can be difficult for the individual, especially those with mental health challenges already. Assisting these patients through the process requires careful documentation and active support from both the military and veteran health systems. Providing evidence-based guidance to prevent injuries can inform the appropriate treatment and ensure optimal physical and mental health outcomes.

To address suicide prevention, the VA has deployed a strategic plan to help veterans transition from military to veteran care. This plan supports return to non-military, private sector employment; improves contact with recently discharged veterans; creates collaborations in the community; and provides education to raise awareness about the storage of weapons, medications, and sharp objects in veteran households (U.S. Department of Veterans Administration, 2018a).

Electronic Health Record. A medical history determines service-related disability and eligibility for VHA benefits. Even though military beneficiaries are now able to be seen at VHA facilities, the MHS and VHA each have distinctly different EHRs, data and information cannot be shared between them, and providing care requires a significant amount of coordination. This lack of EHR access is often identified as a primary source of delays in transitioning patients from the MHS to VHA. To improve communication, a new, commercial EHR system was approved in 2015 and, as of this writing, is undergoing transition.

Health Care for Women and LGBTQ Service Members. The acceptance of LGBTQ service members and the expansion of combat roles for women in the military is anticipated to impact the future health needs of veterans receiving care within the VHA. Historically, a VHA has focused on the health needs of young and older male patients. With an increasing number of women service members, additional services have been added and tailored for women. Both military and veteran health systems will also need to ensure culturally appropriate care for LGBTQ service members, retirees, veterans, and their family members. The VHA may need to take a leading role to determine how best to tailor health care practices for LGBTQ veterans throughout the lifespan.

CONCLUSION

The mission and scope of the MHS and VHA health care surrounds the entire globe and together provides care for over 19 million Americans. It is precisely because of the broad scope and size of the health system that there are numerous policy challenges for both organizations. Despite the difficulties of coordinating care for patients with complex injuries and unique health requirements and the many bureaucratic challenges of such a large organization, the passion to care for military members and veterans remains an important element of the ethos of the MHS and VHA.

DISCUSSION QUESTIONS

1. What is the mission of the Military Health System and the Veteran Health Systems?
2. Who provides oversight of military and veteran health systems and has the ultimate authority for policy changes?
3. What is the impact of changing military policies on the military and veteran health systems, particularly the eligibility of LGBTQ service members and expanding combat roles for women?

REFERENCES

Arnsdorf, I., & Greenberg, J. (2018). The VA private care program gave companies billions and vets longer waits. *ProPublica*. Retrieved from www.propublica.org/article/va-private-care-program-gave-companies-billions-and-vets-longer-waits.

Belmont, P.J., Owens, B.D., & Schoenfeld, A.J. (2016). Musculoskeletal injuries in Iraq and Afghanistan: Epidemiology and outcomes following a decade of war. *JAAOS: Journal of the American Academy of Orthopaedic Surgeons, 24*(6), 341-348.

Campbell, W.R., Jahan, M., Bavaro, M.F., & Carpenter, R.J. (2017). Primary care of men who have sex with men in the U.S. military in the post–Don't Ask, Don't Tell era: A review of recent progress, health needs, and challenges. *Military Medicine, 182*(3-4), e1603-e1611.

Castro, C.A., Kintzle, S., Schuyler, A.C., Lucas, C.L., & Warner, C.H. (2015). Sexual assault in the military. *Current Psychiatry Reports, 17*(7), 54.

Committee on Armed Services. (2016). *The implementation of the decision to open all ground combat units to women.* (S. HRG 114-590). Washington, DC: U.S. Government Publishing Office.

Congressional Budget Office. (2017). *Approaches to changing military health care* (Publication #53137). Washington DC: Congressional Budget Office.

Crum-Cianflone, N.F., Powell, T.M., LeardMann, C.A., Russell, D.W., & Boyko, E.J. (2016). Mental health and comorbidities in U.S. military members. *Military Medicine, 181*(6), 537-545.

Defense Advisory Committee on Women in the Services. (2017). *Defense Advisory Committee on Women in the Services 2017 annual report.* Alexandria, VA: DACOWITS

Defense Health Agency. (2017a). *Accounting for Defense Health Program (DHP) primary care managers (PCMs).* (DHA-IPM 17-003). Falls Church, VA: Defense Health Agency.

Defense Health Agency. (2017b). *Sexual assault medical management with consideration of male service members of the armed forces.* (DHA-IPM 16-004). Falls Church, VA: Defense Health Agency.

Defense Health Agency. (2018). *Standard appointing processes, procedures, hours of operations, productivity, performance measures and appointment types in primary, specialty, and behavioral health care in medical treatment facilities* (DHA-IPM 18-001). Falls Church, VA: Defense Health Agency.

Defense Health Agency Decision Support Division (2018). *Evaluation of the TRICARE program: Fiscal year 2018 report to Congress.* Washington, DC: Office of the Assistant Secretary of Defense. Retrieved from www.health.mil/Reference-Center/Reports/2018/05/09/Evaluation-of-the-TRICARE-Program-Fiscal-Year-2018-Report-to-Congress.

Defense and Veterans Brain Injury Center. (2018). *DOD worldwide number for TBI.* Retrieved from http://dvbic.dcoe.mil/dod-worldwide-numbers-tbi.

Department of Defense. (2017). *Joint health services, joint publication 4-02.* Washington, DC: Joint Chiefs of Staff.

Department of Defense. (2018a). *Construct for implementation of section 702.* Washington, DC: Under Secretary of Defense for Personnel and Readiness

Department of Defense. (2018b). *Department of Defense annual report on sexual assault in the military, fiscal year 2017.* Washington, DC: Under Secretary of Defense.

Department of Defense. (2018c). *DoD healthcare management system modernization MHS GENESIS.* Arlington, VA: DoD Healthcare Management System Modernization (DHMSM®) Program Management Office. Retrieved from www.health.mil/Military-Health-Topics/Technology/Military-Electronic-Health-Record/EHR-Modernization-Interoperability.

Goldbach, J.T., & Castro, C.A. (2016). Lesbian, gay, bisexual, and transgender (LGBT) service members: Life after Don't Ask, Don't Tell. *Current Psychiatry Reports, 18*(6), 56.

Hepner, K.A., Roght, C.P., Sloss, E.M., Paddock, S.M., Iyiewuare, P.O., Timmer, M.J. & Pincus, H.A. (2018). Quality of care for PTSD and depression in the military health system: Final report. *Rand Health Quarterly, 7*(3). Retrieved from www.rand.org/pubs/research_reports/RR1542.html.

House Committee on Veterans' Affairs. (n.d.) *History and jurisdiction.* Retrieved from https://archives-veterans.house.gov/about/history-and-jurisdiction.

Institute of Medicine. (2011). *The future of nursing: Leading change, advancing health.* Washington, DC: National Academies Press.

Isaacs, K., Mota, N.P., Tsai, J., Harpaz-Rotem, I., Cook, J.M., Kirwin, P.D., ... & Pietrzak, R. H. (2017). Psychological resilience in US military veterans: A 2-year, nationally representative prospective cohort study. *Journal of Psychiatric Research, 84*, 301-309.

Kimerling, R., Makin-Byrd, K., Louzon, S., Ignacio, R.V., & McCarthy, J.F. (2016). Military sexual trauma and suicide mortality. *American Journal of Preventive Medicine, 50*(6), 684-691.

Knopf, T. (2017). VA wants to reduce high US veteran suicide rate. *North Carolina Health News.* Retrieved from www.northcarolinahealthnews.org/2017/11/08/va-wants-to-reduce-high-u-s-veteran-suicide-rate/.

Le, T.D., Gurney, J.M., Nnamani, N.S., Gross, K.R., Chung, K.K., Stockinger, Z.T., ... & Akers, K.S. (2018). A 12-year analysis of nonbattle injury among U.S. service members deployed to Iraq and Afghanistan. *JAMA Surgery, 153*(9), 800-807.

Lew H.L., Otis J.D., Tun C., Kerns R.D., Clark M.E., & Cifu D.X. (2009). Prevalence of chronic pain, posttraumatic stress disorder, and persistent post-concussive symptoms in OIF/OEF veterans: Polytrauma clinical triad. *Journal of Rehabilitation Research & Development, 46*(6), 697-702.

Logan, J., Bohnert, A., Spies, E., & Jannausch, M. (2016). Suicidal ideation among young Afghanistan/Iraq war veterans and civilians: Individual, social, and environmental risk factors and perception of unmet mental healthcare needs, United States, 2013. *Psychiatry Research, 245*, 398-405.

Management of Concussion-mTBI Working Group. (2016). *VA/DoD clinical practice guideline for management of concussion/*

mild traumatic brain injury. Retrieved from www.healthquality.va.gov/guidelines/Rehab/mtbi/mTBICPGFullCPG50821816.pdf.

Masini, B.D., Waterman, S.M., Wenke, J.C., Owens, B.D., Hsu, J.R., & Ficke, J.R. (2009). Resource utilization and disability outcome assessment of combat casualties from Operation Iraqi Freedom and Operation Enduring Freedom. *Journal of Orthopaedic Trauma, 23*(4), 261-266.

Military Health System. (2018). *MHS facilities.* Retrieved from www.health.mil/I-Am-A/Media/Media-Center/MHS-Health-Facilities.

Millennium Cohort Study. (n.d.) *About the study.* Retrieved from www.millenniumcohort.org/about.

Nuss, L. (n.d.). Waiting for veterans disability benefits: How long does it take? *Disability Advisor.* Retrieved from www.disabilityadvisor.com/veteran-disability-benefits/.

Rank, M.G., & Heroux, E.F.J. (2018). Military women and veterans. *Military Behavioral Health, 6*(1), 1-2.

Reger, M.A., Smolenski, D.J., Skopp, N.A., Metzger-Abamukang, M.J., Kang, H.K., Bullman, T.A., … & Gahm, G.A. (2015). Risk of suicide among US military service members following Operation Enduring Freedom or Operation Iraqi Freedom deployment and separation from the U.S. military. *JAMA Psychiatry, 72*(6), 561-569.

Robbins, T.L. (2018). What the military health system can learn from private sector mergers and acquisitions. *Military Medicine, 183*(7-8), 146-150.

Saturno, J.V., Heniff, B., Lynch, M.S., & Tollestrup, J. (2012). *Introduction to the federal budget process (Publication 98-721).* Washington, DC: Congressional Research Service.

Sinclair, G. (2009). Homosexuality and the military: A review of the literature. *Journal of Homosexuality, 56*(6), 701-718.

Smith, D.J., Bono, R.C., & Slinger, B.J., (2017) Transforming the military health system. *JAMA, 318*(24), 2427-2428.

Soble, J.R., Cooper, D.B., Lu, L.H., Eapen, B.C., & Kennedy, J.E. (2018). Symptom reporting and management of chronic post-concussive symptoms in military service members and veterans. *Current Physical Medicine and Rehabilitation Reports, 6*(1), 62-73.

Straits-Troster, K. Gierisch, J.M., Strauss, J.L., Duck, D.G., Dixon, L.B., Norell, D., & Perlick, D.A. (2013). Multifamily group treatment for veterans with traumatic brain injury: What is the value to participants? *Psychiatric Services, 64*(6), 541-6.

U.S. Army Medical Department. (2018). *History of the Office of Medical History.* Retrieved from http://history.amedd.army.mil/history.html.

U.S. Congress. (2016). *National Defense Authorization Act for fiscal year 2017, Pub L 114-328, Title VII.* Retrieved from www.congress.gov/114/plaws/publ328/PLAW-114publ328.pdf.

U.S. Department of Veterans Affairs. (2015) *Rehabilitation and prosthetic services, amputation system of care, ASoC special programs: Rehabilitation and prosthetic services.* Retrieved from www.prosthetics.va.gov/asoc/ASoC_Special_Programs.asp.

U.S. Department of Veterans Affairs. (2016). *VA proposes to grant full practice authority to advanced practice registered nurses.* VA Office of Public and Intergovernmental Affairs. Retrieved from www.va.gov/opa/pressrel/pressrelease.cfm?id=2793.

U.S. Department of Veterans Affairs. (2018a). *MIRECC/CoE: Lethal means safety and suicide prevention.* Retrieved from www.mirecc.va.gov/lethalmeanssafety/.

U.S. Department of Veterans Affairs. (2018b). *The VA Mission Act of 2018.* Retrieved from www.va.gov/oei/docs/MISSION_Act_2018_FAQs.pdf.

U.S. Department of Veterans Affairs. (2018c). *Veterans annual benefits report, fiscal year 2017.* www.benefits.va.gov/REPORTS/abr/.

U.S. Department of Veterans Affairs. (2018d). *Veterans Benefits Administration, appeals modernization: Veterans Appeals Improvement and Modernization Act of 2017.* Retrieved from www.benefits.va.gov/benefits/appeals.asp.

U.S. Government Accountability Office. (2018). *Veterans Choice Program: Improvements needed to address access-related challenges as VA plans consolidation of its community care programs.* Retrieved from www.gao.gov/assets/700/692271.pdf.

VA Suicide Prevention Program. (2016). *Facts about veteran suicide.* Retrieved from www.va.gov/opa/publications/factsheets/Suicide_Prevention_FactSheet_New_VA_Stats_070616_1400.pdf.

Wojtowicz, M., Silverberg, N.D., Bui, E. Zafonte, R., Simon, N., & Iverson, G.L. (2017). Psychiatric comorbidity and psychosocial problems among treatment-seeking veterans with a history of mild traumatic brain injury. *Focus, 15*(4), 384-389.

Wood, E.J., & Toppelberg, N. (2017). The persistence of sexual assault within the U.S. military. *Journal of Peace Research, 54*(5), 620-633.

ONLINE RESOURCES

Military Health System
www.health.mil
National Center for PTSD
www.ptsd.va.gov/about
Veterans Health Administration
www.va.gov/health

37

Contemporary Issues in Government

Grant R. Martsolf

> *"Our keen sense of our own unease does not mean that we are stuck. It means that we are already moving. But where, and how?"*
>
> **Yuval Levin**

As we enter the third decade of the 21st century, we face a time of great turmoil and uncertainty. Our country has never seemed more sociologically and politically divided. Policymakers face enormous challenges related to immigration, the economy, education, and, not least, health care. Six issues that will or should be central priorities for health care policymakers at all levels of government across the United States are opioids, the primary care crisis, health insurance coverage, health care expenditures, health care as a job creator, and social determinants of health. But there are significant political and sociological barriers that make addressing these issues especially difficult, including political polarization, inequality, and loneliness and loss of meaning—all of which reflect America's weakening social fabric.

SIX KEY HEALTH ISSUES CHALLENGING POLICYMAKERS

Opioids

Opioids are a class of drugs that include prescription pain relievers such as morphine, fentanyl, codeine, oxycodone, and hydrocodone as well as the illegal drug heroin. The increasing use and abuse of opioids in recent decades is leading to significant morbidity and mortality across the United States. One cannot watch the evening news or cruise social media for long without being confronted with new and depressing information about the *opioid epidemic*. In 2015, approximately 2 million Americans were addicted to prescription painkillers and 591,000 were addicted to heroin (Center for Behavioral Health, 2016). That year, there were 20,101 overdose deaths related to prescription opioid pain relievers and 12,990 overdose deaths involving heroin (American Society of Addiction Medicine, 2016). Overdose deaths increased 200% between 2000 and 2016 (Rudd et al., 2016). Although all of society is feeling the effects of the epidemic, the demographic hit the hardest has been middle-aged Whites without higher education living in predominantly rural areas (Henry J. Kaiser Family Foundation [KFF], n.d.-b).

Although there are many theories about what is "causing" the opioid crisis, it is important to understand the social history of pain medication prescribing in the United States. In the early 1990s, evidence that physicians were underprescribing and nurses were underadministering pain medication led to a significant push among health care providers to focus on identifying and treating pain in patients. Pain became the "fifth vital sign" and was assessed along with blood pressure, pulse, temperature, and respirations (Morone & Weiner, 2013).

At the same time, pharmaceutical companies were heavily marketing opioid pain relievers to health care providers. The amount of opioids prescribed quadrupled between 1999 and 2010. Since 2010, it has decreased, though the rate in 2015 was still three times as high as in 1999 (Guy et al., 2017). Opioid pain relievers became widely overused before it became evident to the public and health care providers that they were, in fact, highly addictive (Zee, 2009). As addiction to opioid painkillers increased, states began developing policies to make it more difficult for individuals to acquire the painkillers (Markus & Thomas, 2016–2017). So, many of those addicted to painkillers turned to heroin, which was often cheaper and more readily available (The Economist, 2017).

It is also important to recognize that the opioid crisis is deeply connected to other troubling trends across the United States. Economists and demographers are identifying dramatic increases in what is often referred to as the *deaths of despair*—deaths due to suicide, drugs, and alcohol. Researchers have noted a marked increase in the rate of suicide that largely parallels the opioid death rate. Although of lower magnitude compared to opioid death rates, suicide rates grew by an estimated 25% from 1999 to 2014 (Curtin, Warner, & Hedegaard, 2016). These deaths of despair tend to hit middle-aged, working class Whites the hardest. In fact, deaths of despair have led to an unprecedented decrease in life expectancy among middle-aged non-Hispanic Whites in the last few decades (Stein et al., 2017).

Primary Care Crisis

Primary care providers are often the first point of contact for patients. Ideally, they provide care that is comprehensive, focus on the entirety of the patient, and manage the patient across the continuum of care (Starfield, 1998). Primary care is the backbone of a well-functioning health care system. Those systems that are oriented toward primary care and the delivery of a specific set of primary care functions as a source of usual care often enjoy favorable levels of quality, outcomes, and costs (Friedberg, Hussey, & Schneider, 2010).

The current primary care system in the United States faces significant challenges. First, estimates suggest that there will be a deficit of up to 23,640 primary care physicians by 2025 (IHS Markit, 2018), with the greatest shortage in rural communities (U.S. Department of Health and Human Services, 2016). This largely can be attributed to an aging workforce (Cherry et al., 2010) and fewer physicians choosing primary care over specialty areas of practice (Schwartz et al., 2011).

Second, chronic conditions account for seven of the top 10 leading causes of death in the United States and the rates of chronic conditions are growing (Anderson, 2010). Primary care is the predominant setting for management of chronic conditions. The current health care system,

designed for acute conditions that require short but intensive periods of care, is built on face-to-face diagnostic encounters with a physician. Treatment of chronic conditions, however, requires frequent, low-intensity consultations and care management that often occurs outside of face-to-face clinical consultations and can be delivered using alternative forms of consultation via telephone or email, and other providers, including registered nurses, social workers, community health workers, nurse practitioners (NPs), and physician assistants (Martsolf, Kandrack, Gabbay, & Friedberg, 2016; Martsolf, Kandrack, Schneider, & Friedberg, 2015).

Challenges affecting the primary care system have myriad causes but much of the problem can be traced to the approach that the United States has taken to reimburse primary care providers. Currently, primary care providers are paid by a fee-for-service system with the rates based on relative-value units. This system primarily rewards providers for supplying high volumes of procedural services that are delivered face-to-face in an office. This payment system has a number of important implications (Berenson & Rich, 2010). First, relative to specialty physicians, primary care providers receive lower payment rates, which compels an increasing number of physicians and NPs to choose specialty practice. Second, because the reimbursement system pays primarily for care that is delivered face-to-face within the office, providers are not paid for the care that may be most effective for improving care for patients with chronic conditions such as care coordination and management (Bujold, 2017). There have been new payment models that have recently emerged that are attempting to pay for these non–face-to-face services. For example, the Medicare program issues new codes that could be used to reimburse practices for delivering chronic care management (Centers for Medicare and Medicaid Services [CMS], 2016). Furthermore, the Medicare Comprehensive Primary Care+ demonstration program is experimenting with alternative payment methods that provide practices with fixed monthly care management fees intended to help practices pay for providing care management services (CMS, 2016). (For more on primary care, see Chapter 31.)

Health Insurance Coverage

The United States has one of the highest percentages of uninsured citizens among comparable high-income countries. Currently, approximately 10% of the entire population of those who are not older adults is uninsured, and this rate has been as high as 18% within the last 10 years (KFF, n.d.-a).

Many policymakers and advocates have proposed a major overhaul of the U.S. health insurance system that relies heavily on private, employer-based insurance, and instead implement a single-payer, publicly-funded health insurance option modeled after countries like France, England, and Canada (Friedman, 2013). This approach, however, underestimates the unique history of private health insurance in the United States, which has fundamentally shaped the current system (see Chapter 17). As such, efforts to expand insurance coverage in the United States have had to include some combination of private and public health insurance. In 2010, Congress passed the Patient Protection and Affordable Care Act (ACA), which attempted to increase coverage through a combination of an expansion of the public Medicaid program and private insurance subsidies coupled with a requirement to purchase health insurance through state-sponsored exchanges. The states began expanding Medicaid and the exchanges opened in January of 2014. Uninsurance rates fell rapidly after the passage of the ACA, from 44 million citizens in 2013 to less than 28 million by the end of 2016 (KFF, n.d.-a).

Although it has undoubtedly contributed to a reduction in uninsurance rates, the ACA has faced a number of challenges to achieving full insurance. First, extending coverage relied on states to expand their own Medicaid program to include all of the working poor who are not generally offered health insurance. To entice states to expand, the federal government attempted to withhold all Medicaid funding from states that refused to expand the program. This move was declared unconstitutional, and states were allowed to decide on their own, without compulsion. However, the federal government did offer to cover nearly all of the costs of the expansion. Still, only 33 states including the District of Columbia have expanded their Medicaid program (KFF, n.d.-c). This has been a major blow to the goal of full coverage.

A second challenge was that success in expanding private health insurance coverage rested on requiring every individual in the United States to certify that they had purchased health insurance. Those that chose not to purchase insurance were required to pay a penalty. This provision was known as the *individual mandate* and ensured that healthy people would enter the market, offsetting the costs of the sicker patients. Unfortunately, the penalty for not buying insurance was set extremely low, nearly seven times less than the price of an average plan. Therefore, many younger and healthier patients chose not to participate. This and various other factors have contributed to a drastic increase in insurance premiums between 2017 and 2018, leading to significant decreases in insurance coverage during that same period as many are choosing to forego health insurance altogether and instead simply pay the penalty (Collins et al., 2018).

Republican lawmakers have been lobbying for the repeal of the individual mandate, citing that it is a violation of individual liberty to compel individuals to purchase health insurance and that the penalty is an unfair tax on the working class. On December 22, 2017, President Donald Trump signed the Tax Cuts and Jobs Act of 2017, which repealed the individual mandate. As he saw it, the penalty was "an especially cruel tax that fell mostly on Americans making less than $50,000 a year" (Chia, 2018). As a result, the future of health insurance coverage is still uncertain.

Health Care Expenditures

The United States spends more on health care than any country in the world. At $9403 per capita, U.S. expenditures are nearly double the mean spending per capita of economically similar countries ($5419) (Papanicolas et al., 2018). In 2016, the United States spent 17.8% of its gross domestic product (GDP) on health care, whereas similar high-income countries spent an average of 9.6% to 12.4%. Since the 1980s, the difference in health spending as a percentage of the economy between the United States and economically similar countries has widened dramatically (Sawyer & Cox, 2018).

Such significant health care spending has a number of important implications. First, high health care spending can have a significant effect on U.S. commercial interests. Approximately 50% of the population is covered by employer-sponsored health insurance, and the average employer contributions for health insurance premiums has tripled from 1999 to 2015 (KFF, 2015). These significant expenditures for employers are not paralleled in other similar countries, which inevitably affects the international prices for American products, threatening American competitiveness in the global economy. Second, such spending is likely crowding out other important public spending. Public spending for health care as a percentage of the GDP has increased approximately 5% from 2010 to 2016, whereas public spending on education has decreased by 11%, housing by 48%, and social protection by 13% (Organization for Economic Cooperation and Development, 2018).

Many theories exist about which factors drive high U.S. health care expenditures, including lower investment in social services, the fee-for-service system, the weakened primary care system, defensive medicine, and higher input costs. Research has found that higher service prices and increased administrative costs seem to be the most important drivers of cost differences between the United States and comparable countries (Anderson et al., 2003; Dieleman et al., 2017). These differences are likely to be accounted for primarily by higher provider salaries and higher technology and administrative costs (Papanicolas et al., 2018). Specifically, physicians and other health care professionals in the United States receive significantly higher salaries than their counterparts in other similar countries (Baker, 2017). Furthermore, the United States appears to pay more per service despite similar levels of utilization for various services, including testing and pharmaceuticals (Anderson et al., 2003).

Health Care as a Job Creator

In 2018, health care overtook retail as the largest job sector in the United States, having long passed manufacturing (Thompson, 2018). Health care is projected to continue to grow, accounting for an ever-greater percentage of all U.S. jobs from 10.2% in 2006 to 13.8% in 2026 (Bureau of Labor Statistics, 2017). An added advantage is that health care jobs appear to be recession-proof; health care was one of the few industries that added jobs (428,000) during the 2008 recession, while the national economy lost 7.5 million jobs (Wood, 2011).

Best estimates suggest that the future growth in health care will be largely due to various entry-level jobs that do not require much advanced education, many requiring no more than a high school diploma or a general educational development (GED) certificate. As noted by Frogner, Spetz, Parente, and Oberlin (2015), the "future health care workforce will be increasingly female, young, racially/ethnically diverse, not U.S.-born, at or below the poverty level, and at a low level of educational attainment."

In many ways, this is a promising prospect, as new jobs will increasingly be open to lower-skilled workers. However, the health care industry is not suitably structured to help low-skilled workers advance to better, higher-paying jobs, compared to other industries such as manufacturing. Historically, someone with a high school education could get an entry-level manufacturing job and then advance to a higher-paying position, acquiring any necessary skills on the job. This allowed low-skilled workers to eventually achieve solidly middle-class careers. Health care jobs, on the other hand, often only allow for limited advancement. Some employers do offer on-the-job training, internships, or further education through the workplace, but advancement often requires returning to school and taking on debt (Frogner, 2017). Therefore, many are excluded from the higher paying jobs in the industry, and there is little potential for advancement. It is also difficult to transition between positions within health care. Most positions require specialization, and there is no clear pathway to transfer from one specialty to another. Many entry-level workers leave health care entirely because they are unable to advance (Frogner, 2017; Snyder et al., 2018).

Addressing the Social Determinants of Health

Despite the trillions of dollars spent each year on health care in the United States, health care services contribute only 10% to 20% of the variance in health outcomes. Seventy percent of the variation can be explained by the patients' social conditions, including housing, physical environment, social circumstances, education level, and economic stability (Health Affairs, 2014).

Many prominent policymakers and researchers are exploring ways in which health care professionals might intervene to address various social and cultural factors that affect health, rather than simply treating their results. The Robert Wood Johnson Foundation (RWJF) has made a significant financial and institutional commitment to advancing a national *culture of health* (Plough, 2015). The RWJF's drive to address social and cultural issues related to health is applied in emerging innovative approaches to health care finance. Championed and expanded by major payers such as Medicare, global payment models pay health care organizations to become accountable for the access to, quality, and costs of care for a designated group of patients (Muhlestein et al., 2017). These accountable care models shift away from traditional fee-for-service models (that incentivize service delivery) in favor of payment models that incentivize population health management, explicitly and implicitly prompting health care professionals to intervene on social determinants of health such as housing and food availability as well as addressing patients' health care needs.

Despite the increasing focus on addressing the social determinants of health, there is still relatively little information available regarding specific interventions that would improve these social determinants on a meaningful scale. Furthermore, it is difficult to determine the relative role of public policy in addressing the social determinants of health or how health care professionals, community organizations, and businesses might interact to make the desired progress.

POLITICAL AND SOCIOLOGICAL BARRIERS TO ADDRESSING KEY ISSUES

The issues outlined above are extremely complicated and will require significant public action to address. At the same time, policymakers must be keenly aware of a number of important political and or sociological barriers that will make addressing these issues especially difficult.

Public Policy and Civic Governance

Public policy plays a key role within the broader context of civic governance and the social fabric of society. For the purposes of this analysis, *public policy* is defined as the "authoritative decisions made in the legislative, executive, or judicial branches of government that are intended to direct or influence the actions, behaviors, or decisions of

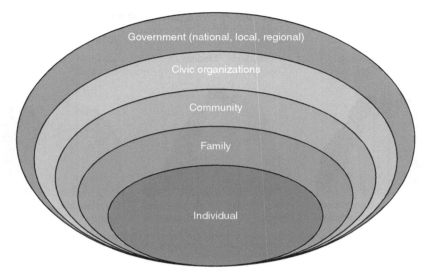

Fig. 37.1 Layers of social fabric.

others" (Longest, 2006, p. 7). Although public policy is a key influencer of the actions, behaviors, and decisions of individuals within a state, it is only a part of a broader system of civic governance. The governance of a society is executed through a complex network of individuals and institutions that exert influence over the actions, behaviors, or decisions of others, forming a sort of social fabric (Levin, 2016).

This social fabric can be thought of as concentric layers of governance, starting with the individual and moving out through the family, community, civic organizations, local and regional government, and finally, national government (Fig. 37.1). The layers that exist between the individual and government have been referred to as the *middle layers* or the *intermediate institutions* (Joint Economic Committee [JEC], Vice Chairman's Staff, 2017; Levin, 2016). The family, community, and civic organizations (e.g., voluntary service organizations, religious organizations, or clubs) that make up these layers are considered to be America's associational life or how we live together.

These middle layers provide governance in a number of ways. The manner in which individuals interact with these layers forms the conventions, habits, virtues, and affections that build the foundation for how they make decisions and regulate their actions. Furthermore, these organizations can be an important source of material assistance to individuals through community services such as job training, food and housing assistance, and pregnancy support. Through interactions with these middle layers, individuals build what Robert Putnam (2000) refers to in his landmark

book, *Bowling Alone*, as *social capital*, defined as the "connections among individuals—social networks and norms of reciprocity and trustworthiness that arise from them" (p. 19). Such social capital has been linked to a number of positive outcomes in areas ranging from health and child welfare to economic prosperity (Frazen, 2006; Putnam, 2000).

The late modern age has been marked by a significant weakening of the middle layers of society. Over the last 50 years, the United States has experienced a notable reduction in family size, marriage rates, connections between extended families, altered patterns of workforce participation, and reduced participation in religious and voluntary civic organizations (JEC, 2017)—paradoxical and simultaneous forces that make us more dispersed yet more consolidated, with the result being autonomous, liberated individuals co-operating with a strong centralized bureaucratic government (Deneen, 2018; Levin, 2016). This has led to a remarkably diffuse society of unconnected individuals whose actions are regulated by a remote and strong central government. The weakening of these middle layers of society has important implications for the stability and prosperity of the United States.

Political Polarization

Over the past several decades, the United States has experienced an incredible polarization in political opinion and commitments (Fig. 37.2; Political polarization, 2014). The mediating institutions must be considered an important contributor. Mediating institutions are often broad, and

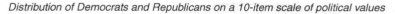

Distribution of Democrats and Republicans on a 10-item scale of political values

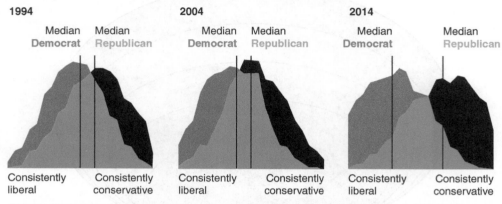

Ideological consistency based on a scale of 10 political values questions. The gray area in this chart represents the ideological distribution of Democrats; the black area of Republicans. The overlap of these two distributions is shaded green. Republicans include Republican-leaning independents; Democrats include Democratic-leaning independents.

Fig. 37.2 Democrats and Republicans more ideologically divided than in the past. (Reprinted from Pew Research Center. [June 12, 2014]. *Political polarization in the American public.* Washington, DC: Author. Retrieved from www.people-press.org/2014/06/12/political-polarization-in-the-american-public.)

include individuals of different political and philosophical commitments. They create a context in which citizens are able to socialize and interact with those who hold opinions different from their own. For example, although a majority of Roman Catholics have historically identified as Democrats, there has always been strong Republican representation within the community. It would not be unusual for a Republican and a Democrat to share a table at the annual church bazaar. The weakening of these mediating institutions makes this sort of interaction far more difficult and unlikely.

While drifting increasingly apart socially, individuals are not eschewing all social interactions. Many are replacing these interactions within formal institutions such as family and churches with smaller networks of affinity. As Francis Fukuyama notes in *The Great Disruption*, "As people [are] liberated from their traditional ties to spouses, families, neighborhoods, workplaces, or churches, they [think] they [can] have social connectedness at the same time, this time the connections being those they [choose] for themselves" (Fukuyama, 2000, p. 15). These new social networks tend to be voluntary, small, temporary, and easily discarded. As people are able to choose new social networks, they tend to form more homogenous groups with people who share similar political, recreational, and philosophical commitments. This phenomenon is often referred to as the *big sort* (Bishop & Cushing, 2008), which has been

escalated in the age of the Internet. In fact, many would argue that the purpose of Facebook and other social media platforms is just this—to sort people into small units of consumptive affinity.

This sort of political and ideological sorting has not been confined to the public, but extends to policymakers who are becoming increasingly partisan. Current party polarization among federal legislators is the worst in history (figure_threeLevin, 2016). The bipartisan committee process that in the 1960s allowed the passage of the Civil Rights Act and the implementation of Medicare and Medicaid no longer works. Major legislation in the last 10 years has been passed primarily along partisan lines, and continued partisan polarization will make it increasingly difficult to pass meaningful and lasting health policy legislation.

Inequality

In addition, over the last 30 years, income inequality has grown substantially in the United States (Fig. 37.3). The overall level of inequality in 2018 is approaching levels seen during the Great Depression and has a number of roots. Globalization has contributed to the elimination of many low-skilled jobs in the United States. Furthermore, many of the income gains attributed to the rapid rise of technological innovation in the 21st century have been accrued within a small group of economic elites. Income for college

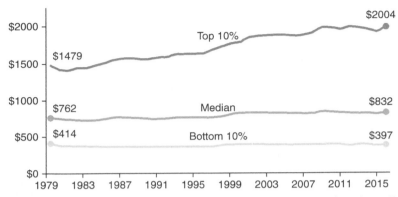

U.S. Real Weekly Wages, 1979–2016

Fig. 37.3 U.S. real weekly wages. (From Bureau of Labor Statistics. Retrieved from https://inequality.org/facts/income-inequality/.)

graduates is the only group for which real income has increased since 1979 (Donovan & Bradley, 2018).

All of these changes are occurring in conjunction with the weakening of the middle layers of society. Mediating institutions provide opportunities for networking with potential employers or learning important "soft" skills such as interpersonal interactions and social norms. They also serve as a system of support and encouragement, helping to bolster individuals' participation in work, education, politics, and civic and religious organizations (Levin, 2016). However, the weakening of the middle layers is not evenly distributed across society. For example, it is widely recognized that the rates of marriage and out-of-wedlock births are divergent between those with and without college degrees (Wilcox & Wang, 2017). Furthermore, it is plausible that the poor and the lower skilled are more vulnerable to the loss of mediating institutions than those with higher incomes who can use financial capital to replace lost social capital.

These trends should be especially concerning for the health care industry, as many of the newest jobs within the industry are entry-level and require no college education. In addition, the highest paying jobs in the industry often exclude those without advanced degrees. Society is further reinforcing the inequality that has been exacerbated in this globalized, diffused, and technological society. At the same time, any approach to address the social determinants of health must recognize that many of the most intractable social determinants are deeply affected by fraying social fabric.

Loneliness and Loss of Meaning

Epidemic levels of loneliness are coinciding with rapid increases in depression, anxiety, and suicide (Klinenberg, 2018; Routledge, 2018). Nearly half (46%) of Americans report sometimes or always feeling alone or left out (Cigna & Ipsos, 2018). It has become such a significant public health priority in the West that the United Kingdom appointed a Minister of Loneliness in 2018 to address this crisis (Yeginsu, 2018).

There is no definitive link between loneliness, depression, anxiety, suicide, and the weakening of mediating institutions, but many commentators have made the implicit connection (Levin, 2016). Studies repeatedly find that communal interaction, family structure, and social relationships benefit physical, emotional, and mental health (Brody, 2017; Umberson & Montez, 2010). Mediating institutions and this middle layer are also an important source of companionship and meaning. Work, family, and religious observance have historically been institutions that have provided structure to people's lives and have given them a means to contribute to the lives of others. In his book *The Quest for Community*, Nisbet (2010) speaks eloquently to this point:

> The quest for community will not be denied, for it springs from some of the powerful needs of human nature—needs for a clear sense of cultural purpose, membership, status, and continuity. Without these, no amount of material welfare will serve to arrest the developing sense of alienation in our society, and the mounting preoccupation with the imperatives of community. (p. 64)

This sense of loneliness and meaninglessness must have some effect on health and challenges our efforts to improve population health outcomes. For example, in the case of opioid abuse, although the causes and solutions are multifactorial, it is difficult to deny the effect increased loneliness and meaninglessness has played in the epidemic. The metaphysical root of our opioid epidemic cannot be denied and likely is not a condition that can be changed by centralized governments, despite the UK's best efforts to do so.

CONCLUSION

The challenges presented in this chapter are significant and will require significant intervention at all levels of civic governance. They will test our nation's ability to identify important issues, determine policy solutions, and implement them. They are not easily overcome, as they are closely tied to deep philosophical, political, and sociological reflexes within the United States and the broader West. Addressing these challenges will require strong public policy to be sure, but may also require the re-enlivening and engagement of the middle layers of civic governance.

DISCUSSION QUESTIONS

1. What important challenges facing policymakers did the author exclude from his list? Why would you include these challenges?
2. How does the weakening social fabric impede policymakers' efforts to address the key challenges facing the United States?

REFERENCES

American Society of Addiction Medicine. (2016). *Opioid addiction 2016 facts & figures.* Retrieved from www.asam.org/docs/default-source/advocacy/opioid-addiction-disease-facts-figures.pdf.

Anderson, G. (2010). *Chronic care.* Robert Wood Johnson Foundation. Retrieved from www.rwjf.org/en/library/research/2010/01/chronic-care.html.

Anderson, G.F., Reinhardt, U.E., Hussey, P.S., & Petrosyan, V. (2003). It's the prices, stupid: Why the United States is so different from other countries. *Health Affairs, 22*(3). Retrieved from www.healthaffairs.org/doi/full/10.1377/hlthaff.22.3.89?url_ver=Z39.88-2003&rfr_id=ori%3Arid%3Acrossref.org&rfr_dat=cr_pub%3Dpubmed.

Baker, D. (2017). The problem of doctors' salaries. *Politico.* Retrieved from www.politico.com/agenda/story/2017/10/25/doctors-salaries-pay-disparities-000557.

Berenson, R.A., & Rich, E.C. (2010). U.S. approaches to physician payment: The deconstruction of primary care. *Journal of General Internal Medicine, 25*(6), 613-618.

Bishop, B., & Cushing, R.G. (2008). *The big sort: Why the clustering of like-minded America is tearing us apart.* Boston, MA: Houghton Mifflin.

Brody, J. E. (2017). Social interaction is critical for mental and physical health. *The New York Times.* Retrieved from www.nytimes.com/2017/06/12/well/live/having-friends-is-good-for-you.html.

Bujold, E. (2017). The impending death of the patient-centered medical home. *JAMA, Internal Medicine, 177*(11), 1559-1560.

Bureau of Labor Statistics. (2017). *Employment by major industry sector.* U.S. Department of Labor. Retrieved from www.bls.gov/emp/tables/employment-by-major-industry-sector.htm.

Center for Behavioral Health Statistics and Quality. (2016). *Key substance use and mental health indicators in the United States: Results from the 2015 national survey on drug use and health.* Substance Abuse and Mental Health Services Administration. Retrieved from www.samhsa.gov/data/report/key-substance-use-and-mental-health-indicators-united-states-results-2015-national-survey-0.

Centers for Medicare and Medicaid Services. (2016). *Chronic care management services.* Retrieved from www.cms.gov/Outreach-and-Education/Medicare-Learning-Network-MLN/MLNProducts/Downloads/ChronicCareManagement.pdf.

Cherry, D., Lucas, C., & Decker, S.L. (2010). *Population aging and the use of office-based physician services.* National Center for Health Statistics, Data Brief No. 41. Retrieved from www.cdc.gov/nchs/products/databriefs/db41.htm.

Chia, J. (2018). Trump heralds the end of "disastrous" Obamacare mandate in State of the Union address. *NY Daily News.* Retrieved from www.nydailynews.com/news/politics/trump-heralds-disastrous-individual-mandate-article-1.3789350.

Cigna, & Ipsos. (2018). *Cigna U.S. loneliness index.* Retrieved from www.multivu.com/players/English/8294451-cigna-us-loneliness-survey/docs/IndexReport_1524069371598-173525450.pdf.

Collins, S.R., Gunja, M.Z., Doty, M.M., & Bhupal, H.K. (2018). *First look at health insurance coverage in 2018 finds ACA gains beginning to reverse.* The Commonwealth Fund. Retrieved from www.commonwealthfund.org/blog/2018/first-look-health-insurance-coverage-2018-finds-aca-gains-beginning-reverse.

Curtin, S.C., Warner, M., & Hedegaard, H. (2016). *Increase in suicide in the United States, 1999-2014.* National Center for Health Statistics Data Brief No. 241. Retrieved from www.cdc.gov/nchs/data/databriefs/db241.pdf.

Deneen, P.J. (2018). *Why liberalism failed.* New Haven, CT: Yale University Press.

Dieleman, J.L., Squires, E., Bui, A.L., Campbell, M., Chapin, A., Hamavid, H., ... & Murray, C.J.L. (2017). Factors associated with increases in U.S. health care spending, 1996-2013. *JAMA, 318*(17), 1668-1678.

Donovon, S.A., & Bradley, D. (2018). Real wage trends, 1979 to 2017. *Congressional Research Service.* Retrieved from https://fas.org/sgp/crs/misc/R45090.pdf.

The Economist. (2017). A selective scourge: Inside the opioid epidemic. *The Economist.* Retrieved from www.economist.com/united-states/2017/05/11/inside-the-opioid-epidemic.

Frazen, A. (2006). Social networks and labour market outcomes: The non-monetary benefits of social capital. *European Sociological Review, 22*(4), 353-368.

Friedberg, M.W., Hussey, P.S., & Schneider, E.C. (2010). Primary care: A critical review of the evidence on quality and costs of healthcare. *Health Affairs 29*(5), 766-772.

Friedman, G. (July 31, 2013). *Funding HR 676: The expanded and improved Medicare for All Act: How we can afford a national single-payer health plan.* Department of Economics, University of Massachusetts at Amherst. Retrieved from www.pnhp.org/sites/default/files/Funding%20HR%20676_Friedman_7.31.13_proofed.pdf

Frogner, B. (2017). The health care job engine: Where do they come from and what do they say about our future? *Medical Care Research and Review, 75*(2), 219-231.

Frogner B., Spetz J., Parente S., & Oberlin S. (2015). The demand for health care workers post-ACA. *International Journal of Health Economics and Management, 15*(1), 139-151.

Fukuyama, F. (2000). *The great disruption: human nature and the reconstitution of social order.* New York: Free Press.

Guy, G.P., Zhang, K., Bohm, M.K., Losby, J., Lewis, B. Young, R., … & Dowell, D. (2017). Vital signs: Changes in opioid prescribing in the United States, 2006-2015. *Center for Disease Control and Prevention Morbidity and Mortality Weekly Report, 66*(26), 697-704.

Health Affairs. (2014). The relative contribution of multiple determinants to health. *Health Affairs Health Policy Brief.* Retrieved from www.healthaffairs.org/do/10.1377/hpb20140821.404487/full/.

Henry J. Kaiser Family Foundation. (2015). *2015 Employer health benefits survey.* Retrieved from www.kff.org/report-section/ehbs-2015-section-six-worker-and-employer-contributions-for-premiums/.

Henry J. Kaiser Family Foundation. (n.d.-a). *Health insurance coverage of the total population.* Retrieved from www.kff.org/other/state-indicator/total-population/?currentTimeframe=0&sortModel=%7B%22colId%22:%22Location%22,%22sort%22:%22asc%22%7D.

Henry J. Kaiser Family Foundation. (n.d.-b). *State health facts: Opioid overdose deaths.* Retrieved from www.kff.org/state-category/health-status/opioids/.

Henry J. Kaiser Family Foundation. (n.d.-c). *Status of state action on Medicaid expansion decision.* Retrieved from www.kff.org/health-reform/state-indicator/state-activity-around-expanding-medicaid-under-the-affordable-care-act/?currentTimeframe=0&sortModel=%7B%22colId%22:%22Location%22,%22sort%22:%22asc%22%7D.

IHS Markit. (2018). *The complexities of physician supply and demand: Projections from 2016-2030.* Association of American Medical Colleges. Retrieved from https://aamc-black.global.ssl.fastly.net/production/media/filer_public/85/d7/85d7b689-f417-4ef0-97fb-ecc129836829/aamc_2018_workforce_projections_update_april_11_2018.pdf.

Joint Economic Committee, Vice Chairman's Staff. (2017). *What we do together: The state of associational life in America.* Retrieved from www.lee.senate.gov/public/index.cfm/socialcapitalproject?ID=1F27B7E7-6538-4A2D-8A77-538A47558C87.

Klinenberg, E. (2018). Is loneliness a health epidemic? *The New York Times.* Retrieved from www.nytimes.com/2018/02/09/opinion/sunday/loneliness-health.html.

Levin, Y. (2016). *The fractured republic: Renewing America's social contract in the age of individualism.* New York: Basic Books.

Longest, B.B. (2006). *Health policymaking in the United States* (4th ed.). Chicago, IL: Health Administration Press.

Markus, P.A., & Thomas, A.L. (2016-2017). Prudent prescribing: An overview of recent federal and state guidelines for opioid prescriptions. *American Bar Association Health eSource, Opioid Epidemic Special Edition.* Retrieved from www.americanbar.org/publications/aba_health_esource/2016-2017/opioids/prescriptions.html.

Martsolf, G.R., Kandrack, R. Gabbay, R.A., & Friedberg, M.W. (2016). Cost of transformation among primary care practices participating in a medical home pilot. *Journal of General Internal Medicine, 31*(7), 723-731.

Martsolf, G.R., Kandrack, R., Schneider, E.C., & Friedberg, M.W. (2015). Categories of practice transformation in a statewide medical home pilot and their association with medical home recognition. *Journal of General Internal Medicine, 30*(6), 817-823.

Morone, N.E., & Weiner, D.K. (2013). Pain as the 5th vital sign: Exposing the vital need for pain education. *Clinical Therapeutics, 35*(11), 1728-1732.

Muhlestein, D., Saunders, R., & McClellan, M. (2017). Growth of ACOs and alternative payment models in 2017. *Health Affairs Blog.* Retrieved from www.healthaffairs.org/do/10.1377/hblog20170628.060719/full.

Nisbet, R. (2010). *The quest for community: A study in the ethics of order and freedom.* Wilmington, DE: ISI Books.

Organization for Economic Cooperation and Development. (2018). *General government spending (indicator).* Retrieved from https://data.oecd.org/gga/central-government-spending.htm.

Papanicolas, I., Woskie, L.R., & Jha, A.K. (2018). Healthcare spending in the United States and other high-income countries. *The Journal of the American Medical Association, 319*(10), 1024-1039.

Plough, A.L. (2015). Building a culture of health: A critical role for public health services and systems research. *American Journal of Public Health, 105*(Suppl 2), S150-S152.

Putnam, R.D. (2000). *Bowling alone: The collapse and revival of American community.* New York, NY: Simon & Schuster.

Routledge, C. (2018). Suicides have increased. Is this an existential crisis? *The New York Times.* Retrieved from www.nytimes.com/2018/06/23/opinion/sunday/suicide-rate-existential-crisis.html.

Rudd, R.A., Aleshire, N., Zibbell, J.E., & Gladden, R.M. (2016). Increases in drug and opioid overdose deaths—United States, 2000-2014. *Center for Disease Control and Prevention Morbidity and Mortality Weekly Report, 64*(50), 1378-1382.

Sawyer, B., & Cox, C. (2018). *How does health spending in the U.S. compare to other countries?* Peterson-Kaiser Health System Tracker. Retrieved from www.healthsystemtracker.org/chart-collection/health-spending-u-s-compare-countries/#item-start.

Schwartz, M.D., Durning, S., Linzer, M., & Hauer, K.E. (2011). Changes in medical students' views of internal medicine careers from 1990 to 2007. *Archives of Internal Medicine, 171*(8), 744-749.

Snyder, C.R., Dahal, A., & Frogner, B.K. (2018). Occupational mobility among individuals in entry-level healthcare jobs in the USA. *Journal of Advanced Nursing, 74*(7), 1628-1638.

Starfield, B. (1998). *Primary care: Balancing health needs, services, and technology.* New York: Oxford University Press.

Stein, E.M., Gennuso, K.P., Ugboaja, D.C., & Remington, P.L. (2017). The epidemic of despair among White Americans: Trends in the leading causes of premature death, 1999-2015. *American Journal of Public Health, 107*(10), 1541-1547.

Stevens, R.A. (2008). History and health policy in the United States: The making of a health care industry, 1948-2008. *Social History of Medicine, 21*(3), 461-483.

Thompson, D. (2018). Health care just became the U.S.'s largest employer: In the American labor market, services are the new steel. *The Atlantic.* Retrieved from www.theatlantic.com/business/archive/2018/01/health-care-america-jobs/550079/.

Umberson, D., & Montez, J.K. (2010). Social relationships and health: A flashpoint for health policy. *Journal of Health and Social Behavior, 51*(Suppl), S54-S66.

U.S. Department of Health and Human Services, Health Resources and Services Administration, National Center for Health Workforce Analysis. (2016). *State-level projections of supply and demand for primary care practitioners: 2013-2025.* Rockville, MD. Retrieved from https://bhw.hrsa.gov/sites/default/files/bhw/health-workforce-analysis/research/projections/primary-care-state-projections2013-2025.pdf.

Wilcox, W.B., & Wang, W. (2017). *The marriage divide: How and why working-class families are more fragile today.* American Enterprise Institute. Retrieved from www.aei.org/publication/the-marriage-divide-how-and-why-working-class-families-are-more-fragile-today/.

Wood, C.A. (2011). Employment in health care: A crutch for the ailing economy during the 2007-2009 recession. *Monthly Labor Review.* United States Department of Labor. Retrieved from www.bls.gov/opub/mlr/2011/04/art2full.pdf.

Yeginsu, C. (2018). U.K. appoints a minister for loneliness. *The New York Times.* Retrieved from www.nytimes.com/2018/01/17/world/europe/uk-britain-loneliness.html.

Zee, A.V. (2009). The promotion and marketing of OxyContin: Commercial triumph, public health tragedy. *American Journal of Public Health, 99*(2), 221-227.

38

How Government Works: What You Need to Know to Influence the Process

Casey R. Shillam and Sandra Whitley Ryals[a]

> *"Only individuals can desire and act. The existence of an institution such as government becomes meaningful only through influencing the actions of those individuals who are and those who are not considered as members."*
>
> **Murray Rothbard**

Influence capacity in the nursing profession is of paramount importance in advancing health policy to improve health care delivery. Influencing public officials to create policies that improve access to quality and affordable health care for all is the responsibility of every nurse. Nurses are well-positioned to serve as advocates in the development, implementation, and evaluation of policy by virtue of their intimate perspective of the impact of health care policy and government regulations on the daily lives of patients and families. The Institute of Medicine (2011) emphasized the importance of nurse leadership in achieving wide-ranging and sustainable changes in the health care system due to their "close proximity to patients and scientific understanding of care processes across the continuum of care" (p. 23). Despite close relationships with patients and care delivery, influence is an often overlooked and underdeveloped skill for nurses. Opinion leaders ranked nurses as the least likely to influence health reform after government officials, insurance executives, pharmaceutical executives, health care executives, doctors, and even patients (Robert Wood Johnson Foundation, 2010). An ability to persuade or convince others is the broadest definition of influence (National Center for Health care Leadership, 2006). Nurses engaging in actions that guide and direct changes in health care at the organization and systems levels can provide substantial power and guidance in developing policy (Newton, 2016). Nursing influence can create, implement, and evaluate policies and

the impact of policies on workforce performance, costs of care delivery, and improvements in population health that focus on health, wellness, and disease prevention (Salmond & Echevarria, 2017).

Government impacts health care delivery systems in multiple ways. Nurses must understand the functions of government at the federal, state, and local levels. This chapter describes key areas of government and policy function and ways for nurse advocates to engage in both policy and political action. Understanding government oversight of health policy and government influence of health care services is essential for nurses practicing at any care setting.

GOVERNMENT OVERSIGHT OF HEALTH POLICY AND HEALTH CARE

Government operations impact health care delivery in the United States in a variety of ways. The U.S. Department of Health and Human Services (HHS) is centered in Washington, DC, with 10 regional offices located across the country (Fig. 38.1) (HHS, 2014). These regional offices are instrumental in policy implementation at state and local levels, addressing needs of communities and individuals by enhancing access to federal officials for HHS programs and policies.

The HHS (2018) is the primary agency responsible for protecting the health of all Americans. Provision of essential human services occurs through the Office of the Secretary and 11 agencies (Box 38.1) that oversee more than 300 programs such as Head Start, Vaccines for Children, and the Centers for Medicare and Medicaid Services. The HHS is responsible for the distribution of the

---

[a]This chapter updates a previous chapter originally developed by Karrie Cummings Hendrickson, PhD, RN and Christine Ceccarelli Schrauf, PhD, RN, MBA and draws on that work.

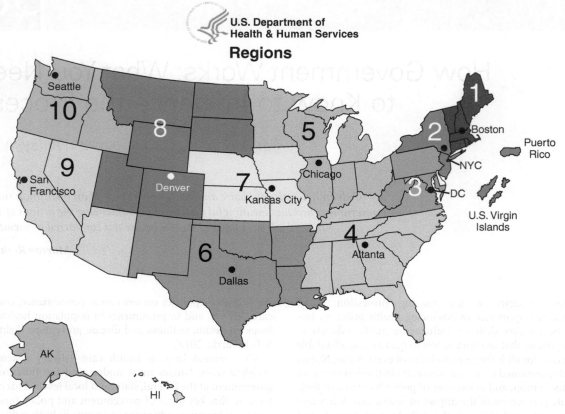

U.S. Department of Health & Human Services

Regions

Fig. 38.1 Regional offices of the HHS. (Source: U.S. Department of Health and Human Services. [2014]. *About: Agencies: Regional offices.* Retrieved from www.hhs.gov/about/agencies/iea/regional-offices/ index.html.)

BOX 38.1   Operating Divisions of the U.S. Department of Health and Human Services

- Administration for Children and Families (ACF)
- Administration for Community Living (ACL)
- Agency for Healthcare Research and Quality (AHRQ)
- Agency for Toxic Substances and Disease Registry (ATSDR)
- Centers for Disease Control and Prevention (CDC)
- Centers for Medicare & Medicaid Services (CMS)
- U.S. Food and Drug Administration (FDA)
- Health Resources and Services Administration (HRSA)
- Indian Health Service (IHS)
- National Institutes of Health (NIH)
- Substance Abuse and Mental Health Services Administration (SAMHSA)

second-largest portion of the federal budget and maintains oversight of implementing new programs or enacting changes to existing health-related programs.

U.S. military spending makes up the largest portion of the federal budget, with a large part going to health care through the U.S. Department of Defense (DoD). The DoD provides care to all active duty military and uniformed services personnel, retirees, National Guard and Reserve members, and their families—approximately 9.6 million people stationed throughout the world (DoD, 2018) (see Chapter 36 on military health care).

The U.S. Department of Education and the Health Resources and Services Administration (HRSA) provide billions of dollars in grants and loans for students to attend college and professional schools, including nursing schools. These departments work with hospitals and other government agencies to provide loan repayment programs which attract nurses to underserved areas (HRSA, 2018).

These are a few examples of the way government operations impact health care delivery in the United States. In each of these departments, opportunities exist for nurses to participate in creating or informing decisions that influence policy development.

FEDERALIST SYSTEM: THREE LEVELS OF GOVERNMENT

The United States government is a federalist system, comprised of multiple tiers of power at federal, state, and local levels of government. A federalist system constitutionally divides sovereignty among the different governmental levels so that the policymakers at each level have final authority in some areas, but not complete authority over all areas. The division of exclusive and concurrent powers of state and federal government, originally designed to ensure no one arm held more power than the others, ultimately provides checks and balances to ensure fair, equal decision-making. The different tiers are intended to act efficiently and independently of one another, but in conjunction with national and local policy agendas. The U.S. Constitution divides governmental authority by prescribing duties and responsibilities of the federal government and withholding both specified and unspecified powers for states.

Despite the different levels of power, the federal government has the capacity to greatly influence state and local policy through government grants, incentives, and federal mandates, while instituting federal requirements for state, local, or tribal governments to expend their own resources to achieve certain goals or receive federal funding (O'Toole & Christensen, 2013). Many powers, such as taxation, law formation, and law enforcement are shared equally among levels of government and may be exercised either in conjunction with one another or independently.

Federal Government

The three branches of the federal government represent a separation of powers and work as a series of checks and balances on one another. The executive, legislative, and judicial branches (Fig. 38.2) require policymakers to work

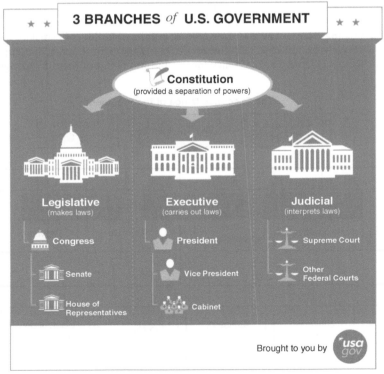

Fig. 38.2 Three branches of federal government. (From USA.gov. [2018]. *Branches of the U.S. government.* Retrieved from www.usa.gov/branches-of-government.)

together to formulate policy that is acceptable to as many people as possible, and they are designed to prevent any individual or small group from making sweeping changes (USA.gov, 2018).

The Executive Branch. The role of the executive branch is to implement laws and oversee enforcement. The executive branch is made up of the Executive Office of the President (EOP), the Executive Cabinet, and many independent agencies, boards, committees, and commissions, the staff of which advise the president and help to oversee programs (USA.gov, 2018). The EOP consists of the president, vice president, and related White House offices and agencies (Fig. 38.3) who develop and implement the policies and programs of the president. The president is the highest ranking, elected federal official and serves as head of the executive branch. The president also serves as the commander-in-chief of all U.S. military forces, and with the approval of the Senate, grants pardons, makes treaties, and appoints high-ranking officials such as Supreme Court justices and Cabinet secretaries.

Some of the president's most notable powers are the veto and executive orders. The veto effectively stops or delays a new piece of legislation from becoming a law. If the president invokes the veto, it can only be overridden by a two-thirds majority vote in both houses of Congress. The executive order, by contrast, has the binding force of law and does not require approval of Congress. For example, an executive order by former President Barack Obama put into policy the

Deferred Action for Childhood Arrivals (DACA) when Congress failed to pass immigration reform laws. This action allowed for certain people who were brought into the United States illegally as minors to have certain protections from deportation. In the first few weeks of President Donald Trump's term, he signed 17 executive orders to impact environmental, health care, and immigration laws.

Some powers of the president are not defined in the Constitution, including the power to set the national policy agenda. Newly elected presidents bring their priority issues to the forefront of the American political agenda, which opens the door for debate of some concerns and closes the door on others. At the beginning of his presidency, President George W. Bush's policy proposals regarding social security, Medicare prescription drug coverage, and homeland security were high on the public and policy agendas. The election of President Barack Obama in 2008 shifted emphasis away from those issues and onto discussions of revitalizing the domestic and worldwide economies, ending the war in Iraq, and providing universal health care. The election of President Donald Trump in 2016 shifted the focus of the American political agenda toward developing domestic industrial infrastructure, implementing immigration reform, and reform of trade policies. A savvy policy advocate must be aware of policymakers' priorities and anticipate how changes in the political climate following an election may affect the politics of health policymaking.

White House staff are appointed by the president but are not confirmed by Congress and are influential in

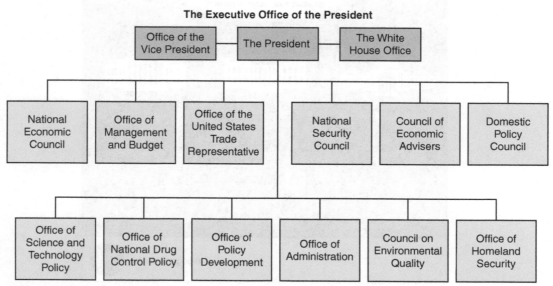

Fig. 38.3 Organizational chart for the Executive Office of the President. (Source: USA.gov. [2018]. *Branches of the U.S. government.* Retrieved from www.usa.gov/branches-of-government.)

setting national agendas and disseminating the president's priorities. They usually hold views similar to those of the president and are instrumental in White House decision-making. Nurses can influence the executive branch of government through several approaches. Most importantly, they can participate in presidential campaigns and by voting. They can also exert influence through petitions aimed at specific departments within the executive branch, including creating new petitions or responding to open petitions.

The Legislative Branch. The legislative branch of federal government consists of the Congress, which is divided into two chambers: the Senate and the House of Representatives. Members of the Senate and House are elected by their constituents for 6-year and 2-year terms, respectively. The Senate, with two members from each state, has 100 seats. The House of Representatives has 435 voting seats and 6 nonvoting seats from U.S. Territories, with each state's number of representatives based on its population. The number of members in each state's delegation may change every 10 years based on the results of national decennial census.

The primary role of the legislative branch is formulation of laws for recommendation to the president. The process of creating such laws can be long and arduous, requiring extensive discussion, debate, and compromise. Once a new topic or bill is introduced into a Congressional chamber, it is assigned to a Congressional committee or subcommittee for further discussion. The Senate consists of 20 standing committees and occasional temporary committees (United States Senate, 2018), and the House of Representatives has 21 standing committees; between the two chambers, they share six joint committees (United States House of Representatives, 2018).

The committee stage of policy development is a critical step for nurse advocates to understand because it provides one of the primary points of entry into the policy arena. The assignment of a bill to a committee signals to those who care about the issue that it is time to act. Policy advocates must be knowledgeable about committee jurisdiction and policy priorities of the committee members. Influential advocates are willing and able to educate committee members and their staff about the issue, and capable of providing persuasive testimony before committee members.

The status of all federal bills can be obtained at one of the most important websites for Congressional information: www.congress.gov. Members of Congressional staff are accessible in Washington, DC, and in the home office within each member's state. Nurses should be familiar with representatives from their home state as well as other legislators who either support their issue or sit on a committee with jurisdiction over the issue.

Congressional caucuses are another way that Congressional members provide a forum for issues or legislative agendas. Caucuses generally exist in the House of Representatives but can consist of both Representatives and Senators interested in diverse health-related topics. As of publication, the 116th Congress has three nurses serving in the House of Representatives: Congresswoman Karen Bass (D-CA-33), Congresswoman Lauren Underwood (D-IL-14), and Congresswoman Eddie Bernice Johnson (D-TX-30) (American Nurses Association, 2018).

The Judicial Branch. The judicial branch of federal government explains and applies the laws of the United States. Article III section 1 of the constitution establishes the Supreme Court of the United States, the highest court of the land. Supreme Court Justices are nominated by the president, confirmed by the Senate, and serve until the time of retirement, death, or impeachment. Court decisions can have a powerful impact on health policy. For example, in 2012, a U.S. Supreme Court ruling made Medicaid expansion optional for individual states in upholding the Patient Protection and Affordable Care Act (ACA). As of publication 34 states, including Washington, DC, have adopted further expansion, with 3 states still considering and 14 states declining expansion (Kaiser Family Foundation, 2018).

State Government

Each state government has its own constitution, which, similar to the federal constitution, defines the roles of each of the three branches of government at the state level. Each state's constitution is unique and is based on the state's history, population, philosophy, and geography. Theoretically, state constitutions and individual state laws cannot conflict with federal law or with the U.S. Constitution. However, conflict arises when states enact laws that go against federal law. For example, 31 states, Washington, DC, Guam, and Puerto Rico currently allow for comprehensive public medical marijuana and cannabis programs. Fifteen states have approved use of "low tetrahydrocannabinol (THC), high cannabidiol (CBD)" products for legal defense or for limited medical situations (National Conference of State Legislatures, 2018). However, under federal government law, marijuana is classified as a schedule 1 drug, which has no legally accepted medical use (Unites States Drug Enforcement Administration, 2018) (see Chapter 81 on medical cannabis).

Although there is much variation in the structure and day-to-day functioning of state governments, there are enough similarities for comparison. For complete information on each state, visit the state government's website or the federal government web portal (www.usa.gov/Agencies/State-and-Territories.shtml).

The Executive Branch. The governor of a state is similar to the president at the federal level. All but three states also have lieutenant governors, whose roles are comparable to that of vice president. The powers of these officials vary widely among the states, but they all are responsible for preparation of the state budget for presentation to the legislature, and management of the approved budget. Also, like the president, governors have the power to veto or approve state-level legislation, and to make appointments to influential positions such as the state board of health. Most lieutenant governors have a leadership position in the legislature (National Lieutenant Governors Association, 2018).

The governor's veto power is slightly different from that of the president. Known as the *line item veto*, it allows governors to cross out or delete sections of a bill before signing it into law. This helps combat *riders*—additional provisions that may be unrelated to the law, but often advance legislators' favorite programs—which may be attached to bills.

Regulatory Function of State Governments. Collectively, 50 states employ about 3.5 million people in state agencies who work to translate the intentions of state legislatures outlined in new laws into sets of rules and regulations (Smith & Greenblatt, 2013). The crafting of regulation language is as important as the law itself, because it determines how it will be implemented. Laws and regulations work together to determine how public policy is implemented (Independence Hall Association, 2018).

One of the most visible roles of the state executive branch with respect to health care is licensing and regulation of health professionals, including nurses. Each state sets both educational and testing requirements for licensure and establishes scope of nursing practice through the state's nurse practice act. Even though some states have entered into compacts allowing nurses to practice in multiple states, practice regulations continue to vary widely among states, particularly regarding scope of advanced nursing practice.

Nursing advocacy and influence in policy is clearly apparent in the work to support advanced practice nurses to practice to the full extent of their education and training. At the time of the release of the Institute of Medicine's *Future of Nursing* report in 2011, 13 states and the District of Columbia had full scope of practice standards. Through a nationally-coordinated campaign to implement report recommendations, the Robert Wood Johnson Foundation and AARP's Center to Champion Nursing in America launched the *Future of Nursing: Campaign for Action* and exerted substantial influence in advancing scope of practice laws (Campaign for Action, 2018) (see Chapter 71). In 2018, 9 additional states had enacted full scope of practice legislation, and 15 states had made improvements.

The Legislative Branch. All 50 states have state legislatures with roles similar to that of the U.S. Congress: create and pass new laws and serve as a check and balance to the executive branch by evaluating the governor's budget and appointments. Beyond this basic structure, aspects of state legislatures may differ. Nebraska has a legislature with a single house, whereas the other 49 states have bicameral (two-house) legislatures. Although most state legislatures meet every year, 4 states have legislatures that meet every other year: Montana, Nevada, North Dakota, and Texas. Just as at the federal level, it is important for nurses to know representatives from their home district, as well as those who support health care issues and committee members with jurisdiction over defined interest areas.

The Judicial Branch. Each state maintains its own court system. Unlike the federal Supreme Court, each state determines the method of appointment of court judges via election, appointment for a specified period of time, or lifetime appointment (Federal Judiciary, 2018). Only certain cases from the state court system are eligible for review by the U.S. Supreme Court (see Chapter 45 for further information on nursing and the courts).

Local Government

There are many types of local governments in the United States, including counties, cities, towns, villages, and school districts. Local governments often have elected executive leaders. They may be referred to as mayors in a county, city, or town. The legislative branch at the local level is often composed of an elected council or board, which creates laws governing the locality. These laws cannot conflict with state or national laws.

Although the structure and function of local-level governments vary more widely compared to the state level, they serve as vital links between local citizens to the state and nation (Donovan, Smith, & Mooney, 2013). Federal health policy can influence local health initiatives through transfer of billions of dollars in grant money to local entities, which disperse funds to community health agencies. These grants are often accompanied by defined health goals such as improved child immunization (Doherty, Buchy, Standaert, Giaquinto, & Prado-Cohrs, 2016).

The increasing responsibility for health care of citizens by local governments offers nurses endless opportunities to influence health policy. Developing and maintaining relationships with local officials is a feasible role that nurses can assume, compared with officials at state or federal levels. Addressing issues and testing proposals at local levels allows for policy development, implementation, and evaluation before scaling to larger populations at state or federal levels.

INFLUENCE AND HOW IT WORKS

Strategies for influence by nurses are built on a core set of competencies and are effective at all levels of government. National organizations have charged nurses and other health care providers to influence policy in the re-design of the U.S. health care system. Interpersonal influence specifically focuses on the ability of one person to guide or encourage another person or group (Adams, 2009). The Adams Influence Model (AIM; Adams & Natarajan, 2016) was developed to describe the attributes, factors, and process of influence by nurse leaders (Fig. 38.4). Signifying a single focus issue and particular moment in time, the AIM distinguishes *influence* from *power*, which is the cumulative result of being able to influence multiple issues.

Principles of influence are the same for influencing policy leaders regardless of government level. One possible

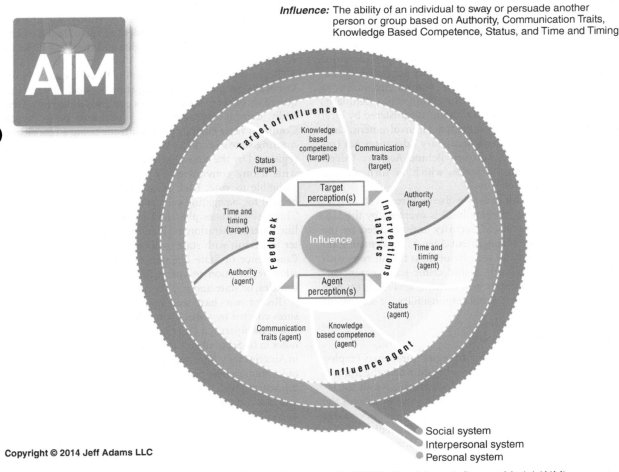

Fig. 38.4 Adams Influence Model. (Source: Adams, J. M. [2009]. *The Adams Influence Model (AIM): Understanding the factors attributes and process of achieving influence*. Saarbruken, Germany: VDM Verlag.)

exception of note may be at the local level. Because of the nature of localities, policy advocates and policymakers may also be neighbors, friends, or colleagues. Such informal relationships must be carefully balanced, but may also aid the advocate in gaining access to influence change.

Influencing the Appropriate Level of Government

The principle of divided powers is a cornerstone of the government level (federal, state, and local) and the government branches (executive, legislative, and judicial). The founding fathers saw this system of checks and balances as key to preventing the accumulation of power by any one group, thereby helping to maintain a democratic nation. Although this organizational structure may present challenges to nurses aiming to influence policy, it is important to understand which issues fall under the jurisdiction of each level of government, and the tasks that are shared responsibilities among the levels.

Many health care initiatives fall to multiple levels of government for both funding and administration. For example, covering the uninsured falls under all three domains, depending on the proposal under debate. Medicaid, which provides insurance for the poorest Americans, is administered by federal and state authorities. Similarly, many education programs, although administered by local education agencies, entail some federal involvement. Laws such as the Elementary and Secondary Education Act (reauthorized as the No Child Left Behind Act) are federal initiatives with grants to states, which in turn allocate funds to local agencies.

Some public health issues involve all three levels of government. Emergency preparedness is overseen by the U.S. Department of Homeland Security and executed by the Federal Emergency Management Agency. Implementation of disaster response and security of mass transit rests with local public health, hospital, and crime enforcement authorities. Federal and state governments retain a great deal of administrative control and responsibility for security of air traffic.

Strategic Use of Influence

There are a variety of specific strategies nurses may employ in making policy change. Depending on where the nurse is employed, the nurse must be knowledgeable about the legal ability to lobby versus educate. Knowing who holds the power, nurses can propose solutions to key policymakers through lobbying, presenting policy briefs, media visibility (see Chapter 12 for media influence), or meeting with legislative aides at the right level of government (see Chapter 40 for more on lobbying). Nurses can also testify at committee hearings or mobilize grassroots support when key votes are approaching.

Influence Through the Electoral Process

The electoral process involves multiple levels: from primaries or caucuses, to the general election by which citizens select candidates to fill an office or position at local, state, or national levels. One important variable influencing national elections is the electoral college, a process established for presidential elections. By a majority of electoral votes, the electoral college determines the election of president and vice president of the United States.

Voting. The most important action for influencing through the electoral process is to register to vote, and then vote! Attention must be given to rules and laws in each state regarding voter requirements including how to register, how to keep registration status current, when and where to vote, and rules of absentee voting. Members of the military, a spouse or dependent of the military, or citizens living overseas still have rights and responsibilities for voting in elections.

Every state requires registration to vote except North Dakota (USA.gov). Contacting state or local offices is required since every state operates elections differently. Generally, citizens may register to vote online or in person. Common voter eligibility rules include being a U.S. citizen, meeting state's residency and age requirements, and being registered by the state's registration deadline. Some people with felony convictions or mental incapacities may be ineligible to vote. Each state's website, and Vote.gov, are helpful for navigating each state's voter registration rules. Thirty-seven states plus the District of Columbia have online voter registration availability or individuals can register in person with state or local election offices (National Conference of State Legislatures, 2018). Many states also allow registration to vote with the department of motor vehicles, or state and county public assistance offices.

Recent years have seen a range of restrictive voting measures enacted by states that could impede people's rights to vote. The bipartisan U.S. Commission on Civil Rights (2018) notes in its September 2018 report on minority voting rights in America that these measures include reducing the number of locations where people can cast their ballot and demanding voters produce specific forms of identification. Thirty-four states request or require some type of identification at the polls before a person is allowed to vote (National Conference of State Legislators, 2018). As of 2018, North Dakota residents are required to present identification with a street address to vote, despite many residents of Native American reservations having post office boxes and not street addresses. Georgia requires an exact match on signatures, has cut back on early voting, and has aggressively purged voting rolls, disproportionately impacting persons of color (Gross, 2018). Noting that "Voting is the foundation of our democracy" and should be accessible, free, and fair for all Americans, the Brennan Center for Justice is proposing automatic voter registration. Proponents believe voting reform would increase accuracy and participation, save money, and add 50 million voters (Brennan Center for Justice, 2018).

Electoral College. Unlike the mantra of "one person, one vote" in local, state, and Congressional elections, presidential elections are determined by the electoral college. The electoral college is a process that includes election of the electors by the states, totaling 538 electors, equaling the numbers in their Congressional delegations (National Archives, 2018). In order to elect the president, a majority of 270 electoral votes is required.

Although the term "electoral college" does not appear in the Constitution, reference is made to "electors" and was known to be a compromise between election of the president by a popular vote and election by a vote in Congress (National Archives, 2018). Although controversial through the years with differences in outcomes between popular vote and electoral vote, it would be necessary to pass a constitutional amendment to change the system. No such amendment has been passed to eliminate or reform the system in over 200 years (National Archives, 2018).

Influencing Campaigns for Public Office

Think of the power and influence of more than four million registered nurses (RNs) nationwide! RNs represent the largest segment of health professionals, representing an incredible force by sheer numbers and expertise. Nurses continue to outrank all other professions as the most trusted profession in Gallup's annual honesty and ethics survey (Brenan, 2018). Yet much work still needs to be done for nurses to extend their influence into all levels of the legislative, political, and policy arenas.

"All politics is local" is a phrase commonly used in political circles, made famous by former U.S. Speaker of the House Tip O'Neill. This statement reflects the importance candidates and elected officials place upon knowing their constituents and what issues are important to them. Candidates and elected officials need and want nurse experts to be an integral part of their campaigns. Nurse advocates need to know the candidates by researching their backgrounds and positions, attending forums, and being involved in community events open to the public.

Nurses know firsthand the impact of being involved upon individuals and communities. Nothing is more compelling than hearing personal stories that capture the care and compassion of nurses. Nurses' knowledge, skills, and abilities make for a meaningful collaboration and powerful influence in public policy decisions. Meeting candidates or legislators at their home office is critical to building relationships with policymakers, providing informed insight on issues, and becoming an influential resource which impacts health policy decisions. Contact must be maintained consistently before, during, and after legislative sessions. These relationships are built on trust and ongoing contact is necessary for maintaining that trust.

Nurses can influence policy and politics by joining professional organizations (see Chapter 67 for more on professional organizations). By lobbying Congress and executive agencies, professional nursing organizations amplify nurses' voices and offer tools and other information, empowering nurses to share expertise and perspectives with policymakers. Professional organizations also maintain policy resources on their website and through listservs to provide updates on nursing and health care–related issues.

DISCUSSION QUESTIONS

1. How does the skill of influence impact nurses' ability to shape health policy?
2. What does policy development entail at the different levels of government?
3. How can nurses influence the development of bills and inform final bill language?

REFERENCES

Adams, J.M. (2009). *The Adams Influence Model (AIM): Understanding the factors attributes and process of achieving influence.* Saarbrüken, Germany: VDM Verlag.

Adams, J.M., & Natarajan, S. (2016). Understanding influence within the context of Nursing: Development of the Adams Influence Model using practice, research, and theory. *Advances in Nursing Science, 39*(3), E40-E56.

American Health Policy Institute. (2015). *How the government as a payer shapes the healthcare marketplace.* Retrieved from www.americanhealthpolicy.org/Content/documents/resources/Government_as_Payer_12012015.pdf.

American Nurses Association. (2018). *Nurses serving in Congress.* Retrieved from www.nursingworld.org/practice-policy/advocacy/federal/nurses-serving-in-congress/.

Brennan Center for Justice. (2018). *Voting rights and elections.* Retrieved from www.brennancenter.org/issues/voting-rights-elections.

Brown, A.R. (2012). The item veto's sting. *State Politics & Policy Quarterly, 12*(2), 183-203.

Campaign for Action. (2018). *Campaign for action dashboard update.* Retrieved from https://campaignforaction.org/wp-content/uploads/2016/02/CCNA-0028_2018-Dashboard-Indicator-Updates_Jul2018_4HR-2.jpg.

Centers for Medicare and Medicaid Services. (2018). *CMS' program history*. Retrieved from www.cms.gov/About-CMS/Agency-Information/History/index.html.

Doherty, M., Buchy, P., Standaert, B., Giaquinto, C., & Prado-Cohrs, D. (2016). Vaccine impact: Benefits for human health. *Vaccine, 34*(52), 6707-6714.

Donovan, T., Smith, D.A., & Mooney, C.Z. (2013). *State and local politics. Institutions and reform* (3rd ed.). Boston, MA: Cengage Learning Wadsworth.

Federal Judiciary. (2018). *Comparing federal and state courts*. Retrieved from www.uscourts.gov/about-federal-courts/court-role-and-structure/comparing-federal-state-courts.

Gross, T. (2018). Republican voter suppression efforts are targeting minorities, journalist says. *NPR: Think out Loud*. Retrieved from www.npr.org/2018/10/23/659784277/republican-voter-suppression-efforts-are-targeting-minorities-journalist-says.

Health Resources and Service Administration. (2018). *NURSE Corps loan repayment program*. Retrieved from https://bhw.hrsa.gov/loansscholarships/nursecorps/lrp.

Independence Hall Association. (2018). *Policy making: Political interactions*. Retrieved from www.ushistory.org/gov/11.asp.

Institute of Medicine. (2011). *The future of nursing: Leading change, advancing health*. Washington, DC: The National Academies Press.

Kaiser Family Foundation. (2018). *Current status of state Medicaid expansion decisions*. Retrieved from www.kff.org/health-reform/slide/current-status-of-the-medicaid-expansion-decision/.

National Archives. (2018). *U.S. Electoral College*. Retrieved from www.archives.gov/federal-register/electoral-college/about.html.

National Center for Healthcare Leadership. (2006). *Health leadership competency model*. Chicago, IL: Author. Retrieved from www.nchl.org/Documents/NavLink/NCHL_Competency_Model-full_uid892012226572.pdf.

National Conference of State Legislatures. (2018). *State medical marijuana laws*. Retrieved from www.ncsl.org/research/health/state-medical-marijuana-laws.aspx.

National Lieutenant Governors Association. (2018). *About NLGA*. Retrieved from www.nlga.us/.

Newton, R. (2016). What great leaders know about influence. *Forbes*. Retrieved from www.forbes.com/sites/rebeccanewton/2016/07/27/six-steps-to-increase-your-influence/#47bd3aac6c58.

O'Toole, L.J., & Christensen, R.K. (2013). American intergovernmental relations: An overview. In L.J. O'Toole & R.K. Christensen (Eds.), *American intergovernmental relations* (5th ed., pp. 1-32). Los Angeles: CQ Press.

Robert Wood Johnson Foundation. (2010). *Nursing leadership from bedside to boardroom: Opinion leaders' perceptions*. Retrieved from www.rwjf.org/en/library/research/2010/01/nursing-leadership-from-bedside-to-boardroom.html.

Salmond, S.W., & Echevarria, M. (2017). Healthcare transformation and changing roles for nursing. *Orthopedic Nursing, 36*(1), 12-25.

Smith, K.B., & Greenblatt, A. (2013). *Governing states and localities* (4th ed.). Washington, DC: CQ Press.

U.S. Census Bureau. (2010). *United States: 2010 to 2050*. U.S. Census Bureau Publication P25-1138. Suitland, MD: U.S. Census Bureau. Retrieved from www.census.gov/prod/2010pubs/p25-1138.pdf.

U.S. Commission on Civil Rights. (2018). *An assessment of minority voting rights access in the United States*. Retrieved from www.usccr.gov/pubs/2018/Minority_Voting_Access_2018.pdf.

U.S. Department of Health & Human Services. (2014). *About: Agencies: Regional offices*. Retrieved from www.hhs.gov/about/agencies/iea/regional-offices/index.html.

U. S. Department of Health & Human Services. (2018). *About: Strategic plan*. Retrieved from www.hhs.gov/about/strategic-plan/introduction/index.html.

U. S. Department of Veterans Affairs. (2018). *Veterans Health Administration*. Retrieved from www.va.gov/health/.

United States Drug Enforcement Administration. (2018). *Drug scheduling*. Retrieved from www.dea.gov/drug-scheduling.

United States House of Representatives. (2018). *House committees*. Retrieved from www.senate.gov/committees.

United States Senate. (2018). *Senate committees*. Retrieved from www.senate.gov/committees.

USA.gov. (2018). *Branches of the U.S. government*. Retrieved from www.usa.gov/branches-of-government.

ONLINE RESOURCES

Future of Nursing Campaign for Action
https://campaignforaction.org
U.S. Bills and Resolutions
www.congress.gov
U.S. Government Official Website
www.usa.gov

39

An Overview of Legislative and Regulatory Processes

Mary Jean Schumann[a]

> *"Law is order and good law is good order."*
>
> **Aristotle**

Policy takes many forms and in the United States is ultimately established or influenced by all three branches of government. The Legislative branch of the Federal Government is assumed to take the lead on policy development and passage in the form of legislation. However, the United States Constitution makes clear that the Executive branch of the Government is responsible for implementation of policy via established laws and rule making. There are many examples of Executive Orders that clearly change the direction of legislation already passed by Congress. The Judicial branch—the court system—has had clear and substantial influence on policy implementation in landmark cases such as *Roe v. Wade* and *Brown v. the Board of Education*. This chapter focuses on the influence of people engaged in policymaking through legislation and the mechanics of the formal legislative process. It will also link the process of legislative passage with the process of legislative implementation once it becomes a law, otherwise known as rule making and regulation. And it will discuss the challenges of regulatory enforcement and the influence of the Justice department in the review of law and regulation. Most of this discussion will focus on the federal level. States have similar processes, although they may structure their legislative bodies and their processes differently.

Chapter 7 provides multiple models for understanding the policymaking process, and Chapter 8 discusses political analysis and strategies. All are essential to the success of policymaking. However, without a concrete and well understood legislative process and coherent rule making, new policy is unlikely to get to the finish line and even less likely to achieve its intended outcomes.

THE POWER STRUCTURE

The U.S. Congress is composed of 435 members in the House of Representatives (based upon population per state) and 100 members in the Senate (based upon 2 senators per state). The Senators are elected for 6-year terms, with one-third being elected every 2 years. Members of the House of Representatives face reelection every 2 years.

Congress completes its business in 2-year terms. That term of service is then referred to as, for example, the 116th Congress. Congress holds legislative sessions throughout the year with periodic recesses in order to complete its business, but most states do not conduct their business the same way. State legislative bodies will typically be in session for 1 to 3 months of the year, but this may vary from fall to winter or spring. Texas conducts its legislative business only every other year.

The Congressional term is important because any legislation introduced during that 2-year session must be enacted upon during that term, or it dies in Congress. Any further interest or action requires new legislation to be introduced in the next Congress. Thus, legislation may be reintroduced repeatedly over many Congressional terms. An example of this is nurse staffing legislation, introduced in some form in Congress each term for nearly 20 years, with no final passage. Types of legislation (bills) that may be proposed by either the House or Senate are included in Box 39.1.

A cautionary note: The discussion of the legislative and regulatory processes is presented here in a straightforward

---

[a]This chapter is an adaptation of one revised by Nancy Ridenour for the 7th edition of this book.

The Bill's number is designated by an "HR" if initiated in the House and an "S" if in the Senate. In certain cases, a bill takes on additional meaning.

- A bill can become a *joint resolution* and the two terms may be used interchangeably in some venues. A joint resolution looks much like a bill, except it contains a preamble, perhaps like the resolutions developed in state nurses' organizations.
- A *concurrent resolution* is used when the matter affects both House and Senate.
- A *continuing resolution*, a variation on this theme, is often used when the Congress cannot come to consensus on a budget, thereby passing a short-term resolution designed to extend the current budget period and approve additional funds for the short term, thus avoiding a government shutdown.
- A *resolution* is used when a matter affects only one chamber and is adopted by the chamber in which it originates.

manner but in actuality is seldom so. Kingdon (2003) proposed that policymaking requires the confluence of problem, political and policy "streams" (see Chapter 7), and the political stream is contingent upon the "national mood." Today, that mood not only reflects the values and beliefs of the current Administration, interest groups' pressures, and turnover of political figures, but also the values and beliefs of the public, as displayed on social media, in the news, and on the streets via protests, marches, and even violence. Political will in the government comes down to people: those who craft the language of a bill that can garner support; those who are willing to sponsor, as well as advocate for it; and who are willing to support compromise to secure its passage. Political will is also engendered by the stories of individuals, families, and organizations who can be positively impacted by a bill's passage or who are negatively impacted because no one has been willing to go to the mat to either generate a feasible solution or solve the problem.

The Power of Committees

The size of Congress makes it quite difficult for it to do the crafting, negotiating, and compromising necessary for any reasonable legislation to emerge. The volume of work and its complexity in both the House and the Senate require a substantial committee structure with staff, an operating budget, guidelines, rules, and procedures. Committees in

the House and Senate each have distinct rules and procedures that differ for each Chamber. Although each may have established guidelines for committees, each committee still chooses to adopt its own rules and procedures under which it will function. There are four types of committees at the federal level: standing, select, joint, and temporary conference committees, which are described in Box 39.2.

The 115th Congress (2017–2018) was composed of 20 standing committees in the House, with 97 subcommittees and one select committee, while the Senate had 16 standing committees, with 68 subcommittees as well as four select or special committees. There were also 4 joint committees (Heitshusen, 2017). The number of subcommittees may be startling to the novice, yet it is where much of the initial review and investigation on the worthiness of the bill takes place. Because few House or Senate or party rules apply to subcommittees, the number, prerogatives, and autonomy of subcommittees vary among committees. Some committees create independent subcommittees with sizeable staff and budgets and regularly refer any proposed bill to its subcommittees for at least initial consideration. In these cases, the subcommittee may play a substantial role by taking the lead in framing issues, drafting reports, and holding hearings and markups. Other committees take on the responsibility for most of the work themselves. In addition, some full committees repeat all actions taken by their subcommittees, whereas others review only major subcommittee work or even forward subcommittee-reported bills to the floor with little change. It is helpful to know where these variations exist if trying to move a bill through committee and the full Chamber.

Ultimately, the choice of seeing a bill make it to the House or Senate floor depends in almost all cases on the determination of the committee to which it has been referred. The committee will vote to refer a bill on for further consideration to other members of the House and Senate or governmental agencies for cost impact or further analysis of its fairness or impact. The committee can also choose to ignore a bill completely if it has no interest in it, or choose to not take up the bill on the recommendation of its subcommittee, or can choose to simply not advance it beyond the committee, or can table it, meaning it cannot come up again. All these approaches essentially cause a bill to die in committee. Of more than 8000 bills initiated by the House and the Senate during each Congress, less than 10% ever get out of committee and moved on for further consideration. Only in a few situations does a bill bypass the committee process—that is, if the leadership of the majority party consents. Thus, the power of the committee is significant to the success or failure of a bill reaching the floor of the House or Senate. And in order for a bill to become law, it must have similar bills reach the floors of

---

BOX 39.2 Types of Committees Supporting Legislative Activities

Heithusen (2017) describes the types and roles of committees:

- A *standing committee* has permanent jurisdiction over bills and issues in its area of business. Most standing committees recommend funding levels—authorizations—for government operations and for new and existing programs.
- *Select or special committees* are generally established by a separate resolution of either the House or Senate. Their purposes may include conducting investigations and studies or even to consider bills. Select committees examine emerging issues that do not fit clearly within existing standing committee jurisdictions or the issue cuts across jurisdictional boundaries.
- *Joint committees* are made up of members of both the House and Senate, currently serving more in the management of housekeeping tasks of the House and Senate.
- A *conference committee* is a temporary joint committee formed to resolve differences between competing House and Senate versions of a bill. Conference committees draft compromises between the positions of the House and Senate, which are then submitted to the full House and Senate for approval.

---

both Chambers. Appointments to committees, particularly to the standing committees, are crucial to individual members' power. The chair of each committee and most of its members represent the majority party, with the chair setting the agenda for committee business. Each party assigns its own members to committees, and each committee distributes its members among its subcommittees. The majority also controls the resources available to the committee, with some portion distributed to the minority committee. The Senate places limits on the number and types of panels any one senator may serve on or chair.

A committee's influence may extend throughout the legislative process to the enactment of bills into law (Heitshusen, 2017). A committee member, often the chair, will play an important role in managing the full Senate's deliberation on the bill. Also, committee members will be appointed as conferees to reconcile differences in the Senate and House versions of a bill. Committees also manage the confirmation or rejection of presidential nominees, consider treaties and international agreements, hold oversight hearings, and launch investigations of suspected wrongdoing.

The Power of Authorizations and Appropriations

As does the senior governance of any large organization, Congress's responsibility is largely to develop and approve decisions related to budgets, funding, and priorities for spending money. Congressional members serve as a Board trying to run one of the largest business enterprises in the world. Given that context, there are any number of opportunities to make sound decisions and poor decisions about spending priorities, investments, and scarce resources. Thus, it makes sense that Congress has a complicated process for determining what agency or entity gets authorization to receive funds, and then how monies will get appropriated to support the work they are supposed to do. Once a bill becomes law, there is a decision about which agency will be tasked to run the program, or if there will be a new agency created for that purpose. If a new agency, a bill authorizing the agency's creation must be passed before any funding can be appropriated to it. That *authorization* creates the legal authority to operate, sets limits on the amount of money it can spend, and guidelines for the program. It also determines how long the agency can be authorized to operate. Existing agencies and programs need periodic *reauthorization*, such as the Children's Health Insurance Program (CHIP) and Temporary Assistance to Needy Families (TANF), or they cannot operate.

Once an authorization is complete or a reauthorization is updated, then an *appropriations* bill is submitted and passed to enable a program or agency to make spending commitments and then actually spend the money. Many nurses have been short-term victims of this requirement, having submitted grant proposals to Health Resources and Service Administration (HRSA) but receiving no confirmation of being awarded a grant until the money is available (often after the anticipated start date of the grant). The date of notification typically coincides with approval of a larger spending bill or approved federal budget or, in recent times, a continuing resolution. It is a reminder that there are many funding issues at stake during the appropriations process.

A summary of the process shows the power of the Appropriations Committee. A committee such as the Senate Health, Education, Labor and Pension (HELP) Committee will have jurisdiction over the issues and the solutions and recommend the amount of funding for its implementation, but it does not decide the final appropriation of funds for the bill's implementation, if passed. Once passed, Congress must also pass a bill authorizing that program or agency to perform the work proposed in the bill. A separate Senate Appropriations Committee will determine the amount of money that will be supported to implement the law once passed. However, it may choose to not fund money for the law or some portion of the law's implementation, rendering that law or provision meaningless. For example, the Patient Protection and Affordable Care Act (ACA) included a National Healthcare Workforce Commission but no funding was provided to support its implementation. The Commission was appointed and a nurse co-chair named, but it never convened because of the lack of appropriations.

In other instances, although the Appropriations Committee may fund a new law or an existing federal agency, it may choose to underfund it sufficiently that, in practical terms, the agency may be forced to choose to fund existing or new provisions, but not both. The Agency for Health Care Research and Quality (AHRQ) experienced this in 2018; the National Guidelines Clearinghouse (NGC), vital for improving health care delivery and quality and used by many health professionals, including nurses, was originally created in 1998 by AHRQ in partnership with the American Medical Association and what is now America's Health Insurance Plans. Although the partnership ended in 2002, AHRQ continued the NGC until 2018 when contract funds ended and it did not have sufficient resources to continue the NGC.

For the most part, nurses receive funding via the HELP Committee or the House Energy and Commerce Committee. It makes good sense to seek out the names and affiliations of the members of these committees to develop relationships that may aid in support of health- and nurse-related programs and services.

Although each state will have its own rules and procedures for proposing bills for acceptance, appropriating funds and other resources, and even ratifying a proposed amendment, the overall principle of representative government prevails. The timeframe for proposing, supporting, and passing legislation is generally much shorter, so the volume of bills and the importance of priorities dictate what gets moved through the process with a chance of adoption. Sometimes this makes governance at the state level very challenging, especially when there is little agreement. Some states, because of lack of movement on the part of state legislators, have chosen to put contentious issues like the expansion of Medicaid on election ballots for citizens to vote for or against expansion, forcing the state to implement what they could not agree to do in legislative session. The power of the legislative branch can be overridden by voters if the citizens believe it has not worked in their best interest, creating another check and balance.

HOW A BILL BECOMES A LAW

Fig. 39.1 demonstrates the legislative process at the federal level, whether in the House or the Senate. Committee action occurs at multiple steps along the way. Alongside the depiction of how a bill becomes a law, there are touchpoints by which nurses can influence the committee process. Even though very few pieces of legislation actually become law, nurses can seize the opportunity to inform members of the committee about a proposed bill, sharing the human stories and key statistics that depict the impact of the legislation's failure or passage.

Only a member of either the House or Senate can introduce or sponsor a bill, although external input into drafts by interest groups and lobbyists is common. In order for a bill to ultimately be successful, similar legislation must be introduced in both the House and the Senate. The writing of an initial piece of legislation, if well written, is actually somewhat complex, and requires its proponents to understand other statutes already in place in order to avoid language that is in conflict with established law, avoid violating basic rights of citizens, minimize confusion on the part of voting members, and limit causes for judicial review. Other members of Congress may volunteer or be asked by lobbyists and interest groups to co-sponsor a bill, which increases the opportunities for support. Getting bipartisan support on a bill increases its chances of passage.

Nurses are key to surfacing health issues that need to be addressed. The direct care experience and management of consumers' health issues and care delivery challenges make the information and stories nurses provide—when well-messaged—quite compelling. Nurses can speak to health care funding and consumer accessibility issues. They can point to the unintended consequences of implemented legislation and shine light on possible solutions based on real-life knowledge of health issues.

Major Actions at the Committee Level

Despite how it might seem, committees rely on expert information from a variety of sources. The way in which Congressional committees engage in the gathering of expert information can be through legislative hearings, markups, and reports. Hearings can be either public or private—they can either allow millions of viewers to hear what is being asked and answered via CNN and other media outlets, or they can be closed to any public communication about the questions and the responses.

Congressional Hearings. Hearings can be *legislative*—held by committees to gather facts, opinions, and perspectives on either a proposed piece of legislation or in advance of any legislative proposal. Experts, special interest groups, and others may be given opportunity to provide information to these committees, usually by request. National organizations like American Nurses Association (ANA) may reach out to known members who have the necessary expertise to speak to a given issue. Often these requests are on short notice, so nurses who are ANA members and have expertise relevant to a bill should reach out well in advance to ANA to let that

HOW A BILL BECOMES A LAW
The Federal level

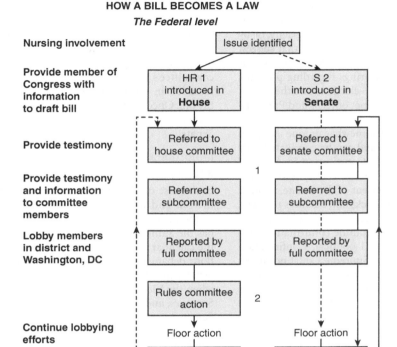

Fig. 39.1 How a bill becomes a law.

Nursing involvement

Provide member of Congress with information to draft bill

Provide testimony

Provide testimony and information to committee members

Lobby members in district and Washington, DC

Continue lobbying efforts

Send telegrams and make phone calls

Send letter to President

Issue identified

HR 1 introduced in **House** — S 2 introduced in **Senate**

Referred to house committee — Referred to senate committee

Referred to subcommittee — Referred to subcommittee

Reported by full committee — Reported by full committee

Rules committee action

Floor action — Floor action

House debate, vote on passage — Senate debate, vote on passage

Conference action

Compromise version voted on — Compromise version voted on

Presidential action

Vetoed — Signed

1 A bill goes to full committee first, then to special subcommittees for hearings, debate, revisions, and approval. The same process occurs when it goes to full committee. It either dies in committee or proceeds to the next step.
2 Only the house has a rules committee to set the "rule" for floor action and conditions for debate and amendments. In the senate, the leadership schedules action.
3 The bill is debated, amended, and passed or defeated. If passed, it goes to the other chamber and follows the same path. If each chamber passes a similar bill, both versions go to conference.
4 The president may sign the bill into law, allow it to become law without his signature, or veto it and return it to Congress. To override the veto, both houses must approve the bill by a $\frac{2}{3}$ majority vote.

expertise be known. Testimony before a Congressional hearing will include prior submission of written copy of the testimony, plus the opportunity to be asked questions once the testimony has been provided orally.

Hearings also can be for *oversight* of the executive branch to review, monitor, or supervise the implementation of a public policy or program and are a means of evaluating a program already implemented. A hearing to decide whether Congress should continue to authorize an active program would fall into this category, and might again call for testimony from those who are most familiar with the program, its success or challenges, or who have benefited from its provisions. Hearings can be *investigative* in nature, particularly if Congress has received allegations of wrongdoing by public officials acting in an official capacity, or by private citizens who have engaged in activities that suggest the need for a legislative solution. The 115th Congress was engaged in such investigative hearings regarding potential Russian interference with the 2016 elections and the behavior of a number of Executive Cabinet officials and Presidential advisors.

Confirmation hearings are a somewhat unique aspect of the committee hearing process and can be conducted only by Senate committees. The U.S. Constitution in Article 7 provides for the President to nominate certain government officials with the advice and consent of the Senate, another opportunity for the system of checks and balances to occur. Although committees are not required to hold hearings before confirmation, a formerly routine confirmation process has become contentious and political. Confirmation hearings tend to be reserved for Supreme Court nominees or nominees to the President's Cabinet—positions with a great deal of authority and where the stakes are high. Since committee rules vary, the confirmation process may vary as well. At times, interest groups and the public express concerns about a confirmation and even hold protests, particularly in the case of appointments of Supreme Court Justices.

Markups in the Committee Process. If the subcommittee or committee decides to move a bill forward for further consideration, there is a process called *markup* that is run by the committee chair. The intent is to vote on amendments to the bill that the members of the Chamber want before recommending that the full Chamber pass the bill. Besides saving time when the bill reaches the floor, markups enable the removal of language that may be vague, unconstitutional, contentious, or otherwise less desirable. The committee concludes a markup not by voting on the bill as a whole, but by voting on a motion to have the bill reported to the Chamber with whatever amendments the committee has approved. A committee must have a majority present when the final vote occurs on the markup. Markups are usually open to the public, except in the case of matters of national security. Lobbyists, special interest groups, and others can be present during most markups and create pressure and tensions to ensure their favorite language is not marked for amendment or removal.

Committee Reports. One of the responsibilities of both House and Senate committees is that they create a report that accompanies each bill to the floor. The report is expected to contain the purpose and scope of the bill, any recommended amendments to the bill, and any changes to current law that would be in effect if the bill was to be adopted. The report provides the cost of the bill to the government (not necessarily to the public), the legislative intent of the bill, and often the position of the dissenting members of the committee. Interest groups and lobbyists have another opportunity in their engagement with the committee's staff to urge that more of their positions be included in the report, whether supporting or opposing the bill. Once the report is complete, the bill is *"reported out of committee"* by sending it to the members of the House or Senate.

Importance of the Speaker of the House and the Senate's President Pro Tempore

In the case of House bills, regardless of the desirability of the bill and its report, the *Speaker of the House* (leader of the majority party and presiding officer of the House) has the authority to determine what priority it receives on the calendar for seeing floor action. He or she controls the floor debate and is even free to speak to the debate. In the Senate, the *President Pro Tempore* is the presiding officer when the Vice President is unavailable, is elected by fellow Senators, and is usually the longest sitting member of the Senate.

A unique feature of the Senate is the ability to filibuster. Unlike the House, Senate rules support the absence of time limits on how long senators can speak to an issue or to a Supreme Court confirmation. Therefore, the strategy of creating a filibuster—a prolonged speech that prevents action but is not technically illegal—can be used to prevent an issue from coming to a vote. The record for speaking at a filibuster is 24 hours and 18 minutes by Senator Strom Thurmond in 1957 speaking against the Civil Rights Act. Current rules say a vote of 60 Senate members are required to stop a filibuster. In recent years, the power of the filibuster has been usurped by Senate majority leaders who have threatened to employ what has become termed the "nuclear option" to eliminate the ability of a minority party to filibuster. This first occurred in 2003 related to President George W. Bush trying to achieve confirmation of appeals court nominees. Since then, it has been invoked by Senator Harry Reid in 2013 on behalf of Senate Democrats for confirmation of lower court nominees, and more recently by Senator Mitch McConnell who required only a simple majority to achieve confirmation of Republican-supported Supreme Court nominees.

Control of a Bill's Progress on the Floor of the Chamber

The committee chair who brought the bill's report to the floor maintains control of the bill on the floor by managing the responses to colleagues' questions, deflecting unwanted amendments, and even building coalitions of support for the bill. At the same time, special interest groups continue to attempt to influence undecided legislators and gather support or opposition for a bill. Constituents of each legislator are urged to write letters, send emails, and otherwise contact them regarding their support or opposition. In a true democratic approach, all voices are heard, weighed, and considered. However, money and power are big influencers, and such factors may cast more weight than rationale and constituent members' opinions.

Once all the attempts to reconcile language and amendments have occurred, there are multiple forms by which members can vote. One may be a *voice vote* with answers "aye" or "nay" with the victory judged by hearing alone. Another is a *division vote*, by headcount. The third and most desirable to special interest groups, lobbyists, and others is a *recorded teller vote*, because it creates a retrievable record by which one can know how each member voted and can hold them accountable to this in future campaigns.

The Power of the Conference Committee

Both the House and the Senate must agree to pass identical bills or at least echo the same language. Usually House and Senate bills are not identical, so members of each Chamber must resolve the differences by meeting together in a *conference committee*. The test of political will to achieve a significant piece of legislation requires both parties to reach compromise, particularly difficult if the House and Senate are controlled by different parties. Appointees to the conference committee are often senior members of each bill's committee and well versed with the markup process. Although Congressional leaders find this frustrating, lobbyists and special interest groups grasp another opportunity to offer language that meets their agenda or to address controversial points such as funding or scope of the program. If and when compromise language is reached, the committee is responsible for a conference report that explains what changed in order to reconcile the differences. Then the identical bills are returned to the respective House and Senate for final votes of approval. The bill then goes to the President's desk, where the President can choose to:

- Do nothing, and after a certain number of days, the bill dies
- Sign the bill into law
- Veto the bill, which then requires an override vote of two-thirds of both the House and Senate voting in favor of the bill in order for it to become law

In most state legislatures, the process of achieving adoption of a bill can be similar. However, in some state legislatures, if the governor does not sign the bill voted on by the legislative body, it becomes law after a certain number of days.

The Impact of Compromise

Like most other compromise situations, the winner will be the lowest common denominator—the least disruptive language to the status quo that suits both House and Senate—or the language that has the greatest likelihood of support. This may mean that the intent of the original bills often gets diluted or that the ability to enforce the law upon implementation gets reduced. Having advocated for a bill, nurses have watched it arrive in front of the legislature and be adopted, only to recognize that the compromise version is overly restrictive, excludes some of the people it was designed to support, or lacks sufficient merit when it becomes law.

In 2018, the Virginia Commonwealth enacted legislation on full practice authority for advance practice registered nurses (APRNs) and particularly nurse practitioners (NPs). The NP community succeeded in getting language into a bill that would eliminate collaborative practice agreements with physicians. However, the physician community, led by a strong state medical society, eroded NP autonomy in the short term, trading those collaborative agreements for a minimum requirement of 10,000 hours of supervised advanced clinical practice before NPs could be deemed independent providers. Some argue that this was worse, whereas others believe that, in the long run, it creates a path to autonomy. Devising strategies to reduce the 10,000 hours in future legislatures will be important to shortening that path.

THE REGULATORY PROCESS

Although Congress may have passed a law, it remains for others to develop the rules and regulations that will provide for a fair and equitable implementation process. The executive and judicial branches become heavily engaged in this process. In many cases, the implementation occurs within one of the many federal agencies designed for that purpose. In some cases, a new agency or program entity will be required in order to initiate a process of implementation. Once authorized, the new agency of program will carry out implementation if funds are appropriated, although Congress can limit the amount to be spent in the rule-making process. Staff and resources are allocated to the rule-making process, in accordance with the spending limits. If a program has been authorized but no money has been appropriated for its implementation, then that program or provision cannot be carried out.

A variety of entities are used to provide oversight for the implementation of a law. Branch level oversight for Implementation includes:

- *Executive oversight*: Central to policy implementation, it includes the Departments of Health and Human

Services (including the U.S. Food and Drug Administration [FDA] and Centers for Medicare and Medicaid Services [CMS]), Justice, and Environmental Protection.

- *Legislative oversight*: The Legislative Reorganization Act of 1946 ensured that implementing organizations adhere to the intent of congressional action. This oversight aims to improve efficiency, effectiveness, and economy of government organizations and assesses the ability of organizations to manage and accomplish implementation, include investigating instances of waste, fraud, dishonesty, or arbitrary actions.
- *Judicial oversight*: Federal Administrative Law Judges (certified by Office of Personnel Management (OPM) serve as referees for many areas of implementation.

What Is a Rule?

The Administrative Procedure Act of 1946 defines a *rule* as "the whole or part of an agency statement of general or particular applicability and future effect designed to implement, interpret or prescribe law or policy" (Longest, 2016, p. 223). Rule making is a complex process which, by law, includes the public. No regulation or rule can be final without a formal proposed set of rules being made public with adequate provisions and timing for the public to access, review, and submit public comment. This is true at both state and federal levels. Proposed rules may be brief (only a few pages) but they may also be extremely lengthy. CMS indicates that it publishes over 10,750 pages of rules and regulations annually. The rule proposed to implement the ACA included over 2000 pages and the number of submitted comments were more than 100,000. CMS read each one and responded within the revised rules to the comments, either collectively or singly, depending upon the frequency of the comment.

The Federal Register Act of 1935 stipulated at the federal level that the responsible agency must post the language in the *Federal Register* (www.federalregister.gov), a daily publication (comment period 30 to 120 days). It includes information on the notice, date of notice, agency providing the notice, comment period, and the proposed or final rule or responses. All Federal proposed rules are also posted at www.regulations.gov. The process for posting public comments is identified there. In addition, the Unified Agenda of Federal Regulatory and Deregulatory Actions (http://reginfo.gov), published twice a year in the *Federal Register*, contains a historical database and searchable tools relative to the proposed rules.

The Rule-Making Process

The overall process for implementation of a statute is shown in Box 39.3. One would think that the finalization of implementation would be straightforward, but it is not.

Challenges in rule making can stall this process. First, new laws often lack sufficient specificity to guide full implementation. In order to get to passage, the process of markup and compromise between House and Senate or state level Chambers may have left a piece of legislation with clauses that remain vague or contentious about what is actually meant or intended. The language may even be in conflict with existing laws, leading to confusion on the part of those they are intended to help, as well as those expected to operate in that space. Second, a new statute may undergo judicial review before proposed rules can be written. That review will include evaluation of language in other statutes that would preclude what has just been passed. For example, amendments to the Constitution will prohibit something passed by Congress that could be constituted as discriminatory. Although one would hope that the review of the legislation before passage would avoid this pitfall, there is no question that many, if not all, final legislation creates unintended consequences. Third, the process of compromise may leave a new law with few teeth in terms of enforcement of the regulation.

Many existing laws and their regulations require either periodic reauthorization of the statute in order for the rules to continue or an annual review and proposed modification of the rules, such as with the Inpatient Prospective Payment System (IPPS) ruling and the Vaccine Injury Compensation Program.

Influencing Rule Making

The importance of nurses providing public comments on proposed rules and revisions cannot be overstated. Nurses can articulate how the rule supports or negates the intent of the legislation; propose alternative language to support inclusion; clarify the operational issues that might confound implementation; let policymakers know that the proposed rule is supported by your group or constituency; provide data that can support the comment; and go on record in support or opposition of proposed language. Attention to the language used to define a provider or a clinician, for instance, can mean the difference between an APRN getting reimbursed for care or allowed to participate as a provider by Medicare or a registered nurse being able to document the presence or absence of vital signs in a terminally ill hospice patient. Nurses with direct care expertise can identify when some details within a rule become obsolete or are no longer applicable; when technology may render language inappropriately restrictive; or when the details of a rule may have the unintended consequence of creating a barrier to those intended to be helped. These may be large or small changes, but they matter to the patients for whom the rule intends to serve.

Even though most nurses focus on comment submissions to federal agencies, there are many other entities with *deemed authority*—that is, they serve as a proxy for the federal agency to extend its reach in order to ensure some level of uniformity of service or performance. These include the National Committee on Quality Assurance; The Joint Commission; The Leapfrog Group; and National Quality Forum. These deemed entities have processes for publishing proposed rules and encouraging health professionals to review and comment on proposed rules that affect the accreditation or other status of the organization applying to them for a credential.

The Enforcement of Regulations

Regulatory enforcement is a key aspect of sound legislation and rule making. Unfortunately, some laws may be passed with little or no enforcement language included. Enforcement becomes a matter of the specificity or vagueness of the law, the consequences for failure to comply, how rules are written, and the criteria and enforceability of deemed entities such as The Joint Commission. Enforcement is dependent upon sound data collection that can demonstrate whether the regulations are being followed and even whether they are enforceable. To the extent that regulations are standard setting, enforcement requires some expectations of compliance and methods for monitoring and measuring such. Health care agencies that take some level of responsibility for the various aspects of enforcement include: Federal Trade Commission (FTC); FDA, Centers for Disease Control and Prevention (CDC); CMS; United States Agency for Toxic Substances and Disease Registry; the Environmental Protection Agency; the Division of Health Care Quality and Outcomes in the Office of The Assistant Secretary for Planning and Evaluation; and deemed authority entities.

Even when agency enforcement has clear authority, it can be complicated to ensure compliance. For example, in May of 2018, the FDA and FTC acted against companies misleading children with e-liquids containing nicotine that resemble children's juice boxes, candies, and cookies. As part of the FDA's new Youth Tobacco Prevention Plan and a joint effort to protect youth from dangers of nicotine and tobacco products, they issued warning letters to 13 manufacturers, distributors, and retailers selling e-liquids used in e-cigarettes with labeling and/or advertising that cause them to resemble kid-friendly food products. Several of the companies receiving warning letters were also cited for illegally selling the products to minors (FDA, 2018).

In other action, the FTC has been called upon by APRNs to weigh in on restraint of trade issues in states such as Florida, where scope of practice statutes are restrictive. Again, warning letters to leaders in medicine and the state medical society were issued, but this has had little effect on Florida's APRN scope of practice and autonomy.

Other examples demonstrate a more effective means of enforcement. Cases of fraud have been successfully addressed by CMS (CMS Report to Congress, June 2014). The Fraud Prevention System (FPS) is the state-of-the-art predictive analytics technology required under the Small Business Jobs Act of 2010 (SBJA). Since June 30, 2011, the FPS has run predictive algorithms and other sophisticated analytics nationwide against all Medicare fee-for-service (FFS) claims prior to payment. In the second implementation year, which aligned with Fiscal Year 2013, CMS took administrative action against 938 providers and suppliers due to the FPS. Reduction in fraudulent charges due to FPS was $210.7 million, almost double the amount identified during the first year of the program. This resulted in more than a $5 to $1 return on investment.

The Role of Courts in Regulation

The U.S. Supreme Court, in *Marbury vs Madison* in 1803, asserted its power to declare a law unenforceable if found to violate the Constitution. The power of judicial review gives courts a role in public policy—the right of courts to affirm or strike down laws. A well-recognized example might be found in the ACA, which called for everyone with an income below 133% of the federal poverty level (FPL) to be eligible for Medicaid. States failing to comply could be excluded from federal Medicaid funding. Instead, the Supreme Court said the penalty was too severe and it could have the effect of coercing states into implementing the Medicaid expansion. As a consequence, Medicaid expansion became voluntary and not all states opted in.

Another influence on regulation and policy by the courts is that of precedence and the concept of *stare decisis*—Let the Decision Stand. Judicial precedence allows for adhering to previous findings in cases with substantially comparable facts and circumstances. The courts can grant deference to their prior ruling, rather than hear a comparable case again. However, courts can overrule prior decisions, but only depart from precedent based upon compelling and clearly articulated reasons. Courts also can define limitations on governmental power to restrict or deny the rights of the citizens. The 14th Amendment has the effect of applying these rights to the actions of the state governments. Laws passed by Congress must be consistent with the Constitution. Laws passed by a state must be consistent with the U.S. Constitution and the state's constitution.

For more information on the role of the courts in policymaking, see Chapter 45.

CONCLUSION

Nurses individually and collectively can influence policymaking, whether through the passage of legislation or the implementation of a law through regulations. Nurses as educators, as direct care providers, and as managers and leaders have great potential to influence what gets on policymakers' agendas, which policy solutions are offered in legislation, the passage of bills, and the implementation of laws. The legislative process is often referred to as "sausage making," as what goes into the process rarely comes out looking the same. It's a reflection of the multiple points influencing what happens to a bill. Once passed, the rulemaking process becomes equally important. Knowledge of both processes is necessary for advancing nursing's policy agenda.

DISCUSSION QUESTIONS

1. Select a health-related bill on the federal or state level that's of interest to you. What is its likely trajectory through the legislature and how might you influence its passage?

2. Identify an unintended consequence of a bill you saw proposed, passed, and implemented.

3. Review a proposed rule (CMS, Joint Commission, or other entity) and the public comments submitted by nurses. Would you agree or disagree with the comments and why?

REFERENCES

Centers for Medicare and Medicaid Services. (2014). *CMS report to Congress: Fraud prevention system second implementation year*. Baltimore, MD: Centers for Medicare and Medicaid Services. Retrieved from www.cms.gov/About-CMS/Components/CPI/Widgets/Fraud_Prevention_System_2ndYear.pdf.

Heitshusen, V. (2017.) *Committee types and roles*. Congressional Research Service, 98-241. Washington, DC. Congressional Research Service. Retrieved from www.senate.gov/CRSpubs/312b4df4-9797-41bf-b623-a8087cc91d74.pdf .

Kingdon, J.W. (2003). *Agendas, alternatives, and public policies* (2nd edition). New York: Addison-Wesley Educational Publishers.

Longest, B.B. (2016). *Health policymaking in the United States* (6th edition). Chicago: Health Administration Press.

U.S. Food and Drug Administration (2018, May 1). *FDA news release: FDA, FTC take action against companies misleading kids with e-liquids that resemble children's juice boxes, candies and cookies*. Silver Spring, MD: Food and Drug Administration. Retrieved from https://www.fda.gov/NewsEvents/Newsroom/PressAnnouncements/ucm605507.htm.

ONLINE RESOURCES

Federal Register
www.federalregister.gov
Federal Regulations
www.regulations.gov
U.S. Congress
www.congress.gov

40

Lobbying Policymakers: Individual and Collective Strategies

Lauren M. Inouye[a]

"Okay, you've convinced me. Now go out and bring pressure on me."

Franklin D. Roosevelt

Known for propelling new social programs and projects comprising The New Deal, President Franklin D. Roosevelt found himself in an era of change for the American people and, with it, throngs of stakeholders urging him to move this new initiative forward. As the story goes, while entertaining an audience of such individuals, he declared, "Okay, you've convinced me. Now go on out and bring pressure on me" (Kaye, 2014, p. 54). Roosevelt's realization that an evidence-based, intellectual case for changing policy often proves to be insufficient in bringing about change on its own. Instead, channeling the political pressures of key stakeholders and wielding the public's passion for change was—in Roosevelt's mind—essential to moving the policy paradigm.

Fast forward to the 21st century: a different timeframe, but one of sweeping change. In late 2016–2017, the landscape of federal health care policy was fraught with uncertainty about the future of the Patient Protection and Affordable Care Act (ACA). This landmark policy of the Obama Administration passed in 2010 and had made significant, albeit imperfect, progress in increasing coverage for individuals across the country. Interest groups including, but not limited to, the insurance industry, the pharmaceutical industry, employers, and health care providers were scrambling to bend the ear of policymakers to ensure that any impending change to the existing law would protect their piece of the policy pie. Lobbyists were essential strategists for these interest groups in navigating the rapid, ever-changing political waters.

Where was the nursing profession in these conversations and negotiations? National nursing organizations, such as the American Nurses Association (ANA), the American Association of Colleges of Nursing, and many representing the advanced practice registered nurse (APRN) community urged Congress to preserve the ability for current law to ensure access to care for patients in all corners of the country. Like their counterparts in the health professions sector, nursing organizations deployed their lobbyists to carry this sentiment to members of the U.S. House of Representatives and Senate. Ultimately, due largely in part to acute, partisan divide and vocal stakeholders (including lobbyists), Congress failed to pass comprehensive legislation to repeal and/or replace the ACA.

In this chapter, we will explore the role of lobbying and compare similarities and differences between advocacy/advocates and lobbying/lobbyists. Athough both entities are critical to the democratic process, there are times when one is more effective than the other. Lobbyists must adhere to strict professional regulations that aim to prevent unsavory practices, particularly when the issues they advance have major societal and economic ramifications. Athough nurses are key advocates who have a professional responsibility to be politically aware and engaged, lobbyists can be instrumental in moving the needle forward on issues that impact our nation's health care and the policies that drive nursing practice.

NURSES: ADVOCATES OR LOBBYISTS?

Nurses advocate for their patients every day. Whether collaborating with the health care team to ensure a patient's plan of care is appropriate, connecting patients and families

---

[a]This chapter updates a previous chapter originally developed by Kenya Beard, PhD, RN, and draws upon that excellent work.

to community resources, or teaching a patient during discharge planning, nurses utilize a set of interpersonal skills that lend them to be natural advocates. So why is it that nurses and the nursing profession often struggle to align themselves with political advocacy and lobbying? Political competence and advocacy are not merely exercised in times of national discourse; rather, they are a professional responsibility that ought to be woven throughout one's nursing career.

Approximately 4 million registered nurses (RNs) and APRNs comprise the largest sector of the health care workforce in the United States (ANA, 2019). Yet, a relatively small proportion engage in political advocacy. An even smaller proportion of those truly "lobby." Nurses who do lobby professionally at the state and federal levels are typically employed under a consulting firm, or are employed as in-house lobbying staff for a professional health care or nursing organization. It should be noted, however, that most the majority of most individuals who serve as lobbyists for state and national nursing organizations do not have a nursing degree, but rather have professional backgrounds in public policy, law, and public affairs/communication, among others. Recognizing that very few nurses become registered lobbyists, the bigger emphasis should be on increasing the number of nurses who serve as advocates (further discussion comparing advocacy to lobbying follows in this chapter).

It should come as no surprise that the public holds the nursing profession in high regard. According to Gallup, from 2002 to 2018, nurses were ranked as the most honest and ethical profession in the eyes of the American people (Brenan, 2018). Although 84% of Americans polled rated nurses as "very high" or "high" in describing their ethics, 58% rated Congress as "very low" or "low." This perception of nurses lends the profession a natural platform on which to advocate for positive changes that improve health. More specifically, nurses should have the ear of legislators who dictate policies that impact health care delivery.

And yet, despite the public's adulation, a chasm exists between the perception of nurses as the trusted backbone of the health care system and the perception of nurses as change agents in the policy arena. In a 2010 Gallup survey commissioned by the Robert Wood Johnson Foundation, opinion leaders' responses regarding nursing as a trusted profession reflected that of the annual public Gallup poll. However, when asked about nurses as agents of change, the sentiment of the opinion leaders pivoted. Only 18% of respondents believed that nurses have a "great deal" of influence in increasing access to primary care, for example (Gallup, 2010, p. 7). When asked what nurses can do in order to increase their influence in transforming health care, respondents rated "making their voices heard/increased input" as the top solution (Gallup, 2010, p. 9).

The call to action for nursing to exert its influence is further echoed in the Institute of Medicine's (IOM's) (now the National Academy of Medicine) 2011 monumental report *Future of Nursing: Leading Change, Advancing Health*, which highlighted a set of recommendations to position the nursing profession to be integral in improving health. More specifically, it includes the recommendations for the profession and its collaborators to "expand opportunities for nurses to lead and diffuse collaborative improvement efforts" and "prepare and enable nurses to lead change and advance health" (IOM, 2011).

IS IT LOBBYING, ADVOCACY, OR BOTH?

Although much of the public dialogue centers on nurses as advocates, it is essential to take a deeper exploration into lobbying. Understanding the relationship between advocacy and lobbying, and how lobbying serves as an effective strategy for influencing policy outcomes, will provide you with a clearer picture on why and when lobbying and employing the services' lobbyists may be an appropriate advocacy strategy.

You may be familiar with the old mathematical adage that based on the characteristics defining a square versus those defining a rectangle, a square is a type of rectangle, but a rectangle cannot be defined as a square (for in order to be a square, a quadrilateral's sides all must be of equal length). Under this conditional framework, we can make the assertion that lobbying (a square) is a form of advocacy (a rectangle), but advocacy is not necessarily lobbying (Fig. 40.1). Advocacy is the broader umbrella term that encompasses multiple strategies to influence policy, including lobbying. Using this logic, all lobbyists are by nature also advocates, but not all advocates can be termed as lobbyists. Although no single definition of "advocacy" serves as the gold standard, phrases such as "supporting a cause," "leveraging political resources," and "the act of influencing an outcome" are frequently used as descriptors.

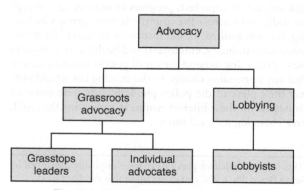

Fig. 40.1 Advocacy can take many forms.

The act of lobbying can also be described using these terms, but the lobbying profession is subject to a set of standards and regulations to which lobbyists, and potentially their clients, must adhere. The U.S. House of Representatives and Senate have a set of policies regulating federal lobbying referred to as the Lobbying Disclosure Act (House of Representatives, n.d.). The law requires regular reporting of lobbying activities and provides clarification around what actions constitute those activities. For the purposes of this chapter, we will examine lobbying at the federal level (it should be noted, however, that many of the skill sets employed by lobbyists apply at both the state and federal levels).

As can be the case with an advocate, there is no single professional track toward becoming a lobbyist. Generally, lobbyists are valued for their ability to network and create relationships, to communicate effectively (both verbally and written), to analyze policy, and strategize on how best to advance legislation, a regulation, or other policy issue while navigating a fluid political environment. Lobbyists must also have an innate understanding of the legislative process so that they know when to act and how strongly.

Both advocates and lobbyists must understand how to "talk the talk" of the policymakers they are attempting to influence. Nursing advocates should be wary of using medical jargon that can detract from the quality of meeting conversation and potentially turn off policymakers from taking action because they do not understand how the issue at hand relates to their constituents. For example, a nursing advocate who is asking their federal Representative to support disease-specific research funding gets too caught up in explaining a complex medical diagnosis rather than making the case as to how the funding will advance research that will benefit that Representative's constituents. Advocates should be aware of how the political climate may advance or hinder their policy request, but their knowledge is usually more "big picture."

Lobbyists, on the other hand, have a more intimate understanding of how relationships between politicians might influence an issue's outcome. For example, through the relationships they have built with members of Congress and their staff, lobbyists often have more first-hand insights into how well a Chairman and Ranking Member of the same congressional committee are willing to work across the aisle to advance a common issue, despite being from different political parties.

PUBLIC SENTIMENT OF LOBBYISTS

A long-favored DC fable tells of the days when President Ulysses S. Grant would find refuge at the upscale Willard Hotel across from the White House, where he would sit and enjoy his favorite brandy and a cigar in the lobby. Petitioners, realizing the President would regularly spend evenings there, would meet with President Grant—hence the origin of the term "lobbyists." Whether or not the story is true, the scenario of an individual representing a special interest appealing to a policymaker is at its core lobbying. Simply put, professional lobbyists are employed as strategists to achieve a desired policy or political outcome.

Today, lobbyists can be found in virtually every industry. Their role in influencing policies that have major social implications has gained greater visibility, and in some instances, drawn even greater criticism. In the same Gallup poll in which respondents ranked nurses as the most honest and ethical profession, lobbyists ranked last (Brenan, 2018). Similarly, part of President Trump's 2016 campaign platform included his promise to "drain the swamp" of the lobbyists he believed had a chokehold over Capitol Hill in DC. Although not a new sentiment from candidates for public office, it has echoed through the media and within citizen groups who warn against the trickle-down effect that lobbyists and campaign contributions have on policy decisions impacting the American people.

In reality, lobbyists are instrumental in building relationships with policymakers in the legislative and executive branches, providing guidance to the interest groups they represent, and serving as a liaison between the two. If they are lobbying Congress or the Administration, their responsibilities may include: attending federal hearings and briefings to gather issue-specific information; working with Congressional staff on the development of legislation; connecting with stakeholders who have a common policy goal and strategize on how to work collaboratively to achieve that goal, such as creating a messaging campaign; responding to calls for public comments on regulations stemming from federal departments and agencies; and preparing clients to have informed, solution-oriented conversations with policymakers. Although certain industries may come under severe public scrutiny for their lobbying efforts, we must not forget that a widerange of professional and business sectors, including health professions, utilize lobbyists. For these reasons, they are an integral part of federal advocacy.

PROFESSIONAL STANDARDS AND REGULATIONS FOR LOBBYING

At the federal level, according to the Lobbying Disclosure Act, the U.S. House of Representatives and Senate require individuals who lobby to register with both chambers of Congress (House of Representatives Office of the Clerk, n.d.) and file quarterly reports detailing the issues they lobby, including any specific pieces of legislation or federal regulations.

Additionally, the Honest Leadership and Open Government Act of 2007 requires lobbyists to file semiannual reports of "certain contributions along with certification that the filer understands the gift and travel rules of both the House and Senate" (House of Representatives Office of the Clerk, n.d.). These regulations are in place to increase the level of transparency and accountability of lobbyists and the legal standards dictating what they may and may not do. For example, lobbyists must report how much, if any, financial contributions they have given to an elected official or candidate for public office twice per year, in January and July (House of Representatives Office of the Clerk, 2017). Any amount totaling $200 or more per reporting period must be included. Even if a lobbyist has not made any contributions, they must still file a report stating no contributions have been made. Moreover, the House and Senate ethics committees outline strict rules on what Representatives and Senators can and cannot receive as gifts from lobbyists (whether monetary or physical), as the act of gift-giving could be construed as trying to influence a legislator's policy actions.

Lobbyists may represent interest groups that operate or interface with a political action committee (PAC). A PAC is a committee that exists for the purposes of raising and spending money to influence political outcomes, namely campaigns and elections. PACs are typically established to "represent business, labor, or ideological interests" (Opensecrets.org, n.d.). For this reason, the money contributed to a particular PAC is solicited from individuals and organizations who have a vested interest in the candidates that PAC aim to have elected or defeated. In this sense, PACs work to ensure that the candidates who are elected are ones who stand the best chance of aligning with the policy interests of the contributors to that PAC. By law, PACs must adhere to regulations set forth by the Federal Election Commission (FEC). The FEC is an independent, regulatory agency charged with administering and enforcing federal campaign finance law with jurisdiction over the financing of campaigns for the U.S. House, Senate, Presidency, and the Vice Presidency. Its mission is "to protect the integrity of the federal, campaign-finance process by providing transparency and fairly enforcing and administering federal campaign finance laws" (FEC, n.d.).

Recent court cases, such as the 2010 Supreme Court case *SpeechNow.org v. Federal Election Commission*, continue to raise the national dialogue on the constitutionality of PACs and whether they disenfranchise interest groups and individuals who do not wield the same level of financial capital (Federal Election Commission [FEC], 2010). The creation of a newer type of PAC known as a super PAC resulted from this case as a workaround to the regulatory limitations of PACs. Super PACs "may raise unlimited sums of money from corporations, unions, associations and individuals, then spend unlimited sums to overtly advocate for or against political candidates. Unlike traditional PACs, super PACs are prohibited from donating money directly to political candidates, and their spending must not be coordinated with that of the candidates they benefit" (OpenSecrets.org, 2018b). In other words, the activities of super PACs may resemble those of regular PACs (developing media campaigns, sending out mailers, calling constituents), but they cannot do these in conjunction with a candidate's own campaign—the money streams must be kept separate. It is important to note that the FEC sets legal contribution limits on how much an individual, a candidate's committee, a PAC, or party committee can contribute in any given spending cycle (a 2-year period that coincides with the House of Representatives elections). Corporations, on the other hand, can raise and spend unlimited amounts to Super PACs (FEC, n.d.).

PAC dollars can also support the ability for lobbyists to advocate on behalf of the PAC's interests. For example, a common tactic that political candidates employ is hosting a dinner, reception, or outing that requires a minimum donation in order to attend. These events typically convene a smaller, selective group of donors. A PAC representing the interests of organization X can allocate money to cover the cost of having organization X's lobbyist attend the event, thus receiving facetime with that candidate in hopes to build a working relationship and discuss the policy issues of importance to organization X.

NURSING AND CAMPAIGN CONTRIBUTIONS

What is nursing's presence in the campaign contribution scene? Table 40.1 highlights the four national nursing organizations with the largest PACs, the amount they each contributed during the 2017–2018 election cycle, and the breakdown where the contributions were allocated by political party (Opensecrets.org, 2018a).

As previously mentioned, there are over 4 million RNs in the United States. With these four national organizations representing only a portion of the nursing workforce (with varying rates of membership actually giving to their organization's PAC), there remains a significant, untapped portion of nurses who do not engage in this form of advocacy. Compared to other health professions, particularly the physician community, nurses do not employ the full strength of their ability to contribute, despite the large size of the workforce.

ADVOCACY AND YOU: CONNECTING WITH YOUR LEGISLATORS

While it is important to understand how professional lobbying impacts the policy process, it is equally, if not more important, for you to understand your role as a constituent

TABLE 40.1 Nursing Organizations' PACs: 2018 Funding Cycle

	Total Amount Spent	Total Contributed to Federal Candidates	% Contributed to Republicans	% Contributed to Democrats
American Association of Nurse Anesthetists	$1,134,579	$718,056	50	49
American Association of Nurse Practitioners	$580,901	$386,500	47	53
American Nurses Association	$479,354	$257,500	18	82
American College of Nurse-Midwives	$78,488	$41,500	37	63

Source: Opensecrets.org, 2018a.
Note: "Total Amount Spent" column includes amounts in "Total Contributed to Federal Candidates" plus other contributions to other PACs, committees, parties, and coalitions.
PAC, Political action committee.

and nursing advocate. Legislative offices are bombarded with constituent requests on a daily basis. This is a pillar of our democracy; citizens hold those elected into public office accountable for making decisions that will improve our society. Members of Congress and their staff make it a priority and pride themselves on being accessible to their constituents. In addition to their legislative responsibilities (e.g., crafting bills, sitting on Congressional committees, voting), Senators and Representatives understand that being responsive to constituents is not just core to their role, but is essential to upholding a positive public image that carries tremendous weight at the voting booth. Recall the discussion earlier in this chapter about the public's perception of nurses as highly ethical and trustworthy? You may or may not be surprised to learn that while 84% of those surveyed rated nurses as "high/very high" in relation to those attributes, only 8% felt the same way about members of Congress (Brenan, 2018). From this vantage point, nurse advocates can wield a respected and powerful voice. Connecting with policymakers affords advocates a number of opportunities to advance their issues.

MEETING IN PERSON

According to the Congressional Management Foundation (2017), in a survey that collected opinions from over 1200 high-ranking Congressional staff over a 10-year period, respondents repeatedly reported that in-person meetings with constituents would have "some" or "a lot" of influence on lawmakers (99% responded this way in 2004; 97% in 2010; 94% in 2015). Face-to-face meetings with legislators or their staff allow advocates to provide the human side of their policy request. Although empirical data and evidence are critical to building a policy case, it is the human story

behind why a policy outcome matters that often tips the scales in an advocate's favor.

Patient-advocacy groups are a great example of stakeholders who understand the power of their presence on Capitol Hill. Patients and their families can make their case first-hand as to why their request, whether increased funding for research and development, changing Medicare and Medicaid policies to cover medical expenses, or raising awareness about a disease/condition, should be adopted. They can relay their personal struggles and elevate the humanity in a policy scenario that could otherwise be reduced to dollars and cents.

WRITTEN COMMUNICATIONS

Since it is not realistic to expect all advocates to make in-person meetings with their legislators, if done well, written materials can serve as powerful tools. These are often referred to as "leave-behind" materials by advocates and Congressional staff. One common leave-behind is a legislative brief, or "one-pager." Because Congressional staff can be overwhelmed by letters, reports, and memos, making your leave-behind materials stand out is a must. Remember, you will want to be clear and concise in your request. If you are asking your Senators or Representative to co-sponsor a bill, they or their staff must be able to understand:
- How this bill would change current law
- What stakeholders, like patient advocacy organizations, support the bill
- Why this bill is worth supporting

The "why this bill is worth supporting" is a natural avenue to offer personal insights or provide the "face" behind the data and evidence.

WRAP-UP

Although both the advocate and the professional lobbyist are instrumental in advancing policies that improve health and health care delivery, it is important to be able to differentiate between the two. Individuals, including nurses, can serve as powerful advocates. Lobbyists, who are also advocates, are beholden to professional standards and federal regulations. Lobbyists and lobbying activities will continue to shape national dialogues on whether current regulations need to be changed and to what extent should lobbying influence the policy process. Nurses are by nature strong advocates for the patients and should be further engaged in political advocacy as a matter of professional responsibility. Understanding how to effectively communicate with policymakers helps achieve desired policy outcomes.

DISCUSSION QUESTIONS

1. How do national nursing organizations help elevate the political voice of the individual nurse?
2. What issues on the national policy agenda are closely tied to lobbying efforts? How do you think policy decisions would differ if lobbying were not an influencing factor?
3. What are some examples of how a lobbyist for a professional nursing organization works with nursing advocates on any given health care–related issue?

REFERENCES

American Nurses Association. (2019). *Practice policy: Workforce*. Retrieved from www.nursingworld.org/practice-policy/workforce/.

Brenan, M. (2018). *Nurses again outpace other professions for honesty, ethics*. Retrieved from https://news.gallup.com/poll/245597/nurses-again-outpace-professions-honesty-ethics.aspx.

Congressional Management Foundation. (2017). *Citizen-centric advocacy: The untapped power of constituent engagement*. Retrieved from www.congressfoundation.org/projects/communicating-with-congress/citizen-centric-advocacy-2017

Federal Election Commission. (2010). *Citizens United vs. FEC (Supreme Court)*. Retrieved from www.fec.gov/updates/citizens-united-v-fecsupreme-court/.

Federal Election Commission. (n.d.) *Contributions limits for 2017-2018 federal elections*. Retrieved from https://transition.fec.gov/info/contriblimitschart1718.pdf.

Gallup. (2010). *Nursing leadership from bedside to boardroom: Opinion leaders' perceptions*. Retrieved from www.rwjf.org/content/dam/farm/reports/reports/2010/rwjf53344.

House of Representatives Office of the Clerk. (2017). *Lobbying disclosure act guidance*. Retrieved from https://lobbyingdisclosure.house.gov/amended_lda_guide.html#section7.

House of Representatives Office of the Clerk. (n.d.). *Lobbying disclosure*. Retrieved from https://lobbyingdisclosure.house.gov.

Institute of Medicine. (2011). *The future of nursing: Leading change, advancing health report recommendations*. Retrieved from www.nationalacademies.org/hmd/~/media/Files/Report%20Files/2010/The-Future-of-Nursing/Future%20of%20Nursing%202010%20Recommendations.pdf.

Journal of Nursing Regulation. (2016). The 2015 national nursing workforce survey executive summary. *Journal of Nursing Regulation, 7*(1), 4-6.

Kaye, H.J. (2014). *The fight for the four freedoms: What made FDR and the greatest generation truly great*. New York: Simon & Schuster.

Opensecrets.org. (2018a). *Nurses*. Retrieved from www.opensecrets.org/industries/indus.php?ind=H1710.

Opensecrets.org. (2018b). *Super PACs*. Retrieved from www.opensecrets.org/pacs/superpacs.php.

Opensecrets.org. (n.d.). *What is a PAC?* Retrieved from https://www.opensecrets.org/pacs/pacfaq.php.

U.S. Department of Labor Bureau of Labor Statistics. (2018). *Occupational employment and wages news release*. Retrieved from https://www.bls.gov/news.release/ocwage.htm.

ONLINE RESOURCES

Gallup Nurses Keep Healthy Lead as Most Honest, Ethical Profession
https://news.gallup.com/poll/224639/nurses-keep-healthy-lead-honest-ethical-profession.aspx

Open Secrets (explore campaign contributions from PACs)
www.opensecrets.org

Oyez (read about *Citizens United vs. FEC*)
www.oyez.org/cases/2008/08-205

41

Political Activity: Different Rules for Government Employees

Kathleen E. Sykes

> *"Government of the people, by the people, for the people, shall not perish from the Earth."*
>
> *Gettysburg Address*

During the birth of our country, following the Revolutionary War, political discussion surrounded how much control the federal government should have over its citizens. Federalists (Alexander Hamilton and James Madison) sought strong central control of government, and Anti-Federalists (Samuel Adams, George Mason, and Patrick Henry) strove to protect personal liberties and rights by limiting a concentration of power at the federal level and advocating for state and local government control (Fuller, 2014).

In 1791, the United States Constitution was adopted along with 10 amendments that constitute the Bill of Rights. The First Amendment was designed to limit government power and to protect individual liberties, including freedom of speech.

> Congress shall make no law respecting an establishment of religion, or prohibiting the free exercise thereof; or abridging the freedom of speech, or the press; or the right of the people peaceably to assemble, and to petition the government for a redress of grievances. (U.S. Const. amend. I)

But despite the broad protection of the First Amendment, government employees have had their rights restricted to protect them from coercion and prevent cronyism and political favoritism. Efforts to restrict political activities by government employees date back to the formation of the United States. President George Washington was among those who were concerned about politicizing the civil service (Bloch, 2005).

HISTORY OF EFFORTS TO RESTRICT POLITICAL ACTIVITIES OF GOVERNMENT EMPLOYEES

Jefferson Executive Order

About a decade after the U.S. Constitution was passed by Congress and ratified by the existing states, President Thomas Jefferson issued an Executive Order that addressed freedom of speech for government employees:

> The President of the United Stated has seen with dissatisfaction officers of the General Government taking on various occasions active parts in elections of the public functionaries, whether of the General or of the State Governments.... The right of any officer to give his vote at elections as a qualified citizen is not meant to be restrained, nor, however given, shall it have any effect to his prejudice; but it is expected that he will not attempt to influence the votes of others nor take any part in the business of electioneering, that being deemed inconsistent with the spirit of the Constitution and his duties to it. (Fuller, 2014)

We do not know how many federal employees were working in the Jefferson Administration. However, one could assume fewer than the first estimate for federal employees in 1940 when there were 699,000 civilian employees (U.S. Office of Personnel Management, 2014).

Pendleton Act: Precursor to the Hatch Act

The first law to restrict government employee political activity occurred with the enactment in 1883 of the Pendleton Civil Service Reform Act. It established that federal government jobs should be awarded based on merit as opposed to political affiliation and made it illegal to fire or demote government employees for political reasons. In addition, it prohibited the solicitation of campaign donations in the workplace on federal property (Pendleton Civil Service Reform Act, n.d.).

The Great Depression began in the U.S. in September of 1929 following the stock market crash on Black Tuesday, October 29, 1929. The unemployment rate rose to 25%, the highest rate in the 20th century (Great Depression, n.d.).

Franklin D. Roosevelt was elected president by a landslide in the fall of 1932 with his pledge for a new deal for the American people. Roosevelt believed that the way out of the depression was by the help of the federal government. The Works Progress Administration (WPA) was "by far the largest employer in the nation—had a payroll of 1.9 million. Other federal work programs provided jobs for another million" (Hamby, 2004, p. 418).

The WPA was the most visible of the relief programs and was criticized by conservatives who charged that the program was a "vote army" (Hamby, 2004, p.418). In the 1930s after the New Deal legislative bills had been enacted, both Republicans and conservative Democrats were angry that President Franklin Roosevelt had acquired too much power through the New Deal and the government jobs it created and that WPA employees were used by Democrats during the midterm election. Among the President's critics was a conservative Senator from New Mexico, Carl Hatch, who would later be the sponsor of the Act to Prevent Pernicious Political Activities (Fuller, 2014).

On January 5, 1939, President Roosevelt recommended that legislation was needed to address "improper political practices" in his request for additional funds for the WPA:

> It is my belief that improper political practices can be eliminated only by the imposition of rigid statutory regulations and penalties by the Congress, and that this should be done. Such penalties should be imposed not only upon persons within the administrative organization of the Works Progress Administration, but also upon outsiders who have in fact in many instances been the principal offenders in this regard. My only reservation in this matter is that no legislation should be enacted which will in any way deprive workers on the Works Progress Administration program of the civil rights to which they are entitled in common with other citizens. (Roosevelt & Rosenman, 1941)

Once the Hatch Act was enacted, it largely depoliticized the WPA (WPA, n.d.).

THE HATCH ACT: WHAT IS IT?

In 1939, Senator Hatch introduced legislation, now known as the Hatch Act, that limited certain political activities of federal employees, as well as some state, DC, and local government employees. At the same time, the Act protects employees from political coercion in the workplace and ensures that employees are promoted based on merit and not political affiliation. The law also ensures that federal programs are administered in a nonpartisan fashion (Hatch Act, n.d.).

AMENDMENTS TO THE HATCH ACT

Throughout the Hatch Act's almost 80-year history, it has been amended only four times—in 1940, 1974, 1993, and 2012. The following summarizes the changes adopted with passage of each of the amendments to the Hatch Act.

1940 Amendments

The 1940 Amendments to the Hatch Act were known as the Clean Politics Act. The Amendments set a limit of $5000 per year on individual contributions to a federal candidate or political committee. The limits apply to primary and general elections. However, the Amendments did not prohibit donations by an individual from contributing to multiple committees all working for the same candidate. Furthermore, individuals and businesses working for the federal government are prohibited from making contributions to federal candidates (Hatch Act, n.d.).

1974 Amendments

In 1974, the Federal Election Campaign Act (FECA) Amendments rolled back the Hatch Act provision with respect to state and local government employees, allowing them to run for office in non-partisan elections. The Hatch Act also revised the laws' prohibition of state and local government employees from taking "an active part in political management or political campaigns." Unlike federal employees, state and local employees were now able to campaign for and hold office in political organizations. A number of Supreme Court decisions (*Mitchell* and *Letter Carriers*) that challenged the constitutionality of the Hatch Act's limitation on free speech and due process and growing protests from the states as well as the Watergate incident may have contributed to the passage of the amendments that loosened restrictions in the Hatch Act for state and local employees (Bloch, 2005, p. 802).

1993 Amendments

President Clinton signed The Hatch Act Reform Amendments (HARA) of 1993, which permit federal employees and postal workers to manage campaigns, fundraise, and hold positions within political parties provided it is on their own time. It still prevents "Hatch Act-covered" employees from running for partisan political office and ensures that the federal workplace would remain off limits to partisan political activity (Bloch, 2005, pp. 805–807).

2012 Amendments

The Hatch Act Modernization Act was signed into law by President Barak Obama on December 28, 2012. The Modernization Act made three major changes: (1) modified penalties under the Act and provided the ability to remove an employee; (2) clarified that the Act applies to the District of Columbia employees (as was already the case for other state and local governments); and (3) prohibited state and local employees from running for public office to only those whose salary is paid entirely by federal loans or grants (Hatch Act, n.d.).

WHAT POLITICAL ACTIVITIES ARE PERMITTED AND PROHIBITED BY THE HATCH ACT?

What a Federal Employee Can and Cannot Do

The Hatch Act applies to all civilian part-time and full-time employees (including the U.S. Postal Service) in the executive branch of the federal government, except the President and the Vice President. Federal and District of Columbia employees are subject to the Act even when they are on annual leave, sick leave, leave without pay, or furlough. There is an exception for employees who work on an occasional or irregular basis or who are special government employees as defined in title 18 U.S.C. § 202 (a; such employees are subject to the restrictions only when they are engaged in government business). Federal employees fall within two categories under the Hatch Act, Further Restricted and Less Restricted. Most federal employees are categorized as "Less Restricted."

"Further Restricted" employees consist of employees in intelligence and enforcement-type agencies (except employees appointed by the President, by and with the advice and consent of the Senate). (U.S. Office of Special Counsel [OSC], 2018a).

Definition of Political Activity

Political activity is defined as "activity directed toward the success or failure of a political party, candidate for partisan office, or partisan political group" (5 C.F.R. Section 734.101) (Brown & Maskell, 2016).

Political Restrictions and Examples of Prohibited Activities

Further Restricted federal employees are prohibited from taking an active part in partisan political management or partisan political campaigns. Specifically, these employees may not campaign for or against candidates or otherwise engage in political activity in concert with a political party, a candidate for partisan political office, or a partisan political group. Such employees:

- May not be a candidate for nomination or election to public office in a partisan election.
- May not take an active part in partisan political campaigns. For example:
  - May not campaign for or against a candidate or slate of candidates.
  - May not make campaign speeches or engage in other campaign activities to elect partisan candidates.
  - May not distribute campaign material in partisan elections.
  - May not circulate nominating petitions.
- May not take an active part in partisan political management. For example:
  - May not hold office in political clubs or parties.
  - May not organize or manage political rallies or meetings.
  - May not assist in partisan voter registration drives.
- May not use their official authority or influence to interfere with or affect the result of an election. For example:
  - May not use their official titles or positions while engaged in political activity.
  - May not invite subordinate employees to political events or otherwise suggest to subordinates that they attend political events or undertake any partisan political activity.
- May not solicit, accept, or receive a donation or contribution for a partisan political party, candidate for partisan political office, or partisan political group. For example:
  - May not host a political fundraiser.
  - May not invite others to a political fundraiser.
  - May not collect contributions or sell tickets to political fundraising functions.
- May not engage in political activity (i.e., activity directed at the success or failure of a political party, candidate for partisan political office, or partisan political group) while the employee is on duty, in any federal room or building, wearing a uniform or official insignia, or using any federally owned or leased vehicle. For example:
  - May not wear or display partisan political buttons, T-shirts, signs, or other items.
  - May not make political contributions to a partisan political party, candidate for partisan political office, or partisan political group.
  - May not post a comment to a blog or a social media site that advocates for or against a partisan political

party, candidate for partisan political office, or partisan political group.

- May not use any e-mail account or social media to distribute, send, or forward content that advocates for or against a partisan political party, candidate for partisan political office, or partisan political group.

Permitted Activities

As discussed, Further Restricted federal employees are prohibited from taking an active part in partisan political management or partisan political campaigns. Specifically, these employees may not campaign for or against candidates or otherwise engage in political activity in concert with a political party, a candidate for partisan political office, or a partisan political group. However, such employees, for example:

- May register and vote as they choose.
- May assist in nonpartisan voter registration drives.
- May participate in campaigns where none of the candidates represent a political party.
- May contribute money to political campaigns, political parties, or partisan political groups.
- May attend political fundraising functions.
- May attend political rallies and meetings.
- May join political clubs or parties.
- May sign nominating petitions.
- May campaign for or against referendum questions, constitutional amendments, or municipal ordinances.
- May be a candidate for public office in a nonpartisan election.
- May express opinions about candidates and issues. If the expression is political activity, however—i.e., activity directed at the success or failure of a political party, candidate for partisan political office, or partisan political group—then the expression is not permitted while the employee is on duty, in any federal room or building, while wearing a uniform or official insignia, or using any federally owned or leased vehicle (U.S. OSC, 2018a).

State and Local and District of Columbia Government Workers

The following are examples of the types of programs that frequently receive financial assistance from the federal government: public health, public welfare, housing, urban renewal and area redevelopment, employment security, labor and industry training, public works, conservation, agricultural, civil defense, transportation, anti-poverty, and law enforcement programs. Hatch Act provisions also apply to employees of private, nonprofit organizations that plan, develop, and coordinate federal Head Start or Community Service Block Grant programs. State, DC, or local employees

subject to the Hatch Act continue to be covered while on annual leave and sick leave, as well as leave without pay, administrative leave, or furlough.

Who Is Not Covered

Hatch Act provisions do not apply to these state and local employees:

- individuals who exercise no functions in connection with federally financed activities; or
- individuals employed by educational or research institutions, establishments, or agencies that are supported in whole or in part by state or political subdivisions thereof, the District of Columbia, or by recognized religious, philanthropic, or cultural organizations (e.g., administrators, teachers).

The law also exempts certain specified employees from the prohibition on candidacy for elective office. These exemptions include:

1. The governor or lieutenant governor of a state or an individual authorized by law to act as governor
2. The mayor of a city
3. A duly elected head of an executive department of a state or municipality who is not classified under a state or municipal merit or civil service system
4. An individual holding public elective office (this exemption applies only when the elective office is the position which would otherwise subject the employee to the restriction of the Hatch Act)

Political Activities and Examples of Prohibited Activities

Covered state, District of Columbia, and local employees may not:

- Be candidates for public office in a partisan election.
- Use official authority or influence to interfere with or affect the results of an election or nomination.
- Directly or indirectly coerce, attempt to coerce, command, or advise a state, DC, or local officer or employee to pay, lend, or contribute anything of value to a party, committee, organization, agency, or person for political purposes.

State, District of Columbia, or local employees subject to the Hatch Act should note that an election is partisan if any candidate is to be nominated or elected as representing a political party (e.g., Democratic or Republican Party).

A note of caution: An employee's conduct is also subject to the laws of the state and the regulations of the employing agency. Prohibitions of the Hatch Act are not affected by state, District of Columbia, or local laws" (U.S. OSC, 2018a).

U.S. DEPARTMENT OF DEFENSE REGULATIONS ON POLITICAL ACTIVITY

Restrictions regarding political behavior of nurses in the U.S. Army, Navy, and Air Force, including those serving in the National Guard or Reserve status, are similar to those in the Hatch Act. The DoD Directive 1344.10 (Department of Defense [DoD], 2008) prohibits any activity that may be viewed as associating the DoD with a partisan political cause or candidate. The Directive further states that activities not expressly prohibited may be contrary to the spirit and intent of the directive.

Nurses in the armed forces may:

- Register, vote, and express a personal opinion on political candidates and issues but not as a representative of the Armed Forces.
- Promote and encourage others to exercise their voting franchise if such promotion does not constitute use of their official authority or influence to interfere with the outcome of any election.
- Join a partisan or nonpartisan political club and attend its meetings when not in uniform, subject to the restrictions of subparagraph 4.1.2.4. (See DoD Instruction 1334.1 (Reference [c]).
- Serve as an election official if such service is not as a representative of a partisan political party, does not interfere with the performance of military duties, is performed when not in uniform, and the Secretary concerned has given prior approval. The Secretary concerned may NOT delegate the authority to grant or deny such permission.
- Sign a petition for a specific legislative action or a petition to place a candidate's name on an official election ballot if the signing does not obligate the member to engage in partisan political activity and is done as a private citizen and not as a representative of the Armed Forces.
- Write a letter to the editor of a newspaper expressing the member's personal views on public issues or political candidates if such action is not part of an organized letter writing campaign or a solicitation of votes for or against a political party or partisan political cause or candidate. If the letter identifies the member as on active duty, the letter should clearly state that the views expressed are those of the individual only and not those of the DoD (or Department of Homeland Security for members of the Coast Guard).
- Make monetary contributions to a political organization, party, or committee favoring a particular candidate or slate of candidates, subject to the limitations under section 441a of title 2, United States Code (U.S.C.) (Reference [d]); section 607 of title 18, U.S.C. (Reference [e]); and other applicable law.
- Display a political bumper sticker on the member's private vehicle.
- Attend partisan and nonpartisan political fundraising activities, meetings, rallies, debates, conventions, or activities as a spectator when not in uniform and when no inference or appearance of official sponsorship, approval, or endorsement can reasonably be drawn.
- Participate fully in the Federal Voting Assistance Program.

A member of the Armed Forces on active duty shall not:

- Participate in partisan political fundraising activities, rallies, conventions, management of campaigns, or debates, either on one's own behalf or on that of another, without respect to uniform or inference or appearance of official sponsorship, approval, or endorsement.
- Use official authority or influence to interfere with an election, affect the course or outcome of an election, solicit votes for a specific candidate or issue, or require or solicit political contributions from others.
- Allow or cause to be published partisan political articles, letters, or endorsements signed or written by the member that solicits votes for or against a partisan political party, candidate, or cause.
- Serve in any official capacity with or be listed as a sponsor of a partisan political club.
- Speak before a partisan political gathering, including any gathering that promotes a partisan political party, candidate, or cause.
- Participate in any radio, television, or other program or group discussion as an advocate for or against a partisan political party, candidate, or cause.
- Conduct a political opinion survey under the auspices of a partisan political club or group or distribute partisan political literature.
- Perform clerical or other duties for a partisan political committee or candidate during a campaign, on an election day, or after an election day during the process of closing out a campaign.
- Solicit or otherwise engage in fundraising activities in federal offices or facilities, including military reservations, for any political cause or candidate.
- March or ride in a partisan political parade.
- Display a large political sign, banner, or poster (as distinguished from a bumper sticker) on a private vehicle.
- Display a partisan political sign, poster, banner, or similar device visible to the public at one's residence on a military installation, even if that residence is part of a privatized housing development.

- Participate in any organized effort to provide voters with transportation to the polls if the effort is organized by or associated with a partisan political party, cause, or candidate.
- Sell tickets for or otherwise actively promote partisan political dinners and similar fundraising events.
- Attend partisan political events as an official representative of the Armed Forces, except as a member of a joint Armed Forces color guard at the opening ceremonies of the national conventions of the Republican, Democratic, or other political parties recognized by the Federal Elections Committee or as otherwise authorized by the Secretary concerned.
- Make a campaign contribution to or receive or solicit (on one's own behalf) a campaign contribution from any other member of the Armed Forces on active duty.

NEW CHALLENGES TO THE HATCH ACT—SOCIAL MEDIA AND TELEWORK

In 2010, Congress enacted the Telework Enhancement Act that requires federal agencies to adopt telework policies (Brown & Maskell, 2016). The U.S. Office of Personnel Management in a report to Congress in November 2015 stated that telework programs had been expanded in both eligibility and participation. These workplace changes raise additional issues and challenges regarding the Hatch Act, which has a limited definition of workplace. For example, the Act prohibits "any political activity while on duty." The U.S. Code that lays out the regulations under the Act—5 U.S.C. Section 7324(a)—states, "Employees may not engage in political activity while (1) on duty, (2) in any room or building or holding of the Government, or any agency, (3) wearing a uniform or insignia identifying the office or position, or (4) using a vehicle owned or leased by the Government of the United States or any agency or instrumentality thereof."

Employees are considered on duty during any "time period when an employee is in a pay status other than leave, compensatory time off, credit hours, time off for an incentive award, or representing any agency of the … United States in an official capacity" (Brown & Maskell, 2016).

A mobile devise used by an employee during the workday may not be used for partisan political activity, even if the employee is on a break when using the device. Although employees are permitted to receive partisan political emails to any account as well as forward an email from a government account to their own personal account, certain email activities are barred under the Hatch Act—for example, forwarding or sending a partisan political email while on duty or in a federal workplace. Employees are barred from sending emails from government accounts or their personal accounts while at work (Brown & Maskell, 2016).

ENFORCEMENT OF THE HATCH ACT

Office of Special Counsel

The OSC Office of Special Counsel (OSC) was created by the Civil Service Reform Act of 1978. The OSC is the government entity responsible for protecting the rights of federal employees and applicants for federal employment and enforces the Hatch Act.

OSC investigates alleged violations of the Act and prepares a report as to its findings and enforces restrictions related to partisan political activity. The OSC also issues advice on the Hatch Act to employees who have specific questions. The Special Counsel, appointed by the President and confirmed by the U.S. Senate, leads the independent federal agency of the OSC.

Penalties

The Hatch Act provides a range of penalties for violating the Act, from a letter of reprimand, to a civil penalty of up to $1000 to suspension or termination or debarment federal employment up to 5 years. Violations committed by White House staff are investigated by the OSC and typically referred to the President for disciplinary action in the event of a violation.

Where to Go to Seek Advice on Questions related to the Hatch Act

Every federal agency has an ethics office. In addition, individuals and employers can contact the OSC and request an "Advisory Opinion" related to political activity under the Hatch Act. For information on how to file a complaint related to the Hatch Act—where to go and what to do—consult the OSC's website at www.OSC.gov.

RECENT VIOLATIONS OF THE HATCH ACT

During the Obama Administration, Secretary of Health and Human Services Kathleen Sebelius violated the Act when she endorsed a candidate while making a speech at a Human Rights Campaign event. The OSC did not recommend that any action be taken against the Secretary (Fuller, 2014).

More recently, during the Trump Administration, allegations of violations of the Hatch Act by Kellyanne Conway, Counselor to the President, were investigated by the OSC. The OSC found Ms. Conway had violated the Act on two occasions during media interviews advocating for and against candidates in the Special election in

Alabama in December 2017. The OSC recommended the President consider appropriate disciplinary action (U.S. OSC, 2018b).

U.S. Ambassador to the United Nations Nikki Haley also violated the Hatch Act when she retweeted Trump's endorsement of a South Carolina candidate, reported the OSC. In addition, the OSC found Dan Scavino, White House Social Media Director, had violated the Hatch Act when he used Twitter to call for the defeat of a Trump critic during the Michigan primary in April 2017 (Gstalter, 2018).

The President's son-in-law, Jared Kushner, has allegedly violated the Hatch Act on two occasions: (1) he used his White House title on a news release for Mr. Trump's re-election bid, and (2) he briefed White House officials during a staff meeting in the West Wing about Mr. Trump's re-election campaign. The OSC has not issued its findings from their investigation on Jared Kushner (Hirschfield Davis, 2018).

DISCUSSION QUESTIONS

1. Do you believe the Hatch Act violates a U.S. citizen's right of free speech? Why or why not?
2. Should there be different rules and regulations regarding political activities of nurses working at the federal level compared to nurses working for the DoD? Discuss the pros and cons.
3. Describe at least three political activities you may engage in as a federal employee and three political activities you may not engage in under the Hatch Act.

REFERENCES

Azzaro, S.D. (2016). The Hatch Act Modernization Act: Putting the government back in politics. *Urban Law Journal*, (42)3, 802.

Bloch, S. (2005). The judgment of history: Faction, political machines, and the Hatch Act. *University of Pennsylvania Journal of Business Law*, 7(2), 225-367.

Brown, C., & Maskell, J. (2016). *Hatch Act restrictions on federal employees' political activities in the digital age*. CRS Report No. R44469. Retrieved from https://crsreports.congress.gov/product/pdf/R/R44469.

5 C.F.R. Section 734.101.

Fuller, J. (2014, July 17). Do you work in government? Have you violated the Hatch Act? Let's investigate. *The Washington Post*. Retrieved from www.washingtonpost.com/news/the-fix/wp/2014/07/17/do-you-work-in-government-have-you-violated-the-hatch-act-lets-investigate/?utm_term=.bd474d13c5d5.

Great Depression. (n.d.). *Wikipedia*. Retrieved from https://en.wikipedia.org/wiki/Great_Depression.

Gstalter, M. (February 27, 2018) *Watchdog: Kushner may have violated Hatch Act with campaign statement* [Web blog post]. Retrieved from https://thehill.com/blogs/blog-briefing-room/news/375847-ethics-group-kushner-violated-federal-law-by-praising-trumps.

Hamby, A.L. (2004). *For the survival of democracy: Franklin Roosevelt and the world crisis of the 1930s*. New York, NY: Free Press.

Hatch Act of 1939. (n.d.). *Wikipedia*. Retrieved from https://en.wikipedia.org/wiki/Hatch_Act_of_1939#Amendments.

Hirschfield Davis, J. (2018, March 12). White House aides blur the legal line between partisans and public servants. *The New York Times*, p. A13. Retrieved from www.nytimes.com/2018/03/12/us/politics/trump-white-house-hatch-act.html.

Lincoln, A. (2017). *The Gettysburg Address* [transcript]. Retrieved from www.nationalarchives.gov/abraham-lincoln.

Pendleton Civil Service Reform Act. (n.d.). *Wikipedia*. Retrieved from https://en.wikipedia.org/wiki/Pendleton_Civil_Service_Reform_Act.

Roosevelt, F.D., & Rosenman, S.I. (1941). A message to Congress on the needs of the Works Progress Administration. In *The Public papers and addresses of Franklin D. Roosevelt, with a special introduction and explanatory notes by President Roosevelt*. New York: Macmillan.

U.S. Const., amend. I.

U.S. Office of Personnel Management. (2014). *Executive branch civilian employment since 1940*. Retrieved from www.opm.gov/policy-data-oversight/data-analysis-documentation/federal-employment-reports/historical-tables/executive-branch-civilian-employmen. rt-since-1940/.

U.S. Office of Special Counsel. (2018a). *How does the Hatch act affect me?* Washington, DC. Retrieved from https://osc.gov/pages/hatchact-affectsme.aspx.

U.S. Office of Special Counsel. (March 6, 2018b). *Report of prohibited political activity under the Hatch Act OSC File No. HA-18-0966 (Kellyanne Conway)*. Retrieved from https://osc.gov/Resources/Conway%20HA-18-0966%20Final%20Report.pdf.

18 U.S.C. §202(a).

Works Progress Administration. (n.d.). *Wikipedia*. Retrieved from https://en.wikipedia.org/wiki/Works_Progress_Administration.

ONLINE RESOURCES

Office of Special Counsel (OSC)
https://osc.gov
OSC Hatch Act
https://osc.gov/Pages/HatchAct.aspx
OSC Frequently Asked Questions
https://osc.gov/Pages/Resources-FAQ.aspx

42

TAKING ACTION: Reflective Musings From a Nurse Politician

Susan L. Adams

"Laws, like sausages, cease to inspire respect in proportion as we know how they are made."

John Godfrey Saxe I

In other words, engaging in politics and creating policy can be a messy and distasteful business. There is a long history of nurses who tackled a variety of messy, distasteful political challenges, from Florence Nightingale who improved the outcomes for wounded soldiers in the Crimean War and Clara Barton who founded the Red Cross, to Dorothea Dix who appealed to Congress for improved treatment for those who were diagnosed with mental illness and Susie King Taylor, a Black nurse who was born into slavery and who cared for Black soldiers during the Civil War. Nurses have been in the trenches and on the front lines of dealing with the messiness and complexities of the human experience within challenging political environments.

Nurses continue to have an important role to play in the political world. As the science has evolved regarding indicators for health, it is becoming more apparent that genetic predisposition and access to health care play a much smaller role in morbidity, mortality, and quality of life than social and environmental factors. Political decisions that are made by legislators who have no background in health and the subsequent narrative about health can have a far greater impact on health outcomes and is the perfect place for nurses to engage.

The California Endowment has built a repository of evidence in their Building Healthy Communities program (2018) that indicates the zip code where people live is a greater predictor of health than genetic code. Dr. Anthony Iton (2016) has been a lead investigator and proponent for closing the gap in health equity based on his work through the California Endowment. Alarming data suggest that zip code affects individuals even as they are gestating in the wombs (Iton & Shrimali, 2016). Living in a community where fast food restaurants and liquor and convenience stores outnumber full service grocery stores or farmers markets is one example of a zip code disparity. High incarceration rates and lack of access to affordable, safe housing; convenient, affordable transportation; quality schools; employment opportunities; public recreational facilities; clean air; and safe drinking water are other examples. In other words, accessing quality health care in and of itself only predicts a small portion of morbidity, mortality, and quality of life. Other factors, including racism, misogyny, and disparities play a much larger role, and there is an important place for nursing in addressing these problems within the policy arena.

The nursing process provides a map toward maneuvering through the most daunting of situations and nurses are well suited to take on the role of elected policymaker and to have an impact on the socioeconomic factors that influence health and quality of life. Having a nursing lens on policy creates the opportunity to significantly benefit the health in our communities. In this chapter, two examples will be provided about how a nurse's lens helped to improve the determinants of health. This chapter is intended to inspire a future generation of nurse leaders to pick up the standard, run for public office, bring a health lens to all policies, and tackle the public health issues that will prevent death by zip code.

ENGAGE! MOUNTAINS CAN BE MOVED WITH THREE VOTES

As a motivated solitary citizen, being able to access policymakers in person about an issue can take weeks if not months. Being able to secure an appointment does not always guarantee a meeting with the elected policymaker. That's not necessarily disadvantageous as legislative staff people are typically knowledgeable and versed in specific policy issues. Although it is desirable to meet with the legislator who casts the deciding vote, not being able to meet with the legislator does not automatically doom the lobbying effort.

Email and social media allow for communication to legislative offices, which may or may not be seen by the elected representative. Methods to personally and directly access legislators include attending town hall meetings and working on their election campaigns and fund-raising events where candidates and legislators are present. Of course, with fund-raising events, there is an expectation that a contribution will be made. But another possible answer to the access dilemma is to become the legislator.

Most nurses likely do not consider political life as a career option. However, a nurse in elected office is akin to being a public health or community health nurse with a broader perspective. As an example, county governments typically expend a third to a half of their annual budgets on health and human services–related issues. Many of the decisions about how that money is spent fall into the hands of the elected officials. Being one of five votes on a local county governing body is powerful. Typically, it only takes a simple majority to pass policy, which means one member only has to convince two other members to agree with a proposed initiative. With three out of five in agreement, amazing things can happen!

THE GENDER FACTOR

The Center for Interdisciplinary Health Workforce Studies at the College of Nursing, Montana State University (2017) reported that nursing is still predominantly a profession of women (89%) in comparison to men (11%). Although there are no reported differences in how men and women function once elected to public office (Lawless & Fox, 2008), women in the United States are less likely than men to run for office in the first place. The result is a national body of elected officials that has less than 25% women (Boschma, 2017) and that currently ranks the United States in 103rd place out of 193 countries for women in national legislatures (International Parliamentary Union, 2018). The United States falls below countries such as Cuba, Ethiopia, and Uganda (Lawless & Fox, 2008; International Parliamentary Union, 2018).

Boschma (2017) reported that as early as childhood, messages about women and girls occupying positions of power contribute to the gender discrepancies and that young men are more likely to be encouraged to run for office by family and friends than young women are. She also reported that by the time a woman enters college, political ambitions that she may have entertained have faded. Factors for the fading interest of women to enter political life include: (1) obligations to work and/or family, (2) not believing they are qualified to do the job if elected, (3) not being actively encouraged to run for public office, and (4) an unwillingness to engage in tough and possibly nasty races in which they may not be treated fairly.

The lack of gender balance in public offices limits a diversity of perspectives on a number of complicated issues facing the country, especially as related to women's and children's issues. This is not to say that we should only encourage women nurses to run for office—men who are nurses can also clearly bring a health perspective to the policy table. However, women may need more encouragement, supportive relationships, and mentorship than men. Women have yet to fully realize their power, in no small part as a result of the narrative in this country about a woman's place (Leonhardt, 2018). When highly qualified women run for office, women will still vote for an equally or less qualified man (Jaffe, 2018). Although policy positions of a candidate play a role in election outcome, misogyny and racism may also be factors.

Women can fail to recognize that feminine power is not a liability. Women are successful when attributes of the feminine, or a woman's heart, are used to direct policy. In 1992, John Gray raised the issue about gender differences when he highlighted how men and women engage in relationships and problem solving in his popular book, "Men Are from Mars, Women Are from Venus." Although academics have questioned and criticized the science (or lack of science) behind his work, the book reached the popular media and the conversation about how men and women approach problems was launched. Goman (2016) highlighted communication differences between men and women and focused on the top three strengths and the top three weaknesses for each gender. Women were identified as being empathetic and able to read people and be good listeners, whereas men were identified as being direct and to the point while displaying command. The case can be made that gender balance is needed.

Organizations such as Emerge America and Emily's List have been created to encourage, support, and train women as they consider running for public office. These organizations also assist with building a campaign team. Nursing organizations such as the American Nurses Association and the American Association of Nurse Practitioners have political action committees (PACs) that support nurses who are running for office.

HEALTH IN ALL POLICIES!

As stated in the opening, the California Endowment identified that the zip code where people live is more predictive of health outcomes than genetic code. By the time patients enter an emergency department with an end-stage disease, it is likely too late to have much of an impact on the long-term health trajectory. Moving further upstream into the zip code arena is the perfect setting for an elected person to affect change. Health care clinicians who are on the front lines can bring a wealth of experience and knowledge to these upstream policy discussions.

If the zip code is truly more predictive of health outcome than genetic code, then how do we expand our public health lens to include the variables that contribute to healthy zip codes, including eliminating food deserts; improving neighborhood assets and aesthetics; creating and improving recreational, educational, and employment opportunities; and investing in affordable housing and transportation options (Iton & Shrimali, 2016). The bottom line is that all issues can be viewed through the lens of healthy people, healthy communities, and a healthy planet. Nurses are well suited to this view. Two examples will be presented from my own experiences as a nurse and as an elected county supervisor that demonstrate the importance of a health care perspective on public policy decisions.

EXAMPLE #1: CREATING A HEALTH AND WELLNESS CAMPUS

Marin County is among the top three wealthiest counties of the 58 counties in California (U.S. Census Bureau, 2010–2015) and in the top five wealthiest counties in the country (U.S. Census Bureau, 2009–2013). Prior to the implementation of the Patient Protection and Affordable Care Act, even in wealthy Marin, approximately 20% of the children living in the county were not enrolled in a health insurance program nor did they have access to health services. The only health care service available to those without insurance or those who had public medical coverage, such as Medicaid, was located in a small portable trailer in the parking lot of the main hospital in the county. The location of the clinic was many miles from the communities that used the service, and it was not easy to access via public transportation or via walking or bike riding. The hours of operation were limited.

At the same time, Marin County, in a joint effort with other counties, won a multimillion-dollar settlement from the tobacco industry to address the tax payer burden that was paying for the care of people who smoked and developed tobacco-related illnesses and death. There were no mandated requirements about how that money could be spent by counties. There were reports that some counties were using the funds to pay for non–health-related infrastructure repairs, such as filling pot holes and to backfill employee salaries. With a nursing lens and through working with the director of health and human services and the chief administrative officer in the county, Marin took a different approach.

Questions that were posed to the full board of five members included: (1) How do we best direct tobacco settlement funds? (2) What would the rationale be for each possible pathway decision? These were easy enough questions for a board member who was a nurse and who viewed policy through the health lens. The nursing perspective was that the funds should be directed toward improving the long-term health in the community. Data and evidence were presented to support this assertion. The advocacy work was to build a coalition of community members who supported the idea and then to convince at least two other board members that the funds should be directed toward improving the health access and care for our residents. One of the most convincing rationales was reasserting that the county had this money only because the people living in the county were becoming ill and dying from tobacco use. The logical line of thought was that the funds should be redirected in a way that improved access to care and further prevented and reduced tobacco use. The full board supported the idea of a comprehensive health program in the county.

The next set of questions addressed what an investment of funds into Marin County health would look like. A number of constituency groups presented their request and rationale for considering investments into anti-tobacco use programs, children's Head Start programs, expansion of the children's health initiative, development of programs to end homelessness and address mental illness and addiction, veteran's health programs, and many others. Public meetings were held to review a variety of proposals, and these meetings were webcast and archived on the county website (www.marincounty.org/depts/bs/meeting-archive).

The fund was a one-time allocation, which meant that ongoing costs for programs or personnel would not be sustained once the money was spent. The final decision was made to develop a capital project for a central health and wellness center that would provide a cadre of coordinated comprehensive services for primary care, women's health, children's health, mental health, and recovery programs. The decision was also made that the new campus should embody the principles of healthy communities by being environmentally sound, community serving, and incorporating health principles throughout each stage of development. Examples of community-serving programs included placement of the campus within a challenged community and with the availability of workforce development; community access for events; gardens and meditation areas; walkable and bike- and transit-friendly location; and availability of organic and healthy food options in the café.

Serendipitously, at the time the decision was made to move ahead with a campus, a major business interest in Marin was moving out of a facility that included five large warehouse buildings in the heart of a low-income community. The property was purchased, and plans were approved to renovate the buildings and create a gold-level Leadership in Energy and Environmental Design (LEED) certified facility, which gained the attention of the architectural profession (Lubell, 2009). A LEED certification is internationally recognized and demonstrates that the building is using the healthiest and most environmentally friendly building elements. Rankings of silver, gold, and platinum are assigned to the project based on the number of criteria that have been fulfilled. As an example, solar and geothermal energy infrastructure was installed. Preferential parking was allocated for carpools, and plug-in stations were installed for electric vehicles. Recycled building materials were used. Natural and light-emitting diode (LED) lighting was placed throughout the campus, low volatile organic compound (VOC) or low toxic fume–emitting paints were used, and carpets and furniture were also low VOC rated. Composting and recycling containers were included, paper records were converted to electronic records, drought-resistant plants were used, permeable outdoor walking surfaces were created, low-flush toilets were installed, and the food that was served at the Blue Skies Café was locally grown and organic. Clients from the mental health programs were mentored as they developed retail and service skills at the café, which helped them with job placements in the restaurants and cafés in the broader community.

The Marin Health and Wellness Center continues to work in collaboration with the non-profit, Federally Qualified Health Center, Marin Community Clinics to this day and has become a central focus for the community. Previously, the community was filled with fast food chains and convenience stores and was identified as a food desert with no access to a full-service grocery store with fresh foods. As a result of the vibrant campus, a full-service and culturally appropriate grocery store moved to the neighborhood. The grocery owners hired residents from within the community, which elevated the incomes for many families. Community and school food gardens were created. Public transportation and bike-friendly access was improved. The goal of covering children was achieved with 99% of all children in the county being able to access affordable health care. The Marin Community

Clinics also established clinical facilities in other geographic locations within the county where low-income and Medicaid clients could easily access services. A nurse's lens in the policy arena helped improve the zip code!

EXAMPLE #2: BUILDING A THERAPEUTIC JUSTICE SYSTEM

During the 1960s and 1970s hospitals and institutions for people with a diagnosed mental illness closed their doors with the promise of more humane, community-based therapeutic programs. When these promised programs failed to appear, American jails and prisons became the de facto institutional warehouses for mentally ill people who broke the law as a result of their untreated mental illness. In the early part of the millennium, the cost for incarcerating an inmate was $22,000 to $31,300/inmate/year in the United States (Treatment Advocacy Center, 2016). However, if the inmate was mentally ill, the cost increased to an average of $30,000 to $50,000/year. The *New York Times* reported the highest costs of incarceration at $168,000/inmate/year for New York City (Santora, 2013). Adults diagnosed with mental illness represent about 10% to 20% of the incarcerated population, and Wilper, Woolhandler, and Boyd, et al. (2009) reported that many people with severe mental illness fail to receive minimally adequate treatment while in prison. The treatment of mentally ill offenders has been ripe for political reform and for placing a health lens on the challenge. Mental health advocacy is a prime area for nurses in representing those who are marginalized and without a voice.

In 1998, California State sheriffs lobbied for Senate Bill 1485, which was created to provide 3 years of funding for a few selected pilot demonstration programs geared toward reducing recidivism in mentally ill offenders housed in jails. The possibility for funding provided an incentive and the opportunity to think creatively about the treatment of mentally ill offenders. Crafting the plan with the assistance of an interprofessional team of stakeholders, obtaining a majority of board members to support and vote for the plan, and finally implementing and evaluating the plan was a major policy issue process that benefitted from having nursing expertise involved.

As a result, Marin County received one of the three-year grants for its Support and Release After Treatment (STAR) program (Austin, Ware, Ocker & Stewart, 2010; Fay & Kramer, 2001). A Criminal Justice and Behavioral Health (CJBH) committee was created and included the county sheriff; a city police officer who was also a psychologist; the district attorney; public defender; probation chief; a superior court judge; the director of health and human services; directors from social services, mental health, and addiction divisions; members of the community who had a diagnosis of mental illness; non-profit providers of care for the mentally ill; neighborhood leaders; the director of the county housing authority; and a representative from the workforce development board. As a member of the board of supervisors, the chair of the task force, and a nurse, the first step was to develop a common language with task force members. The sheriff and the district attorney were elected for their positions on being tough on crime, and they were reluctant at first to embrace a program that had the potential to demonstrate a soft-on-crime approach. The director of health and human services had a harm reduction philosophy in which every door was viewed as the right door to care whether through the jail, a homeless shelter, a library, or a traditional clinic. Neighborhood residents were reluctant to have "those people" (people with mental illness) housed in their community and expressed concerns about possible criminal activity, and the judges were reluctant to pack their busy dockets with a "boutique court" (or a narrowly focused court catering to one specific type of crime). Perhaps most important, the consumers of mental health services stated that they were tired of seeing programs developed without input from them, the users.

In their classic work, *Getting to Yes!*, Fisher, Ury, and Patton (2011) provided practical suggestions for how to build consensus through (1) separating people from the problem; (2) focusing on interests, not positions; (3) inventing options for mutual gain; and (4) using objective criteria. One of the most productive early CJBH sessions included leading the task force through a series of questions that produced unanimous agreement and created a baseline of common beliefs and values. Finding at least five questions on which all could agree laid down a foundation for building a successful team and ultimately a successful program. Questions included: Do we support creating safe communities? Do we believe that jail is NOT the best place to treat mentally ill offenders? Are we frustrated with seeing the same people with mental illness repeatedly moving in and out of our court system? Has a large portion of our county budget been allocated toward adjudicating and incarcerating mentally ill offenders? If current strategies are not working, should a new approach be tried? Do we believe that improvements can be made with our community services for the mentally ill?

As the group found areas of agreement, a running log was kept, reminding the team about core beliefs and values and also about the elements that would be important for the success of the program. All members provided important solution-oriented ideas. The program was designed to divert non-violent mentally ill offenders into treatment under court supervision rather than jail. Entry into the STAR program was voluntary. A specialty STAR court was created with a specially appointed judge, members from the district attorney's office, the public defender's office, the probation office, and from health and human services. The mentally ill participants were supervised by the courts for at least 1 year. Frequent appearances by the client and the STAR team were made before the judge. Over the course of the year or two that STAR clients were under supervision of the courts and case management, they were assisted with securing stable and supportive housing, access to community-based treatment, employment mentoring and assistance with employment placement, and maintaining their medical regimen. Once the STAR clients successfully completed the program, they could petition the court to expunge their record of the offense.

Over a 10-year period, Marin County demonstrated a long-term reduction in recidivism by approximately 80% and a reduction in psychiatric emergency visits by more than half. Marin County became one of the few places in California that could boast of empty jail beds through a therapeutic and humane approach to dealing with mentally ill offenders. The chief justice of California, Ronald M. George, convened an interdisciplinary task force in 2008 with the mission to develop recommendations for changing the paradigm for persons with mental illness in the California criminal justice system. I had the privilege of being invited to represent the county perspective, and I brought my nursing lens to the discussion. The final report was released by the California Judicial Council in 2011 and has provided a template for counties and courts throughout California as they develop therapeutic courts.

In 1999, there were only four mental health courts in the United States, and by 2018 more than 300 have been reported nationally (The Council of State Governments Justice Center, 2018). The California state legislature voted to release funds to support the continuation of successful programs. The therapeutic model of justice has been incorporated into at least 40 of the 58 counties in California, and articles have been published that provide templates for creating successful programs (DeMatteo, LaDuke, Locklair, & Heilbrun, 2012; Lamberti, 2016).

PERSONAL REFLECTIONS

Running for office is not a solo operation. As an unknown underdog who ran against an extremely well-funded and much-liked city council member, I was predicted to lose the race by pundits well in advance of election night. I had three assets. The first was being a nurse, the most trusted profession in the country (Brenan, 2017). Voters believe that if nurses are elected, they will look out for the best interests of the people and their communities. My second asset was the amazing coalition of family members, friends, and believers who helped me raise funds, knock on hundreds of doors, review and critique my policy documents, build my website, and basically be the wind beneath my wings. My third asset was not being attached to the outcome. Whether I won or lost was not as important as building support for improving the quality of life for the residents in my county. In fact, I believed the pundits about my chances. I worked hard with my team and ran a great campaign, however, my main impetus for engaging was to take advantage of every newspaper interview, every public forum and debate, and every door-knocking opportunity to meet with the community, to listen to the issues that were important to them, and to articulate possible solutions to challenging problems. As a result of my being a candidate and participating in the process, the other candidates modified their positions toward the "Healthy People—Healthy Planet" lens. On election night, when I won the seat for county supervisor, I was in shock. My first thought was, "What???" and my second thought was "Wow, now I have to roll up my sleeves and do the job. Am I ready?" Because I am a nurse, the answer was that I was more than ready.

As a young girl and later as a young woman, I never imagined that I would spend 12 years of my adulthood in political life. I did not receive the message from my teachers, family members, or friends that public life was a place for a woman, and especially for me. I did not see myself as a politician, but rather a nurse who was engaging in a political effort to improve the public health of a community that I loved. Those 12 years that I served as a county supervisor were challenging, exciting, and fulfilling. The good news is that there are a number of organizations that mentor and support women who are running for public office. The better news is that nurses do well at the polls just by being a nurse, meaning that men who are nurses also share the goodwill toward the profession.

There is a documented legacy that I was able to leave as a result of being a member of the board of supervisors and as demonstrated by the two examples in this chapter. The county has a comprehensive health and wellness campus; a vibrant therapeutic justice program for mentally ill offenders; a clean energy program; tighter laws on tobacco use, alcohol sales, and gun shows; laws prohibiting the use of toxic pesticides in parks and public buildings; an investment into walkable, bike-friendly, and disability–accessible pathways; an improved public transit system using clean-burning fuels; creation of a disaster medical reserve volunteer corps; a winter sheltering program for homeless residents; and many others. I was able to work with community members and with county staff to create proposals that received the support from at least two members of my board. On a state and national level, I was appointed to boards, commissions, and committees on which the health perspective was valued and incorporated into final policies.

It is my hope that nurses will ask questions of themselves, such as, "What would it take for me to run for public office? Who do I need on my team? Who can mentor me?" I stand ready to help support my nurse colleagues who are ready to take that leap!

REFERENCES

American Association of Nurse Practitioners. Retrieved from www.aanp.org/legislation-regulation/federal-legislation/pac.

American Nurses Association. Retrieved from http://ana.aristotle.com/SitePages/HomePage.aspx.

Austin, J., Ware, W.N., Ocker, R., & Stewart, P. (September, 2010). *Marin County, California jail population projections and assessment of the mental health care system.* Denver: The JFA Institute. Retrieved from http://egovwebprod.marincounty.org/depts/BS/Main/sups/sdistr1/docs/Jail-Study-Marin-Final-Report.pdf.

Boschma, J. (June 12, 2017). Why women don't run for office. *Politico.* Retrieved from www.politico.com/interactives/2017/women-rule-politics-graphic/.

Brenan, M. (December 26, 2017). Nurses keep healthy lead as most honest, ethical profession. *Gallup: Economy.* Retrieved from https://news.gallup.com/poll/224639/nurses-keep-healthy-lead-honest-ethical-profession.aspx?g_source=CATEGORY_SOCIAL_POLICY_ISSUES&g_medium=topic&g_campaign=tiles.

The California Endowment. (2018). *Building healthy communities—How long will you live? Your zip code matters.* Retrieved from www.calendow.org/building-healthy-communities/.

California State Senate. (1998). Senate Bill 1485: Chapter 501. Retrieved from www.leginfo.ca.gov/pub/97-98/bill/sen/sb_1451-1500/sb_1485_bill_19980915_chaptered.pdf.

Center for Interdisciplinary Health Workforce Studies. (2017). *2017 Data brief update: Current trends of men in nursing.* Montana State University. Retrieved from http://healthworkforcestudies.com/publications-data/data_brief_update_current_trends_of_men_in_nursing.html.

Council of State Governments Justice Center. (2018). *Mental health courts.* Retrieved from https://csgjusticecenter.org/mental-health-court-project/.

DeMatteo, D., LaDuke, C., Lockair, B., & Heilbrun, K. (2013). Community-based alternatives for justice-involved individuals with severe mental illness: Diversion, problem-solving courts, reentry. *Journal of Criminal Justice, 41,* 64-71.

Emerge America. Retrieved from https://emergeamerica.org.

Emily's List. Retrieved from www.emilyslist.org.

Fay, J., & Kramer, M. (2003). Restorative policing: A community wide response to mental Illness. *Law Enforcement Executive Forum, July,* 39-50.

Fisher, R., Ury, W., & Patton, B. (2011). *Getting to yes. Negotiating agreement without giving in.* London: Penguin Books, Ltd.

Goman, C.K. (March 31, 2016). *Is your communication style dictated by your gender?* Forbes Leadership. Retrieved from www.forbes.com/sites/carolkinseygoman/2016/03/31/is-your-communication-style-dictated-by-your-gender/#6ad5c998eb9d.

Gray, J. (1992). *Men are from Mars, women are from Venus: The classic guide to understand the opposite sex.* New York, New York: HarperCollins Publishers.

International Parliamentary Union. (May, 2018). *Women in national parliaments.* Retrieved from http://archive.ipu.org/wmn-e/arc/classif010518.htm.

Iton, A. (2016). *Change the odds for health [video].* TEDx San Francisco. Retrieved from www.youtube.com/watch?v=0H6yte4RXx0.

Iton, A. & Shrimali, B. P. (2016). Power, politics, and health: A new public health practice targeting the root causes of health equity. *Maternal Child Health Journal, 20,* 1753-1758.

Jaffe, S. (2018). Why did a majority of White women vote for Trump? *City University of New York: New Labor Forum.* Retrieved from http://newlaborforum.cuny.edu/2018/01/18/why-did-a-majority-of-white-women-vote-for-trump/.

Judicial Council of California. (2011). *Task force for criminal justice collaboration on mental health issues: Final report. Recommendations for changing the paradigm for persons with mental illness in the criminal justice system.* Retrieved from www.courts.ca.gov/documents/Mental_Health_Task_Force_Report_042011.pdf.

Lamberti, J. (2016). Preventing criminal recidivism through mental health and criminal justice collaboration. *Psychiatric Services, 67*(11), 1206-1212.

Lawless, J.L., & Fox, R.L. (2008). Why are women still not running for public office? *Issues in Governance Studies.* Retrieved from www.brookings.edu/wp-content/uploads/2016/06/05_women_lawless_fox.pdf.

Leonhardt, D. (May 13, 2018). Opinion column: I am not quoting enough women. *New York Times.* Retrieved from www.nytimes.com/2018/05/13/opinion/women-sexism-journalism-conferences.html?rref=collection%2Fsectioncollection%2Fopinion-columnists

Lubell. S. (July 27, 2009). Marin health and wellness campus. *Journal of the American Institute of Architects.* Retrieved from www.architectmagazine.com/design/buildings/marin-health-wellness-campus_o.

Marin Health and Wellness Center. Retrieved from www.marinhhs.org/marin-health-wellness-campus.

Santora, M. (August 23, 2013). City's annual cost per inmate is $168,000, study finds. *New York Times.* Retrieved from www.nytimes.com/2013/08/24/nyregion/citys-annual-cost-per-inmate-is-nearly-168000-study-says.html.

Saxe, G.S. (March 29, 1869) Quote from *The Daily Cleveland Herald. Wikipedia.* Retrieved from https://en.wikipedia.org/wiki/John_Godfrey_Saxe.

Treatment Advocacy Center. (September, 2016). *Serious mental illness (SMI) prevalence in jails and prisons.* Office of Research and Public Affairs. Retrieved from www.treatmentadvocacycenter.org/storage/documents/backgrounders/smi-in-jails-and-prisons.pdf.

U.S. Census Bureau. (2009-2013). List of United States counties by per capita income. *Wikipedia.* Retrieved from https://en.wikipedia.org/wiki/List_of_United_States_counties_by_per_capita_income.

U.S. Census Bureau. (2010-2014). List of California locations by income. *Wikipedia.* https://en.wikipedia.org/wiki/List_of_California_locations_by_income

Wilper, A., Woolhandler, S., Boyd, W., Lasser, K.E., McCormick, D., Bor, D.H., & Himmelstein, D.U. (2009). The health and health care of US prisoners: Results of a nationwide survey. *American Journal of Public Health, 99*(4), 666-672.

43

TAKING ACTION: Running Against the Odds: There's a Nurse in the Assembly

Dawn Marie Adams

"Communication and communication strategy is not just part of the game—it is the game."

Oscar Munoz

I've heard many women discuss the moment they decided to run. Many recount stories of anger, grief, and frustration that resulted from the presidential election of 2016. These emotions led them to step out of their comfort zone to run for a government office they'd never considered before.

My run for the Virginia State House was the culmination of the last 5 years—and perhaps the last 30 years—of my life and my career as a nurse. Between 2013 and 2018, I obtained my doctorate and developed a love for the policy aspects of our profession, taught health policy in that same program, and took a newly created position as the Director for the Office of Integrated Health at Virginia's Department of Behavioral Health and Developmental Services, where I was charged with designing and implementing community-based health services for people with developmental disabilities across the Commonwealth.

As part of this role within state government, I was able to make both policy and programmatic changes that required a great deal of persistence and strong communication skills. These necessary skills have revealed how much my background as a nurse prepared me to effectively mobilize change in a bureaucracy. It's been said, and I believe true, that the quality of our communication directly affects the intensity and quality of our influence and relationships. As nurses, we spend much of our time honing our communication skills as we translate medical jargon, explain difficult concepts and procedures, listen intently, and provide understanding while offering support and guidance to patients and families.

During my 4 years in this administrative position in state government, I observed the poor communication at the intra- and inter-agency levels, the struggles to have "the people's" message translate to the General Assembly in a way that would result in meaningful action, and regular miscommunications with the general public—all of which seemed unnecessary and an easy fix if only there were better communicators in place. I believed that I could help improve this communication challenge. At some point while working as a government official I realized I wanted to have a bigger impact and that the best way to do so was to become a member of the General Assembly.

It was definitely because of the 2016 election that the opportunity for me to run arose. Some would say that this was a lucky break, but I believe it was preparedness for the task, borne of education and experience along with the post-election enthusiasm of many women that provided the leverage enabling an unknown, lesbian nurse practitioner (NP) to win a seat in the Virginia General Assembly. Earning a baccalaureate degree in nursing enabled me to think critically and expand my worldview. My master's degree in community health and organizational planning and my work experience as a nurse manager in critical care, as an educator, and as a home health nurse afforded me the ability to appreciate the interconnectedness of people and systems. Becoming a NP forced me to think more deductively, and earning my doctorate after working for more than a decade as an NP harnessed all of my knowledge and experience in such a way that I see the role of nurses and our potential impact on the health care system as the primary resource for healing our country's health care crisis.

When I first entered my name, I met with the Democratic representative who was scouting for candidates. He was unimpressed with me and clearly had no interest in whether or not I ran. There were two other candidates who

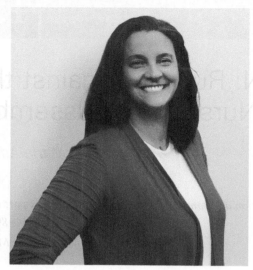

Virginia Delegate Dawn Adams, DNP, RN.

were also interested in the position, and fortunately our district's regional chairs elected to hold a *primary* and not a *caucus* to determine the Democratic nominee. *Primaries* are similar to the general election: voters go to the ballot box to vote for all candidates running in a *primary* on the ticket. For my race this meant I would be on the same ballot as the candidates for Governor, guaranteeing a higher turnout at the polls. A caucus on the other hand, operates more like a popularity contest, and if you're an outsider within the party and unable to get people motivated to turn out for the caucus vote at the one or two designated locations, victory is unlikely. The *primary* afforded me time to do the work that would get my name in front of the public and explain why I would be a better candidate. Although the other candidates were both educated, I believed completely that I was the best of the three to take on a 15-year incumbent. I have no idea why I believed this. I only know that I was *called* to run this race, and that always fortified me. I also believed that, because I was a nurse, I had a stronger work ethic and had spent a lifetime paying attention to what people need and want.

I worked full time while running to win the *primary* election. And running in a *primary* is a full-time job; in fact, party insiders admonished me for not quitting my paid job to dedicate more time to the campaign. Neither of my opponents worked outside of their campaign, and yet somehow we out-worked them. Communicating a well-crafted, concrete message around building a healthier community through better policy allowed me to leverage Democratic enthusiasm and ultimately run an effective campaign without utilizing the typical and often wasteful standard campaign infrastructure. I built a team of volunteers rather than feeding a system that requires hiring many people and forces candidates to raise money to support the people hired. We were able to use raised funds strictly for printed messaging-mailers, leave-behind cards, digital media, radio, yard signs, and billboards.

There were several false starts in my campaign in which I attempted to do what I was told by party insiders. I hired a campaign manager, more than once, but their beliefs and work ethic did not align with my own. Early on a friend told me, "Lose on your own terms." That stuck with me, and that's what I decided to do. I did not embrace the insider party advice and did not hire a marketing company for branding or mailers. My team and I designed and printed them ourselves. All of my team volunteered their time. We had volunteers who knocked on thousands of doors, and I sat in many living rooms answering questions and explaining how I would be helpful in the General Assembly. Fortunately, despite the excellent qualifications of my opponents, I won 23 of 26 precincts. Nobody thought it was possible—nobody but my inner voice and the team of volunteers that believed in me.

Going forward to the general election, I maintained the same strategy, despite criticism that I needed to run a "real campaign." We worked around the clock, knocked on thousands of doors, and had genuine conversations with those who were solid Democrats and Independents alike. Retrospectively, I believe my opponent failed to anticipate and appreciate the importance of real communication. The communication skills that I had developed as a nurse, the lens of a nurse, and the work ethic of a nurse, were vastly underestimated. My opponent was convinced, like many other people within the Democratic and Republican parties, that I did not have a shot at winning, and subsequently he miscalculated how the power of a nurse might manifest. Although the enthusiasm of our community in response to the new federal administration had a great deal to do with the outcome, it was not the only thing that enabled me to win—it was the more than 30 years of education and health care training, relationship building, and human connectedness.

In our district in particular, we had the highest voter turnout in the state. More people voted for the House race (39,168) than they did for the Governor (37,855). Election night was a nail biter, much like a horse race—the vote count swung back and forth; first me, then him and he sustained a small lead for a bit, then me. The final count was 19,427 for the incumbent and 19,774 for the challenger—a mere 347-vote victory was mine and it was both stunning and immensely satisfying. I believe that because of the effort we put into this campaign and the productive communication delivered while canvassing, we had support not only from Democrats but also from Independents.

Going into this new role, I had many new descriptors besides Delegate. I am the first openly lesbian member and the first NP in the entire General Assembly (both the House and the Senate)—and only the second nurse to ever be elected in Virginia for any state position. Although I had hoped I would be appointed to the health care committee and the education committee, I found it to be unnecessary to serve on these committees to have influence within the Democratic caucus and even the larger House on health and education matters. Committee appointments are made by the Speaker of the House. Having beaten the Speaker's candidate, there was no incentive to put me on committees that would allow me to provide direct influence despite what might be in the best interest of developing state policy. Instead, I serve on the Agriculture, Natural Resources and the Chesapeake Bay Committee and the Militia, Police and Public Safety Committee.

I think it's extremely important to bring a health lens to both of these committees, and I have seized the opportunity to speak out on behalf of health-promoting policies. For example, there were many members of the Democratic caucus who were against expanding the Nurse Practice Act toward full-practice authority in Virginia. I was able to influence their votes after speaking out in a caucus meeting. We had little opposition on the Democratic side and even less on the Republican side when we voted on the bill. The bill passed the House and unanimously passed the Senate. Still, the Governor's decision to veto the bill or sign it into law remained unknown for weeks after it was passed by the General Assembly. Ultimately, the Governor did sign the bill and NPs began to apply for independent practice in January of 2019.

There are many other opportunities where I believe I will be able to be influential because of my background, and I think it is really necessary. We have too many other voices that really are serving their profession rather than the needs of the people. For example, I'm very concerned about the direction we are going regarding pharmaceuticals and health care access. It is extremely important that we have people outside of physicians and pharmacists who are helping to shape the policies of Virginia.

To date the biggest challenge for me is raising money. Personally, I hate it—frankly, no one loves it. But as a nurse, I find asking for help in this way monumentally difficult. Most people don't understand how vital it is both as a constituent representative and a candidate. People don't realize that, even though officials are elected to represent and inform them, there is very little money provided by the state for Delegates. In fact, the Commonwealth gives us less than one penny per person to communicate with all of the roughly 80,000 constituents in our districts. That is why we must raise money if we are to do a good job. Yet, there is a great deal of wasteful spending associated within the campaign finance infrastructure, so it is a challenge all the way around.

I was pleased to see 13 bills for which I was chief copatron be signed into law—more than any other freshman delegate. I was able to change access to free voter identification (ID) cards by convincing Virginia's Department of Motor Vehicles (DMV) to advertise and link the State Board of Elections voter ID application on their website. I expect to bring back legislation that would enable people to get these free IDs at the DMV offices. In order to fund this I am also submitting legislation to pass a law supporting the very first "I Have a Dream" license plate. To do this I must have a minimum of 450 pre-ordered plates before the bill is heard in subcommittee.

I'm optimistic about making inroads toward better conversations between the various members of the state house, irrespective of party, because again, as a nurse, I believe I have developed a sincere appreciation for what people have to say and can express an understanding of what they are saying, even while disagreeing. These hard and deep conversations are essential to making better policy. The most important things I can offer as a member of the Virginia General Assembly are a genuine willingness to have difficult conversations and a commitment to being proactive. I'm a nurse and that's formidable as a candidate and as a policymaker.

44

Political Appointments

Amy L. Anderson and Alexia E. Green[a]

"Only a life lived for others is a life worthwhile."

Albert Einstein

Public service is not just a job, it is a calling: one requiring great sacrifice, sound character, integrity, ethical and moral direction, and hard work. Political appointment is one route to public service. Our government provides many opportunities for political appointment at the federal, state, and local level, yet nursing is underrepresented in positions of leadership within all levels of government. With over 7000 federal appointments available at the start of each new presidential term, and hundreds of thousands of positions at various levels of government available across the United States, surprisingly few nurses hold political appointments (Office of Personnel Management [OPM], n.d.).

The Institutes of Medicine (IOM) (2011) identified a lack of nursing influence in health care decision-making and called for a renewed effort for nurses to lead through policy and leadership in the landmark report "The Future of Nursing: Leading Change, Advancing Health." To meet this need, the Robert Wood Johnson Foundation (RWJF) in conjunction with AARP and the AARP Foundation created the *Future of Nursing: Campaign for Action* (the Campaign) to advance the IOM recommendations (Campaign for Action, n.d.). The Campaign has held strategy and educational sessions around the country to further prepare nurses for leadership roles and expanded the support with stakeholders and policy engagement. In addition, the Nurses on Boards Coalition (NOBC) was developed to support nurses obtaining leadership roles on boards, establishing a goal of 10,000 nurses on boards by 2020 (NOBC, 2018). Although significant strides have been made, there is more work to be done. While nurses are seen as the most trusted and honest profession, thought leaders have stated that nurses need more influence in leading health care systems, planning, and reform efforts (RWJF, 2010).

Government needs representation from diverse professions, including nurses, to effectively legislate and govern the people. Nurses must use their power as the largest profession in health care to effect change. Nurses with political appointments can directly and indirectly influence policy decisions in legislative or executive branches of local, state, or federal government. If nurses are to nurture a "culture of health," it is critical that the sphere of influence include policies, structures, and systems and that a unified voice is exhibited. Political appointment provides a significant pathway for influencing decision-making at all levels of government. As political appointees, nurses can directly and indirectly influence policy decisions of local, state, or federal government. The current national health care reform debate, coupled with a heightened political environment around a multitude of other policy issues (e.g., national debt, immigration, environmental concerns) presents nurses with an opportunity to lend their unique expertise and system knowledge to decision-making at the policy table and contribute to the public policymaking process.

CONSIDERING POLITICAL APPOINTMENT?

Political appointment is not for the faint of heart. Nurses seeking appointment must have resilience, composure, the

[a]This chapter builds on work originally developed by Judith Leavitt, RN, MEd, FAAN and Andrèa Sonenberg, PhD, WHNP, CNM. The authors would like to thank them for their excellent work.

BOX 44.1 Identifying Political Appointments

State Government

- **State websites for secretary of state or the office of the governor:** Online search examples: "California secretary of state" or "Governor's office for the state of Texas."
- **Professional organizations (nursing and non-nursing):** often track available positions and seek out potential appointees active within the organization.
- **State government agencies and state employment website:** host information about state-based opportunities.

Federal Government

- **Official Plum Book:** information about U.S. government policy and supporting positions listed after each presidential election.
- **Office of the Federal Register:** hosts information about federal government agencies including information about positions and appointments.
- **Federal government agency websites:** provide information regarding currently open positions.

ability to communicate effectively, and a deep understanding of the system of government in which they are hoping to serve. The appointee must be well-versed in strategy, debate, negotiation, and be intuitive and patient with the political process. Understanding the types of interactions between the different branches of government is essential for success. Appointees should have technical knowledge of stakeholders in the policy area of the appointment (Peters, 2015). While nurses tend to view the world from the lens of their profession, nurse leaders in appointed roles must consider the health care sector in terms of how economics, markets, labor, regulation, and legislation impacts people, and consider the historical context of social, political, legal, and economic domains to engage effectively in the decision-making process. Those that choose this path will often find political appointments both challenging and gratifying. Furthermore, appointees often move to lucrative and powerful positions outside government once the appointment term has ended, opening additional opportunities to influence the future of nursing and advance health.

IDENTIFYING POLITICAL APPOINTMENTS

Determining the purpose of seeking an appointment is important when looking for positions. Whether the goal is to influence a focused area of health care or impact a larger system through legislative change, appointment opportunities are present at the local, regional, state, or national level. The nurse would need to determine which position criteria best fits their expertise.

Federal Appointments

Federal appointees serve at the pleasure of the administration. In 1952, the Eisenhower administration developed what is known as "The Plum Book" (OPM, n.d.). The book is a comprehensive list of federal, non-competitive appointments that is published every four years after the Presidential election. There are four types of federal appointments: Presidential Appointments requiring Senate confirmation, Presidential Appointments not requiring Senate confirmation, Non-Career Senior Executive Service, and Schedule C Appointments (Piaker, 2016). All appointed positions are published and considered open after each election regardless of whether or not the incumbent wins. More than 7,000 positions are typically listed including heads of agencies, high-level supportive positions, policy experts, aides, and advisors (OPM, n.d.). The Senate Committee on Homeland Security and Government Affairs and the House Committee on Government Reform alternate the publication (OPM, n.d.) (see Boxes 44.1 and 44.2). Two nurse leaders who have knowledge and experience with federal appointments are Sylvia Trent Adams and Sheila Burke.

Sylvia Trent-Adams. Growing up in a rural community, Rear Admiral (RADM) Trent-Adams liked helping people, but she never anticipated being in the job she holds today, Deputy Surgeon General of the U.S. Public Health Service (USPHS). RADM Trent-Adams had seen her mother and grandmother care for members of the community and this early exposure to health care resulted in her volunteering as a candy striper at the age of 12, and she knew that her path would include caring for people. She became an Army nurse after attending Hampton University on a scholarship, later working at Walter Reed Medical Center. At Walter Reed, Trent-Adams gained an interest in public health and working with underserved populations. She went on to complete a Master of Science in Nursing and Health Policy and a Doctor of Philosophy from the University of Maryland.

BOX 44.2   Non-Health Care Political Appointments for Nurses

Commerce and economic development: Nursing perspective could benefit industrial development, tourism, and businesses relocating to the region, state, or nation.

Conservation: Experience with public/population health is critical for work on issues such as clean water, air pollution, green technology, and waste removal.

Corrections: Expertise for public/private institutions enacting policies benefitting incarcerated persons at risk of chronic conditions and poor health outcomes.

Education: Valuable insights needed regarding policies guiding school health programs, health care service delivery, and teaching health curriculum in schools.

Higher education: Nurses can advise higher education priorities, improve health outcomes, social change, and influence nursing education.

Licensure and regulatory boards: Advise regarding environmental protections, public health, drinking water, health inspections, and provider licensure impacts.

Public safety: Offer important perspective on public safety focused on domestic violence, motor vehicle safety, gun laws, immigration, and human trafficking.

Transportation: Offer important perspective on highway safety/transportation and effect of location/access to transportation impacting health access and outcomes.

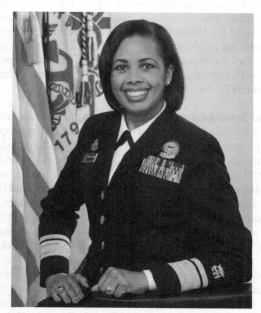

Rear Admiral Sylvia Trent-Adams. (Photo provided and approved by the Office of the Surgeon General.)

In 1992, Trent-Adams left the Army and transferred into the USPHS Commissioned Corps. In her rise to the Office of the Surgeon General, Trent-Adams held various positions in the Department of Health and Human Services (HHS) including Deputy Associate Administrator of the HIV/AIDS Bureau at the Health Resources Services Administration (HRSA). Her experience with the USPHS has included two internships in the U.S. Senate, with work focused on prospective payment systems and scope of practice for nurses and psychologists. She served as the USPHS Chief Nurse Officer from 2013 to 2016, advising the Office of the Surgeon General and HHS on nursing workforce recruitment and retention.

As Deputy Surgeon General, Trent-Adams is the administrator for the USPHS Commissioned Corps, working to support the communication efforts of the Office of the Surgeon General, advising policy, and mentoring USPHS officers. At times, Trent-Adams is the only nurse, only woman in uniform, and the only person of color in the room. She helps bring discussions back to pragmatic, feasible solutions with reasonable expectations of outcomes, but found it can be difficult to build consensus and make tough decisions which impacts people's health and lives. Trent-Adams indicates the job is never done and, while leadership may not always make perfect decisions, "the best decisions are made with the best information available" (Trent-Adams, personal communication, August, 2018).

The office of the Deputy Surgeon General works in direct partnership with other uniformed services, advises on Department of Defense (DoD) policies, and works with other countries on major health concerns such as smoking, tobacco, and obesity. She has consulted with the World Health Organization on workforce and immigration issues, and has led emergency responses, such as the first Commissioned Corps team to West Africa during the 2014 Ebola outbreak. In April 2017, after Vice Admiral Vivek Murthy was relieved of the office following the change of administration, RADM Trent-Adams was selected as U.S. Acting Surgeon General.

For nurses seeking political appointment or high-level government positions, RADM Trent-Adams recommends three key areas to know: policy, operations and finance, and administration. She advises maintaining excellence and never compromising one's integrity. Trent-Adams wants nurses to know and value their unique experiences, use that expertise to translate knowledge into action, and recognize their value to their communities, their nations, and the world. In her vision for health care, she sees nurses as game changers that significantly improve access, increase quality, and reduce the costs of health care. Trent-Adams looks forward to seeing the achievements of the profession over the next 20 years as nurses gain a greater voice in the policy arena and hold more elected offices, and believes "It is not about nursing, it is about the impact of nursing on people" (S. Trent-Adams, personal communication, August 2018).

Shelia P. Burke. Shelia Burke served for 19 years on Capitol Hill, first as legislative assistant to Senator Bob Dole, then as deputy staff director of the Senate Finance Committee. Later as deputy chief of staff, then chief of staff for then Senate Majority Leader Bob Dole, Burke was involved with numerous major health-related policy changes including Medicare, Medicaid, the Maternal and Child Health programs, welfare reform, and budget reconciliation. In 1995, she was elected as the secretary of the Senate, an officer of the Senate. After working on Capitol Hill, Burke moved to academia and held faculty positions at the Harvard University John F. Kennedy School of Government and the Georgetown University O'Neill Institute for National and Global Health Law. During her initial appointment at Harvard, she served as Executive Dean of the Kennedy School of Government and later was appointed deputy secretary and chief operating officer of the Smithsonian Institution. Currently, Burke holds positions at Baker Donelson as a Strategic Advisor, serves on that faculty at the Kennedy School, is a well-known health care author and active speaker, and holds prestigious honors and awards for her service.

Burke indicates that her interest in government started as an active member of the California Student Nurses Association. She started her nursing career at Alta Bates Hospital in Berkeley, California before moving to New York City to serve as the Director of Program and Field Services for the National Student Nurses Association (NSNA). Her move to public service was facilitated by a connection made while advocating for NSNA. Burke credits her early connections on Capitol Hill for her advancement to high-level positions as a public servant.

For those desiring appointment, Burke advises defining what the requirements and skills are for the position being sought, and determining if the position is self-nominated or nominated, which would require seeking out individuals or organizations with authority to nominate someone. Burke suggests that nurses make themselves available to their elected legislators to consult regarding health care and public policy issues, seek support from their professional association, align with other groups that can influence nominations, and volunteer for political campaigns. Finding a mentor in public service to help with the transition into the appointment is important, as creating relationships with those in government can be the difference in finding and obtaining a position. Burke also recommends applying for internships and fellowships and serving on local or state committees and boards (S.P. Burke, personal communication, April 2018).

State and Local Appointments

Nurses can serve on commissions, committees, state boards of health, and task forces. At the state level, many appointments are made by the secretary of state or governor, and information about available positions can usually be found on their respective websites. Various local and regional appointments with agencies and boards might include not only health-focused issues, but also school, police, and animal control. A local mayor's office and/or regional government agency office would be the ideal place to begin a search. Not all appointments held by nurses are health care related, but all are influential in public decision-making for our communities, states, and nation. Two examples of nurse leaders at the state level are Sue Birch from Washington state, and Cynthia Crone from Arkansas.

Sue Birch. Sue Birch currently serves as Director of the Washington State Health Care Authority (HCA), the state's largest health care purchaser. Birch was appointed to the position by Governor Jay Inslee in 2018. As Director, she oversees purchases of health care for two million residents through Washington Apple Health (Medicaid) and the Public Employees Benefits Board Program. In 2020, the School Employees Benefits Board Program will be added to the HCA, further expanding Birch's impact.

Birch was previously the executive director of the Colorado Department of Health Care Policy and Financing where she led Colorado's implementation of the Affordable Care Act. Birch also completed an appointment to the National Advisory Committee on Rural Health and Human Services, a HHS advisory panel to HHS. She has held two leadership-focused fellowships: the Boils-Stanton Foundation Livingston Fellowship and the Robert Wood Johnson Foundation Executive Nurse Fellowship.

Birch's advice for nurses seeking an appointment is threefold:
1. always assert that nurses bring a unique and important perspective to policy conversations, and can drive policy toward embracing social determinants of health;
2. get involved in the community through boards and volunteering to provide a deeper understanding of the issues and challenges facing those being represented, and help build a network; and
3. embrace opportunities to improve public speaking skills (S. Birch, personal communication, April 2018).

Cynthia Crone. In 2010, Cynthia Crone was appointed as Arkansas' Deputy Insurance Commissioner. Crone worked with Governor Mike Beebe and his cabinet to plan and implement the state's new Health Insurance Marketplace during Arkansas' expansion of Medicaid. This involved working directly with a newly elected state legislature, the Centers for Medicare and Medicaid (CMS) officials, consultants, private insurance companies, consumer advocates, and other stakeholders. The state included an innovative "private option" allowing new Medicaid beneficiaries to choose health coverage from private health insurance plans in the Health Insurance Marketplace. Like many states, final implementation in Arkansas was impacted by many factors, including a U.S. Supreme Court ruling which resulted in restrictions and elimination of some programs developed under her leadership. Due to her work as Arkansas Deputy Insurance Commissioner, Crone was appointed to the Health Care Industry Council in Arkansas, where she is serving a second 3-year term. This advising committee provides input from individuals and business interests to accompany economic projections, providing a deeper understanding of community challenges.

Crone previously served as president of the Arkansas Nurses Association, and was appointed by Governor Mike Huckabee to the Arkansas Commission on Nursing. She has also held appointments to legislative task forces on neglected and abused children, substance abuse treatment, and domestic violence. Crone's policy-related work stemmed from her recruitment by state legislators to provide input on health-related issues because of her experience in health care. Crone completed the Robert Wood Johnson Foundation Executive Nurse Fellowship, a position that prepared her for these respected positions. She says that effective health policy should be consumer-focused and evidence-based, and acknowledges that legislative work requires knowledge, risk-taking, networking, coalition-building, negotiation, compromise, and hard work (C. Crone, personal communication, May 2018).

SUPPORT FOR APPOINTMENT

Political appointees are often selected for their unique expertise, previous work, and/or relationships with elected officials. Nurses considering appointment should seek support from professional organizations such as the American Nurses Association (ANA), National League for Nursing (NLN), American Association of Colleges of Nursing (AACN), or academic institutions. Often, political party support is necessary to obtain a political appointment.

Appointments typically require an application or nomination; connections with political transition teams or officials within an administration can increase political parties receiving an appointment. Political appointments may also be a direct result of previous positions held at the local, regional, state, or federal level that provided a vital connection and/or awareness of interest in public service. Nurses

seeking an appointment should remain active in their communities, engaged with professional organizations, apprised of the current political landscape, and aware of current policy and legislative issues.

NETWORKING: POWER OF CONNECTIONS

Appointments are often due to political connections or experiences made throughout one's career. Being visible and expressing interest is often the first step. Legislators and government officials are often looking for individuals with skills and expertise unique to a specific public sector to ensure their decision-making is informed by a greater understanding of the underlying issues. The decision to appoint an individual is often left to the discretion of those making appointments in an agency, allowing for connections to come into play (Tuutti, 2012). Networking is an important part of making beneficial connections in government, such as unexpected introductions made by colleagues or planned interactions with government officials or legislators. Those seeking connections can reach out to other nursing leaders, professional organizations, political parties, and/or community organizations to help them communicate their expertise and interest in public service.

POLITICAL PARTY AFFILIATION

When a new administration or leader takes over, political party affiliation can impact an individual's ability to obtain an appointed position. If an individual has been supportive of an administration or party, such as Republicans or Democrats, then appointment may be a direct result of expressing that support (Tuutti, 2012). However, for someone highly critical of a political party or administration, appointment may be more difficult, as appointments are often a reward for loyalty to a party or administration. Simply volunteering for a campaign, organizing fundraising, making phone calls, handing out signs, writing letters, or financially contributing can enhance the possibility of political appointment.

Administration officials usually seek individuals for appointment that support the agenda and/or ideology of their political party, but that does not exclude experts from other political parties. However, if an appointee does not align with the administration's values and beliefs, political polarization can cause disruption and poor progress on promises made during the election process. Political affiliation can be key to acquiring an appointment, but it is not a requirement.

PREPARING FOR APPOINTMENT

Political appointment typically requires identifying opportunities and strategies to gain support, providing evidence

BOX 44.3 Are You Ready for Political Appointment?

Consider the following questions:

1. What is my motivation for seeking this appointment?
2. Why do I want to enter public service?
3. Does my background, expertise, and experience fit the position I am seeking?
4. Do I have support from professional colleagues, political organizations, and/or professional organizations?
5. Should I seek a full- or part-time position?
6. Does my party affiliation align with the current administration?
7. Can I remain bipartisan while holding this position if my values do not align with the administration?
8. Am I able to look beyond nursing and see the bigger picture?
9. Is my financial situation stable and how does a change of income impact my financial goals?
10. Do I have any potential concerns with past or present social media posts, media presentations, and/or publications?
11. Can I obtain support from multiple stakeholders to advance my nomination?
12. Do I meet the qualifications required and can I clearly articulate how I fit the position?
13. Am I ready for intense scrutiny of my private and public life?
14. Will I be prepared to take on the stress and pressure of the position?
15. Do I enjoy influencing decision-making?
16. Am I able to spend time away from family and friends?
17. Will my family and friends support this decision?
18. Can I expect support from my employer for time away if I plan to return to my old job?

of expertise, and political awareness. Seeking political appointment is arduous and political appointees are highly scrutinized through the vetting process. Individuals with interest in appointment should reflect on personal motivation and complete an assessment of potential issues that could arise during vetting (see Box 44.3).

Organizations Supporting Nurse Appointees

Professional nursing organizations, such as the ANA, NLN, AACN, and the American Academy of Nursing, often support nurses seeking political appointment. However, nurses can seek support from organizations outside of nursing that may align with the candidate's expertise and experience such as AARP, academic colleagues or institutions, or even organizations such as the Small Business Association. Stratifying support by engaging organizations or individuals outside of nursing can demonstrate additional depth and provide important perspective on a potential nominee's qualifications. Broad support is often necessary to receive an appointment (Box 44.4).

Strategy to Gain Appointment

Nurses seeking appointment should consider short- and long-term strategies to earn an appointment. Now is the time to shore up any knowledge deficits about government or the political process. Seeking a review of the nurse's experience and expertise by other nurses that have held political appointment is useful in ensuring a robust portfolio is presented. Garnering support from multiple organizations will add to the strength of a candidate's position demonstrating an expansive network of contacts. In many

BOX 44.4 Organizations With Additional Resources for Political Appointment

In addition to well-known professional nursing organizations such as the ANA, NLN, and state nurse's associations, other organizations aid in identifying, supporting, and providing valuable information for individuals seeking political appointment, including:

- Partnership for Public Service: www.ourpublicservice.org
- The Brookings Institute: www.brookings.edu
- The Heritage Foundation: www.heritage.org
- The National Women's Political Caucus (NWPC): www.nwpc.org
- The Rutgers Center for American Women and Politics (CAWP): www.cawp.rutgers.edu

ANA, American Nurses Association; *NLN*, National League for Nursing.

ways, gathering support for appointment is like coalition building, identifying and bringing together organizations with aligning principles to support and advance a common cause. In this case, the "cause" is to support an appointee who is willing and eager to serve.

Seeking Nomination

Individuals may be sought for or may seek an appointment through application for positions. Political transition teams of newly elected political officials typically work with external advisors to identify potential appointees.

Individuals may be asked to develop a portfolio for consideration by the transition team, which is then reviewed and assessed by transition team members tasked with identifying appointees. Individuals under consideration may be contacted to ascertain their interest in a specific position, or clarify qualifications/expertise related to the appointment. Some positions are filled directly through this process and others are filled after applications are received. For local or state positions, a candidate may apply much like the employment process, may be directly appointed by a government official, or may be recommended by an advocate or organization. Reviewing qualifications and position information is important to gain understanding of the process unique to an appointment.

Vetting Process

Those seeking appointment will be vetted to carefully check the candidate's background. At the federal level, Executive Branch candidates are selected, cleared, and then nominated for positions (Hogue & Carey, 2015). This process can include scrutiny of financial and personal history, social media, credentials, business transactions, taxes, personal and public relationships, a national security questionnaire, or other areas deemed required for the position (The Heritage Foundation, n.d.). Appointees should be prepared for invasive dialogue and questioning. With social media now providing a wealth of information for the vetting process, those seeking a position should carefully review and avoid potentially inappropriate or questionable social media posts. Public and private life are open for examination.

Many appointees withdraw from consideration during vetting, especially when questionable or unfavorable information is discovered through the process. Withdrawals for Presidential appointments are more common than rejection by Senate vote. In fact, only three nominations have been rejected in a recorded Senate vote in the last 100 years (The Heritage Foundation, n.d.). While confirmation proceedings may seem harsh, the government has a duty to protect the public from unethical individuals serving in powerful positions. Vetting is one way to identify potential issues and ensure a qualified candidate is moved forward for appointment.

HOLDING AN APPOINTED POSITION

Relationships

After appointments, appointees should maintain their individual and organizational relationships that were instrumental during the appointment process. Recognition of this support can be done through phone calls, meetings, and letters of appreciation. Political appointees should acknowledge the efforts made on their behalf through correspondence and public expressions of gratitude, as additional support may be needed for the policy work ahead.

Duty to Serve

While recognizing the work and support to get an appointee a position is key to advancement and success, it is also critical to understand who is being served. For a government position, the appointee is serving the constituents or public. For an organizational appointment such as a board of directors, the appointee may be representing a community or group of patients. Some committee appointments require the viewpoint of specific groups of people, and the appointee would be a voice for that population. Maintaining autonomy for decision-making is vital to protect the integrity of the position and the appointee. The duty of the appointee should be to prioritize those being served over those that contributed to their successful appointment.

Compensation

Compensation of political appointees can vary depending on the level of appointment. At the federal level, it is based upon federal schedules of compensation, the "general schedule" employee pay grades (OPM, n.d.). Candidates for federal appointment should look at the payment schedule to determine fair compensation for the position (OPM, n.d.). For those with appointments at the state or local level, compensation may be determined by statute, which should be readily available in public record. Individuals may request information about compensation prior to appointment, including salary, benefits, and reimbursement for expenses. While some positions in government are paid well, pay is not typically the motivating factor for appointment. Many appointees earn less in the public sector working for the government than they may have earned in the private sector (Keefe, 2016). In place of high compensation, public service, problem solving, and the power and influence of the position are often attractive to potential appointees. A position in the private sector following a high-level appointment can be quite lucrative.

CONCLUSION: INFLUENCING PUBLIC POLICY

The opportunity to influence and the power associated with a political appointment can be exciting. Nurses that are looking for an opportunity to make a difference through government or legislation should consider the many open, political appointments. Those who are interested in seeking election to public office can also gain experience working as a political appointee prior to running for office. Nurses are instrumental in making change that positively influences public policy. The nursing profession needs more leaders in government to advance policies that impact health and health care delivery (IOM, 2016). By achieving political appointment, a nurse can have substantial and meaningful impact on the future of the U.S. health care system and our nation.

DISCUSSION QUESTIONS

1. What types of appointed positions are available for nurses to seek?
2. How would an individual seeking appointment prepare for the process?
3. When nurses participate in government, what impact can they have on health care systems?

REFERENCES

The Brooking Institute. (2000). *Staffing a new administration: A guide to personnel appointments in a presidential transition.* Retrieved from www.brookings.edu/wp-content/uploads/2016/06/20000711staffing.pdf.

Campaign for Action (n.d.). *Campaign for action: About us.* Retrieved from https://campaignforaction.org/about/.

The Heritage Foundation. (n.d.). *The confirmation process for presidential appointees.* Retrieved from www.heritage.org/political-process/heritage-explains-the-confirmation-process-presidential-appointees.

Hogue, H.B., & Carey, M.P. (2015). *Appointment and confirmation of executive branch leadership: An overview.* Retrieved from https://fas.org/sgp/crs/misc/R44083.pdf.

Institute of Medicine. (2016). *Assessing progress on the Institute of Medicine report: The future of nursing.* Retrieved from www.nap.edu/resource/21838/AssessingFON_release-slides_2.pdf.

Keefe, J. (2016). *Public sector workers are paid less than their private sector counterparts—and the penalty is larger in right-to-work states.* Retrieved from www.epi.org/publication/public-sector-workers-are-paid-less-than-their-private-sector-counterparts-and-its-much-worse-in-right-to-work-states/.

Nurses on Boards Coalition. (n.d.). *About: Our story.* Retrieved from www.nursesonboardscoalition.org/.

Office of the Federal Register. (n.d.). *Federal Register: The daily journal of the United States government.* Retrieved from www.federalregister.gov/documents/current.

Office of Personnel Management. (n.d.). *The plum book.* Retrieved from www.govinfo.gov/collection/plum-book?path=/GPO/United%20States%20Government%20Policy%20and%20Supporting%20Positions%20%2528Plum%20Book%2529 .

Peters, B.G. (2015). Policy capacity in public administration. *Policy and Society, 34*(3-4), 219-228.

Piaker, Z. (2016). Help wanted: 4,000 presidential appointees [Web blog comment]. Retrieved from http://presidentialtransition.org/blog/posts/160316_help-wanted-4000-appointees.php.

Robert Wood Johnson Foundation. (2010). *Groundbreaking new survey finds that diverse opinion leaders say nurses should have more influence on health systems and services.* Retrieved from www.rwjf.org/en/library/articles-and-news/2010/01/groundbreaking-new-survey-finds-that-diverse-opinion-leaders-say.html.

Tuutti, C. (2012). *How to become a presidential appointee.* Retrieved from https://fcw.com/articles/2012/11/09/hire-presidential-appointees.aspx.

ONLINE RESOURCES

American Nurses Association
www.nursingworld.org
Campaign for Action
https://campaignforaction.org/about/
National League for Nurses
www.nln.org
Nurses on Boards Coalition
www.nursesonboardscoalition.org
Office of Personnel Management
www.opm.gov/policy-data-oversight/classification-qualifications/

45

Nursing and the Courts

David M. Keepnews and Virginia Trotter Betts

"Power concedes nothing without a demand. It never did and it never will."

Frederick Douglass

The courts are an important source of health policy. Their decisions hold significant implications for nurses and for the patients, families, communities, and populations they serve. This chapter provides an overview of the legal and judicial systems and the role of the courts in shaping policy. It is not a comprehensive overview; rather, it aims to provide the reader with a general understanding of this policy arena and its critical importance for nursing. Although this chapter uses several examples to illustrate the relationships between law and policy, it is important to keep in mind that the policy landscape can change rapidly and unpredictably.

THE JUDICIAL SYSTEM

The United States has two parallel court systems: federal and state. The federal courts have jurisdiction over matters that involve federal law (generally speaking, those that pertain to the U.S. Constitution, federal statutes, and/or the actions of federal agencies). The trial courts for the federal system (the entry point for most federal cases) are called district courts, and there are 94 located throughout the United States and its territories. Federal courts of appeal, also referred to as circuit courts, are organized into 12 geographic circuits plus the Federal Circuit Court (Administrative Office of the U.S. Courts, n.d.). The U.S. Supreme Court is the federal court of last resort; there is no higher court to which its decisions can be appealed.

Each state has its own court system. State courts generally rule on issues arising under the state's constitution and laws. They may also hear some claims that arise under federal law or the U.S. Constitution. The state court systems include trial-level and appellate courts, with a high court as the court of last resort. The high court is known as the Supreme Court in most states, but not all; in New York State, for example, its highest court is known as the Court of Appeals.

THE ROLE OF PRECEDENT

An important legal doctrine, *stare decisis* ("let the decision stand"), sets the course for judicial precedents by adhering to previous findings in cases with substantially comparable facts and circumstances. Thus courts grant deference to their prior rulings. Courts are not completely bound by precedent; they sometimes overrule prior decisions, but they are expected to depart from precedent based only on compelling and clearly articulated reasons. Lower courts are expected to follow the rulings of a higher court (Administrative Office of the U.S. Courts, 2010). Thus, for example, a federal district court in California or Oregon would look to rulings of the Ninth Circuit Court of Appeals (which includes those states) for guidance; the Ninth Circuit would look to the U.S. Supreme Court as well as the Ninth Circuit's own prior rulings.

THE CONSTITUTION AND BRANCHES OF GOVERNMENT

The U.S. Constitution sets out the basic structure of the federal government. State constitutions do the same for each state government. A key element of this structure is a system of checks and balances between the three branches of government: legislative branch, executive branch, and judicial branch. Each branch carries out specific functions, but no branch is completely autonomous. The federal courts act independently of the President and Congress, but judges are nominated by the President, subject to confirmation by the U.S. Senate.

The Constitution is the fundamental source of U.S. law. All government action and laws must be consistent with it. This is true of the U.S. Constitution (which applies to the actions of the federal and state governments) and each state constitution (which applies to the actions of each state). Laws passed by a state legislature must be consistent with both the U.S. Constitution and the state constitution.

Although much of the Constitution is concerned with the structure and functions of the federal government, the first 10 amendments to the Constitution, known as the Bill of Rights, define the basic rights of all people in the United States, including: freedom of speech; freedom of assembly; freedom of religion; freedom from unlawful searches and seizures; and protection against being deprived of life, liberty, or property without due process. In the United States, the rights outlined by the Bill of Rights are defined primarily as limitations on government's power to restrict or deny them. Thus, for example, the First Amendment reads as follows:

> Congress shall make no law respecting an establishment of religion, or prohibiting the free exercise thereof; or abridging the freedom of speech, or of the press; or the right of the people peaceably to assemble, and to petition the Government for a redress of grievances.

Although the language of the Bill of Rights specifically focuses on the federal government, the 14th Amendment has had the effect of applying these rights to actions by state governments.

Because the Bill of Rights applies to government action, it does not directly limit the behavior of private individuals (including employers). Other laws may apply to actions by employers and individuals, for example, civil rights laws, which protect people from discrimination based on race, gender, national origin, or other factors, and whistleblower laws that protect employees' rights to report illegal conduct or unsafe practices.

Rules or regulations issued by the executive branch must be consistent with the Constitution. There must also be some statutory (legislative) source of authority for an executive agency to act. For example, the U.S. Secretary of Health and Human Services is authorized by federal law to issue rules and regulations to carry out the functions of his or her department, including the administration of the Medicare program (see, for example, Home Health

Services Act, 42 U.S. Code, Section 1302, 2011); this is the basis for that agency to adopt regulations spelling out Conditions of Participation that health care organizations must meet to participate in the Medicare and Medicaid programs (see, for example, Medicare Conditions of Participation for Hospitals, 2018.) Federal law Administrative Procedure Act (5 U.S. Code, Chapter 5, 2011) and parallel state laws also spell out the procedures that government agencies must follow in issuing regulations, such as how much notice must be provided to the public and how members of the public can provide comments on any proposed regulations.

JUDICIAL REVIEW

A major role of the judicial branch is to review actions of the legislative and executive branches if those actions are challenged. This power of judicial review has given the courts a significant role in public policy because they have the power to affirm or strike down laws or other government action.

Review of Legislative Action

In *Marbury v. Madison* (1803), the U.S. Supreme Court first asserted its power to declare a law unenforceable if it is found to violate the Constitution. A significant illustration of this power was the U.S. Supreme Court's decision in *National Federation of Independent Business v. Sebelius* (2012), in which the constitutionality of major sections of the Patient Protection and Affordable Care Act (ACA) was challenged. (Legal issues related to the ACA are discussed in Box 45.1.)

Review of Executive Action

The actions of an executive agency may be challenged on the basis that it has acted without legal authority or failed to comply with procedural requirements.

In *Spine Diagnostics Center of Baton Rouge, Inc. v. Louisiana State Board of Nursing* (2008), a Louisiana appellate court upheld a challenge to a Board of Nursing advisory opinion that interventional pain management is within the scope of practice of Certified Registered Nurse Anesthetists (CRNAs), finding that it constituted a regulation authorizing CRNAs to perform a service that is "solely the practice of medicine." Because this rule had not been issued in accordance with the state's Administrative Procedures Act (including advance notice and an opportunity for public comment), it was found to be an improper attempt at rulemaking. The state supreme court subsequently declined to hear an appeal of the decision (Louisiana Supreme Court, 2009), thus allowing it to stand.

BOX 45.1   The Patient Protection and Affordable Care Act: Continuing Legal Issues

In *National Federation of Independent Business v. Sebelius* (2012), the Court heard challenges to provisions of the Patient Protection and Affordable Care Act (ACA) and upheld the law's minimum coverage provision (often referred to as the individual mandate), that is, the requirement that most people who are not covered through their employer or through a government program such as Medicare or Medicaid must purchase health insurance. Opponents argued that Congress does not have the authority to compel people to purchase something. This case was closely watched by opponents and supporters of the ACA since the outcome would determine whether a key component of the ACA could go into effect.

The Court found that the individual mandate, which is enforced by requiring people without insurance to pay a financial penalty that will be levied by the Internal Revenue Service, was within Congress' power to lay and collect taxes.

In the same decision, the Court struck down another important part of the ACA. The ACA included an expansion of the Medicaid program. Medicaid, which provides health insurance to many poor and disabled people, is administered by the states with joint federal and state funding. States are not required to participate in the Medicaid program although all states currently do. The ACA called for making everyone with incomes below 133% of the Federal Poverty Level eligible for Medicaid. States that failed to comply with this provision could be excluded from federal Medicaid funding altogether.

The Court, by a 7-2 majority, found that this penalty was too severe and over-reaching and that it would coerce states into implementing the ACA's Medicaid expansion. Justices Ginsberg and Sotomayor wrote a strong dissent from the majority opinion, arguing that the penalty was within Congress's power, especially since state participation in the Medicaid program itself is voluntary. The impact of this ruling was to make states' implementation of the Medicaid expansion voluntary. As of 2019, 14 states have opted not to implement it, thereby excluding millions of potential Medicaid recipients from health care coverage (Kaiser Family Foundation, 2019).

Other Supreme Court decisions have had an impact on the implementation of the ACA. In 2015, the court turned back a challenge that would have weakened the ACA by limiting the states in which individuals could receive federal tax subsidies to assist with paying insurance premiums. In *King v. Burwell*, by a vote of 6-3, the Court found that subsidies could be available in all states and not just those that operated their own health exchanges. Ruling

otherwise could have eliminated subsidies for people in three dozen states.

Subsequently in yet another challenge to the ACA, the Supreme Court ruled in the case of *Burwell v. Hobby Lobby* (2014) that corporations could opt for a religious exemption to the ACA's requirement that employers cover women's contraception.

Political developments have sparked new legal issues regarding the ACA, which continue to be debated in the federal courts.

Challenging the Constitutionality of the Individual Mandate and the Affordable Care Act

As part of its large-scale changes in the federal tax system in 2018, Congress eliminated the penalty for failure to purchase health insurance, effective in 2019. Thus, although the individual mandate provision remains in place, Congress removed the mechanism for enforcing it. A federal lawsuit filed by 20 attorneys general argues that eliminating the penalty rendered the individual mandate unconstitutional since the Supreme Court, in the *National Federation of Independent Business* case, found that the mandate's penalty was allowable under the Constitution's taxing clause; thus, eliminating the penalty also eliminated the basis for the individual mandate *(Texas v. U.S., 2018)*. The Trump Administration's Justice Department filed a brief in support of the plaintiffs. That brief also argues that the other provisions of the ACA—including guaranteed issue (restricting insurer's ability to refuse coverage) and community rating (limiting insurers' ability to charge higher rates to different groups)—should also be eliminated. (It is rare for the federal government to support a court challenge to one of its own laws.)

Many critics of the Trump Administration's position have pointed out that this would also end restrictions on insurer's ability to refuse coverage or charge markedly higher rates for individuals with pre-existing conditions. The case has been appealed to the 5th Circuit; its outcome remains to be seen.

Medicaid Work Requirements

In January 2018, the Trump Administration issued guidance to state Medicaid directors "support[ing] state efforts to test incentives that make participation in work or other community engagement a requirement for continued Medicaid eligibility" and encouraging states to seek waivers to allow such requirements. Kentucky, the first state to receive approval, required that Medicaid recipients devote 80 hours per month to work or "community engagement." (Exceptions to this requirement included pregnant women, full-time students,

---

BOX 45.1   The Patient Protection and Affordable Care Act: Continuing Legal Issues—cont'd

people who are "medically frail," and primary caregivers of a dependent minor or a disabled adult). Notably, Kentucky had previously decided to participate in the ACA's Medicaid expansion for low-income individuals.

Kentucky's work requirement was struck down by the federal district court for the District of Columbia which ruled that, in approving Kentucky's work requirements, the Administration did not give adequate consideration to whether it was in keeping with the Medicaid program's purpose of providing health care to low-income and other vulnerable populations (*Stewart v. Azar, 2018*). The court also struck down Medicaid work requirements in Arkansas (*Gresham v. Azar, 2018*). Additional federal lawsuits have challenged other states' Medicaid work requirements. At this time, the outcome of these legal challenges remains to be seen.

IMPACT LITIGATION

Advocates have developed a tradition of using the courts strategically to establish, affirm, or clarify rights. Litigation that is "focused on changing laws or on the rights of specific groups of people" is often referred to as *impact litigation* (Harvard Law School, 2018).

A major example of such litigation is *Brown v. Board of Education*, the 1954 case in which the U.S. Supreme Court struck down school segregation and mandated that states begin a process of desegregating their public schools. The Court unanimously found that segregated public school education constituted a state policy of inferior education, that "separate educational facilities are inherently unequal," and that it thus violated the Equal Protection Clause of the Fourteenth Amendment to the U.S. Constitution.

Laws passed at the federal or state level often create rights or remedies that can be legally enforced through the courts. For example, the Americans with Disabilities Act of 1990 (ADA) provides for equal treatment for disabled Americans and bars discrimination in a number of areas including employment and public accommodations. The ADA applies principles of equality and fair play that are basic to American law and public life, but it also created specific rights that can be enforced through government action and litigation.

ENFORCING LEGAL AND REGULATORY REQUIREMENTS

The courts are often used as a means to seek enforcement of existing regulatory requirements. Nursing organizations sometimes turn to the courts to challenge practices they believe violate state nurse practice acts. For example, the California School Nurses Organization, the American Nurses Association (ANA), and ANA\California sued the California Department of Education (CDE) challenging a CDE directive authorizing insulin injection in public schools by unlicensed personnel. The CDE had issued this directive in connection with its settlement of a suit by parents of diabetic students who, the parents had charged, were being denied needed care by the lack of school personnel qualified to administer insulin (CDE, 2007). The nursing groups challenged this practice as a violation of California's Nursing Practice Act and questioned the authority of the CDE to issue a directive on nursing practice. The trial court and appellate court ruled in favor of the nurses but the state supreme court later ruled that the CDE directive did not violate the Nursing Practice Act and allowed it to stand (*American Nurses Association v. Torlakson*, 2013).

ROE V. WADE AND ACCESS TO ABORTION

Women's reproductive rights, including the right to choose abortion, have long been a focus of political and legal controversy. In 1973, the Supreme Court's landmark *Roe v. Wade* decision found a constitutional right to choose abortion, overturning state laws prohibiting or unduly restricting abortion before the third trimester of pregnancy. Since that time, the Court has ruled on numerous state laws seeking to place restrictions on access to abortion. The continued evolution of the legal environment for abortion rights is too complex to cover in this chapter. However, it is important to emphasize that the right to choose abortion continues to be an active issue in the federal courts. In 2016, the Supreme Court struck down a Texas law that required abortion providers to have admitting privileges at a hospital within 30 miles and held abortion clinics to the regulatory standards required of ambulatory surgical centers. This law had been framed by its proponents as necessary to protect women's safety. Opponents of the law argued that the law placed unnecessary burdens on clinics that provided abortion (many of which had closed as the law took effect) and restricted women's right to choose abortion. In *Whole Woman's Health v. Hellerstedt* (2016), the Court agreed, finding the law unconstitutional.

The right to choose abortion remains a polarizing political issue, with opponents openly calling for the Court to overturn *Roe*. That goal has been stymied by the composition of the Court, which for many years has consisted of four Justices viewed as generally liberal on major social issues, four Justices viewed as generally conservative, with one Justice—Anthony Kennedy—serving as a swing vote on many issues. Recent changes in the Court's membership (see "Influencing and Responding to Court Decisions," below) have changed the court's composition, tilting it to what many expect will be a more consistently conservative direction. Although the doctrine of *stare decisis* means most Justices are hesitant to break with precedent, it does not rule out overturning precedent if Justices find a compelling reason to do so. Thus, proponents of abortion rights remain concerned that the change in the makeup of the Court puts *Roe* at risk.

If *Roe* were to be overturned, it would not have the effect of outlawing abortion; it would leave decisions about access to abortion to each state. Many states would continue to allow abortion, but states that chose to restrict abortion or even outlaw it outright could do so within whatever standard (if any) the Supreme Court might set.

CRIMINAL COURTS

Most of the court decisions that have an impact on health policy and nursing practice are civil actions. In some prominent instances, however, actions in criminal courts have resulted in significant policy implications for nursing as well. For example, although negligent acts or omissions that lead to patient injury or death are usually addressed in civil suits, on occasion they have led to criminal prosecution.

In 2006, 10 nurses simultaneously resigned their positions at a Long Island nursing home. These nurses were among a larger group, all of whom were recruited from the Philippines, working in facilities owned by the Sentosa Care nursing home chain. These nurses had complained that many of the promises made to them when they were first hired regarding wages and working and living conditions had been broken. The nurses, fearing retaliation by their employer, resigned with minimal notice. The facility, whose patients included ventilator-dependent children, covered their shifts with other nurses. After receiving a complaint from the nursing home, the state's board of nursing found no basis to proceed with a patient abandonment complaint. An investigation by the state Department of Health later yielded a conclusion that no patients had been put at risk. Nonetheless, the local county District Attorney filed criminal charges against the nurses, indicting them for conspiracy and for putting children and disabled patients at risk.

The case raised significant concerns not only about mistreatment of immigrant nurses but also about the rights of all nurses (Keepnews, 2009). Nursing organizations including the ANA, the New York State Nurses Association, and the Philippine Nurses Association of America supported the nurses' call for charges to be dropped. The trial court judge refused to drop the charges; however, the nurses filed an appeal of this decision. A state appellate court issued an order that the trial be stopped. The court found that "criminalizing [the nurses'] resignations" would have the effect of unjustifiably "abridging the nurses' Thirteenth Amendment rights," referring to that constitutional amendment's prohibition on involuntary servitude (*Vinluan v. Doyle*, 2009).

INFLUENCING AND RESPONDING TO COURT DECISIONS

Although judges are expected to rule based on facts and law, several other factors may influence the outcome of court decisions. Judges often take changing social attitudes and standards into account in their rulings. Judges also differ in their own judicial philosophies. The views of federal judicial appointees and their judicial records are factors in a president's judicial nominations and in the Senate's decision whether or not to confirm the nominations. Thus, the outcomes of presidential and Senate elections can have an important impact in the composition of the federal courts, including the Supreme Court. Judges' views may shift over time and cannot always be reliably predicted or neatly categorized. Supreme Court Justice Harry Blackmun, often characterized as a liberal Court member, and who wrote the majority opinion in *Roe v. Wade*, had been nominated to the Supreme Court by President Richard Nixon. Chief Justice John Roberts, a conservative appointed by President George W. Bush, wrote the majority opinion in *National Federation of Business v. Sebelius*, upholding the ACA individual mandate.

However, the appointment of federal judges—all of whom hold lifetime appointments—has increasingly taken on an overtly partisan character. President Trump has boasted of his efforts—largely successful—to appoint younger, staunchly conservative judges at all levels of the federal judiciary who can shape the judicial landscape for decades to come (Kaplan, 2018). In particular, he has stated his goal to seek repeal of *Roe v. Wade*. His administration has utilized conservative think-tank organizations to screen potential judicial appointees for their political views (Baker, 2018).

In February 2016, conservative Supreme Court Justice Antonin Scalia died, creating a vacancy on the Court. Then-President Obama nominated Merrick Garland, a moderate appellate court judge, to fill that vacancy. The Senate's Republican majority, however, refused to let

Garland's appointment move forward, arguing that Obama, as a "lame duck" (with 11 months left to his term), should not be permitted to appoint a new Justice. President Trump, shortly after his inauguration, nominated Neil Gorsuch, a conservative appellate judge, to fill the Supreme Court vacancy; Gorsuch was quickly approved by the Senate. In June 2018, Justice Anthony Kennedy announced his retirement. Trump's nomination of conservative appellate court judge Brett Kavanaugh to replace him sparked considerable controversy, first because of his voting record, judicial philosophy, and partisan history and then because of his alleged conduct as a high school and college student, including charges of sexual assault. His conduct during a Senate Judiciary Committee hearing, which many viewed as belligerent and at times openly partisan, sparked further controversy and questions regarding his judicial temperament. The impending 2018 midterm elections served to heighten partisan differences over Kavanaugh's nomination. Ultimately, the Senate confirmed him on a 51-49 vote, along almost entirely partisan lines.

Persuading the Courts: *Amicus Curiae* Briefs

An important route for influencing courts' decisions is through filing *amicus curiae* (friend of the court) briefs. Amicus briefs provide an important tool for advocacy groups to make their views known on a relevant case. When (with the court's permission) groups and/or individuals file an amicus brief, they bring their perspectives, data, and beliefs about the issues before the court to persuade it on how to rule.

Examples of cases in which nursing organizations have filed amicus briefs include:

- *National Federation of Independent Business v. Sebelius* (2012). The ANA, joined by five other health professional groups, filed an amicus brief in support of the ACA minimum coverage provision. The ANA also filed amicus briefs in other federal cases regarding the ACA.
- *Obergefell v. Hodges*, 576 U.S. ___ (2015). The American Academy of Nursing joined with GLMA: Health Professionals Advancing Health Equality and Sullivan & Worcester LLP in an amicus brief in support of marriage equality.
- *Olmstead v. L.C.* (1999). The American Psychiatric Nurses Association joined other organizations in an amicus brief before the U.S. Supreme Court to support the right of disabled persons to receive care in noninstitutional settings.
- *Commonwealth Brands Inc. v. U.S.* (2010). The Oncology Nursing Society joined with 10 other organizations in support of the U.S. Food and Drug Administration (FDA) regulation of tobacco manufacturing, sales, and advertising.

Appealing Unfavorable Decisions

When faced with an unsatisfactory court ruling, a party may be able to appeal the decision to a higher court. Generally, there must be grounds to appeal beyond simply not being satisfied with the outcome. For example, the losing party may argue that the court made an error in how it applied the law or in refusing to consider relevant evidence. There is no guarantee that an appellate or higher court will agree to hear an appeal. If a court declines to review the decision of a lower court, that decision stands.

A request to the U.S. Supreme Court to consider an appeal of a lower-court decision is called a petition for writ of certiorari. Four out of the nine Justices must agree to grant certiorari in order to hear an appeal. The Court only does so for about 100 of more than 7000 cases submitted for appeal each year (Supreme Court of the U.S., n.d.).

Repudiating the Court

When a court's decision is based on its interpretation of a statute, another option is to seek a change in that statute. Of course, this requires a political strategy to secure passage of new legislation, which may or may not be a viable option.

In *Ledbetter v. Goodyear Tire & Rubber Co., Inc.* (2007), the U.S. Supreme Court interpreted the equal-pay provisions of Title VII of the Civil Rights Act of 1964 as meaning that a violation occurs only at the time that a biased pay scale is instituted, not each time workers are paid unequally as a result of that pay scale. This had the effect of sharply limiting employees' ability to file discrimination claims. In response, Congress passed and President Obama signed the Lilly Ledbetter Fair Pay Act of 2009. The preamble to the bill explicitly criticizes the Court's *Ledbetter* decision, stating that "[t]he limitation imposed by the Court ... ignores the reality of wage discrimination and is at odds with the robust application of the civil rights laws that Congress intended" (Lily Ledbetter Fair Pay Act of 2009).

Amending the Constitution

Another potential means of responding to an unsatisfactory court decision, particularly if the decision is based on an interpretation of the Constitution, is to amend the Constitution. This is much easier said than done. Amending the U.S. Constitution requires approval by not only a two-thirds majority of both houses of Congress but also by three-quarters of the states. The Constitution has been amended only 27 times in its history.

Amending state constitutions, however, is often more readily achievable. States differ in their procedures for amending their constitutions, generally including approval by popular vote. In contrast to the U.S. Constitution's 27 amendments, several state constitutions have been amended hundreds of times (Bowser, 2015).

CONCLUSION

Health care practice and health policy continue to change rapidly in often chaotic and unpredictable ways. Successful policy strategies must include being knowledgeable about the role of the courts in health policy and being prepared to respond to and, when possible, seek to influence the outcome of court decisions.

DISCUSSION QUESTIONS

1. What impact do court decisions have on policy issues related to nursing and health care?
2. How can nurses have an impact on the outcome of legal issues related to nursing and health care?

REFERENCES

Administrative Office of the U.S. Courts. (2010). *Understanding the federal courts.* Retrieved from www.uscourts.gov/uscourts/educational-resources/get-informed/understanding-federal-courts.pdf.

Administrative Office of the U.S. Courts. (n.d.). *The federal court system in the U.S.* Retrieved from www.uscourts.gov/uscourts/FederalCourts/Publications/English.pdf.

Administrative Procedure Act, 5 U.S. Code, Chapter 5 (2011).

American Nurses Association v. Torlakson, 57 Cal.4th 570 (2013).

Americans with Disabilities Act of 1990, P.L. 101-336, 42 U.S.C. § 12101 et seq.

Baker, P. (2018). A conservative court push decades in the making, with effects for decades to come. *New York Times.* Retrieved from www.nytimes.com/2018/07/09/us/politics/supreme-court-conservatives-trump.html.

Bowser, J. (2015). *Constitutions: Amend with care.* Retrieved from www.ncsl.org/research/elections-and-campaigns/constitution-amend-with-care.aspx.

Brown v. Board of Education of Topeka, 347 U.S. 483 (1954).

California Department of Education. (2007). *Children with diabetes win assurance of legally required services at school.* Retrieved from www.cde.ca.gov/nr/ne/yr07/yr07rel97.asp.

Commonwealth Brands Inc. v. U.S., 678 F. Supp. 2d (2010).

Gresham v. Azar, Civil Action No. 18-1900 (2018). Retrieved from https://ecf.dcd.uscourts.gov/cgi-bin/show_public_doc?2018cv1900-58.

Harvard Law School, Bernard Koteen Office of Public Interest Advising. (2018). *Litigation: Impact.* Retrieved from https://hls.harvard.edu/dept/opia/what-is-public-interest-law/public-interest-work-types/impact-litigation/.

Home Health Services, 42 U.S. Code, Sections 1302 and 1395 (2011).

Kaiser Family Foundation. (2019). *Status of state action on the Medicaid expansion decision.* Retrieved from www.kff.org/health-reform/state-indicator/state-activity-around-expanding-medicaid-under-the-affordable-care-act/?currentTimeframe=0&sortModel=%7B%22colId%22:%22Location%22,%22sort%22:%22asc%22%7D.

Kaplan, T. (2018). Trump is putting indelible conservative stamp on judiciary. *New York Times.* Retrieved from www.nytimes.com/2018/07/31/us/politics/trump-judges.html.

Keepnews, D. M. (2009). Welcome news in the Sentosa nurses case. *Policy, Politics, & Nursing Practice, 10*(1), 4–5.

Ledbetter v. Goodyear Tire & Rubber Co., Inc., 127 S, Ct. 2162 (2007).

Lily Ledbetter Fair Pay Act of 2009, Pub.L. 111–2, S. 181.

Louisiana Supreme Court. (2009). *News release #019.* Retrieved from www.lasc.org/news_releases/2009/2009-019.asp.

Marbury v. Madison, 5 U.S. 137 (1803).

Medicare Conditions of Participation for Hospitals, 42 CFR Chapter IV, Subchapter G (2018).

National Federation of Independent Business v. Sebelius, 567 U.S. 519 (2012).

Obergefell v. Hodges, 576 U.S. ___ (2015)

Olmstead v. L.C., 527 U.S. 581 (1999).

Roe v. Wade, 410 U.S. 113 (1973),

Spine Diagnostics Center of Baton Rouge, Inc. v. Louisiana State Board of Nursing, Louisiana Court of Appeal (First Circuit). No. 2008 CA 0813, December 23, 2008.

Stewart v. Azar, Civil Action No. 18-152, D.D.C. (2018). Retrieved from https://ecf.dcd.uscourts.gov/cgi-bin/show_public_doc?2018cv0152-74.

Supreme Court of the United States. (n.d.). *The Supreme Court at work.* Retrieved from www.supremecourt.gov/about/courtatwork.aspx.

Texas v. United States, N.D. Texas, Civil Action No. 4:18-cv-00167-O (2018). Retrieved from www.courtlistener.com/recap/gov.uscourts.txnd.299449/gov.uscourts.txnd.299449.1.0.pdf.

Vinluan v. Doyle, 2009 NY Slip Op. 219. New York State Supreme Court, Appellate Division, Second Department (2009). Retrieved from www.courts.state.ny.us/courts/ad2/calendar/webcal/decisions/2009/D20723.pdf.

Whole Woman's Health v. Hellerstedt, 579 U.S. ___ (2016).

ONLINE RESOURCES

American Association of Nurse Attorneys
www.taana.org
Centers for Disease Control and Prevention (CDC) Public Health Law Program
www.cdc.gov/phlp/index.html
Network for Public Health Law
www.networkforphl.org
Public Health Law Research
http://publichealthlawresearch.org
SCOTUSblog
www.scotusblog.com

46

Nursing Licensure and Regulation

Edie Brous

> *"[A] nursing license is a revocable privilege. It, much like a license to practice medicine and dentistry, represents a property interest, not a fundamental right."*
>
> **Supreme Court of Mississippi, Mississippi State Board of Nursing v. John Wilson, 624 So.2d 485, 494 (1993)**

The application process for nursing educational programs has become progressively more competitive. In 2017, nursing schools turned away more than 56,000 qualified applicants from undergraduate nursing programs (Knowles, 2018). Accepted students must meet the stringent academic rigors of a challenging curriculum, followed by successful completion of state board examinations, before being licensed to practice. The extensive qualifications for licensure have led some to believe they have earned the *right* to practice professional nursing. The practice of nursing, however, is not an unqualified right. It is also a *privilege*, and privileges must be preserved. To maintain one's license in good standing and continue practicing, nurses must understand that rights are always accompanied by responsibilities.

This chapter provides an overview of the regulatory processes, both those that are internal to nursing and those that impose obligations from outside the profession. Although external regulatory schemes impact all health care providers, it is the internal process of self-regulation that greatly influences nursing practice and defines nursing as an autonomous profession.

THE PURPOSE OF PROFESSIONAL REGULATION

The government has an obligation to protect its most vulnerable citizens. This social contract with the public is the reason that nursing is a regulated profession. Those who are sick, infirm, young, of the older population, disabled, or in any manner unable to advocate for themselves may be endangered by unqualified practitioners. Nursing regulation provides public accountability. A member of the lay public may not have the ability to recognize and protect himself or herself from incompetent providers. Government oversight of licensed nurses by a body of nursing experts is intended to keep patients safe by ensuring competence.

SOURCES OF REGULATION

Nursing Boards

The initial qualifications for licensure, continuing educational requirements, disciplinary procedures, complaint resolution processes, professional misconduct or unprofessional conduct definitions, mandatory reporting requirements, and specific scopes of practice are determined at the state level. Some states have separate licensing boards for registered nurses (RNs) and licensed practical nurses/licensed vocational nurses (LPNs/LVNs), although other states have unified boards for regulating all nurses. Boards of nursing (BONs) are given their authority through state laws or administrative procedure acts.

Health and Human Services and the Center for Medicare and Medicaid Services

Through various administrative agencies, the U.S. Department of Health and Human Services (HHS) regulates issues such as civil rights, privacy, food and drug safety, the Medicaid and Medicare programs, health care fraud, medical research, technology standards, and tribal matters. It serves as the umbrella organization for such agencies as the Centers for Medicare and Medicaid Services, the Food and Drug Administration, the Centers for Disease Control and Prevention, and the Office for Civil Rights, among others. The integrity of all HHS programs is protected by the Office of the Inspector General (OIG) through audits and other means.

Health care providers must be compliant with regulations and criteria called Conditions of Participation and Conditions for Coverage to be eligible for Medicare or Medicaid reimbursement. The OIG may place a provider on a List of Excluded Individuals/Entities, designed to protect the health and welfare of recipients of Medicaid or Medicare. Nurses placed on the exclusion list may not be employed by any employers receiving state or federal funding.

Federal, State, and Local Law

Public health codes are laws enacted at the local, state, or federal level to promote community health and safety. They address emergency preparedness, communicable diseases, environmental controls, use of health care facilities, staff credentials and competency, policies and procedures, mental health issues, food safety, and other elements related to nursing care. These laws may be enforced by civil or criminal penalties.

Organizational Policy

Nurses are responsible for being familiar with their employer's policies and procedures and to adhere to them. An organization's protocols may be used to establish the practice standards to which the nurse will be held. They exist to provide standardization and consistency. Failure to abide by an institution's rules may endanger patients and expose the nurse and the employer to liability.

LICENSURE BOARD AUTHORITY AND RESPONSIBILITIES

Nursing is regulated at the state level. Laws referred to as Administrative Procedure Acts or Civil Procedure Codes vary by state and determine the structure and authority of the BON. In some states, the BON is an independent agency, although in others the BON operates under a larger state agency. BONs that are consolidated under larger agencies are functionaries of the Secretary of State, the Department of Health, the Division of Consumer Affairs, Education Departments, or other regulatory and licensing agencies. BONs may also be hybrid organizations, functioning as institutions that are partially independent and partially affiliated with other agencies. Rules and regulations for

nursing practice may also be found in public health and general business laws. The court system generally supports the exclusive authority of the BON but will consider conflicts between employment practices and BON directions.

The primary function of a BON is to protect the health, safety, and welfare of the public and to maintain the public's trust in the profession by ensuring that those individuals who engage in the conduct described in the Nurse Practice Act (NPA) or other nursing statutes are properly trained and licensed. The state in which an applicant seeks licensure by reciprocity or endorsement must confirm that the applicant is in fact a licensee in good standing in another jurisdiction. To confirm that this is the case, state boards will perform licensure verification. Approximately 53 nursing boards in all jurisdictions except Michigan, Alabama, California, and Pennsylvania participate in NURSYS, an online process for providing immediate verification information to the requesting board (National Council of State Boards of Nursing [NCSBN], 2019).

Issue and Renew Licenses

In some jurisdictions, an initial professional license issued by a nursing board is valid for the licensee's lifetime. The licensee must periodically register that license to continue practicing and meet the board's registration requirements to be issued a registration certificate. Such requirements typically include continuing education, clinical practice, the absence of a criminal record, and continued good moral character. The cyclical process of reregistering a license is commonly referred to as a renewal process. In some states, licenses that have not been renewed can be categorized as null and void, and then are ineligible for renewal. Nurses must reapply for licensure in these jurisdictions.

To comply with their legislative mandate to protect the public, BONs define the required elements of nursing education. Graduation from a school that is accredited in one state may not meet the requirements for licensure in another state.

Investigation and Prosecution of Complaints

BONs are statutorily mandated to investigate all complaints against health care providers covered by the state's administrative procedure act or NPA. Some cases may be resolved through informal procedures, although others require formal hearings. Licensees against whom a complaint has been lodged should be advised of the allegations and of their rights. Although nurses may represent themselves, it is strongly advised that they seek legal counsel when responding to Board inquiries, even when the allegations appear baseless.

LICENSURE REQUIREMENTS

Candidates for entry into nursing practice as an RN or LPN/LVN must apply for licensure to a BON and receive an Authorization to Test. They then may be allowed to schedule an appointment to take the National Council Licensure Exam (NCLEX-RN or NCLEX-PN), which they must pass to be granted an initial licensure.

A nurse licensed in one jurisdiction may be granted a license in another jurisdiction without retaking the NCLEX upon meeting certain conditions. Additionally, the nurse may be required to explain criminal activity or any disciplinary actions in the home state. Interstate compact agreements may also allow a multistate privilege.

Enhanced Nursing Licensure Compact

The enhanced nursing licensure compact (eLNC) was implemented on January 19, 2018. This multistate compact, referred to by the NCSBN (2012) as a "mutual recognition model," allows RNs or LPN/LVNs to work across state lines in certain circumstances. Nurses residing in compact member states, known as residency or home states, may practice in other compact member states, known as remote states. Nursing practice must be compliant with the NPA and the nursing licensure compact administrative rules of each state. Nurses must remain within the specific scope of practice in the state in which they are practicing (the state in which the *patient* is located). Home states and remote states communicate through a coordinated database and both may take disciplinary action against a licensee when indicated (NCSBN, 2018a). A separate licensure compact for advanced practice nurses was approved on May 4, 2015 but will not be implemented until 10 states have enacted the necessary legislation (NCSBN, 2018n).

NURSE PRACTICE ACTS

Sets of laws enacted to protect the public specify the scope of practice for nursing attendants, LPN/LVNs, RNs, and advanced practice registered nurses; outline the authority of the Board; define professional misconduct; and detail the investigation and disciplinary processes for resolving complaints. The scope of practice for all levels of nursing has evolved and expanded considerably since the first NPA was enacted, and nurses should periodically review the scope and standards of practice in every jurisdiction in which they practice.

Advisory Opinions and Practice Alerts

Many nursing boards publish opinions regarding scope of practice, professional misconduct definitions, or delegation questions to clarify the board's position. These advisory opinions may be published independently or in conjunction with other organizations. Practice alerts may also be published advising the nursing community and the public at large of any rule changes or urgent issues. Nurses should go to their BON's website periodically to monitor such communications.

DISCIPLINARY OFFENSES

BONs investigate all complaints they receive. Although gross negligence and unsafe practice are obvious sources of disciplinary action, many actions not directly related to patient care may fall within the definition of professional misconduct and result in disciplinary action. Failure to advise the BON of name or address changes, failure to repay student loans, failure to pay child support, driving under the influence, failure to file or pay taxes, dishonesty in licensure or job applications, falsified or deficient documentation and record-keeping, improper delegation, diversion of controlled substances, or criminal convictions are some examples of actions that may result in BON disciplinary action.

Conflict Between the Nursing Board and Other Entities

Employers who ask nurses to practice outside their legal scope are placing those nurses at risk of licensure discipline. Similarly, employers who ask nurses to violate professional ethics or clinical standards of practice also expose them to licensure discipline. Nurses must know their NPA and nursing board expectations and refuse to violate nursing law or professional standards.

In the *Matter of Emery*, Nurse Jean Emery worked as a per diem nurse in a presurgical unit at Memorial Sloan Kettering Cancer Center (MSKCC). MSKCC implemented a 2007 policy requiring nurses to confirm that they had witnessed patients signing a consent form, whether they had actually witnessed the patient signing the form or not. Nurse Emery correctly believed that complying with this policy could subject her to professional discipline and addressed her concerns to management. When MSKCC responded that the policy would not be changed and instructed her to continue following it, she asked to be taken off the schedule, then resigned. She applied for unemployment benefits, which were initially denied. The Department of Labor determined that she had left her job without good cause, thus disqualifying her for the benefits of unemployment insurance. An Administrative Law Judge (ALJ) reversed this decision, finding that she was entitled to benefits because MSKCC had failed to respond to her valid concerns. When the ALJ's decision was upheld by the Unemployment Insurance Appeal Board, MSKCC appealed to the court. The Third Department of the Appellate Division of the Supreme Court of New York affirmed the decision, finding that Nurse Emery did have good cause to leave her employment because, "Under the circumstances here, substantial evidence exists to support the determination that the employer failed to respond to claimant's concerns within a reasonable time, even though the employer's general counsel admitted that a professional disciplinary complaint could be filed against an employee who adhered to the policy" (*Matter of Emery v. Memo. Sloan Kett. Cancer*, 2010).

Conflict can also exist between state or federal law and professional nursing responsibilities. An example is the Religious Freedom Restoration Act (RFRA)—a federal law that is mirrored by some state laws. The original purpose was to protect free exercise of religion from substantial burdens imposed by the government (RFRA, 1993). In enacting this legislation, Congress was responding to a 1990 United States Supreme Court (USSC) decision in which the Court held that First Amendment rights were not violated when unemployment benefits were withheld from Native Americans who had been dismissed from their jobs for ingesting peyote.

In *Employment Division v. Smith* (1990), two Native American men ingested peyote as part of a religious ritual. They were terminated from their employment for work-related misconduct and the state of Oregon denied their application for unemployment benefits. The men brought their case to court, arguing that the use of peyote for religious purposes was protected by their First Amendment right to exercise their religion. The USSC concluded that there was a *rational basis* for the Oregon law outlawing the use of peyote, and thus those who used it for religious purposes were not exempt from that law. Prior to the *Employment Division v. Smith* decision, religious minorities were considered exempt from laws that infringed upon their exercise of religion unless the government demonstrated a *compelling government interest*—a much more rigorous standard than the *rational basis* test. RFRA was an attempt to restore the *compelling government interest* standard. Since its passage, RFRA has been used as a defense to violations of anti-discrimination laws.

In January 2018, the Division of Conscience and Religious Freedom was created under the Department of Health and Human Service's Office of Civil Rights. Under this new division, nurses and other health care professionals can deny health care to some patients if providing that care violates their moral or religious beliefs (HHS, 2018). Even before passage of RFRA or the creation of the Division of Conscience and Religious Freedom, nurses were justified in refusing to participate in abortions, sterilizations, sex-reassignment surgery, or other procedures to which they had moral or religious objections. Nurses must be cautious in exercising their right to express conscience-based objections, however. Nurses cannot refuse, deny, or withdraw from patient care for reasons that reflect discrimination or prejudice, rather than moral or religious objections. And nurses must exercise their rights in a manner that does not constitute patient abandonment. The ANA issued a response to the creation of the Division of Conscience and Religious Freedom (Box 46.1).

BOX 46.1   Response of the American Nurses Association (ANA) to the Creation of the Division of Conscience and Religious Freedom

The ANA Code of Ethics for Nurses with Interpretive Statements states that a nurse has a duty to care. It also states a nurse is justified in refusing to participate in a particular decision or action that is morally objectionable, so long as it is a conscience-based objection and not one based on personal preference, prejudice, bias, convenience, or arbitrariness. Nurses are obliged to provide for patient safety, to avoid patient abandonment, and to withdraw only when assured that nursing care is available to the patient. Nurses who decide not to participate on the grounds of conscientious objection must communicate this decision in a timely and appropriate manner, in advance and in time for alternate arrangements to be made for patient care. Nurses should not be discriminated against by employers for exercising a conscience-based refusal.

However, we must take care to balance health care professionals' rights to exercise their conscience with patients' rights to access a full range of health care services. Discrimination in health care settings remains a grave and widespread problem for many vulnerable populations and contributes to a wide range of health disparities. All patients deserve universal access to high quality care, and we must guard against erosion of any civil rights protections in health care that would lead to denied or delayed care (ANA, 2018).

Source: American Nurses Association. (2018). *ANA responds to the HHS announcement of the New Conscience and Religious Freedom Division.* Retrieved from www.nursingworld.org/news/news-releases/2018/ana-responds-to-the-hhs-announcement-of-the-new-conscience-and-religious-freedom-division/.

Complaint Resolution

The BON may offer the nurse an opportunity to settle the matter informally rather than conducting a full hearing. A settlement called a Consent Order may be reached in which the nurse stipulates to certain findings and agrees to a disciplinary action that has been negotiated. Informal settlement conferences offer the advantage of lower legal costs and more rapid resolution of the complaint. The nurse may elect to attend a formal hearing rather than agree to a Consent Order if the settlement agreement offers a disciplinary action the nurse considers too harsh. A formal hearing may also be preferred when the disciplinary action of a proposed Consent Order would trigger an OIG exclusion.

Disciplinary Actions

The BON may close the file if its investigation finds no violations. The complainant will be advised that the investigation is complete and the matter is resolved. No action is taken against the nurse. Alternatively, the BON may find violations that can be addressed by issuing a letter of reprimand, but no other action. Letters of reprimand may be publicly posted as disciplinary actions. Nurses may also be fined and/or ordered to attend corrective education.

For more serious practice or ethical issues, the BON may impose practice restrictions and place the nurse on probation. During the probationary period, the nurse may be required to submit periodic employer reports, demonstrate attendance in an impaired provider program, and comply with other terms. Licenses may also be suspended, during which time the nurse is not permitted to work, or the suspension can be stayed (temporarily set aside), during which time the nurse is permitted to work while remaining on probation.

The most severe penalty, revocation, is reserved for cases in which the BON believes the nurse presents a serious danger to the public and cannot be rehabilitated to practice safely. A revocation permanently terminates a nurse's license, prohibiting practice and the use of nursing titles. The individual may no longer represent himself or herself as a nurse. The BON may entertain a petition for reinstatement after revocation in certain cases where the individual can demonstrate rehabilitation and competence. Mandatory waiting periods may be imposed before requests for restoration will be entertained, and formal restoration hearings may be required.

When faced with formal disciplinary hearings, some nurses may agree to voluntarily surrender their nursing licenses. In doing so, the nurse must understand that the forfeiture of the license is permanent. Such surrender still constitutes a disciplinary action tantamount to revocation.

The surrender process, sometimes referred to as Discipline by Consent, is an application that the BON may or may not accept. Temporary surrenders may be negotiated for nurses who agree to enter professional assistance programs for impaired providers. Entry into such programs may provide immunity from further disciplinary action if the licensee meets all other required criteria.

Nonpunitive peer assistance programs may provide an alternative to discipline but have not been uniformly adopted in all jurisdictions. Those states and territories that have adopted such alternatives to discipline programs may require the absence of patient harm for nurses to qualify for participation. The NCSBN (2018c) states that, "[A] lternative to Discipline programs for Substance Use Disorder enhance a BON's ability to quickly assure public protection by promoting earlier identification and requiring evidence-based intervention for nurses with substance use disorder. The benefits to the nurse include the opportunity to demonstrate to the BON in a non-disciplinary and non-public manner that they can become safe and sober and remain so, while retaining their license." The NCSBN website also provides links to individual state programs.

Alternatives to discipline programs may address impairment from mental illness as well as from chemical addiction, using a medical model as opposed to a punitive model and allowing the nurse to be rehabilitated and support reporting systems. Nurses working in states without such programs should become active in lobbying for their adoption. Some states have an additional category of license surrender called Voluntary Relinquishment. This is a form of surrender unrelated to disciplinary action in which the licensee is retiring, moving out of state, or for other reasons choosing not to practice nursing in the state.

Appealing board decisions is difficult, expensive, and frequently unsuccessful. All internal administrative steps must be completed before seeking redress in the courts. The court will only reverse BON decisions if the licensee can prove that the BON has violated the constitution or the law and has exceeded its authority under the statute; that it took actions that were an abuse of discretion or were arbitrary and capricious; or that the actions taken by the BON were unsupported by the evidence.

Collateral Impact

The emotional, financial, legal, and professional impact of BON disciplinary action can be profound. Evidence of board disciplinary action may be admissible in medical malpractice lawsuits or in criminal prosecution. OIG exclusions and data bank listings may render a nurse unable to work, even when holding a license in good standing. Subsequent licensure in another profession or jurisdiction may be difficult or impossible to obtain. Reputation damage is very difficult to overcome. The emotional distress can be considerable, even disabling.

REGULATION'S SHORTCOMINGS

Although professional licensing boards are entrusted with keeping the public safe, there is no evidence that the current regulatory system for BONs is effective in improving nursing practice. Some BON practices may in fact be antithetical to patient safety goals. Punitive cultures undermine patient safety by deterring essential reporting of errors. BONs that fail to distinguish between intentional misconduct and inevitable human error perpetuate an ineffective response to adverse events by blaming the end-user or direct provider for the error. This sharp-end focus fails to account for the dangerous systems in which nurses practice and compromises the error-analysis process necessary to prevent recurrence. A latent-error focus—on less apparent failures of organization or design that contributed to the occurrence of errors or allowed them to cause harm to patients—positively impacts patient safety, as opposed to the active-error focus that has a paradoxical and perverse effect on patient safety initiatives.

The level of penalty imposed may be determined by the level of injury to the patient, which is both inequitable and counterproductive. Outcome-oriented discipline results in inconsistency from one licensee to another for the same infraction. Safety experts recommend evaluating processes, not outcomes. The public is not kept safe by imposing a harsher penalty on a nurse because the patient was injured. The nurse whose patient is not injured by the identical error may be a less cautious provider and actually pose a greater risk to patients but would receive a lighter penalty with this approach.

Lengthy suspensions create rusty practice skills. The technical competence and knowledge required for safe practice are not enhanced by removing a clinician from the workforce. Practice deficiencies are not corrected by levying fines or publishing disciplinary actions on the Internet. Without addressing the underlying root causes and contributing factors of nursing errors, they will persist and endanger patients.

Patients cannot be kept safe unless their providers are adequately supported. BON advisory opinions are often unavailable or inadequate. Statements such as "Nurses should work collaboratively with their employers" or "Until the matter is resolved nurses are advised to use their best judgment" offer no direction to the practitioner faced with questionable work situations. Although the NCSBN could provide significant guidance, much of its published materials are restricted to board members and unavailable to the practicing nurse. Many NPAs use generic language when addressing "professional misconduct" or "unprofessional conduct" and do not provide definitions to guide practice or educate nurses regarding potential violations.

The defense of a licensee may be compromised when the BON has information which the licensee is unable to access. Privacy and confidentiality provisions of the administrative statutes are sometimes written or interpreted in such a manner as to prevent even the target of the investigation from obtaining all evidentiary materials. The discovery rights to which a criminal or civil defendant would be entitled may not be afforded to licensees in an administrative action. The collateral impact of disciplinary action may be ultimately more destructive than the actual disciplinary action itself. Onerous practice restrictions compromise employment opportunities. A temporary suspension may be all that is required for OIG exclusion. The inability to practice for several years may make an eventual return to practice logistically impossible, regardless of licensure status. This undermines efforts to rehabilitate motivated professionals.

Board members may not be selected by members of the nursing profession. They are frequently appointed by the governor or some other state-based selection method. As such, appointees may be selected more by political motivations than qualifications the regulated community would find essential. BONs are bureaucratic structures, many of which are underfunded and understaffed. Levels of efficiency vary. Due process rights in agencies differ substantially from due process rights in a court of law. The right to a speedy trial in the criminal system, as well as the standards and goals that move civil suits forward on mandated schedules, do not exist in the administrative setting. The investigative and hearing process can take months or even years from initial complaint to final resolution. This lengthy process is traumatizing even to those nurses who are ultimately vindicated.

Most people understand the need for legal representation to protect their freedom and physical possessions in criminal or civil lawsuits, yet many nurses try to represent themselves with the BON. Licensure defense requires skilled advocacy. Some BONs make telephone calls to licensees. In these circumstances, nurses may unknowingly make statements against their interests. Nurses may also sign agreements with the BON without understanding the long-term collateral impact of doing so. BONs do not always advise licensees that they can and should seek legal representation at all stages of the process. Nursing board investigators and prosecutors may discourage nurses from being represented by counsel or not inform them that their professional liability insurance may provide for licensure defense.

CONCLUSION

A professional license is considered a property right. It is not a right that can be taken for granted, however, and nurses can only protect their licenses by fully understanding the responsibilities that accompany them.

DISCUSSION QUESTIONS

1. Do you consider your license to practice nursing a right or a privilege? What is the difference?
2. Why is nursing a regulated profession? How is it regulated in your state(s)?
3. What are the strengths and weaknesses of the current regulatory scheme for licensed professions?

REFERENCES

Employment Division v. Smith, 494 U.S. 872, U.S.S.C. (April 17, 1990). Retrieved from www.law.cornell.edu/supremecourt/text/494/872.

Knowles, M. (May 2, 2018). Nursing schools reject thousands of applicants amid shortage. *Becker's Hospital Review*. Retrieved from www.beckershospitalreview.com/workforce/nursing-schools-reject-thousands-of-applicants-amid-shortage.html.

Matter of Emery v. Memo. Sloan Kett. Cancer, 508585 [3d Dept 8-5-2010], 2010 NY Slip Op 06333, Appellate Division of the Supreme Court of New York, Third Department. (June 9, 2010.) Retrieved from https://law.justia.com/cases/new-york/appellate-division-third-department/2010/2010-06333.html.

National Council of State Boards of Nursing. (2012). *NCSBN Model Act*. Retrieved from www.ncsbn.org/14_Model_Act_0914.pdf.

National Council of State Boards of Nursing. (2019). *Nursys*. Retrieved from www.nursys.com/NLV/NLVJurisdictions.aspx.

National Council of State Boards of Nursing. (2018a). *Enhanced Nurse Licensure Compact (eNLC) implemented Jan. 19, 2018*. Retrieved from www.ncsbn.org/11945.htm.

National Council of State Boards of Nursing. (2018b). *APRN Compact*. Retrieved from www.ncsbn.org/aprn-compact.htm.

National Council of State Boards of Nursing. (2018c). *Alternative to discipline programs for substance use disorder*. Retrieved from www.ncsbn.org/alternative-to-discipline.htm.

Religious Freedom Restoration Act. (1993). Retrieved from www.law.cornell.edu/uscode/text/42/2000bb.

U.S. Department of Health and Human Services. (2018). *HHS takes major actions to protect conscience rights and life*. Retrieved from www.hhs.gov/about/news/2018/01/19/hhs-takes-major-actions-protect-conscience-rights-and-life.html.

ONLINE RESOURCES

American Nurses Association
www.nursingworld.org
National Council of State Boards of Nursing
www.ncsbn.org/index.htm
Nurses Service Organization
www.nso.com

47

TAKING ACTION: Nurse, Educator, and Legislator: My Journey to the Delaware General Assembly and as Lieutenant Governor

Bethany Hall-Long

"I have come to the conclusion that politics are too serious a matter to be left to the politicians."

General Charles de Gaulle

MY POLITICAL ROOTS

I am a nurse and I became the first registered nurse and health care professional elected into the Delaware General Assembly and more recently as the State's 26th Lt. Governor. The roots of my public service began in a farming community in Delaware, where I volunteered to help others in my church and at neighborhood organizations. At the age of 12, I was a candy striper in a local hospital and continued my civic work during my teen years. When I entered college, I joined a political party. Though my parents were not politically active, my great-grandfather was a member of the Delaware House of Representatives in the 1920s, and I am a descendent of Delaware's 15th governor.

My interest in politics began while working with underserved residents at the same time I was completing my master's degree in community health nursing in the late 1980s. I used an earlier edition of this book, *Policy & Politics in Nursing and Health Care*, in my graduate program, and I vividly recall reading the chapters about becoming involved in politics. I began working with my local city government, the League of Women Voters, and a federal health clinic that served the homeless. Before these experiences, I had thought that public policy was remote to nursing and somewhat dry. These experiences changed my perspective.

VOLUNTEERING AND CAMPAIGNING

I went on to volunteer with nonprofit and civic organizations, join professional associations, and to complete my doctoral degree in nursing administration and public policy. During this time, I served as a United States Senate Fellow and as a U.S. Department of Health and Human Services policy analyst for the Secretary's Commission on Nursing. These experiences exposed me to national policy work, federal officials, leaders in the nation's health associations, and international researchers. I became actively involved with veterans' organizations because my husband was on active duty in the military. I also became a volunteer on political campaigns with the Democratic Party. I had excellent mentors to assist me with both my nursing and political career paths. All these experiences helped me to understand the policy process and the importance of building relationships.

I began my work in politics to make a difference in the lives of many citizens who lack life's necessary resources. As a public health nurse, I had an interest in improving the services available to vulnerable populations. I continue to work to advance issues important to the residents I represent. These include health care, the environment, land preservation, social and criminal justice, education, and economic development.

THERE'S A REASON IT IS CALLED "RUNNING" FOR OFFICE

A number of factors influenced my decision to run for public office in 2000, including my desire to make a significant contribution to the public's health. As a university faculty member, I assigned students to various public health and health policy assignments. During these experiences, I witnessed the need for expert health knowledge in the Delaware General Assembly. The time was ripe within the political party and within my district to run for the Delaware legislature. I ran for office for the first time in 2000 and lost by a mere 1%. I had run against a long-term male incumbent and learned some important political lessons. In 2002, political redistricting left a vacant seat and I ran again. This time I won in a tough election against the president of the local school board. After serving 6 years in the House, I campaigned for, and won, a state senate race in 2008. After serving 9 years as a Senator and earning the reputation as one of Delaware's most prolific legislators with over 1000 pieces of legislation, I decided to run for the executive branch. My focus was on the physical, mental, and economic health of Delaware with the goal of making Delaware healthier and stronger. In a crowded 6-way primary in 2016 and a general election, I won and took the oath of Office for Lt. Governor in January 2017. The *NLN Reporter* (National League for Nursing [NLN], 2017) featured my story (Fig. 47.1).

A DAY IN THE LIFE OF A NURSE-LEGISLATOR AND LT. GOVERNOR

No 2 days in politics are alike. Each elected official's experiences and perceptions are linked to his or her beliefs, the district's

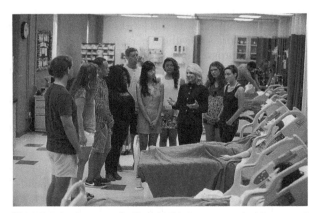

Fig. 47.1 Lt. Governor Bethany Hall-Long appeared with some of her students at the University of Delaware School of Nursing on the cover of the National League for Nursing's newsletter. Dr. Hall-Long's campaign literature identifies her as a nurse and educator.

beliefs, the state's legislative rules, and external economic or social pressures. In Delaware, serving as a legislator and Lt. Governor are part-time jobs. The Lt. Governor's duties, per Delaware's Constitution, are to preside over the Senate, Chair the Board of Pardons, and assume the seat of the Governorship should there be a vacancy. Delaware's bicameral legislative session is active for a total of 45 days/year. Session convenes each January, and the legislature must pass the budget bill and recess by July 1. We meet 3 days a week: Tuesday, Wednesday, and Thursday. I spend the remaining days on executive branch work, in meetings, delivering speeches, assisting with statewide constituent needs, and conducting my job as a nursing faculty member. Between July and January, my days are filled with at least 8 to 12 hours of meetings, community work, board of pardons, engagements for the Governor and, in election years, campaign activities. On occasion, there are Special Sessions in the fall when the senate convenes.

Much of a state legislator's time is spent on the capital and operating budgets of the state, as well as handling senate confirmations. These activities need to be completed by the end of the state's fiscal year: July 1. First as a legislator and now as the state's Lt. Governor, an important role of mine is to represent my constituents at committee meetings, public hearings, and on task forces. The State is both rural and suburban and has numerous policy needs: addiction, smart growth, transportation, education, health care, and economic development.

I juggle caring for my family, legislative work, and nursing education. I'm up at 5 to 6 AM to exercise and then I have breakfast meetings with constituents or campaign committee members. Following the meetings, I usually put on my other hat and spend time with my nursing students. I return phone calls in my car as I head into meetings or the state capital. When I arrive in my office, I'm greeted with phone messages, e-mail, and the pressing issues of the day. As Lt. Governor, I preside over the Senate as that begins at 2 PM. One day a week there are committee hearings. In the afternoons, I squeeze in more phone calls, RSVPs, research with the lawyers, and then head back to the floor to preside.

After each legislative day, there are usually receptions sponsored by interest groups. These provide time for lobbyists and members to review issues and concerns and highlight state funding efforts or programs. Typically, I attend several civic or association meetings each evening after the session in my district (I balance these with my son's sporting and school events.). These meetings are important for gathering community input, staying current on issues, and leading public policy such as Delaware's Behavioral Health Consortium, focusing on mental health and substance abuse issues that are a current public health epidemic. It all takes a lot of time, energy, and a few cups of coffee.

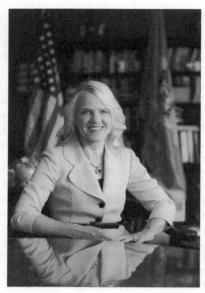

Lt. Governor Bethany Hall-Long, State of Delaware.

WHAT I'VE BEEN ABLE TO ACCOMPLISH AS A NURSE-LEGISLATOR AND LT. GOVERNOR

I sponsored or cosponsored over 1000 bills as a member of the Delaware House and Senate that covered broad policy areas of health, education, transportation, veterans' affairs, agriculture, natural resources and the environment, homeland security, community and county affairs, insurance, and more. As the only health care professional in the Delaware General Assembly and first elected nurse Lt. Governor and second female, I have been the prime sponsor of some important health bills and on task forces such as the necessary code changes for the state's Health Exchange as a result of the federal Patient Protection and Affordable Care Act (www. heatlthcare.gov), Governor's Cancer Council, and the Health Fund Advisory (Master Tobacco Settlement Committee). As Lt. Governor I am pleased to have spent over a year on the Action Plan for Behavioral Health. This is based on statewide community forums of lived experience of over 600 persons impacted by mental health issues or addiction. Delaware will be a national model to address the fractured mental health and substance use system. There is much work with a plan that resembles the nursing care plan process with a timeline and measureable objectives, including expanded prevention, harm reduction, and access and treatment measures. In turn, I have worked with nursing leaders and policymakers on many licensure/scope of practice and public health and environmental policies. These policy issues have included occupational health, disability service expansion, cancer, minority health, dental care access, women's health, environmental justice, chronic illness, mercury removal from the environment, school health, early childhood education, prescription assistance, and end-of-life care decisions. I have found that having a nursing background is extremely valuable in influencing a wide variety of policy issues.

Since I was raised on a farm, I have used this knowledge to advance agriculture and farming policies. I was pleased to sponsor, as my first piece of legislation, the farmland preservation license tag. In addition, I have sponsored land use legislation that helps with county, municipal, and state communication. Only 1% of the U.S. population consumes more than 20% of all health care expenditures, and 5% of the population accounts for more than 50% of the total expenditure (National Institute for Health Care Management [NIHCM] Research and Educational Foundation, 2015). Chronic illness is a major issue for Delaware, as it is for the nation. I sponsored legislation to establish a blue-ribbon task force to analyze the problem of chronic illness in Delaware and to develop policy recommendations. The task force identified strategies including disease standards of care for health professions, improved communication between insurers and providers, outreach to the at-risk, and the use of a disease management approach with Medicaid patients and among the business community.

I was the prime sponsor of legislation creating a cancer consortium for Delaware. This group has completed a comprehensive assessment and plans to tackle our high cancer mortality rates. I am pleased to say that the cancer incidence and cancer rates have dropped since the creation of this body. The state has implemented the consortium's many recommendations, including establishing a free treatment program for cancer patients who lack insurance, adding statewide caseworkers, enforcing indoor tanning bans for teens without parental consent, and creating screening programs. As previously mentioned, we have recently created the Behavioral Health Consortium modeled after the Cancer Consortium's approaches.

The opioid and heroin crises are a national public health epidemic. As the Chair of Delaware's Behavioral Health Consortium, I was pleased to recently give the Governor a 3-year Action Plan. This came from over 600 community members statewide from public forums where goals, actions, cost, and deadline for the gaps and duplications for the fractured system were attacked. These include expanded access and treatment, harm reduction, family support, and drug diversion with law enforcement. All these examples of sponsored legislation and policy actions involve a team effort. Nurses must collaborate with officials, individuals, lobbyists, and organizations or advocates.

TIPS FOR INFLUENCING ELECTED OFFICIALS' HEALTH POLICY DECISIONS

What have I learned as a legislator and Lt. Governor as to who can help other nurses seeking to influence policy? You must communicate well to influence policy, and nurses are naturally gifted communicators and problem solvers. In a study of nurse leaders in federal politics, I found that the political strategies used most frequently by nursing organizations are direct contacts, grassroots efforts, and coalition formation (Hall-Long, 1995). Nurses should not be intimidated by the need to call, write, or visit their elected officials. It is important when meeting with elected officials that you are prepared. Have a one-page fact sheet to leave behind (as opposed to a binder of information) and be prepared to summarize your issue and offer solutions in less than 5 minutes.

If nurses don't speak up on health care issues, who will? Physicians? Hospital associations? Insurers? If nurses don't speak up, legislators will only hear from other groups. Given health reform and a push for a nursing consensus model, advanced practice nurses are expected to take on a broader scope of practice and must be engaged in state-level policy discussions. You have heard the expression, "It's not whether you win or lose but how you play the game."

Well, in politics, how you play the game can determine whether you win or lose an issue. Increasing your influence by working in a group or coalition is an extremely effective strategy.

IS IT WORTH IT?

Life as an elected official has been better than I could have imagined. Although it has taken some time away from my family and my scholarship, it has been worthwhile. I encourage other nurses to consider how they might serve the public, including running for elected office.

REFERENCES

Hall-Long, B. (1995). Nursing education at political crossroads. *Journal of Professional Nursing, 11*(3), 139–146.

National Institute for Health Care Management Research and Educational Foundation. (2015). *The concentration of health care spending* (data brief). Retrieved from www.nihcm.org/categories/publications/the-concentration-of-health-care-spending-data-brief?showall=1.

National League of Nursing. (2017, Fall). For Nurse educator Dr. Bethany Hall-Long, public service is a birthright and passion, *NLN Reporter, 28,* 3-7.

48

Policy and Politics in Health Care Organizations

Rhonda Anderson and Mary Beth Kingston

"Were there none who were discontented with what they have, the world would never reach anything better."

Florence Nightingale

As our politicians continue to discuss health care needs and coverage in America, the health care organizations work to transform themselves from:

- Volume- to value-driven organizations
- Illness to effectively managing populations with chronic illnesses
- Single hospitals to mergers and acquisitions
- Hospital-based clinicians to clinicians coordinating care across the continuum
- Hospital-focused technology to continuum management with use of technology
- Fee-for-service to assuming risk
- Patient experience to shared decision making
- Hospital-centric focus to community health and addressing social determinants
- Hospital nursing to a variety of nursing opportunities across the continuum

FOLLOW THE MONEY

The political climate around health care access and financing continues to be as intense and uncertain as it was in 1965 when President Lyndon B. Johnson's focus was to make sure the older population had access to health insurance. If we "follow the money" through the past 50 plus years, we find legislative and commercial changes in philosophy,

reimbursement, and practice based on the payment incentives or disincentives.

The social security amendments of 1965 provided hospital and medical coverage to older adults at age 65. Medicaid was also added by the Kerr-Mills Amendment to support the needy (Woods, 2016). As the country experienced this new way of funding care for the aged, needy, blind, and disabled, hospitals seemed to be admitting more patients and health care costs began to grow exponentially. The ordering of tests, procedures, interventions, and hospitalizations seemed to dominate the practice of medicine in the years after the inception of Medicare. Payment was received and there was no incentive to order only those procedures and tests necessary to provide appropriate care. As the volumes of tests and hospitalizations grew and the costs to the government and insurers grew, many government leaders became concerned about the ability to fund the rising cost of health care for older adults.

By the early 1980s, Congress and President Ronald Reagan mandated Medicare controls through implementing the Prospective Payment System (PPS). From 1967 to 1983, the cost of Medicare rose from $3 billion to $37 billion (Office of Inspector General, Office of Evaluations and Inspections, 2001). The PPS created Diagnostic Related Groups (DRGs) that were a case rate or flat rate paid for each of the 467 covered diagnoses. This was an abrupt shift from paying the hospital for all that was done for the patient to a specific amount for the diagnosis no matter the number of tests, x-rays, days in the hospital, etc.

Changes to practice were not rapid but many early adopters created "care pathways" to address this transition of incentives. Health care multidisciplinary teams began reviewing best practices and costing those practices. Nurses were integral to the process as these pathways were designed and implemented. In some organizations, the finance team member would cost the proposed path and help determine how cost effective the path was compared to the DRG payment. Some organizations would place the reimbursement amount on the front of the chart (before electronic health records), along with the pathway, as a reminder to the physicians and other clinicians about the new clinical management approach. Other organizations created a companion patient pathway document to guide their patients' day by day through their acute hospital stay. Whiteboards in patient rooms began to be part of the new patient engagement and communication tools. These tools were to help the patient and other clinicians align patient goals and expectations for their acute care hospitalization with the reality of the evidence-based pathway.

Because there was no differentiation of a Medicare patient from a commercial patient, all patients were placed on the pathway. This shift to PPS and DRG payments caused some patient dissatisfaction. Nursing's interventions, and education of their patients, were more important than ever. Increased time in patient education and discharge transitions were required. The nurse case manager role became more prevalent due to the expected focus on efficient patient management in the acute care setting and the improvement in efficient transitions to outpatient management. There was a major issue and conflict for case managers due to them being expected to focus more on utilization and not as much on care coordination (Frater, 2018). Expansion of Medicare benefits continued in the 1980s and 1990s to cover home health, hospice, and low-income Medicare beneficiaries. Under President George W. Bush, an additional enhancement added prescription drug options through private insurers (Rogers, 2018).

In 2010 under President Barack Obama, the Patient Protection and Affordable Care Act (ACA) was signed into law. The concepts brought forward with the ACA were moving from an illness system of care to a health-focused system of care; improving access to care; volume (fee-for-service) to value (global payments linked to key outcome indicators); population health focus; and consumers being engaged in their health care decisions. Between the 1990s and 2010, costs continued to escalate even with the PPS. For over 50 years, the changes to reimbursement incentives, enhancements to Medicare and Medicaid, and partisan differences in

philosophy about government's role in health care, caused the industry to change their care processes but cost escalation continued. From 1960 to 2016, health care spending rose from $147 per person to $10,348 per person (Rogers, 2018).

The ACA legislation provides a roadmap of expectations for consumers, health care organizations, and Centers for Medicare and Medicaid Services (CMS). One legislative requirement is developing and implementing measures that will lead to the long-term goal of comprehensive pay for performance, or value-based care. That work continues today through the National Quality Forum (NQF) as a contracted group with CMS. Experts from the field are members of NQF workgroups and they review and recommend to support, conditionally support, or do not support metrics that CMS requests for various CMS programs. With the Trump administration, the President and the Republicans continue their repeal-and-replace threats and actions. If the approach is to repeal pieces of the ACA without understanding what the new philosophy, concepts, and financing incentives are, there will be severe consequences for health care organizations and major confusion for the consumers. There must be a set of principles built on a philosophy of health and illness care in our country if a transition of the ACA to a new law takes place.

Despite attempts to thwart the ACA, health care systems are proceeding with their transition from volume to value. CMS with their NQF partner is continuing their pay for performance work under the ACA legislation. The U.S. Department of Health and Human Services (HHS) has clearly stated that value-based payment goals can improve health care in the United States.

The three primary strategies (Burwell, 2015) are:
- Incentivizing hospitals, health care systems, physicians, and providers to deliver high quality at decreased costs by the use of alternative payment models (accountable care organizations [ACOs], bundled payments)
- Improving delivery of care, including greater coordination of care and population health efforts
- Accelerating the availability of information to guide decision making and improve communication with consumers

Under the ACA, additional outcome measures will continue to be established. In 2018–2019, Medicaid child and adult workgroups will be reviewing and recommending measures for states to implement. This will affect what health care organizations measure and report to both public and private payers.

The American Hospital Association (AHA) has also supported the transition to value from volume. However, they have been vocal about not having large numbers of measures, but that there is now a measurement system. The AHA is focused on measures that are most meaningful, provide the most value to patients, and support efficient care management and patient engagement. Balancing the value philosophy with meaningful work that is not an excessive burden and doesn't add excessive expense to the health care organizations is what the health care providers and systems are supporting.

It is difficult, expensive, and burdensome to have more and more measures added to providers and provider organizations if they may not be making a difference in quality patient outcomes and encouraging a healthier group of citizens. The AHA identified that approximately $709,000 is the annual amount spent on the administrative aspects of quality reporting and $7.6 million annually is the cost of meeting Federal mandates for quality reporting, record keeping, meaningful use compliance, and the implementation of electronic health records (Dickson, 2017).

Hospitals serving low-income populations have additional concerns about the measures, especially measures around readmission. The social determinants causing readmission of this population post-acute discharge put the hospital in financial jeopardy because they can't control the environment in which these patients live. The hospitals can, however, work with their community to try to improve housing, food insecurities, and other social determinants issues. In 2019, the 21st Century Cures Act should help adjust the financial effects to the hospital for the social determinants issue.

HEALTH AND SOCIAL DETERMINANTS

As a condition of maintaining their tax-exempt status, nonprofit hospitals are required to conduct a Community Health Needs Assessment (CHNA) to access the health, chronic illness, top community health issues, and social issues affecting the health of their community. From that assessment, strategic goals are developed, community partnerships solidified, and 3-year plans for improvement are implemented. These goals and plans are submitted to the Internal Revenue Service (IRS). Even if the CHNA was not in place, hospitals and health care providers should be reaching into their communities to identify the level of health of their communities. Our schools are a great place to start. Many children don't have access to the care of a pediatrician. At Banner Health, they found many children with chronic illness were not receiving primary care and were admitted to the emergency departments when their disease was not appropriately managed. Banner Children's School-Based Health Director applied for and received a federal grant to purchase and equip a mobile health unit. The Banner Health Foundation raised funds for the nurse practitioners and the director evaluated where in the Phoenix metropolitan area there was excessive emergency department use by these children, scheduled the mobile unit to work with the school districts in those areas, and partnered with the schools and the school nurses to encourage families to schedule appointments with the Nurse Practitioner as the primary care provider. The results were a significant decrease in emergency department use, improved health of the children, decreased numbers of days absent from school, and increased access to primary care providers.

Health care systems have accelerated preventive screening and immunization programs and have worked to move some of these programs into the community as a way of reaching more people. The consumer's workplace and community centers are two sites that can be used to improve access for the consumer to receive these primary care services. Increasing the number and involvement of social workers in all health care settings can assist in increasing focus on social issues and barriers to health. In the health systems' new model of care in some inner cities, new roles for nurses and other providers were created to fulfill the 3-year CHNA plan. Some of those roles are community health worker, nurse practitioner, and health coach. Many health systems have made significant investments in this type of community work. Geisinger Health System employs community health assistants to visit people who have specific social needs, including social isolation (Lee & Gorba, 2017). Hennepin Health in Minneapolis has partnered with a local organization, Rise, Inc., that offers patients employment resources (Schrag, 2014), and ProMedica, serving Ohio and Michigan, screens all patients for food insecurity and provides a 3-day supply of food and nutrition counseling on discharge (Health Research and Educational Trust, 2017). These types of programs are promising, but not yet incorporated into many health care delivery systems. A survey conducted by Deloitte, Lee and Gorba (2017) noted that hospitals that were moving more quickly into value-based care models reported higher levels of investment in addressing social needs. Some nurses have also begun to address these social issues. Cadmus et al. did just that as part of the New Jersey Action Coalition. The action Coalition encouraged nurses to become involved in improving the health of their communities. They developed a website that displayed the projects needing nurse volunteers. Nurses were encouraged to join or lead a project with community partners (Cadmus et al., 2018).

Successful coalitions are being formed in many communities across the United States. The AHA, American Organization of Nurse Executives, The American College of Healthcare Executives (ACHE), and other national organizations are educating and encouraging their members to reach beyond their hospital walls and help build healthy communities.

POPULATION HEALTH

In order to be successful in this "new world order," the models of care that are mainly illness focused must change. James Begun (Healthcare Executive, September/October 2017) has clearly stated all work on improvement of the population's health must start upstream. If there are unhealthy environments, excess chronic illness, or lack of access to care, populations are going to receive episodic urgent/emergent interventions. If systems and models of care coordinate care of chronically ill populations and address unhealthy community needs, these populations are more likely to manage their health/illness continuum more effectively.

Populations can be defined in many ways. As health care organizations and insurers evaluate its members for high-risk, high-cost illnesses, they may select the top 6% to 10% who are in this category as their population health challenge. Case managers may be assigned to those groups with like illnesses and develop plans of care with them to keep them as healthy as possible. Other ways a population may be defined might be by location. An example may be those living in inner city housing projects with gang violence causing rape and other traumatic injury. Assessment, plan for intervening, addressing public policy issues, and measuring improved outcomes are important parts of the population health process.

As the federal monies flow to health care organizations based on performance, value, and efficiencies, the commercial insurers pressure these organizations at the contract negotiating table. The commercial insurers aren't going to issue contracts that have generous revenue streams for the organization or allow for the excess costs from caring for Medicare and Medicaid patients to be shifted to them. Fee-for-service, case rates, shared risk, ACO models, capitation, and other arrangements are being brought to the negotiation tables at contract renewal time. Insurers are pursuing various options based on their company's performance, risk assessment of those they insure, and the performance of the health care organization. They, however, still do pay better than Medicare and Medicaid. This reality causes a concern that some health care organizations may focus on contracting for commercial business only (MedPAC: Hospitals' Medicare margins continue to drop, 2018).

DISRUPTION TO THE INDUSTRY

There are also many new non-traditional entrances into the health care space. Disrupters to the past insurance model are those large employers that directly contract with health care systems and organizations for care of their employees. Many of them have corporate wellness programs and incentives for their employees to stay healthy or to manage their chronic illnesses more effectively.

Others, like Amazon, Berkshire, and JP Morgan, formed their joint ventures with the intent to cut the health care costs of their employees. Dr. Atul Gawande, as Chief Executive Officer (CEO) of this new joint venture, states, "I have devoted my public health career to building scalable solutions for better health care delivery that are saving lives, reducing suffering, and eliminating wasteful spending. Now I have the backing of these remarkable organizations to pursue this mission with even greater impact for more than a million people. The system is broken and better is possible" (Rege, 2018). This model as it is implemented could be a seismic disruption to the industry.

Are health care organizations positioned to directly contract with employers? Is the speed of change by disrupters so rapid that health care organizations can't compete? How agile are they or can they be with the regulatory burden they experience? How well can health care organizations provide all levels of care necessary when their focus has been acute care for so many years?

These large employers, nontraditional providers like CVS, Walgreens, Costco, etc., and the tech-savvy younger consumers, are expecting a lot from new models and the use of technology. Savvy retail companies are listening and acting on these customer-focused solutions (Manis, 2018). Nurse practitioners, health coaches, and pharmacists have been involved in the care of adults and children in these new locations and through some telehealth interventions. As these sites expand, needs and opportunities for nurse practitioners, nurses, and pharmacists have grown. A growing opportunity is for speech therapists with stroke patients and psychiatrists and psychologists with mental health issues. All can have far-reaching interactions with their patients through use of telemedicine interventions. There will be more opportunities and need for these and other clinicians in the future.

Some health care systems are also becoming disrupters to the traditional models. Over the past 50 years, they have tried to adapt, redesign, and adjust to the changing incentives and current disrupters. Some have been early adopters, some laggards, and some have just tried to modify their contracting strategies and models of care with no major shift in their illness and volume philosophy.

ACHE President and CEO Deborah Bowen encourages health care leaders to be courageous and bold as they lead disruption (Bowen, 2018).

As these organizations develop and implement bold, courageous strategies, they must be agile, nimble, resilient, and manage rapid change. They also must develop new models of care and invest in technology that supports telehealth, artificial or augmented intelligence, analytics, and informatics. Many health care systems have pursued a population health strategy in the quest to transform care delivery, improve overall health, and decrease health care costs. Population health has been defined in many ways. Kindig and Stoddart introduced the term population health in 2003 and defined it as "the health outcome of a group of individuals, including the distribution of such outcomes within the group." A workforce strategy needs to be developed to support this transition strategy. The following points can guide the system nurse leaders to develop and implement a successful plan:

- Participate in developing the system transformation strategy.
- Create the model of care and define the workforce needs in that new model of care.
- Lead the comprehensive workforce strategic plan as part of the overall planning.
- Know system timeline for transitioning each component of the strategy.
- Partner with each "C" suite member to identify his or her workforce needs for the new strategy.
- Collect state and national comprehensive workforce data and use with each partner; especially involve the human resource leader.
- Develop and implement education plan for all leaders/managers on the strategy, timeline, and their role in the process.
- Develop and implement communication plan for all employees.
- Create formal transition plan for each area of the strategic continuum of care; be specific about timeline and budget.
- Update and use talent map to identify internal potential staff transitions.

As the disruptors enter the market, there are important lessons for health care systems—specifically, knowing more about what is important to the consumer. For many consumers, convenience rises to the top of the list. This has spurred expansion of clinic hours, ability to schedule an appointment online, scheduled urgent care visits, and increased ambulatory sites, remote monitoring, e-visits, and consults. Information technology plays a role, as consumers want access to their information and the ability to communicate with their provider. Patient portals, single or integrated electronic health record, and portability of information among clinicians are a few examples of responding to this need. Being consumer centric and always understanding what they want/need is key to success. Being nimble and agile in timely creation of those needs is essential. Health care clinicians and organizations are usually slow in making changes. Their future success depends on being faster at changing processes and protocols.

OPPORTUNITIES FOR NURSING

The changing health care landscape and climate for innovation and disruption are providing new opportunities for nurses to practice. Lack of coordination of care has received intense scrutiny, as it results in confusion for the consumer and poor outcomes. Coordination, navigator, and transition roles have been and continue to be developed to address gaps in care and the need for ongoing health coaching. A screening or risk stratification tool, identifying those at high risk for complications or disease progression, is often used to tailor the coordination effort to the individual. Nurses fill many of these roles and lead and participate in teams that may be comprised of community health workers, social workers, and others.

eICU and eMed/Surg nursing have been implemented in many systems across the country and across the world. Nurses, as knowledge workers with the use of telemedicine and analytics, have a great opportunity to improve patient outcomes through remote monitoring of intensive care unit and Medical/Surgical patients and alerting the bedside clinicians to intervene earlier than they might have without this intervention. This role has also allowed experienced nurses who may not be able to physically provide direct patient care to continue to practice and remotely help other nurses via analytics, coaching, and mentoring.

The virtual interprofessional teams provide another opportunity for nurses and nurse practitioners. These teams can include the nurse, nurse practitioner, health coach, and pharmacist who have a daily virtual check-in with the patient. These teams have been successful in post-acute care and patient support. Outcomes related to decreased readmissions, decreased emergency department visits, and effective chronic care management are the goals of these virtual teams.

Nurses are inextricably engaged and involved in every aspect of a health care system's population health approach. As Lindrooth et al. (2015) noted, "Nursing is a fundamental driver of both outcomes and costs in most health care organizations." It is certainly critical to have nursing representation in national, regional, and local forums where health policy decisions are made. It is equally important that nurses be engaged and involved with strategy and program development, implementation, and evaluation in the health care system where they practice.

MERGERS AND ACQUISITION

As a result of these fundamental changes in payment and reimbursement systems, there has been a significant increase in merger and acquisition activity in hospitals, health care systems, insurers, and several for-profit health care–related businesses. Federal legislation and policy typically set the stage for significant change in reimbursement nationally, with other payers aligning their programs and practices. Health care systems and other entities are seeking partners as they face increasing financial pressure, ongoing competition, and increased labor costs. In the past, these relationships were primarily pursued to increase size and scope, which had the potential to lower administrative, fixed, and supply costs. In today's environment, mergers and acquisitions are being utilized to gain a strategic advantage in an increasingly complex health care environment.

Although significant change accompanies both mergers and acquisitions, there are financial and operational differences between the two transactions. In a merger, both organizations' assets and liabilities are combined. The organizations mutually agree to collaborate to expand and improve their services. As organizations merge, there is typically discussion about governance, policies, procedures, and processes. For example, decisions may be jointly made to adopt one organization's approach to compensation and benefits. Often, there is an opportunity to examine current practices and create a new approach. In an acquisition, one organization essentially purchases the other and the acquired entity usually adopts the policies and practices of the "buyer" who is the responsible entity for overall governance, operation, and finances.

Although the reasons for the acceleration in health care M&A seem clear, there are many examples of flawed or failed efforts in this area (Roos and Postma, 2016). Each merger or acquisition has its own set of internal and external variables, but meticulous planning, preparation, execution, and evaluation can mitigate some of the risk. Nurses are pivotal members of the health care team, and knowledge of the overall concepts and potential strategies for success can assist nurses at all levels to provide leadership throughout the process.

KEY MERGER AND ACQUISITION ACTIVITIES

The following discussion explains the key activities during the merger and acquisition process.

Due Diligence

Due diligence is a time when organizations considering a merger assess the viability and probability of achieving the value of the proposed transaction (Grauman et al., 2017). The timeframe for due diligence begins with the execution of the letter of intent and ends with the closing or finalization of the agreement. It is a legal process that includes a comprehensive assessment of financial and clinical risk, technology, human resource issues, current contracts, and outstanding

compliance/regulatory issues. Additionally, savvy health care organizations know that a cultural assessment can be invaluable, as significant differences can create major barriers to success. The process involves key internal subject matter experts and, often, external guidance. Nurses play a key role in providing and evaluating current state information, particularly relating to clinical quality risks, workforce issues, and cultural norms. Identifying and understanding key relationships in both organizations is essential in developing communication strategies and laying the foundation for collaborative decision making moving forward.

Regulatory Process

There are also federal regulatory hurdles that will impact whether a merger or acquisition can proceed, including the Federal Trade Commission (FTC) and the Antitrust Division of the Department of Justice (DOJ). These agencies enforce antitrust laws and believe that consumers benefit from competitive health care markets in terms of quality of care, cost, and innovation. The FTC also considers whether the merger or acquisition will result in increased efficiency or improved quality of care. Although there are examples of the FTC successfully challenging selected mergers, often in areas of market overlap, the effects have been modest when compared with the total number of M&As (Glied and Altman, 2017). There are also state approvals to be obtained, though these processes do vary by state.

The FTC and DOJ acknowledge that merging entities typically have a legitimate need to share information. However, before the M&A transaction is complete and during the process of federal and state review, there are limitations of areas of information-sharing and activity.

The organizations:
- Must act like independent competitors
- Can plan activities but cannot implement them
- Cannot present as a combined entity to customers or suppliers
- May not cooperate on sales efforts or seek to influence one another's sales, marketing strategies, or geographic expansion

It is important for nurses to have a clear understanding of the guardrails governing specific communication, particularly as companies and suppliers may reach out to them before finalization of the merger. Organizations should establish a monitoring process for information sharing early in the M&A process.

Integration

Planning for integration begins early in the M&A process. The initial work of bringing organizations together is one of leadership—creating a shared future vision and clearly articulating the benefits of the merger or acquisition.

Communication plans are developed for internal and external stakeholders, including the community and press, and are carefully coordinated with the formal closing date. Objectives and metrics that will define a successful merger are agreed upon and clearly articulated. It is critically important to have a planned change management approach for all integration activities, including culture differences.

In the initial process of integration, there is often a focus on system functions, such as finance, human resources, and information technology that provide support for centralized administrative functions and operations. Identification of key executive leaders is best determined in early stages to facilitate decision making and development of functional integration teams. The work is focused on standardizing, reducing redundancy, identifying cost savings, developing workflow processes, as well as creating new and innovative approaches in a variety of areas. Examples of functional teams include nursing, medical groups, pharmacy, operations, supply chain, risk, culture, quality, legal, and many others. The work of the teams is essential if the economies of scale, structure, scope, skill, and risk are to be realized. In an acquisition, limited time will be spent on these activities, and the acquiring organization will often quickly move to implement the already standardized processes (Piper & Schneider, 2015). The pace of change, at this point, is rapid and accelerates once the transaction has been finalized.

Impact on Nursing

The impact on nursing varies at the initial M&A stages and may be perceived differently in a merger versus an acquisition. Nursing leaders play a pivotal role in communicating the benefits of the merger or acquisition to all nurses in the organization. Changes in leadership can precipitate general anxiety about job security and uncertainty about the future. The nursing functional teams provide a great opportunity to engage nurses from different entities to align cultures, share best practices, and potentially create new and innovative clinical and workforce strategies.

There may be a perceived loss of organizational identity, which is certainly stronger in acquisitions, but also present in mergers (Giessner et al., 2016). Nurses and other team members identify with the unique culture and norms of their "home" hospital or health care system and may have difficulty relating to a new entity (Brodbeck, 2012). A well-executed integration plan and ongoing communication about the progress of the merger or acquisition are strategies that may alleviate these issues (Bradley, 2016).

POST-MERGER CONSIDERATIONS

The work of integration truly begins once the merger or acquisition is finalized. Planning continues, but there is considerable pressure to implement those plans to deliver on the pre-determined goals and metrics. Successful mergers and acquisitions focus on the patient populations to drive service and program planning, as well as new and expanded models of care. Ongoing internal and external communication is critical to dispel rumors, clearly demonstrate leadership, and build pride in the new organization. Many will look to the leaders' behavior as a barometer of the M&A success and, therefore, confidence, clear direction, and collaboration must be visible.

One of the most common reasons for failure in M&As is lack of attention to culture differences. Individuals cite culture concerns as a major reason for leaving an organization during an M&A (Sung et al., 2016). Culture can be defined in many ways, but it is basically the shared values, beliefs, and behaviors that determine how people do things in an organization. Initially, considerable time should be spent in developing relationships and building trust to set the stage for successful execution of the integration plans. A cultural assessment should yield information that highlights key similarities and differences that provide a starting point for factoring in culture to the integration process. Leaders of the new organization work with others to define the desired culture and then develop intentional plans to build this new way of being.

Health care policy, including reimbursement in a value-based care environment, has spurred this increase in M&A activity. Many focus on horizontal integration in which health care entities combine to form larger systems. Health care systems are also pursuing vertical integration strategies, such as merging, acquiring, or developing partnerships that expand their continuum of care and services, including purchasing physician practices and partnering with post-acute care providers. Vertical integration is an essential component for successful population health models of care.

CONCLUSION

Rising costs of care, the move from volume to value, workforce shortages, and many other factors have combined to create tumultuous changes in health care delivery in the United States. One result is the relatively recent acceleration of mergers and acquisitions in efforts to meet these challenges. The present work, and the work that lies ahead, will focus on developing new and innovative processes and care models that can improve outcomes and reduce costs for populations. This requires moving beyond the traditional care settings, focusing on health and wellness, managing chronic disease, coordinating care, partnering to address social determinants of health, and engaging consumers.

Nursing leadership and engagement in identification of strategies, as well as development and evaluation of key initiatives, are essential. Partnerships with education to prepare nurses to work in non-traditional roles; focus on care coordination and population health; attention to workforce issues (looming retirements of nurses, potential shortages); and facilitation of research to evaluate models are top priorities for nursing in a value-based, consumer-oriented health care environment.

DISCUSSION QUESTIONS

1. How are the moves to value-based reimbursement and major industry disruptors impacting nursing practice and the delivery of health care services?
2. What key strategies should nurses and nurse leaders develop to ensure a successful merger or acquisition occurs in their organization?

REFERENCES

Booske, B.C., Athens, J.K., Kindig, D.A., Park, H., & Remington, P.L. (February, 2010). *County health rankings working paper: Different perspectives for assigning weights to determinants of health.* Retrieved from www.countyhealthrankings.org/sites/default/files/differentPerspectivesForAssigningWeights ToDeterminantsOfHealth.pdf.

Bowen, D. (May/June, 2018). Leading for disruption. *Healthcare Executive, 3*(33), 89.

Bradley, C. (2016). Executing on integration: The key to success in mergers and acquisitions. *Nursing Administration Quarterly, 40*(4), 316-320.

Brodbeck, K. (2012). Merger destiny: Synthesizing organizational and executive leadership change. *Nurse Leader, 10*(3), 29-32.

Burwell, S.M. (2015). Setting value-based payment goals—HHS efforts to improve us health care. *New England Journal of Medicine, 372*(10), 897-899.

Cadmus, E., Raja, N., Polahowski, J., Lewis, T., & LoGripp, M. (October, 2018). Leading with the community. *Nurse Leader, 16*(5), 331.

Dickson, V. (November 27, 2017). Slumping Medicare margins put hospitals on precarious cliff. *Modern Healthcare.* Retrieved from www.modernhealthcare.com/article/20171125/NEWS/171129969/slumping-medicare-margins-put-hospitals-on-precarious-cliff.

Frater, J. (2018). *The history and evolution of case management.* Retrieved from www.teshealthcare.com.

Giessner, S.R., Horton, K.E., & Humborstad, S.I.W. (2016). Identity management during organizational mergers: Empirical insights and practical advice. *Social Issues and Policy Review, 10*(1), 47-81.

Glied, S.A., & Altman, S.H. (2017). Beyond antitrust: Health care and health insurance market trends and the future of competition. *Health Affairs, 36*(9), 1572-1577.

Grauman, D.M., Bangs, D., & Looby, S. (2017). Using due diligence to optimize post-transaction benefits. *Healthcare Financial Management, 71*(11), 68-75.

Jacobson, R.M., Isham, G.J., & Rutten, L.J.F. (November, 2015). Population health as a means for health care organizations to deliver value. *Mayo Clinic Proceedings, 90*(11), 1465-1470.

Kern, H. (May 11, 2018). Sentara CEO Howard Stern: 5 strategies that will define mergers of the future. *Becker's Hospital Review.* Retrieved from www.beckershospitalreview.com/hospital-management-administration/sentara-ceo-howard-kern-5-strategies-that-will-define-mergers-of-the-future.html.

Lee, J., & Korba, C. (2017). *Social determinants of health: How are hospitals and health systems investing in and addressing social needs?* Deloitte Center for Health Solutions. Retrieved from www2.deloitte.com/content/dam/Deloitte/us/Documents/life-sciences-health-care/us-lshc-addressing-social-determinants-of-health.

MedPAC: Hospitals' Medicare margins continue to drop. (March 26, 2018). *Modern Healthcare.* Retrieved from www.modern-healthcare.com/article/20180319/NEWS/180319896/medpac-hospitals-medicare-margins-continue-to-drop.

Office of Inspector General, Office of Evaluations and Inspections. (August, 2001). Medicare hospital Prospective Payment System. Retrieved from https://oig.hhs.gov/oei/reports/oei-09-00-00200.pdf.

Piper, L.R., & Schneider, M. (2015). Nurse executive leadership during organizational mergers. *Journal of Nursing Administration, 45*(12), 592-594.

Quality metrics and reporting in value based care. (October, 2017). *Hospitals and Health Networks.* Retrieved from www.hhnmag.com.

Rege, A. (June 20, 2018). *Dr. Atul Gawande tapped to Lead Amazon, Berkshire, J.P. Morgan venture.* Retrieved from https://www.beckershospitalreview.com/hospital-management-administration/let-s-stop-talking-about-digital-disruption.html (April 9, 2018) Jonathan L Manes Sr. VP & CEO Sutter Health.

Rogers, A., (Summer, 2018). The changing landscape of senior health care. *AMAC Advantage.* Retrieved from http://digitaledition.qwinc.com/display_article.php?id=3132888&view=511026.

Roos, A.F., & Postma, J. (2016). Getting cold feet? Why health care mergers are abandoned. *Health Care Management Review, 41*(2), 155-164.

Schrag, J. (October 24, 2014). Social determinants of health: Homelessness and unemployment, *America's Essential Hospitals.* Retrieved from https://essentialhospitals.org/quality/the-social-determinants-of-health-homelessness-and-unemployment/.

Sung, W., Woehler, M.L., Fagan, J.M., Grosser, T.J., Floyd, T.M., & Labianca, G.J. (2017). Employees' responses to an organizational merger: Intraindividual change in organizational identification, attachment, and turnover. *Journal of Applied Psychology, 102*(6), 910.

Woods, R.B. (2016). *Prisoners of hope: Lyndon B Johnson, the great society, and the limits of liberalism.* New York: Basic Books.

49

Taking Your Place at the Table: Board Appointments and Service

Kimberly J. Harper and Laurie S. Benson

"Some questions have no good answer...one such question is why the participation of nurses on hospital and health agency governing boards is the exception, rather than the rule."

John Lumpkin

All across America and beyond, decisions are being made every day that affect health and health care. Some of those decisions are good, resulting in improved health outcomes of our communities. Others, sadly, are not. Some strategy and policy decisions are made in absence of a voice that, if included in the discussion, would result in better decisions and improved health outcomes. That is the voice of a nurse. The Institute of Medicine (IOM) (2011) recognized the importance of this voice and recommended that "Public, private, and governmental health care decision makers at every level should include representation from nursing on boards, on executive management teams, and in other key leadership positions."

Nurses, despite being by far the largest health profession with nearly 4 million registered nurses in the United States, comprise less than 1% of voting members on hospital and health system boards (Benson & Harper, 2017). Additionally, according to a 2014 study that examined a dozen successful community health partnerships, nurses comprise only 4% of the direction-setting bodies (Benson & Harper, 2017). In addition to the absence of the nursing voice and vote at the hospital and health care system level, the number of nurses in governmental appointments is extremely low.

WHY NURSES?

Nurses are expert at managing clinical patient care and are the most trusted profession by the public (Brenan, 2018). Through their education and practice, nurses develop a set of skills and competencies that are extremely useful at policy tables that are not necessarily possessed by other professionals: assessing quality and safety, balancing financial costs with outcomes, and communicating at all levels (Robinson, Harper, & Benson, 2017).

Then why aren't nurses at these tables? Curran (2015) suggests five reasons: (1) Nurses do not realize that boards present an opportunity to address their personal and professional passions and missions; (2) Nurses are not sure what governance is and how boards work; (3) Many nurses do not think they have the skills to serve in governance roles at the board level; (4) Boards are often unaware of the skills and abilities that nurses possess; and (5) Nurses who wish to develop board-ready skills do not know where to begin.

COMPETENCIES REQUIRED OF BOARD MEMBERS

Boards typically create a skills matrix to identify skill sets and experience represented by current board members and strategic gaps to be filled by new board members, but most also look for individuals who possess these competencies:

- Strategic orientation
- Organizational awareness
- Systems thinking
- Personal effectiveness
- Community focus
- Innovative thinking
- Collaboration
- Advocacy

Most nurses possess all these skills making them excellent candidates for open board seats! They require little orientation and can make a seamless transition to immediately contribute to the work of the board. These same skills and competencies also create board environments in which new nurse board members are able to engage at a deeper level of understanding more rapidly than some board members who have not developed such skills prior to board service. Susan Reinhard, Senior Vice President and Director of AARP's Public Policy Institute and Chief Strategist of AARP's Center to Champion Nursing in America, notes (American Hospital Association, 2017):

> Hospitals are part of an increasingly complex health care environment and more than ever seek to form community partnerships. Hospital boards' historical focus on financial strength has shifted as quality of care and patient satisfaction have grown in importance as measures of success. Nurses can add knowledge and insights to all aspects of care, as well as observations other board members might not have about community health, wellness, disease prevention and other public health issues. Nurses also work in community settings such as schools, clinics and businesses and can bring much-needed diversity to the boardroom.

Competencies Nurses Possess

Although nurses may not initially see the value they bring to the boardroom, it is imperative that nurse leaders clearly point out that the skills and competencies they possess make them ideally suited to contribute to the discussions taking place in the boardroom.

> Nurses are often leaders in the shadows. We are most comfortable working behind the scenes to lead change. Some do this well, but when there is a critical mass of shadow leadership, nursing's power and potential are overlooked by others. We must come out of the shadows! (Quote by Diana Mason, in Hassmiller & Mensik, 2017)

Specific high-level competencies that nurses possess include the following:

- **Mission driven.** By nature nurses gravitate toward mission. They have not only the ability, but also the desire, to be committed to advancing the organization's mission and use it as a framework for decisions about the direction of the organization. This allows nurses appointed to a board to easily connect with the mission of that organization, allowing for an "all in" commitment.
- **Financial knowledge.** Though some nurses may not see it as a competency in which the nurse is highly skilled, many nurses possess the ability to review financial statements and interpret the financial condition of an organization. Clearly, nurse leaders are expected not only to review but to manage the budgets of the units and departments for which they have responsibility. This skill set is transferable to their fiduciary responsibilities as

board members. The forms and documents would differ but the set of skills remains the same. Just as importantly, they understand the implications of financial decisions on individuals, the organization, and communities.

- **Communication.** Nurses usually have high-level communication skills. They need to communicate to individuals at all levels within the work environment including patients and families, interprofessional colleagues, organizational leadership, and community stakeholders. Nurses become extremely skillful at not only delivering a message but also at hearing the message. Nurses are great listeners. They ask questions humbly. And nurses are excellent at "teach backs" where they make sure that the message that was meant to be communicated was not only heard but understood. This is an extremely powerful skill in the boardroom.

  Nurses are also able to communicate effectively, professionally, and confidently, using data and information that is helpful to the board in its decision making. And nurses possess a level of emotional intelligence and social etiquette that is often found to be exceptional by other members of boards. Nurses arrive at board meetings well prepared, professional in appearance, respectful, and engage highly in the discussions.

- **Cultural awareness/competence.** Most nurses possess a cultural awareness and competence that is not always well-honed by fellow board members, allowing the nurses to share their important voice in such discussions that increasingly take place as the diversity of our nation changes. Nurses are more likely to lead transformative discussions and processes that not only acknowledge but celebrate the importance of diverse cultures, values, beliefs, and behaviors. This greater understanding, when shared with others at the decision-making table, often results in the recognition of the worth and dignity of individuals and more equitable health care for all.

- **Leadership.** Governance is an extension of leadership. All nurses are leaders, whether or not they see themselves in that light. Nurses lead the care of patients, clinical teams, research projects, and more every day. Nurses gain experience through education, opportunity, and exposure to leadership roles both formally and informally and learn quickly to use that information to guide, support, motivate, and influence the health care of our communities and nation. Nurses are strategic in their actions, consistently envisioning a better way to accomplish the goal, whether it be their personal goal or that of a patient or client. Systems thinking is part of the nurse's skilled thought pattern, creating the ability for nurses to see all sides of multi-faceted situations and utilizing the nursing process in every decision that needs to be made. This type of leadership is an excellent addition to any board, task force, commission, or appointment.

PROCESS FOR IDENTIFYING READINESS FOR BOARD SERVICE

Many organizations have developed tools and questionnaires that help an individual nurse evaluate readiness to serve on a board. Depending on the type of board an individual may need more sophisticated levels of board competencies than others. Novice board members might begin with something comfortable to learn more about board activities, responsibilities, and expectations, such as on boards of nursing organizations at the local or state level. This experience prepares nurses to move onto local or regional non-profit boards of organizations whose missions they are passionate about. See Boxes 49.1 and 49.2 for some questions to consider, or go to the Nurses on Boards Coalition (NOBC) resource page at www.nursesonboardscoalition.org.

BOX 49.1   Types of Boards

Many opportunities exist for nurses to serve on boards, commissions, and other advisory bodies.

Private and Public Corporate Boards

These include corporate industry boards of various structures and sizes ranging from startup companies, entrepreneurs, and corporate enterprises in all industries including insurance, finance, manufacturing, agricultural, food and beverage, technology, medical devices, pharmaceutical, transportation, and other product and service industries. *Private boards* apply to corporations that are privately owned by individuals or families. *Public corporate boards* include those that are publicly owned and often managed by shareholders who own stock in the corporation. Frequently, the members of such boards are carefully selected and well compensated for their participation. Examples include most all types of pharmaceutical, large insurance companies, and organizations that are among the Fortune 500 companies.

Non-Profit Boards

This category is large and includes all types and sizes of non-profit organizations that serve the needs of communities, states, and the nation, as well as global missions. This includes many hospital or health system boards, such as private, public, and non-profit health provider organizations; philanthropic boards and foundations such as United Way and American Red Cross; non-governmental public health boards; local food pantries; literacy councils; poverty advisory groups; elder services; and other organizations that relate to human services.

Advisory Boards

Organizations such as start-up companies, small businesses, and non-profit organizations offer advisory board roles to obtain strategic advice. In most instances the members of advisory boards offer their expertise and assistance by providing data, anecdotal experiences, and expert advice that will assist others in making the strategic decisions. Many health care organizations convene advisory boards to collect input from important stakeholder groups that might otherwise not have their voices heard in such decision making. Examples include a parents advisory board at a children's hospital or an advisory board for a homeless shelter.

Commissions

Numerous and varied, commissions include individuals, frequently selected through a governmental process, to participate in decision making regarding a specific topic or area. Members of commissions are often chosen based on their personal expertise or position, which enables them to present a necessary specific skill set and level of knowledge. This category includes national, state, and local task forces such as the Governor's Commission on the Opioid Epidemic, the Mayor's Council on Charter Schools, or the former Vice President Joe Biden's Blue Ribbon Panel for Cancer Moonshot.

Governmental Appointments

This type of appointment includes any role where an individual is personally selected by a governor, mayor, or member of the legislature to serve on an advisory board, commission, or task force or in a governmental position. These appointments are often connected with one's political views, and individuals may be selected based on which side of the political fence they reside. This category also includes individuals who are elected by the public to serve in roles such as governor, state representative, state senator, member of the school board, and so on.

BOX 49.2 Sample Readiness Evaluation for Board Service Questions

- Am I an effective communicator?
- Am I an effective listener?
- Am I comfortable with inquiry?
- Am I comfortable when challenged?
- Do I possess emotional intelligence?
- Am I accountable?
- Do I possess relationship-building talents?
- Do I have social etiquette?
- Do I possess transformational leadership skills?
- Am I culturally sensitive and competent?
- Am I sensitive to age, gender, social, cultural, and linguistic needs?
- Am I cognizant of organizational cultures?
- Am I a change agent?
- Am I innovative?
- Am I proficient with team functioning and team behaviors?
- Do I possess the ability to direct activities and guide others?
- Do I have the ability to support outcomes even when the decision differs from my own?
- Am I a motivator?
- Am I a systems thinker?
- Am I a visionary?
- Do I possess skills in strategic planning?
- Do I have a community focus?
- Am I a collaborator?
- Do I possess business knowledge?
- Do I possess knowledge in financial operations?
- Do I possess human resources knowledge and skills with talent development?

WHICH BOARDS ARE THE RIGHT FIT?

Selecting which board is right for you is not always easy and it is best to carefully consider before accepting a board appointment. Steps for selecting the right board could include:

- **Start with an open mind.** It is okay to turn down a board opportunity. Be objective in assessing the pros and cons of each opportunity. You are likely qualified to serve on a number of boards, so make sure it is the right opportunity for you.
- **Understand your mission/passion.** One of the best determinants of a good fit is the alignment of your personal interests, values, and passion with the mission of the organization. Think about why and how the role will be meaningful to you personally.

- **Perform a self-assessment and assessment of the organization.** First, conduct a self-assessment to determine what specific strengths you will bring to the board. Write down your skills, qualifications, and experience that will enable you to contribute as a board member. Next, assess the organization's mission, leadership, culture, and values. Access multiple sources to learn everything you can about their strategic direction, financial position, and the reputation of the organization. Make sure you understand the role and composition of the board. From all you have learned, do you have an initial level of trust and confidence in the leadership and direction of the organization? Will you be proud to be associated with the organization? If you can answer yes to these questions, proceed with confidence.
- **Network with colleagues and friends.** Think strategically about who may be willing to help you make relevant connections. Make it easy for them to help you by sharing your specific interests and why you would like to serve on a board. Many board opportunities come to fruition through referrals from colleagues and friends. Always ask how you can help them achieve their goals, too. Great synergies and outcomes are often a result of colleagues helping each other on the journey!
- **Prepare your (one-page) board ready resume.** Make this a high priority *before* you pursue your first board opportunity. The many accomplishments of nurses often result in a multi-page curriculum vitae (CV) that is not ideal for presenting yourself for a board seat. Put yourself in the place of a nominating committee member who is reviewing multiple candidates. Make it easy for them to see you as a "standout" candidate by preparing a one-page bio that captures the strategic highlights of your career, skills, key competencies, experience, and impact. Be sure to include what is most important for them to know about you. It is a best practice to have others read your bio for feedback or engage a professional to do so. Examples and resources for assistance are available on the NOBC website at www.nursesonboardscoalition.org.
- **Contact the organization to declare your interest.** You won't be contacted unless they know you are interested. There is no risk in doing so. Contact the organization's executive leadership and/or board chair, governance or nominating chair to express your interest. Ask about the process for being considered and the appropriate next steps. Each board opportunity is unique and requires a well thought out approach. For non-profit board opportunities, offer to volunteer for a committee to get to know the organization and support their work.
- **Register your interest with the NOBC.** By registering with NOBC online (www.nursesonboardcoalition.org),

you will be included in future board opportunities for which your skills, qualifications, and experience align at the national, state, and local levels. You will also receive updates on new resources available to help you prepare for board service or to further develop your governance skills. For those already serving, register all your board roles on the NOBC website to help us track the number and kind of appointments.

- **Prepare for your interview with the board leadership.** Make sure you understand what the board is looking for in potential candidates, then confirm this at the interview and be able to confidently state your value proposition.

Most governing boards have the expectation that potential candidates should be interviewed for a board seat. Prior to an interview, prepare by spending time on the organization's website, learning the names and backgrounds of the other board members, understanding the mission of the organization, and being prepared to explain how you will be able to contribute to it and to the work of the organization. Make a list of key points that position you as a strong candidate. You do NOT need to have all the competencies; a well-rounded board is made up of members with diverse perspectives, skills, and experiences. Meticulous preparation will allow you to LISTEN during the interview and ask thoughtful questions, which is an important skill set in the boardroom. Before accepting a board role, ask to meet or talk with one or two other board members. This will help you understand the process, culture, and impact of the board, and determine if you are a good fit.

- **Never underestimate your value.** Once you have determined a board is a fit, make sure you are prepared to convincingly communicate your ability and desire to serve. It is important not to dilute your capabilities. Be sure to present yourself with confidence and boldness, yet at the same time, express your humility. Remind yourself why you want to serve on the board in the first place. Then reinforce your commitment to serve, if selected, in a way that not only meets but exceeds expectations!

VALUE OF BOARD SERVICE

The tremendous value of nurses serving on boards is increasingly recognized by many constituents including the organizations, the nurses who serve, communities, and all stakeholders.

Benefit to Boards

All boards can benefit from the nursing perspective. There is much greater awareness of the importance of including the nursing perspective, including hospital boards. John W. Bluford, III, Past Chair of the American Hospital Association and President of the Bluford Healthcare Leadership Institute, says:

> Without exception, nursing representatives on the board has proved to be invaluable. They were not so much an advocate for nursing, but they advocated for the needs of patients. As the board focused on matters of care quality—the voice of nursing was both critical and creditable. (Benson, 2018)

An often-overlooked value is the role nurse leaders play in providing a new source of qualified and committed candidates to expand a slate of candidates for consideration by all types of organizations that are increasingly seeking diverse candidates, including women. Scott Malaney, CEO of Blanchard Valley Health System of Sandusky, Ohio, says,

> In a community our size, it is very difficult to identify a person with extensive experience and education in the nursing field, who isn't already affiliated with our organization. For us, then, the NOBC offered the perfect solution. We had extensive discussions about the type of person and the skill sets we were hoping to attract. Subsequently, three highly qualified candidates were identified for us to interview. We were able to speak with and ultimately attract a person with an impressive background, both educationally and experientially, including significant time spent overseas. In addition, our candidate is the first person to serve on our Board who is not "local." As a result, we have a critically important member of the Board's Quality Committee, as well as a Board member who can bring a rich perspective from outside our immediate geographic area. (Malaney, 2018)

Benefit to Communities

Communities benefit by having nurses present a patient-centered perspective, visibly and powerfully. When nurses serve in community roles outside their formal employment, they expand their influence and impact, as noted by Christine Schuster, RN, MBA, President and CEO of Emerson Hospital in Concord, Massachusetts.

> I have seen the impact that is possible to have by moving beyond the bedside to serve in a broader, more far-reaching capacity. Emerson nurses are working in collaboration with our community agencies, such as Councils on Aging and regional senior care assistance organizations, to develop best practices in reducing readmissions. These collaborations improve patient quality of life, lower costs, and advance patient care quality. I am very proud of our nurses stepping forward to achieve measurable goals in enhancing patient care by working outside the walls of our hospital. (Benson & Harper, 2017)

In many cases, when nurses serve on community boards, they are expanding the influence and reputation of the organization where they work. According to Lawrence W. Vernaglia, Foley and Lardner LLP, one of the NOBC's Founding Strategic Partners (as cited in Benson & Harper, 2017):

> The involvement of their nurse executives in high-profile community boards builds credibility and enhances the reputation for the organizations that employ them. Serving on community boards, nurses are extending the reach and reputation of the hospital beyond the clinical environment in helping shape policy and strategy decisions that impact these critical areas of patient care across the continuum of care. (p. 14)

Benefit to Nurses

The benefits of board service are both tangible and intangible, ranging from monetary compensation in some cases to feeling good about making an impact in support of a mission. The value to the nurse is often on both a professional and personal level. Various board roles, when aligned with the passion of each nurse, provide them with the rewarding experience of making an even greater impact in the communities where they live and work. Board service provides professional development opportunities by building on leadership skills in a board setting, as well as the personal satisfaction that comes from meeting other board members, being a part of a collective voice to influence strategy decisions, and providing an important service.

Board service is a privilege and a responsibility. In short, while nurses bring a valued perspective to the boardroom for the benefit of all they serve, they consistently express they get so much more in return than they had ever imagined.

RESOURCES AVAILABLE THROUGH NURSES ON BOARDS COALITION

In 2014, a dedicated group of 21 national nursing and health care organizations were brought together by the Robert Wood Johnson Foundation and AARP to discuss the issues related to the need for the voice of more nurses at tables where health care decisions were being made. The original group of nursing organizations banded together as the NOBC to bring to life one of the most daunting recommendations in the 2010 *The Future of Nursing* report: "Nurses [...] should serve actively on advisory committees, commissions and boards where policy decisions are made to advance health systems to improve patient care" (IOM, 2011).

Today, NOBC has 28 member organizations (defined as national nursing or health care organizations who join

NOBC and commit to work in collaboration with other member organizations to fulfill the mission and goals of NOBC). In addition, NOBC has over 50 sponsors (defined as an organization that provides financial support to NOBC without a commitment to work on getting nurses appointed to boards) and partners (defined as an organization with whom NOBC has a formal alliance to advance the interests of the NOBC and the partner…specifically, to increase the number of nurses serving on boards), as well as contacts and some type of programming in all 50 states and the District of Columbia.

NOBC, now a not-for-profit organization with 501 (c) 3 status, is overseen by a board of directors and is committed to the belief that the perspective and influence of nurses must be felt more at decision-making tables. Although nurses comprise the largest group of health professionals, they remain vastly underrepresented in board leadership positions. The NOBC has set out to transform this reality. It has created and collated many resources to assure success in the nurses who chose to step up and lead through their service and voice at the table.

The overarching goal of the NOBC is to improve the health of communities and the nation by increasing nurses' presence on corporate, health-related, and other boards, panels, and commissions. By raising awareness that all boards would benefit from the unique perspective of nurses, the NOBC strives to achieve its goal of improved health all across America. The future envisioned by NOBC is one in which every health-related board has at least one nurse member. All nurses in America and across the globe are invited to join in this transformative journey.

Please visit the NOBC (www.nursesonboardscoaliton. org) to find board preparation resources such as articles, webinars, videos, and other publications.

CONCLUSION

Regardless of level of education or experience, there is a place on a board, a commission, or an appointment for EVERY nurse, and nursing must not stop until they are filled. Every such appointment brings America one step closer to our collective goal of healthier communities and a healthier nation. Where will you choose to serve? As Linda Burnes Bolton, Chief Nurse Executive of Cedars-Sinai Medical Center, challenges us:

> Choosing to accept positions and appointments with governing bodies; professional societies; and education, health, and social policy organizations has allowed me to influence a great many people and institutions…Each of you must stand up and call the circle, practice inclusiveness, and remain committed to upholding the value of

nursing...If the doors to quality health care can't be opened, knock the doors down! Step up and lead colleagues! (Cited in Hassmiller & Mensik, 2017).

DISCUSSION QUESTIONS

1. Why is it important for nurses to serve in governance roles?
2. How do nurses identify, prepare, and pursue board opportunities to take their place at the table?
3. What are the benefits of nurses serving in governance roles to boards, communities, and nurses?
4. What skills and competencies make nurses uniquely and ideally suited for board service?

REFERENCES

Benson, L. (2018, August). *Diversity in the boardroom: Consider a nurse.* Directors & Boards. Retrieved from www.directorsandboards.com/articles/singlediversity-board-room-consider-nurse.

Benson, L., & Harper, K.J. (2017). Why your nurses should serve on community health boards. *BoardRoom Press, 28*(1), 1-2. Governance Institute. Retrieved from www.nursesonboardscoalition.org/wp-content/uploads/BRP_2017_02_V28N1_Why-Your-Nurses-Should-Serve-on-Community-Health-Boards_Benson_Harper.pdf.

Brenan, M. (2018). *Nurses again outpace other professions for honesty, ethics.* Retrieved from https://news.gallup.com/poll/245597/nurses-again-outpace-professions-honesty-ethics.aspx.

Curran, C. (2015). *Nurse on board: Planning your path to the boardroom.* Indianapolis, IN: Sigma Theta Tau International.

Hassmiller, S.B., & Mensik, J.S. (2017). *The power of ten* (2nd ed.). Indianapolis, IN: Sigma Theta Tau International.

Institute of Medicine. (2011). *The future of nursing: Leading change, advancing health.* Washington, DC: The National Academies Press.

Malaney, S. (2018, May). *Testimonial.* Nurses on Boards Coalition. Retrieved from www.nursesonboardscoalition.org/testimonial/scott-malaney-ceo-blanchard-valley-health-system/.

Reinhard, S. (2017, March 13). Getting nurses on board. *Trustee Magazine.* American Hospital Association. Retrieved from www.trusteemag.com/articles/1212-getting-nurses-on-the-hospital-board.

Robinson, F.P., Harper, K.J., & Benson, L. (2017). *Nurses on board: The time for change is now* (whitepaper). Minneapolis, MN: Nurses on Boards Coalition, Capella University. Retrieved from www.nursesonboardscoalition.org/wp-content/uploads/2017/06/NursesOnBoardhttps://www.nursesonboardscoalition.org/wp-content/uploads/2017/06/NursesOnBoard-TimeforChange.pdfTimeforChange.pdf.

ONLINE RESOURCES

The Future of Nursing Campaign for Action
www.campaignforaction.org
Nurses on Boards Coalition
www.nursesonboardscoalition.org
Women in the Boardroom
www.womenintheboardroom.com

50

TAKING ACTION: Nurse Leaders in the Boardroom

Linda Burnes Bolton, Catherine Alicia Georges, and Rita Wray

"Leadership is service to others."

Denise Morrison

The number of nurses entering boardrooms across America continues to rise, as discussed in the Nurses on Board Coalition chapter (see Chapter 49). We believe strongly that nurses are obligated to use their knowledge and skill to be of use to others. Serving in the boardroom of America's organizations is an excellent way to demonstrate the passion we as nurses have for human caring. Being willing to serve and to bring other nurses to boardrooms in our cities, counties, states, and across the nation is a true example of being a servant-leader. In this chapter, we share our volunteer and paid experiences serving on local, state, and national boards.

GETTING STARTED

There are many pathways to serving on governing bodies in a leadership position. You may begin by answering the question, "What is my true north?" What am I passionate about and want to actively support?

The first step may be to volunteer for a leadership role in your nursing organization, professional society, parent-teacher group, or family councils within hospital and health care organizations. Select something you care about and to which you are willing to donate your time and efforts. For example, our passion for eliminating health disparities and improving access to social, health, and education services for all led us to pursue leadership positions in our local communities, places of worship, and national organizations. This first step is critical. We have observed nurses join organizations because they want to advance their careers but found themselves feeling burdened by the demands on their time.

Second, discuss your plans with leaders from the organizations you are seeking to serve. Find out if you have the qualifications they seek. If you don't, determine the steps necessary to obtain the qualifications.

Third, broaden your self-assessment and seek stretch opportunities. Go beyond nursing organizations. Consider leading youth sports groups or something entirely different from health care but that contributes to the support of people of all ages, socioeconomic status, ethnicity/race, gender, and health status.

We cite examples from our leadership journeys on boards, beginning with Dr. Catherine Alicia Georges, EdD, RN, FAAN, an educator, community leader, and Volunteer President of AARP. This is followed by the journey of Rita Wray, MBA, RN-BC, FAAN, a leader in society and health care, a medical-legal consultant, and businesswoman whose leadership journey has been in government, hospitals, and communities. We close with the journey of Linda Burnes Bolton, DrPH, RN, FAAN, one of the leading chief nurse executives in the nation, past president of national nursing organizations, and member of the board of trustees of the Robert Wood Johnson Foundation, one of the largest health care foundations in the world.

ALICIA'S JOURNEY

Getting appointed or elected to a board is not an accident. My journey to being elected to the Board of Directors of the AARP in 2010 for a 6-year term started a number of years ago. In 2016, I became the President-Elect of the organization and in June of 2018 I became the National Volunteer President of this consumer organization with 38 million members. I remain a member of its board of directors.

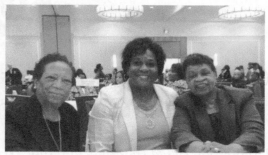

Authors Linda Burnes Bolton, Rita Wray, and Catherine Alicia Georges.

As a graduate nursing student at New York University, I took an elective course in urban planning and development. One of the assignments was to attend a community meeting and to ascertain how decisions were made in such areas as infrastructure projects and zoning policies that would have a potential impact on community development. The first obstacle was to gain access to the community board meeting in my community in the Bronx. After many barriers and challenges to my right to be present at such meetings, I finally got an invitation to attend as a silent observer. What I observed was the vested interests of board members being politically played out during the meeting, with decisions about projects being based on political affiliations. There was no opportunity for community groups to have their voices heard. I left that meeting perplexed and disappointed in the process.

A few years later, the New York City charter was revised and gave communities an opportunity to influence the local governance process. There was a call for those interested in serving on boards to complete an application and submit it to the borough president in one's own borough. My application clearly delineated my specific knowledge and skills, which at the time included teaching nursing at Lehman College and being an active member of the New York Chapter of the National Black Nurses Association (NBNA). I had to undergo a series of interviews, culminating in a brief and final interview with the Bronx borough president. I contacted my city councilperson's office and had a phone interview with him, expressing my interest in serving on the new community boards. I forwarded my resume to his staff and was told a few weeks later that he would support my application. That support was crucial and I was selected by the borough president for the appointment. I served on that board for 18 years and was reappointed by three borough presidents.

During my tenure on that board, I served as secretary, vice chair, and eventually chairperson. As a board member and an officer, I needed to be able to interact with diverse community groups, nongovernmental organizations, governmental agencies, and elected and appointed policymakers; be aware of the issues and have data to support requests for capital and expensive projects; understand public budgets; and be able to interact with the financial experts in the city agencies. Problem solving, negotiation, and conflict resolution were paramount in being an effective community board member, but speaking out and making clear where I stood on issues was also very important.

At the same time, I became active in the local chapter of the NBNA, eventually being elected to the board and then president of the Association. During the time that I served on the boards of my community and the NBNA chapter, I attended various seminars and conferences to expand my knowledge of board governance; improve my performance as a board member; and network with board members from other organizations, which gave me the opportunity to serve on other boards such as CGFNS International (formerly the Commission on Graduates of Foreign Nursing Schools), a credentialing organization for internationally educated nurses and other selected health professionals, and then the Board of Directors of the AARP. I have learned that being a board member requires:

- Being knowledgeable about the issues that the board will have to confront. That means staying abreast of the changing political and social environments.
- Being committed to the mission and vision of the organization.
- Thinking critically and acting strategically as a board member. This requires one to look at facts and evidence and engage in an unbiased analysis of the issue.
- Understanding governance policies of the board.
- Being willing to speak out on issues because they are socially just.
- Always being prepared and having substantive information to share with board members when a contentious issue arises.
- Giving up professional ego and working collaboratively with other board members.

My journey as a board member on these various boards has been challenging, exciting, and educational. I encourage nurses to undertake this journey to board service.

RITA'S JOURNEY

Nurses bring a unique perspective to board service, whether it is visioning, strategic thinking and planning, bringing nursing's values to policymaking, or attention to fiduciary matters. Because of our academic preparation, work experience, and professional expertise, we also make excellent decision makers and leaders. We use a lens of human caring and patient-centeredness when making decisions, whether on behalf of an individual, population, or organization.

The leadership skills learned in the classroom and honed in the clinical and academic settings are the same skills needed to serve effectively on health care–related and non-health care–related boards and commissions; it is merely a transference and translation of core leader skills combined with a deep sense of commitment, experience, and expertise.

My professional clinical career track includes bedside nurse, nurse educator, nurse executive, nurse entrepreneur, and business owner with cumulative leadership skills that I have found highly transferrable in my role as a state government executive, as well as serving on multiple boards and commissions. Many of those skills were cultivated, recognized, and used within nursing circles as the nursing process. With demonstrated knowledge, ability, candor, and tact, I begin with acknowledging the value all bring to the table, actively listening and data gathering (assessing), solidifying the task (planning), engaging bridge builders, and getting the job done (implementing). After group engagement and buy-in is obtained, I close with my trademark charge: "Let's do this." For example, as president of the Greater Jackson Arts Council, I led the board through a visioning exercise where we discerned the need for developing a signature sustainable event (assess). Through our grants program we chose to create new stories with neighborhood associations, emerging artists, community leaders, and major art providers such as museums, symphony, opera, ballet, and theater companies (plan). Begun in 2006, the Storytellers Ball invites all to be a part of the story. It is not only a successful annual black tie fundraiser but a dynamic way of highlighting the collective impact and importance of arts and culture in schools and communities within the capital city (implement).

A snapshot of my board and commission experience is varied and has included:

- Professional organizations—International Women's Forum Mississippi Chapter, president-elect; NBNA, treasurer; and Mississippi Action Coalition, co-lead;
- Private business entities—president of The Capital Club, a 1500-member private business club known for its social and cultural prominence in the capital city of Mississippi; treasurer of the Junior League of Jackson Sustainers Board, an organization of women committed to promoting volunteerism, developing the potential of women, and improving communities through the effective action and leadership of trained volunteers;
- Political organizations—Mississippi Federation of Republican Women, president;

- Religious organizations—National Advisory Council for the U.S. Catholic Bishops, vice chairperson; and Parish Pastoral Council, president;
- Community organizations—Greater Jackson Arts Council, president; and Community Foundation of Greater Jackson, strategic planning committee chairperson;
- Charitable organizations—Susan G. Komen Foundation, president of the Steel Magnolia Chapter; and the American Red Cross, chapter strategic development co-chairperson;
- Gubernatorial appointee—Mississippi Public Procurement Board, vice president; and Mississippi Commission on the Status of Women, commissioner.

The common thread for all of my board and commission service is an identified passion with the board's vision and mission; placement in a marketable pool for consideration when skills in communication, decision making, management, and leadership are sought; and investment in credible mentors or sponsors, all of whom were chosen because they were accomplished leaders with a track record of succeeding. These circumstances are then matched with my time, talent, and treasure (making financial contributions or otherwise raising money for the organization) to the board's mission-driven goals. Skills and attributes such as broad-spectrum credibility, awareness of community needs, and an ability to identify and solve problems will not only bring nurses to the board table but also allow them to ascend as leaders.

If a seat at the boardroom table is your goal, start today to position yourself to be an effective board member and leader. I encourage you to use Rita Wray's Building Blocks of Board Service:

- Identify your passion.
- Network in health care and non–health care settings.
- Educate yourself on governance issues related to your targeted board or commission, as well as board roles and responsibilities often found in an organization's literature.
- Hone, master, and then market your transferable and translatable core leadership skills.
- Locate a sponsor—an influential current or previous board member, a member of the nominating committee, or an appointing authority—to facilitate your entry to board membership.
- Once the board seat is attained, tackle intriguing situations. For example, as a university board member, I have been instrumental in securing a multiyear revenue stream for the Nurses On Boards Coalition to facilitate its mission of improving the health of communities and the nation through the service of nurses on boards and commissions.

Take the initiative and prepare yourself to become an effective leader on various boards and commissions. One initiative I found exceedingly beneficial for board development was through my community (and later state) Chamber of Commerce involvement. In 1987, as the first Black Director of Nursing of a 500+ bed hospital in the state of Mississippi, I was 1 of 40 emerging and existing leaders selected in our metro area to participate in the Leadership Jackson inaugural program. The program is designed to educate participants about major community issues and alternate approaches to solutions to community problems. Participants sharpen their leadership skills while gaining a better understanding of various aspects of the community, and the collective impact has been exponential in Jackson and beyond.

Make a habit of succeeding and realizing the collective impact of board service!

LINDA'S JOURNEY

My first leadership role was as the oldest of nine children in the Burnes family. Learning to lead by listening, demonstrating true concern for another's point of view, and being kind and generous with one's time prepared me to embark upon a leadership journey in society. I began by volunteering for local schools to provide assistance to students struggling to advance their scholarship. Subsequently I continued to hone my leadership skills while working with the local Young Women's Christian Association (YWCA) as a teen volunteer and with a variety of organizations in a college to learn how to be of service to others.

I served on the boards of national and local nursing organizations and was president of NBNA, the American Academy of Nursing, and the American Organization of Nurse Executives. Throughout my career I have mentored hundreds of students, nurses, physicians, deans, hospital executives, and other civic leaders. Using my knowledge of "Circle Calling"—the ancient art of embracing all for their contributions to improving life—I knew the value of being present in the boardroom.

Currently I serve on three national and several local boards including serving as a trustee at Case Western Reserve University where I have the opportunity to influence the lives of students. My role as vice chair of the Academic Association and Student Lives Committee has enabled me to learn about the issues facing young professionals and to work with them to improve their opportunity for giving back to society. Each board member is expected to make a yearly financial contribution as part of their corporate stewardship obligations. My role on the California Health Impact board of directors has helped to advance the attraction, support, and development of diverse individuals into the profession of nursing. I am also a trustee of the Robert Wood Johnson Foundation and have advocated for the organization's efforts to promote a Culture of Health where all have the opportunity to achieve and sustain health. My contributions as a nurse leader on the board include providing important information to the Foundation and my fellow board members regarding nursing's contributions to promoting a culture of health.

I have dedicated much time and financial support to the organizations I serve. The role of giving is very important. It isn't necessary to be a millionaire to serve but it is important that all board members contribute. In *Fortunes of Change*, Callahan (2017) describes the influence of wealth on boards and proposes that boards are better served when they have individuals from all backgrounds as members, not just the wealthy and elite.

Nurses are valuable members of society, as we continue to be identified as one of the most trusted professions by consumers. Society needs our leadership. Step forward and let others know you are willing to serve!

REFERENCES

Callahan, D. (2017). *The givers*. Alfred A. Knopf. New York.

51

Quality and Safety in Health Care: Policy Issues

Jean Johnson, Esther Emard, and Bonnie R. Sakallaris

> *"We want to make sure we incentivize the health care system to be designed to provide you the best quality health care possible."*
>
> *Valerie Jarrett*

Nurses are critical to improving the quality of care but cannot work alone to change a very broken health system. Mortality and morbidity from medical errors are not small problems, and they significantly involve nursing care. In 2000, the Institute of Medicine (IOM; now the National Academy of Medicine) reported that up to 98,000 individuals died per year in hospitals. A more recent study found that over 250,000 hospital deaths per year were due to medical errors, making this the third leading cause of death in the United States (Makary & Daniel, 2016)—and this does not include medical errors in nursing homes, home care, or outpatient care.

Improving quality of care is a national priority with national frameworks that provide a way to think about quality and policy. In *Crossing the Quality Chasm,* the IOM (2001) identified six domains of quality: safe, timely, effective, equitable, efficient, and patient-centered. Performance measures are primarily based on these six domains. In addition, the Institute for Healthcare Improvement has put forward the "triple aim" to improve the patient experience both in outcomes and satisfaction, improve the health of populations, and reduce costs. A fourth aim has been added that reflects health care provider satisfaction with their job. Finally, the Patient Protection and Affordable Care Act (ACA) of 2010 includes important requirements for health care providers to improve the quality of care.

Nurses are at the "sharp" end of care, spending the most time with patients and being involved in all aspects of care, which carries the responsibility of not only protecting our patients through direct care and systems improvement but working with state and federal policymakers to support a safer health system. As such, nurses must be fully knowledgeable about policy issues, as well as the processes for monitoring and improving care, and part of the solution to eliminate medical errors. This chapter is focused on advancing nurses' understanding of key areas of health care quality that are linked to policy including performance measures and public reporting, value-based health care, and regulation.

PERFORMANCE MEASURES AND PUBLIC REPORTING

Performance measurement is foundational to high-value health care. Florence Nightingale had, in fact, recognized the virtues of measurement in her effort to explain inpatient mortality rates following the Crimean War (Nightingale, 1863). It was Nightingale who pioneered the systematic collection and analysis of hospital mortality rates that enabled comparative reporting and quality improvements in Great Britain's health system (McDonald, 2001). Today, hundreds of quality measures have been developed by government agencies (e.g., Centers for Medicare and Medicaid Services [CMS], Agency for Healthcare Research and Quality [AHRQ]), accreditation organizations (e.g., The Joint Commission [TJC], National Committee on Quality Assurance (NCQA]), professional societies and certification boards (American Medical Association-Physician Consortium for Performance Improvement, American Board of Medical Specialties), quality improvement organizations (National Quality Forum [NQF]), and employer-driven organizations (Leapfrog). Quality measures have become deeply embedded in health care policy.

The purpose of health care quality measurement is to assess the quality of care provided in order to identify problems and continually improve care. If health care is not measured, you don't know if you are providing effective and safe care. A quality measure is defined by CMS (2017) as:

Tools that help us measure or quantify health care processes, outcomes, patient perceptions, and organizational structure and/or systems that are associated with the ability to provide high-quality health care and/or that relate to one or more quality goals for health care.

Structure, process, and outcome quality measures were defined by Avedis Donebedian, a physician who worked much of his professional life to integrate quality of care concepts and measures into health care (Donebedian, 1966). The premise of his model was that the right structural aspects of health care needed to be in place to have the right processes and therefore the desired outcomes. An example of this model is having the appropriate number of nurses (structure) in order to provide skin care (process) to prevent pressure ulcers (desired outcome). His work has endured for decades providing the framework for measures and measurement.

Measurement and reporting is intended to provide information to health care institutions, practices, and consumers in order to monitor and improve care and to provide information in order to choose the highest-value providers. *Measures* and *measurement* are important to differentiate, and one should understand *standard* and *benchmark*. See Box 51.1 for definitions. In applying a measure to a specific setting or population, considerations should be given to importance, scientific soundness, and feasibility. Not all existing measures have been endorsed by the NQF. NQF does not create measures; it convenes experts from a variety of stakeholder groups to review measures created by other organizations for scientific

---

BOX 51.2   National Quality Forum Criteria for Measure Selection

Importance: Is the measure relevant to saving lives or preventing debilitating events? Is it relevant to a large population? Does the measure provide important information about health disparities? Who is the measure important to: patients, providers, insurers, employers, government agencies, and/or accreditors?

Scientific soundness: Is there a linkage of clinical logic to structure, process, or outcome of interest? Is the measure valid, measuring what it is intended to measure, and reliable, producing consistent results in similar situations or settings irrespective of who makes the measurement or when it is made?

Feasibility: Are users able to understand and apply specifications of the measure? Can the data be reasonably collected?

From National Quality Forum, n.d.

---

soundness, importance, and feasibility. The review is intended to endorse "best in class" measures for use. See Box 51.2 for the criteria that NQF uses to evaluate quality measures.

An organization may be moving toward meeting a certain standard of care and may set *benchmarks* that move them toward that standard. There are also benchmarks established by external organizations such as CMS that use payment to align performance with benchmarks.

As noted, there are thousands of measures that form many different quality measure *datasets*. These datasets are used for a variety of purposes including quality improvement, payment, and public reporting and for payers, employers, and consumers to make decisions based on meaningful quality information. Table 51.1 provides information on some of the commonly used datasets representing measures that are required for reporting. It does not include datasets related to specific illnesses and clinical issues.

There are many sources of public reporting of quality of health care. CMS has worked to provide consumers with information about different health care settings using a five-star rating to provide a way for consumers to easily interpret complex organizational data and information on individual physicians and advanced practice nurses (Box 51.3). Sources such as Yelp and other social media rely on consumer feedback. *U.S. News & World Report* has rankings for both adult and children's hospitals and several types of specialty care. They base their rankings on a variety of sources, including quality measures and staffing, but they rely most heavily on reputation. Becker's 100 best hospitals are chosen using a combination of rankings from

---

BOX 51.1   Common Terms

Measurement: The process of choosing the appropriate measure, defining how data is to be collected and analyzed, and deciding who needs this information to address a problem.

Measures: Usually interpreted within the context of standards and benchmarks.

Standard: A norm usually established through a consensus process or authority by which others are judged or measured and reflects the structure, process, or outcome that is expected in a specific situation.

Benchmark: Used as a comparison and is sometimes used interchangeably with standard.

TABLE 51.1   Select Performance Measure Data Sets

Measure Data Set Target Audience	Description	How the Measures Are Used	Website
Hospitals			
National Database of Nursing Quality Indicators (NDNQI)	Developed by the ANA and now owned by Press Ganey and combined with measures of patient experience and nursing engagement.	About 2000 hospitals report data to the NDNQI which then provides benchmarking related to unit level data.	www.pressganey.com/solutions/clinical-excellence
CMS Hospital Inpatient Quality Reporting (HIPR)	45 clinical measures (some extracted from chart review) and 16 measures abstracted from EHRs.	Used for consumer information on Hospital Compare and for payment. As of 2017, hospitals can lose one-quarter of a percentage increase in hospital payment updates for nonparticipation.	http://consumerpurchaser.org/files/IQR_Fact Sheet.pdf
AHRQ Quality Indicators	Based on administrative data, there are four measure areas: inpatient (25), prevention (17), patient safety (18), and pediatric care (20).	Used by organizations, health systems, government agencies for internal use, public reporting, payment, and research. Used in AHRQ reports such as *National Healthcare Quality Report* and *National Healthcare Disparities Report*. CMS uses measures for required reporting and on Hospital Compare.	www.qualityindicators.ahrq.gov
ORYX (National Hospital Quality Measure)	Joint Commission integration of performance measures into accreditation process with the use of the ORYX system.	Used for accreditation of hospitals and public reporting of hospital accreditation status.	www.jointcommission.org/specifications_manual_for_national_hospital_inpatient_quality_measures.aspx
CAHPS Hospital Survey (HCAHPS)	Adult hospital and child hospital patient experience survey. Only national database with questions specific about nursing for required reported.	Used for internal quality improvement, payment, and public reporting. Required to be reported to CMS.	www.hcahpsonline.org
Leapfrog	Founded for large employers and purchasers working together to improve care. Categories of measures: inpatient care, medication safety, maternity care, infections, inpatient surgery, and pediatric care, with nearly 2000 hospitals.	Provide information to purchasers to find the highest-value care and give consumers information to make informed choices of providers. Data are publicly reported.	www.leapfroggroup.org/about

Continued

TABLE 51.1   Select Performance Measure Data Sets—cont'd

Measure Data Set Target Audience	Description	How the Measures Are Used	Website
Nursing Facilities			
Resident Assessment Minimum Data Set (MDS)	CMS mandated assessment of residents in Medicare and Medicaid certified facilities identify problems that are the basis for QI at the individual and facility levels.	CMS uses MDS data for quality improvement measures in nursing home assessments. Data from the MDS is integrated in the Nursing Home Compare site.	https://downloads.cms.gov/files/mds-30-rai-manual-v115-october-2017.pdf
Survey and Certification Process	State-based survey using quality measures that feeds into the Certification and Survey Provider Enhanced Reporting (CASPER) system and the Quality Improvement Evaluation System (QIES).	Data used for certification for payment from Medicare and Medicaid and for public reporting on Nursing Home Compare.	www.cms.gov/Medicare/Quality-Initiatives-Patient-Assessment-Instruments/HomeHealthQuality-Inits/downloads/HHQICASPER.pdf
Home Health Agencies			
CMS	CMS requires home health agencies to report outcome and process measures. (1) Data collected in the Outcome and Assessment Information Set (OASIS) submitted by home health agencies; and (2) data submitted in Medicare and Medicaid claims.	Required reporting to CM for Medicare and Medicaid payment, and for public reporting on the CMS Home Health Compare Website.	https://qpp.cms.gov/about/resource-library
Accountable Care Organizations			
CMS	31 quality of care measures (29 individual and 2 composite measures) in 4 domains: Patient/Caregiver Experience, Care Coordination/Patient Safety, Preventive Health, and At-Risk Population.	Required reporting to participate in the ACO Shared Savings Program and measures are embedded in the accreditation processes of NCQA, URAC, and AAAHC	www.cms.gov/Medicare/Medicare-Fee-for-Service-Payment/sharedsavingsprogram/Downloads/2018-and-2019-quality-benchmarks-guidance.pdf

TABLE 51.1 Select Performance Measure Data Sets—cont'd

Measure Data Set Target Audience	Description	How the Measures Are Used	Website
Health Plans	NCQA developed HEDIS measures with currently 92 measures and include required reporting by CMS for many of the measures and many are the bases for publicly reported data	HEDIS measures are integrated into many different data sets and is used for accreditation of health plans.	www.ncqa.org/hedis-quality-measurement
Practitioners CMS	Medicare Incentive Payment System (MIPS) part of Medicare Access and Chip Reauthorization Act (MACRA) passed in 2015 required reporting of six measures including one outcome measure.	MIPS is used for quality assessment for enhanced or reduced payment to physicians and nurse practitioners ranging from +9% to −9% when fully implemented.	www.cms.gov/Medicare/Quality-Payment-Program/Resource-Library/Quality-Performance-Category-fact-sheet.pdf
Core Quality Measures Collaborative— Pediatrics	Pediatric core set of measures include nine measures to align public and private payers intended for individual practitioner or group practices used by CMS and endorsed by NQF.	Seven of the nine measures are the same as for voluntary Medicaid and CHIP reporting, used on a voluntary basis as a set with specific measures being from other datasets.	www.cms.gov/newsroom/fact-sheets/release-core-quality-measures-collaborative-pediatric-core-measure-set
Core Quality Measures Collaborative—ACOs and primary care	These core measures are applied to both ACOs and PCMHs for individual practitioners and group practices.	Required measures for ACOs to CMS with the intention of having private payers also require reporting and use for payment.	www.cms.gov/Medicare/Quality-Initiatives-Patient-Assessment-Instruments/QualityMeasures/Downloads/ACO-and-PCMH-Primary-Care-Measures.pdf
CMS with NCQA, Joint Commission, AHRQ, Pharmacy Quality Alliance, and others	Adult core set of measures to assess care provided to adults enrolled in the Medicaid program.	Voluntary reporting by states to CMS on adult health care quality.	www.medicaid.gov/medicaid/quality-of-care/downloads/medicaid-adult-core-set-manual.pdf

AAAHC; Accreditation Association for Ambulatory Health Care; *ACO,* accountable care organization; *AHRQ,* Agency for Healthcare Research and Quality; *ANA,* American Nurses Association; *CAHPS,* Consumer Assessment of Healthcare Providers and Systems; *CHIP,* Children's Health Insurance Program; *CM,* Certification Maintenance; *CMS,* Centers for Medicare and Medicaid Services; *EHR,* electronic health record; *HEDIS,* Healthcare Effectiveness and Data Information Set; *NCQA,* National Committee on Quality Assurance; *NQF,* National Quality Forum; *PCMH,* patient-centered medical home; *QI,* quality improvement.

BOX 51.3 Centers for Medicare and Medicaid Services Compare Sites

Hospital Compare: Provides a five-star rating based on patient experience, timely and effective care, complications and death, unplanned hospital visits, use of medical imaging, and payment and value of care. Consumers can compare up to three hospitals at a time with a five-star system intended for easy understanding of quality. www.medicare.gov/hospitalcompare/search.html

Nursing Home Compare: Provides a five-star rating based on fire and health inspections, nurse staffing and staffing of other professionals, and results of the state survey related to quality of care provided to residents. www.medicare.gov/nursinghomecompare/search.html

Home Health Compare: Provides information about quality of patient care and patient surveys about their experience of care. www.medicare.gov/homehealthcompare/search.html

Physician Compare: Provides information about physicians and nurse practitioners including where they are practicing, type of practice, and if they accept Medicare. Quality measures will likely be incorporated when the merit-based incentive payment system (MIPS) measures are more evolved. www.medicare.gov/physiciancompare/

U.S. News & World Report's rankings, CareChex, CMS star ratings, Leapfrog grades, and Truven Health Analytics (Becker's, 2018). Leapfrog (2018) publishes quality measure results based on medication safety, infections rates, high-risk surgery, cancer surgery, maternity care, and pediatric care. They rate each area using a four-category rating of fully meets standard, makes substantial progress, some progress, willing to report, and declined to respond.

Efforts in the future related to quality measures will focus on streamlining the number of measures required for reporting, especially when measures related to the same health care issues have different specifications (Berwick, 2016). One effort to do so is the work of the required Core Quality Measures Collaborative. This effort brings together CMS, commercial health plans, Medicare- and Medicaid-managed care plans, purchasers, physician and other care provider organizations, and consumers to identify core sets of quality measures that both public and private payers have committed to using for reporting.

In addition, linking measures to payment will continue to be a priority as will be developing and applying measures reflecting the health of populations, especially minority populations. National Quality Partners (NQP) supported by NQF brings together groups of stakeholders to improve the quality of care through measurement processes and actions. The 2018 goals of NQP for action were the opioid crisis, serious mental illness, and the integration of social determinants of health to improve health outcomes.

VALUE-BASED QUALITY OUTCOMES OF CARE

The main policy strategy, at both a national and state level, has been to drive improved clinical outcomes of care designed to achieve the IOM Six Aims for both individuals and populations. The pathway to this has been through reforming the payment, insurance, and delivery system in this nation. These efforts are operationalized through what is referred to as value-based purchasing, which was primarily initiated by the passage of the ACA—a congressional attempt to address the continued challenges of increasing health care costs, barriers to access, poor clinical outcomes of care, failure to follow evidence-based guidelines, and declining patient satisfaction. Value would be rewarded rather than volume by changing the historic fee-for-service payment system based primarily on the number and type of services/procedures performed, to one based on achieving benchmarked clinical quality outcomes. Since 2008, the Medicare Payment Advisory Commission (MedPAC), a nonpartisan legislative branch agency that provides analysis and policy recommendations to Congress on the Medicare program, has recommended that public reporting begin on hospitals' risk-adjusted readmission rates, accompanied by reduced payments for those with high readmission rates. Up to $12 billion per year is being paid by Medicare for potentially preventable rehospitalizations (Jencks, William, & Coleman, 2018). This became an important focus in the ACA for driving an increase in hospitals' attention and responsibility for patient outcomes after discharge.

Insurance Reform

Ensuring that access to health care is available for all, particularly the uninsured, is critical to address issues of quality. People's out-of-pocket costs have been shown to impact their ability to receive effective high-quality health care. This is also a major concern for accessing primary care. Individuals without health insurance coverage are more likely to delay receiving timely care, seek emergent rather than primary care and preventive and screening services, and die sooner (IOM, 2002). Data from the 2016 National Healthcare Quality and Disparities Report, which is based on 250 measures of a variety of health care services and settings, indicated that, although the quality of health care has improved, the pace of improvement has varied significantly depending on the priority area. Measures of person-centered care improved 80% (2000–2015), whereas measures of the disparity of care across populations did not change significantly for any racial or ethnic group. In addition, uninsured people have worse care than privately insured people (AHRQ, 2016). The ACA attempted to address this aspect of improving access to care through coverage. For more information on the ACA, see Chapter 18.

Payment Reform Driving Delivery System Reform

Payment reform is the main lever being applied to foster delivery system transformation and improve care. Payment reform is intended to impact the high cost of health care, lack of care coordination, poor health care quality outcomes, and the lack of direct patient/consumer engagement in care. The main regulatory efforts to align high-quality outcomes of care to payment methods have been driven primarily by the ACA, the Improving Medicare Post-Acute Care Transformational Act of 2014 (referred to as the IMPACT Act), the Reducing Unnecessary Senior Hospitalization Act of 2018 (referred to as the RUSH Act), and the new Patient-Driven Payment Model (referred to as the PDPM). These approaches toward restructuring payment to reward value rather than volume are occurring across both the acute and post-acute care delivery systems.

One of the main ACA strategies was the establishment of the Center for Medicare & Medicaid Innovations (CMMI) program to test new models of care delivery through the support of numerous demonstration projects. The goal is to reduce health care expenditures and improve clinical outcomes for Medicare, Medicaid, and Children's Health Insurance Program beneficiaries. These demonstration projects are designed to test new approaches of payment and delivery system structures such as accountable care organizations (ACOs); patient-centered medical homes (PCMHs); and global, capitated, and bundled payment for services (National Association of ACOs, 2018).

ACOs are typically groups of providers, hospitals, and/or insurers that align together to provide high-quality care to Medicare beneficiaries. The newest form of an ACO program is the Next Generation model in which the aligned groups agree to accept a higher level of financial risk and/or reward based on their quality-based performance outcomes. Waivers to traditional Medicare benefits can be obtained to provide enhanced services to the beneficiaries such as telehealth, post-discharge home visits, and the three-day skilled nursing facility rule, designed to increase provider and patient engagement in care, care coordination, and care management. Standardized performance measures are used to determine the level of risk or reward for care outcomes as compared to payment that

would be projected in a traditional fee-for-service model of care delivery. The ACO's quality score and final risk or reward share is based on quality measures that compare a ACOs' first year performance to its past and subsequent year's performance against national benchmarks. CMS establishes the number and type of measures on an annual basis.

In the 2018–2019 reporting period, 31 quality measures across 4 quality domains were identified. These domains encompassed Patient/Caregiver Experience, Care Coordination/Patient Safety, Preventive Health, and At-Risk Population. As of the end of the first quarter in 2018 a total of 1011 ACOs participated in the various ACO programs providing care to 32.7 million patients in all regions of this country (Muhlestein et al., 2018). The ACO programs include those ACOs that participated in the Medicare Shared Savings Program (MSSP) which limits the potential downside financial risk and rewards up-side quality performance only.

ACO-type arrangements have also been developed with local Medicaid agencies in 10 states. Although they vary significantly, they all have elements of a value-based purchasing payment design based on achieving a defined level of health care outcomes. In addition most require a focus on addressing the social determinants of health such as living arrangements, transportation, and nutrition in conjunction with local community agencies.

Beginning in 2012 CMS introduced the Hospital Value-Based Purchasing (HVBP) program. This program is designed to financially reward hospitals for improved clinical outcomes and financial performance as determined annually against a specific set of performance measures. For 2019 there were four domains of measures: clinical, person and community engagement, safety and efficiency, and cost reduction. The program also introduced comparative public reporting of results specifically to influence consumer choice through its CMS Compare web sites. There are currently over 4000 hospitals with results in Hospital Compare illustrated with a star rating methodology (1–5 stars, with the average being 3). A recent study by the RAND Corporation indicated that the current approach toward engaging patients to use this type of data has met with limited success (Whaley, Brown, & Robinson, 2018). This research is indicating the need for greater price transparency. Prior to 2019, CMS required hospitals to provide pricing information to consumers upon request. Now, hospitals must post prices on the Internet so consumers and providers can have greater transparency to support their health care decisions.

Efforts to drive reductions in health care expenditures while increasing clinical care outcomes are also focused on the post-acute care delivery systems. CMS has finalized

PDPM, the new payment structure for skilled nursing payments for fiscal year 2019. This model is designed to align payment for therapy visits to the complexity of the patients' clinical need rather than simply to that of the volume or number of hours of service provided, which will increase the focus on the entire patient's needs. The IMPACT Act of 2014 is also focused on improving care coordination and outcomes for the Medicare beneficiaries in any of the post-acute care delivery systems by requiring the use of standardized patient assessment data that will be inter-operable across settings. This goal is to measure, compare, and improve the quality of care across these settings from the analysis, public reporting, and quality payment methods for benchmark performance outcomes.

The RUSH, intended to reduce the unnecessary hospitalization of patients from skilled nursing facilities, is in the first stage of the legislative process (as of July 2018). The act provides support for the use of telehealth in combination with on-site first responders. Qualified provider group practices will be allowed to enter into value-based arrangements for Medicare beneficiaries, with any savings to be shared among the physician group practice, the skilled nursing facility, and Medicare.

REGULATION

The role of regulation is to protect the public from harm and ensure that patients receive safe, high-quality care. Oversight of the health care industry, including practitioners, by federal, state, and local agencies is mandatory, whereas agencies that provide accreditation or certification require voluntary participation. The reality is that clinicians are spending a significant portion of their time on regulatory compliance. The American Hospital Association (AHA) estimated the cost of the administrative aspects of regulatory compliance is approximately $39 billion per year (AHA, 2017). In addition to federal law, clinicians must navigate state, local, and accreditation agency rules. It is important that nurses understand the role regulations play in their individual practice as well as on health care systems and organizations and that they see policy as something they can shape rather than something that happens to them (IOM, 2010).

Individual Practice

Individual practice is strongly influenced by the federal regulations governing payment, privacy, and quality reporting. State law and organizational policy regulate individual practice. The path to practicing nursing is paved with an array of regulatory hurdles implemented by diverse bureaucracies. A potential nurse must attend a nursing school that has received accreditation by one of the

nursing education accreditors, take a national examination (National Council Licensure Examination [NCLEX]) administered by the National Council of State Boards of Nursing (NCSBN), and then obtain licensure from a state board of nursing (BON). The Nurse Practice Act (NPA) of each state outlines the scope of practice, typically for three levels of practice: licensed independent practitioner (LIP) or full practice authority (FPA), advanced dependent practitioner, and dependent practitioner. State legislatures enact the NPA to regulate nursing and delegate authority to the state BON to enforce the NPA. The state BON is responsible to ensure that each applicant has the necessary skills to safely perform a specified scope of practice. Each state BON makes, adapts, amends, repeals, and enforces rules. State BONs set nursing education standards, license qualified applicants, ensure continuing competence, develop nursing standards of practice, implement discipline, and collect and analyze data about nurses. (See Chapter 46 for more on the role of BONs.)

Registered nurses (RNs) hired by health care organizations or medical practices are subject to processes to verify their qualifications to practice. TJC requires primary source verification of an employee's credentials including license, certification, and education. Credentialing is the process of obtaining, verifying, and assessing the qualifications of a practitioner to provide care or services in or for a health care organization. State, local, and institutional rules specify the types of credentials and verification processes that an organization must address in credentialing a practitioner. Credentialing is a major hurdle for hospitals, ambulatory surgical centers, and physician offices; the process can take up to 120 days to complete.

Credentialing is separate from privileging. Privileging allows the practitioner (such as advanced practices nurses) to provide specific clinical services in accordance with the organization's medical staff by-laws. In 2007, TJC introduced its Ongoing Professional Practice Evaluation (OPPE) and Focused Professional Practice Evaluation (FPPE) processes to make the decision of privileging more objective and continuous. Health care insurance companies also credential physicians and advanced practice registered nurses (APRNs) for inclusion in their network.

Health Care Organizations and Systems

Health care's vital role in the health and well-being of U.S. citizens has resulted in thousands of federal, state, local, and non-governmental rules from well-intentioned lawmakers and regulators who are trying to improve on a complex system. Health care regulations and standards are necessary to ensure compliance and to provide safe health care to every individual who accesses the system. The regulatory agencies that protect and regulate public health include the U.S. Departments of Health and Human Services (HHS)

BOX 51.4 National Quality Strategy: Six Priorities

1. Making care safer by reducing harm caused in the delivery of care
2. Ensuring that each person and family is engaged as partners in their care
3. Promoting effective communication and coordination of care
4. Promoting the most effective prevention and treatment practices for the leading causes of mortality, starting with cardiovascular disease
5. Working with communities to promote wide use of best practices to enable healthy living
6. Making quality care more affordable for individuals, families, employers, and governments by developing and spreading new health care delivery models

From Agency for Healthcare Research and Quality. (2018e). *Priorities of the national quality strategy.* Retrieved from www. ahrq.gov/research/findings/nhqrdr/nhqdr15/priorities.html.

and Environmental Protection, the Centers for Disease Control and Prevention, AHRQ, CMS, and the U.S. Food and Drug Administration (FDA). The National Quality Strategy (NQS) outlines three broad aims (better care, healthy people/healthy communities, affordable care) and six priorities that guide the development of HHS and CMS programs, regulations, and strategic plans for new initiatives (Box 51.4). The NQS serves as a critical tool for evaluating the full range of federal health care efforts (AHRQ, 2018b).

Impact of Regulation on Health Care Quality and Safety

The AHRQ update on the 5th anniversary of the NQS indicated that patient safety improved substantially (AHRQ, 2018c):

- *Seventeen percent reduction in hospital-acquired conditions (HACs) between 2010 and 2014.* HACs included falls, catheter-associated urinary tract infections (CAUTIs), pressure ulcers, adverse drug events, and other HACs. Between 2014 and 2016, HACs have declined an additional 8% for a total of 2.45 million HACs avoided since 2010 (AHRQ, 2018d).
- *Eighty percent of the person- and family-centered care indicators showed improvements.*
- *Only about 30% of the indicators of health care disparity have improved* over time.
- *Care coordination improved overall;* however, since 2010, people in poor and low-income families have been less

likely than people in high-income families to have a provider who coordinates care with other doctors.
- *Effective treatment improved, and effective treatment disparities were uncommon.*
- *Priority 5, healthy living, showed little progress.*
- *Priority 6, care affordability, improved* with the enactment of ACA.
- *Affordability disparities have been decreasing.*

UNINTENDED CONSEQUENCES OF POLICIES INTENDED TO IMPROVE CARE

It is important to monitor and mitigate unintended consequences of policies designed to improve health care. The hospital readmissions reduction program (HRRP) is an example of an initiative with mixed outcomes. The HRRP requires CMS to reduce payments to hospitals with excess readmissions. The program started penalizing hospitals with excess readmission rates for acute myocardial infarction, heart failure, and pneumonia in 2012 and expanded to include chronic obstructive pulmonary disease (COPD) and total knee and hip replacement in 2015. Recent studies found broad reductions in Medicare readmission rates for both targeted and non-targeted conditions (Demiralp, He, & Koenig, 2018). However, there have been concerns that these incentives to reduce readmissions could potentially encourage inappropriate care. A study by Gupta et al. (2018) suggested an association between the HRRP implementation and increased mortality in heart failure patients. More research is needed in this area.

Another example is the impact of the TJC pain assessment standard changes in 2001 developed to better meet patients' pain management, documentation of pain management effectiveness, and patient education about pain (Sandlin, 2000). In an attempt to address the issue of undertreated pain, the Pain as the Fifth Vital Sign (P5VS) initiative was established, as well as the implementation of pain-related questions on patient satisfaction surveys. These policies have failed to enhance the treatment of pain and may have unintentionally contributed to the opioid epidemic (Scher, Meador, Van Cleave, & Reid, 2018). In 2018, TJC implemented new and revised pain assessment and management standards for accredited hospitals that called for strategies to decrease opioid use, minimize the risks of opioid use, and provide at least one non-pharmacological pain treatment modality.

CONCLUSION

The U.S. health care system continues to undergo major transitions. Policymakers have emphasized strategies intended to achieve greater value. Transparency and

BOX 51.5   Implications for Nursing

Given our potential political clout, nurses can influence policy to improve the quality and safety of care through:

- Engagement in the national dialogue on access to care, equity, and the socio-determinants of health.
- Advocating for insurance benefit packages that cover preventive and wellness care, maternity and newborn care, and coverage for those with pre-existing conditions.
- Advocating for advanced practice registered nurses to be recognized in all insurance directories as providers.
- Providing the leadership and research that links nursing care directly to the financial state of health care organizations.
- Conducting health services research related to value-based care, quality outcomes, and impact of regulation.
- Expanding the list of nurse-sensitive measures.
- Advancing the translation of research to the practice level.
- Appointment of nurses to boards and committees of organizations that effect policy related to quality.
- Providing expert testimony to decision-making forums.

From Stanik-Hunt et al., 2013; O'Rourke et al., 2017.

accountability are central to these approaches. Broad changes in organizational culture, information technology, payment and delivery models, and health care leadership are necessary to expand health care access, reduce costs, and improve quality.

Despite the role of nursing in delivering high-value care to date, nurses have had limited influence on policy development impacting quality improvement. Box 51.5 suggests ways that nurses can be leaders in shaping the national dialogue around quality improvement. Nurses need to share their first-hand accounts, along with the evidentiary basis and business case, for nursing's role in the quality enterprise. Additionally, nurses need to intensify their involvement in policy development, as well as build leadership and advocacy capacity, to effectively participate in this discourse, collaborate with consumers, providers, other health care professionals, payers, and policymakers in novel ways, and hold themselves accountable for higher-value care.

DISCUSSION QUESTIONS

1. Analyze the fundamental strategies of public reporting, performance measurement, value-based purchasing that policymakers are leveraging to drive the high-value health care.

2. Discuss the leadership role of nursing to influence the quality and safety agenda promulgated by legislation and regulation.
3. Analyze the payment and delivery policy changes that are necessary to drive quality improvement.
4. Discuss how nursing impacts and is impacted by the quality and safety agenda emphasized in regulatory policy.

REFERENCES

Agency for Healthcare Research and Quality. (2016). *2016 National health care quality & disparities report.* Retrieved from www.ahrq.gov/research/findings/nhqrdr/nhqdr16/index.html.

Agency for Healthcare Research and Quality. (2018a). *Quality improvement and monitoring at your fingertips.* Retrieved from www.qualityindicators.ahrq.gov.

Agency for Healthcare Research and Quality. (2018b). *About the National Quality Strategy.* Retrieved from www.ahrq.gov/workingforquality/about/index.html#aims.

Agency for Healthcare Research and Quality. (2018c). *2015 National healthcare quality and disparities report and 5th anniversary update on the national quality strategy.* Retrieved from www.ahrq.gov/research/findings/nhqrdr/nhqdr15/index.html.

Agency for Healthcare Research and Quality. (2018d). *Declines in hospital-acquired conditions save 8,000 lives and $2.9 billion in costs.* Retrieved from www.cms.gov/newsroom/press-releases/declines-hospital-acquired-conditions-save-8000-lives-and-29-billion-costs.

Agency for Healthcare Research and Quality. (2018e). *Priorities of the National Quality Strategy.* Retrieved from www.ahrq.gov/research/findings/nhqrdr/nhqdr15/priorities.html.

American Hospital Association. (2017). *Regulatory overload. assessing the regulatory burden on health systems, hospitals and post-acute care providers.* Retrieved from www.aha.org/system/files/2018-02/regulatory-overload-report.pdf.

Becker's Hospital Review. (2018). *100 Great hospitals in America: 2018.* Retrieved from www.beckershospitalreview.com/lists/100-great-hospitals-in-america-2018.html.

Berwick, D.M. (2016). Era 3 for medicine and health care. *JAMA, 315*(13),1329-1330.

Centers for Medicare and Medicaid Services. (2017). *What is a quality measure?* Retrieved from www.cms.gov/Medicare/Quality-Initiatives-Patient-Assessment-Instruments/MMS/What-is-a-Quality-Measure-SubPage.html.

Demiralp, B., He, F., & Koenig, L. (2018). Further evidence on the system-wide effects of the hospital readmissions reduction program. *Health Services Research, 53*(3), 1478-1497.

Donabedian A. (1966). Evaluating the quality of medical care. *Milbank Memorial Fund Quarterly, 44*(Suppl), 166-206.

Gupta, A., Allen, L.A., Bhatt, D.L., Cox, M., DeVore, A.D., Heidenreich, P.A., ... & Fonarow, G.C. (2018). Association of the hospital readmissions reduction program implementation with readmission and mortality outcomes in heart failure. *JAMA Cardiology, 3*(1), 44-53.

Institute of Medicine. (2001). *Crossing the quality chasm: A new health system for the 21st century.* Washington, DC: National Academies Press.

Institute of Medicine. (2002). *Care without coverage: Too little, too late.* Washington,DC: National Academy Press.

Institute of Medicine. (2011). *The future of nursing: Leading change, advancing health.* Retrieved from http://books.nap.edu/openbook.php?record_id=12956&page=R1.

Institute of Medicine Committee on Quality of Health Care in America. (2000). *To err is human: Building a safer health system.* Washington, DC: National Academies Press.

Jencks, S.F., Williams, M.V., & Coleman, E. (2018). Rehospitalizations among patients in the Medicare Fee-for-Service Program. *New England Journal of Medicine, 360,* 1418-28.

The Joint Commission. (2018). *Specifications manual for national hospital inpatient quality measures.* Retrieved from www.naacos.com/medicaid-acos.

Leapfrog. (2018). *Raising the bar.* Retrieved from www.leapfrog group.org/about.

Makary, M.A., & Daniel, M. (2016). Medical error—The third leading cause of death in the US. *British Medical Journal, 353,* i2139.

McDonald, L. (2001). Florence Nightingale and the early origins of evidence-based nursing. *Evidence Based Nursing, 4*(3), 68-69.

Muhlestein, D., Saunders, R., Richards, R., & McClellan, M. (2018). Recent progress in the value journey: Growth of ACOs and value-based payment models in 2018. *Health Affairs Blog.* Retrieved from www.healthaffairs.org/do/10.1377/hblog20180810.481968/full/.

National Association of ACOs. (2018). *State level ACO activities.* Retrieved from www.naacos.com/medicaid-acos.

National Quality Forum. (n.d.). *Measure evaluation criteria.* Retrieved from www.qualityforum.org/Measuring_Performance/Submitting_Standards/Measure_Evaluation_Criteria.aspx.

Nightingale, F. (1863). *Notes on hospitals.* London: Longman, Green, Longman, Roberts & Green.

O'Rourke, N.C., Crawford, S.L., Morris, N.S., & Pulcini, J. (2017). Political efficacy and participation of nurse practitioners. *Policy, Politics & Nursing Practice, 18*(3), 135-148.

Sandlin, D. (2000). The new Joint Commission Accreditation of Healthcare Organizations' requirements for pain assessment and treatment: a pain in the assessment? *Journal of Perianesthesia Nursing, 15*(3), 182-184.

Scher, C., Meador, L., Van Cleave, J.H., & Reid, M.C. (2018). Moving beyond pain as the fifth vital sign and patient satisfaction scores to improve pain care in the 21st century. *Pain Management Nursing: Official Journal Of The American Society Of Pain Management Nurses, 19*(2), 125-129.

Stanik-Hunt, J., Newhouse, R., White, K., Johantgen, M., Bass, E., Zangaro, G., … & Weiner, J. (2013). The quality and effectiveness of care provided by nurse practitioners. *Journal of Nurse Practitioners, 9*(8), 492-500.

Whaley, C., Brown, T., & Robinson, J. (2018). Consumer responses to price transparency alone versus price transparency combined with reference pricing. *American Journal of Health Economics.* Retrieved from www.mitpressjournals.org/doi/abs/10.1162/ajhe_a_00118.

52

Politics and Evidence-Based Practice and Policy

Sean P. Clarke

"The union of the political and scientific estates is not like a partnership, but a marriage. It will not be improved if the two become like each other, but only if they respect each other's quite different needs and purposes. No great harm is done if in the meantime they quarrel a bit."

Don K. Price

An often-cited definition of evidence-based *practice* is "the conscientious, explicit, and judicious use of current best evidence in making decisions about the care of individual patients" (Sackett et al., 1996). Evidence-based *policy,* by comparison, is an extension, or extrapolation, of the tenets of evidence-based *practice* to decisions about resource allocation and regulation by various governmental and regulatory bodies. Evidence-based policy has been defined as an approach to gathering, interpreting, and applying research findings that "helps people make well-informed decisions about policies, programs, and projects by putting the best available evidence from research at the heart of policy development and implementation" (Davies, 1999) (Box 52.1). The rise of evidence-based policy was influenced by the recognition of the scale of investments in health and social service programs and research around the world, the enormous stakes of providers and clients in the outcomes of policy decisions, and increasing demands for transparency and accountability. Davies (2004) clarified the difference between policy based on evidence versus policy based on opinion:

> This approach [evidence-based policy] stands in contrast to opinion-based policy, which relies heavily on either the selective use of evidence (e.g., on single studies irrespective of quality) or on the untested views of individuals or groups, often inspired by ideological standpoints, prejudices, or speculative conjecture. (p. 3)

Controversies in clinical care and policy development are sometimes very intense—arguably they are becoming more so. Political forces can influence not only the types of research evidence generated, how it is interpreted in the context of other data and values, and, most significantly, how it is used (if at all) in practice or policy. In the United States and internationally, we have witnessed an explosion of access to information online and through social media that have joined more conventional media sources and venues for scientific discourse. These diverse voices compete for the finite attention spans of the public, including health care professionals and policymakers, and contribute to the increasing polarization of political views. This chapter will review the politics of translating research into evidence-based practice and policy, from the generation of knowledge to its synthesis and translation. It will argue that producers and consumers of research of all political leanings should be aware of the political realities of evidence gathering, interpretation, and synthesis, and its use in practice and policy.

THE PLAYERS AND THEIR STAKES

Translating research into practice involves many stakeholder groups (Box 52.2). Their responses to the prospect of applying findings to their work or policies tends to be influenced by several types of forces and motivations.

Health care professionals are often encouraged or pushed to change practices based on evidence. However, their enthusiasm for specific proposed evidence-driven changes in practice will likely vary based on the exact circumstances. Many health professionals are invested in the

BOX 52.2   Stakeholders in the Use of Research in Practice and Policy

- Health professionals
- Health care industry (e.g., manufacturers, vendors, institutions)
- Researchers
- General public/health care consumers/patients
- Politicians and bureaucrats

status quo of treatment approaches and the way care is organized. They often have preferences, pet projects, and passions and may have visions for health care and their profession's role that might be either advanced or blocked by change. Health professionals may seek to protect their working conditions or defend lucrative services or programs from competition from other groups.

There are often direct financial consequences for industries connected with health care when research drives adoption, continued use, or rejection of specific products. Well-known examples include pharmaceutical companies and both consumable (e.g., dressings) and durable (e.g., hospital beds) medical supplies, but also less visible but equally expensive and important products, such as health insurance and human resource consulting services.

Managers, administrators, and policymakers all have stakes in delivering services in their facilities, organizations, or jurisdictions in certain ways or within specific cost parameters. In general, administrators prefer to have as few constraints as possible in managing health care services. Although they may be less enthusiastic about regulations as a method of controlling practice, changes that increase available resources may be better accepted.

For researchers, widespread citation of their findings in various publications, use of their results in practice guidelines and reviews, or having one's work referred to in high-impact policy or legislation are prestigious ways of being recognized. This is especially the case for researchers working in policy-relevant fields, such as health services and outcomes research, where funding and public profile are mutually reinforcing. A separate group of researchers and academics involved in the larger, evidence-based practice movement as specialists in synthesizing and reporting outcomes want to ensure that distilled research in literature syntheses and reviews retains high status.

The general public, especially groups invested and interested in specific types of health care, want safe, effective, and responsive health care. They want to minimize their personal risks, costs, and uncertainties and may or may not have insights or concerns about broader societal and economic consequences of treatments or models of care delivery. For the public, expert opinions and findings tend to carry authority but are often filtered through other sources, such as media and internet outlets.

Finally, elected politicians and bureaucrats are also important stakeholders who want to appear well-informed and responsive to the needs of the public and interest groups while conveying that their decisions balance risks, benefits, and the interests of other stakeholder groups. Elected politicians are usually concerned about voter satisfaction in terms of prospects for reelection. Like the public, they receive research evidence filtered through individuals working with them as government civil servants, and the media. Non-elected bureaucrats inform politicians, manage specialized programs, and implement policies on a day-to-day basis. They may be highly trained and experienced civil servants, and often become very well informed about research evidence in particular fields. As top bureaucrats serve at the pleasure of elected officials, they are sensitive to public perceptions, opinions, and preferences.

THE ROLE OF POLITICS IN GENERATING EVIDENCE

Health care research is often a time- and cost-intensive activity involving competition for scarce resources and rewards. Which projects are pursued, what results are generated, and what is reported from completed studies are all very much affected by political factors at multiple levels.

Research that is likely to influence practice or policy often requires financial support from external funders. Researchers write applications to external funders for grants to cover the resources needed to carry out their work. Before agreeing to underwrite projects, external funders must believe that a research topic is important and relevant to the funding mission, the research approach is viable, and the proposed research team is able to carry out the project. Funders are often governmental or quasi-governmental agencies, but also producers or marketers of specific products or services—pharmaceutical manufacturers would be

BOX 52.3   Stakes in Research for Three Different Types of External Funders

Government Agencies (e.g., National Institutes of Health)

- Preferences for topics, methods, and findings "on message" with government and agency policies and priorities.
- Decisions often seek to ensure that funding arms are wise stewards of public/taxpayer money: important (vs. trivial) findings and outcomes—selection of projects strongly influenced by evaluations of independent experts.

Non-Profit Organizations (e.g., Foundations)

- Aim to fund research projects that fall outside government funding programs' scope.
- Preferences for topics, methods, and findings "on message" with agency priorities and image.
- Ensure that funding arms appear to be wise stewards of donor (endowment) funding, which tends to look more like philanthropic support than government research: programs often ask researchers to look for matching funds (sharing the costs with researchers' employers and/or other funders), as well as evidence that projects will become the seed for something bigger.
- Selection of projects often involves independent, expert evaluation but is heavily influenced by senior officials.

For-Profit Businesses

- Highest priorities for funding outside projects include product development, gathering data that assists in marketing products or services, understanding potential/actual client base, or building company reputation/credibility.
- Decisions about funding are sometimes made exclusively by senior company officials.
- Conflicts of interest and ability of external researchers to retain control of data, data analysis, and report results freely require careful attention.

to industry-researcher partnerships come to light—for instance the undisclosed financial interests in medications and technologies by authors and journal editors (Ornstein & Thomas, 2018). However, not-for-profit and government agencies also have stakes and preferences in what types of projects are funded, and their decisions are also influenced by public relations and political considerations.

Researchers do not always choose projects that are of the greatest personal interest to them or that they believe will best address societal needs. They must please their employers with evidence of their productivity (e.g., successful research grants and high-profile publications) and thus may elect to pursue certain types of projects over others and gravitate toward research topics they believe will help them secure outside funding and prestigious publications. Research topics and approaches go in and out of style over time; topics can become relevant or capture the public or professional imaginations and then fade. As a result, academic departments, funding agencies, institutions, and dissemination venues such as journals and conferences become locales where specific tastes, priorities, and research approaches emerge or disappear. To try and increase their profile and the status of their research area or approach, researchers will often seek positions as reviewers or members of editorial boards of journals, grant review committees, and appointments to positions of real or symbolic power.

Some subject matter or theoretical stances for framing subjects are so inherently controversial that securing funding and collecting data are particularly challenging. For example, anything related to reproductive health or sexual behavior can be potentially volatile, especially in conservative political climates. Research funding for gun safety and violence, health disparities, or the effectiveness or cost-benefit ratio of any health service or program beloved by providers, the public, or both can also be problematic. Examples of the latter could be investigating the usefulness of alternative and complementary health treatments or the appropriateness of widely-used or popular surgeries or diagnostic technologies.

Comparative Effectiveness Studies

Research that evaluates the outcomes of different clinical or public/population health approaches or interventions side by side can be the most relevant for shaping practice and making policy. *Comparative effectiveness research* (CER) was originally defined by the Federal Coordinating Council (2009) for CER as:

> The conduct and synthesis of research comparing the benefits and harms of different interventions and strategies to prevent, diagnose, treat, and monitor health conditions in "real world" settings. The purpose of this research is to improve health outcomes by developing and disseminating

an example of the latter. Examples of factors influencing which projects are funded by different types of funding agencies are presented in Box 52.3.

When research is supported by manufacturers or suppliers of particular medications, products, or services (e.g., drug companies), funders may have overt or implicit interests in the results. Researchers may face pressures around the framing of questions, research approaches, and how, where, and when findings are disseminated. Only recently has the full extent of potential conflicts of interest related evidence-based information to patients, clinicians, and other decision-makers, responding to their expressed needs, about which interventions are most effective for which patients under specific circumstances. (p. 5)

One of the most important sources of CER funding is the Patient-Centered Outcomes Research Institute (PCORI), a non-governmental, non-profit organization that is supported through a levy (tax) on health insurance premiums written into the Patient Protection and Affordable Care Act (ACA) of 2010.

CER can be difficult to carry out. Obtaining access to health care and community settings to ethically conduct research that potentially exposes patients or communities to different interventions requires a willingness of researchers and others to admit they are unsure about a preferable treatment approach over others, at least for some subgroups of patients. To conduct meaningful research, the interventions or approaches need to be sufficiently standardized and researchers must be able to rigorously measure harms and benefits across sufficient numbers of patients, health care organizations, and/or communities (Ashton & Wray, 2013).

CER also can be complicated, demanding, and expensive, often plunging researchers into politically-sensitive policy debates around the area of research they are exploring. Obvious examples include sexual health, health care reform, and substance abuse, but even seemingly politically neutral topics may hit nerves for different stakeholders, as described at the beginning of the chapter. It may not be surprising that, because of the practical challenges and political pitfalls that can be involved in evaluating or testing health care interventions, many health care researchers only engage in research informing the design of interventions, rather than the actual interventions or evaluation themselves. Consequently, when careful evaluations of interventions are subsequently carried out, many widely accepted treatments are shown to be ineffective, needlessly increasing both health care costs and risks to the public (Ioannidis, 2005). This dynamic suggests that more, rather than less, of this difficult research is needed.

THE POLITICS OF RESEARCH APPLICATION IN CLINICAL PRACTICE

As indicated in Box 52.1, the evidence-based policy (and practice) process comprises a number of stages. Here we discuss the second stage: appraisal.

Individual Studies

To stand any chance of influencing practice or policy, research findings must be disseminated to and read by those in position to make or influence clinical or policy decisions. Politically influential audiences will pay more attention to studies on timely topics, those with novel findings, those published by high-profile researchers, and those disseminated in prestigious journals or at large conferences.

A key principle of evidence-based practice and policy during appraisal is that one study alone never establishes anything as incontrovertible fact. In theory, single studies are given limited credence until their findings are replicated. Despite evidence that dramatic findings in landmark studies, especially using non-randomized or observational research designs, are rarely replicated under more rigorous scrutiny (Ioannidis, 2005), there is often an appetite for surprising or "new" findings, and a drive to act on them. As a result, single studies, particularly ones with findings that resonate strongly with one or more interest groups, can receive a great deal of attention and even influence health policy even though their conclusions can only be preliminary.

Journalists try to find newsworthy findings in research reports and make them understandable and entertaining to their audiences. In contrast, for scientists, legitimacy hinges on integrity in reported findings. The use of simplistic language or terminology, or the reworking of complex scientific ideas into layman's terms may result in broad statements unjustified by the data appearing in the popular press. Being seen as a media darling, especially one whose work is popularized without careful qualifiers, can damage a researcher's scientific credibility. Furthermore, given that reactions, responses, and backlashes can be very strong, researchers seeking media coverage of their research must be cautious. It is generally best to avoid popular press coverage of one's results before review by peers and publication and release in a venue aimed at research audiences. Avoiding the overstatement of results and ensuring that key limitations of study findings are clearly described is essential, particularly if a treatment or approach has been studied in a narrow population or context, or without controlling for important background variables.

The Politics of Practice Guidelines and Literature Syntheses

Despite the appeal of single studies with intriguing results, the principles of evidence-based practice and policy dictate that before action is taken, synthesis of research results be carried out where studies with larger representative samples and tighter designs are granted more weight. With an authoritative synthesis of literature in hand, scholars and leaders can move into the third phase of the evidence-based policy process outlined in Box 52.1—identifying organizational and political contexts, and planning implementation.

Conducting and writing up systematic reviews and practice guidelines are labor-intensive and require skill in literature searching, abstracting key elements of relevant research, and comparing findings. The process is expensive and time-consuming, often requiring investments from multiple stakeholders to ensure completion. Synthesis and guideline development are often conducted by teams of content experts to render the work involved manageable, and increase the quality of the products and user perceptions of balance and fairness in the conclusions. Procedures to identify relevant literature are almost always described in detail to permit others to verify (and later update) the search strategy. It is worth noting that except in certain contexts (such as the Cochrane Collaboration where all procedures are clearly laid out in detail and designed to be as bias-free as possible), the grading of evidence and the drafting of syntheses can be somewhat subjective and reflect rating compromises. Reviews commonly deal with high-volume or high-cost services, or services where clients are at high risk and investing in a synthesis is often a strategic and even political decision on the part of a research team and/or a funder: Who prepares synthesis documents, and under what circumstances, reflects research and professional politics as well as input from funders (where syntheses are commissioned by a funder). The credibility of syntheses hinges on the scientific reputation of those responsible for writing and reviewing them.

Interestingly, different individuals tend to be involved in conducting research as opposed to carrying out reviews. Key investigators in the area may not want to take the time away from their research to work on reviews but may feel a need to defend their studies or protect what they believe to be their interests. Even if they were willing to take the work of synthesis, there is debate regarding whether or not subject matter expertise is required of those conducting a synthesis, and to the contrary, whether or not having conducted research in an area creates a vested interest that can jeopardize integrity of a review. However, recognized experts, including noted authors in a field or subfield, are often brought in at the beginning or end of a synthesis to ensure that no relevant studies were omitted and that study results have been correctly interpreted.

Systematic reviews that are disseminated by authoritative sources can be especially influential on both clinical practice and health policy. When the usefulness of a treatment for recipients is brought into question, or it is suggested that some diagnostic or treatment approaches are superior to others, creators, manufacturers, or researchers involved with practices that are unsupported by evidence may bring their resources together to fight, and may even attack, the organizations or agencies that have commissioned the review. For example, in 1995, the Agency for Health Care Policy and Research (AHCPR) released a practice guideline dealing with the treatment of lower back pain that stated spinal fusion surgery produced poor results (Gray, Gusmano, & Collins, 2003). Lobbyists for spinal surgeons and other medical specialist groups were able to garner sympathy from politicians averse to continued funding for the agency. In the face of other political enemies and threats to the AHCPR, the result was the threatened disbanding of the agency. In a gesture of compromise, the AHCPR was reborn in 1999 as the Agency for Healthcare Research and Quality (AHRQ) with a similar mandate, but noticeably *without* the task of practice guideline development in its portfolio. In mid-2018, funding to continue the AHRQ's archives of practice guidelines ended, further suggesting that support for involvement in guideline dissemination remained politically fragile even in AHCPR's reconstituted form (AHRQ, 2018).

Skepticism is warranted when reading literature syntheses involving a particular product or service that has either been directly funded by industry or interest groups, or has had close involvement by industry-sponsored researchers (Detsky, 2006). Guidelines and best practices to reduce bias in literature synthesis and guideline creation are available (Institute of Medicine [IOM], 2009; Palda, Davis, & Goldman, 2007) in much the same way as parameters, checklists, and reporting requirements for various types of research (e.g., the CONSORT guidelines for clinical trials at www.consort-statement.org) were first created and disseminated years ago.

THE POLITICS OF APPLYING RESEARCH IN POLICY FORMULATION

Distilling research findings and crafting messages to support the integration of research evidence into policy can be even more complex and daunting than translating research findings into health care interventions, treatments, or technologies. Direct evidence about the consequences of different policy actions is often sparse, and extrapolation is necessary to link evidence with the policy challenges at hand. There are important political challenges in implementing health policy change including the large sums of money that are often at stake, and great significance is given to health care policy decisions which can accentuate political conflict among stakeholders.

The Robert Wood Johnson Foundation and the Canadian Foundation for Healthcare Improvement are examples of nonprofit foundations seeking to educate the public and policymakers about the links between health services research findings and policy development (see Box 52.4 for "pearls and pitfalls"). Margolis and Haskins (2014) analyzed efforts under the Obama administration

Pearls

- Before linking research with a policy issue, understand the underlying policy issue to determine how results in question add to a debate.
- Consider how opponents of a particular policy stance may interpret study findings and adjust messages accordingly.
- Be aware of major limitations in the study findings (e.g., lack of randomization, a failure to consider an important potential confounding variable), and be prepared to respond to them and explain why results are relevant anyway.
- Refer to bodies of similar or related research rather than individual studies, where possible; acknowledge controversies.

Pitfalls

- Assuming policymakers and journalists are familiar with or interested in research method details.
- Writing research results with needlessly biased or strong language and/or citing such research in policy without reservations.
- Exaggerating the magnitude of effects and ignoring all weaknesses or inconsistencies, particularly those that are easily identified by educated non-specialists.
- Citing research and/or researchers without checking credibility or verifying scientific quality of the results.
- Failing to recognize that research findings are only one component of wider policy debates.

to use rigorously collected research data to inform social policy, including funding of programs to promote parenting competencies, reduce teen pregnancies, and create economic opportunities in communities. They found that political factors, including wrestling over what was considered to be rigorous data, and the precise language about allocating funding to local communities had as much of an influence, if not a more powerful one, on how research was ultimately translated into policy.

Glenn (2002) explained that science can verify statements about reality, but cannot directly address values. Researchers are expected to remain objective and fair: to properly use the rules of scientific inquiry, clearly report facts that contradict impressions or hypotheses, as well as facts consistent with their (and others') leanings and preferences. However, a tendency to resist admitting to incorrect or overly simplified conclusions, as well as social and

political pressures from one's supporters can create problems with these responsibilities.

Researchers may be accused of bias or, worse, promulgating junk science. Journalists have commented on inflated estimates of prevalence or impacts of various diseases or conditions using research data (using loose definitions, questionable assumptions, or data with limited potential to be verified) to lobby for increased funding for research, treatment initiatives, or policy actions (Weissert & Weissert, 2012). Some feel the United States is now in a "post-truth" era where "pronouncements prioritize personal beliefs and feelings, spurn consistency, disregard objective facts, and disdain factual rebuttals and demands for substantiation" (Prado, 2018, p. 7). Not surprisingly, distrust of all authorities has reached an all-time high and researchers have certainly not been spared (Nichols, 2017).

When research findings collide with the interests of stakeholder groups in a policy debate, the responses can be extreme. The researcher's ethical integrity, scientific competence, or motivations can be called into question. High-profile and bitter arguments surround the risks of climate change, potential health hazards associated with genetically-modified crops, nutrition policy, and substance abuse policy. These highly emotional and volatile policy issues can pit scientists, industry, and government stakeholders against each other. After President Trump took office and after multiple attempts by Congress to repeal the ACA in 2017, controversy continues to simmer about the fluctuating public opinion of the ACA, the impact on health insurance premiums, the provisions mandating individual health insurance coverage, penalizing employers who do not offer health insurance, and the creation of health insurance marketplaces in areas where health care access would otherwise be limited (Blendon & Benson, 2017; Chandler, 2017). The next phase of health reform in the United States has yet to unfold: the extent to which evidence is incorporated into policy and is reflected in its provisions remains unknown.

The culture of critique and a media appetite for sensationalism, fueled by rapid dissemination of online news stories have undermined claims of complete objectivity in research and highlighted the political aspects of research. Whether or not the scientific claims or conclusions of any researchers are correct, or whether objectivity can ever exist in research is probably immaterial to the discussion here. Today, many researchers, like politicians, are assumed to have vested interests unless proven otherwise. Furthermore, many in the U.S. general public believe universities and colleges, and the research enterprise, are inherently biased against right-of-center political opinions and policy stances (Turnage, 2017). Good scientific practice is the best defense against claims of bias or worse, but it does not confer immunity from accusations. Instead of attempting to remain distant from the interpretation and use of results in policy debates, researchers would do better to become "honest brokers" of data, presenting the support (or lack of support) that research data provides as completely as possible (Pielke, 2007).

Nurse researchers aspiring to policy relevance and politically-active nurses seeking to use research findings in their endeavors should be aware of the advantages and consequences of the relationship between evidence and policy. It is useful for researchers to identify those who might support and oppose proposed policy changes and anticipate their likely interpretations of research findings. Examples of nursing-related policy issues that have been shaped by research data and their incorporation into lobbying efforts are listed in Box 52.5.

Policy changes supported or defended by research alone can be short lived. Policy victories attributed to research evidence may be more about skill and luck in turning political opinion rather than evidence and how it was presented. The balance between political forces and interest groups can and often do influence policy debates as much as, or more than, thoughtful application of evidence.

Resistance from organized medicine to expanded scope of practice for advanced practice nurses is one example in which a critical mass of evidence supports a change but political forces have conspired against it (Hughes et al., 2010) (see Chapters 60, 62, and 63). The translation of evidence into both clinical practice and policy is a political process. Researchers are most likely to influence policy by designing studies that will yield the clearest possible answers to questions with policy relevance.

DISCUSSION QUESTIONS

1. Think about a familiar clinical practice area where interest groups are attempting to bring about a change in clinical care or systems of service delivery. Assume new, game-changing research findings are published and receive wide attention. Using the list of stakeholder types from this chapter, identify groups that might have an interest in these findings. What are their likely reactions to new research?

2. What are your thoughts regarding the role of political divisions in the United States (and other countries) in which research findings people read and how they interpret them? How should researchers view their work and participation in political debates in a "post-truth" era?

BOX 52.5   Examples of Nursing-Related Health Policy Issues Where Advocates Have Drawn on Research Data

Sharps Safety and the Prevention of Percutaneous Injuries With Used Sharps

- Research data about needlestick incidence and effectiveness of safety-engineered sharps were used by nursing advocacy groups to call attention to the issue, leading to state-level and national policy changes.

Expansion of Autonomous Scope of Practice for Nurse Practitioners and Other Advanced Practice Nurses (APNs)

- Research and evaluation data pointing to acceptability of APNs quality of care and comparability or superiority of outcomes have been cited by advocates of greater APN autonomy; opponents have critiqued the data and their generalizability.

Regulation of Nurse Staffing in Hospitals

- A critical mass of evidence suggests staffing is consistently associated with a variety of hospital outcomes; researchers, clinicians, and managers differ in their opinions regarding the best way to incorporate these findings into the management and regulation of hospitals.

REFERENCES

Agency for Healthcare Research and Quality. (2018). *Clinical guidelines and recommendations*. Retrieved from www.ahrq.gov/professionals/clinicians-providers/guidelines-recommendations/index.html.

Ashton, C.M., & Wray, N.P. (2013). *Comparative effectiveness research: Evidence, medicine and policy*. New York: Oxford University Press.

Blendon, R.J., & Benson, J.M. (2017). Public opinion about the future of the Affordable Care Act. *New England Journal of Medicine, 377*(9), e12. Retrieved from www.nejm.org/doi/full/10.1056/NEJMsr1710032.

Chandler, S. (2017). *Don't use one measure to evaluate Obamacare reform*. Retrieved from www.forbes.com/sites/theapothecary/2017/02/28/dont-use-one-measure-to-evaluate-obamacare-reform/#59e94a1b4b4e.

Davies, P. (2004). *Is evidence-based government possible? Jerry Lee lecture, 2004*. Retrieved from https://webarchive.national archives.gov.uk/20091111094238/http://www.nationalschool.gov.uk/policyhub/downloads/JerryLeeLecture1202041.pdf .

Davies, P.T. (1999). What is evidence-based education? *British Journal of Educational Studies, 47*(2), 108–121.

Detsky, A.S. (2006). Sources of bias for authors of clinical practice guidelines. *Canadian Medical Association Journal, 175*(9), 1033.

Federal Coordinating Council. (2009). *Federal coordinating council for comparative effectiveness research: Report to the*

President and the Congress. Retrieved from https://osp.od.nih. gov/wp-content/uploads/FCCCER-Report-to-the-President-and-Congress-2009.pdf .

Glenn, N. (2002). Social science findings and the "family wars." In J.B. Imber (Ed.), *Searching for science policy*. New Brunswick, NJ: Transaction.

Gray, B.H., Gusmano, M.K., & Collins, S.R. (2003). AHCPR and the changing politics of health services research. *Health Affairs* (Suppl Web Exclusives), W3-283-307.

Gray, M. (2009). *Evidence-based healthcare and public health* (3rd ed.). Edinburgh: Churchill Livingstone Elsevier.

Haskins, R., & Margolis, G. (2014). *Show me the evidence: Obama's fight for rigor and results in social policy*. Washington, DC: Brookings Institution Press.

Hughes, F., Clarke, S.P., Sampson, D.A., Fairman, J., & Sullivan-Marx, E.M. (2010). Research in support of nurse practitioners. In M.D. Mezey, D.O. McGivern, & E.M. Sullivan-Marx (Eds.), *Nurse practitioners: The evolution and future of advanced practice* (5th ed.). New York: Springer.

Institute of Medicine. (2009). Conflicts of interest and development of clinical practice guidelines. In B. Lo & M.J. Field (Eds.), *Conflict of interest in medical research, education, and practice*. Washington, DC: National Academies Press.

Ioannidis, J.P. (2005). Contradicted and initially stronger effects in highly cited clinical research. *Journal of the American Medical Association, 294*(2), 218–228.

Nichols, T. (2017). *The death of expertise: The campaign against established knowledge and why it matters*. New York: Oxford University Press.

Ornstein, C., & Thomas, K. (2018). *Top cancer researcher fails to disclose corporate financial ties in major research journals.*

Retrieved from www.nytimes.com/2018/09/08/health/jose-baselga-cancer-memorial-sloan-kettering.html?action=click&module=inline&pgtype=Article&region=Footer.

Palda, V.A., Davis, D., & Goldman, J. (2007). A guide to the Canadian Medical Association handbook on clinical practice guidelines. *Canadian Medical Association Journal, 177*(10), 1221–1226.

Pielke, R.A., Jr. (2007). *The honest broker: Making sense of science in policy and politics*. Cambridge: Cambridge University Press.

Prado, C.G. (2018). Introduction. In C.G. Prado (Ed.), *America's post-truth phenomenon* (pp. 1-14). Santa Barbara, CA: Praeger.

Sackett, D.L., Rosenberg, W.M.C., Gray, J.A.M., Haynes, R.B., & Richardson, W.S. (1996). Evidence based medicine: What it is and what it isn't. *British Medical Journal, 312*(7023), 71–72.

Turnage, C. (2017). *Most Republicans think college is bad for the country. Why?* Retrieved from www.chronicle.com/article/Most-Republicans-Think/240587.

Weissert, W.G., & Weissert, C.S. (2012). The policy process. In W.G. Weissert & C.S. Weissert, *Governing health: The politics of health policy* (4th ed.) (pp. 279-319). Baltimore: Johns Hopkins Press.

ONLINE RESOURCES

Academy Health (professional association for health policy and health services research)
www.academyhealth.org
Commonwealth Fund
www.commonwealthfund.org

53

The Nursing Workforce

Mary Lou Brunell and Andrea Uitti Bresnahan

"It is truly a unique time to be a nurse. Healthcare reform literally begs for nurses to work to the 'top of their license'—whether a registered nurse or advance practice nurse. It is so critical to deliver comprehensive, compassionate, and coordinated care for our patients and their families. Consumers depend upon our largest and most trusted healthcare workforce members—registered nurses."

Ann Scott Blouin, RN, PhD (from The Power of Ten, *2nd ed., 2017*)

The supply of nurses in the United States is made up of licensed practical/vocational nurses (LPNs), registered nurses (RNs), and advanced practice nurses (APNs). Those with active licenses that are clear (without disciplinary or other limitation) are eligible for employment and represent the potential nurse pool. The actual nursing workforce is composed of those working in the practice of nursing or whose job requires a license. To demonstrate the significance of these distinctions, Fig. 53.1 illustrates the breakdown of licensed LPNs, RNs, and APNs in Florida, compared with those who define Florida's potential nursing workforce, and then with those who are actually working (Florida Center for Nursing [FCN], 2018a, 2018b, 2018c). When considering state-specific data, a nurse must have an address in the relevant state to be included in the potential workforce pool. It is not uncommon for a nurse to be licensed in multiple states, and those serving in the military need only be licensed in a U.S. state or territory to practice wherever they are assigned. Using Florida as an example, more than 47,000 RNs have a Florida license that is either inactive or not cleared to practice and/or do not have a Florida address on record with the state board of nursing.

Successful planning requires knowing the real workforce supply. As shown in Fig. 53.1, there is a difference of more than 80,198 RNs (28%), 5297 APNs (19%), and 13,487 LPNs (21%) between licensees and working nurses. Using the wrong base number could make it appear that a shortage does not exist, on paper, when reality says otherwise. A shortage exists when the supply does not meet the demand. If there is a need for 250,000 RNs, a supply of 289,068 implies a surplus, although a workforce of 208,870 demonstrates a clear shortage of more than 40,000 RNs. Identifying the workforce supply can be achieved by collecting information from nurses or employers. A weakness in seeking the information from employers is their tendency to think in terms of jobs as opposed to people; two full-time jobs could be filled by four part-time nurses. As is the case in Florida, many nurse workforce centers across the country have partnered with their board of nursing to collect supply data during the license renewal process.

The greater challenge is the collection of demand data. The demand for any profession is based on the willingness of employers to hire and pay for their services. Although several national sources of demand data exist, each has limitations and the ideal source is through employer survey (Spetz & Kovner, 2013). The challenges in conducting an employer survey include high cost, low return rates, and inconsistent definitions of terms. Since 2007, the FCN has been collecting and reporting nurse demand by surveying six nurse employing industries that represent approximately 72% of LPNs, 79% of RNs, and 53% of APNs in Florida. The industries surveyed are hospitals, psychiatric hospitals, hospices, public health departments, home health agencies, and skilled nursing facilities. The information

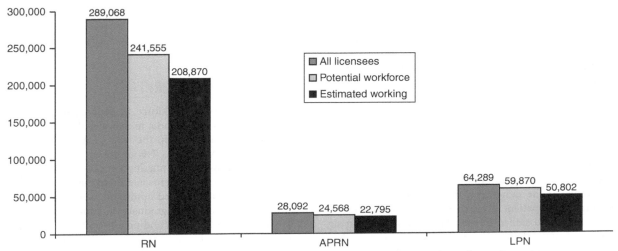

Fig. 53.1 Florida nurse workforce supply as of December 2017. *APRN*, Advanced practice registered nurse; *LPN*, licensed practical nurse; *RN*, registered nurse.

obtained provides turnover rates, vacancy numbers, skill mix information, and projected growth (FCN, 2016). Being able to compare supply to demand at the national, state, and local level is critical for strategic health workforce planning, policy development, and funding decisions.

However, demand is not the same as need. How many nurses are needed to meet the population's health care needs is likely a larger number than that of demand and takes into account future need as well as current demand. Forecasting models project future need based on the supply of nurses and the anticipated demand (employment) for nurses. They factor in changes in supply, such as retirements or expanded nursing education programs, and changes in demand, such as population aging or in-migration. For example, the Health Resources and Services Administration developed the Health Workforce Simulation Model. Using this model, long-term registered nursing jobs from 2015 to 2030 are projected to grow by more than 200,000 full-time equivalent (FTE) positions (46%) nationally. At the same time, licensed practical/vocational nursing jobs in long-term care are projected to grow by nearly 170,000 FTEs (46%) (U.S. Department of Health and Human Services, Health Resources and Services Administration, Bureau of Health Workforce, National Center for Health Workforce Analysis, 2018). Several sources of forecasts and methods to project need exist, however they are not without their limitations and challenges. Though they may be representative of the national level, they often do not take into account the differences in demand at the state level. As a result, some states have developed their own tools to

provide more useful information for planning purposes but this can be an expensive undertaking.

CHARACTERISTICS OF THE WORKFORCE

Nurses are the front-line providers of care for most health care consumers. The U.S. nursing workforce is the largest in the world and remains predominately female and white/non-Hispanic. The National Council of State Boards of Nursing's 2015 National Workforce Study was conducted in partnership with the National Forum of State Nursing Workforce Centers. The results indicated male nurses make up 14.1% of licensed nurses, whereas 19.5% reported a race other than white (Budden et al., 2016).

Researchers have predicted a nursing shortage of over 1 million nurses by 2024 (Kennedy, 2018). A nursing shortage exists because demand, or need, exceeds the supply. Demand is expected to increase more rapidly than the supply as the Baby Boomer cohort of the U.S. population reaches retirement age. There were 77 million Baby Boomers born compared to only 44 million Generation Xers adding to the problems of meeting demand (Underwood, 2017). Currently 50% of all nurses are of or near retirement age and are likely to retire within the next 10 years. The U.S. Bureau of Labor Statistics estimated that registered nursing will create 438,100 jobs by 2026, representing a much faster average growth rate than all other professions (U.S. Department of Labor, Bureau of Labor Statistics, 2018). Even with record-setting growth in the nursing workforce, the increase in supply may not be adequate to keep up with increasing demand. What is more, nurses are increasingly more mobile, a trend that has been noted with Millennials, those born between 1982 and 2000 (Underwood, 2017). Contributing to the mobility, companies have traditionally offered bonuses for new hires when demand is high, often resulting in nurses leaving their positions. As many as 43% of newly licensed hospital nurses in 2016 left their first positions within 3 years of employment. Additionally, many states are part of the multistate compact also increasing the mobility and transiency of nurses (Becker's Hospital Review, 2017).

The U.S. population is living longer and with more chronic conditions, leading to increased demand for RNs and APNs. At the same time, the site for care delivery is shifting from inpatient, acute care settings to home health, community, and skilled nursing facilities resulting in significant demand for LPNs and nursing assistants. New models of care delivery as well as an emphasis on prevention require greater care coordination and underscore the importance of an adequate supply of nurses. It is critical not just to ensure the right number of nurses, but also the correct skillset needed to manage the increasingly complex health care needs of the U.S. population.

Current and future nursing shortages differ due to the fact that they are not driven by the cyclical nature of the economy. During the 1980s, the United States faced two significant nursing labor shortages, caused primarily by wage controls and cost-cutting approaches. Wage increases and increased funding for nursing education rectified the shortages. As supply equaled demand there was a period when new nurse production continued and resulted in an oversupply of RNs. Cuts in education funding followed in an attempt to equalize the workforce thus continuing the cycle of shortages. In addition to the effect of this back and forth of education funding, current and future shortages are affected by nurse retirements and increasing demands of an aging society. Notwithstanding a 2.6% enrollment increase in nursing schools in 2013, a shortage of nurses entering nursing school exists today and those graduating are predominantly in their late 30s (Buerhaus, Skinner, Auerbach, & Staiger, 2017).

Nursing shortages may be contributing to understaffing. Studies since 2002 have corroborated the intuitive idea that when nurses are understaffed, patient safety suffers and medical errors increase. Understaffing also leads to nurse burnout which, of course, causes increased turnover. Even with this knowledge, understaffing and nursing turnover are still prominent issues in 2018. Meaningful work must be done, as the demand for nurses is expected to dramatically increase. Patients require a level of care that is best provided by an appropriate balance of nurses: those with years of hands-on experience and knowledge along with new nurses fresh from the education system (Department for Professional Employees, American Federation of Labor and Congress of Industrial Organizations [AFL-CIO], 2016).

EXPANDING THE WORKFORCE

As with the nursing workforce in general, the educator workforce is also aging, and a mass wave of faculty retirements is anticipated within the next decade. The annual national faculty vacancy is 7%, or about 1565 educators, making it impossible for nursing education programs to accept the number of students needed to meet the demand. More than 50,000 qualified applicants were turned away from baccalaureate and graduate nursing programs in 2016 as a result of limited funding for faculty, lack of clinical sites, and lack of qualified faculty applicants (American Association of Colleges of Nursing [AACN], 2017). Even if education capacity could be expanded to meet demand, there will still be a lapse before an adequately experienced workforce is operational. Policy initiatives must take a multipronged approach by focusing on expanding both the general nursing and faculty education capacity, retaining the current nurse workforce, and increasing the diversity of nurses.

Nursing education programs must be expanded to facilitate growth in the nursing workforce. Successful expansion should be measured not just by increased admissions but also by increased graduations and successful passage of the National Council Licensure Examination. From the employers' perspective, success would also be measured by a graduate's readiness to work and to fill positions of critical need. Lack of funding to hire additional faculty members and lack of qualified faculty applicants are consistently identified as reasons why programs turn away qualified applicants (AACN, 2017). Increased funding for graduate education is an essential first step toward increasing capacity. Government funding for graduate education has been implemented to help expand the faculty pipeline while also expanding the pool of candidates for other hard-to-fill nursing positions. However, programs that only require a 2-year practice commitment do little to address shortage areas long term (Carnevale, Smith, & Gulish, 2015).

A key reason for lack of faculty applicants is the wide discrepancy between industry and academic salaries. Nurses can often earn significantly more in clinical practice than teaching. This salary difference is a significant issue in recruiting new and retaining existing faculty. The average salary of an APN in 2017 was $107,489 whereas an assistant professor makes an average of $77,360 (U.S. Department of Labor, Bureau of Labor Statistics, 2018). Funding aimed at increasing salaries for nurse faculty in entry-level programs would have considerable impact on reducing the faculty shortage. Many employers partner with local colleges to develop faculty-sharing programs; employers pay for salary and benefits and then donate 50% to 100% of the nurse's time to the school. These programs have been very successful, enabling educational institutions to expand admissions while providing faculty who are familiar with the clinical sites and their policies. Employers benefit from the availability of a higher number of nurse graduates. Employers may also offer tuition reimbursement for nurses seeking an advanced degree; this not only serves as a retention strategy for the employer but may also expand the pool of potential nurse educators. Private donations are another source of funding for educational programs.

Strategic use of scarce resources is a critical component of effectively expanding education capacity. Lack of access to clinical sites ranks as a barrier to expansion for all levels of nursing education. In Florida, Deans and Directors of pre-licensure RN programs reported that "limited clinical sites" was the most common barrier to admitting more students (FCN, 2018). As a result, simulation is being used to provide practical experiences.

Critical to expanding the nursing workforce is the successful entry of new graduates into work settings. Over the last decade, programs have been developed to facilitate "transition to practice" after completion of a pre-licensure or advanced practice degree program or when a nurse transitions to a new clinical practice area. Evidence points to residency programs having positive outcomes, easing the transition from education to clinical practice, strengthening commitment to the profession, and improving retention for newly licensed nurses (Altman, Butler, & Shern, 2016). Development of experience and practical knowledge improves the quality of care and patient outcomes. As demand increases for APNs, the expectation that applicants enter graduate education with years of experience as an RN is no longer present. The resulting need for intense practical experience is being met, in large part, through residency programs in hospitals where the majority of APNs are employed. At the same time, the nurse workforce must respond to changing health industry demands as hospital admissions and lengths of stay decline, resulting in increased levels of care required in long-term care settings, outpatient care centers, and home health. Growth is expected to be faster in outpatient areas, telehealth, or treatment centers that provide same-day services. Residency programs should be implemented to transition nurses from acute care to the community setting and telehealth. These programs should provide intensive training for various chronic conditions in America's aging population, such as arthritis, dementia, Alzheimer disease, diabetes, and obesity (U.S. Department of Labor, Bureau of Labor Statistics,

2018). Increasing the availability of specialized training for experienced nurses may also help produce a workforce with qualified applicants to enter hard-to-fill positions such as critical care and front-line management.

INCREASING DIVERSITY

The U.S. population continues to grow and increase in diversity. In fact, the "no majority" America is thriving in 2018 and will be here for the under-18 population by 2020 (Frey, 2018). This makes investing in the next generation of younger minorities a priority to the nursing workforce. To effectively meet patient care needs and ensure cultural competency, nurse leaders, educators, and administrators will need to be more prepared to reach out to diverse populations to fill their current roles. Nursing is a predominately female profession; only 14.1% of the national nursing workforce is composed of men, although men make up nearly 50% of the population. Increasing the visibility of men in nursing is a crucial first step toward attracting more male applicants. The same is true for improving the appeal of nursing to ethnic and racial minorities. Increasing diversity in the nursing workforce also requires increasing diversity in the education pipeline. Diverse nurse faculty are key to attracting and maintaining a diverse student population. Currently, only about 14% of nursing faculty members are from minority backgrounds compared with 39% for the national population.

RETAINING WORKERS

Nursing turnover in 2017 was up to 20.6% from 15.6% in 2010. It is difficult to accurately calculate the full cost of nurse turnover given the range variables, but estimates range from $97,216 to over $104,440 per turnover and up to $8.1 million annually in turnover costs to U.S. hospitals. The costs associated with turnover and understaffing have a powerful impact on the economy (Rosenbaum, 2018).

Policy efforts to address the shortage have included a focus on retention in both the public and private sectors. All of these efforts point to the importance of retaining experienced nurses. Health care leaders must focus on creating a healthy work environment for nurses. Understanding that meeting workforce demand cannot be accomplished through a single effort of expanding the education of new nurses, state workforce centers and professional organizations have implemented nursing leadership development programs to not only enhance the professional image of nursing but also to promote nurses into policy-setting positions. The American Organization of Nurse Executives provides a variety of programs, such as the Emerging Nurse Leader Institute, Nurse Manager Institute, and

Essentials of Nurse Manager Orientation (aone.org). The American Nurses Association, AACN, the American Hospital Association, and the National League for Nursing have made the shortage a priority issue. The Joint Commission has a Nursing Advisory Council on initiatives to resolve the nursing shortage. An important and effective first step toward improving nurse retention is ensuring that the organization's leadership clearly values nurses. The Magnet Recognition Program administered by the American Nurses Credentialing Center is one example of a process that supports nursing work (see Chapter 59). It provides a focus on improved collaboration, increased autonomy/accountability for nurses, improved decision-making abilities, safe staffing levels, effective leadership, and improved access to professional development opportunities.

Effective nurse managers can have a significant impact on turnover. To ensure that front-line managers are both a good fit and adequately trained, some organizations have divided the traditional role into two: one focused on clinical activities and the other on administrative and management functions. Separating the roles not only helps reduce what was previously an overwhelming workload for one person but also enables nurses with strong clinical skills to lead without being responsible for management. Identifying new roles is an important step in developing career pathways, which may improve retention. New roles are increasing opportunities for nurses to move across health care settings, such as patient liaison, attending RN, health coach, or admissions counselor (Robert Wood Johnson Foundation [RWJF], 2015). These are just some of the innovative new roles embraced by nurses as they help transform health care.

To keep a safe mix of new and experienced nurses, nurse employers must implement strategies specifically aimed at retaining older nurses. In addition to the improved benefit to patient outcomes, the expertise that older and experienced nurses bring to the workplace is invaluable. This expertise is particularly beneficial when older nurses are paired with new nurses in mentorship programs. Not only do experienced nurses possess extensive clinical knowledge from years of hands-on experience, but they also possess a strong knowledge of the organizational culture. Mentorship initiatives help organizations facilitate the transfer of the institutional knowledge to new nurses. New graduates in particular benefit from mentorships, to help ease the transition from school to real-life clinical work. Strategies aimed at retaining older nurses may also serve to improve retention among other groups, including working mothers or inactive nurses. These strategies include implementing tools to reduce the physical demands of the job, offering alternative scheduling such as shorter shifts and reduced workweeks, enhancing retirement benefits, and rewarding loyalty by creating incentives for longevity.

ADDRESSING THE NURSING WORKFORCE ISSUES

To address the nursing shortage on a local level, many states have established nursing workforce centers. In general, they focus on collecting, analyzing, and reporting state-level nursing workforce data while also serving as a source of information related to the shortage and identifying strategies for resolution. By collecting data at a state level, they are typically able to produce more accurate information than previously published by national groups. The 2015 FCN survey of primary nurse employers asked responders to identify the top five most difficult-to-fill positions (FCN, 2016). The majority of the most difficult-to-fill positions identified required advanced experience, advanced education, or both (e.g., adult critical care, emergency department, unit manager, nurse practitioners). The surprising result in 2015 was the inclusion of positions that would be open to certified nursing assistants, LPNs, and RNs, potentially as new graduates (e.g., inpatient staff nurse, home hospice staff RN, nurse aide, LPN). The only industry that did not indicate a need for entry-level positions was hospitals, sending a clear message to nurse educators: It is time to stop emphasizing hospital settings as the favored location for new graduate entry into practice. Nursing's academic partners must adjust to change and meet future demands, which indicate decreasing acute care bed use and increasing home health and long-term care needs. Nursing workforce centers also focus on workforce planning within the state, and they serve a key role in presenting recommendations and educating legislators and policymakers.

The National Forum of State Nursing Workforce Centers (the Forum) was established in 2004. With 34 participating states (as of June 2018), the Forum seeks to create a unique dialogue that serves as a medium for wisdom sharing and strategy development in promoting the development of an optimal nursing workforce to meet the health care needs of the population. Centers have established data-collection methods and are producing extremely accurate state-level information. However, there can be substantial differences in both the methods and metrics used for collecting nursing workforce data, making it difficult to produce an accurate national picture of the nursing shortage. After evaluating data-collection practices, the Forum established three datasets—Nursing Supply Minimum Dataset, Nursing Demand Minimum Dataset, and Nursing Education Minimum Dataset—to standardize the collection of state-level nursing workforce data and to create a national repository of data. The goal is to enable state and national workforce planners to identify and implement accurate and timely approaches to resolve the shortage. Planners and policy analysts will be able to benchmark progress and improve accuracy in forecasting the future workforce supply and demand.

As states and hospitals are focused on RN preparation with, in some cases, preference given to Bachelor of Science in Nursing (BSN)–prepared nurses, clinical space is being limited for LPN student nurses because their future role is uncertain in the hospital settings. Having clinical rotations in hospitals is an important component of the LPN's training in preparation to care for patients with multiple chronic conditions. Perhaps more significant is the shortening of patient stays in acute care settings resulting in transfers to skilled nursing facilities. At these facilities, predominantly staffed with LPNs, patients present with acute care and rehabilitation needs previously confined to hospital settings. With a national nursing shortage, LPNs can help fill some of the critical needs in sectors of health care: home health and long-term care. Additionally, LPNs offer a seamless transition to RN if educational institutes work to facilitate educational mobility.

CONCLUSION

The uniqueness of the nursing shortage is related to a variety of factors that require new solutions. It is not a simple issue of supply and demand. It is time to consider what changes and enhancements must be implemented to assure an adequate, qualified nurse workforce to meet the health care needs of the U.S. population. To be successful, planning must be based on a solid foundation of accurate data and information. It is critical to know the nurse workforce numbers, not just the number of licensed nurses. State and national efforts to understand supply data have been successful, although work remains to be done. The critical need is to better understand the demand for nurses of all licensure statuses and locations of work. With this information, nurse workforce researchers can predict the future and evaluate goal achievement. Progress has been made in forecasting at the national level, but the cost of developing state forecasting models may be prohibitive. One thing is clear—the United States is experiencing a nursing shortage that is going to worsen.

What actions are necessary to address the current and minimize the future shortage of nurses? Nurse education programs need to expand production of LPNs, RNs, and APNs who are knowledgeable, culturally sensitive, and capable of achieving required licensure and/or certifications. Barriers to program expansion must be addressed. Nurse faculty salaries should be market competitive. Nurses

should be incentivized to pursue advanced degrees and careers in academia. Creative clinical learning opportunities must be explored including the use of simulation and non-traditional clinical experience locations such as skilled nursing facilities and assisted living facilities. However, increasing production alone will not resolve the shortage.

Improvements in the work environment are essential to retain the workforce. As with the population at large, the nurse workforce is aging and the challenges associated with age must be accommodated. Scheduling options that include shorter work days in environments that require less walking and are not as physically demanding may extend the work life of senior nurses. The employer benefit is immediate—preventing the loss of an employee—and strategic—retaining the experiential knowledge essential to successfully mentor new team members. There are issues to be resolved for the new nurse as well. Providing a positive student-to-work transition in an environment that is free of violence, inclusive in policy discussions, and demonstrates that each nurse is a valued member of the team can significantly reduce turnover and its associated costs.

Although slight progress has been made in the presence of men in nursing, true diversity has not been achieved. The "no majority" America is in force, and nurses must reflect the populations they serve. A necessary starting point is to address the diversity of the nursing faculty. Evidence shows that the more a faculty reflects the student population, the more successful the students will be.

It is time for the nursing profession to respond to the changing health care industry. Just as patients are moving out of hospitals to community settings, nursing student experiences must occur in the settings where health services are being delivered. Including clinical rotations in ambulatory clinics, hospices, skilled nursing facilities, rehabilitation units, assisted living facilities, and patient homes will require creativity but will prepare students for the areas where there will be open positions. Licensed practical nursing educators and industry leaders should unite to address critical curriculum changes such as reducing maternal-child and increasing geriatric learning opportunities.

In summary, strategic solutions to the nursing shortage and nurse workforce issues must include strategies that will (1) increase education capacity by addressing the nurse faculty shortage and clinical space limitations; (2) retain the current nursing workforce by improving the work environment, addressing age-related challenges, and valuing nurses' contributions; and (3) collect necessary data as the base for accurate forecasting, evaluation of interventions, sound health policy development, and allocation of scarce resources. Good policy requires good data, and this is particularly evident in developing policy surrounding the nursing shortage in the United States. Continued sharing of information, collaboration to successfully implement programs, and funding to support the work are critical to effectively address nurse workforce issues.

DISCUSSION QUESTIONS

1. Why do you think the issues presented in this chapter persist in today's workforce culture?
2. What steps can be instituted to resolve the nursing shortage through a partnership between academia and the health industry?
3. In your opinion, who are the biggest stakeholders for addressing the nurse workforce issues? Why?

REFERENCES

Altman, S.H., Butler, A., & Shern, L. (2016). *Assessing progress on the Institute of Medicine report: The future of nursing.* Washington, DC: National Academies Press.

American Association of Colleges of Nursing. (2017). *Annual report: Advancing higher education in nursing.* Retrieved from www.aacnnursing.org/Portals/42/Publications/Annual-Reports/AnnualReport17.pdf.

Becker's Hospital Review. (May 11, 2017). *Hospitals face unprecedented turnover, attrition rates: 4 Survey findings.* Retrieved from www.beckershospitalreview.com/human-capital-and-risk/hospitals-face-unprecedented-turnover-attrition-rates-4-survey-findings.html.

Budden, J.S., Moulton, P., Harper, K., Brunell, M.L., & Smiley, R. (2016). The 2015 National Nursing Workforce Study. *Journal of Nursing Regulation, 7*(1), S1-S90.

Buerhaus, P.I., Skinner, L.E., Auerbach, D.I., & Staiger, D.O. (2017). State of the registered nurse workforce as a new era of health reform emerges. *Nursing Economics, 35*(5), 229-237. Retrieved from www.aaacn.org/sites/default/files/documents/StateoftheRegisteredNurseWorkforce.pdf.

Carnevale, A.P., Smith, N., & Gulish, A. (2015). *Nursing supply and demand through 2020.* Retrieved from http://cew.georgetown.edu/wp-content/uploads/Nursing-Supply-Final.pdf.

Department for Professional Employees, American Federation of Labor and Congress of Industrial Organizations. (2019). *Safe staffing: Critical for patients and nurses: fact sheet 2019.* Retrieved from http://dpeaflcio.org/programs-publications/issue-fact-sheets/safe-staffing-ratios-benefiting-nurses-and-patients/.

Florida Center for Nursing. (2016). *Florida's demand for nurses: 2015 Employer survey.* Orlando, FL: Author. Retrieved from www.flcenterfornursing.org/StatewideData/FCNNurseDemandReports.aspx.

Florida Center for Nursing. (2017). *2015-2016 Education survey results: Pre-licensure RN programs.* Orlando, FL: Author. Retrieved from www.flcenterfornursing.org/StatewideData/FCNNurseEducationReports.aspx.

Florida Center for Nursing. (2018b). *Florida's 2016-2017 workforce supply characteristics and trends: Licensed practical nurses.* Orlando, FL: Author. Retrieved from www.flcenterfornursing.org/StatewideData/FCNNurseSupplyReports.aspx.

Florida Center for Nursing. (2018a). *Florida's 2016-2017 workforce supply characteristics and trends: Advanced registered nurse practitioners.* Orlando, FL: Author. Retrieved from www.flcenterfornursing.org/StatewideData/FCNNurseSupplyReports.aspx.

Florida Center for Nursing. (2018c). *Florida's 2016-2017 workforce supply characteristics and trends: Registered nurses.* Orlando, FL: Author. Retrieved fromDocument74 www.flcenterfornursing.org/StatewideData/FCNNurseSupplyReports.aspx.

Frey, W. (2018). *The US will become "minority White" in 2045, census projects: Youthful minorities are the engine of future growth. Brookings Institute.* Retrieved from www.brookings.edu/blog/the-avenue/2018/03/14/the-us-will-become-minority-white-in-2045-census-projects/.

Hassmiller, S., & Mensik, J. (2017). *The power of ten: A conversational approach to tackling the top ten priorities in nursing* (2nd ed.). Indianapolis: Sigma Theta Tau International Publishing. 153.

Kennedy, M.S. (June, 2018). Nurses wanted almost everywhere. [Editorial]. *American Journal of Nursing, 118*(6), 7.

Robert Wood Johnson Foundation. (2015). *Nurses take on new and expanded roles in healthcare.* Retrieved from www.rwjf.org/en/library/articles-and-news/2015/01/nurses-take-on-new-and-expanded-roles-in-health-care.html.

Rosenbaum, M. (2018). Will 2018 be the year healthcare addresses its turnover problem? *Becker's Hospital Review.* Retrieved from www.beckershospitalreview.com/finance/will-2018-be-the-year-healthcare-addresses-its-turnover-problem.html.

Spetz, J., & Kovner, C.T. (2013). How can we obtain data on the demand for nurses? *Nursing Economics, 31*(4), 203–207.

Underwood, C. (2017). *America's generations: In the workplace, marketplace, and living room.* CreateSpace Independent Publishing Platform.

U.S. Department of Health and Human Services, Health Resources and Services Administration, Bureau of Health Workforce, National Center for Health Workforce Analysis. (2018). *Long-term services and supports: Nursing workforce demand projections, 2015-2030.* Rockville, MD. Retrieved from https://bhw.hrsa.gov/sites/default/files/bhw/nchwa/projections/hrsa-ltss-nursing-report.pdf.

U.S. Department of Labor, Bureau of Labor Statistics. (June 24, 2018). *Occupational outlook handbook: Registered nurses.* Retrieved from www.bls.gov/ooh/healthcare/registered-nurses.htm.

ONLINE RESOURCES

Florida Center for Nursing
www.FLCenterForNursing.org
Health Resources & Services Administration Bureau of Health Workforce
https://bhw.hrsa.gov
The National Forum of State Nursing Workforce Centers
www.NursingWorkforceCenters.org

54

Rural Health Care: Workforce Challenges and Opportunities

Pamela Stewart Fahs and Nicole Rouhana[a]

"Historically, delivery of health-care services in rural settings has been problematic for both public and private institutions, and so it remains..."

Burkett, Mulchahy, and Zahorik (2006)

Rural America is a vast, sparsely populated geographic area where 19.3% of the U.S. population live (Holder, Fields, & Lofquist, 2016). The nation's land mass is currently 97% rural (United States Census Bureau, 2017). A new federal classification system of rural areas, Frontier and Remote (FAR), indicates that 2.3 million Americans live in the most remote areas of the U.S. (U.S. Department of Agriculture, Economic Research Services [USDA, ERS], n.d.). Rural Americans face a combination of factors that create significant disparities in health (Gonzalez et al., 2018). Furthermore, there are unique obstacles that confront rural health care providers and systems (Meit et al., 2014). Professional nurses fill a critical need when responding to challenges distinctive to rural health systems (Box 54.1; Rural Health Information Hub [RHI Hub], n.d.-b).

DEFINING RURAL

Although there is no universally accepted definition of the term *rural*, the need to define rural remains a deceptively complex issue and is a key issue of rural health care policy. Multiple classification systems (Table 54.1) help policymakers to delineate rural places. The U.S. Census Bureau describes the term *rural* as anywhere that is not an urban area or urban core (Ratcliff, Burd, Holder, & Fields, 2016). Rural is most often defined by default, a place that is not otherwise classified as metropolitan, micropolitan, or urban.

---

[a]This chapter updates a previous chapter originally developed by Alan Morgan, MPA and draws on that excellent work.

Use of the variety of rural definitions allows a better fit for policymakers to meet the needs of rural communities, providers, and residents (RHI Hub, n.d.-c). By successfully defining rural, a community may qualify for a specific type of heath care facility, such as a critical access hospital or rural health clinic (Table 54.2).

WHAT MAKES HEALTH AND HEALTH CARE DIFFERENT FOR RURAL POPULATIONS?

Social determinants of health including economic factors and cultural and social demographic differences conspire to impede rural Americans in their struggle to lead healthy lives (Gonzalez et al., 2018). The higher rate of home ownership in rural (81.1%) compared to urban (59.8%) communities (Mazur, 2017) and the lower costs of living are positive rural economic indicators, whereas median household incomes are slightly lower in rural ($52,386) than urban ($54,296) areas (U.S. Census Bureau, 2016). The question of whether rural or urban areas have more poverty depends on factors included in the poverty calculation (Renwick & Fox, 2016). Rural workers experience annual income fluctuations (Ziller, Thayer, & Lenardson, 2018) that may reflect seasonal or part-time work and can affect eligibility for publicly-funded health insurance and other social support.

Education may also influence the economic picture for an area. Rural Americans are better educated than ever before with most now holding a high school diploma or general education development (GED) certificate (USDA, ERS, 2017). Attainment of a bachelor's or higher degree still lags significantly behind the same benchmark in urban populations (Table 54.3).

BOX 54.1 Rural Nursing Practice Challenges

- Increased proportions of older population or chronically ill patients requiring more frequent care.
- Less primary care providers result in less opportunity for preventive screening and education.
- Fewer opportunities for career advancement or continuing education.
- Lower staffing ratios, longer shifts, less flexibility in work schedules.
- Fewer health care facilities limit employment opportunities.
- Lower starting salaries.
- Wide state-to-state variation of advanced practice registered nurse (APRN) scope of practice.
- Lack of personal privacy within the community.

From Goodell, S., Dower, C., & O'Neil, E. (2011). *Primary care workforce in the United States.* Retrieved from www.rwjf.org/content/dam/farm/reports/issue_briefs/2011/rwjf70613; Rural Health. Information Hub. (n.d.-c). *What is rural?* Retrieved from www.ruralhealthinfo.org/topics/what-is-rural.

Rural dwellers may choose rural living for a variety of reasons including strong cultural beliefs, social ties, or a positive sense of place. Two factors predict community attachment: (1) distance to an urban center, and (2) community size small enough to know others by their first name (McKnight, Sanders, Gibbs, & Brown, 2017).

The lack of anonymity discussed in rural literature (Lee, Winters, Boland, Raph, & Buehler, 2018) has a positive side: the familiarity within communities and community organizations can provide a buffer to some of the difficulties that come with rural living. Rural community members tend to be supportive of each other, particularly in times of difficulty such as illness.

Cultural and social differences may influence the way rural Americans view their health and how they interact with health care providers and systems (Lee & McDonagh, 2018). Rural dwellers often define health in terms of being able to function or work. Self-reliance is valued. Any additional support is first sought from lay networks of family and community, and reliance on government may be seen as a last resort or a sign of weakness.

HEALTH DISPARITIES OF RURAL AMERICANS

Rural areas often have a natural beauty; however, a bucolic view is unsupported in the realities of rural life and health. Rural health challenges are significant (Box 54.2), and rural adults have a high chronic disease burden (National Center for Health Statistics [NCHS], 2018; Towne et al., 2017) (Table 54.4).

Obesity and smoking are known contributing factors to chronic illness. The highest obesity rates occur in rural women (40%) and men (35%). Adults from rural counties are more likely to smoke, and rural adolescent smoking is higher (11%) than in urban areas (5%) (Health Resources and Services Administration [HRSA], 2018). Vaping or "juuling"—smoking electronic cigarettes (e-cigarettes)—is a tremendous public health threat in the U.S., including in rural areas (Cullen et al., 2018).

TABLE 54.1 Common Rural Classification Systems

Code	U.S. Department of Agriculture, Economic Research Services				U.S. Census Bureau	Office of Management and Budget
Code	RUCC	RUCA	UIC	FAR		Core Based Statistical Areas
Unit Level	County	Census Track and Zip Code	County	Census Track and Zip Code	Census Blocks	County
Number of Levels	9	10	12	4	3	3
Common Level Groups	1–3 Metro	1–3 Metro	1–2 Metro	1 Least Remote	UA	Metro
	4–9 Nonmetro	4–6 Micro	3–10 Nonmetro		UC	Micro
		7–10 Nonmetro	11–12 Noncore, Not Adjacent	4 Most Remote	Rural	Noncore

FAR, Frontier and remote area; *Metro,* metropolitan; *Micro,* micropolitan; *Nonmetro,* non-metropolitan; *RUCA,* rural urban commuting area; *RUCC,* rural urban continuum codes; *UA,* urbanized area; *UC,* urban cluster; *UIC,* urban influence codes. From United States Department of Agriculture Economic Research Services. (n.d.). *What is rural?* Retrieved from www.ers.usda.gov/topics/rural-economy-population/rural-classifications/what-is-rural.aspx.

TABLE 54.2   Types of Health Care Facilities Seen in Rural Places

Name	Known As	Type	Staffing	Federal Funding	Location	Requirements	Operation Status
Critical Access Hospital (CAH)	CAH	Inpatient—up to 25 beds—may have swing beds Continuous emergency services	On-site or on-call provider for emergency	Yes—special payment	Mainly rural, some urban	Beyond 35 miles to nearest hospital, or 15 miles under special circumstances	Usually larger systems, nonprofit
Small Rural Hospital	Rural	In patient—up to 49 beds		Yes—pass through to states	Rural		
Federally Qualified Health Center (FQHC)	FQHC	Clinic		Yes	Rural and urban	Open 32.5 hr/week, must provide some emergency service arrangement, comprehensive primary care	Nonprofit or public
Federally Qualified Health Center—lookalikes	FQHC lookalike	Clinic		Reduced cost meds or apply for CMS FQHC payment	Rural and urban	Provides comprehensive primary care	Nonprofit or public
Rural Health Clinic (RHC)	Provider-based RHC	Clinic as part of system	At least 1 NP/PA	Yes	Non-urbanized	May be type specific (e.g., primary care)	Primarily health system, nonprofit
	Independent RHC			Special reimbursement	Non-urbanized		Primarily provider, for-profit
Public Health	Health Department	May offer clinics		No	Rural/urban		State
School-Based Health Clinics (SBHC)	SBHC	Clinic			Rural/urban		Schools in partnership with systems, nonprofit

CMS, Centers for Medicare and Medicaid Services; *NP*, Nurse Practitioner; *PA*, Physician Assistant.
From Health Resources and Services Administration. (n.d.). *Rural hospital programs*. Retrieved from www.hrsa.gov/rural-health/rural-hospitals/index.html; Rural Health Information Hub. (n.d.-a). *Rural health clinics (RHCs)*. Retrieved from www.ruralhealthinfo.org/topics/rural-health-clinics.

Lifestyle behaviors and preventative health measures are key components in reducing, delaying, or decreasing the severity of illness. For example, surveys reflecting health measures show lower outcomes on preventive measures for rural Americans (Table 54.5), including dental visits, colorectal cancer screening, and having met physical activity guidelines. Vaccination coverage for rural young children and adolescents is also lower (NCHS, 2018).

Opioid use disorder (OUD) in rural areas is receiving increasing attention. The overall prevalence of metropolitan (urban) and non-metropolitan (rural) drug use shows little variation (Rural Health Research Gateway [RHRG],

TABLE 54.3 Educational Attainment, Rural and Urban Change (2000–2015)

Educational Level	Rural	Urban	Rural Change 2000–2015	Urban Change 2000–2015
Bachelor's degree or higher	19%	33%	+4%	+7%
Associate degree	9%	8%	+3%	+2%
Some college	22%	21%	+3%	+2%
High school or general education development	36%	26%	0%	−1%
Less than high school diploma	15%	13%	−9%	−6%

From U.S. Department of Agriculture, Economic Services Research. (2017). *Rural education at a glance, 2017 edition.* Retrieved from https://drive.google.com/file/d/0B5BdbPm9jpqOQi0teFJyMnNCY0U/view.

BOX 54.2 Rural Health Problems

- Chronic illnesses (diabetes, heart and lung diseases) are higher in rural America.
- Rural residents are less likely to receive annual dental exam (across age groups).
- Increase in opioid drug use (prescription and non-prescription) with non-prescription use outpacing urban communities.
- Age-adjusted death rates are higher for rural populations.
- Distance, geography, and transportation challenges.

From National Center for Health Statistics. (2018). *Health, United States 2017: With special feature on mortality.* Retrieved from www.cdc.gov/nchs/data/hus/hus17.pdf; Rural Health Research Gateway. (2018). *Rural health research recap: Opioid use and treatment availability.* Retrieved from www.ruralhealth research.org/assets/925-3046/opioid-use-and-treatment-availability-recap.pdf.

2018); however, an increase in reported OUD prevalence occurred in 2014–2015. Although there was a spike in the perceived need for drug treatment in 2011–2013 among non-metropolitan individuals, by 2014–2015 treatment use rose to be equivalent to those in metropolitan areas (~24%).

The Comprehensive Addiction and Recovery Act (CARA) of 2016, signed into law to address the opioid epidemic, began a prescription waiver program to allow more physicians to treat drug addiction with a medication-assisted program (Community Anti-Drug Coalition of American, n.d.). As of publication, the final regulations broadened the term "prescriber" to include nurse practitioners (NPs) and physician assistants (PAs) with specific training requirements (Patterson, 2018). However, over 60% of rural counties are without a provider with a prescription waiver, and the vast majority (91%) of waivered providers are in urban counties (Andrilla, Coulthard, & Patterson, 2018; RHRG, 2018). Another provision of CARA allowed distribution of naloxone, or Narcan, to first

TABLE 54.4 Differences in Health Indicators (per 100,000) by Location of Residence

Indicator	Metropolitan	Non-Metropolitan	Difference	Group
Conditions				
Heart Disease	10.2	13.2	Higher	Adults
Cancer	6.1	6.5	Higher	Adults
Stroke	2.5	3.1	Higher	Adults
2–3 Chronic	18.9	22.6	Higher	Adults
4 or more Chronic	4.2	5.1	Higher	Adults
Health Status				
Fair to Poor Health	8.6	11.4	Higher	All ages
Usual Source of Health Care Past Year				
No Usual Source	17.0	15.7	Higher	Adults
No Usual Source	3.2	4.1	Higher	Under 6 years old
No Usual Source	5.4	3.9	Higher	6–17 years old

TABLE 54.4 Differences in Health Indicators (per 100,000) by Location of Residence—cont'd

Indicator	Metropolitan	Non-Metropolitan	Difference	Group
No Usual Source	4.7	4.0	Higher	Under 18 years old
No Office/Clinic Visits	8.4	10.4	Lower	Under 18 years old
No Visits	14.2	16.4	Higher	Age-adjusted
1–3 Visits (Office, Emergency Department or Home)	50.1	45.7	Lower	Age-adjusted
4–9 Visits	23.1	24.0	Higher	Age-adjusted
12–6 Visits	12.6	13.9	Higher	Age-adjusted
Severe Pain				
Headache/Migraine	14.9	19.2	Higher	Adults
Low Back	27.7	32.9	Higher	Adults
Neck	14.6	17.2	Higher	Adults
Mental Health				
Serious Psychological Distress	3.3	5.1	Higher	Adults
Senses—Limitations				
Vision Trouble—without correction	9.7	12.1	Higher	Adults
Hearing-Trouble—without hearing aids	13.3	19.2	Higher	Adults

From National Center for Health Statistics. (2018). *Health, United States 2017: With special feature on mortality*. Retrieved from www.cdc.gov/nchs/data/hus/hus17.pdf.

TABLE 54.5 Disparities in Prevention (per 100,000) by Residence and Age Group

Indicator	Metropolitan	Non-Metropolitan	Difference	Age Group
Dental Visits				
	69.1%	69.3%	Lower	2 years +
	84.3%	83.4%	Lower	2–17 years
	65.7%	56.1%	Lower	18–64 years
	66.6%	53.9%	Lower	65 years +
Colorectal Cancer Screening and Prevention				
Any Colorectal Test or Procedure	63.2%	58.5%	Lower	50–75 years
Colonoscopy	59.8%	56.5%	Lower	50–75 years
Met Physical Activity Guidelines				
Aerobic	53.7%	46.4%	Lower	Adults
Muscle-strengthening	27.4%	18.4%	Lower	Adults

Lower percentage = worse outcome.
From National Center for Health Statistics. (2018). *Health, United States 2017: With special feature on mortality*. Retrieved from www.cdc.gov/nchs/data/hus/hus17.pdf.

responders and law enforcement in the community to reduce opioid-related deaths.

Often, rural law enforcement deals with drug-related behaviors where access to mental health (Andrilla, Patterson, Garberson, & Coulthard, 2018) and drug rehabilitation services are limited. The parameters of reporting a serious mental health illness in the past year worsened for adults as rurality increased (HRSA, 2018).

Finally, suicide is the 10th leading cause of death in the U.S. Rates over a 15-year period were highest in nonmetropolitan counties compared with metropolitan counties (17.32 vs. 11.92 per 100,000). Use of firearms as a means for suicide was twice as high in nonmetropolitan compared with large metropolitan counties (10.53 vs. 5.29 per 100,000) (Ivey-Stephenson, Crosby, Jack, Haileyesus, & Kresnow-Sedacca, 2017).

RURAL HEALTH CARE

Rural America has a distinctive health care environment. Rural health care systems are shrinking in number and scope of services. Generally, there are fewer primary care providers in rural areas and specialty services are particularly scarce. Low volumes of patients present a challenge in delivering care in an economical manner. Patients are often older, have significant underlying health care problems, and are less likely to participate in preventive health care screenings, which may increase complications and health expenditures. This situation leads to a lack of volume purchasing power, greater transportation costs, and higher health care needs (Mueller et al., 2018).

On average, rural residents have a greater distance to travel to access health care than their urban counterparts, a problem compounded by a general lack of rural public transportation. This has a direct impact on patient care, follow-up, and long-term outcomes. Furthermore, Carr et al. (2017) found less rural access to Level I and II trauma care, with more rural locations having the least access. An analysis of national data showed that rural emergency medical services (EMS) response times were significantly longer; whereas seven minutes was an average time from 911 call to EMS arrival, median rural response times were greater than 14 minutes (Mell et al., 2017). A longer EMS response time could affect health outcome, particularly in trauma patients.

Rural health care systems, with small numbers of providers and sparse resources, are tenuously balanced to meet the needs of residents. Rural specialty care requires a greater reliance on utilization of local tenens providers, regionalization of specialists, and limited consultations onsite or via telehealth. Telehealth options are limited by federal and state regulations and to communities with adequate internet infrastructure.

Sixteen percent of registered nurses (RNs) in the workforce are employed in rural areas (HRSA, 2013). Rural nurses are expected to become consummate generalists, functioning at a high level of expertise sooner, in varied situations, and with less resources than their urban counterparts (Fahs, 2017). Rural nursing is rewarding. Rural health care settings' often smaller and more tightly interrelated environments foster collegiality and creative problem solving. Both RNs and advanced practice registered nurses (APRNs) are familiar with the needs of their local community and can implement improvements in the health care system to address the unique needs of rural populations. Rural and urban nurses' characteristics differ and may contribute to rural workforce challenges (Box 54.3).

Although nursing education is producing more graduates than ever, a maldistribution of RNs is predicted. Rural populations will remain disproportionately underserved. Increasing the supply of RNs and APRNs may not address the challenges related to rural workforce retention in terms of adequate wages, start-up bonuses, and benefits. Rural nurses may feel a sense of professional isolation, decreased potential for professional advancement, and limited opportunities for social interactions. Collectively these factors may decrease access to care. Also influencing the rural nursing workforce are the high rates of RN retirement and a shift of responsibility to RNs and APRNs in rural areas (Buerhaus, Skinner, Auerbach, & Staiger, 2017). Spetz, Stillman, and Andrilla (2017) estimate up to three-quarters of rural primary care services could be provided by APRNs and PAs. The role of the APRN includes certified nurse-midwife (CNM), certified registered nurse-anesthetist (CRNA), clinical nurse specialist (CNS), and NP. As NPs are trained to care for a variety of patient populations in

---

BOX 54.3 Characteristics of Rural Nurses Versus Urban Nurses

- Sixteen percent of the U.S. nursing workforce are rural nurses.
- Rural nurses are closer to retirement within the next decade.
- Rural nurses are less racially and ethnically diverse (primarily white).
- Rural nurses are less likely to obtain a bachelor's degree.

Reference: Health Resources and Service Administration. (2013). *The U.S. nursing workforce: Trends in supply and education.* Retrieved from www.ruralhealthinfo.org/assets/1206-4974/nursing-workforce-nchwa-report-april-2013.pdf.

both in-patient and outpatient settings, they are highly effective in addressing the demand for primary care services in rural communities. CNMs are primary care providers of women and help address the shortage of obstetrical providers. Almost 50% of all U.S. counties are lacking obstetrical and gynecological care, or have lost obstetrical services with the closure of rural hospitals (Hung, Henning-Smith, Casey, & Kozhimannil, 2017).

Spetz et al. (2017) found that, despite a greater workload, NPs practicing in a rural setting reported higher satisfaction than urban NPs. Where state regulations allow, rural NPs are more likely to work independently and to their fullest scope of practice. Traczynski and Udalova (2018) found NPs improve utilization of services, increase routine checkups, and decrease emergency department use, with patient-reported improved quality of care.

RURAL POLICY, RURAL POLITICS

Specific components of the Patient Protection and Affordable Care Act (ACA), such as payment system changes from fee-for-service to value-based payments, have been challenging for rural health care systems (Newkirk & Damico, 2014). In rural areas, changes in taxation and health care insurance markets have created an air of uncertainty (Wengle, Blumberg, & Holahan, 2018). The ACA included coverage for pre-existing health conditions, allowed adult children to remain on parental polices until age 26, and permitted expansion of Medicaid. States that did not expand Medicaid were lagging in numbers of insured by 2018. Health care exchanges serving rural areas typically have fewer options available and the cost of insurance is often higher for rural Americans (Williams & Holmes, 2018), even when controlling for factors such as the Medicaid expansion (Wengle et al., 2018). Not all rural populations have embraced the ACA.

Insurance market payment reforms moved hospital reimbursement from a fee-for-service model to one of value-added purchasing and population health, raising concerns that decreased profit margins threaten sustainability. Various types of hospitals and clinics serve rural populations (see Table 54.2) and qualify for special Medicare payment and other types of funding (Freeman, Thompson, Howard, Randolph, & Holmes, 2015).

In Medicaid expansion states, rural hospitals had slim financial operating margins, whereas those in states that did *not* expand Medicaid were more likely to have negative operating margins (Kaufman, Reiter, Pink, & Holmes, 2016). Two-thirds of rural hospital closures have been in non-Medicaid expansion states (Holmes, Kaufman, & Pink, 2017). Between 2010 and 2019, nationally there were 94 rural hospital closures, with a marked increase since 2013 (University of North Carolina, n.d.). In some cases, a closed hospital became an outpatient clinic with limited emergency services (Holmes et al., 2017) that could maintain some access, but employed fewer people. Loss of rural hospitals has a significant adverse impact on the sustainability of the rural community.

THE OPPORTUNITIES AND CHALLENGES OF RURAL HEALTH

Rural communities offer opportunities and challenges to providing health care that best meets the population needs. The federal government's role in supporting innovative systems of care is critical. Because of the nature of rural practice and workforce shortages, federal and state health policies that support rural health care providers need continued attention. The ongoing policy debate centers on whether rural hospitals can continue to provide the appropriate level of care, in a timely manner, with the appropriate providers for the care needed.

Medicare enrollment is anticipated to expand to 80 million by 2030, and about one-quarter (23%) of Medicare beneficiaries live in rural areas (Buerhaus et al., 2017). Rural physicians accept Medicare beneficiaries at a higher rate (81% rural vs. 72% in urban areas) (Boccuti, Fields, Casillas, & Hamel, 2015). The increased enrollment to primary care services coupled with the growing population of senior citizens is challenging the rural health care system. To maintain health care services for rural populations, workforce development, including targeted recruitment and retention efforts, is necessary in rural communities.

Internet conductivity and speed are necessary for telehealth applications to improve access to health care for rural dwellers. Telehealth services require infrastructure for internet access, adequate bandwidth, and technological support. An analysis of national broadband capabilities found a connectivity gap that worsened on measures of speed, despite federal assistance to equalize internet capability in rural America (Whitacre, Wheeler, & Landgraf, 2016). Critical policy work is needed to address issues that hamper implementation of telehealth: state health care professional licensing (Pauli, Bajjani-Gebara, O'Quin, Raps, & DeLeon, 2018), insurance coverage, provider training to utilize telehealth for effective outcomes, technical support, mismatches in equipment, and electronic health records across systems (Schwamm et al., 2017).

The National Health Service Corps provides scholarships and student loan repayments to individuals who agree to a period of service in a federally-designated Health Professional Shortage Area. The ACA also reauthorized and expanded existing health workforce education and training programs under Titles VII and VIII of the Public

Health Service Act and bolstered undergraduate and graduate nursing education and training (Williams & Koslosky, n.d.). Because health care providers most likely to serve in rural areas come from rural areas, workforce development efforts can include increased educational opportunities to allow individuals to remain in their rural communities to prevent outmigration.

ACTIONS THROUGH POLICY AND POLITICS

Nurses can make a difference through policy in multiple areas influencing rural health care. Nurses can work on issues of health disparities by volunteering at local organizations to build community capacity to promote change: volunteer at a local, free clinic; become part of a taskforce to write a community sustainability grant; or work with your local Head Start to teach young children and their families about reducing childhood obesity.

Use the power of professional organizations to address health care disparities or system policies that block the most effective health care delivery. Link with professional organizations such as the American Association of Nurse Practitioners to change the laws regulating advanced practice. Join the Rural Nurse Organization or the National Rural Health Association to stay apprised of issues affecting rural health policy. Rural hospitals and community organization boards, nonprofit board of directors, schools, and health care systems will gain from nurses' wealth of expertise and experience with professional nurse board members.

Finally, to meet the need for new political candidates, nurses can fill a void for needed representation to address issues of injustice and the health care needs of rural populations. Get involved, run for an elected office, support candidates that understand the issues of rural health care, and vote!

DISCUSSION QUESTIONS

1. Describe rural health challenges. What role can nurses play in addressing these issues, including policy actions?
2. What are unique attributes of rural practice?
3. What role does the ACA play in addressing workforce shortages in rural communities?

REFERENCES

Andrilla, C.H.A, Coulthard, C., & Patterson, D.G. (2018). Prescribing practices of rural physicians waivered to prescribe buprenorphine. *American Journal of Preventive Medicine, 54*(6Se) S208–S214.

Andrilla, C.H.A, Patterson, D.G., Garberson, L.A., & Coulthard, C. (2018). Geographic variation in the supply of selected behavioral health providers. *American Journal of Preventive Medicine, 54*(6Se) S199–S207.

Boccuti, C., Fields, C., Casillas, G., & Hamel, L. (2015). *Primary care physicians accepting Medicare: A snapshot.* Retrieved from http://files.kff.org/attachment/data-note-primary-care-physicians-accepting-medicare-a-snapshot.

Buerhaus, P., Skinner, B.A., Auerbach, D.I., & Staiger, D.O. (2017). Four challenges facing nursing workforce in the United States. *Journal of Nursing Regulation, 8*(2), 40–46.

Burkett, G.L., Mulchahy, R.P., & Zahorik, P.M. (2006). Health. In R. Abramson & J. Haskell (Eds.), *Encyclopedia of Appalachia* (pp. 1611–1636). Knoxville, TN: University of Tennessee Press.

Carr, B., Bowman, A., Wolff, C., Mullen, M.T., Holena, D., Branas, C.C., & Wiebe, D. (2017). Disparities in access to trauma care in the United States: A population-based analysis. *Injury, 48*, 332–338.

Community Anti-Drug Coalitions of America. (n.d.). *The Comprehensive Addiction and Recovery Act (CARA), Public Law 114-198.* Retrieved from www.cadca.org/comprehensive-addiction-and-recovery-act-cara.

Cullen K.A., Ambrose B.K., Gentzke A.S., Apelberg B.J., Jamal A., & King B.A. (2018). Notes from the field: Use of electronic cigarettes and any tobacco product among middle and high school students—United States, 2011–2018. *Morbidity and Mortality Weekly Report, 67*, 1276–1277.

Fahs, P.S. (2017). Leading-following in the context of rural nursing. *Nursing Science Quarterly, 30*, 176-178.

Freeman, V.A., Thompson, K., Howard, H.A., Randolph, R., & Holmes G.M. (2015). *The 21st century rural hospital: A chart book.* Retrieved from www.shepscenter.unc.edu/wp-content/uploads/2015/02/21stCenturyRuralHospitalsChartBook.pdf .

Gonzalez, K.M., Shaughnessy, M.J., Kabigting, E-N.R., West, D.T., Robinson, J.C., Chen, Q., & Fahs, P.S. (2018). The healthcare of vulnerable populations within rural societies: A systematic review. *Online Journal of Rural Nursing and Health Care, 18*(1), 112–147.

Goodell, S., Dower, C., & O'Neil, E. (2011). *Primary care workforce in the United States.* Retrieved from www.rwjf.org/content/dam/farm/reports/issue_briefs/2011/rwjf70613.

Health Resources and Services Administration. (n.d.). *Rural hospital programs.* Retrieved from www.hrsa.gov/rural-health/rural-hospitals/index.html.

Health Resources and Services Administration. (2013). *The U.S. nursing workforce: Trends in supply and education.* Retrieved from www.ruralhealthinfo.org/assets/1206-4974/nursing-workforce-nchwa-report-april-2013.pdf .

Health Resources and Services Administration. (2018). *Health equity report 2017.* Retrieved from www.hrsa.gov/sites/default/files/hrsa/health-equity/2017-HRSA-health-equity-report.pdf.

Holder, K.A., Fields, A., & Lofquist, D. (2016). *Rurality matters.* Retrieved from www.census.gov/newsroom/blogs/random-samplings/2016/12/rurality_matters.html.

Holmes, G.M., Kaufman, B.G., & Pink, G.H. (2017). *Financial distress and closure of rural hospitals.* Retrieved from www.ruralhealthresearch.org/assets/540-1584/9212017-financial-distress-closures-of-rural-hospitals-ppt.pdf.

Hung, P., Henning-Smith, C.E., Casey, M.M., & Kozhimannil, K.B. (2017). Access to obstetrics services in rural counties still declining, with 9 percent losing services. *Health Affairs, 36,* 1663-1671.

Ivey-Stephenson, A.Z., Crosby, A. E., Jack, S.P.D., Haileyesus, T., & Kresnow-Sedacca, M-J. (2017). Suicide trends among and within urbanization levels by sex, race/ethnicity, age group, and mechanism of death—United States, 2001–2015. *Morbidity and Mortality Weekly Report Surveillance Summaries, 66*(18), 1–10.

Kaufman, B.G., Reiter, K.L., Pink, G.H., & Holmes, G.M. (2016). Medicaid expansion affects rural and urban hospitals differently. *Health Affairs, 35,* 1665-1672.

Lee, H.J., & McDonagh, M.K. (2018). Updating the rural nursing theory base. In C.A. Winters & H.J. Lee (Eds.), *Rural nursing: Concepts, theory, and practice* (pp 45–62). New York, NY: Springer.

Lee, H.J., Winters, C.A., Boland, R.L., Raph, S.W., & Buehler, J.A. (2018). Concept analysis. In C.A. Winters & H.J. Lee (Eds.), *Rural nursing: Concepts, theory, and practice* (pp 31–44). New York: Springer.

Mazur, C. (2017). *Rural residents more likely to own homes than urban residents.* Retrieved from www.census.gov/library/stories/2017/09/rural-home-ownership.html.

McKnight, M.L., Sanders, S.R., Gibbs, B.G., & Brown, R.B. (2017). Communities of place? New evidence for the role of distance and population size in community attachment. *Rural Sociology, 82,* 291-317.

Meit, M., Knudson, A., Gilbert, T., Yu, A.T., Tanenbaum, E., ... & Popat, S. (2014). *The 2014 update of the rural-urban chartbook.* Retrieved from https://ruralhealth.und.edu/projects/health-reform-policy-research-center/pdf/2014-rural-urban-chartbook-update.pdf.

Mell, H.K., Mumma, S.N., Heistand, B., Carr, B.G., Holland, T., & Stopyra, J. (2017). Emergency medical services response time in rural, suburban, and urban areas. *JAMA Surgery, 152,* 983–984.

Moy, E., Garcia, M.C., Bastian, B., Rossen, L.M., Ingram, D.D., ... & Iademarco, M.F. (2017). Leading causes of death in nonmetropolitan and metropolitan areas—United States, 1999–2014. *Morbidity and Mortality Weekly Report, 66* (No. SS-1), 1–8.

Mueller, K.J., Alfero, C., Coburn, A.F., Lundblad, J.P., MacKinnery, A.C., McBride, T.D., & Barker, A. (2018). *Insuring rural America: Health insurance challenges and opportunities.* Retrieved from www.rupri.org/wp-content/uploads/Insuring-Rural-America.pdf.

National Center for Health Statistics. (2018). *Health, United States 2017: With special feature on mortality.* Retrieved from www.cdc.gov/nchs/data/hus/hus17.pdf.

Newkirk, V.R. II, & Damico, A. (2014). *The Affordable Care Act and insurance coverage in rural areas.* Retrieved from https://kaiserfamilyfoundation.files.wordpress.com/2014/05/8597-the-affordable-care-act-and-insurance-coverage-in-rural-areas1.pdf.

Patterson, R.W. (2018). *Implementation of the provision of the Comprehensive Addiction and Recovery Act of 2016 relating to the dispensing of narcotic drugs for opioid use disorder.* Retrieved from www.gpo.gov/fdsys/pkg/FR-2018-01-23/pdf/2018-01173.pdf.

Pauli, E., Bajjani-Gebara, J.E., O'Quin, C., Raps, S.J., & DeLeon, P.H. (2018). Telehealth: The future for advance practice mental health nursing. *Archives of Psychiatric Nursing, 32,* 327-328.

Ratcliff, M., Burd, C., Holder, K., & Fields, A. (2016). *Defining rural at the U.S. Census Bureau: American community survey and geography brief.* Retrieved from www.census.gov/content/dam/Census/library/publications/2016/acs/acsgeo-1.pdf.

Renwick, T., & Fox, L. (2016). *The supplemental poverty measure: 2015. Current population reports.* Retrieved from www.census.gov/content/dam/Census/library/publications/2016/demo/p60-258.pdf.

Rural Health Information Hub. (n.d.-a). *Rural health clinics (RHCs).* Retrieved from www.ruralhealthinfo.org/topics/rural-health-clinics.

Rural Health Information Hub. (n.d.-b). *Rural healthcare workforce.* Retrieved from www.ruralhealthinfo.org/topics/healthcare-workforce.

Rural Health Information Hub. (n.d.-c). *What is rural?* Retrieved from www.ruralhealthinfo.org/topics/what-is-rural.

Rural Health Research Gateway. (2018). *Rural health research recap: Opioid use and treatment availability.* Retrieved from www.ruralhealthresearch.org/assets/925-3046/opioid-use-and-treatment-availability-recap.pdf.

Schwamm, L.H., Chumbler, N., Brown, E., Fonarow, G.C., Berube, D., Nystrom, K., ... & Tiner, A.C. (2017). Recommendations for implementation of telehealth in cardiovascular and stroke care: A policy statement from the American Heart Association, *Circulation, 135,* e24-e44.

Skillman, S.M., Kaplan, L., Fordyce, M.S., McMenamin, P.D., & Doescher, M.P. (2012). *Understanding advanced practice registered nurse distribution in urban and rural areas of the United States using national provider identifier data.* Retrieved from http://depts.washington.edu/uwrhrc/uploads/RHRC_FR137_Skillman.pdf.

Spetz, J., Skillman, S.M., & Andrilla, H.A. (2017). Nurse practitioner autonomy and satisfaction in rural settings. *Medical Care Research and Review, 74,* 227–235.

Towne, S.D. Jr., Bolin, J., Ferdinand, A.O., Nicklett, E.J., Smith, M.L., Callaghan, T.H., & Ory, M.G. (2017). *Diabetes and forgone medical care due to cost in the U.S. (2011–2015): Individual-level & place-based disparities.* Retrieved from https://srhrc.tamhsc.edu/docs/srhrc-pb1-towne-diabetes.pdf.

Traczynski, J., & Udalova, V. (2018). Nurse practitioner independence, health care utilization, and health outcomes. *Journal of Health Economics, 58,* 90-109.

United States Census Bureau. (2016). *Measuring America: Our changing landscape.* Retrieved from www.census.gov/content/dam/Census/library/visualizations/2016/comm/acs-rural-urban.pdf.

United States Census Bureau. (2017). *One in five Americans live in rural areas.* Retrieved from www.census.gov/library/stories/2017/08/rural-america.html.

U.S. Department of Agriculture, Economic Research Services. (n.d.). *What is rural?* Retrieved from www.ers.usda.gov/topics/rural-economy-population/rural-classifications/what-is-rural.aspx.

U.S. Department of Agriculture, Economic Research Services. (2017). *Rural education at a glance, 2017 edition.* Retrieved from https://drive.google.com/file/d/0B5BdbPm9jpqOQi0te FJyMnNCY0U/view.

University of North Carolina. (n.d.). *94 rural hospital closures: January 2010–present.* Retrieved from www.shepscenter.unc.edu/programs-projects/rural-health/rural-hospital-closures/.

Wengle, E., Blumberg, L.J., & Holahan, J. (2018). *Are marketplace premiums higher in rural than in urban areas?* Retrieved from www.urban.org/sites/default/files/publication/99341/moni-ruralurban_-_final_0.pdf.

Whitacre, B.E., Wheeler, D., & Landgraf, C. (2016). What can the national broadband map tell us about the health care connectivity gap? *Journal of Rural Health, 33,* 284–289.

Williams, D. Jr., & Holmes, M. (2018). Rural health care costs: Are they higher and why might they differ from urban health care costs? *North Carolina Medical Journal, 79*(1), 51–55.

Williams S.D., & Koslosky S.S. (n.d.). *Presentation of Title VIII programs.* Retrieved from www.hrsa.gov/sites/default/files/hrsa/advisory-committees/nursing/meetings/2015/20150728-titleviiiprograms.pdf.

Ziller, E., Thayer, D., & Lenardson, J.D. (2018). *Medicaid income eligibility transitions among rural adults.* Retrieved from https://digitalcommons.usm.maine.edu/insurance/66/.

ONLINE RESOURCES

Federal Office of Rural Health Policy
www.hrsa.gov/rural-health/index.html
National Rural Health Association
www.ruralhealthweb.org
Rural Health Information Hub
www.ruralhealthinfo.org
Rural Nurse Organization
www.rno.org

55

TAKING ACTION: Increasing Specialty Medical Care ACCESS in Rural Communities

Deirdre E. Kearney and Debra A. Banks

> *"I think one's feelings waste themselves in words; they ought all to be distilled into actions which bring results."*
>
> **Florence Nightingale**

NEW MEXICO AT A GLANCE

New Mexico, the 47th U.S. state, is known as the "land of enchantment." It is a largely rural/frontier state, fifth largest in land mass of all 50 states, and with a total population of just over 2 million, covering 121,356 square miles (U.S. Census Bureau, 2012, 2017). As a minority-majority state, 48.8% of the state population identify as Hispanic/Latino and 10.9% as American Indian/Alaska Native (Stepler & Lopez, 2016).

Although both the state and people are enchanting, New Mexico has structural issues that affect health care in general and rural health more specifically (see Chapter 54). Its poverty level ranks second in the nation (20.9%), the household median income ranks 48th out of 50 states (New Mexico Department of Workforce Solutions, 2018), and the Chance-for-Success Index that measures the outcome of education from birth to adulthood ranks New Mexico lowest of all 50 states (Education Week, 2018). More than 40% of the state's population live in federally designated, health care professional shortage areas, contributing to its ranking of 24th in access to health care and 33rd for health care quality for all 50 states. New Mexicans also experience disparities in rates of obesity, smoking, suicide, mental health, and mortality for adults and infants that are higher than national averages (U.S. News, 2018). Although these inequities of poverty, education, and health are vast, New Mexicans have shown considerable resourcefulness and creativity to address these challenges, especially in the rural corners of the state. One example of these innovative efforts was the Access to Critical Cerebral Emergency Support Services (ACCESS) telemedicine program.

ACCESS TELEMEDICINE: "ACCESS TO CRITICAL CEREBRAL EMERGENCY SUPPORT SERVICES"

In 1996, the Institute of Medicine described telemedicine as "the use of electronic information and communication technologies to provide and support health care when distance separates participants" (p. 1). It encompasses a two-way interaction between patient and provider at a distant site through telecommunication equipment that includes at minimum, audio and visual equipment. Telemedicine is key to increasing access to care as our U.S. population grows: the total U.S. population is predicted to increase from 319 to 417 million by 2060, and more than 24% will be older than the age of 65 (Colby & Ortman, 2015). Stroke is one issue expected to impact this growing older population, currently the fifth leading cause of death. Approximately 795,000 people in the United States experience a stroke annually, and stroke reduces physical mobility in more than half of survivors age 65 and older (Benjamin et al., 2017). Additionally, the need for full-time neurosurgeons and neurologists to care for stroke patients is expected to increase between 15% and 20% by the year 2025 (Dall et al., 2013).

ACCESS PROJECT ORIGINS

In response to the growing need for neurological services to serve an older population, between 2007 and 2010 the University of New Mexico (UNM) and the Navajo Area Indian Health Service (IHS) established guidelines for the use of telemedicine neurosurgical consults, including the transmission of pertinent diagnostic images, for patients with mild or minor traumatic brain injury (mTBI). The 2010 data from this project demonstrated that 42% of patients were treated locally, whereas 58% were transferred to UNM or elsewhere. Successfully treating patients at the local, rural hospital presented potential cost savings by keeping patients in their local hospital versus transferring them to a tertiary level of care for emergent, neurologic services.

In 2013 the UNM Department of Neurosurgery received an innovation grant from the Centers for Medicare and Medicaid Services (CMS) to provide access to neurospecialty care via telemedicine consultation. This project, ACCESS, attempted to keep patients in their local hospitals for neurologic care by providing telemedicine consultations for neuroemergency patients, leveraging community-based coalitions to reduce the cost of neuroemergent consultation services to improve outcomes for patients with neuroemergent disorders, such as mTBI and stroke. ACCESS endeavored to meet the Institute for Healthcare Improvement (2018) Triple Aim: improve the patient experience of care, improve the health of populations, and reduce the per capita cost of health care, by providing timely access to specialty care and reduced cost by decreasing preventable transfers (Berwick, Nolan, & Whittington, 2008).

ACCESS NURSING ROLES AND RESPONSIBILITIES

Nursing played a key role in the ACCESS telemedicine program. Four critical nursing roles are described in Table 55.1.

Quality

ACCESS nurses were actively involved with health care quality measures (Table 55.2). A needs assessment tool evaluating hospital readiness to adopt telemedicine was created (Becker, 2015). This "baseline logistic review" interviewed hospital departments and community resources for capabilities to care for neurologic patients (e.g., ability to provide head computed tomography [CT] scan 24/7).

Key issues that rural staff may encounter with telemedicine are equipment malfunction, network interruption, incorrect consultation or assessment requested, clerical/data entry errors, and response delays. To address these quality concerns, the ACCESS nursing team developed site-specific incident reporting tools to track and review incident reports, detailing each event for follow-up, intervention, and outcome.

The ACCESS nurses met bimonthly with a telemedicine-consultant physician from the UNM Neurology or Neurosurgery Department to review cases for appropriate care recommendations. Cases discussed included all stroke patients who received tissue plasminogen activator (tPA), new provider telemedicine consultations, new participating hospitals, and any case with incidents reported. A charter created for the ACCESS Telemedicine Clinical Review Committee supported the meetings, and prepared reports were for peer review purposes, per the New Mexico Peer Review Statute (Health Information and the Law, 2012).

TABLE 55.1 ACCESS Telemedicine Program: Critical Nursing Roles		
Role	**Description**	**Responsibilities**
Rural Telemedicine Registered Nurse (RN) Presenter	Emergency Department (ED) Staff nurse	Provides human connection between patient and telemedicine specialist; teaches patient/family about telemedicine consult; obtains consent; demonstrates equipment; manages clinical data; assists with neurologic examination.
Telehealth Coordinator (THC)	Grant-funded position, RN with ED or quality management experience	Program champion; "superuser" to hospital staff; critical relationship builder, "boots on the ground," connects patients and staff with hospital and community; tracks demographic and clinical data abstraction; coordinates stakeholders.
Nurse Researcher	Manages clinical/financial databases, monitors billing accuracy	Oversight and training of THC; physician credentialing; monthly consult reviews; monitor, measure, report trends; follow-up on telemedicine incidents.
Clinical Nurse Director	Leadership role covering administrative and educational functions	Facilitates hospital-onboarding to project; provides clinical education and support to staff and providers; manages clinical quality metrics; facilitates ACCESS community engagement/education.

TABLE 55.2   ACCESS Telemedicine Program Quality Measures

Clinical Metrics	Clinical data and measures include time metrics, number of consults by hospital (monthly/quarterly/annually), percentage of neurology versus neurosurgery consults, top consulting diagnosis, administration of tPA, and percentage of consults by specific provider and specialist.
Patient and Provider Telemedicine Experience	Collected surveys of telemedicine physician perception of consult experience, provider/staff experience with ACCESS telemedicine and impact on care, and patient perception of the telemedicine encounter.

Clinical Education

The Rural Health Information Hub (2016a) summarizes the importance of education and training for rural health care providers:

> . . . maintaining healthy, rural communities depends on proper preparation of the rural health workforce, which includes professionals living and working in rural communities and distant providers who provide services or support through telehealth. This involves ensuring that physicians, nurses, dentists, and other healthcare professionals are well-educated, well-trained, and have had experiences that expose them to and prepare them for rural practice. (p. 1)

Common barriers for continuing education in rural areas include geographic isolation, distance from tertiary care, lack of financial resources, and inability to take time away from work due to a shortage of staff (Doorenbos et al., 2011). For the ACCESS project, we had to consider and address the confidence and competence of the rural staff in caring for the acute, neurologic patient. The previous impulse from rural providers was to immediately transfer patients with head injuries to a level I trauma center. The innovative approach with ACCESS suggested that if rural staff received education on how to manage patients with head injuries *and* received an appropriate telemedicine consultation, then the patient could be managed effectively in their community hospital, thus decreasing the excessive transfer of patients to other facilities and increasing the potential cost savings for keeping patients in their local, rural hospital.

Program education sought to answer why, who, what, when, and how of neuroemergent patient care management. The 3-year educational plan was layered and targeted toward rural hospital staff, to improve confidence in triage and care for neurologic conditions. In addition, we provided onsite and remote training of telemedicine equipment, orientation to the ACCESS protocols, patient and family education, and reporting of quality issues. From 2015 to 2018, the ACCESS program provided no-cost education to 1597 participants, 477 hours of continuing education and training, and 4458 continuing medical and nursing education credits.

BUILDING BRICK BY BRICK

The ACCESS program facilitated many changes for the rural health care environment. ACCESS increased access to neurology specialists for rural hospital emergency departments (EDs) and encouraged shared-decision making between rural providers and specialists (Whetten, 2018). The program facilitated appropriate diagnosis and triage, provided a convenient and cost-effective delivery of care, maximized timeliness of treatment, decreased transfer rates thus reducing medical costs, and demonstrated positive patient satisfaction. The ACCESS program also engaged the larger health policy environment, advocating with insurance companies and state policymakers for sustainability through changes to the payment and reimbursement structures for telestroke consultations. To date, ACCESS has increased access to specialty care with 15 hospitals active with telemedicine covering the four corners of New Mexico, more than 3400 consults from 2015 to 2018, increased tPA administration for acute ischemic stroke, and significantly decreased rural patient transfers, resulting in a substantial decrease in transportation costs, estimated at more than $100 million.

Key barriers to rural telemedicine continue to be reimbursement, licensure, and broadband internet service (Rural Health Information Hub, 2016b) (Table 55.3). In addition to these barriers, ACCESS programs had to address contract negotiations, credentialing for consultant physicians, adequate specialist resources, technology support and capacity, rural hospital reimbursement, hospital and community engagement, rural staff turnover, and educational needs.

LESSONS LEARNED: IT'S ALL ABOUT RELATIONSHIPS

The success of ACCESS rested on a collaborative relationship with the rural hospital and community. As of 2019, ACCESS neurological and neurosurgical consultations are

TABLE 55.3	New Mexico Telemedicine Policy
Private Insurance Coverage Reimbursement Rates	2013 New Mexico Telemedicine Parity Law: private payers in New Mexico are required to reimburse for telemedicine services in the same way they would cover comparable in-person medical services.
Medicaid	New Mexico Medicaid covers telemedicine for all services under both fee-for-service and managed care plans, including standard consultations, behavioral health, dental care, hospice, home health, rehabilitation, and school-based services.
Kinds of Telemedicine Covered	Services: behavioral, addiction/substance abuse, counseling, social work, home rehabilitation, school-based, dental care, and hospice.
Eligible Providers	No restrictions on which providers can bill for telemedicine.
Cross-State Telemedicine Licensing	Issues telemedicine licenses to out-of-state providers who hold a full license in another state and meet New Mexico standards for "good moral character."
Restrictions on Locations	New Mexico Medicaid has no specific requirement on where the patient needs to be located at the time of service.

From American Telemedicine Association, 2018; Center for Connected Health Policy, 2018.

now covered by Medicaid. Furthermore, the recommendation to CMS from the Physician Technical Advisory Committee was to continue development and implementation of the ACCESS advanced payment model.

DISCUSSION QUESTIONS

1. How do you think that the use of telemedicine can address the goals of the Institute of Healthcare Improvements Triple Aim?
2. What benefits do you think that telemedicine can provide to rural hospitals, providers, and communities?

REFERENCES

American Telemedicine Association. (2018). *State policy resource center*. Retrieved from www.americantelemed.org/policy-page/state-policy-resource-center.

Becker, K.L. (2015). Conducting community health needs assessments in rural communities: Lessons learned. *Health Promotion Practice, 16*(1), 15–19.

Benjamin, E.J., Blaha, M.J., Chiuve, S.E., Cushman, M., Das, S.R., ... & Muntner, P. (2017). Heart disease and stroke statistics—2017 update: A report from the American Heart Association. *Circulation, 135*(10), e146–e603.

Berwick, D.M., Nolan, W.T., & Whittington, J. (2008.) The Triple Aim: Care, health, and cost. *Health Affairs, 27*(3), 759–769.

Center for Connected Health Policy. (2018). *Current state laws and reimbursement policies: New Mexico*. Retrieved from www.cchpca.org/telehealth-policy/current-state-laws-and-reimbursement-policies?jurisdiction=60&category=All&topic=All.

Colby, S.L. & Ortman, J.M. (2015). *Projections of the size and composition of the U.S. population: 2014 to 2060*, P25-1143, Washington, DC: U.S. Census Bureau. Retrieved from https://census.gov/content/dam/Census/library/publications/2015/demo/p25-1143.pdf.

Dall, T.M., Gallo, P.D., Chakrabarti, R., West, T., Semilla, A.P., & Storm, M.V. (2013). An aging population and growing disease burden will require a large and specialized health care workforce by 2025. *Health Affairs, 32*(11), 2013-2020.

Doorenbos, A.Z., Kundu, A., Eaton, L., Demiris, G., Haozous, E.A., Towle, C., & Buchwald, D. (2011). Enhancing access to cancer education for rural healthcare providers via telehealth. *Journal of Cancer Education, 26*(4), 682–686.

Education Week. (2018). *Quality counts 2018: Grading the states: New Mexico earns a D on state report card, ranks 50th in nation*. Retrieved from www.edweek.org/ew/collections/quality-counts-2018-state-grades/highlight-reports/2018/01/17/new-mexico.html.

Health Information and the Law. (2012). *Medical peer review in New Mexico*. Retrieved from www.healthinfolaw.org/state-topics/32,62/f_topics.

Institute for Healthcare Improvement. (2018). *Initiatives: The IHI Triple Aim*. Retrieved from www.ihi.org/Engage/Initiatives/TripleAim/Pages/default.aspx.

Institute of Medicine. (1996). *Telemedicine: A guide to assessing telecommunications in health care*. Washington, DC: The National Academies Press.

New Mexico Department of Health. (2018). *Health equity in New Mexico*. Retrieved from https://nmhealth.org/publication/view/report/2045/.

New Mexico Department of Workforce Solutions. (2018). *New Mexico 2018: State of the workforce report: A report highlighting New Mexico's current and future workforce.* Retrieved from www.dws.state.nm.us/Portals/0/DM/LMI/NM_2018_SOTW_Report.pdf.

Rural Health Information Hub. (2016a). *Education and training of the rural healthcare workforce.* Retrieved from www.ruralhealthinfo.org/topics/workforce-education-and-training.

Rural Health Information Hub. (2016b). *Telehealth use in rural healthcare.* Retrieved from www.ruralhealthinfo.org/topics/telehealth#different-from-telemedicine.

Soo, S., Berta, W., & Baker, G. R. (2009). Role of champions in the implementation of patient safety practice change. *Healthcare Quarterly, 12*(Special Issue), 123-128.

Stepler, R., & Lopez, M.H. (2016). *U.S. Latino population growth and dispersion has slowed since onset of the great recession.*

Retrieved from www.pewhispanic.org/wp-content/uploads/sites/5/2016/09/PH_2016.09.08_Geography.pdf.

U.S. Census Bureau. (2012). *New Mexico 2010: Population and housing unit counts.* Retrieved from www.census.gov/prod/cen2010/cph-2-33.pdf.

U.S. Census Bureau. (2017). *QuickFacts: New Mexico.* Retrieved from www.census.gov/quickfacts/fact/table/nm/PST045217.

U.S. News. (2018). *Best states for health care.* Retrieved from www.usnews.com/news/best-states/rankings/health-care.

Whetten, J., van der Goes, D.N., Tran, H., Moffett. M, Semper, C., & Yonas, H. (2018) Cost-effectiveness of Access to Critical Cerebral Emergency Support Services (ACCESS): A neuro-emergent telemedicine consultation program. *Journal of Medical Economics, 21*(4), 398-405.

56

Nurse Staffing Ratios: Policy Options

Joanne Spetz

"The law of unintended consequences is the only real law of history."

Niall Ferguson

The importance of nursing to the delivery of high-quality health care has been recognized since the inception of the practice of nursing. Various factors contribute to the quality of nursing care, including the expertise of nursing staff, availability of supportive personnel and other health professionals, good communication among the care team, and the nurse staffing ratio. It was not until the early 2000s that high-quality, empirical research found consistent relationships between licensed nurse staffing and the quality of patient care (Kane et al., 2007; Lang et al., 2004). Even prior, some nursing organizations and leaders had raised concerns about declining nurse staffing levels in hospitals from the 1990s (Kilborn, 1999; Wunderlich et al., 1996), and nursing unions were advocating for regulations to ensure adequate staffing.

These concerns, combined with the increasing influence of nursing unions, resulted in the passage of California Assembly Bill (AB) 394 in 1999—the first comprehensive legislation in the United States to establish minimum staffing ratios for registered nurses (RNs) and licensed vocational nurses (LVNs) working in hospitals (Spetz, 2001). This bill required that the California Department of Health Services (DHS) establish the specific, minimum nurse staffing ratios. These were announced in 2002 and implemented beginning in 2004.

Since then, other states and the federal government have considered their own regulations for nurse staffing in hospitals. In September 2014, Massachusetts established a regulation requiring that nurse staffing in intensive care units be no less than one nurse per two patients, and that hospitals establish patient acuity systems to determine when staffing should be more than one nurse per two patients (Buppert, 2017). Other states have implemented two

other approaches to staffing regulations: requiring that hospitals develop and implement nurse staffing plans with input from direct care nurses, and/or requiring public disclosure of staffing levels. As of 2018, seven states require hospitals to have staffing committees responsible for staffing plans (CT, IL, NV, OH, OR, TX, WA), and one state (MN) requires a Chief Nurse Officer (CNO) or designee develop a core staffing plan with input from others. Five states require some form of public reporting (IL, NJ, NY, RI, VT) (Lippincott Solutions, 2018). In recent years, new legislation was introduced in New York, Ohio, and New Jersey to establish specific, minimum nurse staffing ratios (Buppert, 2017). The proposal passed the New York legislature, but was vetoed by the governor, who later announced he would introduce legislation to direct the state department of health to establish staffing regulations, as opposed to staffing ratios being specified in legislation (New York State Nurses Association, 2018). In 2018, Massachusetts voters rejected Ballot Question 1, which would have established specific nurse staffing ratios in hospitals (Bebinger, 2018). At the federal level, multiple bills have been introduced in the U.S. Congress; some of these have specified nurse staffing ratios, whereas others, such as H.R.5052 and S.2446 introduced in 2018, would require staffing committees to develop staffing ratios within each hospital (Kinsella, 2018).

THE ESTABLISHMENT OF CALIFORNIA'S REGULATIONS

California's AB 394 was passed by the California legislature in 1999 as a result of ongoing concern about poor staffing in hospitals and coincident with the emergence of a shortage of RNs (Kilborn, 1999). Previous Republican governors had vetoed similar legislation; union-friendly Democratic Governor Gray Davis signed the bill, which charged the DHS with determining specific, unit-by-unit nurse-to-patient ratios.

The DHS launched an extensive effort to determine the new minimum nurse staffing ratios, with little research to guide them (Spetz et al., 2000). To help develop proposed ratios, the DHS commissioned a study by researchers at the University of California, Davis (Kravitz et al., 2002). The DHS also received recommendations from stakeholders, ranging from the California Hospital Association (CHA) proposal of a ratio of 1 licensed nurse per 10 patients (1:10) in medical-surgical units, and the California Nurses Association (CNA) recommendation of 1 licensed nurse per 3 (1:3) patients in medical-surgical units. The minimum nurse staffing ratios established by DHS fell between those recommendations: 1:6 in medical-surgical units starting January 2004, and 1:5 in medical-surgical units commencing in January 2005. Other units require more nurses per patient. These minimum staffing ratios did not replace the Patient Classification System (PCS) hospital staffing regulations already in existence (Seago, 2002).

WHAT HAS HAPPENED AS A RESULT OF CALIFORNIA'S MINIMUM NURSE STAFFING RATIOS?

The implementation of California's minimum nurse staffing ratio legislation led to legal challenges ending in a court ruling upholding the minimum nurse staffing ratios (Benson, 2005). To support the regulation, California launched a statewide effort to expand RN education, which led to nursing graduations increasing 72% between 2005 and 2010 (Spetz et al., 2013).

ARE HOSPITALS MEETING THE MINIMUM NURSE STAFFING RATIOS?

The California DHS inspection and enforcement mechanisms are relatively weak. The DHS does not have the authority to impose fines or monetary penalties on hospitals found violating the minimum nurse staffing ratios, but instead requests and monitors plans submitted by hospitals to remedy the problem. Other mechanisms exist to ensure that hospitals adhere to the minimum staffing ratios. First, Medicare and Medi-Cal (California Medicaid program) require that hospitals meet all state and federal regulations, and can deny payment to violators. Second, California's cap on malpractice awards does not apply in cases of negligence, and it is possible that a hospital could

be determined negligent if it consistently did not adhere to minimum nurse staffing regulations (Robertson, 2004). Third, unions draw public attention to hospitals that do not meet the staffing requirements, resulting in negative publicity for hospitals and increased scrutiny from DHS inspectors. Fourth, labor organizations representing nurses, such as the CNA and the Service Employees International Union (SEIU), sought to incorporate staffing standards in their contract negotiations, with some success (Gordon, 2005; Osterman, 2005).

It should be noted that enforcement of other types of state nurse staffing regulations, such as staffing committee requirements to oversee staffing plans, is also weak; some states are required to submit staffing plans to a state government agency, but there is generally no process to verify that the staffing plan is adequate or being followed (Serratt et al., 2014). Oregon is the only state that has procedures to audit a random set of hospitals each year for compliance, but the fines for noncompliance have a maximum of only $5000 (Serratt et al., 2014).

Several studies of California hospitals have found that annual average numbers of licensed nurse productive hours and nurse staffing ratios in medical-surgical units increased markedly between 2001 and 2006 (Munnich, 2014; Serratt, 2013; Spetz et al., 2009, 2013). This growth in licensed nurse staffing was primarily the result of increases in RN staffing; no study reported an increase in LVN staffing (McHugh et al. 2012; Serratt, 2013). Spetz and colleagues (2009) found that statewide, average RN hours per patient day increased 16.2% from 1999 to 2006 an average of 6.9 hours per patient day. Interviews conducted with hospital leaders revealed that many CNOs and other managers said they hired nurses in order to meet the minimum nurse staffing ratios, and most noted the challenge to adhere to the minimum staffing ratios at all times, including during scheduled breaks (Chapman et al., 2009).

Aiken and colleagues (2010) surveyed nearly 80,000 RNs in California, New Jersey, and Pennsylvania to learn about their experiences with staffing, the work environment, and patient safety. The researchers found nurse workloads, measured as average patients per shift, were lower in California than in New Jersey and Pennsylvania, and over 80% of California nurses reported their assigned workloads complied with the state's regulation.

A study of mandated nurse staffing committees in Texas from 2000 to 2012 reported a smaller increase in total nurse staffing in Texas (5%) than national trends (13.6%). The researchers found notable variation across hospitals in staffing changes, with the smallest changes among small, rural, government hospitals and among hospitals with the highest pre-regulation staffing levels (Jones et al., 2015).

HAS THE MIX OF STAFF CHANGED?

There has been concern about the possibility that hospitals eliminated support staff positions because of the minimum nurse staffing ratios (Spetz, 2001). Analyses of staffing data collected by the Collaborative Alliance for Nursing Outcomes (CALNOC) suggested the substitution of licensed nurses for unlicensed staff may have been widespread (Bolton et al., 2007; Donaldson et al., 2005). In a series of qualitative interviews, some hospital leaders reported they had laid off ancillary staff to use their personnel budgets to hire more RNs (Chapman et al., 2009), and Aiken and colleagues (2010) found nurses perceived reductions in LVN and nursing assistant staffing. More recent analyses have measured a slight decline in LVN staffing (Cook et al., 2012; Spetz et al., 2013) and aide staffing (Cook et al., 2012; Spetz et al., 2009), and some have found no decline at all (Serratt et al., 2011).

DID WAGES FOR NURSES INCREASE?

In theory, when the demand for workers rises more rapidly than the supply, wages will rise. Three studies have examined whether the increase in RN employment due to the staffing regulations was linked to more rapid growth in RN wages. One study compared wage growth among urban RNs in California to other states and found wages increased as much as 12 percentage points (Mark et al., 2009). Another analysis reported mean RN wages, after adjusting for inflation, rose 9% from 2000 to 2006 (Serratt et al., 2011). Finally, a more recent analysis measured a 4.9% increase in RN wages between 2000 and 2007 with one dataset, yet no increase with a different dataset (Munnich, 2014). Together, these studies suggest RN wages likely increased in California due to the staffing regulation, with the average estimate around 4%.

HAVE HOSPITALS REDUCED SERVICES AND UNCOMPENSATED CARE?

Prior to the implementation of AB 394, the CHA warned that strict minimum nurse staffing ratios would force hospitals to reduce their services. To maintain the minimum staffing ratios, hospitals might reschedule procedures, close selected units and beds, or shut their doors entirely. However, there is no evidence the minimum staffing ratios caused permanent closures of inpatient hospital units or beds. Between 2003 and 2004, one study of an urban teaching hospital emergency department (ED) reported wait times increased significantly, including room time, throughput time (time from registration until discharge, excluding admitted patients), and admission time; however, the share

of patients who left without being seen decreased slightly, and the time-from-written-order to administration of antibiotics in pneumonia patients also decreased (Weichenthal & Hendey, 2011). There is some indication there was lower growth in the provision of uncompensated care services among hospitals for which the regulations had the greatest impact on staffing (Reiter et al., 2011).

HAVE HOSPITALS SUFFERED FINANCIAL LOSSES?

Qualitative evidence reported hospital Chief Executive Officers (CEOs) absorbed costs of the minimum nurse staffing ratios by reducing other budget areas, and some hospitals obtained higher insurance reimbursement rates to cover additional staff expenses (Spetz et al., 2009). One analysis found hospital prices rose even more between 1999 and 2005 than could be explained by labor cost increases that resulted from the minimum nurse staffing ratios (Antwi, Gaynor, & Vogt, 2009).

In an analysis of hospital financial data, Cook and colleagues (2010) found no significant change in total annual labor costs for licensed nurses, annual hospital costs, or hospital prices after implementation of the regulation. Reiter and colleagues (2012) used data from Medicare cost reports to explore whether changes in financial status differed both between California hospitals that had higher versus lower pre-regulation staffing levels, and between California and other states. They found, relative to hospitals outside California, operating margins for California hospitals with lower pre-regulation staffing levels declined, and operating expenses increased significantly.

ARE NURSES MORE SATISFIED?

Advocates of minimum nurse staffing ratio regulations link improved staffing to nurse satisfaction, and argue greater nurse satisfaction will reduce nurse turnover and lead to better patient outcomes (Public Policy Associates, 2004). Seven studies of the California regulation reported mixed results regarding nurse satisfaction, with two producing no change or mixed results (Serratt, 2013). An analysis of statewide nurse survey data found there were significant improvements in overall job satisfaction among hospital-employed RNs between 2004 and 2006, and nurse satisfaction also increased with respect to the adequacy of RN staff, time for patient education, benefits, and clerical support (Spetz, 2008).

Aiken and colleagues (2010) found in their survey of nurses in three states that California RNs were more satisfied with their working conditions. California nurses were significantly more likely to report that their workload was reasonable, allowed them to spend adequate time with patients, and that they were able to take breaks during the workday. Nurses with lower workloads were significantly less likely to report having received complaints from families, faced verbal abuse, were burned out, were dissatisfied, felt quality of care was poor, or were looking for new jobs.

One study examined the effect of the California regulations on occupational injuries experienced by nurses, comparing changes in injury rates among California hospital nurses after 2004 with changes in all other states and the District of Columbia (Leigh et al., 2015). The authors found California's minimum nurse staffing ratios was associated with 55.6 fewer occupational injuries and illnesses per 10,000 RNs per year, 31.6% lower than what would have been expected without the law. A similar rate of injury reduction was found for LVNs.

DID THE MINIMUM NURSE STAFFING RATIOS IMPROVE THE QUALITY OF CARE?

One of the main purposes of California's minimum nurse staffing ratios was to improve quality of patient care. However, to date there is no convincing evidence that patient safety or quality of care improved. Rates of patient falls and hospital-acquired pressure ulcers reported to the CALNOC between 2002 and 2004 analyzed for 68 hospitals found no statistically significant change attributable to the minimum nurse staffing ratios (Donaldson et al., 2005) and a study of data through 2006 confirmed these results (Bolton et al., 2007). These analyses had two main shortcomings: they included only a subset of California's hospitals that voluntarily report to CALNOC, and the two outcomes of patient falls and hospital-acquired pressure ulcers might not be very sensitive to changes in licensed nurse staffing (Agency for Healthcare Research and Quality, 2005).

Aiken and colleagues (2010) linked their survey data from California, New Jersey, and Pennsylvania to secondary data on patient outcomes collected by state government agencies. They found higher nurse staffing levels were associated with lower rates of 30-day inpatient mortality and "failure-to-rescue," defined as mortality following a complication during the hospitalization. These relationships were stronger in California than in other states. However, this analysis cannot say that the staffing regulations directly caused changes in patient outcomes. Research based on a single year of data does not measure the effect of *changes* in policy or practice on *changes* in patient outcomes. Although the responses of nurses regarding the patient safety environment suggest the lower workloads in California are associated with more positive nurse perceptions of patient safety, these perceptions may not lead to true improvements in patient outcomes. The analysis of patient outcomes was limited to the two outcomes of 30-day mortality and failure-to-rescue.

Several studies used multiple years of statewide data and examined a wider variety of outcomes. For example, Spetz and colleagues (2009) examined Office of Statewide Health Planning and Development (OSHPD) patient discharge data for all non-federal, general acute care California hospitals from 1999 to 2006 and could not associate improvements in outcomes to the implementation of the minimum nurse staffing ratios. In a more rigorous analysis of OSHPD data from 2001 to 2006, Cook and colleagues (2012) found no association between changes in nurse staffing and changes in pressure ulcer rates or failure-to-rescue a patient after a complication. Using similar methods, Spetz and colleagues (2013) examined six patient safety indicators using OSHPD data from 2000 to 2006 and found growth in RN staffing was associated with improvement for failure-to-rescue, but not for pressure ulcers, hospital-acquired infections, post-operative respiratory failure, postoperative pulmonary embolism or deep-vein thrombosis, or postoperative sepsis. They also analyzed whether the average length of stay declined among patients who experienced adverse events, to explore the possibility that improved surveillance in hospitals with improved nurse staffing ratios might reduce the severity of complications. However, they found growth in staffing was significantly associated with reduced length of stay for only one patient safety indicator.

Two studies have focused on a single type of hospital service. A study that compared pediatric cardiac surgery programs in hospitals in California versus other states reported California's standardized mortality ratio decreased more than in all other states, but the standardized complication ratio increased in California and decreased in other states (Hickey et al., 2011). A study of two urban hospital EDs reported patient waiting times were 13% to 17% longer when hospitals were adherent to the minimum nurse staffing ratio versus when they were not, and median care time within the ED also was longer when ratios were not met (Chan et al., 2010).

The most comprehensive analysis of the impact of California's regulations on patient outcomes was published by Mark and colleagues (2012). Using patient discharge data from California and 12 comparison states, they examined whether differences in staffing changes between states were associated with different patient outcomes trajectories. Their analysis also considered differences between hospitals with high pre-regulation staffing as compared with low pre-regulation staffing. They found that failure-to-rescue following a complication decreased significantly, and infections due to medical care increased significantly in some California hospitals than in comparison state hospitals. There were no statistically significant changes in either cases of respiratory failure or postoperative sepsis.

Together, this research indicates California's regulations did not systematically improve the quality of patient care. However, the outcomes examined thus far have been relatively limited, and there remains a need for more research on this topic. It is possible patient care improvements occurred in other areas, such as medication safety. It also is possible that the impact of changes in nurse staffing on patient outcomes will occur over an extended period. However, examining data over more time will be complicated by the many health systems and hospitals that have established quality improvement programs in response to other issues, such as increased public attention to medical errors and patient outcomes.

WHAT'S NEXT?

One remaining issue central to the debate about minimum nurse staffing ratios has not been addressed: what was the total cost of minimum nurse staffing ratio regulations? At this time, the total costs of California's ratio regulations have not been quantified. A careful accounting of the extent to which nurse staffing increases were necessitated by the minimum staffing ratios and the cost of such increases is necessary. Moreover, it is important to quantify the value of other investments hospitals might have made if they were not required to adhere to the minimum nurse staffing ratios. For example, a hospital may have delayed implementation of a new infection-control system that would have reduced infection rates; this "opportunity cost" should be included as part of the overall cost of the staffing regulations.

FINANCIAL INCENTIVES FOR NURSE STAFFING IMPROVEMENT

Several studies have found higher nurse staffing levels can produce a positive financial return to hospitals by reducing costs associated with adverse patient events (Twigg et al., 2015; Unruh, 2008). In Maryland, Nevada, and California, higher total nurse staffing (including RNs, LVNs, and aides) was associated with reductions in nursing-sensitive adverse events and patient length-of-stay without any increase in patient care costs (Martsolf et al., 2014). The same study also found increases in the proportion of RNs as a share of licensed nursing staff led to reductions in costs, results supported in three additional studies (Cho et al., 2013; Dall et al., 2009; Shamliyan et al., 2009). In a comparison of 35 nationally recognized hospitals for good

nursing care with 293 other hospitals, the study concluded that better work environments and higher average-staffing levels had lower mortality rates and similar costs (Silber et al., 2016).

Whether hospitals are reimbursed by fee-for-service, diagnosis-related group, per patient day, or through bundled payments covering a full episode of care (including post-hospital care), and whether they are penalized for poor-quality outcomes, is likely to affect whether higher nurse staffing produces a positive financial return (Needleman, 2008). One study concluded that increasing nursing hours and proportion of nurses who are RNs would result in improved quality and fewer deaths but also would lead to small cost increases (Needleman et al., 2006). Under traditional reimbursement methods, this cost increase might be perceived as a poor investment for hospitals and could produce financial benefits in "value-based" payment systems that pay more for high-quality outcomes or bundle payments (Needleman, 2008). Extrapolating from research linking nurse staffing to reductions in mortality found that the cost of nurse staffing increases was $136,000 per life saved (Rothberg et al., 2005). As hospital reimbursement using value-based approaches grows, the positive financial return on investing for higher nurse staffing levels is likely to become more apparent (Keepnews, 2013).

More research on the impact of nurse staffing regulations, patient outcomes, and costs is needed. Any positive impact of minimum nurse staffing ratios should be weighed against the costs of the regulations (Donaldson & Shapiro, 2010). More importantly, changes in how hospitals are paid, with a greater emphasis on high-value care and reducing adverse patient outcomes, may lead to improvements in nurse staffing regardless of established regulations.

DISCUSSION QUESTIONS

1. Although research conducted thus far has not shown whether California's staffing regulations improved patient outcomes, studies have found nurse satisfaction improved, and nurses perceived that they are providing safer care. Is this enough of a reason to establish this type of regulation?
2. Several studies have suggested hospitals responded to the staffing regulations by reducing staffing of non-RN personnel in exchange for increasing their RN staffing. What might be the benefits and consequences of reducing employment of non-RN staffing?
3. Will value-based health care reimbursement provide enough incentive for hospitals to improve nurse staffing ratios?

REFERENCES

Agency for Healthcare Research and Quality. (2005). *AHRQ quality indicators—Guide to patient safety indicators,* Version 2.1, Revision 3. AHRQ Publication No. 03-R203. Rockville, MD: Agency for Healthcare Research and Quality.

Aiken, L.H., Sloane, D.M., Cimiotti, J.P., Clarke, S.P., Flynn, L., Seago, J., ... & Smith, H. (2010). Implications of the California nurse staffing mandate for other states. *Health Services Research,* 45(4), 904-921.

Antwi, Y.A., Gaynor, M.S., & Vogt, W.B. (2009). A bargain at twice the price? California hospital prices in the new millennium. *Forum for Health Economics & Policy,* 12(1). Berkeley Electronic Press.

Bebinger, M. (November 6, 2018). *Mass. voters say 'no' to nurse staffing ballot question.* Retrieved from www.wbur.org/com monhealth/2018/11/06/nurse-staffing-ratio-initiative-loses.

Benson, C. (June 8, 2005). Final ruling backs higher nurse ratio. *Sacramento Bee,* A5.

Bolton, L.B., Aydin, C.E., Donaldson, N., Storer Brown, D., Sandhu, M., Fridman, M., & Udin Aronow, H. (2007). Mandated nurse staffing ratios in California: A comparison of staffing and nursing-sensitive outcomes pre- and post-regulation. *Policy, Politics, & Nursing Practice,* 8(4), 238-250.

Buppert, C. (2017). *What's being done about nurse staffing?* Retrieved from www.medscape.com/viewarticle/877838_4.

Chan, T.C., Killeen, J.P. Vilke, G.M. Marshall, J.B., & Castillo, E.M. (2010). Effect of mandated nurse-patient ratios on patient wait time and care time in the emergency department. *Academic Emergency Medicine,* 17(5), 545-552.

Chapman, S., Spetz, J., Kaiser, J., Seago, J.A., & Dower, C. (2009). How have mandated nurse staffing ratios impacted hospitals? Perspectives from California hospital leaders. *Journal of Healthcare Management,* 54(5), 321-336.

Cho, D., Bretthauer, K.M., & Schoenfelder, J. (2013). *Nurse staffing ratios: A case for higher quality of care.* University of Indiana, Kelley School of Business.

Conway, P.H., Konetzka, R.T., Zhu, J., Volpp, K.G., & Sochalski, J. (2008). Nurse staffing ratios: Trends and policy implications for hospitalists and the safety net. *Journal of Hospital Medicine,* 3(3), 103-199.

Cook, A., Gaynor, M., Stephens Jr., M., & Taylor, L. (2012). The effect of a hospital nurse staffing mandate on patient health outcomes: Evidence from California's minimum staffing regulation. *Journal of Health Economics,* 31(2), 340-348.

Dall, T.M., Chen, Y.J., Seifert, R.F., Maddox, P.J., & Hogan, P.F. (2009). The economic value of professional nursing. *Medical Care,* 47(1), 97-104.

Donaldson, N., Bolton, L.B., Aydin, C., Brown, D., Elashoff, J., & Sandhu, M. (2005). Impact of California's licensed nurse-patient ratios on unit-level nurse staffing and patient outcomes. *Policy, Politics, & Nursing Practice,* 6(3), 1-12.

Donaldson, N., & Shapiro, S. (2010). Impact of California mandated acute care hospital nurse staffing ratios: A literature synthesis. *Policy, Politics, and Nursing Practice,* 11(3), 184-201.

Everhart, D., Neff, D., Al-Amin, M., Nogle, J., & Weech-Maldonado, R. (2013). The effects of nurse staffing on hospital financial performance: Competitive versus less competitive markets. *Health Care Management Review,* 38(2), 146–155.

Gordon, R. (June 22, 2005). Nurses pact ready for vote: Plan would raise pay, offer higher signing bonus. *San Francisco Chronicle,* B4.

Hickey, P.A., Gauvreau, K., Jenkins, K., Fawcett, J., & Hayman, L. (2011). Statewide and national impact of California's staffing law on pediatric cardiac surgery outcomes. *Journal of Nursing Administration,* 41(5), 218-225.

Jones, T., Heui Bae, S., Murry, N., & Hamilton, P. (2015). Texas nurse staffing trends before and after mandated nurse staffing committees. *Policy Politics and Nursing Practice,* 16(3-4), 79-96.

Kane, R.L., Shamliyan, T., Mueller, C., Duval, S., & Wilt, T.J. (2007). *Nursing staffing and quality of patient care.* Rockville, MD: Agency for Healthcare Research and Quality.

Keepnews, D. (2013). *Mapping the economic value of nursing.* Seattle: Washington State Nurses Association.

Kilborn, P.T. (March 23, 1999). Current nursing shortage more serious than those of the past. *New York Times,* A14.

Kinsella, L. (2018). *New safe staffing legislation introduced to Congress.* Retrieved from https://dailynurse.com/new-safe-staffing-legislation-introduced-to-congress/.

Kravitz, R., Sauve, M., Hodge, M., Romano, P., Maher, M., Samuels, S., ... & Lang, T. (2002). *Hospital nursing staff ratios and quality of care.* Davis, CA: University of California.

Lang, T.A., Hodge, M., Olson, V., Romano, P.S., & Kravitz, R.L. (2004). Nurse-patient ratios: A systematic review on the effects of nurse staffing on patient, nurse employee, and hospital outcomes. *Journal of Nursing Administration,* 34(7-8), 326-337.

Leigh, J.P., Markis, C.A., Iosif, A.M., & Romano, P.S. (2015). California's nurse-to-patient ratio law and occupational injury. *International Archives of Occupational and Environmental Health,* 88(4), 477-484.

Lippincott Solutions. (2018). *Update on nursing staff ratios.* Retrieved from http://lippincottsolutions.lww.com/blog.entry.html/2018/03/08/update_on_nursingst-HJoe.html.

Mark, B., Harless, D.W., & Spetz, J. (2009). California's minimum nurse staffing legislation and nurses' wages. *Health Affairs,* 28(2), w326-w334.

Mark, B., Harless, D.W., Spetz, J., Reiter, K.L., & Pink. G.H. (2012). California's minimum nurse staffing legislation: Results from a natural experiment. *Health Services Research,* 48(2), 435-454.

Martsolf, G.R., Auerbach, D., Benevent, R., Stocks, C., Jiang, H.J., . . . & Gibson, T.B. (2014). Examining the value of inpatient nurse staffing: an assessment of quality and patient care costs. *Medical Care,* 52(11), 982-988.

McHugh, M.D., Brooks Carthon, M., Sloane, D.M., Wu, E., Kelly, L., & Aiken, L.H. (2012). Impact of nurse staffing mandates on safety-net hospitals: Lessons from California. *Milbank Quarterly,* 90(1), 160-186.

Munnich, E. (2014). The labor market effects of California's minimum nurse staffing law. *Health Economics,* 23(8), 935-950.

Needleman, J. (2008). Is what's good for the patient good for the hospital? Aligning incentives and the business case for nursing. *Policy Politics and Nursing Practice, 9*(2), 80-87.

Needleman, J., Buerhaus, P.I., Stewart, M., Zelevinky, K., & Mattke, S. (2006). Nurse staffing in hospitals: Is there a business case for quality? *Health Affairs, 25*(1), 204-211.

New York State Nurses Association. (2018). *A breakthrough for minimum staffing standards in hospitals and nurses' working conditions.* Retrieved from www.nysna.org/press/2018/new-york-state-nurses-association-lauds-governor-andrew-cuomo-commitment-safe-staffing#.W_rkwehKg2w.

Osterman, R. (2005, July 13). Hospitals accept nursing ratios. *Sacramento Bee,* D1.

Public Policy Associates. (2004). *The business case for reducing patient-to-nurse staff ratios and eliminating mandatory overtime for nurses.* Lansing, MI: Michigan Nurses Association.

Reiter, K.L., Harless, D.W., Pink, G.H., & Mark, B. (2012). Minimum nurse staffing legislation and the financial performance of California hospitals. *Health Services Research,* 47(3, pt 1), 1030-1050.

Reiter, K.L., Harless, D.W., Pink, G.H., Spetz, J., & Mark, B. (2011). The effect of minimum nurse staffing legislation on uncompensated care provided by California hospitals. *Medical Care Research and Review, 67*(6), 694–706.

Robertson, K. (2004). New nurse law fails to cause emergency. *Sacramento Business Journal, 21*(9), 1.

Rothberg, M.B., Abraham, I., Lindenauer, P.K., & Rose, D.N. (2005). Improving nurse-to-patient staffing ratios as a cost-effective safety intervention. *Medical Care, 43*(8), 785-791.

Seago, J.A. (2002). A comparison of two patient classification instruments in an acute care hospital. *Journal of Nursing Administration, 32*(5), 243-249.

Serratt, T. (2013). California's nurse-to-patient ratios, part 1: 8 years later, what do we know about nurse-level outcome? *Journal of Nursing Administration,* 43(9), 475-480.

Serratt, T., Harrington, C., Spetz, J., & Blegen, M. (2011). Staffing changes before and after mandated nurse-to-patient ratios in California's hospitals. *Policy Politics and Nursing Practice, 12*(3), 133-140.

Serratt, T., Meyer, S., & Chapman, S.A. (2014). Enforcement of hospital nurse staffing regulations across the United States: Progress or stalemate? *Policy Politics and Nursing Practice,* 15(1-2), 21-29.

Shamliyan, T.A., Kane, R.L., Mueller, C., Duval, S., & Wilt, T.J. (2009). Cost savings associated with increased RN staffing in acute care hospitals: simulation exercise. *Nursing Economics, 27*(5), 302-314, 331.

Silber, J.H., Rosenbaum, P.R., McHugh, M.D., Ludwig, J.M., Smith, H.L., Niknam, B.A., ... & Aiken, L. H. (2016). Comparison of the value of nursing work environments in hospitals across different levels of patient risk. *JAMA Surgery, 151*(6), 527-536.

Spetz, J. (1998). Hospital use of nursing personnel: Has there really been a decline? *Journal of Nursing Administration, 28*(3), 20-27.

Spetz, J. (2001). What should we expect from California's minimum nurse staffing legislation? *Journal of Nursing Administration, 31*(3), 132-140.

Spetz, J. (2008). Nurse satisfaction and the implementation of minimum nurse staffing regulations. *Policy, Politics, & Nursing Practice, 9*(1), 15-21.

Spetz, J. (2013). *Forecasts of the registered nurse workforce in California.* Sacramento, CA: Board of Registered Nursing.

Spetz, J., Chapman, S., Herrera, C., Kaiser, J., Seago, J.A., & Dower, C. (2009). *Assessing the impact of California's nurse staffing ratios on hospitals and patient care.* Oakland, CA: California HealthCare Foundation.

Spetz, J., Harless, D.W., Herrera, C.-N., & Mark, B.A. (2013). Using minimum nurse staffing regulations to measure the relationship between nursing and hospital quality of care. *Medical Care Research and Review, 70*(4), 380-399.

Spetz, J., Seago, J.A., Coffman, J., Rosenoff, E., & O'Neil, E. (2000). *Minimum nurse staffing ratios in California acute care hospitals.* San Francisco: California HealthCare Foundation.

Twigg, D.E., Myers, H., Duffield, C., Giles, M., & Evans, G. (2015). Is there an economic case for investing in nursing care—What does the literature tell us? *Journal of Advanced Nursing, 71*(5), 975-990.

Unruh, L. (2008). Nurse staffing and patient, nurse, and financial outcomes. *American Journal of Nursing, 108*(1), 62-71.

Weichenthal, L., & Hendey, G.W. (2011). The effect of mandatory nurse ratios on patient care in an emergency department. *Journal of Emergency Medicine, 40*(1), 76-81.

Wunderlich, G.S., Sloan, F.A., & Davis, C.K. (Eds.). (1996). *Nursing staff in hospitals and nursing homes: Is it adequate?* Washington, DC: National Academies Press.

ONLINE RESOURCES

American Nurses Association: Nurse Staffing
www.nursingworld.org/practice-policy/advocacy/state/nurse-staffing/

National Nurses United: National Campaign for Safe RN-to-Patient Staffing Ratios
www.nationalnursesunited.org/ratios

Robert Wood Johnson Foundation: The Impact of Nurse Staffing on Hospital Quality
http://thefutureofnursing.org/resource/detail/impact-nurse-staffing-hospital-quality

57

The Contemporary Work Environment of Nursing

Deborah Washington

> *"Our ability to reach unity in diversity will be the beauty and the test of our civilization."*
>
> **Mahatma Gandhi**

DEFINITIONS

Organizational policy: An actionable body of rules used as a basis for reasoning and problem solving. Such are considered binding upon the function of a complex system as well as individual conduct and judged in ethical and philosophical alignment with organizational mission and vision.

Diversity and inclusion: The ability to hold multiple perspectives without judgment.

INTRODUCTION

A new frontier—the best phrase for the workplace of the 21st century. Within this context management, leadership and clinical practice furnish new platforms for the active presence of the nursing profession. The workplace can no longer be viewed as so narrow an idea that events of the larger social narrative have no place in the day-to-day experience of work. News headlines and issues of national health policy bring to bear the need for response and reaction that mold the basic tenets of the nursing profession. The former communicates problems rising to the surface and in need of attention. Professional ideology, doctrines, and even dogma undergo clarifying processes as precepts and theories are processed within the context of new research and evolving upstream and downstream narratives of public health, ambulatory, and inpatient care. Strains on old workplace conventions call for a qualitative remodeling. For example, diversity and inclusion, culturally competent care, a multicultural workforce, health disparities, social determinants of health, and inequities in care all combine to invite awareness of how differently a workplace is experienced today compared to one lived through in any previous era. Bullying, incivility, and microaggressions are other dimensions of interpersonal interactions increasingly evident as contributing factors to an adverse work environment. Progressive change is needed. Today, the meaning of personal agency, organizational strategy, corporate responsibility to the community, and patient and family engagement have taken on new significance. Practices conforming to old default standards are no longer adequate to define excellence. Something new is required.

The need for diversity and its increased presence in the contemporary workplace is state-of-the-art discourse in organizational development. Its impact is not yet universally established under the heading of pivotal asset. However, diversity and inclusion are better understood as risk and financial liability within the context of meeting legal obligations and moral responsibility. Attached to the presence of diversity is the need for alignment with issues of employee engagement, culturally competent/culturally and linguistically appropriate care, patient satisfaction, quality and safety, peer-to-peer and clinician-to-patient communication, individualized care, and innovation in the ideals of equity and equality. This list makes for new perspectives on the crafting of organizational culture and policies and guidelines that direct action for a before-diversity and after-diversity difference. The ideal is to develop a work and care environment responsive to the needs of all accessing the healthcare system, those employed by it, and those who need its services. Engagement implies what is created is accepted and acted upon by all involved. There is an inherent challenge in creating policy to address the social history of diverse groups within an organization. Seldom do representatives of those groups as employees of an organization live within and see the same reality.

The workplace coming to light cannot function by ignoring the long-forecasted change in American demographics. The arrival of these changes puts into focus the relative standing of different persons in American society, especially the multidimensional and intersectional aspects of these differences and their effect on workplace relationships. Responsibilities of the employer to meet the needs of a diverse workforce add a watchful response from employees questioning if policies and procedures guiding leadership performance are effective. Compelling issues and various ideas about their importance sharpen discussion about whether the trendsetting workplace operates at its highest level of development. Differing perspectives on the need to adapt and accommodate inspire fresh analysis of answers to questions raised by these discussions. Work-life issues driving creation of the harassment free and equitable work environment is the sought-after goal for the employer of a predominantly White, Christian, heterosexual male lead, able bodied, boomer-prevalent workforce. For such a long-established labor pool, emotions connected to concepts like White privilege create philosophical anxiety. The endemic power of the traditionally dominant is rarely acknowledged as originating where it is found. Often displayed in day-to-day interactions in which the dominant group expresses the need for more *elbow* room, whereas the marginalized are perceived as *elbowing* their way in, this exemplifies the need for policies that promote inclusion and protect the vulnerable. Particularly pertinent is dialogue about replication of the social class system within the organizational structure. This is especially true when mobility within the organizational structure is called into question. Such perceptions present opportunity for discussions about the need for innovation in the status quo. Diversity within the workforce makes actions focused on such change an ambitious undertaking.

DEMOGRAPHICS OF THE NEW WORKFORCE

By 2019, Millennials (born 1981–1996 and 43% non-White) will surpass Baby Boomers (born 1946–1964) as the largest U.S. adult generation. Their social profile depicts them as more likely to be foreign born and to speak other than English as their first language (Cohn & Caumont, 2016). The 2015 report on nursing statistics by the journal Minority Nurse describes the profession as 9.9% Black or African American (non-Hispanic), 8.3% Asian, and 4.8% Hispanic or Latino; 1.3% categorize themselves

as two or more races, and 0.4% claim American Indian or Alaskan native as their heritage. Adding another detail to the profile of the profession, a 2015 fact sheet published by the Department for Professional Employees of the American Federation of Labor and Congress of Industrial Organizations (AFL-CIO), indicates that among registered nurses (RNs) who were 35 years old and younger, 11% were Hispanic or Latino matched by 12% who were Asian or Hawaiian Pacific Islander. When compared with White nurses, data from the 2015 National Nursing Workforce Survey indicate ethnic minorities are better represented in younger age groups and in more recently licensed RNs than in older RNs and RNs licensed prior to 2000. More specifically, 19% of the nursing workforce is represented by ethnic minorities, whereas those groups represent 37% of the overall population in the United States. It is important to note a specific aspect of the Boomer Generation as it relates to age. Boomers will turn 65 at a rate of 10,000 a day over the next 18 years, and 67% of the employed boomers share they are either not engaged or actively disengaged at work; 65% of them feel they are the subjects of ageism (Schawbel, 2017). The Boomer is majority White and often described as aging out of the workforce. On the other hand, it is the current trend that this age group is delaying retirement. This includes the boomer who is a nurse. People in this age group are closely followed by a more ethnically diverse generation. One demographic portrait of that approaching ethnically diverse generation describes them as 19% Hispanic, 14% Black, and 5% Asian with 38% being bilingual. They also account for 1 in every 5 same-sex couple (Marketing Charts, 2014). This demographic narrative holds import for the employer regarding education and training, employee services, and workplace accommodations. Meaningful work, resilience, stress, and demands of physical and emotional strain are all examples of issues that nurse leaders and organizational vision must direct efforts toward managing effectively.

HIDDEN CURRICULUM

Acknowledging prevailing mores opens organizational culture to examination of governing values, beliefs, and practices that form the context for rules and laws that determine policy. This inevitably leads to modification or displacement of the status quo and widens the space occupied by nursing leadership development as it relates to support for diversity. What that leadership actively does in the workplace should demonstrate distinguishing characteristics of nursing leadership at work. This goes beyond labor and into ideas, innovation, thinking, and power. Any specific behavior that indicates this marks the scope of the territory that is uniquely nursing as an influence while providing evidence of its impact. This may require both a concrete and an abstract or ideological shift for the nursing profession in its attention to diversity and inclusion. Understanding the meaning of this shift will expand thinking into the significance of having a broader range of social groups in the workplace. The meaning of this influence gives purpose and direction to leadership behavior and provides a framework for the future. Articulation of the way forward informs vision and provides insight into needed disruptions to the general state of things. Such leadership takes the form of progress through moral and intellectual means leading to momentum in the direction of desired goals. Concepts such as the hidden curriculum come to light and results in codes of organizational culture becoming more apparent and move beyond equivocal perception.

Andarvazh, Afshar, and Yazdani (2017) defined the hidden curriculum as:

> a hidden, powerful, and sometimes contradictory message which is intrinsic in organizational structure and culture. This message is conveyed implicitly and tacitly in the learning environment by structural and human factors. The content of the message would be cultural habits and customs, norms, values, belief systems, attitudes, skills, desires and behavioral and social expectations and could have positive or negative effect on the learners. The educational goals of the hidden curriculum are unplanned, neither planners and teachers, nor learners are aware of it. The final-outcome of the hidden curriculum will be reproducing the existing class structure, socialization, and familiarizing learners for transmission and joining the professional world. (p. 204)

Statements that exemplify the hidden curriculum are:

"That person is not a good fit."
"We don't do that here."
"They usually go elsewhere for their care."
"You still here?"

The hidden curriculum operates to socialize its users to adhere to the written and unwritten rules of the culture. What can be said or done without consequence becomes one method of sharing the conventions of the environment. A case scenario follows, and a model for processing information to inform a policy approach is outlined.

CASE SCENARIO

Carrie came crying to the office of the Director of Diversity and Inclusion. She is a 10-year employee at a large academic medical center on an inpatient unit as a patient care associate. Her job is to help patients with their activities of daily living and do blood draws as needed. She said she didn't know what to do about a recent change in her work schedule. As a Seventh Day Adventist, Carrie did not want to work on Saturday, her Sabbath. Her work schedule had always accommodated her ability to keep the Sabbath. Now there was a new Nursing Director. This recent change in unit leadership now threatened that practice. The new Director in her desire to meet the needs of her staff was now scheduling Carrie to work an occasional Saturday. Carrie wanted to continue to adhere to the principles of her faith tradition and found this change hard to accept. She spoke to her manager and to human resources and received two messages. Patients come first and we must make sure we staff are keeping patient safety a priority. The team is made up of people with various scheduling needs (e.g., school schedules, child and elder care, leaves of absence, and vacations). Carrie reports she offered to work any schedule Monday to Friday and Sunday in return for a consistent sunset Friday to sunset Saturday off. "They made it work for 10 years. What's so different now?" she asked.

PROCESS FOR ORGANIZATIONAL POLICY DEVELOPMENT FOR CASE SCENARIO

Desired Ideal

The ideal is accommodation of religious practices and customs.

Normative Example

In Christian protestant and catholic-dominant organizations, work shifts are typically not impacted by a doctrine of not working on a Sunday Sabbath. A Christian Sabbath-keeping philosophy in conflict with a work ethic is not typical. As a historically Christian-dominant society, the American employer acknowledges formally (federal law) and informally (by custom) secular and non-secular (Christmas, New Year, Thanksgiving, Easter) traditions as part of scheduling principles.

Qualities, Nature, Significance of Desired Ideal

The desired ideal requires modification of the normative example. This modification is the consequence of commitment to inclusion and creates a different management system for decision making and identifying priorities. Strict adherence to rules is problematic in a diverse work environment. Judgment and utilizing experience with diversity provide insights into the resulting dilemma in which a choice based on the normative example automatically rules out an alternative.

Feasible Equivalent to Desired Ideal

What can be done? In this case, the decision maker should determine range of flexibility in religious rules outlined by relevant religious authority as opposed to subjective adherence/interpretation. Ascertain applicable organizational principle (e.g., "patients first"). Ration need for intrusion into subjective adherence to religious practices (i.e., the need to accommodate an emergent issue in contrast to covering scheduled staff vacations).

The ultimate question related to the hidden curriculum is: in what way do systems and clinicians function in the organization such that performance results in disadvantages to diverse groups as defined by members of those groups?

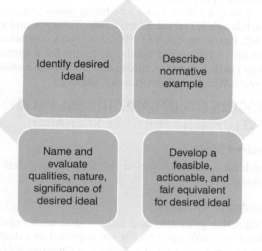

Process for organizational policy development.

HARASSMENT

In 2015, the U.S. Equal Employment Opportunity Commission (EEOC), the federal agency that enforces laws against workplace discrimination, reported that, of the complaints received from employees working for private or state and local government employers:

- 45% alleged harassment based on sex
- 34% alleged harassment based on race
- 19% alleged harassment based on disability
- 15% alleged harassment based on age
- 13% alleged harassment based on national origin
- 5% alleged harassment based on religion

In 2016, EEOC published a report from the Select Task Force on the Study of Harassment in the Workplace. In it, examples of behaviors that constitute harassment are listed as: offensive jokes, slurs, epithets or name calling, undue attention, physical assaults or threats, unwelcome touching

or contact, intimidation, ridicule or mockery, insults or put-downs, constant or unwelcome questions about an individual's identity, and offensive objects or pictures. However, not every work environment identifies the same behaviors as harassment, and therefore no definitive acts of improper conduct exist on this issue. One consequence of this is the troubling response of victims to the list of behaviors mentioned above. Oftentimes worrisome conduct is not reported. Accusations are abandoned due to formidable reporting processes. Choosing not to take prescribed action is problematic and alarming. EEOC specifies that this shortfall in needed response is due to:

- Fear of disbelief
- Inaction on a claim
- Blame
- Retaliation

A well-publicized accountability structure within an organization is the best assurance to employees of a zero-tolerance philosophy related to harassment. The infrastructure for handling complaints may include Human Resources, Employee Assistance Programs, Managers, Office of Diversity, Ombudsman, and Police and Security. A safe and secure work environment results from alignment between stated beliefs and actions. Anti-harassment policies serve as deterrents.

EEOC recommends that a policy include:

- Detailed description of disallowed behaviors.
- Commitment to confidentiality and protection against reprisal.
- Complaint process easy to navigate and progress through.
- Conduct a timely and efficient investigation.

BULLYING AND MICROAGGRESSIONS

Background

The American Nurses Association (ANA) defines bullying as "repeated, unwanted, harmful actions intended to humiliate, offend, and cause distress in the recipient." The National Institute for Occupational Safety and Health (NIOSH) provides more detail in its definition of Workplace violence as the act or threat of violence, ranging from verbal abuse to physical assaults directed toward persons at work or on duty, "the risk for nonfatal violence resulting in days away from work is greatest for healthcare and social assistance workers."

Of those victims who experienced trauma from workplace violence:

- 70% were female
- 67% were aged 25 to 54
- 70% worked in the health care and social assistance industry
- 21% required 31 or more days away from work to recover, and 19% involved 3 to 5 days away from work

Bullying as part of workplace culture is no longer an anomaly. In many ways resulting from dysfunctional power relationships, bullying is especially noteworthy as a phenomenon bracketed with diversity. Groups who do not share social environments but do share strained social histories meet in the workplace as individuals expected to form cohesive relationships as members of the same team. A lack of harmony in relationships in such a scenario interferes with inclusive excellence in the workplace (Dzurec, Kennison, & Gillen, 2017). To members of targeted groups, a social connection message "I like you. I don't care if you're gay" contrasted with a social change message "Homophobic behavior will not be tolerated and this is what we're going to do about it;" the former is less comforting than the latter (Rattan & Ambady, 2014). This points to the need for written policies and guidelines as deterrents to acts that shame and embarrass. Cyberbullying is included as the latest entry into the need for standards. Inappropriate behavior must be detailed and communicated to foster accountability for managing awareness of any inadequacy in organizational response to intimidation or coercion. Factors such as hospital setting, scheduling, workload, withholding needed information, and negative affect can be predictors of disruptive behavior in the form of verbal abuse (Keller, Krainovich-Miller, Budin, & Djukic, 2018).

Microaggressions, a term coined in the 1970s, are forms of bullying defined as "brief, everyday exchanges that send denigrating messages to people of color because they belong to a racial minority group" (Sue, Capodilupo, Torino, Bucceri, Holder, Nadal, & Esquilin, 2007). Pierce (1970) described these messages as incessant and cumulative in effect.

CURRICULUM ON DIVERSITY

Diversity as a concept in the workplace has much to do with understanding organizational culture and the vocabulary used by the organization that supports and upholds the construct. A sustained conversation about the relevant issues is supported by a slate of programs that examine points in question. The purpose of a curriculum on diversity is to bring objectivity, reflection, and a breakthrough toward equity. In this intentional objective, the next evolution of the 21st century workplace is intimately linked with the demographics of the larger social environment and faces the challenge of accomplishing what the overall society failed to. Through organizational development, attending to diversity results in the betterment of skills that advantage praxis, pedagogy, and research because the process serves to release the organization and the way it operates from the deficits of the dominant culture. Unconscious bias, incivility, and inadequate policies and

procedures that fail to terminate harmful practices are factors used by the status quo and with detrimental effect on a psychologically and emotionally healthy work environment. The ultimate purpose is to put into use learning that applies knowledge, experience, and insight to the provision of care and improvement of work place relationships that involve the unfamiliar "other." At its core, this progress actualizes values and enables a move to a new state of belief about who belongs and who constitutes the body that makes that decision.

Such a curriculum must include the following elements:
- A learning methodology based in dialogue and individual narratives demonstrating experiences with race and other "isms"
- Data analysis that tells the organizational story related to diversity in its workforce and patient population (e.g., aggregated data segmented by group identities connected to turnover rates, complaints of discrimination, grievance applications)
- Organizational assessment and climate survey that reveals staff and employee experiences in the workplace as persons from differing backgrounds (e.g., race, gender, gender identity, age, physical/mental range of abilities) sharing the same space
- Inventory of resources that reflect the ombudsman role (e.g., employee relations, employee assistance program, grievance process, diversity officer)
- Listing of resources that identify the organization as a place of opportunity for all employees (e.g., promotions, educational supports, mentoring programs, pipeline programs)

CONCLUSION

Acknowledging prevailing mores opens organizational culture to examination of its governing values, beliefs, and practices. These form the context for rules and laws that determine policy. This inevitably leads to modification or displacement of the status quo, which widens the space occupied by nursing leadership and what that leadership actively does in the workplace. Noting nursing administrators as responsible for direct effect on systems must go beyond nursing as labor and more into nursing ideas, innovation, thinking, and power. Any specific behavior that indicates all this marks the scope of the territory uniquely nursing as a profession of influence with the capacity to design a more civil and bias-free workplace. This may require a concrete as well as an abstract shift into a transformational position for the nursing profession. It should be a steering influence in modernizing organizational culture. Understanding the meaning of this shift expands managing the impact of diversity in the health care workplace.

The meaning of such influence gives purpose and direction to leadership behavior, reasons for actions taken, and articulation of desired goals. In this moment in shaping the future, nursing leadership must take the form of an applied force steering movement in the direction of desired and sought-after goals.

DISCUSSION QUESTIONS

1. What factors would you use to create a strategy for a positive and inclusive work environment?
2. How would you address issues that appear in news headlines that impact employees from diverse communities?

REFERENCES

Andarvazh, M.R., Afshar, L., & Yazdani, S. (2018). Hidden curriculum: An analytical definition. *Journal of Medical Education, 16*(4), 18061-18061.

Cohn, D. & Caumont, A. (2016). *10 Demographic trends shaping the U.S. and the World in 2016. Pew Research Center.* Retrieved from www.pewresearch.org/fact-tank/2016/03/31/10-demographic-trends-that-are-shaping-the-u-s-and-the-world/.

Demographic stats about US millennials. (2014). *Marketing Charts.* Retrieved from www.marketingcharts.com/demographics-and-audiences-40016.

Department for Professional Employees, American Federation of Labor and Congress of Industrial Organizations. (2015).

Nursing: A profile of the profession, fact sheet 2015. Retrieved from http://dpeaflcio.org/wp-content/uploads/Nursing-2015.pdf.

Dzurec, L.C., Kennison, M., & Gillen, P. (October, 2017). The incongruity of workplace bullying victimization and inclusive excellence. *Nursing Outlook, 65*(5), 588-596.

Get the latest nursing statistics and demographics in the US. (2015). *Minority Nurse.* Retrieved from https://minoritynurse.com/nursing-statistics/.

Keller, R., Krainovich-Miller, B., Budin, W., & Djukic, M. (March-April, 2018). Predictors of nurses' experience of verbal abuse by nurse colleagues. *Nursing Outlook, 66*(2), 190–203.

National Institute for Occupational Safety and Health. (2016). *Occupational violence: Fast facts.* Retrieved from www.cdc.gov/niosh/topics/violence/fastfacts.html.

Pierce, C. (1970). Offensive mechanisms (pp. 265-286). In F. Barbour (Ed.), *The Black seventies.* Boston, MA: Porter Sargent Publisher.

Rattan, A. & Ambady, N. (2014). How "It Gets Better": Effectively communicating support to targets of prejudice. *Personality and Social Psychology Bulletin, 40*(5), 555-566.

Schawbel, D. (2017). *53 of the most interesting facts about Baby Boomers.* Retrieved from http://danschawbel.com/blog/53-of-the-most-interesting-facts-about-baby-boomers/.

Sue, D., Capodilupo, C., Torino, G., Bucceri, J., Holder, A., Nadal, K., & Esquilin, M. (2007). Racial microaggressions in everyday life: Implications for clinical practice. *American Psychologist. 62*(4), 271-286.

U.S. Equal Employment Opportunity Commission, Select Task Force on the Study of Harassment in the Workplace. (2016). *Report of Co-Chairs Chai R. Feldblum & Victoria. A. Lipnic.* Retrieved from www.eeoc.gov/eeoc/task_force/harassment/upload/report.pdf.

58

TAKING ACTION: Racism in the Workplace

Kenya V. Beard

"Institutional racism is not the proverbial grit in the machine that conventional programs of race awareness training can remove. Rather, it is organic in nature and function and grows in cunning and resilience with each challenge it successfully overcomes."

Law, Phillips, and Turney (2004)

As a visiting nurse in Long Island, New York in the 1980s, it was routine for me to call patients, introduce myself, and schedule an initial visit. The conversations were brief, yet cordial, and ended with a mutually agreed upon time for me to visit. However, shortly after the call ended, on too many occasions, my beeper would vibrate and the number to my homecare agency would appear on the dimly lit screen. After responding to the page, I was alerted that the patient or family member whom I had just spoken to had suddenly refused our recently arranged visit and requested a different nurse. A feeling of disbelief, coupled with the heaviness of hurt, denied me the ability to deeply consider the role that race might have played in the abrupt request for a change in nurses. I quickly learned the modus operandi and never questioned the "matter of fact" tone of my manager or received an explanation for the affront. My thoughts of race-related discrimination remained a thinly veiled subtext that operated on a subliminal level.

Although I graduated nursing school with the knowledge, attitude, and skills to manage the health care needs of patients, I quickly realized that my training left me ill equipped to effectively respond to what I perceived to be racism in the workplace. Thus, several years later, I turned to the literature to deepen my understanding of racism and join others in the quest to eradicate it.

Currently, racism continues, albeit at times at a less macroscopic level. This chapter describes racism, explores why policies alone have not eradicated racism, illuminates how racism manifests in the workplace, and provides actionable steps to eradicate the remnants of racism.

RACISM

When discussing racism in the workplace, one should consider how racism was used four centuries ago to construct and sustain an atypical form of enslavement in America. Racism, the false "...doctrine of the congenital inferiority and worthlessness of a people" (King, 2010), changed the rules of involuntary servitude by dehumanizing a socially constructed group of individuals who shared certain physical characteristics. The debasing narratives, falsely concocted to support and sustain a rhetoric that viewed people with darker complexions as less than human, intellectually inferior, and violent, were deadly and powerful. Racist ideologies blurred realities regarding which groups were considered human, amplified fear, and fueled rage, cruelty and bigotry. Individuals were overtly discriminated against because of the color of their skin.

In 1967, Martin Luther King Jr. gave a speech at the National Conference on New Politics in Chicago where he discussed racism as one of the three evils of society. Specifically, he stated that

> Racism can well be, that corrosive evil that will bring down the curtain on western civilization. Arnold Toynesbee has said that some twenty-six civilizations have risen upon the face of the Earth, almost all of them have descended into the junk heap of destruction. The decline and fall of these civilizations, according to Toynesbee, was not caused by external invasion but by internal decay. They failed to respond creatively to the challenges impingent upon them. If America does not respond creatively to the challenge to

banish racism, some future historian will have to say, that a great civilization died because it lacked the soul and commitment to make justice a reality for all men.

Sir Winston Churchill's well-known maxim "those who fail to learn from history are doomed to repeat it" is echoed in Dr. King's speech. Indeed, much is being done to address inequities in and around institutions. Yet, policies alone are not enough.

POLICIES TO ERADICATE RACISM

Removing the bars of a prison cell while keeping a falsely accused individual incarcerated does not translate to freedom. Similarly, although the 13th Amendment in 1865 abolished slavery, the law did not dismantle the oppressive remnants of racism (i.e., the discriminatory practices and beliefs that powered slavery). Rather, the pursuit of liberty and justice continues to be constrained by structural racism.

Dr. Tricia Rose, Director of the Center for the Study of Race and Ethnicity in America at Brown University, defines structural racism as "the normalization and legitimization of an array of dynamics—historical, cultural, institutional and interpersonal—that routinely advantage whites while producing cumulative and chronic adverse outcomes for people of color" (Rose, 2015, video). Structural racism has been likened to the base of an iceberg, dangerous and elusive; whereby overt acts, such as lynching, reflect the visible part of the iceberg (Gee & Ford, 2015). Dismantling that which is visible while ignoring its origin supports the pervasive nature of structural racism.

Like the genetic information a child inherits, structural racism gives birth to discriminatory beliefs and unjust practices. Legislative rulings enacted to address or counteract the effects of racism have focused on overt acts and proven impotent in regard to delegitimizing racist narratives and dismantling structural racism. Although the 14th amendment of 1868 attempted to extend "equal protection of the laws" to former slaves (The Library of Congress, 2018), it took *Brown v. Board of Education* (1954) to rule racial segregation in public schools unconstitutional and the Civil Rights Act of 1964 to prohibit discrimination in public schools, colleges, and employment. Likewise, the Fair Housing Act of 1968 intended to ban "racial discrimination in the sale or rental of housing" and improve access for all individuals. However, discriminatory practices in housing have continued (Labert, 1997).

Although legislative rulings make overt racial discrimination illegal, the policies fail to eliminate the negative thoughts and beliefs that stoke irrational fears and give birth to actions that further inequities. Essentially some policies exist to tell individuals what they can and cannot do based on race. However, these policies fail to address or alter mindsets rooted in hate, fear, or misconceptions. Currently, the false doctrine of race-related inferiority continues to taint beliefs, allowing damaging stereotypical beliefs to persist and give way to discriminatory practices in the workplace.

RACISM IN THE WORKPLACE

The roots of racism lie deep beneath the bedrock of institutions limiting the effect that policies and practices have on effectively eliminating America's racial hierarchy. Although numerous policies, whether written as laws, regulations, or voluntary practices, have attempted to eliminate the remnants of racism, racial discrimination persists (Beard & Julion, 2016; Beard & Volcy, 2013; Bowen-Matthew, 2017; Law, Phillips, & Turney, 2004). Racism persists in the workplace as discriminatory policies and practices that overtly and covertly marginalize people of color and sustain negative stereotypes. Indeed in the United States, racism is not only used to disadvantage people who appear to be Black or African American. Individuals who classify as American Indian, Alaskan Native, Pacific Islander, Hispanic/Latino, and Asian are also impacted by the powers of structural racism (Agency for Healthcare Research and Quality [AHRQ], 2017; Bowen-Matthews, 2015; Gee & Ford, 2011).

The inaccurate typifications used to describe melanin-rich individuals in the past continue today, serving to fuel stereotypes that hijack egalitarian values, promote discriminatory practices, and result in inequitable outcomes. One does not have to look far to observe the chameleon-like mutations of racism. Nursing, the largest health care discipline in the United States, is not immune to the effects of racism. Darlene Hine (1989) illuminates in *Black Women in White* that in the early 1900s, Black nurses were marginalized and excluded from nursing organizations such as the American Nurses Association. Hine also reports that the erroneous belief of intellectual inferiority hindered the advancement of Black nurses, prevented them from taking the same licensing examination, branded them as inferior, and contributed to race-based wage discrepancies.

More than 100 years later, nursing remains mainly an institution of whiteness, although a national effort to strengthen diversity has ensued (National League for Nursing 2017; American Association of Colleges of Nursing, Institute of Medicine [IOM], 2017; National Organization of Nurse Practitioner Faculties, 2018). The institutional impediments that continue to limit racial diversity among nursing students, faculty, and administrators are concerning. Researchers have reported that historical barriers such as racism, false beliefs regarding intellect, and discriminatory hiring practices continue to hinder diversity efforts (Kirwan

Institute, 2017). Beard and Julion (2017) conducted a qualitative study among Black nursing faculty and asserted that "race is indeed a factor that hinders the nursing profession from achieving its diversity goals" (p. 593). A reoccurring theme that emerged was the false belief of intellectual inferiority. Several participants "…believed that their skin color perpetuated stereotypes about African-Americans and led to a culture of prejudice." Discriminatory practices and microaggressions, the subtle insults and acts of discrimination, drove some faculty away from academia. However, one participant posited that "…it [institutional racism] is everywhere" (p. 10).

Remnants of racism know no boundaries and flourish inside and beyond the criminal justice system, education, health care, and housing. Race has been implicated as a critical factor in sentencing disparities, the academic achievement gap, and health care disparities (Kirwan Institute, 2017). In health care, the unconscious beliefs about individuals of color could result in death. The 2003, IOM bold and provocative landmark report, *Unequal Treatment; Confronting Racial and Ethnic Disparities in Health Care* illuminates the disparate treatments that racial/ethnic minorities receive. The authors assert that health care systems along with providers contribute to health care disparities and that disparities are associated with worse outcomes and contribute to disability and death. Several years later, the Department of Veterans Affairs (2007) echoed the IOM, stating that sometimes the provider's therapeutic decision making was negatively influenced by a veteran's race. More recently, the AHRQ (2017) has echoed that race and ethnicity remain significant predictors of the quality of health care that is received. The report reveals that inequities in morbidity and mortality are linked to the lower quality of care that some groups are more likely to receive.

Abolishing slavery has not resulted in an eradication of discriminatory practices that stem from and preserve structural racism. Rather, Dr. Bowen-Matthews (2017), in *Just Medicine: A Cure for Racial Inequality in American Health,* asserts that policies like the Civil Rights Act of 1964 allowed covert discriminatory acts to swing to the forefront. Structural racism has escaped the power of policies that sought to promote equality. Sue (2016) posits that the less blatant forms of racism surface nowadays as racial biases—the attitudes, beliefs, and ideas that give way to words or statements that are derogatory, insulting, and defaming. In health care, racism emerges currently as unconscious race-related biases that could influence treatment decisions and contribute to health care disparities (FitzGerald & Hurst, 2017; Hall, 2015; IOM, 2004). Do humans have the capacity to eliminate the implicit thoughts and actions that link to structural racism?

ACTIONABLE STEPS TO ERADICATE STRUCTURAL RACISM

Society has yet to identify a panacea strong enough to eradicate structural racism. Like the air we breathe, structural racism continues to permeate institutional settings and elude legislative policies that seek to annihilate its existence. The evidence suggests that the attacks on racism have aimed above the iceberg. However, attempts to address and eliminate structural racism could be misinterpreted. When United States Senator Elizabeth Warren remarked about racism in the criminal justice system, she was met with an onslaught of criticism (2018). Individuals argued that she was attacking individuals who risked their lives to maintain law and order. Discrepant beliefs regarding racism are likely to challenge efforts to address and dismantle structural racism.

Looking around a room to see which groups are in attendance and missing is not enough to uproot structural racism. Although acknowledging that structural racism persists could advance society one step closer toward social justice, refusing to discuss the historical implications of racism is likely to widen the divide between where America is and could be.

Because discrimination is sometimes implicit, some might argue against its existence. Obliterating the remnants of racism without acknowledging structural racism sounds wishful at best. Thus, to end structural racism in the workplace, one should be willing to explore the extent to which discriminatory practices exist. Leaders should use a race-equity lens to examine policies and determine the extent to which race, power, and privilege influences practices. The structure and processes that intersect with ubiquitous factors that reinforce racism should be examined. Of course, individuals should also be prepared to discuss race and analyze the impact current policies have on eliminating or perpetuating structural racism. The following actionable steps are provided to serve as a guide to recognizing, planning, and dismantling structural racism in the workplace.

Leaders of institutions should:
- Be clear about what structural racism is and how it is perpetuated.
- Be prepared to explain how institutionalized racism operates.
- Discuss how policies address actions and not necessarily beliefs.
- Create a culture that affirms the right to "sense something, say something."
- Create a milieu that invites open and effective racial discourse.
- Examine the extent to which policies perpetuate structural racism.

- Identify the thoughts and beliefs that intertwine and drive institutional practices.
- Determine whether policies seeking to eliminate discrimination are wedded to organizational behaviors.
- Provide trainings that result in institutional changes along a continuum.
- Establish checkpoints to determine the effectiveness of practices.
- Create evaluations that align with institutional values and mission statement.
- Evaluate individuals based on actions and outcomes that reinforce the institutional values and mission.

SUMMARY

The United States continues to struggle in its pursuit to advance to a post-racial society where the tenets of racial equity prevail. Indeed, social justice policies alone have failed to eradicate racism, and individuals could be blindsided by the insidious nature and powerful forces of structural racism. Negative stereotypes surrounding people of color appear deeply engrained as unconscious biases and sometimes undermine explicit intentions. Like cancer, the cure for racism might elude the capacity of a capitalistic society.

Discrimination in the workplace stems in part from America's racist past. The typifications of skin color were intentionally linked, implicitly and explicitly, to corrosive thoughts that resulted in inferior treatment and outcomes. The belief that some humans are insignificant based on the amount of melanin in their skin is absurd. However, as society wrestles with that absurdity, remnants of racism continue to undermine social justice and excellence in the workplace.

Denying structural racism is unlikely to advance the United States toward a remedy. Because some discriminatory practices are rooted around race, how can institutions effectively eradicate structural racism without adequately discussing race? The aforementioned actional steps should strengthen the capacity of leaders to address racism and achieve what has never been accomplished in this country before: the eradication of structural racism.

REFERENCES

Agency for Healthcare Research and Quality. (2018). *2017 National healthcare quality and disparities report*. Retrieved from www.ahrq.gov/sites/default/files/wysiwyg/research/findings/nhqrdr/2017nhqdr.pdf.

American Association of Colleges of Nursing. (2017). *Diversity, inclusion, and equity in academic nursing*. Retrieved from www.aacnnursing.org/Portals/42/Diversity/AACN-Position-Statement-Diversity-Inclusion.pdf.

Beard, K.V., & Julion, W. (2016). Does race still matter in nursing? The narratives of African-American nursing faculty members. *Nursing Outlook, 64*(6), 583-596.

Beard, K.V., & Volcy, K. (2013). Increasing minority representation in nursing: A more diverse faculty is crucial. *American Journal of Nursing, 113*(2), 11.

Bowen-Matthew, D. (2017). *Just medicine: A cure for racial inequality in American health care*. New York: NYU Press.

Department of Veteran Affairs. (2007). *Racial and ethnic disparities in the VA healthcare system: A systematic review*. Retrieved from www.hsrd.research.va.gov/publications/esp/racialdisparities-2007.pdf.

Doalmsavid, E.J. (2013). *Martin Luther King: The three evils of society*. [Video]. Retrieved from www.youtube.com/watch?v=j8d-IYSM-08.

FitzGerald, C., & Hurst, S. (2017). Implicit bias in healthcare professionals: A systematic review. *BMC Medical Ethics*. Retrieved from https://bmcmedethics.biomedcentral.com/articles/10.1186/s12910-017-0179-8.

Gee, C.G., & Ford, C.L. (2011). Structural racism and health inequities. *Du Bois Review, 8*(1), 115-132.

Hine, D.C. (1989). Black women in white: Racial conflict and cooperation in the nursing professions 1890-1950. Bloomington, IN: Indiana University Press.

Institute of Medicine. (2004). *Unequal treatment: Confronting racial and ethnic disparities in health care*. Retrieved from www.nationalacademies.org/hmd/Reports/2002/Unequal-Treatment-Confronting-Racial-and-Ethnic-Disparities-in-Health-Care.aspx

King, M.L., Jr. (2010). *Where do we go from here: Chaos or community?* Boston: Beacon Press.

Kirwan Institute. (2017). *State of the science: Implicit bias review*. Retrieved from http://kirwaninstitute.osu.edu/wp-content/uploads/2017/11/2017-SOTS-final-draft-02.pdf.

Lambert, B. (1997). At 50, Levittown contends with its legacy of bias. *The New York Times*. Retrieved from www.nytimes.com/1997/12/28/nyregion/at-50-levittown-contends-with-its-legacy-of-bias.html.

Law, I., Phillips, D., & Turney L. (Eds.). (2004). *Institutional racism in higher education*. Great Britain: Trentham Books Limited.

Library of Congress. (2018). *14th Amendment to the U.S. Constitution*. Retrieved from www.loc.gov/rr/program/bib/ourdocs/14thamendment.html.

National League for Nursing. (2017). *NLN diversity and inclusion toolkit*. Retrieved from www.nln.org/docs/default-source/professional-development-programs/diversity_toolkit.pdf?sfvrsn=6.

Rose, T. (2015). *How structural racism works: Tricia Rose*. Retrieved from www.youtube.com/watch?v=KT1vsOJctMk&feature=youtu.be.

Sue, D.W. (2015). *Race talk and the conspiracy of silence: Understanding and facilitating difficult dialogues on race*. Hoboken, NJ: John Wiley.

Wyatt, R., Laderman, M., Botwinick, L., Mate, K., & Whittington, J. (2016). *Achieving health equity: A guide for health care organizations*. [IHI White Paper.] Cambridge, MA: Institute for Healthcare Improvement. Retrieved from www.ihi.org.

59

Collective Strategies for Transformation in the Workplace

Toby Bressler and Linda M. Valentino

> *"Let whoever is in charge keep this simple question in her head (not, how can I always do this right thing myself, but) how can I provide for this right thing to be always done?"*
>
> *Florence Nightingale*

This chapter highlights strategic change in the workplace with a focus on what front-line nurses, managers, and administrators should think about transformational change in patient care delivery settings. There are different strategies that can be used whether the setting is a union, non-union, urban, or academic one.

TRANSFORMATION

There are many theoretical discussions of transformational leadership (Anderson & Anderson, 2001; Bass, 1985; Bass & Avolio, 1994, Bass & Reggio, 2006; Burns 1978, 2003), with some common aspects to their transformational leadership theories and some significant differences. One commonality is that leaders who wish to lead in transformational ways must clearly understand the process of transformation. It is important to understand the difference between change and transformation through the lens of leadership. Transformation is described as the emancipatory process of becoming critically aware of how and why the structure of assumptions of the way we see ourselves and our relationships, and reconstituting this structure to allow a more inclusive understanding of our experiences and act upon our new understanding and knowing (Chinn & Kramer, 2011).

Transformational leadership is defined by Fischer (2016) as an integrative style of leadership as well as a set of competencies. Fischer describes transformational leadership style as identified by an enthusiastic, emotionally mature, visionary, and courageous lifelong learner who inspires and motivates by empowering and developing followers (Fig. 59.1).

Transformational leadership is actualized by utilizing structured change management theories and formulas. Change management theories are the tools that leaders use to implement transformational change. There are many change theories used by nursing leaders. Some contemporary models include Appreciative Inquiry (AI) (Cooperrider, Whitney, & Stavros, 2008), Lean Six Sigma, and Kotter's Eight Stages of Change (2012a) (Box 59.1).

One example of a successful large-scale formula for change in nursing organizations is the I_2E_2 model described by Jayne Felgen (2007). The I_2E_2 formula includes the elements of Inspiration, Infrastructure, Evidence, and Education. These aforementioned elements will be described in detail later in the chapter. The I_2E_2 method for Leading Lasting Change is a simple and elegant formula that may be utilized to create both small- and large-scale organizational change nursing. This model supports the tenets of transformational leadership in that the first step in the change process is to establish a vision for the future. This is a unique approach to change management, as it is does not support the recreation of an existing business model; rather, it supports innovative thinking about change grounded in a practical and logical business-like approach. The I_2E_2 model supports the notion that each person involved in the change process has something valuable to offer, thereby creating a culture of inclusiveness integral to supporting sustainable change.

Beginning with the vision in a large-scale organization change or a small-scale change, the I_2E_2 model may be utilized. However, it is not sufficient to have a vision such as "to be the health care organization of choice in our

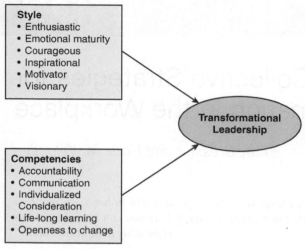

Style
- Enthusiastic
- Emotional maturity
- Courageous
- Inspirational
- Motivator
- Visionary

Transformational Leadership

Competencies
- Accountability
- Communication
- Individualized Consideration
- Life-long learning
- Openness to change

Fig. 59.1 Transformational leadership. (Adapted from Fischer, S. A. [2016]. Transformational leadership in nursing: A concept analysis. *Journal of Advanced Nursing, 72*[11], 2644–2653.)

BOX 59.1 Change Management Theoretical Components

Appreciative Inquiry	Lean Six Sigma	Kotter's Eight Stages of Change
• Define the change	• Define	• Create urgency
• Discover "what works"	• Measure	• Form a coalition
	• Analyze	• Create the vision
• Dream the vision	• Improve	• Communicate the
• Design the plan	• Control	vision
• Deliver and create		• Empower action
the change		• Create short-term
		wins
		• Maintain momentum
		• Anchor the change

---

community;" you must be specific with measurable goals about the changes you set out to achieve. Specific statements that support the actualized vision must be a part of the change process.

Examples of such statements may include:
- Nurse engagement will be at or above national benchmarks by the end of the second year.
- Patient satisfaction will be at or above the 75th percentile ranking within 24 months.
- Physicians and nurses partner in care planning; this is evidenced by an increase in patient perception of nurse and physician communication within 12 months.

- Patient harm is decreased as evidenced by a 50% reduction in falls with injury within 12 months.
- Relationship-based care is evident by the patient experiencing caring as he or she describes it upon admission.

The core elements of the I_2E_2: Leading Lasting Change model is as follows (Felgen, 2007; Fig. 59.2):

1. Vision: "Construct your vision with its end use in mind: It is to be used as a touchstone for all that you do on the way to making your vision *live* in the daily workings of your organization" (p. 44). The vision includes clarity of the common purpose or goal.
2. Inspiration (I1): "Inspiration helps other to see that the benefits of change outweigh the risks of upsetting the status quo" (Felgen, 2007, p. 46). Inspiration includes supporting creativity in others and the exuberance within you.
3. Infrastructure (I2): "Design your organization's Infrastructure so that every role practice, standard, system, and process actively advances the realization of your vision for change" (p. 51).
4. Education (E1): "In order to effectively bring individuals into the change, it is vital to provide for any learning initiatives necessary to ensure their early success" (p. 57).
5. Evidence (E2): "The Evidence element of I_2E_2 assesses how successful our efforts in Inspiration (I1), Infrastructure (I2), and Education (E1) are in advancing the organization's new vision."

The I_2E_2 model is a structured approach to leading lasting organizational change. A key element of any cultural transformational process in nursing organizations is to manage perceptions of those who are involved in the changes. Perceptions of change differ within and external to groups in any organization. One group may view the change as threatening to the status quo, whereas another views it as an opportunity to make things better for patients, staff, and the organization. Unionized environments by nature may present a more polarized culture. However, Cooperrider, Whitney and Stavros (2008) posit the philosophy and methodology of AI (2008) may be utilized as a way of enlightening constituent groups of the other's viewpoint. A practice of AI, "the practice of looking at 'what is' with appreciation for what it has provided for us so far allows us to move forward unencumbered by the ghosts of past failures" (Felgen, 2007, p. 9). AI is a tool that helps us to focus on the success of past experiences and vision for the future, avoiding the perception that barriers to our future vision may be immovable. Transformational leaders focus on the elimination of barriers and utilize AI to consistently deliver an empowering message, to achieve what matters most. For example, "If you have achieved nursing certification, and

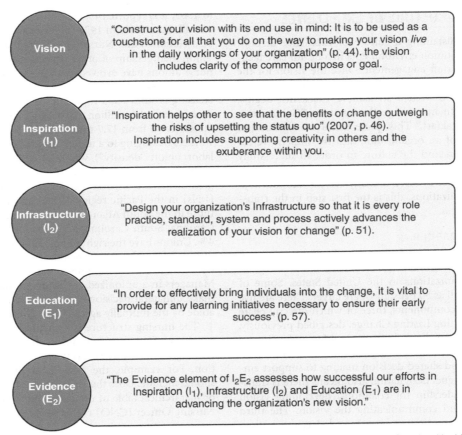

Vision — "Construct your vision with its end use in mind: It is to be used as a touchstone for all that you do on the way to making your vision *live* in the daily workings of your organization" (p. 44). the vision includes clarity of the common purpose or goal.

Inspiration (I_1) — "Inspiration helps other to see that the benefits of change outweigh the risks of upsetting the status quo" (2007, p. 46). Inspiration includes supporting creativity in others and the exuberance within you.

Infrastructure (I_2) — "Design your organization's Infrastructure so that it is every role practice, standard, system and process actively advances the realization of your vision for change" (p. 51).

Education (E_1) — "In order to effectively bring individuals into the change, it is vital to provide for any learning initiatives necessary to ensure their early success" (p. 57).

Evidence (E_2) — "The Evidence element of I_2E_2 assesses how successful our efforts in Inspiration (I_1), Infrastructure (I_2) and Education (E_1) are in advancing the organization's new vision."

Fig. 59.2 I_2E_2: Leading Lasting Change model. (Used with permission. Copyright 2007, Creative Health Care Management. From *I2E2: Leading Lasting Change*. Retrieved from https://shop.chcm.com/I2E2-Leading-Lasting-Change.)

you are competent to care for cardiac telemetry patients, I'm confident you can implement this evidence-based practice change." AI supports the concept of collaborative change rather than the winner/loser paradigm that exists in both unionized and non-union health care environments.

The I_2E_2: Leading Lasting Change embraces AI as a core assumption to igniting the change management process in a positive direction rather than looking at previous practices as failures (Havens, Wood, & Leeman, 2006).

According to the American Hospital Association (AHA), there are 5534 registered hospitals in the United States (AHA, 2019). Of these facilities, 3015 are classified as urban and 1825 as rural (AHA, 2019). The remaining 694 are specialized facilities including psychiatric hospitals, most of which are in urban areas. There are 209 federal government hospitals. The definition of rural and urban is not provided in this resource, but we can surmise that the urban facilities are generally larger and more complex. Most of these hospitals are not unionized. According to the Bureau of Labor Statistics (2017), California and New York have the highest number of unionized health care workers and North Carolina and South Carolina have the lowest. To date, only 8% of all hospitals (482 hospitals) have achieved the Magnet designation from the American Nurses Credentialing Center (ANCC). Administrative leadership in Magnet-designated facilities reflect the management philosophy of the Chief Executive Officers (CEOs) and key executives who embrace a transformational leadership culture and continuously assess the needs of patients, staff, and the communities served. Relationships often will extend into the community where many individuals will know each other through churches, schools, and social activities. These relationships are generally supportive of a high level of trust and clear organizational goals that may make the change process less challenging.

CREATING A CULTURE OF EXCELLENCE

Creating and sustaining a culture of excellence in both union and non-union environments in a health care facility begins with staff engagement. Once the vision for the future has been established, the change process to create the infrastructure needed to achieve excellence begins. Peter Drucker in his change theory states "Culture eats strategy for breakfast." This quote belies the significance of the culture of an organization and the imperative for leaders to understand the culture in order to successfully transform and lead. Although few hospitals have been designated as Magnet by ANCC, many are "on the journey." For many organizations, this is the first step in the transformation process.

Magnet Designation

Magnet designation has been equated with a culture of excellence in nursing and health care. There are 482 Magnet-designated organizations in the United States. Some of these are as small as 50 beds; most are larger. There are five Magnet model components, three of which directly relate to the I_2E_2: Leading Lasting Change, described previously. If an institution has been designated a Magnet facility, we can assume that it has a flat organizational structure with decentralized and shared decision making to support empowerment. Magnet designation also means there is transformational leadership for coalitions, developing vision and strategy, and communicating the vision. The third Magnet model component, new knowledge, innovation, and improvements, reflects the presence of a culture with professional development and the encouragement of the innovations required to design successful change. The ANCC does not keep statistics on how many Magnet hospitals are unionized; however, we know there are more than a few (Moran, 2014).

ASSESSMENT OF SETTING AND STRUCTURE

In order to lead transformational change, it is important for the nurse, manager, or administrator to understand the structure and setting from both the macro and micro perspective of the organization. An urban and/or an academic setting, or union or non-union settings, are elements that influence the structure of the organization.

The Union Setting

Nursing unions are relatively new to hospitals and health care organizations. The first nurses' union was in the 1940s and represented nurses to ensure fair wages. Although there aren't data on nursing union membership rates prior

to 1983, it is reported that health care union membership overall was at 13% in 1974 (Spetz et al., 2011, p. 61); it can be ascertained that Nursing has more than three times the union membership of other private industries. Since then, nurse unions have evolved, with nurse union membership around 18% from 1983 to the mid-1990s, and then increasing around 2005 (Spetz et al., 2011, p. 61). In 2016, there were 14.6 million union members in the United States, down from 17.7 million in 1983. The percentage of workers belonging to a union in the United States (or total labor union "density") was 10.7%, compared to 20.1% in 1983. Union membership also differs according to region, with the highest percentage of registered nurses (RNs) in the Pacific region (43%) and the lowest among those in the South Atlantic region (Florida, Georgia, North Carolina, South Carolina, Virginia, and West Virginia) at 4%. Unions have the right to bargain for benefits and conditions of employment, including an appeal process for decisions related to discipline and termination and layoffs. Managers in a unionized environment may not be able to make unilateral decisions on these key matters and must abide by the mutually agreed upon contract.

The nursing structure is a significant factor of the assessment of an organization, in the composition of the nursing workforce as well as the evolution of the organization. For example, the assessment of the organization should include: Does the department of nursing have a flat or hierarchical table of organization? Who does the Chief Nursing Officer (CNO) report to? Is there a shared governance structure in place?

In a working environment in which there are differing structures, settings, and composition of the nursing workforce, nurses in a management or administrative role need robust leadership skills. Developing skill in emotional intelligence—self-awareness, self-regulation, self-motivation, and social awareness—will be the keys crucial to success.

FORMULA FOR SUCCESS

A deep understanding of the structure and setting of an organization as well as its attributes and characteristics will enable the nurse, manager, or administrator to create a formula for successful navigation to lead transformative change.

There are various methods in which organizations assess and measure a culture. Two of these quantitative methods are the Nurse Engagement Survey through the National Database of National Quality Indicators (NDNQI) and the Culture of Safety Survey through the Agency for Health Care Research and Quality (www.ahrq.gov).

IMPLEMENTING TRANSFORMATIONAL CHANGE

The Case: Pitfalls and Perils, a Transformational Leadership Case Study

Mary Ellen is a Nurse Manager of a 15-bed surgical intensive care unit (SICU) in an academic medical center in San Francisco, California. Mary Ellen has a Master's degree in Nursing Administration and she is Board Certified as Nurse Executive. She has been in her role for the past 3 years. On her team there are 56 RNs, 15 nursing assistants (NAs), and 8 unit secretaries who report to her directly. She manages a $3.6 million salary budget and a $2.5 million non-salary budget. Eighty-six percent of her RN staff have a BSN and 25% are certified Critical Care Nurses. The average tenure of the nursing staff working on this unit is 10 years. The RNs are unionized and belong to the California Nurses Association. The RN turnover on this unit has been not greater than 5% for the past 5 years. The NAs are certified and belong to a different labor union. The unit culture is such that the NAs are not generally considered a strong part of the clinical team. They have not been integrated into shift report with the RNs. Mary Ellen would like to improve communication among the RNs and NAs by implementing bedside handoff that includes the NAs.

Mary Ellen attends a monthly Labor Management meeting along with her Director of Nursing and CNO. A long-term RN delegate is a charge nurse in the SICU and he is the Co-Chair of the Labor Management Committee. At a recent Labor Management meeting, the Director of Nursing shared the most recent Nurse Engagement survey results which revealed that the RNs in the SICU were the least engaged staff by comparison to other units within the hospital and they also fell below the national benchmarks.

Mary Ellen also attends a Council for the NAs that was recently formed by the Director of Nursing. The Nursing Assistants in the hospital expressed a desire to share ideas and concerns across units at the hospital in the hope they could increase their competencies and improve patient and family satisfaction. The Director of Nursing shared her plans for this Council with her management team to re-educate the NAs on the Department of Nursing Relationship-Based Care Model and to understand the concerns they have in the work environment. The Director of Nursing expressed concern over the working relationships between the RNs and the NAs in the ICU and on some other units reporting to her. The CNO acknowledged her concern and stated that this was a theme throughout the hospital, as evidenced by the recently completed Nurse Engagement Survey. The CNO engaged her leadership team and there was a decision along with the hospital president and executive team to transform the hospital and begin a Magnet Journey. Because the issues in the ICU appeared to be most compelling, the CNO decided to begin the transformation in the ICU.

At her agenda meeting with the Director of Nursing, Mary Ellen shares her concerns regarding the working relationships between the RNs and NAs in the ICU. The Director of Nursing advises Mary Ellen that the President and CNO are supporting a Magnet Journey and transformation of the hospital culture. Mary Ellen was informed that her unit would be the first to engage in the transformation process. The CNO and Director of Nursing support Mary Ellen to attend a workshop where she learns how to utilize the I_2E_2: Leading Lasting Change model to transform the culture on her unit.

The first step Mary Ellen takes is to formulate a Vision for Change. The hospital vision states, "The ABC Hospital System's vision is to grow and challenge ourselves to continuously transform health care through exceptional relationship-centered care, leadership, and research for the communities we serve."

The Director of Nursing advises that Mary Ellen organize the creation of a vision for her unit. Mary Ellen understands the value of using her influence with her staff to set the stage for the I_2E_2 change process. She recruits the NA interested in Bedside Handoff and the night RN delegate as change agents. She advises the Unit Physician Chief to join as well. Together they hold an all-staff meeting to review the recent Staff Engagement scores and invites them to join a process of transformation, which will begin with an off-unit retreat and visioning session.

During the meeting, Mary Ellen utilizes AI with her staff when she states, "you are a fantastic team, you have the lowest infection rates in the hospital, now imagine what it would be like if we had the highest nurse engagement scores."

Inspiration (I1). The SICU Surgical ICU team engaged in a visioning process. Their inspiration was drawn from their shared competitive nature to be the unit with the best outcomes and to work together as a team to achieve those outcomes.

The ICU Vision Statement is to provide high quality, relationship-based care to SICU Surgical ICU patients and their families through teamwork and evidence-based practice.

Infrastructure (I2). Mary Ellen and the SICU team gather additional data on high performing work teams, bedside handoff methods, and characteristics of high performing work teams.

They set guiding principles to ensure they remain on course toward their goals. The guiding principles include designing and implementing an RN/NA bedside handoff tool within 1 month, feedback sessions with RNs and NAs to debrief the process, fidelity to the model, and review of patient satisfaction surveys to reveal changes in patient/family perceptions of communication between providers.

Education (E1). All RNs and NAs are educated on the use of the tool and the process for bedside handoff. They complete a learning module and are observed completing handoff by their Manager and the Nurse Educator for a period of 8 weeks.

Evidence (E2). Three months after implementation, the NAs approach Mary Ellen to express that the bedside handoff is working; however, the RNs are still not including them in their daily huddles and they are concerned that their feedback is not being incorporated into the patient plan of care.

At the same time, the RN communication scores on the patient satisfaction survey are improving. The RN delegate raises concern at the Labor Management meeting, and he does not think the project should continue the RN/NA Bedside Handoff.

Mary Ellen and the CNO review the new Patient Satisfaction scores with the Labor Management group, utilizing AI to validate the efforts of the team appear to be working. Upon further discussion, it is revealed that the NAs feel treated as "less than" an equal team member by the RNs.

The Director of Nursing and Mary Ellen work with the Labor Management Committee and both the nursing and ancillary unions commit to support this transformation process by supporting the roll-out of unit-based shared governance models. The union has a strong education base of support for its members and they are aligned with the vision for the future.

A Chair, Co-Chair, and members of the SICU shared governance council were elected by the unit staff. The Chair is an RN and the Co-Chair is an NA. The unit council worked together to evaluate the team-building strategies that would position them for success. Some of these strategies included establishing a unit softball team and a quarterly pizza night out. Mary Ellen and the Union Leadership are included in these team activities.

By the end of year one, the RN/NA bedside report remained a staple of teamwork in the SICU. The success of this was based on a complete transformation of the unit workflow and teamwork. The RNs and NA created a partnership model, the RNs implemented primary nursing, and the team instituted a daily morning phone call to an appointed family member to provide the status of the patient. These interventions yielded an increase in patient/family satisfaction, increased collaboration with the union, and improved teamwork in the SICU.

LESSONS LEARNED

Implementing the Change Decision

The first step of clearly stating the problem to be resolved is crucial or it will not be possible to establish the required sense of urgency. In an organization with a culture of change, problem identification can come from any level. Problems identified by management are clearly their prerogative to solve, ideally with inclusion of key stakeholders. Management should also support problem solving at any level in the organization where steps for successful change are followed and all key stakeholders should be included.

Who will be invited to join the guiding coalition when complex systemic problems are identified? Obviously, those with background information on the issue should be present as well as managers who will have the responsibility of implementing the designated change. Kotter (2012b) emphasizes the need to ascertain commitment from executive-level positions. A change process can be interrupted in the later stages if there is no commitment from the top. Representation from relevant groups that will be affected by the change should also be included. By creating a guiding coalition of thought from leaders from different areas in the organization, there is a stronger ability to define the scope of the problem and to develop strategies for root cause interventions. The implementation of the selected strategies will have greater potential for success when a larger number of stakeholders have a shared understanding of the problem and the rationale for the change. This creates champions for change and increased ability for the problem and strategies to be consistently communicated throughout the organization.

When a union is involved, there will always be an extra voice at the table or, if not present, alert to respond as necessary to any information that is available. The extra voice is that of the elected union leaders within the institution who could be considered ex officio participants in any discussion that may affect their members. They will want to be able to assure the members that they have paid close attention to the protection of their interests. If the issue is one affecting nursing practice, there will be nurses who are union members sitting at the table. The determination of their participation may be defined in the union contract specifying the process for addressing nursing practice issues. Their role is to focus on identifying a best solution to the problem within the union guidelines.

It is important for each working group to understand their level of authority. Does the group have authority to make the decision or are they generating recommendations for change? How will the values of the union and/or the Magnet environments be upheld as groups fulfill their assignments? Although management may feel a sense of urgency in obtaining a solution and/or recommendations for change to the problem, it is important that all possible options be explored. This will be important for union leadership as they communicate the need for the change to their members because they can then assure them that the best possible option was chosen. These steps provide the groundwork for greater acceptance when the change is announced to the entire organization.

Edwards (2017) has identified several reasons why changes may fail, even when the steps of a framework are carefully followed. One reason may be a history of past change initiatives that fell by the wayside for lack of commitment or follow-through. Employees may just decide to wait it out if that tactic has previously been successful in thwarting the outcome. Another factor is trust in the organizational leadership. Trust determines how accurately the change message is perceived, accepted, and actualized.

A lack of trust may be present among those who are resisting the change, and the leaders will need to respect the power of this group. In fact, resistance is a normal part of change. The ability to address the concerns voiced can lead to improved thinking about the problem as well as the interventions. Forums held to discuss a large organizational change should encourage those doubtful of the need for the change or of the interventions to openly discuss their concerns in the hope of increasing buy-in to the change. Often resisters are thought to be leaders who anticipate problems others may have missed and their comments should be heard and evaluated.

EXAMPLES OF CHANGE DECISIONS

Health Care Benefits
Changing the group health insurance carrier for the institution is one example of a change that is a management prerogative. In a nonunion setting, the appropriate executives and managers may search for a new carrier for a variety of reasons. They will review proposals from other companies, compare the benefits, and make a decision. There will likely be staff meetings to announce the decision and explain the rationale. The employees will be more accepting of the changes in their own health care if management has communicated the decision elements clearly.

In a union environment, there will be a separate conversation with the union leaders, who will want to ascertain that no contract violations occur with the change. The employment contract may define what health benefits must be offered to the employee and their family members.

If the union believes contract provisions are violated, grievances may be filed, prolonging the decision-making process. It is therefore better to have the union at the table early in the process.

Changes in Care Delivery
New evidence-based findings are regularly published about health care delivery. When an organization determines that a change in care delivery would be beneficial, the key people at the table must include all the stakeholders affected. Almost all facilities, including those with union contracts, have established practice committees to address patient care issues, and these groups should be key members of the guiding coalition. The union contract may define the composition and qualifications for such committees, although policies and procedures will provide guidelines in nonunion practice environments. The union leaders should be a voice at the table, assuring their members that their interests are being considered and preserved.

CONCLUSION

In conclusion, the implementation of a successful change process is more closely related to the leadership of an organization rather than whether an organization is unionized, a Magnet facility, or, as most acute care facilities are, neither unionized or Magnet. A unionized workplace may add an element of complexity, but it need not be an impediment when there is a known framework for leading or creating organizational change that is consistently followed. The successful implementation of any change builds a foundation to support changes in the future. Organizations that fail to develop that culture will find it difficult to be successful in the evolving world of health care.

DISCUSSION QUESTIONS

1. What limits might management encounter when planning change involving a unionized staff?
2. What do you believe is the most important factor in a successful change initiative?
3. What is the value of using a framework for change in your workplace?

REFERENCES
American Hospital Association. (2019). *Fast facts on US hospitals.* Retrieved from www.aha.org/statistics/fast-facts-us-hospitals.

Anderson, D., & Anderson, L.A. (2001). *Beyond change management.* San Francisco, CA: Jossey-Bass/Pfeiffer,

Bass, B. (1985). *Leadership and performance beyond expectations.* New York: The Free Press.

Bass, B., & Reggio, R. (2006). *Transformational leadership.* Mahwah, NJ: Lawrence Erlbaum.

Blackard, K. (2000). *Managing change in a unionized workplace.* Westport, CT: Quorum Books.

Bureau of Labor Statistics (2017). *Union members—2018.* Retrieved from www.bls.gov/news.release/pdf/union2.pdf.

Burns, G.M. (1978). *Leadership.* New York: Harper & Row.

Burns, G.M. (2003). *Transforming leadership.* New York: Atlantic Monthly Press.

Chinn, P.L., & Kramer, M.K., (2011). *Integrated theory and knowledge development in nursing* (8th ed.). St. Louis: Mosby/Elsevier.

Commins, J. (2012, January 3). Why do nurses join unions? Because they can. *HealthLeaders Media.* Retrieved from www.nationalnursesunited.org/news/why-do-nurses-join-unions-because-they-can.

Cooperrider, D.L., Whitney, D., & Stavros, J.M. (2008). *Appreciative Inquiry handbook: For leaders of change* (2nd ed.). San Francisco, CA: Berrett-Koehler Publishers.

Edwards, M.T. (2017). An organizational learning framework for patient safety. *American Journal of Medical Quality, 32*(2), 148–155.

Felgen, J. (2007). *I₂E₂: Leading lasting change.* Minneapolis, MN: Creative Health Care Management. Retrieved from http://chcm.com/the-i2e2-formula.

Fischer, S.A. (2016) Transformational leadership in nursing: A concept analysis. *Journal of Advanced Nursing, 72*(11), 2644–2653.

Havens, D.S., Wood, S.O., & Leeman, J. (2006, October). *JONA: Journal of Nursing Administration, 36*(10), 463-470.

Koloroutis, M. (2004). *Relationship-based care: A model for transforming practice.* Minneapolis, MN: Creative Healthcare Management.

Kotter, J. (2007, January). Leading change: Why transformation efforts fail. *Harvard Business Review, 85*(1), 96-103. Available from Business Source Complete, Ipswich, MA.

Kotter, J. (2012a). *The 8-step process for leading change.* Kotter International. Retrieved from www.kotterinternational.com/our-principles/changesteps.

Kotter, J. (2012b). *Leading change.* Boston: Harvard Business Review Press.

Moberg, D. (2013, February 20). Are mergers the answer for fractious nurses? *In These Times.* Retrieved from inthesetimes.com/working/entry/14631/are_mergers_the_answer_for_nurses_unions.

Spetz, J., Ash, M., Konstantinidis, C., & Herrera, C. (2011). The effect of unions on the distribution of wages of hospital-employed registered nurses in the United States. *Journal of Clinical Nursing, 20*(1-2), 60-66.

ONLINE RESOURCES

American Hospital Association
www.aha.org
American Nurses Credentialing Center
www.nursecredentialing.org
Find a Magnet Facility
www.nursingworld.org/organizational-programs/magnet/find-a-magnet-facility/

60

Political Context of Advanced Practice Nursing

Andrea Brassard

> *"Politically, NPs have been a force to be reckoned with in demanding legislation for freedom to practice"*
>
> **Loretta Ford, co-founder of the first nurse practitioner program in the United States**

As defined in Chapter 1, "*Politics* is the use of relationships and power to gain ascendancy among competing stakeholders to influence policy and the allocation of scarce resources. Because inevitably there are competing interests for scarce resources, policymaking is done within a political context." Political context includes finding out who is influential among competing stakeholders. Advanced practice registered nurses (APRNs) may avoid politics and the policymaking process because "politics introduces divisive and self-interested agendas into the policymaking process. This resistance to APRNs by organized physician groups is a quintessential definition of politics: the struggle for ascendancy or dominance among groups with different power relationships and agendas" (O'Grady & Ford, 2016, p. 542). This chapter describes how APRNs are navigating the political system and using relationships to influence policy.

ADVANCED PRACTICE REGISTERED NURSE PRACTICE, FEDERAL AND STATE LAWS

As outlined in Chapter 15, the federal government is heavily involved in the organization, financing, and delivery of health care (Hendrickson & Schrauf, 2016, p. 367). Federal laws enacted by Congress include Medicare and Medicaid, both governed by the U.S. Department of Health and Human Services. Other federal agencies that impact APRN practice include the Centers for Disease Control and Prevention, the Federal Employees Health Benefits Program, the Federal Trade Commission (FTC), the U.S. Food and Drug Administration, National Institutes of Health, and

Veterans Affairs. The largest source of dedicated funding for APRN education is Title VIII Nursing Workforce Development. Other sources of federal funding for APRN education and training include the National Health Service Corps and the U.S. Public Health Service (Miyamoto, 2018).

Nurses can refer to Chapter 39 to learn how nurses can be involved at every step of the federal legislative process. The American Nurses Association (ANA) and national APRN organizations include federal advocacy links on their websites and send out action alerts to members detailing how to contact their legislators about specific legislation.

Influencing regulation is as important as influencing legislation. Refer to Chapter 39 to learn the federal regulatory process. In the states, boards of nursing regulate APRN practice through nurse practice acts and other laws and regulations. Although organized nursing has tried to standardize APRN licensure for more than a decade through the APRN Consensus Model (Pappas, Kowalski, & Denholm, 2016), states vary widely in APRN practice provisions. State boards of nursing differ in how they are composed and where they are positioned within the state's regulatory structure (Filipovich, 2018). Nationally, about half of the boards of nursing are part of an umbrella structure of state boards or departments; the other half are independent agencies within state governments, except for North Carolina, which is an independent agency outside of state government. Nebraska has a separate APRN board (National Council of State Boards of Nursing [NCSBN], 2018), and many state boards of nursing have mandated or appointed APRNs to their boards.

ASSESSING PROGRESS ON THE INSTITUTE OF MEDICINE REPORT RECOMMENDATION

The 2011 landmark report by the Institute of Medicine (IOM; now the National Academy of Medicine) titled *The Future of Nursing: Leading Change, Advancing Health* has been a game changer for APRNs. Its first recommendation was to remove scope-of-practice barriers: "Nurses should practice to the full extent of their education and training" (IOM, 2011, p. 4). Federal and state progress toward removing scope-of-practice barriers since the release of the IOM report has been slow but steady, as documented in the 2016 National Academies of Science, Engineering and Medicine (NASEM) report, *Assessing Progress on the Institute of Medicine Report the Future of Nursing* (NASEM, 2016).

The progress report highlighted the anti-discrimination provision of the Patient Protection and Affordable Care Act (ACA) that prohibits health insurers from denying coverage for services provided by APRNs. The ACA also included health service delivery provisions that expanded APRN practice and care. Section 3114 increased the Medicare reimbursement rate for Certified Nurse-Midwives (CNMs) for covered services from 65% of the rate that would be paid were a physician performing a service to the same rate (100%) as physicians ([ANA], 2014). Although Medicare payment for CNM services is relatively small, this is a symbolic victory. Medicare reimbursement for nurse practitioner (NP) and clinical nurse specialist (CNS) services remains at 85% of the rate of physician services.

In 2015, federal legislation known as the "doc fix" included language that removed a major barrier to durable medical equipment authorization by APRNs. This bill also confirmed that Patient Centered Medical Homes led by APRNs can receive incentive payments for managing patients with chronic disease (American Association of Nurse Practitioners [AANP], 2015).

The 2016 Comprehensive Addiction and Recovery Act (CARA) authorized NPs to prescribe buprenorphine (medication-assisted treatment [MAT]) to patients with opioid addictions, but only for a 5-year pilot period (AANP, 2016). The 2018 "SUPPORT for Patients and Communities Act" makes the NP provision permanent and gives temporary authority to CNMs, certified registered nurse anesthetists (CRNAs) and CNSs to provide MAT. This authority expires on October 1, 2023. The APRN authority to provide MAT must be consistent with any APRN state laws (NACNS, 2018).

Turning to progress at the Veterans Health Administration (VHA), Cathy Rick, the former chief nursing officer of the VHA, responded to the IOM report by recommending that APRNs practice to the full extent of their education and training in all VHA facilities in all states and territories. This federal preemption—when federal laws conflict with state laws, federal law prevails—was already in place for APRNs employed by the Department of Defense and Indian Health Services. This recommendation to allow APRNs full practice authority throughout the VHA was added to the revised Nursing Handbook, distributed electronically in 2012. Although this recommendation could have been implemented by VHA leadership, political pressure moved the regulation deeper into the federal regulatory process. Four years later, in 2016, a final regulation was published in the *Federal Register*. The regulation allows VHA NPs, CNSs, and CNMs to practice to the full extent of their education and training without the supervision of a physician, regardless of the practice restrictions in the state where the Veterans Administration (VA) facility is located. CRNAs were excluded. The regulation stated that the CRNA exclusion "does not stem from the CRNAs' inability to practice to the full extent of their professional competence, but rather from VA's lack of access problems in the area of anesthesiology" (U.S. Veterans Affairs Department, 2016, p. 90199). This statement contradicted two reports describing anesthesia shortages that were submitted to the VHA prior to the final regulation (American Association of Nurse Anesthetists, 2017). The VHA decision to deny full practice authority to CRNAs—past and future—is political, arising from pressure from anesthesiologists seeking to protect their supremacy in anesthesia care.

Implementation of full practice authority for the three APRN roles in the VHA has been uneven. The VHA allowed individual health systems to determine whether full practice authority would be implemented in their health system. As of 2018, 70 VA health systems had fully implemented full practice authority, 60 VA health systems were moving toward implementation, and 6 VA health systems had no plans to implement full practice authority (S. Thorne-Odem, personal communication, November 5, 2018). The 2018–19 Department of Veterans Affairs funding bill was passed with language directing the VA Secretary to work with those VA hospitals that have not yet implemented full practice authority for APRNs.

PERSISTENT FEDERAL BARRIERS

The 2011 IOM report had several specific recommendations for removing federal barriers to APRN practice and care. Barriers in two Medicare settings, home health services and skilled nursing facilities (SNFs), greatly impact APRNs. Medicare home health services are only provided upon physician certification. To change this outdated

Medicare regulation, federal legislation is needed. As of 2018, S. 445/H.R. 1825, the Home Health Planning and Improvement bill, had bipartisan Congressional sponsors and strong support from APRN advocates, including AARP, the American Association of Home Care Medicine, and the American Geriatrics Association (American College of Nurse-Midwives [ACNM], 2017). Similar bills have been introduced in prior Congresses but have not moved forward due to the lack of a Congressional Budget Office (CBO) score, with the perception that allowing APRNs to certify Medicare home health services would increase costs as access increased. The Gerontological Advanced Practice Nurses Association is leading a task force of advocacy experts to approach removing this long-standing barrier using several approaches (S. Mullaney, personal communication, November 14, 2018).

In SNFs, APRNs are prohibited from conducting the admission history and physical under Medicare and can only bill for "physician services" every other month. The AANP points out the inappropriate restrictions do not apply to other long-term care nursing facilities, only to Medicare beneficiaries in SNFs (AANP, 2018a). Although legislation is also needed to modernize these arbitrary rules, no bills have been put forward.

In two ambulatory settings that are federally regulated—community health centers and rural health clinics—APRNs provide large numbers of patient visits but are prohibited from serving as medical directors.

FEDERAL TRADE COMMISSION

The FTC has been a strong advocate for removing barriers to APRN practice and care. *The Future of Nursing* report called on the FTC to "review existing and proposed state regulations concerning APRNs to identify those that have anticompetitive effects without contributing to the health and safety of the public" (IOM, 2011, p. 10). Since the release of the IOM report, the FTC provided analyses and comments to legislators in more than a dozen states. In 2014, the FTC released a paper "Policy Perspectives: Competition and the Regulation of Advanced Practice Nurses" that built on the state letters and expanded their recommendations nationwide. The FTC advised state legislators to be mindful when considering legislation that limits access to care provided by APRNs and concluded that "expanded APRN scope of practice is good for competition and American consumers" (FTC, 2014, p. 42). The 2015 Assessing Progress report listed additional states where the FTC provided letters, comments, and/or testimony directed to state legislators (NASEM, 2015), and the FTC continues to respond to proposed state legislation.

STATE PROGRESS IN INCREASING ACCESS TO APRN CARE

As outlined in Chapter 71, the *Campaign for Action* at the Center to Champion Nursing in America at AARP is an initiative of AARP Foundation, AARP, and the Robert Wood Johnson Foundation. The Campaign provides resources to AARP state offices and other advocacy organizations promoting state legislation to modernize APRN practice laws. Since the publication of the IOM report, nine states have modernized their laws to grant NPs full practice authority. Six additional states have made substantial progress toward NP full practice authority, but administrative barriers remain (Fig. 60.1).

The NCSBN tracks progress toward state implementation of the APRN Consensus Model. State implementation of the APRN Consensus Model includes independent practice and prescribing for all four APRN roles. This has been achieved by 15 states to date. Recently, NCSBN has funded research, messaging, and media in several restricted states through their Nursing America campaign (http://nursingamerica.org).

Unfortunately, after state legislation is enacted to modernize APRN scope of practice, other policy barriers continue. Two major policy barriers are not being credentialed by insurance companies and not having hospital privileges. Most state Medicaid programs credential APRNs but Medicaid reimbursement for APRN services differs among states. The reimbursement rate for NP services is equal to the physicians' rate in some states but it is as low as 75% of the physicians' rate in other states (Kaiser Family Foundation, 2012). States that have enacted Medicaid managed care programs may not include APRNs as designated primary care providers. Legislation is needed in several states to designate NPs and CNMs as primary care providers to increase the utilization and reimbursement of APRNs in state Medicaid programs (AANP, 2013).

INSURANCE COMPANY CREDENTIALING

CNMs also have challenges in fee-for-service reimbursement. Although CNMs gained 100% Medicare reimbursement in a provision of the ACA (Walker, Lannen, & Rossie, 2014) and most Medicaid programs now reimburse CNMs at 100% of physician rate (ACNM, 2018a), these payment victories have not improved private insurers' coverage of and reimbursement to CNMs (Walker et al., 2014).

Insurance companies vary greatly in whether or not they credential or contract with APRNs; and if they do,

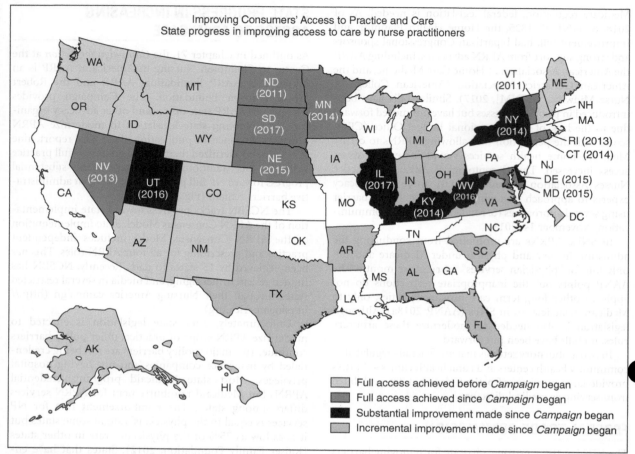

Improving Consumers' Access to Practice and Care
State progress in improving access to care by nurse practitioners

Legend:
- Full access achieved before *Campaign* began
- Full access achieved since *Campaign* began
- Substantial improvement made since *Campaign* began
- Incremental improvement made since *Campaign* began

For more detail about the practice environment for all types of APRNs, see the National Council of State Boards of Nursing's maps: https://www.ncsbn.org/5397.htm.
View definition criteria at https://campaignforaction.org/resource/state-progress-removing-barriers-practice-care.

Updated: September 19, 2018   Years denote when laws were passed.

Fig. 60.1 State progress in removing barriers to practice and care. (Source: *Future of Nursing: Campaign for Action*. Retrieved from https://campaignforaction.org/resource/state-progress-removing-barriers-practice-care/.)

whether APRNs are reimbursed at the same rate as physician providers for the same services, or at a discount rate. Not only is there variation among insurance companies, but the same insurance company may vary in APRN credentialing and reimbursement in different geographic regions and under different insurance plans that it provides. The National Nursing Centers Consortium has tracked whether managed care organizations (MCOs) contract with NPs for several years. Surveys conducted in 2017 found that 25% of MCOs did not credential NPs as primary care providers (Bellot et al., 2017). To help remove insurance barriers, the Advanced Practice Nurse Multistate

Reimbursement Alliance (MRSA) tracks insurance credentialing, contracting, and reimbursement through the AANPs (AANP, 2018b).

HOSPITAL PRIVILEGES

Being able to admit their patients to hospitals is essential for APRNs, particularly CNMs (Brassard & Smolenski, 2011). The 2011 IOM report called on the Center for Medicare and Medicaid Services (CMS) to ensure that APRNs are eligible for clinical privileges, admitting privileges, and medical staff membership. CMS issued a final rule in 2012 that allows "other practitioners (e.g., APRNs, PAs, pharmacists) to perform all functions within their scope of practice" (CMS, Department of Health and Human Services, 2012, p. 29034). Despite this CMS rule, individual hospitals are not prohibited from denying privileges and medical staff membership to APRNs. The ACNM reports on their website that all states except Maryland "have laws or regulations that explicitly or implicitly allow CNMs to admit patients to a hospital. [However] even where state laws allow these actions, individual hospitals may not, or may allow privileging only with physician supervision" (ACNM, 2018b). Hospital privileges are essential for CNMs who practice obstetrics to ensure pregnant women have full and direct access to midwifery care in all settings. ACNM advocates have proposed federal law to remove this barrier, but legislation has not moved.

PHYSICIAN OPPOSITION

The NP role was developed by nurse educator Loretta Ford and pediatrician Henry Silver with mutual respect and collaboration (O'Grady & Ford, 2016). As the numbers of NPs and other APRNs increased, so did physician opposition to APRN autonomy. The release of the 2011 IOM *The Future of Nursing* report was followed by opposition from organized medicine, as medical societies spoke out against the report's recommendation to remove scope-of-practice barriers. Five years later, the *Assessing Progress on the Institute of Medicine Report the Future of Nursing* found that APRNs (1) provide high-quality care to patients, (2) progress has been made toward expanding scope of practice for APRNs, either fully or incrementally, but (3) physician organizations' opposition to expansion of scope of practice for APRNs remains a significant obstacle. The 2016 report recommended that legislative work to remove scope of practice continue through a broad coalition of APRNs, their advocates, and more diverse stakeholders.

O'Grady and Ford (2016, p. 545) called out physician opposition to APRN practice as "tired and sclerotic." Physician organizations claim that APRN practice is harmful to the public, but this has been discredited by decades of research. Physicians testifying at legislative hearings on APRN scope of practice promote outdated, single-setting, physician-authored research studies that question the quality of APRN care. O'Grady and Ford (2016) quote nursing historian Joan Lynaugh, who says, "Declare victory and move on!" (p. 545). No state that has modernized its laws has reported patient safety concerns, increased rates of APRN malpractice, or serious legislative attempts to return to restricted practice. Although physician opposition cannot be ignored in the political arena, broader coalitions and effective messaging can overcome unfounded claims.

MEDIA AND MESSAGING

The term *"independent practice"* has been a rallying cry for physician opponents despite APRN messages that no health professionals practice independently. To counter the rhetoric, the AANP at first substituted "plenary authority" and now uses "full practice authority." The Association's message is that consumers will have full and direct access to NPs.

The consumer voice is powerful in the political arena (White, 2016). By framing scope of practice advocacy as a consumer issue, the Campaign for Action helped eight states achieve NP full practice authority since 2010 and worked with more than a dozen states to remove significant barriers to APRN. In each of these legislative victories, AARP state offices have messaged modernizing APRN scope of practice as increasing access to care for consumers, patients, and family caregivers.

Advocates need to frame messages in line with stakeholder and policymaker values. Frame messages around other state and local issues. For example, in states with large populations of Medicaid and Medicare beneficiaries, the message should focus on improving clinical and financial outcomes for "dual eligible"—those qualifying for both programs. In states with multiple Health Services and Resources Administration (HRSA) primary care shortage areas (HRSA, 2018), the message may be about APRN primary care providers and should weave in data about state health measures. Increasing access to care by removing barriers to APRN practice is a strong message to legislators in states that rank low on United Health Foundation's America's Health Rankings. Indeed, United Health Group's Center for Nursing Achievement found that states with low health rankings were more likely to have required physician oversight of NPs (United Health Group, 2016).

As the political climate nationally and in the states changed directions, the Future of Nursing: *Campaign for Action* promoted coalition building and messaging to conservative-leaning policymakers. Outdated scope of practice laws were framed as government overreach and restraint of free trade. Benefits of modernizing legislation include increasing provider choice, cutting red tape, and reducing regulations. Two examples of states with recent successful legislation, Nebraska and West Virginia, organized broad coalitions of diverse stakeholders such as Americans for Prosperity, Farm Bureaus, Hospital Associations, Rural Health Associations, and School Boards. In West Virginia, AARP West Virginia took the lead to promote legislation as increasing access for consumers and their family caregivers,

BOX 60.1 Messaging Do's and Don'ts	
Do	**Don't**
Keep it simple	Don't complain about physicians or make this about nurses versus physicians
Speak about the impact on patients (consumers, constituents)	Don't be defensive
Use real examples of the benefits of full practice authority (patients, costs)	Don't give complicated explanations or use health care jargon
Use real examples of the burdens of restricted practice (amount spent on contracts, delays/disruptions to patient care)	Don't talk about independent practice or replacing physicians

aligning their messages with a legislature that had flipped from Democratic to Republican control (see Chapter 62). When journalists cast scope of practice legislation as a doctor/nurse turf battle, consumer advocates respectfully praise both physicians and nurses and change the message (Gutman, 2016).

The Future of Nursing: *Campaign for Action* and the AANP organized several in-person meetings to educate APRNs and consumer advocates on "Winning Strategies for Full Practice Authority for Advanced Practice Registered Nurses." Attendees practiced messaging to prospective coalition partners and legislatures. Examples of messaging "do's and don'ts" are featured in Box 60.1.

POLITICAL STRATEGY AND TACTICS

Resources from the FTC and the National Governors Association have strategic significance. As mentioned previously, the FTC has been a source of support for APRN legislative work. When contacted by state legislators, the FTC will review proposed legislation and send a message about how the legislation could impact competition and consumers. The National Governors Association's report "The Role of NPs in Meeting Increasing Demand for Primary Care" (National Governors Association, 2012) offers a positive perspective on NPs. Both Nebraska and West Virginia referred to this report in their successful efforts to improve their states' laws. Support from the governor is vital for advancing state legislation.

A united nursing voice is essential. Legislators assume that the state affiliate of the ANA speaks for the nursing profession in their state. ANA advocates for APRNs and RNs nationally and this is true for most state nurses' associations. In a few states, the state nurses' association has an APRN coalition.

Legislators look to state boards of nursing when APRN scope of practice legislation is in session. State boards of nursing vary in whether they can propose legislation or lobby, but every board of nursing can respond to policymakers' questions about APRN practice and thus function as educators.

National, state, and local membership organizations represent all the APRN roles and specialties, although not every national APRN organization has a state affiliate. One strategy that was successful in Minnesota and is being replicated in Wisconsin and other states is a state-wide APRN umbrella organization. The Minnesota APRN Coalition functioned as the center point of communication for the state's APRNs and charged nominal dues, but the large number of members supported an effective lobbyist. Another key tactic of the Minnesota APRN Coalition was connecting individual APRNs and APRN students with their legislators, as legislators are more likely to respond to constituent contacts.

Because states vary widely in how each APRN role is regulated with or without physician oversight, legislative efforts to remove barriers to APRN practice may focus on just one or two of the four APRN roles. Whether or not all four APRN roles are included in proposed legislation, it is important that all state APRN organizations and their lobbyists communicate positive messages about the other APRN roles.

The state APRN coalition needs to include partners beyond nursing and health care providers. Recruiting and mobilizing diverse coalition partners requires networking, connecting, timing, and sustained effort. Involving students adds energy and creativity. Although organized medicine continues to oppose APRN legislation, a few supportive physicians can be recruited to provide oral or written testimony supporting collaboration in the best sense of the word.

Political advocacy often starts in policy course work and membership in professional organizations. Serving on the organization's government affairs or political action committee is a logical next step. Committee leadership will follow, plus networking with other state and national leaders. Experienced nurse advocates should aspire to political office. The number of nurses serving in local, state, and federal government is small but growing.

All APRNs should take an active role in removing barriers to practice to increase access to high quality, cost effective care. Policy barriers are apparent at the practice, health system, state, and federal levels. Individual APRNs working in coalitions with consumers, businesses, and organizations can use political strategy and tactics to lead change and advance health.

DISCUSSION QUESTIONS

1. Examine the APRN scope of practice laws and regulations in your state. To what extent do these permit APRNs to practice to the full extent of their education and training?
2. What other legal or regulatory barriers do APRNs in your state face, including federal ones?
3. Design a strategy for removing barriers to APRNs in your state being able to have full practice authority, without federal or state or private sector barriers.

REFERENCES

American Association of Nurse Practitioners. (2013). *Fact sheet: Medicaid managed care.* Retrieved from www.aanp.org/68-articles/352-medicaid-managed-care.

American Association of Nurse Practitioners. (2015). *Nurse practitioners applaud SGR repeal in U.S. House of Representatives.* Retrieved from www.aanp.org/press-room/press-releases/166-press-room/2015-press-releases/1697-nurse-practitioners-applaud-sgr-repeal-in-u-s-house-of-representatives.

American Association of Nurse Practitioners. (2016). *Comprehensive Addiction and Recovery Act (CARA).* Retrieved from www.aanp.org/education/2131comprehensive-addiction-and-recovery-act.

American Association of Nurse Practitioners. (2018a). *Improve patient access to Medicare skilled nursing care.* Retrieved from www.aanp.org/images/documents/federal-legislation/issuebriefs/Issue%20Brief%20-%20Improve%20Patient%20Access%20to%20Medicare%20Skilled%20Nursing%20Care.pdf.

American Association of Nurse Practitioners. (2018b). *Multistate Reimbursement Alliance.* Retrieved from www.aanp.org/practice/msra.

American College of Nurse-Midwives. (2017). *Group letter of support for the Home Health Planning Improvement Act.* Retrieved from www.midwife.org/acnm/files/ccLibraryFiles/Filename/000000006638/hhc518.pdf.

American College of Nurse-Midwives. (2018a). *Essential facts about midwives.* Retrieved from www.midwife.org/Essential-Facts-about-Midwives.

American College of Nurse-Midwives. (2018b). *Hospital credentialing and privileging.* Retrieved from www.midwife.org/Hospital-Credentialing-and-Privileging.

American Nurses Association. (2014). *Health care reform.* Retrieved from www.nursingworld.org/~4afc9b/globalassets/practiceandpolicy/health-policy/healthcare-reform-document.pdf.

Bellot, J., Valdez, B., Altdoerffer, K., Quiaoit, Y., Bronzell-Wynder, T., & Cunningham, P. (2017). Does contracting with managed care organizations remain a barrier for nurse practitioners? *Nursing Economics, 35*(2), 57-63.

Brassard, A., & Smolenski, M. (2011). *Removing barriers to advanced practice registered nurse care: hospital privileges.* Retrieved from www.aarp.org/health/doctors-hospitals/info-10-2011/Removing-Barriers-to-Advanced-Practice-Registered-Nurse-Care-Hospital-Privileges.html.

Centers for Medicare and Medicaid Services, Department of Health and Human Services. (2012, May 16). Medicare and Medicaid Programs: Reform of hospital and critical access hospital conditions of participation, *Federal Register, 77*(95), 29034–29076. Retrieved from www.cms.gov/Regulations-and-Guidance/Legislation/CFCsAndCoPs/Downloads/CMS-3244-F.pdf.

Federal Trade Commission. (2014). *Policy perspectives: Competition and the regulation of advanced practice nurses.* Retrieved from www.ftc.gov/system/files/documents/reports/policy-perspectives-competition-regulation-advanced-practice-nurses/140307aprnpolicypaper.pdf.

Filipovich, C.C. (2018). Effective state-level APRN leadership in health policy. In K.A. Goudreau & M.C. Smolenski (Eds.), *Health policy and advanced practice nursing* (2nd ed., pp. 79-92). New York: Springer.

Gutman, D. (2016, February 14). Bipartisan nursing bill could help ease rural health care shortages. *Charleston Gazette-Mail.* Retrieved from www.wvgazettemail.com/business/bipartisan-nursing-bill-could-help-ease-rural-health-care-shortages/article_d31a204e-3e72-5ae3-afe0-042173a8bc09.html.

Health Services and Resources Administration. (2018). *Health professional shortage areas (HPSAs).* Retrieved from https://bhw.hrsa.gov/shortage-designation/hpsas.

Hendrickson, K.C. & Strauf, C.C. (2016). How government works: What you need to know to influence the process in policy and politics. In D.J. Mason, D.B. Gardner, F.H. Outlaw & E.T. O'Grady (Eds.), *Policy & politics in nursing and health care* (7th ed., pp. 356-369). St. Louis: Elsevier.

Institute of Medicine. (2011). *The future of nursing: Leading change, advancing health.* Retrieved from www.nationalacademies.org/hmd/Reports/2010/The-Future-of-Nursing-Leading-Change-Advancing-Health.aspx.

Kaiser Family Foundation. (2012). *Medicaid benefits: Nurse practitioner services.* Retrieved from www.kff.org/medicaid/state-indicator/nurse-practitioner-services/?currentTimeframe=0&sortModel=%7B%22colId%22:%22Location%22,%22sort%22:%22asc%22%7D.

Miyamoto, S. (2018) Funding of APRN education and residency programs. In K.A. Goudreau & M.C. Smolenski (Eds.), *Health policy and advanced practice nursing* (2nd ed., pp. 141-160). New York: Springer.

National Academies of Sciences, Engineering, and Medicine. (2016). *Assessing progress on the Institute of Medicine report The Future of Nursing.* Washington, DC: The National Academies Press.

National Association of Clinical Nurse Specialists. (2018). *Nurse leader applauds enactment of opioid bill.* Retrieved from https://nacns.org/2018/10/nurse-leader-applauds-enactment-of-opioid-bill-calling-it-a-measure-the-country-urgently-needs/.

National Council of State Boards of Nursing. (2018). *Member boards*. Retrieved from www.ncsbn.org/member-boards.htm.

National Governors Association. (2012). *The role of nurse practitioners in meeting increased demand for primary care*. Retrieved from https://classic.nga.org/cms/home/nga-center-for-best-practices/center-publications/page-health-publications/col2-content/main-content-list/the-role-of-nurse-practitioners.html.

O'Grady, E.T., & Ford, L.C. (2016). The politics of advanced practice nursing in policy and politics. In D.J. Mason, D.B. Gardner, F.H. Outlaw & E.T. O'Grady (Eds.), *Policy & politics in nursing and health care* (7th ed., pp. 542-560). St. Louis: Elsevier.

Pappas, S., Kowalski, K., & Denholm, E.M. (2016). Policy and politics in health care organizations. In D.J. Mason, D.B. Gardner, F.H. Outlaw & E.T. O'Grady (Eds.), *Policy & politics in nursing and health care* (7th ed., pp. 469-477). St. Louis: Elsevier.

United Health Group. (2016). *Correlation between nurse practitioner (NP) scope of practice and overall health rankings, by state*. Retrieved from www.unitedhealthgroup.com/content/dam/UHG/PDF/About/CFCA-Practice-Environment-Health-Rankings-Correlation.pdf.

U.S. Veterans Affairs Department. (2016, December 14). Advanced practice registered nurses, *Federal Register*, 81 FR 90198, pp. 90198-90207. Retrieved from www.federalregister.gov/documents/2016/12/14/2016-29950/advanced-practice-registered-nurses.

Walker, D., Lannen, B., & Rossie, D. (2014). Midwifery practice and education: Current challenges and opportunities. *Online Journal of Issues in Nursing, 19*, 2.

White, K.M. (2016). Political analysis and strategies. In D.J. Mason, D.B. Gardner, F.H. Outlaw & E.T. O'Grady (Eds.), *Policy & politics in nursing and health care* (7th ed., pp. 80-90). St. Louis: Elsevier.

ONLINE RESOURCES

Future of Nursing: Campaign for Action
https://campaignforaction.org
Nursing America
https://nursingamerica.org

61

TAKING ACTION: Never Underestimate the Power of a Personal Story

Danielle Howa Pendergrass

At the age of 16, I realized that my rural Utah community desperately needed women's health services. My friends and I would travel over 100 miles to reach the nearest provider. At my first visit, I met a women's health nurse practitioner (NP) who changed the trajectory of my life. It was then I decided I wanted to be "that nurse" and vowed to open a practice to care for the women in my community.

Fast forward 20 years. I was living and working in California as a women's health NP, and I wanted to return home to raise my son with family and the social cohesion that small towns bring. At the time, my community was devoid of a single women's health care provider due to difficulties in recruitment and retention of physicians in my designated health care provider shortage area (HPSA). I started reaching out to local providers and the hospital, only to discover they were not accepting the NP role and refused to hire a "mid-level provider." Faced with this opposition, the implementation of the Patient Protection and Affordable Care Act (ACA), and an article about the future of nursing, I returned to my community and became the first woman and first NP in the history of our area to own a practice solely dedicated to women.

Eastern Utah Women's Health opened in late 2012 and currently offers services to over 20,000 vulnerable and underserved women spanning three large rural counties. With the mission statement of "Healthcare for ALL Women," I contracted with insurance companies and secured local, state, and federal funding to ensure *all* women had access to affordable health care. I understood that it "takes a village" and as part of my business plan began to build bridges between health and other factors that influence the lives of women. I partnered with the health department, behavioral health, the Children's Justice Center, corrections, parks and recreation, our local university, and the business community. My community of diverse partners embraced this new way of working together to better the lives of women and girls.

THE PROBLEM

One aspect of setting up a practice is contracting with insurance companies. My practice was rapidly growing, and it was not long before I encountered a significant policy and payment barrier that would shape my career and NP practice. I was unable to get paneled with Medicaid. I started researching and discovered that Utah's Medicaid Policy contained language that only recognized pediatric and family NPs, certified nurse midwives, and certified registered nurse anesthetists as eligible Medicaid providers. The policy excluded NPs with a specialty in adult, acute care, geriatric, neonatal, psychiatric/mental health, and women's health.

Although Utah's laws and regulations allow NPs to practice independently, except for a required consultation and referral agreement to prescribe controlled substances II and III, the Utah Medicaid Policy did not parallel the Utah Nurse Practice Act (2013). Utah's Medicaid policy included language that required a collaborative practice agreement for eligible NPs. The policy went on to require NPs to bill "under a physician" (Medicaid.gov, 2012, p. 2–3), thus preventing NPs from directly billing and reimbursement by Medicaid.

I knew I had to do something about this policy barrier. After all, my mission statement was "Healthcare for ALL Women," and my county had the most Medicaid-eligible citizens in the state. Knowing this demographic, I realized this was going to be detrimental to the women who needed it most. But I had never changed a policy before.

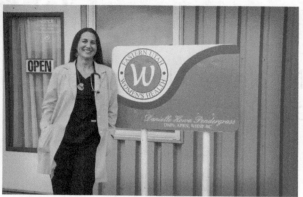

Danielle Howa Pendergrass welcoming women to her clinic in Price, Utah.

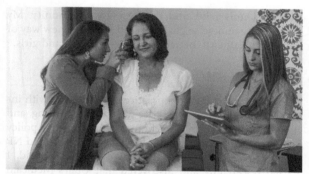

Danielle Howa Pendergrass and her team providing high-quality, cost-effective, person-centered care.

BACKGROUND

In an attempt to recognize NPs as viable providers for the increasing numbers of Medicaid beneficiaries, the Balanced Budget Act (BBA) of 1997 (BBA, P.L. 105-33) made changes to Medicaid law and inadvertently created new barriers to NP practice (American Nurses Association, 2011). The BBA only recognized certified nurse midwives, family, and pediatric NPs as eligible Medicaid providers (Department of Health and Human Services, Office of the Inspector General, 2001). The rationale for choosing three types of NPs is not detailed in the laws or literature. The exclusionary 1997 BBA has not changed but now asserts states have their own discretion to "open up" provider enrollment to all providers, including NPs (American Nurses Association, 2011).

In its 2011 landmark report, *The Future of Nursing: Leading Change, Advancing Health*, the Institute of Medicine (IOM) makes several recommendations regarding NP payment practices. The IOM recommends that states "Require third-party payers that participate in fee-for-service

payment arrangements to provide direct reimbursement to advanced practice registered nurses who are practicing within their scope of practice under state law" (2010, p. 1). The IOM also recommends "Extending the increase in Medicaid reimbursement rates for primary care physicians included in the ACA to advanced practice registered nurses providing similar primary care services" (2010, p. 1).

COMMITMENT TO CHANGE

In 2010, the Utah Medical Education Council (UMEC) reported that 23 of Utah's 29 counties met the criteria for Primary Care HPSA designations (Association of American Medical Colleges [AAMC], 2012). Yet, physician participation in Medicaid was already low, and with fewer physicians practicing in lower income, rural, and underserved communities, the health care needs of Medicaid beneficiaries were continuing to go unmet (Garcia, 2013). There was an acute need for more primary care providers, particularly in my currently underserved area where many newly eligible Medicaid beneficiaries were likely to reside (Muller, Coburn, Lundblad, MacKinney, McBride, & Watson, 2012).

I was turning away several Medicaid beneficiaries on a daily basis due to my inability to get paneled. Like many nurses, I tried to find a workaround. The language in the policy states that I could hire a supervising physician to "bill under." In my attempt to find one, everyone I approached refused because of the wording in the Medicaid manual. The physician had to "supervise" and be available to consult. Many physicians felt that they were taking on an "added risk" in supervising me because they did not know enough about women's health. This rebuff was the final deciding factor in taking action!

WHY HASN'T THIS POLICY BEEN CHANGED?

I started by contacting everyone who was connected to this issue to offer insight as to why this policy had not been resolved. I discovered that it had been addressed and readdressed over a 10-year period by many diligent NPs from various organizations. Although progress was made, previous efforts had never resulted in policy change. In discussing this policy with my colleagues who have been pursuing the issue, I heard everything from "the computer system was not capable of making changes" to the offering of a "pilot project" in a rural area to determine the impact of NPs billing Medicaid directly.

None of these rationales seemed reasonable, yet I took what they conveyed to me and used it to start thinking about what might seem equitable. I knew the solution, and it became clear that this issue had to be addressed.

WHAT IS NEEDED FOR CHANGE?

Policies are ideas that are generated to address problems. To my astonishment, this policy change did not require lengthy legislation but was a simple rule change to the state plan. The Director of Medicaid can suggest the rule change to be voted on by the Medical Care Advisory Committee (MCAC). The MCAC is required by federal regulation to provide the state Medicaid agency with recommendations on the operation and planning of Medicaid programs. The committee is comprised of medical professionals familiar with the needs of low-income population groups, consumer stakeholders, and state department of health members (Utah Department of Health, n.d.).

I had never viewed myself as a "policy person." There seems to be a negative connotation when addressing policy in that it is difficult, disappointing, and ultimately impossible to make a change. After some research, it looked like changing this policy may be within reach. This being realized, I was compelled to at least try.

WELCOME TO POLICY

Being on the cusp of implementing the ACA along with continued governmental and public attention to the option of Medicaid expansion, Utah's Medicaid program was already attracting a considerable amount of attention. With the addition of the media coverage on national, state, and local levels, both public officials and their constituents were engaged in identifying what efforts were being made to ensure that Utah was ready to meet the challenge of the ACA.

Coupled with a new understanding of what was needed to change this policy and a personal story, I scheduled a meeting with the policymakers. I met with the Executive Director of the Utah Department of Health (UDOH) and the Director of Medicaid and articulated how the Medicaid policy was impacting access to care for Medicaid beneficiaries in rural Utah. I was able to frame the problem using my experience and expertise from both a provider's and a business owner's perspective.

The Director of Medicaid's resistance was felt immediately. He expressed that this issue had been brought up before, and a pilot project was suggested, but there was lack of follow through on the NP side. Acknowledging his frustration, I explained that many NPs do not own and operate their own practices and they may not have had the ability to execute the pilot project.

In listening to his concerns, three main areas were identified for which policymakers needed more information to understand the impact of this policy fully. These areas included access to care, quality of care, and physician opposition. I assured him that I would not "drop the ball" and would get him the information he needed to make an informed decision about changing this policy. I left the meeting feeling slightly hopeful, knowing I had just crossed the line into the policy arena.

RELATIONSHIP BUILDING

The process of relationship building had begun. I immediately went to work and was in constant communication with the Director of Medicaid. I gathered data, referenced the County Health Rankings, which my county ranked last for several consecutive years, and benchmarked off other states that have implemented this policy change. Although he welcomed the information, I perceived that more was needed to influence this change.

Having never called, emailed, or even approached an elected official, I found myself on the phone with my senator. I explained that there was a policy issue that I would like his help with and he offered to meet me at my office. This key meeting proved to be advantageous. He could see the benefit of this policy change for his constituents. He believed this was a rural health as well as a small business issue and agreed to call the policymakers in support of this change. In a chance encounter, shortly after his call with the policymakers, the Senator verbally reinforced his support of this policy change to the Executive Director of UDOH. The communication and follow up with my senator was effortless.

I also made appointments with my community partners and explained the situation and solicited their support. Each partner composed a letter to the policymakers in favor of the policy change. The letters of support, along with a White Paper from the Utah NPs entitled "The Role of Nurse Practitioners in Improving Access to Care for Utah Medicaid Beneficiaries," were sent via email.

I continued to network with my colleagues and follow through on leads. Emails were sent and calls were made to organizations such as Utah NPs, American Association of NPs, Utah Action Coalition for Health (UACH), Utah Health Policy Project, and UMEC requesting their support.

JOINING FORCES

A colleague who had been guiding and mentoring me through this process connected me by way of an "electronic introduction" to the project manager of the UACH. This coalition is comprised of many of the state's leaders interested in improving access to health care. The UACH is charged with implementing the IOM recommendations in Utah in collaboration with *The Future of Nursing: Campaign for Action* funded by the Robert Wood Johnson Foundation and AARP.

The project manager and I set up a time to talk. To my great fortune, she happened to be the former Director of Medicaid and former nurse lobbyist and was willing to mentor me. I welcomed the coaching and was eager to learn everything I could from her.

It was at this critical juncture we began to devise a solid strategy to move this policy change to completion. I shared what I had learned from my meeting with the policymakers at the UDOH. She shared that they were comprising a letter in support of this policy change. I sent her the information I had exchanged with the policymakers along with the studies to support this policy change. She sent me the letter that was endorsed by several key stakeholders, including hospitals, statewide integrated health care organizations, university-based nursing and medical education programs, national nonprofit organizations, community health centers, nurse leaders, and several NP organizations.

Voicing concern over physician opposition, I was assured that the physicians had been approached in a private meeting and their organizational leaders provided their signature. The letter was hand-delivered to the policymakers by the AARP state representative.

THE MEETING

The UACH had yet to get an appointment to discuss the letter they had sent. I was already in the process of setting up a follow-up meeting, and we thought it was wise to go in together.

The pivotal meeting that brought key stakeholders together with policymakers took place at the UDOH. Along with the Director of Medicaid and the Executive Director of the UDOH, influential stakeholders including the Co-Chair of the UACH (who was also the Dean of the University of Utah College of Nursing), the project manager from the UACH, a Certified Nurse Midwife representative from the Utah NPs organization, and myself were in attendance. After a thorough discussion, the Director of Medicaid announced that he was willing to change this policy. The recommended written solutions were furnished to provide the policymakers with specific reference to current rules along with the suggested changes.

DECISION AGENDA

The agreement to support a change to Medicaid policy was monumental, but the process was not over. Now the policy had to be placed on the MCAC decision agenda for discussion and vote.

It took several months before the proposed policy change was placed on the MCAC agenda. A group of policy advocates, including myself and the UACH program manager, were in attendance to monitor the meeting and provide information if needed. After a brief discussion of the issue, the MCAC members unanimously voted to remove restrictive language and change Utah's Medicaid policy to allow all NPs to directly bill and be reimbursed by Medicaid.

CONCESSIONS

Now that the policy was changed, it was time to focus on reimbursement. We were anticipating the fee schedule to mirror the current schedule at 85% of the physician rate. To our surprise, the Director of Medicaid proposed to pay the newly eligible NPs at 75% of the physician rate and keep those already eligible at 85%.

A follow-up meeting was scheduled, and I began researching. Armed with data and a calm demeanor, the UACH project manager and I met with the Director of Medicaid. He expressed his concerns about the cost of adding the newly eligible NPs. I reassured him that the cost would be negligible because most NPs are already billing "under a physician." We then discussed the logistics of having to manage three different fee schedules (two for NPs and 1 for physicians). With reimbursement moving toward payment based on quality, it is essential to be transparent regarding which provider is actually providing care. Medicaid needed to be ready for this paradigm shift and having one fee schedule positions them to participate in emerging alternative payment models.

After exchanging information and discussing different scenarios, the Director of Medicaid agreed to one fee schedule, and now all NPs are paid at 100% of the physician rate.

THREE KEY FACTORS

I have identified three key factors that I believe explain the success of this policy change.

The Timing Was Right

In previous attempts to change this policy, there was no national push for health care reform. Nothing was looming that was going to put additional stress on an already fragile system. In the wake of health care reform, the creation of a state insurance exchange, and the Medicaid eligibility expansion option, Utah needed to prepare for an influx of people who had not previously had health insurance due to the ACA requirements that went into effect in 2014. Utah had to be ready to meet this challenge.

Having a Powerful Personal Story

If I had not opened my own practice and learned about this policy issue from a business perspective, my story might not have been as compelling. This issue was brought up in the past, but there was no actual personal story to help explain the gravity of the situation.

It All Comes Down to Relationships

The relationships that were built along the way taught me the most about policy. Mentors and colleagues were generous with their time and expertise and patiently guided me through the process. They nurtured my interest by providing me with the insight and encouragement to keep moving forward.

The nature of any relationship is both exhilarating and exhausting. It is a constant back and forth of exchanging information and ideas, which takes commitment to continue to build your network and keep everyone in the loop. Meeting face to face with colleagues and policymakers creates a human connection that can be more powerful than emails and telephone calls combined.

Building and maintaining relationships takes a considerable amount of time and effort. There are countless players in policy, and it is crucial that you know the players on both sides of the issue. You must pursue and maintain relationships with as many players as possible. Keeping your word and providing credible information aids in establishing trust. Policy hinges on the relationships you have had in the past and those you are developing in the present, all of which influence the future.

CALL TO ACTION

The ACA has provided NPs with the opportunity to be the "superstars" of health care. It is our time to shine! Although numerous evidence-based studies consistently support NPs providing high-quality, cost-effective care, we have to get involved in policy to be eligible to provide that care. I did not know a lot about policy but chose to dive in headfirst out of necessity to care for the women in my community. The point is you do not have to know policy to get involved in policy; you just have to get involved. Together, we can reshape health care!

REFERENCES

American Nurses Association. (2011). *Medicaid coverage of advanced practice registered nurses.* Retrieved from https://secure3.convio.net/ana/site/Advocacy?cmd=display&page=UserAction&id=373&ct=1.

Association of American Medical Colleges. (2012). *Recent studies and reports on physician shortages in the U.S.* Retrieved from www.aamc.org/download/100598/data/recentwork forcestudies.pdf.

Institute of Medicine. (2011). *The future of nursing: Leading change, advancing health.* Retrieved from www.iom.edu/~/media/Files/Report%20Files/2010/The-Future-of-Nursing/Future%20of%20Nursing%202010%20Recommendations.pdf.

Muller, K.J., Coburn, A.F., Lundblad, J.P., MacKinney, A.C., McBride, T.D., & Watson, S.D. (2012). *The current and future role and impact of Medicaid in rural health.* U.S. Department of Health and Human Services, Federal Office of Rural Health Policy Health Resources and Services Administration, Rural Policy Research Institute. Retrieved from www.okoha.com/AM/Template.cfm?Section=Home&Template=/CM/ContentDisplay.cfm&ContentID=23329.

U.S. Department of Health and Human Services, Office of the Inspector General. (2001). *Medicare coverage of non-physician practitioner services* (OEI-02-00-00290). Retrieved from https://oig.hhs.gov/oei/reports/oei-02-00-00290.pdf.

Utah Department of Health. (n.d.). *Medical care advisory committee.* Retrieved from http://health.utah.gov/mcac/.

Utah Division of Professional Licensing (2013). *Nurse practice acts,* (Title 58, Chapter 31b-102[13]). Retrieved from www.dopl.utah.gov/laws/58-31b.pdf.

Utah Medicaid Program. (2012, October 25). *Utah Medicaid provider manual.* Retrieved from www.health.utah.gov/medicaid.

Utah Medical Education Council. (2012). *Utah's physician workforce: A study on the supply and distribution of physicians in Utah.* Retrieved from www.utahmec.org/uploads/files/75/2012-Physician-Workforce-Report.pdf.

62

TAKING ACTION: Removing APRN Regulatory Barriers in West Virginia

Toni DiChiacchio

"Leaders must pick causes they won't abandon easily, remain committed despite setbacks, and communicate their big ideas over and over again in every encounter."

Rosabeth Moss Kanter, Harvard Business School professor

The Future of Nursing: Leading Change, Advancing Health (2011) by the Institute of Medicine (now the National Academy of Medicine) was a catalytic document for advanced practice registered nurses (APRNs) across the country, as it included a recommendation for removing barriers to full practice authority (FPA). For me, as a family nurse practitioner (NP), it was an endorsement of what I had been examining as part of earning my Doctorate of Nursing Practice. I had explored the literature, looking for differences in quality and outcomes between physicians and NPs with the intent of a doctoral project to narrow the differences I expected. However, study after study showed there was no significant difference. In several instances, outcomes such as patient satisfaction were actually better for patients receiving care from APRNs.

The Patient Protection and Affordable Care Act (ACA) had just become law. Anticipating an increased demand for primary care from the ACA extending health coverage and certain that the APRN regulatory barriers in West Virginia (WV) would soon be removed, I opened a primary care practice focused on the chronic health conditions of those previously underserved. Because WV law required a collaborative agreement for NPs to prescribe medications, I searched for months and found a collaborative physician willing to support me—for remuneration—for the short time I anticipated needing him. Little did I know when I opened the practice in 2012 that changing policy would take more than just presenting strong evidence—it would take strategic action, time, and patience.

HISTORY OF ADVANCED PRACTICE REGISTERED NURSE REGULATION IN WEST VIRGINIA

West Virginia recognized APRNs formally in the code of state rules in 1991 through an announcement of advanced practice (WV Board of Examiners for Registered Professional Nurses, 1991) that permitted NPs and clinical nurse specialists (CNSs) to *practice* without supervision or collaboration. Certified nurse midwives (CNMs) were required to be supervised to practice per another WV Code at that time (W. Va. Code § 30-15-7, 1991), and that changed to a collaborative relationship the following year (W. Va. Code § 30-15-7, 1992). The nurse practice act (NPA) has required certified registered nurse anesthetists (CRNAs) to administer anesthesia in the presence and under the supervision of a physician or dentist qualified to administer anesthesia (W. Va. Code § 30-7-15, 1992). The WV Board of Nursing (BON) has been the sole regulatory body for APRNs since statutory recognition. In 1992, statutory limited prescriptive authority was granted (W. Va. Code § 30-15-7a, 1992; W. Va. Code § 30-7-15a, 1992), but all APRNs were limited by restrictions on types of medications they could prescribe and the length of time certain medications could be prescribed. Schedule II drugs were forbidden, Schedule III drugs and benzodiazepine were limited to a 72-hour supply, and anticoagulants were prohibited. All prescribing was required to be done under a collaborative agreement with a licensed WV physician.

The collaborative agreement requirements were vague and did not require on-site availability of the collaborating physician.

FPA bills were regularly introduced starting in the late 1990s. Although unsuccessful, incremental changes were made over time. For example, during the 2012 regular legislative session, the restriction on prescribing anticoagulants was removed and a separate APRN licensure was instituted (W. Va. Code §30-7-15a; W. Va. Code §30-7-1). In addition, a new law went into effect that requires any individual or professional organization that desired a revision or expansion of their regulatory scope of practice to file an application with the Joint Standing Committee on Government Organization to explore the request (W. Va. Code §30-1A-2). In 2013, the West Virginia Nurses Association (WVNA) filed an application—well over 100 pages—requesting removal of regulatory barriers that limited APRNs from FPA or practicing to the full extent of their education and training. At the time, APRNs in 17 other states enjoyed FPA. Although the legislative auditor's office did complete their analysis by the due date, they did not finish their final recommendations before the December 31st statutory deadline. Thus, it was not presented to the legislature by the end of the year, effectively preventing the legislature from considering the issue during the regular 2014 legislative session.

A month later, the auditor released the report with recommendations (West Virginia Legislative Auditor, 2014). The body of the report was quite favorable regarding APRNs' safety, efficacy, and cost-effectiveness, but the auditor's recommendations to the legislature were disappointing. They included removing the collaborative agreement for prescribing only after 5 years, requiring CNMs to maintain a collaborative agreement to practice, and shifting APRN regulation from the BON to the Board of Medicine. The WVNA rebutted these recommendations. In 2014, the legislature heard testimony from both the legislative auditor in support of their recommendations and from the WVNA in support of FPA. There was no certainty of what would be recommended to the Legislature in 2015. Over a year of hopefulness that FPA could be achieved through the aforementioned mechanism was quashed and the disappointment was palpable. But historic changes were on the horizon in West Virginia that would provide renewed hope.

HISTORIC SHIFT OF POWER PROVIDES NEW OPPORTUNITIES

For the first time in 83 years in West Virginia, the 2014 election resulted in a shift of the majority to Republicans. This produced opportunities and challenges. One of the primary benefits was the requisite change in legislative committee leadership. The prior leadership had long-seated Health Committee chairs in both the House and Senate who were strongly opposed to FPA for APRNs and had never placed FPA bills on their committees' agendas. With a new majority and new committee chairs, getting an FPA bill on the Health Committees' agenda for debate was suddenly plausible.

The new power shift also expanded the potential of building coalitions with other powerful stakeholders who had been pragmatic in past years and avoided actively working with nurses on the issue. Although those groups may have been interested in and seen the benefits of APRN FPA, many recognized the futility at that time and chose not to deplete political capital on an issue that would never be heard in committee.

A short 2-month transition from the general election in November, 2014, until the 60-day session began, found nurse advocates scurrying to provide a more in-depth education on the FPA issue and reframe the message on the importance of changing the law to better align with the Republican philosophical view. Historically, we had framed the issue largely around access to care and health disparities for rural, vulnerable, and underserved citizens of the state. Prior to the passage of the ACA, we had focused on the number of uninsured West Virginians who could not afford health care and suggested APRNs as a more affordable access point if regulatory barriers were removed. After West Virginia decided to expand Medicaid under the ACA, we discussed the large number of newly insured patients who would now have insurance but due to a physician shortage, particularly in primary care, would still remain unable to receive timely care. With the new majority, we shifted the frame to "excessive regulation." Specifically, the message focused on how excessive occupational regulation can be detrimental to job creation and private-sector economic development; it adds costs to employers related to compliance adherence, translating to additional cost of health care for consumers; and that competition in general tends to increase quality, expand available services, and reduce prices as multiple providers attempt to entice patients to use their services. Finally, empowering consumers to make the ultimate selection of which health care provider can best meet their needs—otherwise known as freedom of patient choice—was emphasized.

We also needed to find specific champions, educating them and finessing the messaging, so they could adeptly speak of the benefits of FPA. Prior to the beginning of the legislative session, WV nursing leaders and nursing constituents of the new Senate Health Chair, Senator Ryan Ferns (R-01) met with him to discuss the regulatory impediments APRNs faced in his district and across the state.

The meeting included several physician constituents of the new Chair, who were conceptually supportive of removal of barriers. We also discussed the recommendations and the discordance within the Legislative Auditor's report. During the first week of the 2015 Legislative Session, Senator Ferns arranged a stakeholder meeting, including the new House Health Committee Chair, nurse and physician stakeholders, and members of the Legislative Audit team to discuss how to handle a potential FPA bill on their respective agendas.

We also had to quickly identify new legislators in the majority party to sponsor FPA bills. A group of nurse leaders organized a post-election, bipartisan congratulatory reception and invited all winning candidates from the area. Most attended. FPA was discussed and two new majority party legislators were identified as potential sponsors: Delegate Amy Summers (R-49), a registered nurse obviously familiar with nurses' capabilities to provide quality advanced care; and Senator Kent Leonhardt (R-2), a retired Marine whose father was a physician and who had seen how non-physicians in the combat theater were trained to provide excellent care.

A bipartisan FPA bill was introduced in the 2015 session. The Health Committee chairs from both chambers subsequently crafted what they envisioned as a compromise amendment to the bill, addressing some of the barriers to APRN practice. The amended bill included the ability for APRNs to prescribe without a regulatory physician collaborative agreement after 5 years; removing CNMs' regulatory collaborative agreement to practice; the ability to sign death certificates; a separate APRN Board, which did have physician representation but the majority would be APRNs (similar to Nebraska's APRN Board); Schedule IIIs limited to 30 days rather than 72 hours; and Schedule II medication prescribing permissible for only hydrocodone combination products limited to a 72-hour supply. We showed a willingness to compromise and supported the bill, recognizing that it was not FPA but an incremental improvement in regulation. APRNs went into the Senate Health Committee in unenthusiastic support of this bill, but when an amendment was made to have us regulated by the Board of Medicine, all nursing support was withdrawn and the nursing community had the bill "killed." Ultimately, the amendment nursing could not accept would provide momentum in the future.

COALITION BUILDING

The WVNA was the primary organization advocating for FPA and the central organizer of a coalition of partners to share how amending the law would provide wide benefit. Through the years, a number of organizations had become supporters of FPA including Our Children, Our Future Campaign; West Virginians for Affordable Health care; and the WV Center on Budget & Policy. Some organizations supported FPA and historically sought to join the coalition prior to 2015, but had not been vocal supporters, fearing that doing so could jeopardize their important legislative goals. The new political landscape changed that. A strategy was developed to build the coalition of supporters with diverse political perspectives.

The Future of Nursing West Virginia (FONWV) is the state action coalition associated with the national Campaign for Action and its mission is implementation of the *Future of Nursing* recommendations. The foundational sponsors of the FONWV are the WVNA, the West Virginia Hospital Association (WVHA) and the West Virginia Organization of Nurse Executives (WVONE). Many influential individuals serve as strategic advisers to the FONWV. For some stakeholders involved in the FONWV, legislative advocacy was uncomfortable, so some agreed to meet quietly with their respective legislators to discuss the benefits of FPA for their constituents. Other stakeholders had extensive and regular involvement in the legislative arena. AARP in West Virginia was one such organization and is well-respected. AARP became a central and integral coalition partner bringing operational strength to the coalition and demonstrating that FPA was not an attempt for the nursing profession to garner power for singular gain, but rather a true benefit to healthcare consumers and their caregivers.

From a political perspective, we continued to work to align our strategy with the philosophical views of the new majority. We approached the WV affiliate of Americans for Prosperity (AFP), an organization whose mission includes limiting government and regulatory interference with free markets. Nebraska nurses had worked successfully with their state affiliate of the organization on FPA. The WV affiliate quickly affirmed that removing APRN regulatory burdens aligned with their goals, particularly since there was a shortage of primary care physicians and the costs of health care significantly outpaced inflation. They joined as a coalition partner and, together with WVNA and AARP, became the "core team" coordinating activities at the Capital.

No stranger to the FPA issue, the Federal Trade Commission (FTC), which had provided a written position supporting FPA during the 2012 Interim session, was again contacted (FTC, 2012). During the 2015 session, an attempt was made to place APRNs under the regulatory authority of the Board of Medicine, so the FTC's analysis on the economic effect of having the nursing profession regulated by a Board of Medicine was requested by Senator Leonhardt. As before, they provided legislative testimony in the form of a letter on the likely positive benefit of having only as many regulatory restrictions as necessary to protect the public. The FTC also noted that, because of the strong evidence supporting APRN safety, FPA appears to have competitive benefits that outweigh any associated costs. They concluded that having the Board of Medicine as the regulatory body in charge of oversight of APRNs would be an anticompetitive tactic and could be detrimental to consumers (FTC, 2016).

STRATEGIC EFFORTS

Strategic efforts to prepare for the January start of the 2016 Legislative Session began in mid-2015. The core team of leaders from WVNA, AARP, and AFP, along with the primary sponsors of the 2016 FPA bill from the House and Senate, held meetings to discuss in which chamber we would try to pass the bill initially, expected positions of each legislator, and what key evidence would be most important to present during testimony. We also discussed who could most likely gain support from legislators who were ambivalent on the issue. Potential influencers included nurses with particularly strong relationships with their legislators, legislator champions whose opinion held significant weight with their colleagues, and particular coalition members whom ambivalent legislators looked to frequently for guidance and insight on issues.

We briefed AARP volunteers who regularly advocate at the Capital so they would have a working knowledge of the FPA issue, evidence supporting our position, and messaging. We wanted them to be able to answer questions and express why the bill was important. For continuity, I was selected as the nurse content expert who would regularly be present at the Capital to answer specific questions of legislators, as well as deliver testimony at each committee hearing as needed through the entire process.

A lobbyist was hired by the WVNA. We wanted someone with a strong and relevant professional history; candor yet poise; an understanding of the potential animosity involved with "scope of practice" bills, but ready for the challenge; and ideally known and respected by legislators and legislative staff, regardless of party affiliation. The lobbyist selected had an extensive work history at the state level in both the legislative and executive branch. She was well liked by legislators of both parties. She was willing and enthusiastic about working in a team fashion with our core coalition's lobbyists from AARP and AFP.

WVNA organized a legislative leader in each senatorial district. These leaders in swing vote districts sponsored dinners with those legislators and nurse constituents to discuss the bill, provided education on FPA merits, and addressed any concerns. Legislative leaders were used throughout the session to rally nurses in their districts when key votes were coming up or strong messaging needed to be delivered. Communication was done only with a directive from our lobbyist to ensure our efforts were concerted and noticeable but not irritating or spread thinly. We didn't "pull the trigger" on phone calls and emails without appropriate timing, and those times were used to show our strength and unity.

Timing was paramount for everything, including publication of op-eds, media appearances, and sponsored dinners with legislators. All were done with intention and immediately before important votes. For example, the aforementioned letter from the FTC was released to us the evening immediately before a public hearing and the first committee meeting in which the bill, HB4334, was heard. Only those closest to our mission knew of its existence, making its distribution at the first hearing most impactful.

On the night prior to committee hearings, sponsored dinners for key legislators on each committee were held to educate them, in a relaxed environment, on the importance of the bill. Attendance at the meetings always included AARP, the WVNA lobbyist, and the WVNA content expert. Some dinners included other experts. One included a former nurse fellow from the conservative Heritage Foundation who spoke on her research related to FPA and its benefits. Another guest who spoke about the bill and attended several private meetings with legislators was a WV political science professor whose expertise was in health policy. He spoke to the impact on affordability and access that the FPA would provide consumers. An important element throughout all these points of exposure for legislators on the bill was that a nurse was not the primary deliverer of messages. Consistently present but typically quiet, I was used to answer specific questions the other supporters did not know and to provide committee testimony. Using advocates other than nurses showed that the issue was not "nurse versus physician" but rather a patient-centered consumer choice issue.

The same tactic carried over generally to media appearances. There were three local television segments done on different shows during the session and in none was a nurse the voice of the issue. One included the AARP communications director for the protagonist view of the bill alongside a physician senator as the antagonist. The others included AARP and WVNA lobbyists describing benefits of the bill.

A public hearing was requested by Delegate Summers immediately before the first committee meeting in which the bill was heard. Twenty-one individuals presented. Seventeen spoke in support of HB4334 and four in opposition. The four opposing were all representing physicians. The 17 in support included: AARP, APRN patients, a public health nurse, the Heritage Foundation Graduate Policy analyst, WV Citizens Action Group, the WV Social Workers Association, WV for Affordable Health Care, AFP, the WV Funeral Home Directors Association, the WV Center on Budget & Policy, APRNs who had lost their independent practices because of over-regulation, and other APRNs who explained barriers to care experienced by patients caused by over-regulation. A summary of the FTC's response to Senator Leonhardt regarding the anticompetitive effects of restricted APRN practice was also presented.

This broad range of bipartisan support was noticed by the media and legislators themselves reported it was a very enjoyable bill to work on because of its bipartisan support during a very contentious session filled with political wedge issues. The largest newspaper in the state covered the bill with a focus on the irony of having support of both the Citizens Action Group and AFP (Hindman, 2016). The article began:

> The West Virginia Citizens Action Group is a progressive organization that fights for things like environmental protection, consumer advocacy and reducing the influence of money in politics. Americans for Prosperity is a conservative group that fights for things like less environmental regulation, pro-business policies and lower taxes. Founded and largely funded by the Koch brothers, it is a veritable poster child for the role of money in politics. Safe to say, the two groups agree on little. But they both agree that highly trained nurses in West Virginia should have more power to treat patients and prescribe medication without a doctor's supervision.

TRAJECTORY OF THE BILL

The 60-day session of the WV Legislature in 2016 convened on January 13th. House Bill 4334 was introduced in the House of Delegates on January 29th and included: retiring the collaborative agreement to prescribe after 2 years and the agreement could be with an experienced APRN or a physician; repeal of the requirement that CNMs have a collaborative agreement to practice; ability to prescribe 72 hours of Schedule II medication with no refills with the exception of attention deficit hyperactivity disorder (ADHD) medication which could be prescribed for 30 days with no refills; ability to prescribe 30 days of Schedule III medication with no refills; no additional state limits on medication prescribing; and global signatory authority for forms and documents.

The bill required testimony at three hearings: House Health, House Government Organization, and Senate Health Committees. The most contentious testimony was in Senate Health, where I fielded questions for over 90 minutes. Opponents of the bill who were questioned at committee meetings were from organized medicine and the prominent arguments were: the education and training of APRNs are much less than that of a physician; quality of educational programs for APRNs are not uniform or reliable, with particular emphasis on distance learning programs; West Virginia was in the throes of an opioid crisis, and permitting "lesser trained" prescribers of Schedule II medications would be a threat to public safety; APRNs do not go to rural areas when they are granted full practice; and the BON was not stringent enough to oversee APRNs "practicing medicine." No significant evidence was provided to substantiate these arguments, and ample evidence that does exist was cited to overcome each argument during testimony.

Regarding the rural presence of primary care APRNs in full practice states, one initial tactic by opponents was to point out the federal government's defined Health Provider Shortage Areas (HPSAs) had not been shown to decline when full practice had been granted in other states. When subsequently called to testify, I explained to the committee that the HPSA designation for primary care only includes a ratio of the population of an area to the physicians in said area (U.S. Department of Health & Human Services, 2018). APRNs are not considered in that ratio, thus that is an invalid method to measure the rural impact of full practice for APRNs. That quieted the argument. Ultimately, the bill was about consumers' options to choose a provider in their own community whom they trusted and could conveniently access.

When APRNs and their patients were faced with dilemmas from the collaborative agreement requirement or other regulatory barriers, we would have them contact their legislators and tell their story. The team at the Capital then would emphasize community impact to those legislators, should they fail to modernize outdated language.

Both House Committees passed the bill easily with no amendments despite some being offered in House Government Organization Committee. The bill was sent on to the full House of Delegates and two amendments were offered from the floor. The first would have required that during the collaboration period of the first 2 years, the collaborating provider must be at the same facility as the APRN. It failed. The second added a clause to the global signature language clarifying that only forms that are within the APRNs' scope and specialty can be signed by the APRN. It passed.

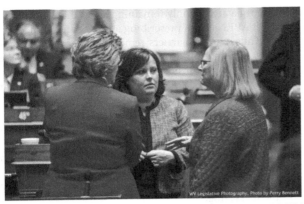

From left to right: Delegate Amy Summers (R-49), AARP-WV lobbyist Angela Vance, and AARP-WV State Director Gaylene Miller discuss strategy prior to final vote by the WV House of Delegates on HB4334.

The day of the final vote in the House, physician opponents of the bill were present in the galleries, but nurses made the strategic decision to not make a mass presence. This was to emphasize that this was not a "nurse versus physician" issue, and it was thought that having both groups of professionals staging an opposing presence would contribute to that appearance. The primary sponsor of the bill, Delegate Summers, spoke eloquently to the need for the bill and the positive impact it would have on West Virginia. As an RN and primary sponsor, she added a powerful touch at the beginning of the floor session that day: she introduced her mother, also a nurse, who was present in the gallery, saying that she was proudly visiting to watch the vote on what had been commonly dubbed "the nurse bill." The bill, which was intact as an FPA policy, passed with overwhelming support: 72 voted in favor, 20 against, and 8 abstained or were not present.

In the Senate, the bill went first to Senate Health and Human Resources Committee and then was assigned to Senate Government Organization Committee. This was a favorable assignment, as the Senate Health Committee was the biggest hurdle for the bill and, if any negatively perceived amendments were made in the Health Committee, we were confident they would be corrected in the Senate Government Organization Committee.

Our primary goal for the Senate Health Committee's deliberations was just to keep the bill moving regardless of amendments. Changes were made that were not favored by nursing, including: reinsertion of a regulatory collaborative agreement perpetually, reinserting limits on the drug formulary that APRNs would be allowed to prescribe, a requirement for joint promulgation of rules for APRNs by the Board of Medicine and Nursing, and the creation of an Advisory Council to the BON that included APRNs, physicians, and a pharmacist. But with the Senate Health Committee passing the amended bill, it met our goal of moving forward.

Anxiety ramped up when the second reference to the Government Organization Committee, which had committed to "fixing" the bill by removing the amendments adopted by the Senate Health Committee, was withdrawn. The impetus of this was unknown and came as a surprise. It was speculated that either it was a suggested strategy by opponents from organized medicine agreed upon by the chamber's leadership or a mechanism to force compromise. Regardless, removal of the unsavory amendments now would be required on the Senate floor and thus involve a likely contentious debate, not typically favored by the Senate.

The bill was in front of the full Senate and, on the reading when amendments could be offered, they were not. But a motion was made and adopted to allow the bill to move to final reading the following day and to retain the right to amend. Later that day, the Senate Majority Leader requested the team at the Capital meet with physician senators to discuss possible negotiations. Several concessions by nursing and our team were agreed to but no final negotiated bill emerged that all could accept. We were back to anticipating a Senate floor debate to amend the bill to what the House had passed and expected a very tight vote but remained hopeful our position would prevail.

The next morning, 20 minutes prior to the scheduled Senate floor session and 2 days before the regular session would end, an unscheduled conversation with the senator physicians, the AARP state director, and me occurred and agreeable terms emerged. The final bill drafted included the following compromises:

- The length of the required collaborative agreement went from 2 to 3 years with a physician.
- APRNs wouldn't be able to sign a certificate of merit for a malpractice claim against a physician and must receive training on death certificate completion.
- Schedule II drugs would remain excluded for APRN prescribing.
- A Joint Advisory Council on Limited Prescriptive Authority would be formed to advise the BON regarding APRN collaborative agreements and prescriptive authority with four physicians, six APRNs, a pharmacist, a consumer, and a representative from a School of Public Health. It would hold no disciplinary power but could examine barriers and issues related to APRN prescribing including negative impacts on consumer care and access.

The amendments were made to bring the compromise bill to the Senate. Both physicians serving in the Senate at the time spoke in favor of the bill, as did several other senators. It passed, 34-0. The House approved the Senate version of the compromised bill along with other technical amendments in a vote of 91 in favor, 5 opposed, and 4 absent/not voting. With all amendments, technical changes and votes cast, the bill was completed with only 4 hours left in the session.

From the time the bill passed the House and entered the Senate, the lobbyist team from AARP and WVNA had been monitoring the pulse of the Governor's office regarding any hesitancy he may have had about signing the bill. Because of significant addiction and overdose rates in West Virginia, there was some minimal concern that the Governor may have an issue with the limited 72 hours of Schedule II prescribing authority. However, because that particular section of the bill was removed in the Senate, there was confidence that it would be signed. Although some opponents did put forth a final effort to get the bill vetoed, advocates for the bill were organized to call the Governor's office in a coordinated fashion to encourage his approval. In West Virginia, the Governor has three options. He could sign the bill. He could take no action and, within 5 days if the Legislature is still in session or 15 days if they are adjourned, the bill would become law. If he vetoed the bill and the legislature is still in session, they could override the veto with enough time and enough votes. We would have had the votes to override a veto but not the time because the bill ultimately passed and was received by the Governor after session adjourned. Within 6 days of receipt, the Governor directly affirmed his approval of the bill by signing it. It became law in June 2016.

LESSONS LEARNED

Despite having signatory authority, APRNs continue to face certain challenges to their ability to execute documents that are addressed on a case-by-case basis. Payment by third-party health insurance payers is also a challenge. WV Medicaid, covering one third of our population, prohibited APRNs from being paid for services delivered in hospitals or nursing homes. With great collegiality, the Bureau of Medical Services removed that limit in 2018. Another bill was passed in the 2018 session with unanimous support that prevents health insurance companies from requiring a collaborative agreement to provide APRNs payment for services (HB4175).

The remaining element that prevents West Virginia from being considered a full practice state is the ability to prescribe Schedule II medications. West Virginia, Oklahoma, and Georgia are the only remaining states that completely prohibit APRNs from prescribing any Schedule II medications. Thus, patient barriers remain and are felt particularly by children in rural areas with ADHD who see APRNs, as well as for hospice, palliative care, and nursing home patients cared for by APRNs. This will be brought back to the legislature at the appropriate time to discuss.

Important lessons learned during this process include:
- Incremental change is better than stagnation if it is a move forward.
- Make the issue consumer-centered and get away from the "nurse versus physician" argument.
- Nurses may have to relinquish some level of controlling the messaging.
- Develop excellent grass-roots nursing organization connected closely to their local legislators.
- Be strategic when "pulling the trigger" on mass nurse communication with legislators to deliver a common message with noticeable volume and vigor.
- A respected lobbyist is key.
- Frame the message to the targeted audience or person.
- Nurse content experts should be available at the Capital nearly continuously during the session but not always as the primary messenger.
- Build a strong bipartisan coalition, including consumer advocacy groups with well-established legislative influence.
- Be focused and maintain a rational, strategic approach despite a likely roller-coaster of ups and downs.
- Before agreeing on concessions, assure that all coalition partners find them acceptable.
- Be ready to work tirelessly. It took commitment and long hours at the Capital, as we were often the first to arrive in the morning and the last to leave at night. As one coalition partner stated at the outset, "They may beat us, but it won't be because they outwork us."

It was more than a decade from the introduction of an FPA bill and the removal of significant regulatory barriers for APRNs in West Virginia. Some barriers to FPA remain, and implementation of the new law has also faced challenges. Thus, the most important message is never relinquish attempts at forward progression despite defeats along the way. Patience and perseverance will ultimately reap just rewards.

REFERENCES

Federal Trade Commission. (September, 2012). *Advocacy filings*. Retrieved from www.ftc.gov/sites/default/files/documents/advocacy_documents/ftc-staff-testimony-subcommittee-wv-legislature-laws-governing-scope-practice-advanced-practice/120907wvatestimony.pdf.

Federal Trade Commission. (February 10, 2016). *Advocacy filings*. Retrieved from www.ftc.gov/system/files/documents/advocacy_documents/ftc-staff-comment-senate-west-virginia-concerning-competitive-impact-wv-senate-bill-516-regulation/160212westvirginiacomment.pdf.

Hindman, T. (February 14, 2016). Bipartisan nursing bill could ease rural healthcare shortages. *Charleston Gazette*. Retrieved from www.wvgazettemail.com/business/bipartisan-nursing-bill-could-help-ease-rural-health-care-shortages/article_d31a204e-3e72-5ae3-afe0-042173a8bc09.html.

Institute of Medicine. (2011). *The future of nursing: Leading change, advancing health*. Washington, DC: National Academies Press.

U.S. Department of Health and Human Services. (2018). *Designated health provider shortage area statistics*. Washington DC: Author.

West Virginia Legislative Auditor. (January 30, 2014). *Performance Evaluation & Review Division*. Retrieved from www.wvlegislature.gov/legisdocs/reports/perd/APRN_1_2014.pdf.

WV Board of Examiners for Registered Professional Nurses. (July 1, 1991). *19CSR7*. Charleston, West Virginia. Retrieved from http://apps.sos.wv.gov/adlaw/csr/readfile.aspx?DocId=19087&Format=PDF.

63

TAKING ACTION: Full Practice Authority: A Tale of Two States

Carolyn Montoya and Gale Adcock

"The secret of change is to focus all of your energy not on fighting the old but on building the new."

Socrates

New Mexico and North Carolina have different regulatory climates for advanced practice registered nurse (APRN) practice. Since 1993, New Mexico has had full practice authority (FPA), whereas North Carolina has been engaged in a multiyear effort to pass FPA legislation. It seems that these two states have very little in common. However, each struggles with fully realizing one of the key recommendations of the *The Future of Nursing* report from the Institute of Medicine (IOM, 2011): "Nurses should be full partners, with physicians and other health professionals, in redesigning health care in the United States" (p. 4). As long-time activists in advancing APRN practice at the state level, we discuss the differences and surprising similarities between our two states: Carolyn Montoya in New Mexico and Gale Adock in North Carolina.

A MOMENT IN TIME: NURSE PRACTITIONER PAST PORTENDS ITS FUTURE

New Mexico

The "first" family nurse practitioner (NP) provided care in a rural community in New Mexico in 1969 ("New Mexico Hamlet," 1969). In 1989, NPs' practice included prescriptive privileges, excluding controlled substances, under written protocols, and physician supervision was required (Pearson, 1989). In 1991, the Nursing Practice Act was revised to define advanced practice as being in collaboration with, rather than under the supervision of, a physician. In 1993, NPs were successful in obtaining FPA under a statute allowing APRNs to:

> . . . practice independently and make decisions regarding health care needs of the individual, family community and carry out health regimens including the prescription and distribution of dangerous drugs, and controlled substances in Schedules II through V of the Controlled Act; and serve as primary acute, chronic long-term and end of life provider and as necessary collaborate with licensed medical doctors, osteopathic physicians or podiatrists. (New Mexico Nursing Practice Act, 2014, p. 16)

How was New Mexico able to achieve independent practice in such a short time? With 33 counties and a population of 2.2 million, New Mexico has approximately 17 individuals per square mile (U.S. Census Bureau, 2017). Given the rurality of the state, low population, and shortage of primary care providers, state legislators were generally open to expanding the role of the NP to ensure that their constituents were able to receive health care.

North Carolina

North Carolina does not have FPA and is referred to as a "supervisory state." Legislation establishing NP practice was passed in the mid-1970s after pilot programs showed that experienced registered nurses overseen by physician preceptors could bring primary care to underserved rural areas of the state. However, the NP role was unambiguously tied to medicine, establishing joint regulation between the boards of medicine and nursing, and requiring physician supervision for "the performance of medical acts." After a decade of "supervised practice," cracks in the logic and practicality of the model surfaced. Experienced NPs had the same supervisory requirements as new NP graduates, and NPs relocating to North Carolina from FPA states were frustrated by supervision of what they previously did independently. Ironically, the compelling reason for establishing NP practice—to increase access to primary care in underserved areas—was being hampered by the requirement for physician supervision.

When I began NP practice in 1987, there was a general atmosphere of respect among the state's physicians and NP leaders, and progress was made through carefully negotiated regulatory changes. The most significant breakthroughs occurred between 1994 and 1996: replacement of a restrictive formulary with a "drug and device agreement" specific to an NP's practice setting and patient population; addition of prescriptive authority for controlled substances mirroring the physicians' Drug Enforcement Administration regulations (except for 90-day supplies of Schedule II drugs); and elimination of the "supervising physician" signature on patient visits performed by NPs.

In the 1990s, the collegial relationships between NP and physician leaders began to fray as managed care reimbursements tightened, marketplace competition increased, and more NPs opened successful private practices. The American Medical Association (AMA) became displeased with what they perceived as physicians' participation in expanding NP scope of practice. Several physician champions were publicly shamed at the 1995 AMA House of Delegates for offering a resolution on collaborative practice with NPs and other APRNs. As a result, NPs lost leverage with previously supportive physician leaders. Having exhausted all regulatory avenues to improving practice, in 2001 they filed a bill in the state legislature to amend the Medical Practice Act to remove physician supervision, eliminate collaborative practice agreements, and authorize the North Carolina Board of Nursing to solely regulate NPs. With this one action, what had once been achieved through respectful consensus became fodder for debate in the state legislature.

A NEW DAY: THE NURSE PRACTITIONER MOVEMENT MATURES

New Mexico

In 1993, as President of the New Mexico Nurse Practitioner Council (NMNPC) and with our community partners, we were successful in the passage of the legislation that provided FPA for NPs in our state. Naively, I believed that all our practice problems were solved with this legislation.

Passage of legislation is different from implementation of policy. Although some health care organizations embraced the ability to have NPs work without being supervised by physicians, others circumvented the legislation by implementing organizational policies requiring physician supervision. Health insurance companies, many located out of state, would not directly reimburse NPs for their services. To

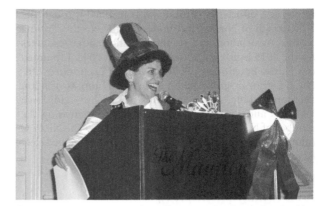

Carolyn Montoya leading the efforts to raise funds for the National Nurse Practitioner Political Action Committee.

address these challenges, the NMNPC began a concentrated effort to meet with executives from local health care organizations and insurance companies to discuss the legislation and advocate for organizational policies that would embrace the legislative intent. The most successful strategy was to have NPs in these organizations become executive team members or be appointed to the board of directors. The importance of NPs having a positive relationship with, or being members of, organizational leadership is a key strategy for successful implementation of NP legislation, a conclusion also reached by Poghosyan, Norful, and Laugesen (2018).

North Carolina

Our unsuccessful bid for FPA, plus attempts by North Carolina anesthesiologists to impose joint regulation, physician supervision, and collaborative practice agreements on certified registered nurse anesthetists (CRNAs), led to renewed efforts by NPs, CRNAs, clinical nurse specialists and certified nurse-midwives to work together. Adopting an "all for one and one for all" philosophy, the four APRN groups began *for the first time* to pool their resources and efforts. This circling of the APRN wagons was challenging and time-consuming, but essential for our mutual struggle for autonomy. Regular conference calls and in-person meetings to share information, perfect policy language, and devise strategies resulted in strong personal and professional relationships across APRN groups and leaders. The foundation of this deepening trust was built on a commitment not to sacrifice any APRN group for the benefit of any other group's FPA progress.

The Modernize Nursing Practice Act was first introduced in 2015 and again in 2017, with a substantial portion of the bill establishing FPA for all APRNs. This time, two unrelated decisions proved to be NPs powerful tools. First, in 2008, NPs agreed to pay an extra $25 with each annual association dues renewal to build an "advocacy fund" for future FPA efforts. This fund was controlled through the NP Council of Nurse Practitioners of the North Carolina Nurses' Association and resulted in substantial resources for the 2015 legislative session. Second, in 2005, I founded the Nurse Practitioner Political Action Committee (NP PAC), a strategic group with independent, non-association decision making. Advocacy funds helped hire additional lobbyists and staff members dedicated to increasing the number of NPs engaged in political advocacy. The NP PAC funds raised our profile as political players and helped elect legislators who supported FPA.

LESSONS LEARNED: FINDING AND USING YOUR VOICE

New Mexico

Given the battles that other states continue to encounter to achieve FPA, one has to ask, "Why were New Mexico NPs successful in their efforts over 25 years ago?" Although state legislators were open to independent practice, there was opposition from the New Mexico Medical Society and NPs themselves who were concerned about the increased responsibility of independent practice. Key strategies to success included presenting a united front from all state nursing associations, accurate health care data, a strong lobbyist who was an NP, meetings between NP advocates and members of the state medical society, and a willingness to compromise with physicians on policy language (Birkholz & Walker, 1994).

Since 1993, more states have achieved FPA and are disseminating their experiences in the literature, many of which mirror strategies described by Birkholz and Walker (1994). Rigolosi and Salmond (2014) used the Kingdon model of policy analysis to conduct a qualitative study of key informants from six states that passed independent legislation between 2007 and 2012. Two major themes emerged that led to legislation change: (1) driving factors for the change and (2) process approach strategies to advocate and secure change. Driving factors included problems finding collaborators, exorbitant fees and payment for a signature of a provider rather than a health care service provided, shortage of physicians, limited access to care, and sunset laws, all leading to the "perfect storm of opportunity." Strategies used to move the legislation forward included coalition support, identifying coalition opposition, and grassroots activities with legislators, such as providing patient stories and face-to-face meetings (Box 63.1).

North Carolina

Joining forces across APRN practice lines and ditching the "silo thinking" of separate groups were critical steps for North Carolina and are core to many states' successful

---

BOX 63.1   Tips for Legislative Success

- Assess the health care status of the state, including access to care.
- Involve APRN and health-related professionals early in the process.
- Cultivate APRN community and legislative champions.
- Gather succinct evidence-based health outcomes of care provided by APRNs.
- Identify opposing groups and opposing views and prepare counterpoints.
- Educate legislators regarding APRNs as partners in solving health care problems in the state.
- Recruit articulate APRNs to tell their stories regarding the care they provide in their communities.
- Assemble an experienced and respected team of lobbyists, APRNs, and professional staff.

APRN, Advanced practice registered nurse.

FPA initiatives. Our most transformative lesson was the fundamental change in group mindset: we stopped viewing each state legislative session without passage of an FPA bill as a loss and instead, adopted the view that each session was a separate skirmish in a larger, lengthier campaign. By redefining success in this way, our messaging is positive, our optimism contagious, and our momentum sustained. We haven't come this far to only come this far.

MOVING FORWARD: IT TAKES A VILLAGE TO BUILD A BENCH

New Mexico

Advocacy for patients and the NP profession has continued in New Mexico since the passage of independent practice in 1993. New Mexico is part of Medicaid expansion, with an approximate enrollment of 843,729—almost half of our population (New Mexico Medicaid Advisory Board, personal communication, August 6, 2018). We continue to have a shortage of primary care providers, particularly in rural settings, and face the "silver tsunami" of an aging population and aging health care workforce.

The NMNPC continues to emphasize political advocacy by supporting our lobbyist and monitoring each legislative session for bills that affect our patients' health and bills that could possibly impact our ability to maintain our FPA. Recent legislative successes include the ability to declare and sign death certificates, continuation of a $3000 tax credit for NPs working in rural areas, and defeat of legislation that would have created a physician-controlled "super board" tasked with providing recommendations to legislators regarding changes in the Nursing Practice Act or any other health profession practice act. We continue to support the American Association of Nurse Practitioners and participate in regional meetings to learn from other states and offer advice based on our experiences. Nurse educators, nurse researchers, and APRNs need to remain united in their advocacy for improving health outcomes and obtain the necessary political skills to effect positive changes for our patients and our profession.

North Carolina

One result of increasing the ranks of knowledgeable and engaged NP advocates is the growing interest of many to run for office. I am the first NP to be elected to our state legislature, elected just in time to participate in renewed FPA efforts in 2015 and 2017. I was reelected in 2018 and will support the FPA bill reintroduction in 2019.

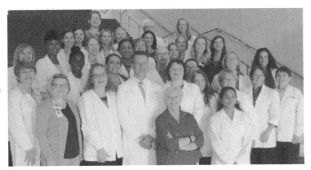

Gale Adcock and North Carolina NPs advocate for full practice authority at the state legislature

Having more NP elected officials will move important policy conversations forward, not just FPA. Building a bench requires mentoring a large number of NPs to become effective advocates and positioning them before critical issues are on the table. Energized by their policy experiences, NPs can develop a growth mindset that can lead to running for elected office at the local, state, or national levels. Box 63.2

BOX 63.2   Groundwork for Running for Office

- Figure out your passions and interests.
- Add community and political involvement to your nursing resume.
- Attend campaign school.
- Let others know you are interested in running.

---

provides fundamental considerations for NPs interested in seeking office (also see Chapter 43).

CONCLUSION

Dr. Loretta Ford, co-founder of the NP profession, stated, "We're going to survive—and thrive. But we do have to do it politically, and we cannot do it unless we unite" (Ford & Gardenier, 2015, p. 577). Although these two states are different in terms of population, economy, and culture, the story of their collective challenges can be used when trying to improve health care legislation. Whether a state has enjoyed FPA for 25 years like New Mexico or is engaged in a multiyear lobbying effort to achieve FPA like North Carolina, FPA is not the end point. It is the foundation for APRNs to acquire the power necessary to fulfill the goal of equal partnership as leaders in redesigning health care.

DISCUSSION QUESTIONS

1. Discuss the advantages and disadvantages of collaborating with physician organizations when pursuing FPA legislation.
2. Provide a personal example of an experience you have had where you were unable to provide a service to a patient due to the limits of your state practice authority.

REFERENCES

Birkholz, G., & Walker, D. (1994). Strategies for state statutory language. Changes granting fully independent nurse practitioner practice. *Nurse Practitioner, 19*(1), 54-58.

Ford, L.C., & Gardenier, D. (2015). Fasten your seat belts—It's going to be a bumpy ride. *Journal for Nurse Practitioners, 11*(6), 575-577.

Institute of Medicine. (2011). *The future of nursing: Leading change, advancing health.* Washington, DC: The National Academies Press.

New Mexico hamlet avoids medical isolation. (1969). *Journal of the American Medical Association, 207*(10), 1808-1809.

New Mexico Nursing Practice Act, NM Statue § 61-3-23.2 (2014).

Pearson, L.J. (1989). How each state stands on legislative issues affecting advanced nursing practice. *Nurse Practitioner, 14*(1), 27-34.

Poghosyan, L., Norful, A.A., & Laugesen, M.J. (2018). Removing restrictions on nurse practitioners' scope of practice in New York State: Physicians' and nurse practitioners' perspectives. *Journal of the American Association of Nurse Practitioners, 30*(6), 354-360.

Rigolosi, R., & Salmond, S. (2014). The journey to independent nurse practitioner practice. *Journal of the American Association of Nurse Practitioners, 26*(12), 649-656.

U.S. Census Bureau. (2017). *QuickFacts: New Mexico.* Retrieved from www.census.gov/quickfacts/nm.

64

Policy and Politics in Nursing Academia

Ellen Frances Olshansky

"If the structure does not permit dialogue the structure must be changed"

Paulo Freire

The intent of policies is to clarify, provide direction and structure, and ultimately improve a system of government or an organization. There is controversy, however, about what policies advance a society and what policies deter progress. Much of this controversy is due to differing political views, with politics having a direct influence on policies.

In academia, the mission is to generate knowledge in the spirit of improving society. Politics and policies can be barriers (interferences) or facilitators (constructive change agents) to advancing academic nursing and ultimately improving society. Academic institutions are not immune to political influence. In fact, many academic policies are developed based on the larger political context. This chapter describes how internal and external politics and policies influence nursing academia. Examples of internal and external policies are presented with discussion of how they act as barriers or facilitators for advancing academic nursing (Box 64.1).

Our educational programs dictate and influence our professional practice, and policies dictate our educational programs. Understanding the relationship between policies, nursing education, and nursing practice is key to improving and creating more constructive policies that are conducive to outstanding educational programs.

ACADEMIC FREEDOM AS CENTRAL TO NURSING EDUCATION

It is crucial that nursing leaders advocate for maintaining an environment in which academic freedom thrives, supporting policies that facilitate nursing education. A recent American Academy of Nursing position statement (Taylor, Olshansky, Woods, et al., 2017) describes the basic tenets of academic freedom. It is a fundamental commitment by a university that all members are able, with the broadest latitude, to speak, write, listen, challenge, and learn. It provides the ability to express one's views at the broadest scope through research, analysis, and discourse. This right is protected by legal principles upheld by the American Association of University Professors (AAUP, 1940) and the American Association of Colleges and Universities.

Despite this strong history over the past 7 decades, threats to academic freedom continue. Many policies may either facilitate or interfere with academic freedom, affecting academia in general and nursing academia specifically. The following section presents examples of internal and external policies, influenced by politics, that ultimately can affect nursing academia.

INTERNAL POLITICS AND POLICIES

Academic freedom and free speech are significant issues in educational institutions (Chemerinsky & Gilman, 2017). When social or political events heighten a community's awareness of social justice issues, nursing academics often feel ethically bound to support efforts to address the issues. Grassroots organizations, such as Black Lives Matter, raise awareness of important issues. However, faculty involvement in controversial issues is not always well received by societal and academic organizations. Instead, organizations may attempt to censor new ideas or perspectives that may be perceived as threatening to the status quo.

For example, in Arizona, politicians wanted to ban ethnic studies and social justice courses on campus. A bill introduced in 2017 by state representative Bob Thorpe followed an earlier Arizona law banning a Mexican American studies

BOX 64.1   Summary of Internal and External Forces on Nursing Academia Policy

Internal	External
Academic freedom	Professional organizations
Tenure process	Grassroots organizations
Recognition of nurses as academicians	Government organizations
Governance within colleges and universities	Non-profit organizations
Sources of revenue/ priorities for spending	

class in the Tucson Unified School District, eventually thrown out after a federal judge ruled this ban as racist (Galvin, 2017). Specifically, the proposed legislation prevents all courses, classes, activities, and events that promote "social justice toward a race, gender, religion, political affiliation, social class or other class of people" from being presented in public schools in Arizona (Levin, 2017). Although this is targeted to public schools in K-12, the potential censuring at public colleges and universities, and therefore nursing education centrally concerned with cultural diversity and sensitivity is important to understand. Academic freedom, or lack of freedom, is an important issue for nursing education. This bill is an example of both external and internal political factors and has implications for how academic organizations address free speech and academic freedom. The major tenets of academic freedom are important in understanding where interference with or barriers to academic freedom persist.

Within academia itself, political context is reflected in governance issues…how decisions are made and who influences decisions…that in turn impact development of academic policies. Traditional academic priorities affect nursing education. In academic research institutions, the acquisition of major research funding is a requirement for faculty looking to achieve tenure. As the nursing discipline has developed its own body of scientific research (evidenced by its own institute within the National Institutes of Health [NIH]), and more nursing faculty have been awarded research funding and achieved tenure, they have strengthened their political influence in academia. Tenure provides secure employment, giving both clout and empowerment to speak up. Having more tenured nursing professors within academic research institutions contributes a voice in these settings.

This empowerment has not been without a struggle. Only within the past several decades has nursing been recognized as an equal member of traditional academic

institutions. For example, in 1965 at the University of California San Francisco (UCSF) School of Nursing, the UCSF Academic Senate and the California state legislature approved a doctoral program in nursing but refused to call the degree from this program a Doctor of Philosophy, or PhD. Instead, it was a Doctor of Nursing Science, or DNSc, despite the curriculum being a rigorous research degree like other PhDs. This refusal reflected reticence on the part of Academic Senate members as well as state legislators to recognize nurses as researchers with an equal voice in academic settings. In the 1980s, the state legislature and the Academic Senate were more supportive of nurses as academicians and researchers; with Academic Senate approval, the UCSF School of Nursing changed its doctoral program to a PhD for incoming students. Several years later, the Academic Senate, through pressure from UCSF nursing alumni, granted retroactive PhDs to DNSc graduates. They recognized that the curriculum for the PhD program was the same as the DNSc program and the potential gender bias in the original 1960s decision. Although many DNSc graduates have contributed in remarkable ways to the body of nursing science, it is an example of how academic and state legislative politics are reflective of the time and context. It is important to recognize that some DNSc graduates opted to keep their DNSc, demonstrating pride in their original, outstanding degree. Although this issue raises the question of why a PhD matters, in the larger world of academia, the PhD is understood across disciplines. This issue represents power, gender, and hierarchical issues in academia.

Governance within educational institutions affects policies. Is there shared governance? To what degree? How is representation in decision-making from faculty assured? Academic institutions tend to be organized on a hierarchy of tenured and non-tenured faculty, staff, students, and alumni and each group has a relative voice. There are varying degrees of shared decision-making/shared governance within different institutions.

Another internal factor influencing academic politics is the source and internal distribution of revenue within an academic setting. Funding for nursing education will vary depending on the priorities of individual institutions and the allocation of funding to specific programs, departments, and schools. Although some universities have a strong faculty governance, it is usually the provost of a university who is the final decision-maker regarding allocation of resources.

EXTERNAL POLITICS AND POLICIES

Although external to academic/educational organizations, many organizations and government politics have significant influence on academic policies. The examples described here specifically relate to influence on nursing academic organizations.

Professional Organizations

Professional organizations provide strong influence on academia. For example, the American Academy of Nursing issued a position statement in opposition to political interference in nursing research and practice, with a specific focus on sexual and reproductive health (Olshansky, Taylor, Johnson-Mallard, et al., 2018; Taylor, Olshansky, Woods, et al., 2017; Reproductive Health in Nursing, 2017). This position statement was responding to attempts by the federal government administration to create policy barriers to academic research on sexual and reproductive health. The proposed policies created unnecessary restrictions on clinics that provided abortion services, limiting access to Food and Drug Administration-approved contraceptives, limiting Title X funding (which provides services for sexual and reproductive health), and proposed a ban on students conducting research related to contraception and abortion. By attempting to limit nursing research and practice in controversial areas (such as abortion), these policies impede knowledge generation in academia. More specifically, students will be precluded from gaining important and needed clinical experience.

The American Nurses Association (ANA) is the largest nursing professional organization in the United States and has tremendous influence on policy. Much of its focus is on nursing workforce development and policies that have a direct effect on the health and health care of citizens. The ANA identified 2018 as the "Year of Advocacy" (ANA, 2018) and has focused lobbying to support its priority issues: (1) local advocacy, (2) advocacy through influence on elected officials, (3) advocacy to ensure that all citizens vote in elections, and (4) global advocacy (Table 64.1).

One specific example of an educational program/degree issue advanced by the ANA is the bachelor of science in nursing (BSN) degree as the entry into practice for registered nurses (RNs). In 1965, the ANA called for the BSN degree to be the entry educational level into nursing practice. Today, we are still working to make that recommendation policy. Ideally, this would be a national policy; however, individual states issue RN licenses. Therefore, policy change must occur at the state level. In order to be strategic and make constructive changes, we need to work within our complex political environments that include numerous interrelated factors. For example, New York state passed the "BSN in Ten" policy (Mensik, 2017), mandating that all RNs working in New York state have a BSN in ten years in order to continue practicing

TABLE 64.1 Priorities for the Year of Advocacy at the American Nurses Association	
Priority Area	**Description**
Nurses need to advocate locally	Advocating for patients at the bedside, on boards; advocating for nursing profession
Nurses need to become proactive in influencing elected officials	Becoming involved in advocating for political candidates who support nursing's values to promote health of patients, health care providers, communities
Nurses need to influence the public to vote in elections	Nurses have a big role in ensuring that people exercise their right to vote; nurses, themselves, are also encouraged to run for public elected office
Nurses need to become involved globally	Nurses can have an impact on our global environment by participating in global organizations and being aware of global issues

Source: American Nurses Association, 2018.

nursing. This political activism and advocacy by nursing organizations in collaboration with legislators made a concrete difference. The debate regarding the BSN degree as entry into practice continues across the country, but New York set an important precedent that will directly affect academic programs that prepare nurses for licensure.

New York state's success is just the beginning. The American Association of Colleges of Nursing (AACN), which represents baccalaureate and graduate nursing education and is one of the credentialing bodies for nursing education programs, has consistently supported the BSN degree as the entry into practice. However, other organizations, specifically the American Association of Community Colleges (AACC) and the Association of Community College Trustees (AACCT) (Smith, 2017) continue to oppose the BSN as entry into practice, as they represent the interests of colleges that offer associate nursing degree programs. This issue is an example of how external factors can promote or inhibit policies that directly affect nursing education. This is also an example of how what is considered facilitating and what is considered interfering is dependent upon the views of various organizations. In other words, which side of a policy debate a person supports will determine whether a factor is considered a facilitator or a barrier. These differing views of the BSN as the entry into practice often reflect differing political opinions and perspectives.

Another example of an educational degree program influenced by policies and politics is the AACN's 2006 proposal for the Doctor of Nursing Practice (DNP) degree, with the goal of making the DNP the entry into practice for advanced practice nurses (APNs) by 2015. The debate about the DNP encompasses two issues. One is whether the nursing profession should adopt the DNP at all and the other is if the DNP should replace the master's degree as the entry into practice for APNs. As with the debate surrounding the BSN degree, many differences of opinion exist, even within the nursing profession itself. Cronenwett, Dracup, Grey, and colleagues (2011) presented concerns about the DNP issue related to workforce development, especially because this was proposed during a time of economic distress in the country. Taking a supportive position of the DNP, Danzey and colleagues (2011) proposed it would contribute to alleviating the nursing faculty shortage. Even as more DNP programs have been established, this graduate degree has not become the required entry into advanced practice. The National Organization of Nurse Practitioner Faculties (2015) developed a white paper recommending the DNP for entry into practice for APNs.

Sigma Theta Tau International (STTI) and International Council of Nurses are examples of international professional nursing organizations that have global impact while also influencing nursing education in the United States. The position statement supporting the use of evidence-based nursing issued by STTI (2002) is relevant to academic freedom in that in order to generate knowledge, freedom of investigation and exploration of data is essential.

The AACN's Commission on Collegiate Nursing Education (AACN, 2018) and the National League for Nursing (NLN) (Jackson & Halstead, 2016) both contribute to policies that guide credentialing of nursing education programs, including developing education standards and curricular design and requirements. In order to be accredited, nursing education programs must comply with the education standards and requirements developed in these organizations. Nursing educators contribute to the creation of these standards through collaborative participation in these accrediting organizations.

Many state organizations also attempt to influence practice and educational issues. The California Association of Nurse Practitioners (CANP) worked to support the California legislature in granting APNs a more independent scope of practice. In 2015, California State Senator Ed Hernandez championed Senate Bill 323 to propose full practice authority for APNs in California (California Legislative Information, n.d.). However, this legislation was not successful two years in a row, with much of the opposition coming from the California Medical Association (CMA), the largest professional organization representing physicians in California. As of this publication, California still does not grant full practice authority to APNs.

There is also a myriad of specialty nursing organizations that focus on specific areas of nursing and health and have implications for nursing academia. For example, the Association of Women's Health, Obstetrics, and Neonatal Nursing (AWHONN) has developed policies related to reproductive justice as well as to nursing education and issued a statement of support for the BSN as entry-level education (AWHONN, 2014).

In describing how organizations are influential in policy development, the politics of the organizations are important to understand. For example, the American Medical Association and the CMA have strong views about the place of medicine in the hierarchy of health care, as noted earlier in the description of the attempt to change legislation to increase the scope of practice of APNs. These two very strong organizations often oppose policies recommended by nursing professional organizations.

Non-Profit Organizations

Non-profit philanthropic organizations also exert influence within nursing education. For example, The Hartford Foundation, a non-profit foundation that supports gerontology, funds the National Hartford Center of Gerontological Nursing Excellence, which prioritizes and supports gerontological nursing education (Perez, Mason, Harden, & Cortes, 2018). Leaders in nursing and health policy worked with the Hartford Foundation to create resources that emphasize the importance of focusing on gerontological nursing as a major portion of nursing academia. This is an example of a facilitator of nursing education.

The Robert Wood Johnson Foundation has had strong influence on nursing education through its Nurse Faculty Scholars Program (Gillespie et al., 2018), underwriting of the Institute of Medicine's *The Future of Nursing* report (Perez, Nichols, & Quinn, 2018), and Culture of Health programs (Montavlo & Veenema, 2015). The Jonas Philanthropies Foundation has also supported nursing doctoral education, nursing education for veterans, and created the Jonas Policy Scholars program in partnership with the American Academy of Nursing to develop health policy expertise in nurse educators (Oerther, Hallowell, Rossiter, & Gross, 2018).

Grassroots Organizations

Many grassroots organizations address specific social determinants of health, such as homelessness, violence against women, and immigration. Their work may overlap with the mission of many academic nursing programs. Grassroots organizations bring awareness to important political issues that are a part of the social determinants of health and have a strong impact on health outcomes (Olshansky, 2017).

Garcia and Sharif (2015) implore us to consider and embrace the public health aspects of racism and the importance of the message of Black Lives Matter. Structural racism is a social determinant of health and academic nursing must be able to openly discuss and teach about these issues. How have these organizations facilitated and intersected with nursing academia? The answer to this question is intertwined with academic freedom, free speech, and lack of censorship in order to bring new ideas to the academic setting.

The Orange County Women's Health Project (OCWHP) is an example of how grassroots organizations and nursing education intersect. The OCWHP (www.ocwomens health.org/) is a fiscally-sponsored organization founded by five women (Allyson Sonenshine, Ellen Olshansky, Stephanie Kight, Sue Bryant, and Karol Gottfredson) to serve as an advocacy organization for women's health in Orange County, California. OCWHP selected three priority areas for their work based on data that showed need in: (1) domestic violence, (2) breast and cervical cancer, and (3) prevention of unintended pregnancies. Through a partnership with the University of California, Irvine (UCI), California State University at Fullerton, and Chapman University, academic programs were influenced by emphasizing domestic violence as part of nursing curricula.

Similar to the OCWHP, MOMS of Orange County (MOMS OC, 2018) is a nonprofit, grassroots organization that addresses the needs of under-resourced pregnant and postpartum women. UCI School of Nursing has partnered with MOMS OC in conducting clinical research. Policies and priorities set by MOMS OC influences the focus of nursing education toward home care of ethnically diverse women of lower socioeconomic status.

Government Organizations

Governmental organizations and agencies at all levels, and the politics and policies within them, can have tremendous influence on nursing education. At the national level, the Title VII Nursing Workforce: Nurse Workforce Reauthorization Act (S. 1109/H.R. 959) is a policy that provides financial support for nursing workforce programs and grants. Currently, this particular bill proposes an amendment to the Public Health Service Act by extending its support through fiscal year 2022, and by expanding eligibility for such support for Clinical Nurse Leaders and Clinical Nurse Specialist programs. This bill also proposes to extend support for loan repayment and scholarships for nurses, loans for nursing faculty with a specific focus on geriatric nursing care, and for programs that expand diversity in nursing educational institutions until 2022. Nursing education initiatives such as nurse-managed clinics and nurse-residency programs are also mentioned in the bill, with financial support also extending through 2022.

For many years, gun violence and gun safety research was banned at the federal level through the Dickey Amendment (Rostron, 2018). In the wake of increased incidence of high-profile gun violence, in 2017 the Gun Violence Research Act (HR1478) was proposed by Representative Stephanie Murphy (D-FL) to re-authorize research on gun safety and prevention of gun violence. This bill amends the Consolidated Appropriations Act of 2016, allowing research on gun violence and how to achieve gun safety. This legislation directly affects what research will be funded by governmental organizations, like the Centers for Disease Control and Prevention (CDC). This could, in turn, influence the research funding available for nurses and nursing programs involved in public health research and it directly affects the basic tenets of academic freedom as outlined earlier.

Also, at the federal level, the U.S. Department of Health and Human Services (HSS) created a new Office of Conscience and Religious Freedom that is part of the Office of Civil Rights (HHS, 2018). This office is directed to "protect" practitioners from being forced to care for patients who conflict with their own conscience/moral views. Although such a policy can be debated as being in direct conflict with nursing's ethic of caring for all people, the fact that it exists at the federal level can and will affect nursing education. We are already witnessing a decrease in the focus on health care issues such as abortion, which is protected by federal law, but experiencing fewer and fewer providers who learn how to care for women choosing abortion. Another example of federal political interference is the 2018 warning sent to UCSF from the HHS, indicating that the federal government will end funding for research involving fetal tissue. The research being conducted was using fetal tissue to create "humanized mice" as a way of developing potential vaccinations against human immunodeficiency virus (HIV) (Grady, 2018).

Finally, at the state level, numerous policies in various states were recently introduced that could affect nursing education and the availability of clinical education sites. As of this printing, Planned Parenthood has withdrawn from federal Title X funding rather than comply with what is referred to as the "gag" rule, wherein clinicians who even discuss abortion as an option will be precluded from receiving Title X funding. Litigation is continuing on who is eligible for Title X funding. This funding began in 1970 and is the mainstay of funding for Planned Parenthood. Even before this recent decision, states were chipping away at funding. The state of Missouri ended contracts with Planned Parenthood, leading to a dearth of nursing education/clinical sites for nursing students to learn about women's health (Taylor, Olshansky, Woods, et al., 2017). In 2018, the Supreme Court ruled a California law was unconstitutional that compels anti-abortion pregnancy centers to tell clients about their pregnancy options, including abortion (Savage, 2018). The consequences of this ruling are that these clinics will be able to withhold information about all the reproductive choices available to women. This may limit clinical services that offer or inform women about abortion, resulting in fewer and fewer clinical sites available for nursing students to learn about all aspects of reproductive health. On the other hand, California recently passed two bills (CA 154 and 980) that allow nurse practitioners, certified nurse midwives, and physician assistants to perform first-trimester abortions (Taylor, Battistelli, & Anderson, 2017). This ruling affects nursing academia in California by potentially providing additional clinical sites for nursing students.

SUMMARY: INFLUENCE OF POLITICS AND POLICIES ON ACADEMIC NURSING

In considering both external and internal politics and policies, the effects on academic nursing can be witnessed in each of the tripartite aspects of academic nursing: education, practice, and research.

In nursing *education*, the profession of nursing has continued to embrace the explosion of knowledge and technology. Advanced nursing education programs must keep up with the complexity of nursing and health care. Yet, this increased complexity and knowledge has not always directly led to changes in nursing education. Resistance to change has existed simultaneously with progress. As noted at the beginning of this chapter, creating policies that support the BSN as the entry into practice for RNs has been an ongoing debate since 1965. The more recent debate over the DNP as the entry into practice for APNs is also evidence of simultaneous progress and resistance. Our educational programs will dictate our professional practice, and policies dictate our educational programs.

Nursing *practice* is a key and critical factor in nursing academic programs. One essential factor for learning the professional nursing role is the availability of clinical sites for students. As noted previously, some current policies make it difficult, if not impossible, for students to work in quality clinical sites where they can learn to care for women seeking abortions. Despite scientific evidence on the safety of abortions, efforts continue to try to limit or outright ban abortion and consequently prevent clinical training for APNs and other nurses in abortion care (Taylor, Safriet, & Weitz, 2009). This interference with clinical practice sites in nursing education is a direct result of policies based on politics.

Nursing *research* is another key factor in nursing academic programs. Academic programs can be facilitated or constrained depending on research conducted by nurse scholars. Prior to 2018, the amendment to the rule that banned research on gun violence and gun safety precluded such research. As health policy leaders influence legislators to view gun violence as a public health issue, there may be more funding and fewer obstacles to research in this area (Zhang, 2018). Funding agencies often make it difficult to study certain topics. For example, NIH is less eager to fund research on abortion or contraception, thereby precluding or severely limiting nursing research in these areas. Thus, research that is "fundable" will influence the actual research conducted in academic settings, and decisions about what is fundable are based on policies and politics.

Nursing academia functions within a larger political context, and nursing education does not occur in a vacuum or in an isolated institution. Nursing leaders must be aware of and sensitive to the influence of politics and policies in the academic setting.

DISCUSSION QUESTIONS

1. Discuss the difference between internal and external factors that influence policy, and describe examples of both.
2. Why is it important for nurse educators to be aware of and understand the implications of policies that may affect nursing education? How can nursing educators influence health policy?

REFERENCES

American Association of Colleges of Nursing. (2018). *About CCNE accreditation*. Retrieved from www.aacnnursing.org/CCNE-Accreditation/About.

American Association of University Professors. (1940). *1940 Statement of principles on academic freedom and tenure*. American Association of University Professors and of the Association of American Colleges. Retrieved from www.aaup.org/report/1940-statement-principles-academic-freedom-and-tenure.

American Nurses Association (ANA). (2018). *Year of advocacy: 2018*. Retrieved from https://ana.aristotle.com/sitepages/yearofadvocacy.aspx.

Association of Women's Health, Obstetric, and Neonatal Nursing. (2014). Position statement: Nursing education. *Journal of Obstetric, Gynecologic and Neonatal Nursing, 43*(1), 130-131.

California Legislative Information. (n.d.). *SB-323 nurse practitioners: scope of practice (2015-2016)*. Retrieved from https://leginfo.legislature.ca.gov/faces/billNavClient.xhtml?bill_id=201520160SB323.

Chemerinsky, E., & Gillman, H. (2017). *Free speech on campus*. New Haven, CT: Yale University Press.

Cronenwett, L., Dracup, K., Grey, M., McCauley, L., Meleis, A., & Salmon, M. (2011). The Doctor of Nursing Practice: A national workforce perspective. *Nursing Outlook, 59*(1), 9-17.

Danzey, I.M., Ea, E., Fitzgerald, J.J., Garbutt, S.J., Rafferty, M., & Zychowicz, M.E. (2011). The Doctor of Nursing Practice and nursing education: Highlights, potential, and promise. *Journal of Professional Nursing, 27*(5), 311-314.

U.S. Department of Health and Human Services. (2018). *HHS announces new conscience and religious freedom division*. Retrieved from www.hhs.gov/about/news/2018/01/18/hhs-ocr-announces-new-conscience-and-religious-freedom-division.html.

Galvin, A.G. (2017). Judge: Racism behind Arizona ban on Tucson Unified School District's Mexican-American studies. *Tucson.com News*. Retrieved from https://tucson.com/news/local/judge-racism-behind-arizona-ban-on-tusd-s-mexican-american/article_468a9280-bf80-5df8-82d3-dadb5b608cf7.html.

Garcia, J.J., & Sharif, M.Z. (2015). Black lives matter: A commentary on racism and public health. *American Journal of Public Health, 105*, e27-e30. Retrieved from https://ajph.aphapublications.org/doi/pdf/10.2105/AJPH.2015.302706.

Gillespie, G.L., Gakumo, A., Von, A.D., Pesut, D.J., Gonzales-Guarda, R.M., & Thomas, T. (2018). A summative evaluation of productivity and accomplishments of Robert Wood Johnson Foundation Nurse Faculty Scholars Program partici pants. *Journal of Professional Nursing, 34*(4), 289-295.

Grady, D. (2018). Fetal tissue research is curtailed by Trump administration. *New York Times*. Retrieved from www.nytimes.com/2018/12/12/health/fetal-tissue-research-trump.html?rref=collection%2Ftimestopic%2FHealth%20and%20Human%20Services%20Department&action=click&contentCollection=timestopics&region=stream&module=stream_unit&version=latest&contentPlacement=1&pgtype=collection.

Jackson, A., & Halstead, J. (2016). National League for Nursing commission for nursing education accreditation. *Nurse Educator, 41*(6), 303.

Levin, S. (2017). Arizona republicans move to ban social justice courses and events at schools. *The Guardian*. Retrieved from www.theguardian.com/us-news/2017/jan/13/arizona-schools-social-justice-courses-ban-bill.

Mensik, J. (2017). *New York governor signs BSN in 10 into law for nurses*. Retrieved from www.nurse.com/blog/2017/12/20/new-york-governor-signs-bsn-in-10-into-law-for-nurses/.

MOMS of Orange County. (2018). *About MOMS of Orange County*. Retrieved from www.momsorangecounty.org.

Montavlo, W., & Veenema, T.G. (2015). Mentorship in developing transformational leaders to advance health policy: Creating a culture of health. *Nurse Leader, 13*(1), 65-69.

National Organization of Nurse Practitioner Faculties. (2015). *The Doctorate of Nursing Practice NP preparation: NONPF perspective*. Retrieved from https://cdn.ymaws.com/www.nonpf.org/resource/resmgr/DNP/NONPFDNPStatementSept2015.pdf.

National Organization of Nurse Practitioner Faculties. (2016). *Background paper: Transitioning to a seamless, integrated DNP NP curriculum*. Retrieved from https://cdn.ymaws.com/www.nonpf.org/resource/resmgr/Docs/DNPSeamlessTransitionNONPFFi.pdf.

Oerther, S., Hallowell, S., Rossiter, A., & Gross, D. (2018). The American Academy of Nursing Jonas Policy Scholars Program: Mentoring future nurse leaders to advance health policy. *Journal of Advanced Nursing, 75*(10), 2253-2257.

Olshansky, E. (2017). Social determinants of health: The role of nursing. *American Journal of Nursing, 117*(12), 11.

Olshansky, E., Taylor, D., Johnson-Mallard, V., Halloway, S., & Stokes, L. (2018). Sexual and reproductive health rights, access and justice: Where nursing stands. *Nursing Outlook, 66*, 416-422.

Perez, A., Nichols, B., & Quinn, W.V. (2018). Growing diverse nurse leaders: The current progress of the future of nursing campaign for action. *Nurse Leader, 16*(1), 38-42.

Perez, G.A., Mason, D., Harden, J.T., & Cortes, T. (2018). The growth and development of gerontological nurse leaders in policy. *Nursing Outlook, 66*(2), 168-179.

Reproductive Health in Nursing. (2017). *Nurses oppose political interference in research and health professional education*. Retrieved from https://rhnursing.org/resource/policy-nurses-academic-freedom/.

Rostron, A. (2018). The Dickey Amendment on federal funding for research on gun violence: A legal dissection. *American Journal of Public Health, 108*(7), 865-867.

Savage, D.G. (2018). Supreme court rules for faith-based pregnancy centers, blocks California disclosure law. *The Los Angeles Times*. Retrieved from www.latimes.com/politics/la-na-pol-court-pregnancy-abortion-20180626-story.html.

Sigma Theta Tau International 2005-2007 Research and Scholarship Advisory Committee. (2002). Position statement on evidence-based practice. *Worldviews Evidence Based Nursing, 5*(2), 57-59. Retrieved from www.sigmanursing.org/why-sigma/about-sigma/position-statements-and-resource-papers/evidence-based-nursing-position-statement.

Smith, A. (2017). Debate continues on nursing degrees. *Inside Higher Education*. Retrieved from www.insidehighered.com/news/2017/12/22/battle-over-entry-level-degree-nursing-continues.

Taylor, D., Battistelli, M., & Anderson, P. (2017). *Fact sheet summarizing the HWPP aims and background, study methods and findings, and policy strategy for durable change*. Retrieved from https://rhnursing.org/resource/hwpp-fact-sheets/.

Taylor, D., Olshansky, E.F., Woods, N.F., Johnson-Mallard, V., Safriet, B.J., & Hagan, T. (2017). Position statement: Political interference in sexual and reproductive health research and health professional education1. *Nursing Outlook, 65*(2), 242-245.

Taylor, D., Safriet, B., & Weitz, T. (2009). When politics trumps evidence: Legislative or regulatory exclusion of abortion from advanced practice clinician scope of practice. *Journal of Midwifery and Women's Health, 54*(1), 4-7.

Zhang, S. (2018). Why can't the US treat gun violence as a public health problem? *The Atlantic.* Retrieved from www.theatlantic.com/health/archive/2018/02/gun-violence-public-health/553430/.

ONLINE RESOURCES

American Academy of Nursing Jonas Policy Scholars
www.aannet.org/initiatives/academy-jonas-policy-scholars
American Nurses Association practice and policy overview
www.nursingworld.org/practice-policy/
California Association of Nurse Practitioners advocacy
   overview
https://canpweb.org/advocacy/

65

The Intersection of Technology and Health Care: Policy and Practice Implications

Carol A. Romano[a]

> *"Technology is a useful servant but a dangerous master."*
>
> **Christian Lous Lang**

The invasion of information technology into the information-intensive area of health care has evolved together with the intent to improve access to care, enhance quality and safety, and reduce administrative and operational costs. Information technology holds great promise to improve a health care system in which patients cannot be assured they will receive the right care at the right time and in which coordination and communications related to care are lacking. Despite the introduction of information technology into the health care environment over half a century ago, in 2010 remote monitoring and telehealth technologies were not commonly used (The National Ambulatory Medical Care Survey, 2010). A 2016 study using national hospital data reported increases in adoption of electronic health records (EHRs) among hospitals eligible for policy-driven incentive programs, but not for others (Adler-Milstein & Jha, 2016). A surge of national policies in the past 2 decades has emerged to protect health information and facilitate and incentivize improved health outcomes and access to care through enhanced use of information technology.

This chapter presents an overview of critical policies related to health information technology (HIT) and addresses the implications that each pose to clinical practice. The chapter also presents considerations and concerns related to the unintended consequences of the technology-health care intersection.

The 1999 Institute of Medicine (IOM) report *To Err Is Human: Building a Safer Health System* catalyzed a revolution to improve the quality of care and triggered the demand for a new direction and approach to health care. HIT is viewed as a necessary tool to aid the health reform process (Berwick, Nolan, & Whittington, 2008; Hebda & Czar, 2013). HIT encompasses a wide range of electronic tools that can help to access up-to-date evidence-based clinical guidelines and decision support and provide proactive health maintenance for patients. HIT can also facilitate better coordination of patient care with other providers through the secure and private sharing of clinical information. Given these benefits, concerns arise over the need to protect the privacy of personal health information in electronic form. There are also concerns about financial, technical, and social barriers to the implementation of HIT that may limit the benefits for improving care, access, and efficiency. In 2004, the government addressed these concerns and spawned public policy focused on HIT as a necessary tool to reform health and health care. The federal government's official website for HIT is www.healthit.gov.

PUBLIC POLICY SUPPORT FOR HIT

Public policy can be generally defined as a system of laws, regulatory measures, courses of action, and funding priorities concerning a given topic promulgated by a governmental entity. A major aspect of public policy is laws that formalize funding and give statutory authority to initiatives (Kilpatrick, 2000). Several laws have formalized government support for HIT.

Health Insurance Portability and Accountability Act

Patients and providers hold a long-standing concern over the privacy and unprotected access to personal

---

[a]The views expressed in this chapter reflect those of the author and do not represent opinions or positions of the U.S. government, Department of Defense, or the Uniformed Services University.

health information (Hebda & Czar, 2013). In 1996, Health Insurance Portability and Accountability Act (HIPAA) not only provided health insurance coverage protection, it included privacy and security rules that describe what information is protected, how it can be used and disclosed, who is covered by the protections, and what safeguards must be in place. HIPAA also requires the establishment of national standards for electronic health care transactions. The law named specific code sets for all Medicare transactions, including the International Classification of Diseases (ICD) version 10 and the Clinical Modification component (ICD-10-CM), which provide more codes for the more detailed information available in electronic transactions. This classification system is periodically updated and the ICD-11 version was released by the World Health Organization (WHO) in 2018 (WHO, 2018).

The new 2009 standards required conversion of the alphanumeric designations given to every diagnosis, description of symptoms, and cause of death attributed to human beings and significantly increased the amount of data to more accurately describe clinical conditions. However, the conversions to ICD-10-CM are expensive and expectedly posed hardship to providers and institutions in meeting the standards (Hebda & Czar, 2013; Torrey, 2013). Federal policy was needed to help support nationwide implementation.

Health Information Technology for the Economic and Clinical Health Act (HITECH)

Title XII of the American Recovery and Investment Act of 2009 (Pub. L. 111-5) is known as the Health Information Technology for Economic and Clinical Health (HITECH) Act (www.healthit.gov/sites/default/files/hitech_act_excerpt_from_arra_with_index.pdf). The provisions of this act are viewed not as investments in technology, but as efforts to improve the health of Americans and health care system performance (Blumenthal, 2010). The law promotes the use of HIT to improve health care quality, safety, and efficiency by setting the "meaningful use" of interoperable EHR adoption as a critical national goal and by financially incentivizing the meaningful use of EHRs. In health care, *interoperability* is the ability of different information technology systems and software applications to communicate, exchange data, and use the information that has been exchanged. The Act defined privacy and security provisions to protect electronic health information. The Act also funded programs to support training and consulting needs of health care providers seeking to adopt EHRs. To achieve EHR adoption, the Office of the National Coordinator for Health Information Technology (ONC) was formalized within the U.S. Department of Health and Human Services (HHS) and charged with coordination of national efforts to implement and use the most advanced HIT and the electronic exchange of health information. The ONC defined a 2015–2020 strategic plan (ONC, n.d.) and certification processes to ensure EHR technologies meet standards to achieve certain quality and quantity goals to qualify for financial incentives.

HITECH Privacy and Security Provisions. Electronic health information exchange cannot reach its potential benefit unless patients and providers are confident that patient data are private and secure. Thus the HITECH Act also provides new improved privacy and security provisions that have major implications for providers, hospitals, and health insurance plans. This law requires health care entities to report data breaches affecting 500 or more individuals to the HHS and the media and to notify affected individuals within 60 days of any breach. In addition, patients can restrict some disclosures in certain circumstances and can request an accounting of any disclosures made. Penalties for violation of these requirements can be as high as $1.5 million.

HITECH Meaningful Use of EHR: Promoting Interoperability. Sections 4001 to 4201 of the HITECH Act established the Medicare and Medicaid EHR Incentive Programs to provide incentive payments for eligible professionals, hospitals, and critical access hospitals to adopt, implement, upgrade, or demonstrate meaningful use of certified EHR technology. ONC works with the Centers for Medicare and Medicaid Services (CMS) to establish the criteria for certified EHR technology. Section 4101 of the HITECH Act defines "meaningful use" as e-prescribing, engaging in health information exchange, and submission of information regarding quality measures. The goal is to change provider behavior by increasing the use and reporting of outcome measures and increasing the exchange of electronic patient information. The CMS sponsors the programs to incentivize the meaningful use of certified EHRs (www.healthit.gov/topic/meaningful-use-and-macra/promoting-interoperability).

MEDICARE AND MEDICAID ELECTRONIC HEALTH RECORD INCENTIVE PROGRAMS AND HIT

In 2011, CMS established the Medicare and Medicaid Electronic Health Record (EHR) Incentive Programs to encourage adoption and demonstrate meaningful use of certified EHR technology. Incentive Programs were designed to measure meaningful use of EHRs in three stages: first, to establish requirements for electronic capture of clinical data and provision of electronic copies to patients; second, to focus on advancing clinical processes and quality improvement; and then to focus on improved health outcomes (www.athenahealth.com/knowledge-hub/meaningful-use/stages). Between 2009 and 2012, EHR adoption nearly doubled among physicians and more than tripled among hospitals. In October 2013, progress on adoption of electronic records reported that 85% of eligible hospitals and greater than six in ten eligible providers had received federal EHR incentive payments (Reider & Tagalicod, 2013).

In 2015, the Medicare Access and Children's Health Insurance Program (CHIP) Reauthorization Act (MACRA) replaced meaningful use incentive programs and changed how Medicare pays clinicians. This law required providers to report on meaningful use (stage 3) measures of improved health outcomes but allowed them to choose which measures were suited to their practice. Under MACRA, the EHR Incentive program was transitioned to become a component of the new Merit-Based Incentive Payment System (MIPS). MIPS streamlined multiple quality programs and linked payment to quality, defined by a performance score.

A score is used for performance-based payment adjustment and is based on four weighted categories: quality, resource use, clinical practice improvement activities, and advancing care information through use of certified EHR technology (CMS, n.d.-b). The provider's performance score in the category of using EHRs to advance care information includes six objectives: protecting patient health information, electronic prescribing, patient electronic access, coordination of care through patient engagement, health information exchange, and public health and clinical data registry reporting. The MACRA incentive/bonus payment adjustments were effective January 2019 and are based on 2018 data. CMS continues to work to improve interoperability and patients' access to health information. To better reflect this focus, the EHR Incentive Programs were streamlined and later renamed the Promoting Interoperability (PI) Programs, intended to reduce the time and cost required of providers (CMS, n.d.-a).

POLITICAL AND CLINICAL IMPLICATIONS OF HIT POLICY FOR NURSING

HIPAA, the HITECH Act, and other policies are important to the clinical practice of nurses and affect the information handling practices of all clinicians. Standards for transmission of electronic information allow for seamless exchange and communication of information across providers. The ICD-10-CM requirements (and the successive revised versions) foster continuity and coordination through detailed clinical documentation and accurate communications. The new standards and coding systems affect the documented information that reflects the care provided by nurses. The incentives for EHRs increase the use of HIT and require all nurses to have knowledge and understanding of electronic information management. Skill in the effective use of EHRs is also required and affects how we prepare nurses in the academic and practice settings for such systems. Also, the advocacy role of nurses is critical to provide vigilance in advocating and monitoring privacy practices. The new requirements for incentive payments for the meaningful use of technology that promotes interoperability emphasize the need for informatics nurses to direct the development and implementation of EHRs to meet certification standards and support clinical outcomes. Hebda and Czar (2013) cite political issues related to the implementation of technology-related laws. Benefits of HIT are based on the assumption that health care practices and hospitals will have fully functioning, effective EHRs and supporting information systems in place. The reality is that many EHRs are not fully implemented, the technology infrastructures fall short of full support, and security measures are imperfect. Absent perfect systems, few hospitals or practices are paperless. Those with some EHR capacity need to expand their infrastructure, increase skilled personnel, and redesign their systems of care.

Critics of EHRs say they slow down providers, limit flexibility in care, and may increase opportunities for fraud. In addition, there is a delicate balance between free exchange of information and privacy protections. There are parties with vested interests in information access who pose potential problems for the protection of health information. Informed policy requires good information, and no perfect or complete information exists regarding outcomes or effectiveness of EHRs. The HITECH Act may trigger purchases without the due diligence of site visits, preparing staff, exploring decision support tools, and assessing compatibility with certification standards. It is also not clear which of these costs are covered by the HITECH Act. There is also concern that loss of Medicaid dollars may eliminate funding streams that supported health care IT (Halamka, 2017).

Although the nation has turned to widespread use of HIT to improve patient safety, there is a concern that poorly designed and implemented HIT can actually create new hazards in the complex care delivery system. Technology can only maximize safety and minimize harm if it is more usable, interoperable, and easier to implement and maintain than was previously the case.

To address this concern, the IOM (renamed the National Academy of Medicine) was asked by HHS to evaluate HIT safety concerns.

SAFETY AND HIT

HIT can improve patient safety in some areas such as medication safety; however, there are significant gaps in the literature regarding how HIT impacts patient safety overall. In 2011, the IOM report *HIT and Patient Safety* acknowledged that the information needed for an objective analysis and assessment of the safety of HIT and its use is not available. There is little published evidence on quantifying the magnitude of the risk posed by HIT. Although specific types of HIT can improve patient safety under the right conditions, those conditions cannot be replicated easily and require continual effort to sustain. The report asserts that although some studies in the literature suggest improvements in patient safety, others have found either no effect or instances of harm. Examples of harm include medication dosing errors, failure to detect fatal illnesses, and treatment delays caused by poor human-computer interactions or loss of data. These have led to several reported patient deaths and injuries. The degree to which existing literature concerning the health care system can be generalized is limited, and the magnitude of harm is unknown because of the heterogeneous nature of HIT products, the diverse impact on different clinical environments and workflow, legal barriers and vendor contracts, and inadequate evidence in the literature. The absence of a central repository to collect and analyze information and the nondisclosure and confidentiality clauses that prevent users from sharing information about adverse events contribute to the lack of safety.

Many problems with HIT relate to usability, implementation, and how software fits with the clinical workflow. It is acknowledged that an EHR, or any software, is neither safe nor unsafe because safety is a function of how software is used by clinicians. The IOM report concluded that safety is the product of the larger sociotechnical system. The safe use of HIT is contingent on multiple factors that include the interplay of people, processes, and technology and the involvement of government, the private sector, and users and vendors of the technology. There is no single cause for safety problems or errors; however, poor user-interface design, poor workflow, and complex interfaces (or lack of interfaces) between systems threaten patient safety. Similarly, lack of system interoperability limits the availability of data and poses a barrier to improving clinical decisions and patient safety.

Creating safer systems begins with user-centered design principles and continues with quality assessments and adequate testing at each stage of design and implementation. Each of these areas should involve nurses, who are the largest users of HIT. A consistent commitment to safety is needed and all users of HIT bear the responsibility for diligent surveillance of any mismatches between user needs and system performance, unsafe conditions, adverse events, and unintended consequences. To build upon the recommendations made in the 2011 IOM safety report and to affirm the commitment to safety, HHS issued the Health IT Patient Safety Action and Surveillance Plan in 2013. This plan is available online along with evidence-based tools and interventions for various stakeholders and can be retrieved from www.healthit.gov/sites/default/files/safety_plan_master.pdf.

UNINTENDED CONSEQUENCES OF HIT

Although there are high expectations for HIT to achieve quality, safety, and cost benefits, studies have shown that unplanned and unexpected consequences have resulted from major policy and technology changes (Ash, Berg, & Coiera, 2004; Bloomrosen et al., 2011). Bloomrosen et al. (2011) differentiate "unintended consequences," which implies lack of purposeful action or causation, from "unanticipated consequences," which implies an inability to forecast what actually occurred. These consequences can be positive, negative while achieving the desired effect, or negative without achieving what was originally intended. Ash et al. (2004) categorized two types of unintended consequences of patient care information systems related to silent errors: those occurring during the process of entering and retrieving information and those in the communication and coordination process that the HIT is supposed to support. Harrison, Koppel, and Bar-Lev (2007) view these unintended consequences from an interactive sociotechnical analysis (ISTA) perspective with recursive processes that effect second-level changes in social systems. The ISTA model refers to the influences of sociotechnical forces that shape work processes, the effects of work technologies and physical environments on individuals, the interactions among technology users, technology-in-practice as shaped by practitioners yet mediates practice, and social informatics that acknowledges the embedding of IT in organizations and society.

The implementation of HIT and information systems results in changes to clinical practices and workflows and triggers emotions such as uncertainty and resentment. These can affect the clinician's ability to carry out complex physical and cognitive tasks. Patient safety is also impaired by the failure to quickly fix technology when it becomes counterproductive and when dangerous workarounds are developed to address unresolved problems. Safety is also compromised when health care information systems are not integrated or updated consistently. If not carefully planned and integrated into workflow processes, new technology can create new work and complicate or slow clinical care.

Front-line clinicians need to be involved in the HIT planning processes to consider best practices and the costs and resources needed for ongoing maintenance and to consult product safety reviews or alerts. Learning to use new technologies takes time and attention and places strain on demanding schedules, yet needs to be addressed in HIT implementation to enhance safety in the longer term. Unintended consequences result from complex interactions between technology and the surrounding work environment even when HIT is well planned. The Joint Commission (2008) offers recommendations for safely implementing health information and converging technologies to avoid a range of adverse unintended consequences that can occur with daily use of HIT.

FUTURE DIRECTION FOR NATIONAL HIT POLICY

There are many challenges in the implementation of HIT as it intersects with health care and the trajectory of policy continues to evolve at a rapid pace. Halamka (2017) reflected on key areas where HIT developments will demand responsive policy in the future. He posits there is a strong stakeholder consensus that technology and policy need to enhance usability and interoperability to support the coordination of care, population health, precision medicine, research, and patient engagement. Strategies to address patient identity is also an issue of concern to government, industry, and academia as biometric strategies and voluntary national identifiers issued by some authority or creative software solution are explored. The protection of patient privacy continues to be a high priority, and some believe that the convergence of heterogeneous state privacy policies that focus on the patient as a steward of their data may be a fertile area for policy development. Finally, the future direction of IT policy needs to be more aligned with value-based care with a focus on outcomes to be achieved by HIT, such as reduced errors, decreased readmissions, or redundant testing.

CONCLUSION

Policy can and does shape the intersection of technology in health and health care by removing barriers to the adoption and use of HIT, ensuring technology is designed and implemented to meet national standards for exchange through certifications, protecting the privacy and security of health information, and fostering and incentivizing new systems of care delivery to enhance coordination of care through the effective, interoperable exchange of information. As leaders in shaping health care reform and the policies that support it, nurses are critical to ensuring quality, safety, and cost-effective care. Nurses need to understand the role of technology as it intersects the health and health care systems as well as the power of policy to influence its use. Nurse involvement at the policy level is important so that issues related to care and reimbursement for advanced practice nurses can be included in the regulations.

DISCUSSION QUESTIONS

1. How can nurses inform/influence the development of health policy related to HIT?
2. How does the use of HIT affect reimbursement for nursing care, evidence-based practice, and the use of data for population health?
3. What are recommended practices for avoiding unintended consequences of EHR?

REFERENCES

Adler-Milstein, J., & Jha, A.K. (2016). HITECH Act drove large gains in hospital electronic health record adoption. *Health Affairs, 36*(8). Retrieved from https://www.healthaffairs.org/doi/full/10.1377/hlthaff.2016.1651.

Ash, J.S., Berg, M., & Coiera, E. (2004). Some unintended consequences of information technology in health care: The nature of patient care information system-related error. *Journal of the American Medical Informatics Association, 11*(2), 104–112.

Berwick, D., Nolan, D., & Whittington, J. (2008). The Triple Aim: Care, health, and cost. *Health Affairs, 27*(3), 759–769.

Bloomrosen, M., Starren, J., Lorenzi, N.M., Ash, J.S., Patel, V.L., & Shortliffe, E.H. (2011). Anticipating and addressing the unintended consequences of health IT and policy: A report from the AMIA 2009 health policy meeting. *Journal of the American Medical Informatics Association, 18*(1), 82–90.

Blumenthal, D. (February 4, 2010). Launching HITECH. *New England Journal of Medicine, 362,* 382–385.

Blumenthal, D., & Tavenner, M. (2010). The "meaningful use" regulation of electronic health records. *New England Journal of Medicine,* Retrieved from www.nejm.org/doi/full/10.1056/NEJMp1006114.

Centers for Medicare and Medicaid Services. (n.d.-a). *Electronic health records (I) incentive programs.* Retrieved from www.cms.gov/regulations-and-guidance/legislation/EHRincentivePrograms/index.

Centers for Medicare and Medicaid Services. (n.d.-b). *MACRA.* Retrieved from www.cms.gov/Medicare/Quality-Initiatives-Patient-Assessment-Instruments/Value-Based-Programs/MACRA-MIPS-and-APMs/MACRA-MIPS-and-APMs.html.

Halamka, J. (July 18, 2017). *Reflections on the US HIT policy trajectory.* Retrieved from www.hitechanswers.net/reflections-us-hit-policy-trajectory/.

Harrison, M.I., Koppel, R., & Bar-Lev, S. (2007). Unintended consequences of information technologies in health care—An interactive sociotechnical analysis. *Journal of the American Medical Informatics Association, 14*(5), 542–549.

Hebda, T., & Czar, P. (2013). *Handbook of informatics for nurses & health professionals* (5th ed., pp. 379–407). Upper Saddle River, NJ: Pearson Education Inc.

Institute of Medicine. (1999). *To err is human: Building a safer health system.* Washington, DC: National Academy Press.

Institute of Medicine. (2011). *HIT and patient safety: Building safer systems for better care.* Washington DC: National Academy Press.

The Joint Commission. (2008). Safely implementing health information and converging technologies. *Sentinel Event Alert, 42.* Retrieved from www.jointcommission.org/assets/1/18/SEA_42.pdf.

Kilpatrick, D.G. (2000). *Definition of public policy and the law.* Retrieved from www.musc.edu/vawprevention/policy/definition.shtml.

The National Ambulatory Medical Care Survey. (2010). *American Hospital Association IT Supplement 2010.* Retrieved from www.cdc.gov/nchs/data/ahcd/namcs_summary/2010_namcs_web_tables.pdf.

Office of the National Coordinator. (n.d.) *Federal Health IT Strategic Plan 2015-2020.* U.S. Department of Health and Human Services. Retrieved from www.healthit.gov/sites/default/files/9-5-federalhealthitstratplanfinal_0.pdf.

Reider, J., & Tagalicod, R. (2013). *Progress on adoption of electronic health records.* Retrieved from www.healthit.gov/buzz-blog/electronic-health-and-medical-records/progress-adoption-electronic-health-records/.

Torrey, T. (2013). *What are ICD-9 or ICD-10 codes? How ICD codes affect your care.* Retrieved from www.verywellhealth.com/what-are-icd-9-and-icd-10-codes-2615312.

World Health Organization. (June 18, 2018). *WHO releases new International Classification of Diseases (ICD 11).* Retrieved from https://www.who.int/news-room/detail/18-06-2018-who-releases-new-international-classification-of-diseases-(icd-11).

ONLINE RESOURCES

Federal government's official website for Health Information Technology
www.healthit.gov
HHS Health IT Patient Safety Action and Surveillance Plan
www.healthit.gov/sites/default/files/safety_plan_master.pdf
Medicare and Medicaid Promoting Interoperability Program Basics
www.cms.gov/Regulations-and-Guidance/Legislation/EHRIncentivePrograms/Basics.html

66

Interest Groups in Health Care Policy and Politics

Joanne Warner

> *"Politics isn't about big money or power games; it's about the improvement of people's lives."*
>
> **Paul Wellstone**

Gun violence provides a riveting intersection of challenges in framing policy problems and competing interest groups' interventions. Nurses, physicians, and public health professionals declare gun deaths as a health crisis (Jimenez, 2018); however, the National Rifle Association (NRA) lobbies to defend gun ownership and oppose most all forms of gun regulation or potential remedies for gun violence (Center for Responsive Politics, 2018a). Although an average of 100 Americans dies each day as a result of gun violence, we have not reconciled the support for the right to bear arms with the quest for public safety and violence prevention (Bauchner et al., 2017). In 2018, 17 students and staff lost their lives during the school shooting in Parkland, Florida. Public pressure for legislative action soared, and President Trump suggested that lawmakers were "too fearful of the National Rifle Association [NRA] to act" (Associated Press, 2018, first paragraph).

Interest groups like the example above play a significant role in public health policy. They are a paradox within our governing system. We need and value them but, at the same time, they annoy and distract us. We embrace them as empowered citizen involvement, and we resent the perception of buying elections and votes. The love-hate ambivalence is born, in part, from the way a 1787 notion has translated into today's Washington-centric political era. Democracy within our individualistic society presents inherent tensions that are both our genius and our burden.

An interest group is a collection of people who pursue their common interests by influencing political processes. They are also known as factions, special interests, pressure groups, or organized interests. The original definition depicted them as "united and actuated by some common impulse of passion, or of interest, adverse to the rights of other citizens, or to the permanent and aggregate interests of the community" (Madison, 1787, paragraph 2). Today, federal, state, and local political arenas experience the activity of organized groups who influence elections, votes, societal opinion, and the policy process itself.

This chapter gives context to the duality of distrust and appreciation for interest groups and portrays them as a significant feature of our governing system. It traces the historical roots of interest groups, describes their functions and methods, and concludes that they embody the good and the bad of governance. It also describes the contemporary terrain of health care interest groups as well as a discernment framework for interest group involvement.

DEVELOPMENT OF INTEREST GROUPS

James Madison's *The Federalist No. 10* (1787) forms part of his treatise on the preferred structure of a republic. He proposes that rather than removing the causes of factions, the best wisdom is to control the effects of interest groups. To do otherwise is to undermine liberty. The legitimate roots of interest group organizing are therefore traced to the framers of the Constitution and the birth of the American version of democracy. Later, the French philosopher Alexis de Tocqueville observed the country from an outsider's view. His *Democracy in America* (1835) endures as a classic description of our inclination to form associations for common purpose and to create a vibrant political structure independent of the state (de Tocqueville, 1835/2010).

The impetus to organize exists not only within the American people but also within the political structure. Groups can influence policy through elections, lobbying the legislature, and pressuring the executive branch of any level of government. This diffusion of power presents many opportunities for persuasion. It also allows interest groups to shop for a different level of government if they are unhappy with policy; for example, federal versus state government (Anderson, 2014).

Historically, groups formed around interests such as slavery and alcohol prohibition. At the turn of the 20th century, interest groups based in Washington blossomed. The social activism of the 1960s generated more groups focused on civil rights, the environment, and specific economic and humanitarian causes (Nownes, 2013). As the power and money of interest groups grew, Congress acted to restrict their influence and limit direct contributions to candidates. However, the reforms that grew from the Watergate scandal of the 1970s inadvertently enhanced their power by promoting the formation of political action committees (PACs). The Bipartisan Campaign Reform Act of 2002 (the McCain-Feingold Act) revised the Federal Election Campaign Act of 1971 to control soft money contributions—that is, funds funneled through political parties to candidates and the funding of issues ads (Federal Election Commission, n.d.). For good or ill, special interest money continues to grease electoral and political wheels.

From this historical perspective, more categories of interest groups exist today: business, labor unions, professional associations, intergovernmental groups, and public interest groups (Hayes, 2017). Within the latter group, there are interest groups that provide information and are active in the health policy. Examples include the U.S. Public Interest Research Groups (USPIRG), which stand "up to powerful interest on behalf of the American public, working to win concrete results for our health and our well-being" (USPIRG, 2018); Essential Action, which wages campaigns on topics not visible in the mass media or on political agendas, including examples of large finances altering policy decisions that harm citizens (Essential Information, 2018); and the Center for Science in the Public Interest (CSPI), whose advice and advocacy focuses on nutrition and a healthier food system through research and information sharing (CSPI, 2018). These examples sample the diverse public interest groups advancing health.

There are at least two cautionary notes for citizens and policymakers as they evaluate interest groups' messages and integrity. There are front groups whose public persona is that of an unbiased group but whose funds and agendas are from an industry or political party. For example, the Center for Consumer Freedom has a message of individual choice but is a front group for the restaurant, alcohol, and tobacco industries. This group opposes public health messages of science, health, and environmental groups, calling them a "growing fraternity of food cops, health care enforcers, anti-meat activists, and meddling bureaucrats who 'know what's best for you'" (Source Watch, 2017). Secondly, Holyoke (2016) highlights the lack of ethical standards for lobbyists and whether there is accountability and transparency to truly represent the collective interests of those they represent. For instance, NRA membership polls found two-thirds supported background checks and a requirement to report lost or stolen guns following the 2012 Sandy Hook school shooting, but the NRA took a hard-line opposition to any such legislation. These two issues call consumers and policymakers to vigilance about the bias and representation of groups who advocate and provide information toward the goals of influencing thinking and policy.

FUNCTIONS AND METHODS OF INFLUENCE

How do interest groups function within a complicated governance system? What methods can they use to advance their causes, and how do they determine which to use? Their methods are lobbying, grassroots mobilization, influencing elections, shaping public opinion, and litigation.

Lobbying

Lobbying involves the direct influence of public officials and their decisions. Wolpe (1990) presented a concise and classic description of lobbying as "the political management of information" (p. 9) because it involves educating, shaping opinions, and offering data and analyses. Lobbyists also often assist in bill drafting and revision. By hiring full-time Washington- or state-based lobbyists, groups have a more enduring presence; this also allows for ongoing relationships between staff, officials, and lobbyists to be the foundation of influence. Lobbyists become adept at the nuances of the legislative process and can provide nimble responses.

The largest number of registered federal lobbyists recorded to date is 14,842 in 2007 and the total lobbying expenditure exceeded $3.1 billion each year from 2008 through 2017. In 2017, 11,592 federal lobbyists were a part of

$3.37 billion lobbying spending (Center for Responsive Politics, 2018b). Of the top seven lobbying industries in 2017, four are related to health: pharmaceuticals, insurance, hospitals, and physicians, in order of size, spending a total of $93.8 billion (Center for Responsive Politics, 2018c). Lobbying is a substantial business.

Grassroots Mobilization

Grassroots mobilization involves indirectly influencing officials through constituency contact. With the evolution of new political technologies, the creation of grassroots infrastructure is increasingly possible and complex. Benefits of grassroots coordination include the strong persuasion inherent in face-to-face contact, the efficiency of targeting a specific audience through social media, and the energizing and amplifying effect of contact with those who share values and goals. Most interest groups employ some version of grassroots mobilization (Riordan, 2018).

Electoral Influence

Electoral influence can be considered the primary prevention of policymaking because it is an important activity that precedes policy work. It determines who is elected to shape future policies (Warner, 2002). Successful electoral campaigns need three resources: time, money, and people. Interest groups can provide the last two. Just as interest groups provide a collective voice, PACs provide the collective financial support. For example, the American Nurses Association (ANA) formed the ANA-PAC in the 1970s to support federal candidates who are aligned with the ANA agenda and values, with the ultimate intent of improving the health care system. The 2015 ANA Code of Ethics provides the basis for nursing's ethical obligations to advocate and influence policies that promote health (ANA, 2018a). PACs contributed about one-third of campaign cash for U.S. House races and 16% for Senate races. During 2017 to 2018, PACs can only donate $5000 per election (primary, general, or special) and $15,000 annually to a national party, although individuals can give up to $2700 per year to each candidate (Center for Responsive Politics, 2018d).

Shaping Public Opinion

Shaping public opinion overlaps with electoral influence and grassroots mobilization; it involves issue advocacy and public persuasion, similar to campaigning for an issue. It is similar to an infomercial that sells an issue or to direct mail with information promoting a particular perspective. The impression of societal consensus could, in turn, persuade policymakers as they create policy. These initiatives either cost money or are free media in the form of news coverage.

Litigation

Lastly, litigation can shape governance toward the goals of the group. The *Brown v. Board of Education of Topeka, Kansas* is a classic example of years of strategic effort culminating in a significant judicial ruling changing the landscape of society. The National Association for the Advancement of Colored People (NAACP) was the interest group championing social justice and the elimination of racial discrimination that organized 200 plaintiffs in five states to bring cases of racial segregation and discrimination in schools to the Supreme Court. This ruling affected racial discrimination throughout society and inspired interest groups to pursue their proposed change through the court system (Brown Foundation for Educational Equity, Excellence and Research, n.d.).

To create their action plans, each interest group develops a distinct identity that originates in its methods, resources, and purpose. This discussion of function and method illustrates that their influence within the governance process, whether nuanced or bold, can span the entire process and can range from superficial to substantial.

Related to the scope of influence is the question of interest group effectiveness, especially when compared to average citizens or economic elites. Effective influence ranges from molding public opinion, to shaping the agenda of issues under consideration, to determining the policy outcomes. When compared directly, Gilens and Page (2014) concluded that interest groups have substantial impact on policy, more than average citizens and less than the economic elite.

Narrowly defined interest groups, including business- and professional-related groups, wielded more influence than mass-based groups. The context for this research reveals the complexity of the legislative dance and the evolving nature of American democracy yet recognizes interest groups as an actor in policy formation.

LANDSCAPE OF CONTEMPORARY HEALTH CARE INTEREST GROUPS

Citizen action waxes and wanes according to the prioritized topics on the political agenda, but there are always challenges for either health policy or "healthy" public policy. Who are the health players, what money is involved, and what is nursing's place and relative effectiveness in the context of federal lobbying groups?

Funds from interest groups are predominantly spent on lobbying and on campaign contributions, and the health industry is heavily involved in both. The Center for Responsive Politics (a nonpartisan research group that tracks money in politics) ranked the health sector as the sixth largest interest group contributor. During the 2016 election cycle, the health sector contributed a record $561.2 million to federal candidates, with the pharmaceutical industry leading with donations of $247.6 million (Center for Responsive Politics, 2018e). The American Medical Association dominated the health professionals sector in 2017 by contributing $21.5 million and ANA contributing $1.56 million to earn it the tenth largest donor among health professionals (Center for Responsive Politics, 2018f). Stakeholders concerned with health care also include those outside the health industry (e.g., insurance corporations, labor unions, and myriad business and consumer groups). In fact, from an ecological perspective, most topics eventually trace back to health and the human potential it impacts.

Table 66.1 presents campaign contributions made by health professionals from 2000 to 2016, including both health professional PACs and individual contributions. It demonstrates dramatic increases in contributions and variation in the partisan allocations, usually related to whatever party is in power. Clearly, health professionals are engaged in electoral politics.

Nursing has experience and success with collective involvement in campaigns through ANA-PAC and other involvement by nurses. Decisions to endorse candidates are made by the ANA-PAC Board of Trustees. It is important to realize that endorsement decisions are based on agreement with ANA's policy stands and not on the candidate's party. In the 2016 cycle, 82% of their $208,561 contributions went to Democrats and 18% to Republicans (Center for Responsive Politics, 2013g). Table 66.2 lists contributions of nursing PAC contributions to federal candidates in 2016.

Trended data provide interesting information about the choices that nurses make for their collective electoral

TABLE 66.1 Health Sectors' PAC and Individual Contributions to Campaigns

Election Cycle	Total Contributions	% to Democrats	% to Republicans
2016	$204,005,395	52	48
2014	$133,590,519	43	57
2012	$210,306,593	44	56
2010	$145,352,871	51	48
2008	$181,757,288	55	45
2006	$107,744,626	38	62
2004	$128,297,931	39	61
2002	$67,696,224	35	65
2000	$74,353,934	40	60

Adapted from Center for Responsive Politics. (2018). *Health professionals: Long-term contribution trends.* Retrieved from www.opensecrets.org/industries/totals. php?cycle=2018&ind=H.

TABLE 66.2 Nursing PAC Contributions to Federal Candidates: 2016

Nursing PAC	Amount Contributed
American Association of Nurse Anesthetists	$650,150
American Nurses Association	$208,561
American Academy of Nurse Practitioners	$183,650
American College of Nurse Midwives	$48,500

Adapted from Center for Responsive Politics. (2018). *Health Professionals: PAC contributions to federal candidates.* Retrieved from www.opensecrets.org/pacs/industry. php?txt=H01&cycle=2012.

influence. The ANA-PAC raised and spent over $1 million in one election cycle (1994) but has not reached that amount since. Contrast this to trended data about the American Association of Nurse Anesthetists whose PAC has exceeded $1 million in every election cycle since 2000, with a record high of $1.6 million in 2008 (Center for Responsive Politics, 2013g, 2013h). A simplistic assumption is that nurses donate closer to their specialty, yet the fuller explanation is likely more complex and not yet explained.

When the campaign dust settles and policymaking continues, lobbyists base their advocacy on the values and positions of the group. The ANA, for example, has a long history of supporting universal access to quality, cost-effective health care, and advocating for a well-staffed system that serves the interests of both patients and nurses (ANA, 2018a).

The landscape for health care reform, therefore, is populated with many interest groups, some in the health industry and many with vested interests in the cost and structure of the reform efforts. Significant money goes into elections and lobbying; nursing is involved in both. Although it may not be ranked as one of the most powerful groups, its political currency is trust, integrity, and a reputation for championing quality care for all within an equitable and accessible system.

ASSESSING VALUE AND CONSIDERING INVOLVEMENT

Most choices involve a "what's-in-it-for-me?" appraisal. In addition to that discernment, the robust ambivalence surrounding interest groups heightens the need for evaluation criteria. How can nurses and other health care providers assess the qualities of an interest group? Where should they allocate their finite resources of time, energy, money, and reputation?

Table 66.3 presents a framework for discernment to assess an interest group and determine the extent of involvement. The framework also provides language and justification for decisions. This approach matches the spirit, though not the rigor, of the scientific evidence-based nature of the health care profession. The ten queries are not listed by priority, as the weight of their importance will differ per individual. Nurses can engage in the discernment and defend their involvement in terms of the guiding principles, which may prove more thoughtful than replicating our parents' choices or simply following the crowd.

CONCLUSION

In a democracy, interest groups are integral to the governing process. They are sanctioned by our Constitution and valued as a vehicle for citizen participation but are also despised as an underhanded wielding of influence through money. Despite societal ambivalence, they are likely here to stay. Perhaps the best approach is to intentionally discern our own involvement, maximize the collective voice of our profession, know the rules of the game, and use interest group power to further the causes and values we treasure.

TABLE 66.3 Framework for Assessing Interest Groups	
Factor	**Queries to Assess Characteristics of an Interest Group**
Efficiency	What portion of the group's budget supports advocacy, education, or the social interest represented, compared with the portion that supports the group's infrastructure, overhead, or administration?
Effectiveness	What is the track record of accomplishments related to education, awareness, legislation, or cultural change? What outcomes can be credited to the group, either individually or in coalition?
Values	Do the values of the group align with your personal, political, and professional values? Do your beliefs match the values that inspire the group's work? Does this work stir some passion in you?
Tactics	Do you support the methods used by the group? Do the tactics match your preferred approach to social change, including options such as violence, protesting, nonviolent resistance, media campaigns, or organized action?
Visibility and responsiveness	Does the group have the level of public visibility that you prefer? Do they employ the level of outreach to their members that you prefer? Do they communicate clearly and consistently with the constituency?
Social norms	Does the group match your local culture and the social norms of the people with whom you associate? Would your involvement in this group change the way people perceive you personally or professionally? Does that perception matter to you?
Perception	What is your perception of the leaders and key stakeholders of the interest group? Does that perception matter to you?
Accountability transparency	Does the group disclose issue positions and tactics used? Can you provide feedback and input on the positions proactively or during the process?
Costs	What would involvement require of you? Are there dues or voluntary financial commitments? Can you contribute the amount of time required? Will they ask to use your name, title, or reputation, and will any unintended implications involve professional cost? Does your employer prohibit or discourage involvement with this group?
Benefits	What's in it for you? Will you obtain any profit, professional advantage, or membership benefits? Do you value the social benefit of association? Are you willing to be involved for altruistic intentions? Are you willing to be involved if the benefits go to others, for example, an underrepresented population, the environment, or a cause beyond your immediate life?

DISCUSSION QUESTIONS

1. In what ways is, or is not, the nursing profession a special interest group in American democracy?
2. What strategies would enhance the effective influence of nurses as a collective special interest group in policy advocacy and electoral politics?
3. What role does the nonpartisan stance of nursing PACs play in the broad engagement of nurses in electoral politics and policy advocacy?

REFERENCES

American Nurses Association. (2018a). *ANA-PAC*. Retrieved from https://ana.aristotle.com/SitePages/pac.aspx.

American Nurses Association. (2018b). *Policy and advocacy: Health care reform*. Retrieved from www.nursingworld.org/MainMenuCategories/Policy-Advocacy/HealthSystemReform.

Anderson, J.E. (2014). *Public policymaking: An introduction* (8th ed.). Boston: Cengage.

Associated Press. (March 1, 2018). *Trump says lawmakers too fearful of NRA to act on guns*. Retrieved from www.snopes.com/ap/2018/03/01/trump-says-lawmakers-fearful-nra-act-guns.

Bauchner, H., Rivara, F.P., Bonow, R.O., Bessler, N.M., Disis, M.L., Heckers, S., ... & Robinson, J.K. (2017, October 9). Death by gun violence: A public health crisis [Editorial]. *Journal of American Medicine Association Network Facial Plastic Surgery, 318*(18), 1763-1764. Retrieved from https://jamanetwork.com/journals/jamafacialplasticsurgery/fullarticle/2657424.

Brown Foundation for Educational Equity, Excellence and Research. (n.d.). *Brown v. Board of Education: Background, overview and summary*. Retrieved from brownvboard.org/content/background-overview-summary.

Center for Responsive Politics. (2018a). *National Rifle Association*. Retrieved from www.opensecrets.org/orgs/summary.php?id=d000000082.

Center for Responsive Politics. (2018b). *Influence and lobbying: Lobbying database*. Retrieved from www.opensecrets.org/influence/.

Center for Responsive Politics. (2018c). *Lobbying: Top spenders*. Retrieved from www.opensecrets.org/lobby/top.php?indexType=s&showYear=2013.

Center for Responsive Politics. (2018d). *2018 Campaign contribution limits*. Retrieved from www.opensecrets.org/overview/limits.php.

Center for Responsive Politics. (2018e). *Industries: Health*. Retrieved from www.opensecrets.org/industries/indus.php?ind=H.

Center for Responsive Politics. (2018f). *Influence and lobbying: Health professionals*. Retrieved from www.opensecrets.org/lobby/indusclient.php?id=H01&year=2017.

Center for Responsive Politics. (2018g). *PACs: American Nurses Association*. Retrieved from www.opensecrets.org/pacs/lookup2.php?strID=C00017525&cycle=2016.

Center for Responsive Politics. (2013h). *PACs: American Association of Nurse Anesthetists*. Retrieved from www.opensecrets.org/pacs/lookup2.php?strID=C00173153&cycle=2014.

Center for Science in the Public Interest. (2018). *Mission*. Retrieved from https://cspinet.org/about/mission.

de Tocqueville, A. (1835/2010). *Democracy in America*. New York: Penguin Group.

Essential Information. (2018). *Essential action*. Retrieved from www.essentialinformation.org.

Federal Election Commission. (n.d.). *Bipartisan Campaign Reform Act*. Retrieved from www.fec.gov/pages/bcra/bcra_update.shtml.

Gilens, M. & Page, B.I. (2014). Testing theories of American politics: Elites, interest groups, and average citizens. *Perspectives on Politics, 12*(3), 564-581. Retrieved from www.cambridge.org/core/journals/perspectives-on-politics/article/testing-theories-of-american-politics-elites-interest-groups-and-average-citizens/62327F513959D0A304D4893B382B992B/core-reader.

Hayes, R.A. (2017). *The role of interest groups*. Retrieved from https://web-archive-2017.ait.org.tw/infousa/zhtw/docs/demo-paper/dmpaper9.html.

Holyoke, T.T. (2016). *The ethical lobbyist: Reforming Washington's influence industry*. Washington, DC: Georgetown University.

Jimenez, S. (March 5, 2018). *Health professionals declare gun violence a public health threat*. Retrieved from www.nurse.com/blog/2018/03/05/health-professionals-declare-gun-violence-a-public-health-threat/.

Madison, J. (November 22, 1787). *The Federalist No. 10: The utility of the union as a safeguard against domestic faction and insurrection*. Retrieved from constitution.org/fed/federa10.htm.

Nownes, A.J. (2013). *Interest groups in American politics: Pressure and power*. New York: Routledge.

Riordan, C.O. (2018). *Campaign strategy: Grassroots mobilization*. Retrieved from www.ecanvasser.com/blog/campaign-strategy-grassroots-mobilization/.

Source Watch. (2009). *Center for Consumer Freedom*. Retrieved from www.sourcewatch.org/index.php?title=Center_for_Consumer_Freedom.

U.S. Public Interest Research Groups. (2018). *Mission statement*. Retrieved from https://uspirg.org/page/usp/about-us-pirg-0.

Warner, J.R. (2002). Campaign management: Policy's primary prevention strategy. In D. Mason, J.K. Leavitt, & M.W. Chaffee (Eds.), *Policy and politics in nursing and health care* (4th ed., pp. 579–583). Philadelphia: WB Saunders.

Wolpe, B.C. (1990). *Lobbying Congress: How the system works*. Washington, DC: Congressional Quarterly.

ONLINE RESOURCES

American Nurses Association: ANA-PAC
https://ana.aristotle.com/SitePages/pac.aspx
Center for Responsive Politics
www.opensecrets.org
The Federalist Papers 10: The Utility of the Union as a Safeguard Against Domestic Faction and Insurrection (by James Madison)
www.congress.gov/resources/display/content/The+Federalist+Papers#TheFederalistPapers-10

67

Policy Issues in Nursing Associations

Ramón Lavandero[a]

> *"Associations are formed by people who share a common interest in [a profession] and who are able to identify others with the same interests. In many cases, individuals are not aware of others who share their interest or concern until the association's founders articulate it and make it known."*
>
> **Alexis de Tocqueville**

Nursing associations intersect with policy issues in many situations. An association then chooses with which issues, if any, it will engage. This chapter explores what associations are, where associations are likely to intersect with policy issues, and why associations may or may not choose to engage.

WHAT IS AN ASSOCIATION?

In the early 21st century, associations are considered essential threads in the fabric of American society. They were unusual in the early days of the republic. French scholar Alexis de Tocqueville marveled at the uniquely American inclination to counter individualism by "constantly joining together in groups" (Zunz, 2015). In *Democracy in America*, his masterful analysis of life in early 19th century American life, he described associations as helping people accomplish what their members could not do as individuals. Associations are types of organizations, and this chapter uses use the two terms interchangeably.

DEVELOPMENTAL PHASES

Associations generally develop in phases resembling the life cycles of the human beings that create them (Fig. 67.1) (Thompson & Lavandero, 2001). During the start-up phase, a few individuals discover a shared interest. Their informal conversations gain traction to frame a purpose that will attract resources. Others contribute time and money as they join the effort. The founders soon discover that volunteered time will not be enough to grow the fledgling association, so they begin paying some of the volunteers or hire a management agency to do the work.

This growth phase evolves as the organization attracts paying members, offers them services, then requires more human and financial resources to deliver them. Tension often marks this period, as the volunteer founders and paid staff members clarify their roles. When roles are sufficiently clarified to support accelerated member growth, programs expand, and financial assets accumulate to support the association's strategic goals.

The cycle isn't always linear. Unresolved conflicts may lead to splintering or even cause the association to disband. Shared interests that brought the founders together morph, requiring a change in focus or rendering the association irrelevant. Programs and services—even very successful legacy offerings such as in-person conferences and print publications—may become irrelevant, outdated, or too expensive to support.

The path to renewal or decline and dissolution depends on how successfully an association addresses new challenges. Where policy is concerned, the dynamics of its current developmental state influences each time an association intersects with a policy issue and discerns which direction to take.

DEVELOPMENT OF AMERICAN NURSING ORGANIZATIONS

New York City's Bellevue Hospital Training School for Nurses adopted the principles of Florence Nightingale

---

[a]This chapter updates a previous edition chapter originally developed by Glenda Christiaens, PhD, RN, AHN-BC.

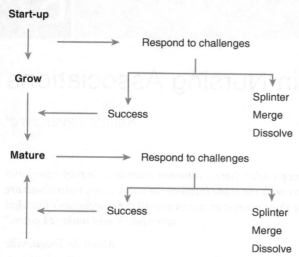

Fig. 67.1 Developmental phases of an organization. (Source: Thompson & Lavandero, 2001.)

when it opened in 1873 as the first nursing school in the United States (Bradley-Sanders, 2012). Similar schools followed at hospitals in major cities. Student nurses provided the direct care in those hospitals and graduates who remained as employees moved into leadership and education. From their beginning, American nursing organizations grouped into two broad categories: general and special interest. It's not surprising that, in 1893, the American Society of Superintendents of Training Schools for Nurses—today's National League for Nursing—began as the country's first special interest nursing association (National League for Nursing, n.d.). In 1897, graduate nurses followed suit, creating the Nurses' Associated Alumnae of the United States and Canada—today's American Nurses Association (ANA) (ANA, 2016a).

A general association trains its mission and vision on issues that affect nurses regardless of their role or where they practice. The ANA is the pre-eminent, general association for nurses with the mission of advancing the profession to improve health for all, and a vision of nurses as a powerful, unified force engaging consumers and transforming health and health care (ANA, 2017).

A special interest organization focuses on a specific aspect of nursing, such as clinical specialty, workplace, ethnicity, or role. The American Association of Critical-Care Nurses (AACN Critical Care), National Association of School Nurses, National Association of Hispanic Nurses, and American Organization for Nursing Leadership are examples. Table 67.1 shows a list of many current American nursing associations.

A few, such as the American Academy of Nursing, could be considered hybrids. The Academy is a general association because accomplished leaders in education, management, practice, and research from every area of nursing are elected as fellows. It is also a special interest organization because its mission is to serve the public and the profession by advancing health policy, practice, and science, issuing policy briefs and position statements (American Academy of Nursing, n.d.-a). An association's presence may be national, regional (including by state), and/or local depending on its focus and scope. Its presence may be formal or informal and shift over time depending on the organization's maturity and needs. Most nursing associations have individuals as members. The American Association of Colleges of Nursing (AACN Colleges) is an exception because its members are the schools and colleges of nursing that offer undergraduate and graduate degrees and postgraduate programs such as a certificate in informatics or educational technology.

ALLIANCES

In the same way that an association brings together people with common interests, nursing associations create formal and informal alliances of multiple nursing organizations based on common interests such as policy issues, leveraging economies of scale, and strength in numbers. With nearly 60 member associations, the Nursing Organizations Alliance (NOA) was formed in 2001 when two, long-standing coalitions—the National Federation for Specialty Nursing Organizations and the Nursing Organizations Liaison Forum—created a single alliance to advance the profession through cohesive action and a strong voice. This developed into programs designed to inspire and develop association leaders by identifying, educating, and building collaboration around issues of common interest (NOA, n.d.c).

Created in 2008, the Nursing Community Coalition promotes efforts that advance health through nursing care. The coalition focuses on policy advocacy guided by the belief that American health care should promote wellness, advance research through scientific discovery, and provide timely access to care across the continuum. The 60+ member associations represent a cross section of education, practice, research, and regulatory organizations (Nursing Community Coalition, n.d.).

In 2010, the ANA Organizational Affiliates Program began to offer an organizational-level membership option for specialty associations interested in a formal relationship with ANA. Program members maintain their autonomy while collaborating with ANA and each other to address issues facing the profession as a whole.

TABLE 67.1 Nursing Associations and Alliances

Organization Name	Website
Academy of Medical-Surgical Nurses	www.medsurgnurse.org
Academy of Neonatal Nursing	www.academyofneonatalnursing.org
Academy of Spinal Cord Injury Professionals, Spinal Cord Injury Nurses Section	www.academyscipro.org/aboutscin
Air and Surface Transport Nurses Association	www.astna.site-ym.com
Alliance of Nurses for Healthy Environments	www.envirn.org
American Academy of Ambulatory Care Nursing	www.aaacn.org
American Academy of Nursing	www.aannet.org
American Assisted Living Nurses Association	www.alnursing.org
American Association for Men in Nursing	www.aamn.org
American Association for the History of Nursing	www.aahn.org
American Association for Respiratory Care	www.aarc.org
American Association of Colleges of Nursing	www.aacnnursing.org
American Association of Critical-Care Nurses	www.aacn.org
American Association of Diabetes Educators	www.diabeteseducator.org
American Association of Heart Failure Nurses	www.aahfn.org
American Association of Legal Nurse Consultants	www.aalnc.org
American Association of Managed Care Nurses	www.aamcn.org
American Association of Moderate Sedation Nurses	www.aamsn.org
American Association of Neuroscience Nurses	www.aann.org
American Association of Nurse Anesthetists	www.aana.com
American Association of Nurse Assessment Coordination	www.aanac.org
American Association of Nurse Attorneys	www.taana.org
American Association of Nurse Life Care Planners	www.aanlcp.org
American Association of Nurse Practitioners	www.aanp.org
American Association of Occupational Health Nurses	www.aaohn.org
American Cannabis Nurses Association	www.cannabisnurses.org
American College of Nurse-Midwives	www.midwife.org
American Heart Association-Council on Cardiovascular and Stroke Nursing	www.professional.heart.org
American Holistic Nurses Association	www.ahna.org
American Medical Informatics Association, Nursing Informatics Working Group	www.amia.org/programs/working-groups/nursing-informatics/
American Nephrology Nurses Association	www.annanurse.org
American Nurses Association	www.nursingworld.org
American Nursing Informatics Association	www.ania.org
American Organization for Nursing Leadership	www.aonl.org
American Pediatric Surgical Nurses Association, Inc.	www.apsna.org
American Psychiatric Nurses Association	www.apna.org
American Public Health Association, Public Health Nursing Section	www.apha.org/apha-communities/member-sections/public-health-nursing
American Society for Pain Management Nursing	www.aspmn.org
American Society of Ophthalmic Registered Nurses	www.asorn.org
American Society of PeriAnesthesia Nurses	www.aspan.org
American Thoracic Society, Assembly on Nursing	http://www.thoracic.org/members/assemblies/assemblies/nur/
Army Nurse Corps Association	www.e-anca.org
Association for Nursing Professional Development	www.anpd.org

Continued

TABLE 67.1   Nursing Associations and Alliances—cont'd

Organization Name	Website
Association for Radiologic and Imaging Nursing	www.arinursing.org
Association of Black Nursing Faculty, Inc.	www.abnf.net
Association of Camp Nursing	www.campnurse.org
Association of Child Neurology Nurses	www.childneurologysociety.org/acnn
Association of Community Health Nursing Educators	www.achne.org
Association of Faculties of Pediatric Nurse Practitioners	www.afpnp.org
Association of Nurse Practitioners in Business, Inc.	www.anpbfl.org
Association of Nurses in AIDS Care	www.nursesinaidscare.org
Association of Pediatric Gastroenterology and Nutrition Nurses	www.apgnn.org
Association of Pediatric Hematology/Oncology Nurses	www.aphon.org
Association of periOperative Registered Nurses	www.aorn.org
Association of Public Health Nurses	www.phnurse.org
Association for Radiologic & Imaging Nursing	www.arinursing.org
Association of Rehabilitation Nurses	www.rehabnurse.org
Association of Women's Health, Obstetric and Neonatal Nurses	www.awhonn.org
Baromedical Nurses Association	www.hyperbaricnurses.org
Chi Eta Phi Sorority, Inc.	www.chietaphi.com
Coalition for Nurses in Advanced Practice	www.cnaptexas.com
Commissioned Officers Association, U.S. Public Health Service	www.coausphs.org
CGFNS International	www.cgfns.org
Dermatology Nurses' Association	www.dnanurse.org
Dermatology Nurses' Association, Nurse Practitioners Society	www.dnanurse.org/aboutdna/np-society/
Developmental Disabilities Nurses Association	www.ddna.org
Eastern Nursing Research Society	www.communities.enrs-go.org
Emergency Nurses Association	www.ena.org
Endocrine Nurses Society	www.endo-nurses.org
Federal Nurses Association	www.dnpprogramsonline.com/federal-nurses-association
Gerontological Advanced Practice Nurses Association	www.gapna.org
Home Healthcare Nurses Association	www.hhna.org
Hospice and Palliative Nurses Association	www.hpna.org
Infusion Nurses Society	www.ins1.org
International Academy of Nursing Editors	www.nursingeditors.com
International Association of Clinical Research Nurses	www.iacrn.memberlodge.org
International Association of Forensic Nurses	www.forensicnurses.org
International Nurses Society on Addictions	www.intnsa.org
International Society of Plastic and Aesthetic Nurses	www.ispan.org
Long Term Care Nurses Association	www.ltcna.org
Midwest Nursing Research Society	www.mnrs.org
Minnesota Nurses Peer Support Network	www.nursespeersupport.nonprofitoffice.com
NANDA International	www.nanda.org
National Association for Practical Nurse Education and Service, Inc.	www.napnes.org
National Academy of Dermatology Nurse Practitioners	www.nadnp.net
National Association of Clinical Nurse Specialists	www.nacns.org
National Association of Directors of Nursing Administration in Long Term Care	www.nadona.org
National Association of Hispanic Nurses	www.nahnnet.org
National Association of Licensed Practical Nurses	www.nalpn.org

TABLE 67.1   Nursing Associations and Alliances—cont'd

Organization Name	Website
National Association of Neonatal Nurses	www.nann.org
National Association of Nigerian Nurses in North America	www.nannna.org
National Association of Nurse Practitioner Faculties	www.nonpf.org
National Association of Nurse Practitioners in Women's Health	www.npwh.org
National Association of Orthopaedic Nurses	www.orthonurse.org
National Association of Pediatric Nurse Practitioners	www.napnap.org
National Association of School Nurses	www.nasn.org
National Association of State School Nurse Consultants	www.schoolnurseconsultants.org
National Black Nurses Association, Inc.	www.nbna.org
National Coalition of Ethnic Minority Nurse Associations	www.ncemna.org
National Council of State Boards of Nursing	www.ncsbn.org
National Flight Nurses Association	www.astna.site-ym.com
National Forum of State Nursing Workforce Centers	www.nursingworkforcecenters.org
National Hospice and Palliative Care Organization	www.nhpco.org
National League for Nursing	www.nln.org
National Nurses in Business Association	www.nnbanow.com
National Organization of Nurse Practitioner Faculties	www.nonpf.org
National Student Nurses' Association	www.nsna.org
Navy Nurse Corps Association	www.nnca.org
Nurses Christian Fellowship	www.ncf-jcn.org
Nurses Organization of Veterans Affairs	www.vanurse.org
Nursing Ethics Network	www.nursingethicsnetwork.org
Nursing Network on Violence Against Women International	www.nnvawi.org
Nutrition Support Nurses Practice Section of ASPEN	www.nutritioncare.org
Oncology Nursing Society	www.ons.org
Organization for Associate Degree Nursing	www.oadn.org
Pediatric Endocrinology Nursing Society	www.pens.org
Philippine Nurses Association of America	www.mypnaa.org
Respiratory Nursing Society	www.respiratorynursingsociety.org
Rheumatology Nurses Society	www.rnsnetwork.org
Sigma	www.sigmanursing.org
Society for Vascular Nursing	www.svnnet.org
Society of Gastroenterology Nurses and Associates, Inc.	www.sgna.org
Society of Nurses in Advanced Practice	www.snapaprn.org
Society of Otorhinolaryngology and Head-Neck Nurses	www.sohnnurse.com
Society of Pediatric Nurses	www.pedsnurses.org
Society of Trauma Nurses	www.traumanurses.org
Society of Urologic Nurses and Associates	www.suna.org
Transcultural Nursing Society	www.tcns.org
Visiting Nurse Associations of America	www.vnaa.org
Wound Ostomy & Continence Nurses Society	www.wocn.org

Source: Nurse.org, n.d.; Nursing Organizations Alliance, n.d.-a.

The Nurses on Boards Coalition (NOBC) convened in 2014 at the invitation of the Robert Wood Johnson Foundation and AARP in response to the Institute of Medicine (IOM) report *The Future of Nursing: Leading Change, Advancing Health* (IOM, 2011). The coalition seeks to increase nurse representation on corporate, health care, and other boards, panels, and commissions—many of which either create or influence policy (see Chapter 49). NOBC set a goal of placing nurses in at least 10 000 seats by 2020 (NOBC, n.d.). Individual associations have developed initiatives such as the Academy's Institute for Nursing Leadership to help reach this goal (American Academy of Nursing, n.d.-b).

Nursing organizations, especially specialty organizations, often join other professional groups outside nursing and health care to create special interest alliances. Interprofessional alliances that include a nursing organization can exert considerable influence because consumers have repeatedly considered nurses as highly trustworthy (McCarthy, 2018).

CREDENTIALING ORGANIZATIONS

Credentialing refers to activities such as certification, certificate programs, accreditation, licensure, and regulation (Institute for Credentialing Excellence [ICE], n.d.a). State licensing boards are examples of public credentialing organizations. Private organizations include specialty certification and program accreditation. Although these organizations do not have individual members, their work has significant policy implications at national, state, and institutional levels and affects the members of nursing associations because of its impact on academic preparation, practice privileges, scope of practice, job mobility, and payment for services.

Nursing credentialing organizations often join the ICE, which develops standards and serves as an information clearinghouse and education hub for the credentialing industry. Many credentialing organizations become accredited by the National Commission for Certifying Agencies, an ICE-affiliate. Assessment-based certificate programs may be accredited through the ICE 1100 Standard program (ICE, n.d.b).

The more than 40 nursing specialty credentialing organizations shown in Table 67.2 belong to the American Board of Nursing Specialties (ABNS). Established in 1991, ABNS creates uniformity in nursing certification and raises public awareness about its value (ABNS, n.d.).

TABLE 67.2   Nursing Credentialing Organizations

Organization Name	Website
Addictions Nursing Certification Board	www.intnsa.org/certification
American Holistic Nurses Credentialing Corporation	www.ahncc.org
American Academy of Nurse Practitioners National Certification Board	www.aanpcp.org
American Association of Critical-Care Nurses Certification Corporation	www.aacn.org/certification
American Board for Occupational Health Nurses	www.abohn.org
American Board of Certification for Gastroenterology Nurses	www.abcgn.org
American Board of Neuroscience Nursing	www.abnncertification.org
American Board of Nursing Specialties	www.nursingcertification.org
American Board of Perianesthesia Nursing Certification, Inc.	www.cpancapa.org
American Legal Nurse Consultant Certification Board	www.aalnc.org
American Midwifery Certification Board	www.amcbmidwife.org
American Nurses Credentialing Center	www.nursecredentialing.org
American Organization for Nursing Leadership	www.aonl.org
American Society for Metabolic & Bariatric Surgery	www.asmbs.org
Board of Certification for Emergency Nursing	www.bcencertifications.org
Certified Nurse Life Care Planners	www.camedlink.com
CGFNS International (foreign education credentials assessment)	www.cgfns.org
Competency and Credentialing Institute (perioperative certification)	www.cc-institute.org
Dermatology Nursing Certification Board	www.dnanurse.org/education/certification
Gerontological Nursing Certification Commission	www.gapna.org
Hospice and Palliative Credentialing Center	www.goHPCC.org
Infusion Nurses Certification Corporation	www.ins1.org
Institute for Credentialing Excellence	www.credentialingexcellence.org

TABLE 67.2 Nursing Credentialing Organizations—cont'd	
Organization Name	**Website**
Medical-Surgical Nursing Certification Board	www.msncb.org
National Board for Certification of School Nurses	www.nbcsn.org
National Certification Board for Diabetes Educators	www.ncbde.org
National League for Nursing	www.nln.org
National Board of Certification and Recertification for Nurse Anesthetists	www.nbcrna.com
Neonatal Nursing Specialties	www.nccnet.org
Nephrology Nursing Certification Commission	www.nncc-exam.org
Oncology Nursing Certification Corporation	www.oncc.org
Orthopaedic Nurses Certification Board	www.oncb.org
Pediatric Nursing Certification Board	www.pncb.org
Plastic Surgical Nursing Certification Board	www.psncb.org
Radiologic Nursing Certification Board	www.certifiedradiologynurse.com
Rehabilitation Nursing Certification Board	www.rehabnurse.org
Wound Ostomy and Continence Nursing Certification Board	www.wocncb.org

Source: American Board of Nursing Specialties, 2016.

THE WORK OF NURSING ASSOCIATIONS

An association's mission, vision, and resources determine its program of work, which generally involves setting standards, professional development, recognition, and group benefits.

Setting Standards

Standards set by nursing associations may be broad or narrow and apply to individual nurses, what they learn, what they do, and where they do it. Broad standards, such as the ANA (2015) *Code of Ethics for Nurses with Interpretive Statements*, will affect every nurse regardless of role or setting. Narrow ones, such as the American Nephrology Nurses Association *Nephrology Nursing Scope and Standards of Practice* (Gomez, 2017), focus on an individual nursing specialty.

Scope and standards of practice documents can influence policy at every level. For example, they can determine the requirements for national certification and state licensure. State agencies rely on these documents when framing regulations to expand or limit clinical practice. These regulations in turn will inform the payment criteria for clinical services, which impact services available to consumers and nurses' financial income, especially in advanced practice. Locally, employers use scope and standards of practice documents to delineate practice privileges, job descriptions, and performance reviews.

The *AACN Procedure Manual for High-Acuity, Progressive, and Critical Care* (Wiegand, 2017) is an example of standards for what nurses do—specifically, clinical procedures. Nursing is no longer part of the title because, over seven editions, the book has become widely accepted by mandatory and voluntary accreditation agencies as the standard for clinical procedures regardless of who performs them.

Professional Development

Many nursing associations—especially those focused on clinical practice or specific roles—were created to fill the need for continued learning while generating revenue. Learning opportunities usually offer continuing nursing education credit or units to meet credentialing, licensing, and employment requirements. Associations develop learning opportunities for any interested learner, although members remain the primary audience. Associations develop learning content for individual and group learning that can be delivered live or via delayed online feeds and recorded media such as webinars and podcasts.

Recognition

Associations recognize individual and group accomplishments with awards often sponsored by companies that provide products and services used by nurses—usually members—engaged in the organization's area of focus. An association may consider scholarships as professional development initiatives that also recognize the achievements of those who receive them. Research and project grants also provide evidence to develop and implement standards. Certification and certificate credentialing programs may be an organization's most visible, far-reaching, and enduring recognition initiative. The link to standards-based practice and professional development furthers more than one organizational goal. The ICE defines certification—for example, Critical Care Registered Nurse (CCRN) certification in acute and critical care nursing—as professional recognition for meeting established knowledge, skills, or competencies and usually requires successfully completing an exam.

A certificate program, such as one in nursing education, builds "capacity and recognition of a specialty area of practice or set of skills" (ICE, n.d.). Board certification represents the nursing profession's commitment to protect the public. Certification "demonstrates to patients, employers and the public that a nurse's knowledge reflects national standards and a deep commitment to patient safety" (AACN Certification Corporation, 2018).

Group Benefits

Professional associations often offer through third-party vendors group benefits such as various forms of insurance (liability, disability, long-term care, auto, and vision), travel discounts, financial planning, and student loan solutions. This service to members allows associations to meet member needs at discounted rates from vendors while also generating funds for the organization to fund mission-focused initiatives that do not generate revenue.

POLICY ISSUES AFFECTING NURSING ASSOCIATIONS

Associations continuously intersect with a wide range of national, regional, state, and local policy issues. Specific issues may change over time, but they will typically involve three factors: being an association, having non-profit tax status, and carrying out a focused mission.

Being an Association

A wide range of policy issues affects the association industry. Issues may range from incorporation, financial management and taxation, workforce development, intellectual property rights, to internet usage. Professional associations advocate for policy changes that will benefit their organization's work and seek to modify or defeat changes that create barriers. Associations ensure their own governing rules and operating procedures align with approved policy. The American Society of Association Executives' (ASAE) Center for Association Leadership supports association groups by representing the industry at national, regional, state, and local policy tables including meetings with individual policymakers and their staff, legislative forums, and lobbying initiatives. The ASAE Foundation conducts industry-related research and supports the development of association professionals (ASAE, n.d.).

Tax Status

An association's tax status—and policy changes in tax law and regulations—can affect the organization and its individual members. Most nursing associations receive federal non-profit tax designation. The type of designation—usually based on sections 501(c)(3) or 501(c)(6) of the Internal Revenue Code (IRC)—determines its scope of activities including those for which it is exempt from paying taxes. It also allows the association to support its work by retaining excess revenue (Internal Revenue Service, 2018). The mission of advancing education or science generally qualifies for 501(c)(3) status but restricts how much political lobbying and activity the association may conduct, including financial contributions to political organizations and support of candidates. 501(c)(6) status offers narrower tax exemptions but expanded policy-related and political options that allow some engagement in political activity and lobbying for issues related to the organization's mission.

State legislation and local tax regulations also may create policy issues for associations. For example, proposed changes to sales and property tax exemptions based on non-profit status may affect not only where an association is headquartered, but wherever it does business. This can include chapters, educational programs, and product sales across state and city lines. Policy changes to group plans also affect associations offering benefits to members.

Credentialing

Credentialing organizations face policy issues at every level. They also engage in policy development about scope of practice, education, credentialing, and reimbursement for new roles such as advanced practice nurses and clinical nurse leaders. Individual nurses interact most often with state boards of nursing and the organizations listed in Table 67.2. State boards, regulatory agencies themselves, belong to the National Council of State Boards of Nursing (NCSBN), a non-governmental organization without regulatory authority that develops shared processes that ensure regulatory excellence for patient and public protection (NCSBN, n.d.). NCSBN develops and administers the National Council Licensure Exam (NCLEX) used by every nurse licensing board to ensure a psychometrically sound and legally defensible licensure process. The council also develops standards to address related processes such as criminal background checks, verification of licensure by endorsement, and reporting of disciplinary actions. NCSBN was instrumental in developing the Nurse Licensure Compact which "allows a nurse to have one multistate license with the ability to practice in the home state and other compact states" (NCSBN, 2018).

CHALLENGES WHEN ADDRESSING POLICY ISSUES

Associations face philosophical and resource challenges when confronting policy issues.

Philosophical

Once an association chooses to engage in policy issues and identifies the financial and human resources it can make available, it must select the issues and decide how involved to become. Philosophical challenges may include determining the widest possible audience for the organization to represent and whether to collaborate with others or go it alone.

An association's work reaches beyond its members. For this reason, nursing associations often describe themselves as representing the interests of all nurses involved in the association's focus area. For example, ANA describes itself as "representing the interests of the nation's 4 million registered nurses." AACN Critical Care represents "the interests of more than half a million acute and critical care nurses" and AACN Colleges represents "814 member schools of nursing at public and private universities nationwide."

Associations are showing increased flexibility adopting blended approaches to achieve policy agendas, experimenting with the NOA and the Nursing Community Coalition as practical alternatives to all-or-nothing solutions.

Nursing Community Coalition. Since 2008, the Nursing Community Coalition has continued refining the elusive goal of speaking with one voice for all of nursing. Collectively, coalition members represent more than one million registered nurses, advanced practice registered nurses, nurse faculty and executives, researchers, and students. The actual number of nurses supporting a policy issue will vary because each organization chooses which issues to endorse. This nimble approach allows for rapid responses that leverage aggregate membership numbers without demanding unanimity and allow associations with both general and special interests to participate.

Nursing Organizations Alliance. Learning from the experience of its predecessor organizations, NOA organizations replaced the "one voice" goal with two collaborative programs to strengthen their members' skills in policy advocacy and volunteer leadership (NOA, n.d.b). The Nursing Alliance Leadership Academy provides newly elected and emerging leaders the knowledge and skills needed to effectively govern and lead their organizations. Volunteer leaders learn how to fulfill leadership roles and develop strong networking relationships with fellow leaders from a wide range of organizations.

NOA's Nurse in Washington Internship is open to any registered nurse or nursing student at every level of education who is interested in an orientation to the legislative process. Participants learn how to become involved and influence policy at all levels by understanding the legislative process and grassroots advancement of legislative issues.

Resources

As a non-profit organization, an association does not have investors with vested interests such as profit sharing. Instead, all excess revenue must be used to support the association's work. This includes accruing adequate financial reserves to support operations for a designated period of time—usually at least 3 to 6 months—in the event of an unexpected shortfall. However, even the best managed and most financially stable association is not likely to enjoy the financial health of a successful for-profit company. This means even modest goals for policy engagement will always compete for financial and human resources with all other organizational initiatives.

Volunteers. Engaging volunteer members to help carry out policy activities expands an organization's reach and creates new challenges. Volunteers may reduce the direct cost of compensation and even expenses such as travel and lodging, if the member agrees to underwrite those. However, their work will need to be coordinated and they will require training—including those with policy experience to ensure they understand the scope of the policy agenda, how it relates to the association's mission, and how its tax status may limit what can be done.

Social Media. Wide availability and limited expense of social media can extend the reach of an association's policy agenda. Volunteers with social media expertise can further reduce expense. But using social media—whether by volunteers or paid staff members—also requires careful management to ensure messaging does not inadvertently tarnish the association's image or jeopardize its tax status.

CONCLUSION

Associations are uniquely positioned within nursing to address policy because their representation of a full range of general and special interests affords access to numbers and experts based on individual association missions. Associations also face challenges because of limited resources and competing priorities. Collaborative approaches such as the NOA, Nursing Community Coalition, and the ANA Organizational Affiliates Program offer alternatives to the frequent dogged insistence on all-or-nothing solutions instead of seeking practical compromise.

DISCUSSION QUESTIONS

1. How are nursing associations uniquely positioned to influence national, regional, state, and local policy?
2. What unique challenges do associations face when framing their policy agenda?
3. How does a blended strategy offer flexibility in achieving an association's policy agenda?

REFERENCES

American Academy of Nursing. (n.d. a). *About the academy.* Retrieved from www.aannet.org/about/about-the-academy.

American Academy of Nursing. (n.d. b). *Institute for Nursing leadership.* Retrieved from www.aannet.org/initiatives/institute-for-nursing-leadership.

American Association of Critical-Care Nurses. (2018). *Board certification.* Retrieved from www.aacn.org/certification?tab=First-Time%20Certification.

American Board of Nursing Specialties. (2016). *Membership directory.* Retrieved from www.nursingcertification.org/membership/membership-directory.

American Board of Nursing Specialties. (n.d.) *About us.* Retrieved from www.nursingcertification.org.

American Nurses Association. (2015). *Code of ethics for nurses with interpretive statements.* Silver Spring, MD: Author.

American Nurses Association. (2016a). *Historical review.* Retrieved from www.nursingworld.org/~48de64/globalassets/docs/ana/historical-review2016.pdf.

American Nurses Association. (2016b). *Organizational affiliates.* Retrieved from www.nursingworld.org/~48e2b9/globalassets/ana/ana-organizational-affiliates/org-affiliates-obligations-2016.pdf.

American Nurses Association. (2017). *Strategic plan.* Retrieved from www.nursingworld.org/~48daea/globalassets/docs/ana/2017-2020-anastrategicplan.pdf.

American Society of Association Executives. (n.d.). *About us.* Retrieved from www.asaecenter.org/about-us.

Bradley-Sanders, C. (2012). *Bellevue school of nursing.* Retrieved from https://archives.med.nyu.edu/collections/bellevue-school-nursing.

Christiaens, G. (2015). Current issues in nursing associations. In D. Mason, D. Gardner, F.H. Outlaw, & E. O'Grady (Eds.), *Policy & politics in nursing and health care* (7th ed., pp. 588-595). St. Louis: Elsevier.

de Tocqueville, A. (1945). *Democracy in America* (vol. 2, p. 117). New York: Random House. (Original work published 1835 [volume 1] and 1840 [volume 2]. London: Saunders and Otley.)

Gomez, N.J. (2017). *Nephrology nursing scope and standards of practice.* Pitman, NJ: American Nephrology Nurses Association.

Institute for Credentialing Excellence. (n.d.a). *About ICE.* Retrieved from www.credentialingexcellence.org.

Institute for Credentialing Excellence. (n.d.b) *Certificate vs. certification.* Retrieved from www.credentialingexcellence.org/p/cm/ld/fid=4.

Institute of Medicine. (2011). *The future of nursing: Leading change, advancing health.* Retrieved from www.nationalacademies.org/hmd/Reports/2010/The-Future-of-Nursing-Leading-Change-Advancing-Health.aspx.

Internal Revenue Service. (2018). *Tax information for charities and other non-profits.* Retrieved from www.irs.gov/charities-non-profits.

McCarthy, N. (2018). *America's most and least trusted professions.* Retrieved from www.forbes.com/sites/niallmccarthy/2018/01/04/americas-most-and-least-trusted-professions-infographic/#793628cd65b5.

National Council of State Boards of Nursing. (2018). *Nurse licensure compact.* Retrieved from www.ncsbn.org/nurse-licensure-compact.htm.

National Council of State Boards of Nursing. (n.d.). *About NCSBN.* Retrieved from www.ncsbn.org/about.htm.

National League for Nursing. (n.d.). *Overview.* Retrieved from www.nln.org/about/overview.

Nurse.org. (n.d.). *Organizations: List of nursing organizations.* Retrieved from https://nurse.org/orgs.shtml.

Nurses on Boards Coalition. (n.d.) *Our story.* Retrieved from www.nursesonboardscoalition.org/about/.

Nursing Community Coalition. (n.d.). *Core principles.* Retrieved from www.thenursingcommunity.org/core-principles.

Nursing Organizations Alliance. (n.d.a) *About us: Member organizations.* Retrieved from www.nursing-alliance.org/dnn/About-Us/Our-Members.

Nursing Organizations Alliance. (n.d.b) *Nursing alliance leadership academy.* Retrieved from www.nursing-alliance.org/Events/NALA-Nursing-Alliance-Leadership-Academy.

Nursing Organizations Alliance. (n.d.c). *Our history.* Retrieved from www.nursing-alliance.org/dnn/About-Us/Our-History.

Thompson, P.E., & Lavandero, R. (2001). Professional associations for the millennium. In N.L. Chaska (Ed.), *The nursing profession: Tomorrow and beyond* (pp. 101-108). Thousand Oaks, CA: Sage Publications.

Wiegand, D.J. (2017). *AACN procedure manual for high-acuity, progressive, and critical care.* Philadelphia: Saunders.

Zunz, O. (2015). *Alexis De Tocqueville on associations and philanthropy.* Retrieved from https://histphil.org/2015/07/13/alexis-de-tocqueville-on-associations-and-philanthropy/.

ONLINE RESOURCES

American Board of Nursing Specialties
www.nursingcertification.org
Nursing Community Coalition
www.thenursingcommunity.org
Nursing Organizations Alliance
www.nursing-alliance.org

68

TAKING ACTION: School Nursing at the Intersection of Health and Education

Donna Mazyck and Nina R. Fekaris

> "…nurses can drive transformations in effective care delivery; they can open the door to innovation that heals our patients and advances health and well-being across our communities. It is the power behind the voice of nursing."
>
> *Angela Patterson, DNP, FNP-BC, NEA-BC*

When Lillian Wald brought together public health and education to put nurses in New York public schools in the early 1900s, school nursing emerged as a specialty practice rooted in public health and safety. The actions of those nurses in schools decreased communicable diseases among children, increased student attendance, and were so successful they soon became an integral part of the public school's mission (Wald, 1915). Today, the connection between health and learning is still recognized, and the role of the school nurse, although greatly expanded, continues to provide for the health and safety of all children attending schools. The definition of school nursing encompasses this foundation:

> School nursing, a specialized practice of nursing, protects and promotes student health, facilitates optimal development, and advances academic success. School nurses, grounded in ethical and evidence-based practice, are the leaders who bridge health care and education, provide care coordination, advocate for quality student-centered care, and collaborate to design systems that allow individuals and communities to develop their full potential. (American Nurses Association [ANA] and National Association of School Nurses [NASN], 2017, p. 1)

School nurses are the first provider delivering health care and health education to children without their parents/guardians being present. The lessons taught during these interactions potentially have a lifetime impact. When the school nurse teaches a child how to properly use an asthma inhaler, the nurse empower the child to take control over one aspect of his or her physical health. When children are taught how, when, and why they need to wash their hands, they begin to understand disease prevention and how to live a healthy lifestyle. School nurses influence the health of generations by supporting students' opportunities to learn about and practice healthy behaviors, providing school health services, creating safe and positive school environments, and engaging families and community (Michael, 2015) (Box 68.1).

WHOLE SCHOOL, WHOLE COMMUNITY, WHOLE CHILD MODEL

The Centers for Disease Control and Prevention (CDC) recognizes the importance of a coordinated approach to school health. In collaboration with the Association for Supervision and Curriculum Development (ASCD), the CDC developed the Whole School, Whole Community, Whole Child (WSCC) model depicting the importance of collaboration between schools, health agencies, parents, and communities in working toward supporting the health and academic achievement of all children (ASCD, 2014). It recognizes the important connection between education and health, emphasizing a school-wide approach that acknowledges learning and health as an integral foundation of the local community.

The WSCC model identifies 10 components:
- Social and Emotional Climate
- Counseling, Psychological, and Social Services
- Physical Environment
- Employee Wellness
- Family Engagement
- Community Involvement

"One morning, Samuel, an academically-struggling, third grade student, came into the office carrying his new inhaler. He experienced frequent illness and missed over 20 days of school during first and second grades. After helping his grandmother find a pediatrician, I learned Samuel received an asthma diagnosis. Over the course of the school year, Samuel learned how to manage and live with asthma. His attendance improved dramatically and by the end of third grade he was catching up academically. Even with severe asthma, we were able to manage most exacerbations at school. Last year, Samuel graduated from high school with honors, and he was very excited to share with me his plan to pursue a career in respiratory therapy. He said he wants to help kids just like him." (Christy M., School Nurse, Elementary)

- Health Education
- Physical Education and Physical Activity
- Nutrition Environment and Services
- Health Services

School nurses focus their practice within the Health Services component where "school health services connect school staff, students, families, community, and health care providers to promote the health care of students and a healthy and safe school environment." (Lewallen et al., 2015, p. 733).

FRAMEWORK FOR 21st CENTURY SCHOOL NURSING PRACTICE

NASN created the *Framework for 21st Century School Nursing Practice* (Framework) to better describe the role and function of the school nurse (Fig. 68.1). The Framework aligns with the WSCC model by identifying a collaborative and coordinated approach to health and learning. The

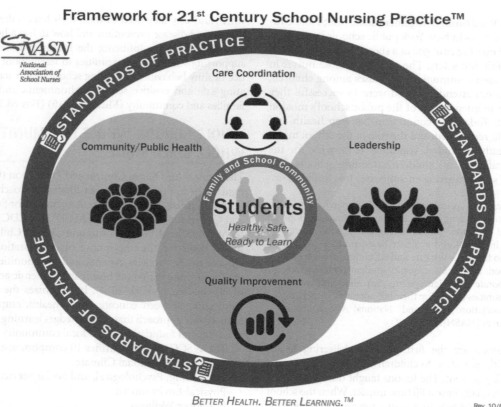

Fig. 68.1 Framework for 21st Century School Nursing Practice. (Source: NASN, 2016.)

principles of the Framework describe foundational skills for school health services that promote student health, safety, and academic success (NASN, 2016). The overarching structure includes concepts integral to the complex, clinical practice of school nursing, depicted with five, non-hierarchical principles surrounding students as listed here:

- *Students* are at the center of school nursing practice, surrounded and supported by relationships and connection with families and school communities.
- *Care coordination* is critical to the daily work school nurses do connecting health care and education. School nurses base care on student-centered assessment and promote self-empowerment. They provide chronic and acute disease management, transition planning utilizing motivational interviewing, collaborative communication, and trauma-informed care. With interdisciplinary teams, they develop student-specific plans: individualized health care, 504, and Individualized Education Programs.
- *Leadership* encompasses school nurse advocacy based on student, school, and community needs, education that promotes problem solving, effective communication, collaboration with others, and students' efficacy in self-management and life skills. Leadership includes policy development, funding and reimbursement, systems-level approaches, and advocacy for health care and education reform.
- *Quality improvement* encompasses consistent evaluation whereby school nurses implement student outcome improvement measures and interventions. The evidence base for school nursing practice is founded by continuous data collection and analysis.
- *Community/public health* components focus beyond the individual student to community and populations, delivering health promotion and disease prevention. School nurses provide primary, secondary, and tertiary public health services including screenings, referrals, disease prevention, and follow-up access to care, while addressing the social determinants of health and health equity that impact the school community.
- *Standards of practice* surround and support all other principles: they delineate clinical competencies for school nurses, providing foundation for evidence-based practice, the scope of school nursing practice, clinical guidelines, code of ethics, evidence-based practice articles, and position documents.

OPPORTUNITIES AND CHALLENGES WITH EDUCATION POLICY

In December 2015, the federal legislation Every Student Succeeds Act (ESSA) reauthorized the federal Elementary and Secondary Education Act (P.L. 114-85, 2015), allowing state and local policy changes that advance health, well-being, and learning for all students.

School Health in ESSA

ESSA defines *specialized instructional support personnel* (SISP) to include school counselors, school social workers, school psychologists, school nurses, speech language pathologists, and school librarians (ESSA, 2015, Sec. 8101, paragraph 47). The law lists school nurses as leaders in chronic disease management and describes programs and activities to support safe and healthy students and school conditions, including (1) drug and violence prevention, (2) school-based mental health services and partnerships, (3) integration of health and safety practices in school and athletic programs, (4) support for a healthy, active lifestyle, and (5) bullying, harassment, coercion, and abuse prevention, along with other programs and activities (ESSA, 2015, Sec. 4108, 120 USC 7118).

State and Local Needs Assessments and Non-academic Indicator

ESSA requires states to select a non-academic, accountability indicator of school and student success; 36 states and Washington, DC selected chronic absenteeism (Jordan & Miller, 2017). School nurses bring critical skills in identifying and mitigating health and other factors that present barriers to student attendance (McClanahan & Weismuller, 2015). They advocate for students and influence policies developed to address chronic absenteeism and ESSA implementation on state and local levels.

HEALTHY AND SAFE SCHOOLS

The school nurse office is one of several places in schools where students can avoid being graded, tested, or judged, and offers a place of healing, support, and care. School nurses help support healthy and safe schools in multiple ways (Box 68.2).

School Violence

Schools aim to provide students with the knowledge and tools they need to succeed in a safe and engaging environment. However, recent acts of violence occurring in schools dominate news headlines. For school year 2015–2016, close to 69% of schools recorded one or more violent incidents of crime, and 15% recorded one or more serious violent incidents (Musu-Gillette et al., 2018). Violence—experienced or witnessed—and subsequent trauma impacts health and a child's ability to succeed in school (Finkelhor, 2015).

"One Friday afternoon, about 5 minutes prior to school dismissal, a 10th grade girl came into my health office. Based upon my first assessment (her hoodie was pulled up hiding a pale face with dark circles under her eyes, her hands were shaking, her posture was stooped), this was a student in crisis. She soon revealed that she had been staying with a friend because she had run away from home, she hadn't been eating because her stomach was 'in knots all the time,' and she had been cutting. We talked about her home life and both determined that was not a healthy place for her to go. She identified she had an aunt she felt safe with. She came and met with us at school and agreed to provide care for my student. Over the next several months and through Children's Protective Services support, we were able to get her the mental health services she needed. The student completed that school year, however never returned to school in the fall." (Lori P, School Nurse, High School)

Adverse Childhood Experiences

Adverse childhood experiences (ACEs) are stressful or traumatic childhood events, including abuse, neglect, and household dysfunction, witnessing domestic violence, or growing up with family members who have substance use disorders. In addition to violence, ACEs influence a child's ability to learn and are determinants to adult success. Although more research is needed on intervention strategies and violence prevention, school nurses identify and provide care for students who have experienced violence and ACEs (Giovanelli, 2016).

Mental/Behavioral Health

Mental and behavioral health conditions present a challenge for children. Currently, the global prevalence of mental health disorders in children and adolescents is 13.4% (Polanczyk, 2015). School nurses, educators, and mental health professionals collaborate to support student mental health (Bohnenkamp, 2015).

The school nurse is often the first person to recognize symptoms of poor mental health. Children with anxiety and poor coping skills visit school nurses with vague complaints such as headaches or stomach aches. School nurses provide a safety net for students and their families to access appropriate interventions in schools.

OPPORTUNITIES AND CHALLENGES WITH HEALTH POLICY

The NURSE Act

Many children and youth arrive each school day without the critical presence of school nurses. In the United States, 25.2% of schools have no school nurses: disparities exist in health services provision for students within and across states (Willgerodt, 2018).

On March 12, 2018, U.S. Senator Jon Tester (D-MT) and U.S. Congresswoman Dina Titus (D-NV-1) introduced the NURSE (Nurses for Under Resourced Schools Everywhere) Act (NURSE Act, S 2532 and HR 5251, 2018), proposing federal grants from the U.S. Department of Education to place or increase the number of registered school nurses in Title I schools. In June of 2018, NASN launched a "Virtual Hill Day" to advocate for student health and create momentum for this legislation. School nurses tweeted, emailed, and called members of Congress to voice support for health and well-being of all students.

Opioid Crisis

In 2015, the NASN Board of Directors published a policy statement about harm reduction related to the opioid crisis. Safe and effective management of opioid overdose in schools is part of school emergency preparedness and response (NASN, 2015). When naloxone is available in schools, overdose deaths can be prevented. A toolkit for school nurses provided information about the opioid crisis and prevention education for students.

KEY TAKEAWAYS

Schools have the opportunity and responsibility to teach students how to stay healthy and productive in a safe, supportive learning environment. School nurses possess skills and expertise to support safe, healthy students who are ready to learn; they influence school policies by advocating with clear, concise, and consistent messages.

Creating a culture of school and community health requires a coalition of teachers, school nurses, other SISP, school administrators, students, families, and policymakers working together to reduce barriers to learning, improve mental and behavioral health supports, and promote an environment of health, safety, and engagement. The WSCC model and the *Framework for 21st Century School Nursing Practice* provide structure for a coordinated school health program, with school nurses linking school health services with health care, community, families, and school.

DISCUSSION QUESTIONS

1. How can school nurses leverage their role in chronic disease management to influence district policies related to chronic student absenteeism?
2. With increased focus on student mental health needs, what enables school counselors, nurses, psychologists, and social workers to address student needs and connect with community-based mental health providers?

REFERENCES

American Nurses Association, & National Association of School Nurses. (2017). *School nursing: Scope and standards of practice* (3rd ed.). Silver Spring, MD: Author.

Association for Supervision and Curriculum Development. (2014). *Health and learning: Whole school, whole community, whole child.* Retrieved from www.ascd.org/programs/learning-and-health/wscc-model.aspx.

Bohnenkamp, J.H., Stephan, S.H., & Bobo, N. (2015). Supporting student mental health: The role of the school nurse in coordinated school mental health care. *Psychology in the Schools, 52*(7), 714-727.

Every Student Succeeds Act. (2015). Pub. L. No. 114-95. Retrieved from www2.ed.gov/documents/essa-act-of-1965.pdf.

Finkelhor, D., Turner, H.A., Shattuck, A., & Hamby, S.L. (2015). Prevalence of childhood exposure to violence, crime, and abuse. *JAMA Pediatrics, 169*(8), 746.

Giovanelli, A., Reynolds, A.J., Mondi, C.F., & Ou, S. (2016). Adverse childhood experiences and adult well-being in a low-income, urban cohort. *Pediatrics, 137*(4), 1-11.

Jordan, P.W., & Miller, R. (2017). Who's in: Chronic absenteeism under the every student succeeds act. *FutureEd.* Retrieved from www.future-ed.org/wp-content/uploads/2017/09/REPORT_Chronic_Absenteeism_final_v5.pdf.

Lewallen, T.C., Hunt, H., Potts-Datema, W., Zaza, S., & Giles, W. (2015). The whole school, whole community, whole child model: A new approach for improving educational attainment and healthy development for students. *Journal of School Health, 85*(11), 729-739.

McClanahan, R., & Weismuller, P. (2015). School nurses and care coordination for children with complex needs: An integrative review. *Journal of School Nursing, 31*(1), 34-43.

Michael, S.L., Merlo, C.L., Basch, C.E., Wentzel, K.R., & Wechsler, H. (2015). Critical connections: Health and academics. *Journal of School Health, 85*(11), 740-758.

Musu-Gillette, L., Zhang, A., Wang, K., Zhang, J., Kemp, J., Diliberti, M., & Oudekerk, B.A. (2018). *Indicators of school crime and safety: 2017.* National Center for Education Statistics, U.S. Department of Education, and Bureau of Justice Statistics, Office of Justice Programs, U.S. Department of Justice. Washington, DC. Retrieved from https://nces.ed.gov/programs/crimeindicators/.

National Association of School Nurses. (2015). *Naloxone use in the school setting: The role of the school nurse.* [Position statement]. Silver Spring, MD: Author. Retrieved from www.nasn.org/nasn/advocacy/professional-practice-documents/position-statements/ps-naloxone.

National Association of School Nurses. (2016). Framework for 21st Century School Nursing Practice. *NASN School Nurse, 31*(1), 45-53.

Nurses for Under-Resourced Schools Everywhere (NURSE) Act. (2018). 115th Congress, Senate 2532, House of Representatives 5251. Retrieved from www.congress.gov/bill/115th-congress/senate-bill/2532/text.

Polanczyk, G., Salum, G., Sugaya, L., Caye, A., & Rohde, L. (2015). Annual research review: A meta-analysis of the worldwide prevalence of mental disorders in children and adolescents. *Journal of Child Psychology & Psychiatry, 56*(3), 345-365.

Wald, L.D. (1915). *The house on Henry Street.* New York: Henry Holt and Company.

Willgerodt, M.A., Brock, D.M., & Maughan, E.M. (2018). Public school nursing practice in the United States. *Journal of School Nursing, 34*(3), 232-244.

69

TAKING ACTION: The Alliance of Nurses for Healthy Environments Promoting Environmental Health

Ruth McDermott-Levy and Katie Huffling

"Unless someone like you cares a whole awful lot, nothing is going to get better. It's not."

Dr. Seuss, The Lorax

It may seem unusual for nurses to be concerned about public policies that impact the environment such as chemical regulations, our energy use, or our changing climate, but the truth is, more than likely, you have or will care for a patient, family, or community whose health has been affected in some way by these environmental exposures. Regardless of your practice setting, an essential role of the nurse is to prevent health risks, illness, and disease. Understanding and engaging in environmental policy is an important way to protect the health of the population the nurse serves.

As nurses caring for adult patients in home care (Ruth McDermott-Levy) and women during their pregnancy (Katie Huffling), we always saw the relationship between our patients' environment and their health. We advocated on a patient-by-patient level regarding the existing evidence of environmental exposures to promote health and prevent illness within our respective patient populations. But we always believed we needed to do more—we needed to move into the policy arena in order to maximize our impact.

ENVIRONMENTAL HEALTH NURSING IN CONTEXT

Historically, nursing has always included care of the environment. Florence Nightingale noted the importance of a clean patient care environment for healing (Nightingale, 1860). Nightingale was influenced by the environmental health (EH) theories of her time (Johnson, 2006), which have since evolved with greater scientific knowledge on the origin of disease (Leffers, Smith, Huffling, McDermott-Levy, & Sattler, 2016). One of Nightingale's greatest accomplishments was that she collected data related to sanitary conditions and mortality among patients in military hospitals. She created charts to make the evidence clear to policymakers. She used the evidence and collaborated with military, royal, and health officials to improve the health outcomes related to an environmental issue: sanitation in hospitals (Kopf, 1916). Nightingale's influence of improving patient care environments and relying on the evidence to promote healthy environments continues to be an important function of the nurse. Today, nurses rely on toxicological, epidemiologic, public health, biological, chemical, and nursing sciences to advocate for healthy environments.

Despite the fact that care for the environment is part of our nursing history, a 1995 report of the Health and Medicine Division of the National Academies (formerly the Institute of Medicine), *Nursing, Health and the Environment* (Pope, Snyder & Mood, 1995) identified that most nurses are not adequately prepared to address environmental hazards in the workplace, home, and in the community. This has led to nurses' inability to engage in and advocate for health protective environmental regulation, policies, and legislation. The report suggested that nurses at all levels be knowledgeable in EH nursing research, education, advocacy, and practice.

Concern about the findings of the 1995 report led to a group of committed nurses to seek funding and address the shortcomings of nurses engaging in EH advocacy

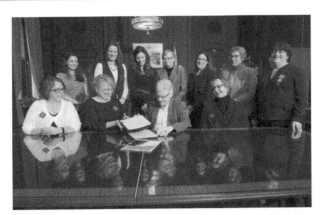

ANHE nurses meet with EPA Administrator Gina McCarthy in 2017.

and policy by offering educational programming in EH for nurse educators and practicing nurses (Leffers, McDermott-Levy, Smith, & Sattler, 2014). For example, in the late 1990s, with financial support from the Kellogg Foundation and the National Environmental Education and Training Foundation, 217 nursing faculty were trained in principles of EH and toxicology. These trained faculty returned to their schools of nursing and integrated EH into their existing curricula, with EH woven throughout undergraduate nursing education (Department of Health and Human Services, Agency for Toxic Substances and Disease Registry, 2002).

Although more nurses were now prepared to support EH for their patients or work settings, there was no central place for nurses to engage in, learn about, share, and support EH issues. In December 2008, 50 U.S. nurses representing a broad array of nursing practice areas came together to establish the Alliance of Nurses for Healthy Environments (ANHE), the only professional nursing organization devoted solely to EH. ANHE was organized to address the EH needs identified in the *Nursing, Health and the Environment* (1995) report with workgroups in research, education, advocacy, and practice. The formation and work of ANHE galvanized nurses to engage, share information, conduct research, and advocate for healthy environmental policies at the institutional, local, state, and national levels.

A group of ANHE nurses also addressed the gap in EH at the nursing organization level. In the summer of 2009, ANHE members met to develop nursing competencies for EH in nursing. Those competencies were shared with the American Nurses Association (ANA) and in 2010, the ANA published the revised ANHE EH competencies that became an EH standard in the Nursing Scope and Standards for Practice (now Standard 17 [ANA, 2010, 2015]). ANHE has provided the tools and connections among EH nurse experts to advance EH evidence through research,

knowledge of the latest science, and best practice related to EH through education; advance EH policies through advocacy, and implement EH into nursing practice to protect population health.

A core component of nursing practice is advocacy, and within the EH arena, advocacy moves beyond the bedside and into the policy realm. Nurses are trained to be advocates for their patients to ensure they receive the best care. Nurses are also skilled at taking complex scientific information and translating the science into everyday language that is understandable by the general public. These skills make nurses very effective advocates in the public policy arena.

Through the ANHE Policy-Advocacy Work Group, hundreds of nurses have been trained to be effective advocates for EH policies. ANHE has brought nurses from around the country to Washington, DC to speak with their elected officials about EH legislation, such as climate change, safer chemicals, and clean air and water legislation. Nurses can provide an effective mix of science and personal stories concerning the EH impacts they are seeing in their patients and communities.

In a recent example, Sarah Bucic, MS, RN, a resident of Delaware, discovered that lead paint was still legally being used in her state to paint outdoor structures such as bridges and water towers, without the public living near these structures being notified when paint removal or repainting was occurring. There is no safe level of lead and its use in this paint created a risk of exposure to the children and families living in surrounding homes. Her nursing voice was an essential component to a coalition that worked with the Delaware legislature to successfully pass HB 456, with significant bipartisan support, which bans the use of lead paint on outdoor structures.

Nursing Collaboration

Just as Nightingale used the evidence and collaboration with others to advance patient care environmental conditions, ANHE nurses have relied on the support from one another and collaboration with other organizations to advance the role of EH in the nursing profession. As nurses increase their expertise in EH, they have become a necessary force to collaborate with other nursing organizations and other professional, environmental, labor, and advocacy groups. The work of these initiatives is highlighted in the following examples of nurse advocacy.

Chemicals

More than 25 years ago, an environmental activist knocked on Kathleen Curtis's door in upstate New York. Kathleen was surprised to learn from the environmental advocate that there were toxic-waste dumps near her home. As a young mother and nurse, Kathleen listened to the advocate and then she set out to investigate the health risks of the dumps to her family and community. She was surprised to learn that there were health risks from the dumps located so close to her. She soon understood that, as a nurse, she needed to advocate for the health of her community. From that early encounter with environmental activism, Kathleen realized she could make a difference for the health of communities through engagement in EH policy. Kathleen took the time to learn about the issues and science that placed her community at risk.

She has become such an effective EH leader and advocate that she was awarded the prestigious "Charlotte Brody Award" from Health Care Without Harm in 2015 for her ability to influence environmental policy. She frequently visits policymakers in Albany, New York and Washington, DC to advocate for safer chemical regulations to reduce health risks such as firefighters' health risk from flame-retardant exposure and the elimination of toxic chemicals in children's products. In 2017, the strong collaborative efforts of firefighters and nurses provided support for a successful petition to the Consumer Product Safety Commission to ban toxic organohalogen flame retardants in children's products and certain electronics. Kathleen was also instrumental in the successful passage of several NY state laws to regulate chemicals, including the nation's first ban of bisphenol A (BPA). She used her nursing expertise to develop policy skills and is nationally recognized as a chemical policy expert. Nurse colleagues and other health advocates seek her expertise. Currently, Kathleen is the executive director, chief lobbyist, and organizer of Clean and Healthy New York.

Pennsylvania's Fossil Fuel Legacy

When Ruth McDermott-Levy was studying to be a nurse in Wilkes-Barre, PA, she was familiar with occupational health policies to protect Pennsylvania's coal miners from respiratory disease. But she was primarily concerned with learning about nursing care related to those respiratory illnesses and getting the patients well and home to their families. Later, as a home care nurse serving the oil refinery areas near Philadelphia, Ruth saw clearly how one's environment influenced health. So, when Pennsylvania State Nurses Association (PSNA) began an EH task force in 2007, she quickly joined. By 2009 she was a co-Chairperson of PSNA's Environmental Committee; this coincided with the unparalleled expansion of unconventional gas development, or fracking, in Pennsylvania. Ruth's role as PSNA's Environmental Health Committee Co-Chair led to reviewing research related to the health impacts of natural gas development and educating other nurses of those impacts of this growing industry in Pennsylvania. In 2012, Ruth and two other nurses authored an ANA environmental resolution that called for a ban for

new fracking wells in the United States. The ANA's House of Delegates unanimously approved the resolution. In addition, she worked with gas development community members to develop a community-based participatory study to address their EH education needs.

As an ANHE member, Ruth also collaborated with other organizations such as PennEnvironment, Philadelphia Physicians for Social Responsibility, and the Southwest Pennsylvania Environmental Health Project to address policies to put public health first. Initially, working with an environmental advocacy group such as PennEnvironment seemed contrary to her role as a nurse, educator, and researcher, but she soon learned the value of this collaboration. The advocacy groups knew the policymakers and their staff and they provided valuable advocacy strategies beneficial to health advocacy. The strength of these collaborative efforts is exemplified in their work to hold the Pennsylvania Department of Health accountable when it was discovered that they had not been responding to health complaints related to fracking. Having nurses, physicians, and public health professionals speaking out publicly against this practice quickly brought about change in the state government addressing health complaints. Pennsylvania ANHE nurses, with their collaborating organizations, continue their work in this area by addressing methane leaks from the gas industry, pipeline safety, and supporting a statewide health registry to monitor the health impacts of fracking on the population.

Climate Change: Nursing Collaborative

In May 2016, ANHE and the Obama Administration organized the first of its kind roundtable on Climate Change, Health, and Nursing at the White House. This roundtable was attended by representatives from 16 diverse, national nursing organizations. There was a robust discussion

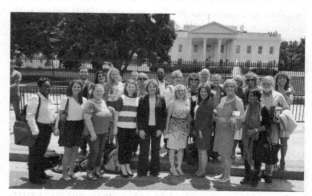

Representatives from nursing organizations meet at the White House for a roundtable on Climate Change, Health, and Nursing in 2014.

regarding nursing's role on climate change mitigation and adaptation. One of the outcomes of this meeting was a consensus that a unified nursing voice was needed to elevate this critical public health issue within the nursing profession, the public's consciousness, and with policymakers. With almost 4 million nurses in the United States, the group recognized the strength and power that our collective action could bring to the climate challenge. This led to the formation of the Nursing Collaborative on Climate Change and Health.

The Nursing Collaborative was launched in 2017 with support from Climate for Health, a national initiative that brings together leaders and institutions across the health sector to advance climate solutions to protect the health and well-being of Americans. Currently, the Collaborative is comprised of nine national nursing organizations and continues to grow. These organizations have committed to: (1) elevating climate change as a visible health priority within their organization; (2) creating a climate-literate nursing community through webinars, articles in their publications, and presentations at their annual meetings; (3) engaging all stakeholders on the intersection of climate change and human health; and (4) working together for climate solutions that will have a positive impact on the health of all.

Engaging in Environmental Health Policy in Times of Political Challenges

Having clean air, clean water, and access to safe products should not seem controversial, yet in today's political climate, there are constant attacks on environmental protection policies. These issues are seen as politically partisan. But for nurses, environmental issues are not partisan issues; they are matters of health. Having nurses actively engaged and addressing the health implications of maintaining critical environmental protections is part of nursing practice. As trusted messengers without a biased agenda, nurses' perspectives are very creditable to policymakers. Nurses speak authoritatively regarding environmental protections on health and are able to highlight the economic benefit of environmental regulations due to decreased health care costs from exposures. For example, during the debate over the introduction of the Clean Power Plan, the landmark regulation of carbon emissions from power plants, ANHE nurses spoke with their legislators and officials at the U.S. Environmental Protection Agency on the significant cost savings in health care due to decreased costs of treating chronic illnesses, such as asthma and cardiovascular disease, that are projected with the Plan implementation.

Even when new administrations may not appear to support environmental protections, we have found it essential to have areas of common interest in order to keep moving health protective policies forward and have some wins that keep morale high. For example, the Trump Administration has expressed a great interest in supporting infrastructure improvements. There are many communities throughout the United States with aging water infrastructure that can result in drinking water contaminated with lead and other toxic compounds. By working on this common interest of updated infrastructure, we can significantly improve the health of those living in those communities.

As ANHE looks forward in the policy arena, we have recognized the vital importance of having a thread of diversity, equity, and inclusion (DEI) throughout our work. Many of the communities and populations most vulnerable to environmental exposures are communities of color and low-income communities. Without addressing DEI within our own organization and throughout nursing, we will not be able to effectively meet the needs of the most vulnerable populations. In May 2018, ANHE along with representatives of the National Association of Hispanic Nurses, National Black Nurses Association, and the National Alaska Native American Indian Nurses Association came together and updated our commitment to meaningfully and equitably address EH so that all nurses can guide their practice and prevent harm to those most vulnerable.

REFERENCES

American Nurses Association. (2010). *Scope and standards of practice: Nursing* (2nd ed.). Silver Spring, MD: Nursebook.org.

American Nurses Association. (2015). *Nursing: Scope and standards of nursing practice* (3rd ed.). Silver Spring, MD: Nursebook.org.

Department of Health and Human Services, Agency for Toxic Substances and Disease Registry. (2002). *Nurses and environmental health: Success through action.* Washington, DC: National Environmental Education and Training Foundation.

Johnson, S. (2006). *The Ghost map.* New York: Riverhead Books.

Kopf, E.W. (1916). Florence Nightingale as statistician. *Publications of the American Statistical Association. 15*(116), 388-404. Retrieved from www.jstor.org/stable/2965763.

Leffers, J., McDermott-Levy, R., Smith, C., & Sattler, B. (2014). Nursing education's response to the 1995 Institute of Medicine report: Nursing, health and the environment. *Nursing Forum. 49*(4), 214-224.

Leffers, J., Smith, C., Huffling, K., McDermott-Levy, R., & Sattler, B. (Eds). (2016). *Environmental health in nursing.* Alliance of

Nurses for Healthy Environments. Retrieved from https://envirn.org/e-textbook/.

Nightingale, F. (1860). *Notes on nursing: What it is and what it is not.* New York: D. Appleton and Company. Retrieved from http://digital.library.upenn.edu/women/nightingale/nursing/nursing.html.

Pope, A.M., Snyder, M.A., & Mood, L.H. (1995) *Nursing, health and the environment: Strengthen the relationship to improve the public's health.* Washington, DC: Institute of Medicine.

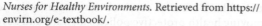

ONLINE RESOURCES

Alliance of Nurses for Healthy Environments
https://envirn.org
Clean and Healthy New York
www.cleanhealthyny.org
Environmental Protection Agency
www.epa.gov
Health Care Without Harm
https://noharm.org

70

Coalitions: A Powerful Political Strategy

Rebecca (Rice) Bowers-Lanier

"When spider webs unite, they can tie up a lion."

Ethiopian proverb

Coalitions are always a work in progress, and they can be very powerful. At the same time, they are complex and sometimes complicated to manage and lead. This chapter explores works in progress toward creating effective coalitions around two vexing health-related issues: (1) Medicaid expansion as a component of the Patient Protection and Affordable Care Act (ACA), and (2) obtaining support services for individuals with developmental disabilities, mental illness, and/or substance use disorder. These are collaborative efforts from Virginia; however, the case examples are universal, regardless of jurisdiction and focus.

BIRTH AND LIFE CYCLE OF COALITIONS

The power of coalitions lies in their ability to bring people together from diverse perspectives around clearly defined purposes to achieve common goals. Strength lies in numbers—in working together and in strategizing for success. What factors contribute to success or failure of coalitions? How do we go about forming and maintaining coalitions? What are the ingredients? How do we know when or whether coalitions achieve their goals? This chapter describes the factors associated with each of these questions.

In simplest terms, coalitions are created to bring about collective action at the local, state, or national level. Energy Efficiency for All (EEFA) (n.d.) defines a coalition as "any group of organizations and individuals who come together to improve policy, programs, and/or practice" in one area, such as environmental preservation.

Why form coalitions? The answer lies in "strength in numbers." When an individual or one association works on an issue, it, like the spider, creates a small web; working with other similar-minded organizations creates a powerful network that can capture much more than an individual or association working alone. Coalitions create

their effectiveness by empowering individual organizations to pool their resources and creativity to foster more strategic and effective action; enabling and enhancing communication and collaboration among members; increasing diversity by bringing together new and alternative voices; and increasing their impact through greater numbers.

Coalitions arise out of challenges or opportunities, and the key for all coalitions is to maintain their effectiveness until they achieve their goals. For some coalitions, the work may be completed within a matter of weeks; for others, like our two case examples, the work may persist for years.

After Medicaid expansion under the ACA was deemed optional by a Supreme Court decision in 2012 (Rosenbaum & Westmoreland, 2012), Virginia failed to pass legislation to expand its Medicaid program each subsequent year until 2018. One can trace final passage to several turning points, including election of a new governor, loss of substantial opposition seats in the Virginia House of Delegates, popular support of Medicaid expansion, economic realities, and the efforts of stakeholder groups working together to advocate for expansion. Chief among the stakeholder groups is the Healthcare for All Virginians (HAV) coalition (http://havcoalition.org), convened in 2007 to improve Medicaid, and in 2010, to advocate for Medicaid expansion. By 2018, over 110 state and community-based organizations belonged to this coalition.

In 1983, a group of disability advocates joined forces to form the Coalition for Mentally Disabled Citizens of Virginia (MH coalition). The original purpose of the coalition was to develop annually a common legislative agenda and to hold a unitary advocacy day at the Virginia General Assembly. The MH coalition's ongoing mission was to increase state funding for services. The coalition disbanded in 2013.

BUILDING AND MAINTAINING A COALITION: THE PRIMER

Essential Ingredients

To build and maintain effective coalitions requires five ingredients: purpose or reason for being, leadership, membership, resources, and serendipity or the ability to "seize the moment." Each of these is discussed below.

As discussed above, coalitions are formed to serve a *purpose* to achieve one or more goals. Because coalitions bring together people and organizations centered on their own interests, each member brings his own perspective to the table. Organizations and individual members are invited to become part of a coalition because they have a stake in the general context of the problem or issue to be solved. For example, the MH coalition formed for the purpose of increasing funding for services to individuals with mental disabilities. It began out of a commonly heard story that lawmakers were growing weary of hearing from advocates representing similar interests but seeking funding for their own "slice of the pie." When that happens, typically lawmakers will say something like, "You all need to get together and come back to us when you are organized about what you really want."

The second ingredient is *leadership*. Leadership is fundamentally about relationships that integrate deep listening, inclusion, and connecting divergent ideas and non-traditional allies. It is less about certainty of progress and more about imagining and creating solutions. Most importantly, it honors those who might not be in the room or in the conversation, understanding that a path forward must be respectful of divergent views (EEFA, n.d.).

Two types of leaders are critical to coalition work: inspirational and organizational. Inspiring leaders use personal strengths and power to constructively and ethically influence others to an endpoint or goal. They motivate others to participate and meet their obligations; they encourage new ideas, problem solving, and risk taking. They know when to steer forward, when to idle, and when to back up, if necessary. Organizational leaders possess the skills to keep members on track between meetings, ensure that communication methods are in place, and follow through on coalition assignments. Inspiration and organization may coexist in one person, but frequently two leaders are needed to serve the coalition (Coalitions Work, 2007).

The HAV coalition has been led since 2007 by a poverty law center lawyer who is widely acknowledged as an expert on Medicaid. In the past several years, she has been joined in leadership by a policy analyst for a nonprofit that works on the fiscal impact of social justice issues. The lawyer serves as the inspirational leader, the fiscal analyst, the organizer.

Coalition members comprise the third ingredient. Members increase the productivity of the coalition. They also increase the visibility of the coalition, because they represent diverse constituencies and networks. Members must commit to the purpose and goals of the coalition, attend meetings, and communicate outcomes to their constituencies. The EEFA (n.d.) lists five membership criteria:

- Alignment—agreeing with the goals of the coalition
- Contribution to diversity—embracing different ideas and solutions
- Complementary methodology—adding to the mix of needed expertise such as legal, technical, community engagement, and advocacy
- Relationships/influence—knowing people outside the coalition who can help or challenge coalition work
- Capacity—contributing to funding and resource allocation

The MH coalition members represented a core of advocates for each of the three disability groups—developmental, mental health/illness, and substance use disorder. Membership grew over the years, then subsided in the final years of the coalition.

The fourth ingredient for coalitions is *resources*, the tools for the leaders and members to accomplish the coalitions' goals. They include money and in-kind donations from members and others, such as support for developing marketing materials, purchasing supplies, putting on educational sessions, and developing and maintaining websites. Coalitions need to have clear guidelines for seeking funding from outside sources that may be soliciting explicitly or implicitly quid pro quo arrangements. Therefore, coalitions must be transparent in sources of funds and how these are utilized (EEFA, n.d.).

The HAV coalition was particularly well resourced in 2017–2018 for its final push to obtain Medicaid expansion. Once the results of the November 2016 election were known, work began on developing a grassroots campaign funded by four organizations to conduct phone-banking of targeted legislators, to hold regional town hall meetings, and to support a series of marches on the capitol in Richmond. The coalition's work was just one component of the multi-pronged effort to finally pass Medicaid expansion, but clearly the coalition's members turned out in large amounts when and where the leadership directed. The bottom line is that when resources were needed to achieve a result, having them was a game changer.

The last ingredient for coalition success is *serendipity*—a mysterious phenomenon often thought of as a "happy accident." Serendipity occurs when unexpected circumstances produce an "aha" moment that leads to a valuable and unanticipated outcome (University College London, 2012). In order to effectively seize the moment, leaders and members must obligate themselves to conduct continual environmental scans, such as tracking current events, connecting with many different kinds of people, and spending time thinking creatively. These coalitions utilized serendipitous happenings to gain their intended outcomes. For the HAV coalition, it was the political turn of events; for the MH coalition, we will discuss the events leading to its initial success in the section below on "evaluating effectiveness."

Coalition Structure

Structure refers to the organization of the coalition, and it defines the procedures by which the coalition operates. The structure serves the members, not the other way around. It also includes how members are accepted, how leadership is chosen, how decisions are made, and how differences are mediated.

Coalition structure, although necessary, is dynamic, depending upon the purpose, resources, and the members. Some coalitions are highly structured, with formal committees, task forces or work groups, and communication mechanisms; others are more loosely structured, with shared leadership and work done by ad hoc groups. Highly structured coalitions may be necessary if the coalition work is complex and multifaceted, involving more than one goal. Committees and/or task forces may be established around the goals.

Coalition structure should make provisions for governance. This is especially true if the size exceeds 15 people. Beyond this number, the group becomes too large for effective, efficient decision-making. The governance committee should, at the very least, include all committee and work group chairs to facilitate communication. The committee should represent the diversity of the members.

No matter what coalitions call themselves or how they structure themselves, an important factor to achieving goals is to engage appropriate support systems. Someone must agree to do a task, and that someone should have the means to get the task done. The work may be done by volunteers, as it is in many coalitions. Often, paid staff can deliver on the tasks and move the coalition along more effectively, especially when the work is complex and multifaceted. For example, because over 100 members comprise the HAV coalition, the work was primarily spearheaded with a steering committee and volunteers who took on various responsibilities, such as developing promotional materials, following up on calls to action in regions, etc. (Community Tool Box, 2018).

Decision-Making

Decision-making is a source of great concern, usually at the beginning of a coalition's life. Because members represent different constituencies and perspectives, they will often not trust one another, thus leading to conflict. Everyone wants to protect his or her own interests.

Optimally, decisions are made by consensus without voting; members simply agree or disagree. When decisions are controversial, coalition members should step back and discuss the situation again. By operating on consensus, coalition members must come to a decision with which all are comfortable. What frequently happens is that alternative solutions are offered until one is made to which all can agree. The journey to consensus requires leadership skill and finesse.

Coalition work can be tricky. Member groups are bound to disagree on specific priorities or tactics. When challenges arise, coalition leaders should consider dialing back coalition expectations and/or shifting duties to other willing participants. Effective coalition leaders recognize the importance of creating a space for the disagreements to be discussed in an honest and forthright fashion behind "closed doors." In other words, "what happens in Vegas, stays in Vegas." Divisions within coalitions should not become public, because advocacy requires a single message and a unified front (EEFA, n.d.).

Both the HAV and MH coalitions utilized consensus decision-making. The HAV coalition sought to gain passage of Medicaid expansion, and its decision making centered on advocacy strategies to deploy advocates and deliver messages to targeted lawmakers. The MH coalition, on the other hand, sought increased funding for delivery of services, meaning some would gain whereas others might lose in a particular funding cycle. However, in the background was the clear knowledge that members would have to agree; otherwise, all would lose. Consensus was difficult, but not impossible, given that alternative.

Meetings

Coalitions must meet; otherwise, the work doesn't get done. Meetings take place in a variety of modes: face-to-face, conference call, and/or through web-based connections. At least initially in the forming stage, face-to-face meetings are preferable because they facilitate conversation and getting to know one another. As coalitions mature, other types of communication may replace face-to-face venues. Coalition leaders should remember, however, that much of the cache and strength of coalitions comes from the interpersonal connections that members have with one another. In rural areas, this may be through web-based video conferencing. Regardless of the venue, meetings must take place regularly and in an organized fashion to keep members engaged.

The interval between meetings and the time of meetings is very important. The interval should be long enough for members to accomplish their assignments. Meetings should consist ideally of presenting alternatives for action and making decisions. If the interval between meetings is too long, little interim work will get done, as human nature in our busy world is to wait until right before a meeting to complete an assignment. Leaders should confirm with members the amount of time each will need to get the work accomplished in the interim and then schedule the next meeting accordingly.

The content of the meeting should be focused on problem-solving and decision-making. There should be a sense among members that work is being done and decisions made; otherwise, results-oriented members will soon stop attending meetings. A good meeting has energy. If the meeting is primarily conducted to exchange information, some members will see this as a waste of their time, and they may drop out. Alternatives such as e-mail and electronic bulletin boards exist for disseminating information. Coalition leaders and members should regularly assess the content of the meetings to see what works and what doesn't and make necessary adjustments (Community Tool Box, 2018).

Both the HAV and MH coalitions matured over the years and settled into a meeting schedule that was parsimonious and productive. The HAV coalition met twice between legislative sessions and depended on frequent email updates. During the legislative sessions, advocates met weekly to check in and modify legislative contacts as needed. The MH coalition met monthly in the several months leading up to the legislative session to revise its legislative agenda and plan its annual advocacy day.

Promoting the Coalition

What good is a coalition if no one knows it exists? Coalitions are formed to advance a common agenda, and communication is the vehicle with which that agenda is advanced. From the beginning, coalition members must develop and implement a communications plan aimed at getting the coalition's message out to the broader community of interest. The plan should include branding (i.e., logo and tag line), ways to reach intended audiences (i.e., website and social marketing venues, such as Facebook and Twitter), and assigning individuals to keep the communication up to date and vibrant (Spitfire Strategies, 2014).

Funding

Coalition work takes money. Some coalitions run on little or no money, using the time and talent of their members. Coalitions will need to look for additional funds to stay solvent and accomplish their work. How much money is needed depends on several factors. First are the mission and aims of the coalition. Second, the strategic plan will define the resources needed; then members can decide how to best obtain the funds. Third, members should develop a fund-raising plan that includes tailoring the message to prospective funding sources, assigning people to make the contacts, communicating the mission and aims of the coalition, and seeking funding (Campaign for Action, 2016).

PITFALLS AND CHALLENGES

Coalitions usually start out with a flurry of excitement and activity. Sustaining the excitement and guiding the activity are ongoing challenges. Coalition work is difficult and complex. Following are some common pitfalls and challenges, with suggestions for overcoming them.

Failure to Get the Right People to Participate

Coalitions should attract those who are most interested in seeing that the work gets done, and these members will commit to participating in the coalition. At regular intervals, coalitions should assess who is "at the table" and who is not. The following three common membership errors exist.

First is the error of exclusion of an entire group of stakeholders. In examining the purpose of the coalition, members should ask themselves these questions: "Who have we excluded?" "Whose expertise do we need?" "Who may work to derail the coalition's work if not invited to become a member?"

The *second* error is not achieving buy-in from major players like the "800-pound gorillas." These may be major players because of their positioning within well-resourced hierarchy, such as health systems. But they most assuredly include those who will be the end-users of the coalition's work, including patients and people living in economically depressed circumstances, for example. Coalition members should identify these individuals/organizations and seek their buy-in. Occasionally, these large players may agree to serve as participants without signing on for political or other reasons. Coalition members will have to determine whether their "silent" participation is satisfactory.

The *third* error involves participation in the coalition by the "wrong" members. When organizations send participants who do not have the authority to speak and represent the organization in coalition decision-making, they hinder the work of the coalition. Organizations sometimes use this approach as a passive-aggressive way to derail the coalition. This problem may be solved by communication with the organizational leadership about the importance of consistent participation by members who can speak for the organization (EEFA, n.d.).

Cultural and Language Differences Among Coalition Members

Because coalition members represent different perspectives on the goals and mission of the coalition, all must learn the meaning of significant words used by coalition members. Sometimes simple words carry completely different connotations. For example, in nursing coalitions, the word *time* connotes entirely different interval spans for nurse administrators (who operate day-to-day) and nurse educators (who operate by semesters). Consequently, coalition leaders and members must continually be attuned to words that have different connotations, and they should agree on a common definition (if possible) or agree to understand the differences in the meaning of words.

Cultural differences among coalition members are to be expected. Depending on the purpose of the coalition, these cultural differences may be paramount, such as coalitions formed in response to racial or ethnic injustices. Often, cultural differences may serve as barriers to starting a coalition—for example, if some participants perceive that others are dominating the coalition's work because the others are "professionals" or some other elite. There are no easy solutions to cultural differences, but there are rewards for learning about them and embracing them as part of the work of the coalition. To do so requires building relationships among members, one by one, during each meeting (Coalition building, 2018).

Persistent Distrust Among Coalition Members

Like cultural differences, distrust is one of the thorniest challenges that coalition leaders face, because much of the success of coalitions comes from the ongoing interaction among members that allays misperceptions and builds trust. When members become disengaged from coalition work, their absence can derail progress, especially if they fail to keep their own constituencies informed. Another source of distrust emanates from long-standing perceived inequalities among members. To overcome distrust, leaders and members must work diligently on including these potentially disenfranchised members. In the end, people must feel valued and treasured for their participation and contributions to the enterprise.

In the several years preceding the dissolution of the MH coalition, two coalition members grew to distrust the motives of the other. One thought the other represented a member organization that should not have been invited to join in the first place, and this distrust helped erode the work of the coalition. Unfortunately, the situation did not rectify itself. Although this example of distrust did not in and of itself doom the coalition, it certainly contributed to its dissolving.

Control Freaks and Protecting Turf

The tendency to control and protect turf can happen at the individual member level and at the coalition level. At the individual level, there are those in whom coalition success

breeds a type of person—one who knows "the truth" and is always willing to share it. Competing coalitions may form, leading to turf protection and dysfunctional competing coalitions. One of the most unfortunate outcomes of competing coalitions aimed at the same outcome is that policymakers will disregard the petitions of both coalitions, and nothing will be gained.

Poor Handling of Different Perspectives

Coalition leaders and members have an obligation to recognize points of contention and determine how they will be handled. In fact, some worthy goals of a coalition might need to be postponed or shelved altogether if the members cannot agree on a selected outcome. That is not to say that the work will never be achieved, but that more time will be needed to come to consensus on strategies and goals.

Failure to Act

Coalitions begin with fire in their bellies. Going from words to action is sometimes more difficult than members had originally thought. Some coalitions formulate and reformulate action plans ad infinitum without getting to action. Without action, there will be no resources to support the work.

At least two factors contribute to failure to act. One is weak leadership, and the other is the inability for the coalition to coalesce around solutions. To resolve the leadership issue, new leaders will have to emerge, and in this case, the coalition members may need to lead a quiet coup to replace leadership. Resolving the consensus issue requires a regrouping and reexamination of the purposes of the coalition and an analysis of whether consensus can be achieved. Coalition members should adhere to working by consensus, as messy as the process is.

Losing Balance

Coalition leaders and members wear out. Managing, leading, and working in coalitions drain energy. Each person must assess his or her readiness to step aside and support the leadership and membership activities of new recruits. Coalitions should set in place a means for leadership succession planning at regular intervals.

POLITICAL WORK OF COALITIONS

Should coalitions speak out on issues that matter to them? Of course they should, because advocating is the vehicle by which coalitions achieve their goals; otherwise, why do they exist? However, advocacy work has its downsides and upsides.

Reasons Not to Advocate

When coalitions advocate for certain positions, they run into opposition from stakeholders who diverge from those positions. The further coalitions go out on the limb, the more people line up to saw off the limb. In fact, coalitions stand to lose their financial support if they veer out too far. In addition, there are legal restrictions on advocacy by tax-exempt groups in lobbying, so coalitions whose members may be from tax-exempt organizations may be forced to pull back if they become too forcefully active in lobbying. Therefore, coalitions should choose their battles carefully, making certain that they are willing to accept the consequences of winning or losing (Bowers-Lanier, 2010).

Reasons to Advocate

Nursing and other health care coalitions that are established to advocate for specific legislative or policy initiatives will be successful if the initiatives are enacted into law or become established policies. When that happens, the coalition will have met its goal, and it may disband or reformulate and start on another goal.

How to Advocate With Grace

The solution, of course, is to proceed with care. By its very nature, advocacy involves risk. Coalition members should work out their differences and carefully select the words they will use when advocating for positions. Coalition members should agree in advance on the advocacy approaches they will take that will not jeopardize their legal status or disenfranchise funders and members. Developing and adhering to a common message are essential for all coalition members.

EVALUATING COALITION EFFECTIVENESS

Coalitions should evaluate their effectiveness on a regular basis. Evaluation helps to keep members on track, determine strengths and areas for improvement, and, in the final analysis, determine whether the coalitions' goals are met or if further work is needed. Evaluation should be both formative (assessing the progress of the coalition on a continual and regular basis such as after each meeting) and summative (assessing the status of coalition deliverables after a defined period such as annually) and should occur at regular intervals. Table 70.1 lists the questions governing formative and summative coalition evaluation.

For most of this chapter, we have been following the work of two coalitions as they were formed and, in the case of the HAV coalition, as they continue their work. Now that Medicaid expansion has been enacted into law, what are the next steps? The coalition has agreed to continue to advocate for the provisions of Medicaid expansion. The budget bill, signed into law, contains a work requirement provision. Researchers have posited that taking coverage away from recipients who fail to adhere to work reporting requirements will result in poorer health outcomes (Katch, Wagner, & Aron-Dine, 2018; Garfield et al., 2018). The HAV coalition will be working to derail the work requirements as antithetical to the goal of improved health to support improved lives.

The MH coalition, formed in 1983, was at least partially responsible for an increase in state funding of $83M for

TABLE 70.1	Coalition Formative Evaluation
Evaluation Type	**Questions to Be Answered**
Formative	**Questions to be asked on a regular basis (by meeting, monthly, quarterly at maximum):**
	Membership
	1. Are the right member organizations at the table? Who is missing?
	2. Are members fully engaged? If not, why not?
	3. Are all equal players? Why or why not?
	Coalition work
	1. Are goals realistic?
	2. How is the work being accomplished? By committees? By one person?
	3. Is there a better way to do the work?
	4. What are the barriers and facilitators to goal achievement?
	5. Are strategies in place for minimizing barriers? Maximizing facilitators?
	6. Is the work plan on schedule?
Summative	**Semi-annually or annually: Goal achievement**
	1. Have the goals been achieved? Why or why not? Should any strategies be changed?
	2. Are the goals still relevant to the mission of the coalition? Why or why not?
	3. Has the coalition achieved its stated goal? Should it be disbanded? Why or why not?
	4. Is there additional work to be done and the will to do it?

mental health, developmental disability, and addiction treatment. The work was certainly not done, but over time, leadership became an issue. Leading and belonging take energy, and sometimes the work cannot be sustained, at least in its current format.

Coalition work can be extremely exciting and fulfilling. By bringing together individuals who represent varying perspectives, coalitions can achieve their goals.

DISCUSSION QUESTIONS

1. Select a policy issue of interest. How could a coalition help to move the policy forward?
2. What "stakeholder" groups should you consider asking to join the coalition? Who are the "800-pound gorillas" that need to be at the table?
3. What challenges might confront the coalition, and how would you prevent or address them?
4. How would you know whether your coalition is effective in reaching its goal?

REFERENCES

Bowers-Lanier, R. (2010). Advocacy in the public arena. In K.A. Polifko (Ed.), *The practice environment of nursing* (pp. 565-592). Clifton Park, NY: Delmar Cengage Learning.

Campaign for Action. (May, 2016). *Fundraising and coalition building*. Retrieved from https://campaignforaction.org/webinar/fundraising-coalition-building/.

Coalitions Work. (2007). *Coalition membership*. Retrieved from http://coalitionswork.com/resources/tools/.

Community Tool Box. (2018). *Improving organizational management and development*. Retrieved from https://ctb.ku.edu/en/improve-organizational-management-and-development.

Energy Efficiency for All. (n.d.). *EEFA coalition cookbook*. Retrieved from http://networkecology.org/eefa/.

Garfield, R., Rudowitz, R., Musumeci, M., & Damico, A. (2018). *Implications of work requirements in Medicaid: What does the data say?* Kaiser Family Foundation. Retrieved from http://files.kff.org/attachment/Issue-Brief-Implications-of-Work-Requirements-in-Medicaid-What-Does-the-Data-Say.

Katch, H., Wagner, J., & Aron-Dine, A. (August 13, 2018). *Taking Medicaid coverage away from people not meeting work requirements will reduce low-income families' access to care and worsen health outcomes*. Center on Budget and Policy Priorities. Retrieved from www.cbpp.org/research/health/taking-medicaid-coverage-away-from-people-not-meeting-work-requirements-will-reduce.

Rosenbaum, S., & Westmoreland, T.M. (2012). The Supreme Court's surprising decision on the Medicaid expansion: How will the federal government and states proceed? *Health Affairs*, 1663-1672. Retrieved from www.healthaffairs.org/doi/10.1377/hlthaff.2012.0766.

Spitfire Strategies. (2014). *Working with coalitions: Getting agreement on messages that work*. Retrieved from www.spitfirestrategies.com/working-with-coalitions-getting-agreement-on-messages-that-work/.

University College London. (2012). *Researchers discover serendipity is more than a "happy accident."* Retrieved from www.ucl.ac.uk/news/news-articles/1210/121004-serendipity-more-than-a-happy-accident.

ONLINE RESOURCES

Community Tool Box
https://ctb.ku.edu/en
Developing Effective Coalitions: An Eight Step Guide
www.countyhealthrankings.org/sites/default/files/eightstep.pdf

71

TAKING ACTION: Campaign for Action

Susan B. Hassmiller

"Be the change you wish to see in the world."

Mahatma Gandhi

Nurses can tackle many of the challenges confronting U.S. health care, including managing chronic diseases, promoting prevention and wellness, and coordinating care across settings. The Robert Wood Johnson Foundation (RWJF) has invested more than $663 million in programs designed to support and strengthen the nursing workforce. In 2008, RWJF partnered with the esteemed Institute of Medicine (IOM), now known as the National Academy of Medicine, to support a major study on the future of nursing. The IOM convened experts from diverse fields to define U.S. health care challenges and the role of nurses in meeting them. Chaired by former U.S. Secretary of Health and Human Services Donna Shalala, the IOM committee reviewed the scientific literature and talked to diverse experts about the nursing workforce.

THE FUTURE OF NURSING REPORT

In 2011, the IOM committee released *The Future of Nursing: Leading Change, Advancing Health* (2011), a landmark report that envisioned new roles for nurses in the rapidly evolving U.S. health and health care landscape. The report noted the essential roles played by nurses, who are the health professionals and who spend the most time directly caring for people, families, and communities, and, at four million, make up the largest segment of the health workforce. The report made a compelling case to build a nursing workforce that is diverse, well-educated, and prepared to practice to the full extent of its education and training in order to meet the U.S. population's current and future needs. The report recommended strengthening nursing education, removing barriers to practice, promoting nursing leadership, fostering interprofessional education and collaboration, and improving workforce diversity.

IMPLEMENTING THE FUTURE OF NURSING REPORT

RWJF partnered with AARP, the nation's largest nonprofit, nonpartisan organization dedicated to empowering Americans 50 and older, and its Center to Champion Nursing in America (CCNA), to establish the *Future of Nursing: Campaign for Action*, a national initiative of AARP Foundation, AARP, and RWJF, to implement the report's recommendations. (See Fig. 71.1 for a photo of the *Campaign* leaders.) CCNA coordinates the *Campaign* with its vision that everyone in America can live a healthier life, supported by a system in which nurses are essential partners in providing care and promoting health equity and well-being. The *Campaign* (Box 71.1) has advanced the IOM recommendations by mobilizing the nursing community and engaging partners from business, consumer organizations, government, health care, philanthropy, academia, and other sectors. Because much policy change happens at the state level, the *Campaign* created Action Coalitions in every state and the District of Columbia, each co-led by a nurse and a partner from outside the nursing field. Action Coalitions have raised more than $54 million in funding (independent of RWJF) from numerous outside organizations, stakeholders, and individuals.

STRENGTHENING NURSING EDUCATION

More BSN-Prepared Nurses

The IOM report's call for 80% of the nursing workforce to attain a baccalaureate degree or higher by 2020 helped quiet

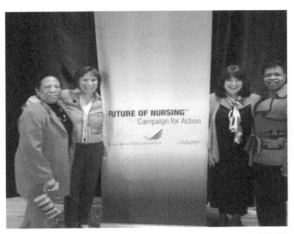

Fig. 71.1 (From *right* to *left*) Linda Burnes Bolton, DrPH, RN, FAAN, RWJF Trustee and Vice President for Nursing, Chief Nursing Officer and Director of Nursing Research at Cedars-Sinai; Susan Hassmiller, PhD, RN, FAAN, RWJF senior adviser for nursing and director of the *Future of Nursing: Campaign for Action*; Susan Reinhard, RN, PhD, FAAN, a senior VP at AARP and chief strategist, Center to Champion Nursing in America; and Catherine Alicia Georges, EdD, RN, FAAN, president-elect of AARP and professor and chair of the Department of Nursing at Lehman College and the Graduate Center of the City University of New York, attend a *Future of Nursing: Campaign for Action* Summit.

BOX 71.1   **Join the Campaign for Action!**

Join the *Future of Nursing: Campaign for Action* by visiting www.CampaignForAction.org. The site includes accomplishments, state activity, and resources. Follow the *Campaign* on Facebook (www.facebook.com/Campaign ForAction) or Twitter (@Campaign4Action).

---

the longstanding debate over whether an associate degree or baccalaureate degree was preferable for practice. Following the report's release, the Magnet Recognition Program—which recognizes health care organizations for quality patient care, nursing excellence, and innovations in professional nursing practice—required hospitals to adopt a plan that advances the goal of having 80% of their nurses holding baccalaureate degrees before applying for Magnet status.

To increase the number of nurses with baccalaureate degrees, the *Campaign* promoted academic progression. It convened experts in education, business, and government to reduce the costs and complications for those seeking higher degrees. A decade ago, a nurse with an associate

degree often was required to retake courses to earn a baccalaureate degree, wasting time and money. To remove these hurdles, RWJF launched from 2012 to 2016 the *Academic Progression in Nursing* (APIN) program in nine states. APIN established partnerships and tailored specific nursing education models to local needs, offering flexible, streamlined options for nursing students. In 2012, for the first time, more nurses graduated with a bachelor's degree than an associate degree (Buerhaus, et al., 2014). By 2017, the number of registered nurses (RNs) obtaining a bachelor's degree in nursing through RN-to-BSN programs increased to more than 62,725—up 178% since 2010 (American Association of Colleges of Nursing, 2018). RWJF also launched the *State Implementation Program* (SIP) from 2013 to 2017 to provide funding for Action Coalitions to focus on one or two IOM recommendations; 21 chose nursing education. The National Education Progression in Nursing Collaborative (NEPIN) builds on APIN's and SIP's momentum. Its goals are one million incumbent nurses and 90% of new graduates earning a BSN or higher by 2025. Joanne Spetz, PhD, the associate director of research at Health Workforce Research Center at the University of California-San Francisco, projected that about two-thirds of RNs will have a bachelor's degree or higher by 2025 (Spetz, 2018).

Double the Number of Doctorates

The *Campaign* achieved a milestone in 2015 when it met the IOM recommendation to double the number of nurses with doctorates by 2020. Since then, the *Campaign* has called for more nurses to attain research-focused doctoral degrees to advance nursing science, translate research into practice, and to teach future nurses. In 2014, RWJF launched the *Future of Nursing Scholars*, a three-year, expedited PhD funding program that supports 200 nurse scholars' education and leadership development. The program is developing a best-practices model that graduate schools can tailor to create a 3-year option for nursing PhD students.

Scope of Practice

The IOM report recommended that advanced practice registered nurses (APRNs) be able to practice to the full extent of their education and training. Since the *Campaign* began, nine states (Connecticut, Maryland, Minnesota, Nebraska, Nevada, North Dakota, Rhode Island, South Dakota, and Vermont) have removed statutory barriers that restricted nurse practitioner (NP) practice. These victories expanded access to high-quality health care and increased consumer choice. In addition, more than a dozen states have made incremental improvements (Fig. 71.2). Nationally, the Veterans Administration (VA) in 2016

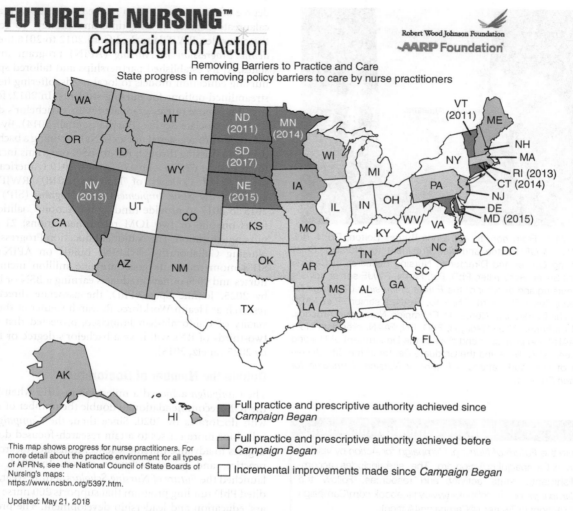

FUTURE OF NURSING™
Campaign for Action

Robert Wood Johnson Foundation
AARP Foundation

Removing Barriers to Practice and Care
State progress in removing policy barriers to care by nurse practitioners

Full practice and prescriptive authority achieved since *Campaign Began*

Full practice and prescriptive authority achieved before *Campaign Began*

Incremental improvements made since *Campaign Began*

This map shows progress for nurse practitioners. For more detail about the practice environment for all types of APRNs, see the National Council of State Boards of Nursing's maps:
https://www.ncsbn.org/5397.htm.

Updated: May 21, 2018

Fig. 71.2 Since the *Campaign* began, nine states have removed barriers to practice that prevented APRNs from practicing to the full extent of their education and training.

agreed to allow certified NPs, clinical nurse specialists, and certified nurse-midwives to practice to the full extent of their education and training without the supervision of a physician, regardless of the practice restrictions in the state where the VA facility is located. The *Campaign* continues to work to remove barriers to APRN practice and care and support research showing that APRNs improve access to high-quality care.

Nurse Leadership

The IOM report stressed that policymakers should expand opportunities for nurses to lead. A study by Marilyn Szekendi and Lawrence Prybil found nurses only made up 2% of voting members on hospital, health system, and academic medical center boards (Szekendi et al., 2015). As a result, AARP's CCNA created and launched the Nurses on Boards Coalition, a 501(c)(3) organization, to place 10,000 nurses on health and community boards by 2020. As of August 2019, 6516 nurses report serving on boards. Many Action Coalitions offer leadership institutes, mentoring programs, and "40-under-40" awards for emerging leaders. The *Campaign* emphasizes the importance of nurses acting as leaders regardless of title, participating in interdisciplinary teams, and volunteering to serve on committees. RWJF also expanded its renowned *Clinical Scholars* leadership program to nurses and other providers.

Fostering Interprofessional Collaboration

Studies have demonstrated that effective coordination and communication among health professionals can enhance the quality and safety of patient care. The *Campaign* promotes a team-based approach to education and practice to improve the quality and coordination of health care. Since 2010, eight of the 10 top nursing schools have increased the number of required clinical courses and/or activities that include both RN students and graduate students of other health professions (Fig. 71.3).

Promoting Diversity

The *Campaign* works to recruit and prepare the nursing profession to provide culturally competent care in a variety of settings. Most Action Coalitions are incorporating diversity plans into their education and leadership efforts. A National Academy of Medicine report that assessed the progress on the 2010 report recommended that the *Campaign* continue to prioritize and promote diversity (NAM, 2015).

CONCLUSION

By advancing the IOM recommendations, the nursing profession is prepared to take on one of the greatest challenges

Campaign progress

Indicator 4: Interprofessional Collaboration

IOM Recommendation: Expand opportunities for nurses to lead and disseminate collaborative improvement efforts

Number of required clinical courses and/or activities at top nursing schools that include both RN students and graduate students of other health professions

School	2011	2012	2013	2014	2015
Duke Univ.	2	2	2	1	3
Yale Univ.	0	0	1	1	1
Univ. of California, San Francisco	0	1	1	1	0
Univ. of North Carolina	0	0	0	0	0
Univ. of Washington	2	2	5	4	5
Univ. of Pennsylvania	0	1	4	7	9
Univ. of Michigan	0	0	0	0	2
Univ. of Pittsburgh	1	1	3	4	4
Oregon Health and Science Univ.	0	1	2	2	2
Johns Hopkins Univ.	1	1	3	3	6

Data Source: Top nursing schools (as determined by *US News and World Report* rankings) that also have graduate-level health professions schools at their academic institutions. Course offerings and requirements include clinical and/or simulation experiences.

Updated: December 6, 2017

Fig. 71.3 Since 2010, 8 of the 10 top nursing schools have increased the number of required clinical courses and/or activities that include both registered nurse (RN) students and graduate students of other health professions.

of our time: building a Culture of Health to enable all people to experience greater health and well-being. Poverty; inequity; violence; poor housing; and lack of a good education, jobs, access to healthy food, and safe places to play are responsible for an estimated 80% of all illnesses; only 20% can be attributed to biological causes alone (Braveman and Gottlieb, 2014).

The RWJF white paper *Catalysts for Change: Harnessing the Power of Nurses to Build Population Health in the 21st Century* explores how nurses can help the United States to reverse course on the declining health of its citizens and promote population health. The report includes recommendations in the areas of nursing education, practice, leadership, research, and advocacy. RWJF is also collaborating with the National Academy of Medicine on a second *Future of Nursing* report that will span the years 2020 to 2030 and focus on nursing's role in building a Culture of Health and health equity. The report, planned for release at the end of 2020, will spotlight population and community-based care.

The initial *Future of Nursing* report enabled the field to live up to its promise of "leading change, advancing health." During the next decade, the profession will take leading roles in enabling more people to live healthier lives and to experience greater well-being.

REFERENCES

Academic Progression in Nursing. (n.d.). Retrieved from https://campaignforaction.org/our-network/grantee-and-award-programs/academic-progression-in-nursing/.

American Association of Colleges of Nursing (2018). *2017-2018 Enrollment and graduations in baccalaureate and graduate programs in nursing.* Washington, DC: Author.

Braveman, P., & Gottlieb, L. (2014). The social determinants of health: It's time to consider the causes of the causes. *Public Health Reports, 129*(1, Suppl 2), 19-31.

Buerhaus, P.I., Auerbach, D.I., & Staiger, D.O. (2014). The rapid growth of graduates from associate, baccalaureate, and graduate programs in nursing. *Nursing Economics, 32*(6), 290–295, 311.

Institute of Medicine. (2011). *The future of nursing: Leading change, advancing health.* Washington, DC: National Academies Press. Retrieved from http://nationalacademies.org/hmd/reports/2010/the-future-of-nursing-leading-change-advancing-health.aspx.

National Academy of Medicine. (2015). *Assessing progress on the IOM study report The Future of Nursing.* Washington, DC: National Academies Press. Retrieved from www.nationalacademies.org/hmd/reports/2015/assessing-progress-on-the-iom-report-the-future-of-nursing.

Robert Wood Johnson Foundation. (n.d.). *Catalysts for change: Harnessing the power of nurses to build population health in the 21st century.* Retrieved from www.rwjf.org/en/library/research/2017/09/catalysts-for-change—harnessing-the-power-of-nurses-to-build-population-health.html.

Spetz, J. (2018). Projections of progress toward the 80 percent BSN recommendation and strategies to accelerate change. *Nursing Outlook, 66*(4), 394-400.

Szekendi, M., Prybil, L., Cohen, D.L., Godsey, B., Fardo, D.W., & Cerese, J. (2015). Governance practices and performance in US academic medical centers. *American Journal of Medical Quality, 30*(6), 520-525.

ONLINE RESOURCES

Future of Nursing: Campaign for Action
www.CampaignforAction.org
Institute of Medicine: The Future of Nursing: Leading Change, Advancing Health
www.nationalacademies.org/hmd/Reports/2010/The-Future-of-Nursing-Leading-Change-Advancing-Health.aspx
Nurses on Boards Coalition
www.nursesonboardscoalition.org
Nursing Education and a Decade of Change: Strategies to Meet America's Health Needs
https://campaignforaction.org/resource/nursing-education-and-the-decade-of-change/
Robert Wood Johnson Foundation Catalyst Report
www.rwjf.org/content/dam/farm/reports/reports/2017/rwjf440286
Robert Wood Johnson Foundation Nursing Information
www.RWJF.org/Popfocusednursing

72

TAKING ACTION: Why Not Minot? The Battle Over North Dakota's First Smoke-Free Ordinance

Kelly Buettner-Schmidt, Mary Muhlbradt, and Lori Brierley

"Let whoever is in charge keep this simple question in her head (not, how can I always do this right thing myself, but) how can I provide for this right thing to be always done?)"

Florence Nightingale, Notes on Nursing: What It Is, and What It Is Not

"PROTECT YOUR RIGHTS—SUPPORT FREEDOM OF CHOICE," screamed the full-page ad urging voters to reject an ordinance prohibiting smoking in public eateries. "Who's Next? What's Next?" went the slippery-slope line of reasoning.

Minot, a mid-sized city (pop. 35,000) on the Upper Great Plains, like many western North Dakota communities, is steeped in the traditions of rugged individualism and Scandinavian stoicism. As with most efforts to pass clean indoor air legislation, Minot's campaign split along familiar themes: public health vs. the rights of business owners-smokers' rights vs. the right of workers and patrons to breathe clean air. That Minot citizens came down on the side of public health is a testament to the work and energy that went into sustaining the ordinance, but it was an unexpected achievement nevertheless. It was not culturally inclined to extend government's regulatory power to control behavior traditionally left to individual choice. Minot's success, therefore, is cause for optimism. If it could be done here, it can be done anywhere.

MINOT'S STORY

In 2001, the Minot City Council passed by a vote of 10 to 4 an initiative called the Smoke-Free Family Dining Ordinance, the first smoke-free ordinance in North Dakota at the time. Passage on second reading came after three hours of contentious debate focusing on individual rights and fears of a negative economic impact. But legislative victory was merely a beginning. Barely a month later, the City Auditor's office certified signatures, forcing the ordinance to a referendum. An election was held and the ordinance was upheld by a margin of 55% to 45%.

LAYING THE GROUNDWORK

Educate Before You Legislate

This maxim is a good reminder that public policy does not change overnight. It requires a long-term effort to educate community leaders and the public. In the case of Minot, smoke-free dining was not the first step toward greater protection against tobacco. A coalition of health, education, and youth advocates, Stop Tobacco's Access to Minors Program (STAMP), came together with the aim of reducing tobacco sales to minors. This group achieved a number of legislative successes over the course of several years:

- Local ordinance restricting cigarette vending machines.
- Local ordinance providing for local licensing of tobacco retailers with penalties imposed for those caught selling tobacco to youth under 18. Penalties ranged from fines to ultimate revocation of the retailer's license.
- City policy prohibiting smoking in city-owned buildings.
- Local ordinance restricting access to self-serve displays of tobacco products requiring photo ID of anyone under age 27 purchasing tobacco and creating a system of mandatory compliance checks to facilitate enforcement.

Then STAMP expanded its focus to include clean indoor air. It used the annual Great American SmokeOut as a "hook" to recognize restaurants that had voluntarily gone smoke-free and to encourage others to do the same the day of the smoke-out. Public education events included a symposium with secondhand smoke expert James Repace (www.repace.com).

Next, STAMP and the First District Health Unit launched a "Blue Ribbon" restaurant campaign to reward eating establishments that not only met standards of cleanliness, but also provided patrons with a smoke-free dining experience. Billboards and decals were distributed promoting the value of eating at a Blue Ribbon restaurant.

All the while, we pondered what further steps our community was "ready for" and willing to take. Our answer came in the form of a telephone call from the President of the Minot City Council—a call prompted by—of all things—the birth of his daughter.

A LEGISLATIVE CHAMPION

Though previously opposed to smoke-free legislation, Minot's council president began to have second thoughts. How great it would be, he thought, to take his new daughter to a nice, sit-down restaurant without exposing her to secondhand smoke. Thus, he was interested in doing something to promote smoke-free environments, especially in restaurants. A meeting between this official and members of the STAMP coalition resulted in consensus on a bold vision: together we would craft North Dakota's first smoke-free ordinance and place it before the City Council.

Pros and Cons

Having a legislative champion is a welcome windfall. However, it also entails certain risks. Instant credibility and clout with other members of a legislative body are the obvious advantages. But it also means giving up a certain amount of control. The legislative process always involves compromise. Questions that must be asked at the outset are: What compromises are acceptable and which aren't? At what point will compromise so severely weaken the legislation that it is no longer effective? It is better to not have an ordinance than to have an ineffective one. At one critical point in working with our champion, an issue arose over the timetable for implementing the ordinance. The coalition had to take a stand and say we would have to pull our support if the provision he sought was adopted. He then respected the coalition's stance and did not introduce the provision.

Defining the Bottom Line

Using the Americans for Non-Smokers Rights' (n.d.) model ordinance as a starting point, we tailored Minot's ordinance to suit our community and its residents. Experts recommend against replicating the language of other local ordinances, as most previously enacted ordinances include local legal requirements, norms, and compromises made during the legislative process. Thus, using previously passed laws may weaken the potential public health protections of your law (American Cancer Society et al., 2009).

LEGISLATIVE PROCESS

Getting Your Ducks in a Row

Grassroots. A full year before the ordinance was formally introduced, STAMP and our legislative sponsor developed a plan for rolling out the ordinance and lining up support. Building grassroots support became an early priority. A public opinion survey, already in the pipeline, showed that most people surveyed would go out to eat more often or in about the same frequency if Minot restaurants were smoke-free. The results of the survey were coordinated with the ordinance roll-out. Using a large database of supporters developed over a period of years, the coalition was able to activate its membership for letters to the editor, calls to council members, and attendance at council sessions.

Business/Community Leaders. Other activities included meeting with key stakeholders (i.e., restaurant owners, Chamber of Commerce officials, and others in the hospitality industry). Our legislative sponsor and individual coalition members met one-on-one with council members and several key restaurant owners. In this way, we were able to gain a clear picture of where our support stood and to whom we needed to provide more education prior to the council vote.

Chamber officials were supportive, agreeing to remain officially neutral on the issue. (Interestingly, a straw poll among members of the Chamber board produced a strong vote in favor of the ordinance!) Minot's Convention and Visitors Bureau also maintained official neutrality but raised concerns during legislative debate about a possible negative impact on convention business, travel, and tourism to the city.

Restaurant Owners. Restaurant owners themselves were curious and skeptical, but most were not adamantly opposed. Opposition eventually came, but from relatively few numbers of restaurant owners. Their arguments centered on predictions of economic harm and the right of business owners to run their enterprises with as little government interference as possible.

Staying Sharp

Our day-to-day efforts during this period involved assessing our legislative support, gathering resources, educating the public, and responding to critics and the media. Our primary goal was to answer council members' concerns and make sure that whenever the ordinance came up for consideration before the council (i.e., for hearings, first and second readings, etc.), we were able to pack the council chambers with our supporters. This show of support was crucial; at each meeting it was "standing room only," with our backers overflowing into the lobby and down the stairwell.

Also critical during this period was staying in close contact with our legislative champion to monitor and get a jump on any legislative maneuvering. At the final reading of the ordinance, several amendments were proposed— among them, exemptions for very small restaurants and truck stops. These amendments were defeated and North Dakota's first smoke-free restaurant ordinance passed on a vote of 10 to 4.

THE REFERENDUM PROCESS

Immediately after the Council vote, a small group of restaurant owners began circulating petitions to refer the measure to a citywide vote. The referred measure was placed on a citywide ballot just two months after passage. This crunched time frame meant the coalition and its supporters had a very short period to mount a credible campaign. Although we knew we had most of the public on our side, a vote in mid-summer—so close to the Independence Day holiday when many people are vacationing and tuned out to politics—presented us with a daunting challenge.

Strategies and Tactics

A public attitude survey indicated broad public support for smoke-free dining. However, the history of special elections shows that a small but passionate minority (i.e., smokers and restaurant owners), can sway a small-turnout election. There was another risk factor: an assumption that *because* most people are nonsmokers, the ordinance would pass without much effort. This overconfidence had the potential of depressing turnout amongst those sympathetic with our cause.

We also knew that supporters of the tobacco industry's position typically have plenty of resources with which to mount a campaign. (Although there was some indication of tobacco industry involvement in the election, it was largely under the radar.) We determined that to win the referendum, we would have to rely on time-honored methods for identifying a sufficient number of favorable voters and getting them to the polls to vote. Specifically, our objectives were:

- Identify and turn out a "Yes" majority sufficient to achieve a 60% victory at the polls.
- Conduct an aggressive educational media campaign to promote a "Yes" victory at the polls.

As essential as broad public support and a determined coalition were to our efforts, the help we received from state and national partners was equally crucial. The American Cancer Society, American Heart Association, American Lung Association of North Dakota, Smokeless States, North Dakota Medical Association, Campaign for Tobacco-Free Kids, and American for Non-Smokers' Rights all came through with the advice and financial backing that enabled our Coalition to conduct a six-week "textbook" campaign focusing on message development and media advocacy, voter identification, and get-out-the-vote (GOTV) efforts (Table 72.1).

TABLE 72.1 Referendum and Get-Out-The-Vote (GOTV) Workplan									
			COUNTDOWN TO VOTE BY WEEKS						
Referendum and GOTV Workplan	**May**	**June**	**5**	**4**	**3**	**2**	**1**	**0**	**Aug to Dec**
		6/1 to 6/2	6/3 to 6/9	6/10 to 6/16	6/17 to 6/23	6/24 to 6/30	7/1 to 7/7	7/8 to 7/10	
Activity									
Hire project coordinator			X						
Campaign kick-off event			X						
Random Telephone Survey									
Develop questions			X						
Survey completed				X					
Message developed				X					

Continued

TABLE 72.1   Referendum and Get-Out-The-Vote (GOTV) Workplan—cont'd

Referendum and GOTV Workplan	May	June	COUNTDOWN TO VOTE BY WEEKS						Aug to Dec
			5	4	3	2	1	0	
Earned Media									
Power Against SHS Award	X								
World No Tobacco Day	X								
Relay for Life		X							
Paid Media									
Pre-vote: print, TV, radio, mail, billboards							X	X	
Post-vote: print, billboards								X	X
Media Advocacy									
Preemptive media visit on TI strategies				X					
Suggest stories to daily news				X	X	X	X	X	
General Public Education									
Service club presentations				X	X	X	X		
Special events: to be scheduled									
Increase Voter Turnout									
Obtain voter list	X								
Add phone #s to list	X	X	X						
Phone for campaign office			X	X	X	X	X		
Poll voters			X	X	X				
Educate community on absentee voting			X	X	X	X	X		
Direct mailing							X		

Media Advocacy

Breathing someone else's smoke is more than a nuisance; it's a serious health hazard. But if we want to keep the right to dine out without breathing someone else's cigarette smoke, we must Vote YES July 10th.

Most people know from experience that contact with secondhand smoke is unpleasant. If presented with the knowledge that such smoke is also dangerous to their health, most people will be inclined to support smoking restrictions.

With help from Campaign for Tobacco-Free Kids, we commissioned a five-question telephone survey to update our level of support and test the most persuasive arguments for upholding the city's new smoke-free restaurant ordinance. The result was the key message italicized above,

which we drove home to voters utilizing the following vehicles:

- Paid ads, including print, television, and radio (Fig. 72.1)
- Direct mail, in the form of postcards and flyers
- Four-page, four-color tabloid insert into the Minot Daily News

Voter Identification

Voter identification, or Voter ID, involves contacting people, either by telephone or door-to-door, to determine whether they favor, oppose, or are undecided about the issue at hand. Figures from the city election office indicated the previous six special elections in Minot had generated turnouts ranging from 3716 to 7318. Our instinct was that a smoking issue, due to its emotional nature, would produce

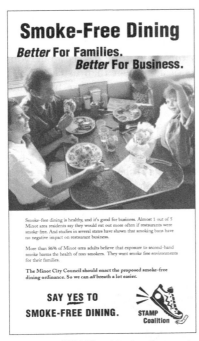

Fig. 72.1 STAMP paid advertisement.

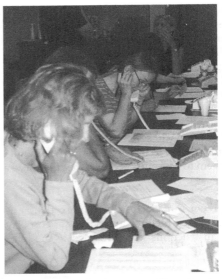

Fig. 72.2 Volunteers conducting get-out-the-vote phone calls. (Photo courtesy of the STAMP Coalition.)

a higher-than-normal turnout for a special election. (This assumption proved correct.) Therefore, assuming a larger-than-normal turnout of 10,000 voters, we would need to identify and turn out 6000 supporters.

Voter List. Since the people most likely to vote in any given election are those who have voted in previous elections, a supporter purchased the list of people who voted in the 2000 General Election within the Minot city limits (approx. 15,000 voters). These lists are available in every state and locality, although formats may differ. North Dakota is one of the few states without any form of voter registration. Our voter lists did not include telephone numbers, which meant volunteers had to be recruited to match names on the voter rolls with names in the local phone book. This was a time-consuming task and one we were able to complete only with the help of numerous individuals—adults, youth, and health care advocacy groups and foundations (Fig. 72.2). Given our tight time frame and because the resources were available, we hired a tele-marketing firm to identify half of the phone numbers needed.

Concise Question. Again with help from our national partners, we crafted a clear and concise question which we used in our telephone conversations to glean how the

voters on our list felt about the referral measure. Approximately 60% were amenable to our cause. This group was then targeted with direct mail, which included our key message and instructions for how to vote absentee. In addition, a postcard was sent just before Election Day reminding them to cast their ballots.

Absentee Voting. Because our election occurred in July, it was essential to provide our supporters with information on how to vote absentee. Conferring closely with city election officials, we obtained accurate information about the absentee voting process and mailed this to those identified as sympathetic to our cause. The effort proved worthwhile—absentee voting was unusually heavy.

Getting Out The Vote

Every battle needs soldiers. Ours came from every corner of North Dakota. The education community and health advocacy groups proved our most valuable allies locally. But tobacco coalition leaders from throughout the state poured into Minot to help staff phones, check lists, and the like.

GOTV is a science that involves a myriad of tasks. Of course, the function of a GOTV effort is to ensure that each individual supporter casts a vote on Election Day. This begins days and even weeks in advance with voter and absentee ballot information. In our campaign, we mailed postcards to our supporters within a few days of the election. And we made plans to call all our voters on Election Day utilizing two phone banks.

A thorough GOTV effort usually involves an extra step—using poll watchers at the voting sites to make sure the voters on our favorable list actually cast their ballots. Our poll watchers positioned themselves as close to the voter registration desk as possible with their voter list in hand. They listened as each voter announced his/her name. If the voter was on the poll watcher's list, the name was marked as having voted. At specified intervals, these lists were retrieved so that the callers back at the phone banks would know which supporters had already voted and which ones needed to be called, perhaps a second time, to remind them to vote and check whether they need a ride to the polls.

Training. On our election eve, more than a hundred volunteers assembled for a training session (Fig. 72.3). Detailed instructions were provided to the phone bank callers and poll watchers. When Election Day dawned, we had poll watchers at each polling site. Our callers began phoning later in the morning. Our phone banks buzzed with activity throughout the day as we nervously monitored reports of a "heavier than usual" turnout. By the time the polls closed, we knew we had done our jobs (Fig. 72.4).

"PUBLIC HEALTH IMPROVED"

Thanks to the organizational support and hundreds of volunteers, the totals broke in our favor. In a record turnout for a special election, North Dakota's first smoke-free ordinance prevailed 55% to 45%, prompting the Minot Daily News Editorial Board to proclaim "Public Health Improved."

If it can be done here, it can be done anywhere (Fig. 72.5)!

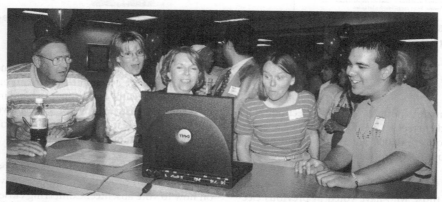

Fig. 72.3 Volunteers watching poll results come in on the eve of the election. (Photo courtesy of the STAMP Coalition.)

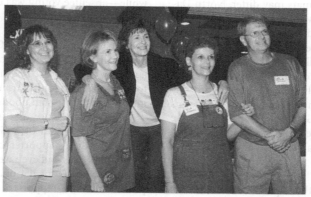

Fig. 72.4 Campaign leaders celebrating on the eve of the election. (Photo courtesy of the STAMP Coalition.)

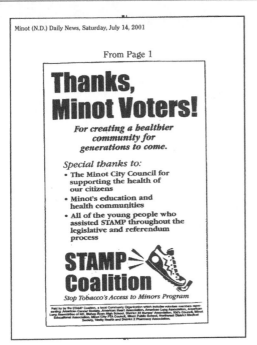

Minot (N.D.) Daily News, Saturday, July 14, 2001

From Page 1

Thanks, Minot Voters!

For creating a healthier community for generations to come.

Special thanks to:
- The Minot City Council for supporting the health of our citizens
- Minot's education and health communities
- All of the young people who assisted STAMP throughout the legislative and referendum process

STAMP Coalition

Stop Tobacco's Access to Minors Program

Fig. 72.5 A thank-you advertisement published in the Minot Daily News thanking voters, Minot City Council, Minot's education and health communities, and young people for voting for the smoke-free ordinance, thereby creating a healthier community for generations to come.

DISCUSSION QUESTIONS

1. Discuss a public health problem that would benefit having nurses focus on and lead policy solutions.

2. What health-related issue sparks your passion? Discuss existing organizations that advocate for this issue and the pros and cons of joining the organization or developing a new entity.

3. Do you think tobacco prevention and control is an important issue to nursing? Why or why not?

REFERENCES

American Cancer Society, American Heart Association, American Lung Association, Americans for Nonsmokers' Right, American Public Health Association, APPEAL, ... & Tobacco Technical Assistance Consortium. (2009). *Fundamentals of smokefree workplace laws: Executive summary and index.* Retrieved from https://nonsmokersrights.org/sites/default/files/2018-03/CIA_Fundamentals.pdf.

Americans for Nonsmokers' Rights. (n.d.). *Model ordinance prohibiting smoking in all workplaces and public places (100% smokefree).* Retrieved from https://nonsmokersrights.org/sites/default/files/2018-06/modelordinance.pdf.

ONLINE RESOURCES

American for Nonsmokers' Rights Foundation
https://no-smoke.org/
Americans for Nonsmokers' Rights
https://nonsmokersrights.org
Campaign for Tobacco Free Kids
www.tobaccofreekids.org
Centers for Disease Control and Prevention: Best Practices for Comprehensive Tobacco Control Programs
www.cdc.gov/tobacco/stateandcommunity/best_practices/index.htm
Centers for Disease Control and Prevention: Secondhand Smoke
www.cdc.gov/tobacco/basic_information/secondhand_smoke/index.htm

73

Where Policy Hits the Pavement: Contemporary Issues in Communities

Elizabeth Dickson and Monica R. McLemore

"Real, sustainable community change requires the initiative and engagement of community members."

Helene D. Gayle

The effects of public policy in the community take many forms: health insurance company regulations to ensure access to and payment for health care, housing and transportation policy, public smoking regulations to minimize exposure to second-hand smoke, and immunization requirements for elementary schools to lower rates of preventable diseases. Regardless of the policy focus, most people experience the personal effects of public policy in their own communities within their own daily lives.

Recent community and public involvement in the provision of health care and promotion of health has gained important and necessary attention as a significant factor that may improve outcomes for communities and populations (Franck et al., 2018). This chapter will define what "community" is, examine community engagement, explore how communities are shaped by contemporary policy issues, and consider how nurses engage communities around policy issues in practice, education, and research.

COMMUNITY DEFINED

Although Merriam Webster (2018) describes a *community* as "a unified body of individuals; a group of people with common interests/characteristics living in a particular area," the meaning of *community* is much more complex. No single definition applies to every group in every situation. We cannot delineate a role for ourselves or, more importantly, understand the assets of a community, without a shared definition. It can be an experience, a feeling, a set of relationships among people who share not only experiences, but a common history (Davis & Lee, 2015). However, it is important to note in a globally connected world these definitions are not static, but rather flexible and subject to interpretation. MacQueen et al. (2001) offer a more comprehensive definition of community as "a group of people with diverse characteristics who are linked by social ties, share common perspectives, and engage in join action in geographical locations or settings" (p. 1932). When trying to understand the impact of policy on community, it is important that the definition of *community* be flexible and allow us to clarify what nurses mean when we talk about our relationship with communities.

When considering the health of members of a community, the location or *place* of the community matters. The infrastructure that surrounds and supports a community (i.e., businesses, government, transportation, housing, schools, recreation, and communication) is foundational to understanding the sources of support to which members of that community have access. The quality, availability, and accessibility of the infrastructure impacts the lives of the individuals who live there. Members of communities may share and engage in relationships with one another within that infrastructure, creating social responsibility for building a healthy environment.

Several national initiatives have sought to help support healthy communities, examine the conditions within communities that can lead to poor health outcomes, and support community-led interventions that can change the larger community. Many local and state foundations have embraced and supported this priority as well (Table 73.1).

These initiatives also seek to understand how to partner in communities to spur the innovations that can help improve community health. They define communities as

places that enable people to live the healthiest lives possible, with access to healthy food, quality schools, stable housing, good jobs with fair pay, and safe places to exercise and play. The physical and socioeconomic conditions of a person's environment can be of tremendous importance in their health, as "the health risk conferred by place is above and beyond the risk that individuals carry with them" (Institute of Medicine [IOM], 2003, p. 68).

As discussed in Chapter 1, the social determinants of health (SDOH) are "conditions in which people are born, grow, work, live, and age, and the wider set of forces and systems shaping the conditions of daily life" (World Health Organization [WHO], 2018a)

TABLE 73.1 National Initiatives to Advance Community Engagement in Health Policies

American Public Health Association (APHA)	Creating Healthy Communities/Healthiest Cities & Counties Challenge: www.apha.org/what-is-public-health/creating-healthy-communities	Partnership with Aetna Foundation and National Association of Counties to support cities, counties, and federally-recognized tribes to show measurable changes in health and wellness by being "economically competitive, inclusive, and equitable" (American Public Health Association, 2018).
Joint Center for Political and Economic Studies	Place Matters Initiative: http://jointcenter.org/content/our-purpose	Place Matters teams with community-based leadership across the country, who receive technical assistance (grants, access to data, facilitation) to address social determinants of health (SDOH) and environmental conditions in their communities to eliminate health disparities (Joint Center for Political and Economic Studies, n.d.).
Robert Wood Johnson Foundation	Culture of Health: www.rwjf.org/en/our-focus-areas/focus-areas/health-leadership.html	Supporting health care providers, individual scholars, and interdisciplinary research teams (community and academia) to build healthier communities, spark community action, and address root causes of health disparities to achieve health equity (Robert Wood Johnson Foundation, 2018).
Federal Reserve	Community development resources promoting people, place, policy and practice, and small business: www.fedcommunities.org	These community resources include applied research, public programs, outreach, and technical assistance to "promote economic growth, financial stability" in low- and moderate-income communities across the country (FedCommunities.org, 2019).
Kellogg Foundation	Equitable Communities and Mission-Driven Investments: www.wkkf.org/what-we-do/mission-driven-investments	Focused grant making to prioritize "lasting, transformational change" for children, working families, and equitable communities; commit to communities for an entire generation. Support of private-sector, for-profit organizations to work for social change, with equal emphasis on social and financial returns (W.K. Kellogg Foundation, n.d.).
Center for Medicare & Medicaid Innovation	Accountable Communities for Health: https://nam.edu/elements-of-accountable-communities-for-health-a-review-of-the-literature/	Blending community funds and resources, integrate across health care sectors to address the health and social needs of individuals and communities to improve population health outcomes and reduce costs (Mongeon, Levi, & Henirich, 2017).

(see Chapter 1 for more detail). The systems surrounding individuals and their communities are shaped by the distribution of resources at national, state, and local levels. However, it is important to note that SDOH were first described by sociologists and critical race theorists when attempting to understand health disparities many decades before (Du Bois, 2003), and therefore are not new phenomena, nor unsolvable. If SDOH are to be managed toward optimal outcomes for all citizens, communities need to be supported to identify and advance solutions that would be most effective, based on their unique perspectives, setting, and circumstances. Common terminology is critically important to ensure clarity in the goals of individuals involved in work with, in, and for communities.

COMMUNITY ENGAGEMENT

Community engagement can take place at multiple levels and includes consultation, involvement, and shared leadership and decision-making (Fig. 73.1; Ocloo & Matthews, 2016). *Consultations* with communities often look like invitations to participate in exchange of information, surveys of patients' care experiences, and/or focus groups about specific health issues. *Community involvement*, however, is a deeper level of engagement which can involve rich discussions to elicit

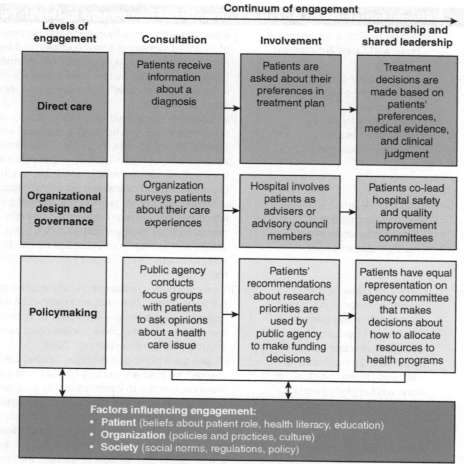

Fig. 73.1 Continuum of engagement. (Source: Carman, K.L., Dardess, P., Maurer, M., Sofaer, S., Adams, K., Bechtel, C., & Sweeney, J. [2013]. Patient and family engagement: A framework for understanding the elements and developing interventions and policies. *Health Affairs, 32*[2], 223–231.)

community preferences, or forming and working with a community advisory board to advise on health-related projects or research. Finally, the highest level of engagement is *shared leadership and decision-making* that affords communities the opportunities to actively engage in defining their own development, research, and policy priorities and needs, including funding decisions, according to their strengths, assets, and needs—as defined by the members of the community and not by outside groups (Carman et al., 2013).

From a policy perspective, it is important that nurses understand how to work with communities. It is also critical to assess what level of engagement is being used—specifically when policies are being developed, implemented, or evaluated—because it is in the community where policy hits the pavement.

CONTEMPORARY POLICY ISSUES AFFECTING COMMUNITIES

One only needs to watch the daily news headlines to get a sense of the multitude of contemporary policy issues facing communities today. Although some headlines are driven by political party politics, other health policy issues are ongoing concerns regardless of politics, geographic location, or demographics. While not an exhaustive list, examples of some of those issues include access to health care, the gap in health insurance coverage, and ongoing threats to the Patient Protection and Affordable Care Act (see Chapter 18); disaster and pandemic preparedness and emergency response (see Chapter 30); domestic and sexual violence (see Chapter 79); prescription drug pricing; current and future health care workforce shortages (see Chapter 53); lack of access to mental substance use disorder health care (see Chapter 25); housing/homelessness; changing demographics of populations (urban and rural); equity issues; and disparities across populations (see Chapter 22).

Another evidence-based way nurses can keep current in policies that affect communities is to use the dashboard tool developed in partnership with the Robert Wood Johnson Foundation that shows county rankings state by state (see www.countyhealthrankings.org). These interactive maps and databases that are publicly available provide data on health outcomes and health factors including length of life, quality of life, health behaviors, clinical care, socioeconomic factors, and the physical/built environment at the county and state level.

NURSES ENGAGING CONTEMPORARY POLICY IN COMMUNITY

It is the members of any community that need to define and prioritize the policy issues of most importance to them, not individual or groups outside of the community or part of powerful bureaucratic institutions in the community itself (e.g., members of academia or health services). When partnering with community members to prioritize policy issues, nurses have a wealth of experience and skills to contribute, but none as important as the skill of active listening. Listening to community concerns, trying to understand community members' lived realties, and working with them to prioritize issues for action are critical to building relationships and trust, and fundamental to any interventions or policy work (Falk, Rafael, & Betker, 2012; Martsolf, Sloan, Mason, Sullivan, & Villarruel, 2017; Martsolf, Sloan, Villarruel, Sullivan, & Mason, 2018). Additional considerations to keep in mind when working with a community are that community members may need to meet outside of "normal" business hours, may prefer alternative methods of communication (such as text messages and social media), and may need to be offered childcare, food, and remuneration for their time.

Nurses have been leading multiple efforts to develop, test, and expand community engagement models with policy implications in both acute and community and public health care settings. Chapter 1 describes the Stephen and Sandra Sheller 11th Street Family Health Services in North Philadelphia that was founded by Patricia Gerrity and affiliated with Drexel University. When she began her work, she asked the community leaders of a public housing project if she could have a room to put a nurse to be available to tenants with health concerns. The community leaders told her that they didn't need or want her there, and they were tired of "university people" coming into their community to "do their thing" and then leaving. Gerrity told the community that she was there to stay and asked them what they thought they needed and wanted. They told her they needed a stop sign on the corner because cars would speed down the street and run unto their children and elders. As an insightful public health nurse, Gerrity knew that she had to deliver on the stop sign—and she did. The community took note and gave her the room. She invited the community members to be part of a community advisory committee to guide the work. They accepted and the committee remains an integral part of what is now an endowed, modern, federally qualified health center that serves over 2500 people annually.

Specific to community engagement and policy work in public health, nurses have been leading several innovative programs specific to maternal and child health (MCH). Long considered a barometer of a nation's health, MCH programs have sought to improve outcomes for and with communities. Some of the seminal work toward understanding the role of attachment, bonding, breastfeeding, and the determinants of readiness for school has been developed by nurses (Beck, 2008; Mercer, 2004), illustrated by the Centering Pregnancy program developed by Certified Nurse Midwife Sharon Rising (1998). Rising brings women into groups for their prenatal care, education, and support. She sees her work as community building, as the women build connections that continue after their deliveries and are empowered to take actions in support of their own health and that of their newborns and families. She subsequently extended her work to Centering Parenting and used the model for other conditions such as diabetes. She developed the Centering Healthcare Institute for training and policy advocacy to support group models of care. Additional examples of nurses working to advance community policy issues are included in Table 73.2. All of these programs have been nurse-led and/or nurse-designed with an exclusive focus on building on the community assets and engaging communities to work in partnership with nurses to develop community-defined problems and place-based solutions.

Advocacy

Advocacy is a core concept to nursing practice. An advocate is often described as an individual or group who argues for or supports an individual, common cause, or issue, or someone who works for a cause or group as an advocate (Gardner & Brindis, 2017). Anyone can advocate for something they care about. Most nurses, however, would identify it as an essential skill to their practice as patient advocates and a core competency of their nursing education (American Academy Colleges of Nursing [AACN], 2008). Not all nurses are aware that advocacy extends beyond an individual patient or family for whom they are

caring. Nursing's role in advocacy, whether at the bedside in a hospital setting or in a legislative statehouse as an elected policymaker, is well documented in the literature (Hanks, Starnes-Ott, Stafford, 2018; Shillam & MacLean, 2018). Spenceley, Reutter, & Allen (2006) provide an epistemological review of advocacy in nursing while framing nursing advocacy within the community, policy, and system levels of impact. Although advocacy for policy issues at the community or policy level can seem less tangible than advocating for an individual patient, it is no less critical, and is considered a population health intervention increasingly expected of nurses, particularly nurses with a Doctor of Nursing Practice (DNP).

Local policy decisions can deeply impact communities. Israel et al. (2010) emphasizes that policy advocacy must have engagement of community members at the local level. It is important that nursing knowledge and experience be expressed in *collaboration* with other individuals from other professional disciplines and community groups. As stated before, community consists of many different voices and experiences. Nurses involved with community advocacy can develop the ability to reflect critically about how they contribute their nursing experience to advocacy efforts while also supporting the experience and voice of others within community. (See Chapter 3 for more on advocacy for policy.)

Coalition Building and Support

It is important to highlight how Nursing (capital "N" meaning collectively as organizations and as an institution) works with community-driven and/or community-led coalitions to support important health policy issues. Professional associations and organizations that represent nurses (see Chapter 67) have specific policy agendas and work to sign letters of support, amicus briefs

TABLE 73.2   Nursing Role/Education for Engaging in Contemporary Policy in Community

Project Name or Theme	Outcome Impacted by Policy	Website
American Academy of Nursing—Edge Runners Program	Tobacco cessation, care coordination, global health, aging and chronic disease, integrated care	www.aannet.org/initiatives/edge-runners
Native American Nursing Learning Collaborative	Improve wellbeing of native communities and address health inequities through nursing.	https://campaignforaction.org/resource/native-american-nursing-learning-collaborative/
Nurse Family Partnership	Improving maternal and child health outcomes	www.nursefamilypartnership.org
Minnesota Prison Doula Project and Roots of Labor Birth Collective	Carceral health improvement	www.mnprisondoulaproject.org/ www.rootsoflaborbc.com/

to the Supreme Court of the United States, and national proposals to ensure Nursing's voice is heard in policy debates. For example, in the summer of 2018, 33 of the 60-member organization of the Nursing Community Coalition (2018) signed a letter to the Secretary of the U.S. Department of Homeland Security to express extreme concern about the separation of families and the health and well-being of immigrant children at the U.S. border. A second example of Nursing's coalition action involved efforts by the International Council of Nurses and other national and international nursing organizations to reinstate the Chief Nursing Officer position within WHO (2018b). Director General Tedros Adhanom Ghebreyesus subsequently appointed Elizabeth Iro to that position and her presence in WHO ensures that nurses will again have a voice in health policy development and implementation within the world's leading health organization.

As the largest group of health care professionals, nurses must remember two important factors that strengthen their ability to support and engage coalition building: (1) the trust the public has continuously maintained for the profession of nursing (Gallup, 2018), and (2) the perspective of being a health care provider that gives nurses an important contribution to community discussions about health policy. The potential impact of a collective Nursing voice to any policy issue addressing health of communities cannot be understated.

Engaging the Community in Research

There are great opportunities for nurses to work with community partners to develop and engage in research that can inform evidence-based policy related to the community's concerns and priorities. Nurses and health care teams can partner with communities to set research agendas (Ulm, Crowe, Dowling & Oliver, 2014) and allocation of research funding (Franck et al., 2018). Community-Engaged Research (CEnR) and Community-Based Participatory Research (CBPR) are two approaches for partnering with community around research. Professionals from clinical, academic, and nongovernmental groups often reach out to community members, wanting to learn more about an issue or test the effectiveness of an intervention. However, the approach with which they engage individuals or groups within community must be thoughtful and respectful. Historically, many communities have been overlooked and/or subject to unethical research methods (Morello-Frosch, Brown, & Green Brody, 2017). For these reasons, the relationships and trust between partners working together is critical.

CBPR is not a method of research, but rather an approach and orientation to research. Instead of engaging

on, in, or for community, this orientation engages research with community (University of New Mexico [UNM], 2018). This approach requires a central belief of consciously challenging the power relationship between researcher and community, so that the distinction between who decides what or who gets studied is removed (Wallerstein, et al., 2017). The CBPR conceptual model (Fig. 73.2) (Wallerstein & Duran, 2010; UNM, 2018) helps explain the necessary domains for partnerships working together to impact health or policy outcomes and has demonstrated psychometric validity (Oetzel et al., 2015).

USING HEALTH EQUITY AND SDOH FRAMEWORK FOR EVERY POPULATION

In working with any individual, nurses must ask key questions beyond chief complaints and signs and symptoms presented: Where is this individual from? Where is the community within which they live and work? Do they have a social support system? Do they have adequate access to food, transportation, health care, education? These questions not only provide context for the structures that shape an individual's life, and the choices they make about their health, they also provide the basis for understanding population-level data to guide the needs and concerns of the community based on evidence. These questions also make up key components of the SDOH framework (see Chapter 1). Understanding that the choices we all make are determined by the choices we have is a critical perspective to understanding community concerns about health equity and policy.

Although identifying these concerns is key to begin conversations about health disparities, it does not always emphasize the inequities in distribution of income, power, and resources that can result in health inequities in the first place (Ford & Airhihenbuwa, 2018). A political and policy example of this issue is wealth and income inequality, or the growing disparity and gap between those who possess a larger share of money and wealth compared with those who do not. This dynamic creates inequity in available resources to afford health care services, medicine, food, transportation, and other life essentials that can have severe health consequences (Arcaya & Figueroa, 2017; Elgar, et al., 2017). This can result in the increasing rates of chronic disease in what Dickman and colleagues (2017) call a "predictable pattern of rising prevalence with declining income" (p. 1431).

Whether a nurse cares for an individual, family, or population, these all exist within the community, and surrounding that community are policies that shape health on every level. Good health for individuals and

CBPR Conceptual Model

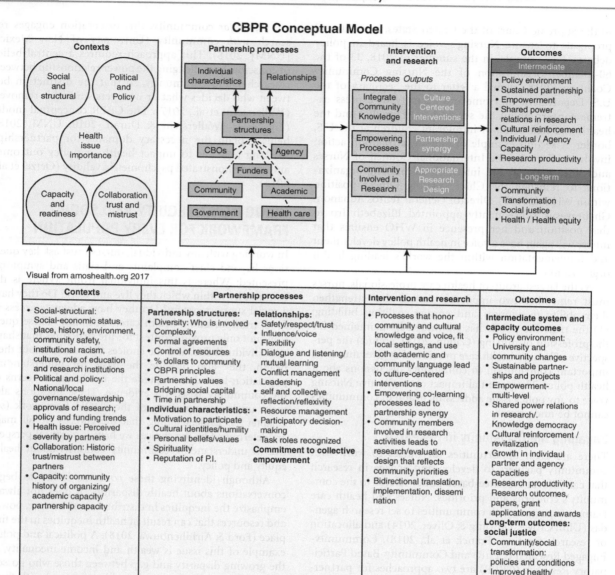

Fig. 73.2 Community-based participatory research (CBPR) conceptual model. (Adapted from Wallerstein & Duran [2010]. Retrieved from https://cpr.unm.edu/research-projects/cbpr-project/cbpr-model.html.)

communities requires policies that are actively created for and support health (WHO, 2012). Although the best of nurses' skills and gifts are amplified in the struggle for health and wellbeing for each person in every community, there is ample opportunity and need for nurses to become involved with and contribute their knowledge and experience as a partner of the community to advance health-promoting policies.

DISCUSSION QUESTIONS

1. What are the most effective levels of engagement that nurses can provide communities?
2. What are the most important factors for nurses to consider prior to conducting community-engaged work?
3. In your clinical area of expertise, what would policy advocacy at the community level look like?

REFERENCES

American Academy Colleges of Nursing. (2008). *The essentials of baccalaureate education for professional nursing practice.* Retrieved from www.aacnnursing.org/Portals/42/Publications/BaccEssentials08.pdf.

Arcaya, M.C., & Figueroa, J.F. (2017). Emerging trends could exacerbate health inequities in the United States. *Health Affairs, 36*(6), 992-998.

Beck, T. C. (2008). State of the science on postpartum depression. *Maternal Child Nursing: American Journal of Maternal Child Nursing, 33*(3), 151-156.

Carman, K.L., Dardess, P., Maurer, M., Sofaer, S., Adams, K., Bechtel, C., & Sweeney, J. (2013). Patient and family engagement: A framework for understanding the elements and developing interventions and policies. *Health Affairs, 32*(2), 223-231.

Davis, C., & Lee, K. (2015). What is community anyway? *Stanford Social Innovation Review.* Retrieved from https://ssir.org/articles/entry/what_is_community_anyway.

Dickman, S.L., Himmelstein, D.U., & Woolhandler, S. (2017). Inequality and the health-care system in the USA. *The Lancet, 389*(10077), 1431-1441.

Du Bois, W.E.B. (2003). The health and physique of the Negro American, 1906. *American Journal of Public Health, 93*(2), 272-276.

Elgar, F.J., Gariépy, G., Torsheim, T., & Currie, C. (2017). Early-life income inequality and adolescent health and well-being. *Social Science & Medicine, 174*, 197-208.

Falk-Rafael, A., & Betker, C. (2012). The primacy of relationships: A study of public health nursing practice from a critical caring perspective. *Advances in Nursing Science, 35*(4), 315-332.

FICare, F.I.C. (2018). *Family integrated care: About FICare.* Retrieved from http://familyintegratedcare.com/about-ficare/.

Ford, C.L. & Airhihenbuwa, C.O. (2018). Commentary: Just what is critical race theory and what's it doing in a progressive field like public health? *Ethnicity & Disease, 28*(1), 223-230.

Franck. L.S., McLemore, M.R., Cooper, N., De Castro, B., Gordon, A.Y., Williams, S., ... & Rand, L. (2018). A novel method for involving women of color at high risk for preterm birth in research priority setting. *Journal of Visualized Experiments, 131*, 56220.

Gallup. (2018). *Honesty and ethics in professions.* Retrieved from https://news.gallup.com/poll/1654/honesty-ethics-professions.aspx.

Gardner, A., & Brindis, C. (2017). *Advocacy and policy change evaluation: Theory and practice.* Stanford, CA: Stanford University Press.

Hanks, R.G., Starnes-Ott, K., & Stafford, L. (2018). Patient advocacy at the APRN level: A direction for the future. *Nursing Forum, 53*(1), 5-11.

Institute of Medicine. (2003). *The future of the public's health in the 21st century.* Washington, DC: National Academies Press.

Israel, B.A., Coombe, C.M., Cheezum, R.R., Schulz, A.J., McGranaghan, R.J., Lichtenstein, R., ... & Burris, A. (2010). Community-based participatory research: A capacity-building approach for policy advocacy aimed at eliminating health disparities. *American Journal of Public Health, 100*(11), 2094-2102.

MacQueen, K.M., McLellan, E., Metzger, D.S., Kegeles, S., Strauss, R.P., Scotti, R., & Trotter, R.T.(2001). What is community? An evidence-based definition for participatory public health. *American Journal of Public Health, 91*(12), 1929-1938.

Martsolf, G., Sloan, J., Mason, D.J., Sullivan, C., & Villarruel, A. (2017). *RAND report: Nurse-designed models of care and culture of health: Three case studies.* Santa Monica, CA: RAND Corporation. Retrieved from www.rand.org/pubs/research_reports/RR1811.html.

Martsolf, G., Sloan, J., Villarruel, A., Sullivan, C., & Mason, D.J. (2018). Promoting a culture of health through cross-sector collaborations. *Health Promotion Practice, 19*(5), 784-791.

Mercer, R.T. (2004). Becoming a mother versus maternal role attainment. *Journal of Nursing Scholarship, 36*(3), 226-232.

Merriam-Webster. (2018). *Community: Definition of community.* Retrieved from www.merriam-webster.com/dictionary/community.

Morello-Frosch, R., Brown, P., & Green Brody, J. (2017). Democratizing ethical oversight of research through CBPR. In N. Wallerstein, B. Duran, J. Oetzel, & M. Minkler (Eds.), *Community-based participatory research for health: Advancing social and health equity* (pp. 215-225). San Francisco: Jossey-Bass.

Nursing Community Coalition. (2018). *Recent news: Nursing community coalition sends letter to Department of Homeland Security, June 19, 2018.* Retrieved from https://docs.wixstatic.com/ugd/148923_2fccec4d555c418aad70bd66bf971248.pdf.

Ocloo, J., & Matthews, R. (2016). From tokenism to empowerment: Progressing patient and public involvement in healthcare improvement. *BMJ Quality & Safety, 25*(8), 626-632.

Oetzel, J.G., Zhou, C., Duran, B., Pearson, C., Magarati, M., Lucero, J., ... & Villegas, M. (2015). Establishing the psychometric properties of constructs in a community-based participatory research conceptual model. *American Journal of Health Promotion, 29*(5), e188-e202.

Rising, S.S. (1998). Centering pregnancy. An interdisciplinary model of empowerment. *Journal of Nurse Midwifery, 43*(1), 46-54.

Shillam, C.R., & MacLean, L. (2018). Leadership influence: A core foundation for advocacy. *Nursing Administration Quarterly, 42*(2), 150-153.

Spenceley, S., Reutter, L., & Allen, M.N. (2006). The road less traveled: Nursing advocacy at the policy level. *Policy, Politics, & Nursing Practice, 7*(3), 180-194.

Ulm, S., Crowe, S., Dowling, I., & Oliver, S. (2014). The process and outcomes of setting research priorities about preterm birth—A collaborative partnership. *Infant, 10*(6), 178-181.

University of New Mexico. (2018). *NM CARES health disparities center: Community engagement core: Health equity and policy making: Community-based participatory research (CBPR) and reducing health disparities.* Retrieved from https://hsc.unm.edu/programs/nmcareshd/cec.shtml.

Wallerstein, N., & Duran, B. (2010). Community-based participatory research contributions to intervention research: The intersection of science and practice to improve health equity. *American Journal of Public Health, 100*(Suppl 1), S40-S46

Wallerstein, N., Duran, B., Oetzel, J., & Minkler, M. (2017). On community-based participatory research. In N. Wallerstein, B. Duran, J. Oetzel, & M. Minkler (Eds.), *Community-based participatory research for health: Advancing social and health equity* (pp. 31-46). San Francisco: Jossey-Bass.

World Health Organization. (2012). *Gender, equity and human rights: Understanding social determinants of health.* Retrieved from www.who.int/gender-equity-rights/understanding/sdh-definition/en/.

World Health Organizations. (2018a). *Social determinants of health: What are social determinants of health?* Retrieved from www.who.int/social_determinants/en/.

World Health Organization. (2018b). *Health workforce: WHO reaffirms commitment to nursing and midwifery.* Retrieved from www.who.int/hrh/news/2018/WHO-reaffirms-commitment-to-nursing-midwifery/en/.

ONLINE RESOURCES

American Public Health Association
www.apha.org
Healthy People 2020
www.healthypeople.gov
World Health Organization: Social Determinants of Health
www.who.int/social_determinants/en/

74

An Introduction to Community Activism

DeAnne K. Hilfinger Messias and Robin Dawson Estrada

> *Never doubt that a small group of thoughtful, committed citizens can change the world. Indeed, it is the only thing that ever has.*
>
> **Margaret Mead, anthropologist**

Community activism is the means through which individuals, groups, and organizations work together to bring about specific, often radical, changes in social, economic, environmental, and cultural policies and practices. The broad goal of community activism is to enact social transformation that contributes directly to improving living conditions, enhancing community environments, and eliminating health and social disparities. Community activists engage in collaborative, sustained actions aimed at changing or removing underlying structures and barriers, be they political, social, economic, environmental, or cultural, with the ultimate aim of improving the lives of individuals or groups subjected to disparate, discriminatory, or oppressive conditions (Table 74.1). The primary focus on changing underlying or contributing structures, practices, or policies distinguishes community activism from both community service and community development. Community service involves the provision of goods or services for underserved or underprivileged individuals or groups (Jennings et al., 2006; Jennings, Hardee, & Messias, 2010; Nam, 2012), whereas the primary focus of community development is to enhance existing social and economic infrastructures through the creation of new service programs, leadership training, and innovative partnerships (Larsen, 2004; Dale & Newman, 2010). Another distinguishing characteristic of community activism is that the primary commitment and motivation for change are generated from within the community of interest. In contrast, the motivation, expertise, and resources for community service and development often originate outside the local community.

KEY CONCEPTS

The concepts of social justice, community, consciousness-raising, critical reflection, praxis, and empowerment are integral to community activism (Fig. 74.1). Social justice is a philosophical, political, and public health concept rooted in the ideal of human rights and social equity (Reichert, 2007). The equitable distribution of resources and opportunities for a productive and fulfilling life is a human rights concern. Prerequisites for social justice include the establishment and assurance of equal treatment under the law, equal access to opportunities, and fair and equitable distribution of resources. Yet in many communities around the globe, the availability of basic resources (e.g., safe drinking water, clean air, adequate housing, secure neighborhoods) and access to opportunities and resources (e.g., education, employment, health care, and fair and equal treatment under the law) are not distributed equitably across diverse groups (Braveman, 2006). Rather, factors such as social privilege or market forces determine the distribution of these key resources and opportunities, resulting in social injustices and health inequities. Health inequities are avoidable differences in health status between groups, both within regions or countries and between countries (World Health Organization, n.d.). Overcoming health inequities and social injustice requires collective action and solutions on multiple fronts. Community activism is one way the ideal of social justice is translated into practice.

Community is a dynamic and fluid concept, conceptualized and practiced in diverse ways. In relation to activism, community implies the actual involvement of

TABLE 74.1 Types and Definitions of Community Actions

Type of Community Action	Definition
Community Activism	Collaborative, sustained actions focused on changing structures or removing barriers with the ultimate aim of improving the lives of individuals or groups subjected to disparate, discriminatory, or oppressive social, economic, political, cultural, or environmental conditions.
Community Development	The creation of new programs and services to improve and enhance local social and economic infrastructures.
Community Service	The provision of goods or services for underserved or underprivileged individuals or groups.

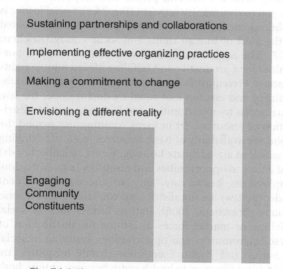

Fig. 74.1 Key concepts of community activism.

Sustaining partnerships and collaborations

Implementing effective organizing practices

Making a commitment to change

Envisioning a different reality

Engaging Community Constituents

individuals and groups directly impacted by the specific issues or conditions that are the focus of change. In a more traditional sense, community, or grassroots, activism is both locally generated and locally focused. Many community activists are located within and focused on creating change in a specific geographic location, such as the neighborhood, school district, or city where they live,

study, or work. Neighborhood activists frequently mobilize around issues related to public safety, environmental health, education, land use, zoning, and economic development. The focus may be location-specific (e.g., getting traffic signs installed at busy intersections, organizing a neighborhood watch or clean-up effort, eliminating the presence of alcohol and tobacco advertising in low-income and minority neighborhoods) or may address broader structural issues such as economic development or environmental pollution.

In the United States, education is a common focus of activism involving students, parents, teachers, and the broader community. The implementation of bilingual education programs in southwest Chicago public schools came about in response to Mexican American community activism (Stovall, 2006). In 2013, education cuts to the North Carolina state budget led to demonstrations by students, parents, teachers, community and religious leaders, and members of national organizations including the National Education Association (NEA) and the National Association for the Advancement of Colored People (NAACP). The movement, which became known as Moral Mondays, included protests and rallies at the North Carolina Legislative Building, voter registration drives, and legal opposition to the proposed budget changes (Blythe, 2013). Violence can be a powerful impetus for activism, as exemplified by the Black Lives Matter movement and the student activism in response to the school shooting at Marjory Stoneman Douglas High School in Parkland, Florida (Freelon, McIlwain, & Clark, 2016; Witt, 2018).

Historically, community activists have participated in broader social movements including the women's rights, civil rights, workers' rights, and environmental health movements. Grassroots activists often mobilize across geographical and social communities, as exemplified by mothers who effectively rallied against the use of bisphenol A (BPA) in baby bottles and other food and beverage containers (Smith & Lourie, 2009; Brewer & Ley, 2011). Activism also may occur within the context of communities formed through a shared sense of political responsibility or affiliation with a collective social identity (e.g., cultural or ethnic group, race, religion). The increasingly widespread availability and decreased costs of devices that share written and visual information through the internet and cellular phones have allowed activists to construct a concept of community defined by connectedness with a common issue of concern rather than by physical location (Tufekci & Wilson, 2012).

Collective social identities related to specific health issues (e.g., human immunodeficiency virus/acquired immunodeficiency syndrome [HIV/AIDS], cancer, mental health, tuberculosis, women's reproductive health) have given rise to significant community activist movements. Over the past 30 years, what is now a global HIV/AIDS movement began as local activism within gay communities in the United States, Canada, Western Europe, and Australia. These early activists mobilized to educate their own communities around HIV prevention and, at the same time, demand responsive public action from governments, medical researchers, health care providers, pharmaceutical companies, and legal systems (Piot, 2006). Subsequent HIV/AIDS grassroots mobilizations have involved diverse communities, including persons living with AIDS in Brazil, Uganda, and South Africa; sex workers in Thailand; religious and community leaders in Senegal; and impoverished mothers of childhood AIDS victims in Romania. Through relentless advocacy and demands for changes in public policy as well as local health care systems, HIV/AIDS community activists have provoked governmental and industry responses, resulting in more effective prevention and access to treatment and significantly impacting the global HIV/AIDS epidemic (Marcolongo, 2002; Piot, 2006; Gulaid & Kiragu, 2012).

Consciousness raising, critical reflection, and praxis are three interrelated components of community activism. Underlying liberatory approaches to community activism is the premise that empowerment emerges from engagement in focused dialogue, listening, critical reflection, and reflective action (Freire, 1970/1997, 1973/1993). One of the first steps to engaging participants in activist endeavors is to increase public awareness of specific issues and the associated root causes. Consciousness-raising goes beyond simply presenting others with information, to actually engaging with others in critical reflection. Popular educator and community activist Paulo Freire originally defined and applied the concept of *conscientização* (Portuguese for conscientization) in his community-based work with illiterate Brazilian peasants. *Conscientização* is a reflective process in which individuals and groups examine their own particular situations and contexts to identify social, economic, cultural, political, and environmental forces contributing to those situations. Critical awareness arises through the reflective processes of problem-posing and interpretive decoding of lived experiences (Freire, 1970/1997).

Critical reflection is integral to understanding the linkages and connections between a local community's issues and problems and those of other communities across the globe. By engaging in critical dialogue and reflection, community activists begin to envision possibilities for collective action leading to transformation (Jennings, Hardee, & Messias, 2010). Critical reflection also involves attention to the political processes and actions necessary to challenge inequalities and effect change. Praxis is purposeful, reflective action arising out of individual and collective

conscientization and theorizing, and grounded in a commitment to building a more just society through diverse means, including culture circles, critical pedagogies, action research, and community activism (Freire, 1970/1997, 1973/1993; Stovall, 2006; Hesse-Biber, 2007). Community activism is a form of critical social praxis, an iterative cycle of conscientization-reflection-reflective action in which relations of power and inequality are identified, challenged, and changed.

Empowerment is a multilevel construct that incorporates processes and outcomes of social action through which individuals, families, organizations, and communities gain control and mastery within the social, economic, and political contexts of their lives to attain greater equity and improve the quality of life (Jennings et al. 2006). At the individual level, empowerment may result from the generation of new knowledge and understanding of issues, and the development of new skills among community activists. Subsequently, individual empowerment can lead to individual self-protective and other socially responsible behaviors and also may be linked to community organizing to support social action and political change (Wallerstein, Sanchez-Merki & Velarde, 2005). Collective empowerment occurs within families, organizations, and communities. It involves processes and structures that enhance members' skills, provides them with the mutual support necessary to effect change, improves their collective well-being, and strengthens intra- and inter-organizational networks and linkages to improve or maintain the quality of community life.

The process of making connections between personal experience and broader social issues is integral to personal and community empowerment and to effective action. In describing a youth empowerment program at an alternative high school for youth unable to succeed within the traditional educational system, Mitra (2008) reported an adult advisor's observation that "the kids involved are changing [from] delinquent into activists. [They can see] how they got sucked into being delinquent and into the criminal justice system through their upbringing—not just their family, but the community and the policies" (p. 210). The purpose of empowerment education is to develop the requisite knowledge and skills for community activism, particularly among the youth. By participating in community action projects (peer teaching, the production of murals, cultural institutes, the creation of videos for use in educational efforts, or photo-voice projects), young people and other potential activists develop the requisite knowledge and skills for community activism as they engage in collective conscious-raising, critical reflection, and reflective action (Messias et al., 2008; Ivashkavich, Hilfinger Messias, Soltani, & Cayir, 2020).

TAKING ACTION TO EFFECT CHANGE: CHARACTERISTICS OF COMMUNITY ACTIVISTS AND ACTIVISM

Activists not only recognize injustice but also are willing to take action to correct it (Sherrod, 2006). Situated across the social, economic, and political spectrum, activists share a desire to contribute to the collective welfare and create a more just and equitable society. Motivation and commitment of personal time and energy to social involvement, a willingness to take risks, and belief in the power and efficacy of groups to effect change are common characteristics among community activists. The motivation may be rooted in personal or professional experience, empathy, or solidarity (Lewis-Charp, Yu, & Soukamneuth, 2006; Montlake, 2009). Because of the risks embedded in social justice work, activists must individually and collectively assess the potential harm that may come from actions, help each other prepare if they choose to take calculated risks, and take steps to protect themselves and others as best as possible when they do (Cohen, de la Vega, & Watson, 2001).

Community activism grows out of the desire to change existing social, political, or environmental conditions. In their commitment to change and transform the way power is distributed or controlled, activists draw on the power of the people and the community (power within) and exert pressure on those who hold institutional power (power over). Characteristics of successful community activism include the ability to frame issues and envision a different reality, a clear commitment to change at various levels, the implementation of effective organizing practices and actions, and the ability to develop and sustain collaborative partnerships and relationships (Fig. 74.2).

Envisioning Change and Possibilities for Different Realities

New ways of collective seeing, perceiving, and acting are essential for change (Jennings, Hardee & Messias, 2010). To create the momentum and sustain progress toward social change, activists may need to refocus issues around commonalities rather than fuel polarization around differences. When working toward the goal of a new and different reality, the processes of consciousness-raising and critical reflection can result in collective redefinition and reframing of issues. For instance, in addressing problems such as educational inequality, activists may need to rethink commonly held wisdom and redirect the focus of their actions. Lightfoot (2008) provided an example of such rethinking and reframing, citing the case of local education activists changing the focus from replacing school

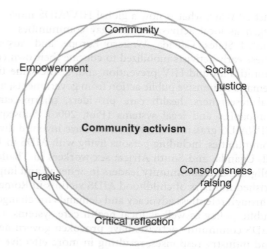

Fig. 74.2 Characteristic processes of effective community activism.

segregation with integration to actively addressing the underlying racism that had fostered and perpetuated segregation in the first place. In the case of transnational activism to improve the lives of marginalized Filipino bar girls working in a country where prostitution is illegal, the commitment to change was informed by activists' understanding of the social and political context (Ralston & Keeble, 2009). Rather than framing the issue as eliminating prostitution, the activists focused on alleviating sex workers' legal, financial, and social hardships, by changing the minds and practices of exploitative bar owners and clients, an unsympathetic community, and an insensitive court system.

Taking Action

Beyond critical conceptualization and framing of issues, creating change requires action on multiple fronts and the participation of individuals with a wide range of skills, talents, and competencies. Activists work to create change in social norms, public policies, legislation, or environmental practices. Effecting change in policies, practices, and social structures entails integrated information, mobilization, relationship building, and communication work. This requires extensive research and analysis of complex issues; monitoring of local power dynamics; and ongoing planning, implementation, and evaluation of the effectiveness of strategies and approaches.

Community activists organize and act to call attention to their issues, communicate and disseminate information, develop and maintain networks, and engage others in problem-solving and policy change strategies. Communication and information dissemination actions include door-to-door soliciting; writing letters to the editor; creating and distributing flyers, posters, and leaflets; and producing and disseminating print, radio, and television ads. Increasingly, activists employ Internet formats (e.g., websites, email, blogs, social networking sites) to communicate within and across their existing networks and to reach new audiences. In tailoring their messages for specific audiences, community activists use a range of media from art, storytelling, songs, theater, photography, videos, and multimedia presentations to expert panels, research reports, and policy briefs.

To engage community members and policy-makers policymakers employ a variety of mobilization and organizing actions. These include conducting public meetings and forums; planning and carrying out mass demonstrations, rallies, and marches; supporting and participating in boycotts and strikes; collecting signatures on petitions and carrying out letter-writing campaigns, both in-person and on-line; conducting teach-ins, trainings, and workshops; and engaging in community-based participatory research. The production of documentary films is another strategy to both expand the number of activists and mobilize them for further action (Whiteman, 2009).

Creating and Sustaining Collaborations

Less visible but clearly as important is the behind-the-scenes work of networking, building relationships, and sustaining coalitions. Everyday social networks through home, school, and work provide potential connections and opportunities for activism (Martin, Hanson, & Fontaine, 2007). Collaboration is a key process within community activism and is necessary to develop and implement policies and practices to effect the desired changes. Collaboration requires considerable time, energy, skill, and the involvement of multiple stakeholders, but the power of collaboration is that by working together, concerned individuals and groups can create the synergy needed to produce a desired change that could not be generated by individual action alone.

Partnering with like-minded individuals and organizations strengthens activist movements, but to effect real change, activists often must build bridges and create collaborative relationships that cross differences in age, race, class, social position, location, or nationality and bring together groups with differing perspectives on the issues. Productive collaborations contribute to capacity building among individuals, groups, and organizations, resulting in enhanced ability to achieve mutual goals. At its core, activism is relational work, as exemplified in the life and work of Ella Baker. Although not as widely known or well recognized as Martin Luther King, Jr., Baker was an instrumental visionary and community organizer within the civil rights movement who dedicated her life to organizing and mentoring students and community members. Born and educated in the Jim Crow South, in 1927 Baker moved to New York City, which became the base for her activist career over the next 50 years. Ella Baker worked on social justice issues ranging from child welfare, youth services, school reform, and consumer education to police brutality, desegregation, and voting rights. Through her collaborative associations with other activists, educators, and policymakers in various organizations (including Parents in Action, NAACP, Southern Christian Leadership Conference, In Friendship, and the Student Nonviolent Coordinating Committee), Baker's activism was essential in developing the groundwork for legal and institutional changes of the civil rights movement and eventual de facto racial desegregation. Baker's approach to furthering human rights was to build *strong people* rather than to support a *strong leader* (Ransby, 2003).

CHALLENGES AND OPPORTUNITIES IN COMMUNITY ACTIVISM

Community activists in the 21st century face numerous challenges and opportunities, including advocating for incremental or radical change, addressing local issues within the context of an increasingly globalized world with widening social and economic gaps within and across countries, effectively harnessing the potential of new technologies, and encouraging and empowering new activists. A major strategic challenge is the decision to pursue incremental or radical change, concomitantly balancing the potential costs with prospective gains of either strategy. Ralston and Keeble (2009) provided an example of this challenge in their assessment of transnational collaborative efforts to improve the lives of Filipino prostitutes. Despite the fact that several of the partner activist organizations were steadfast in their commitment to the eradication of prostitution as a way to end sexual exploitation, Ralston and Keeble recognized that to have begun with the explicit goal of "eliminating prostitution in such an exploitative context … would have prevented the germination of a project like ours, where the process of harm reduction to women in the sex trade began" (p. 161). Although making some headway in their collaborative effort to build the capacity of Filipino groups working directly with prostitutes, these activists also came to recognize the significance of actions and change at the individual level, arguing that transcending differences to work for social justice involved both standing with others and changing individual minds, one person at a time.

The forces of globalization and its concomitant movement of people, goods, services, technology, information, and ideas across geographical and political borders have influenced both the form and focus of community activism. Today's community activists address local issues within the context of an increasingly globalized and interconnected world. There are enormous opportunities for ongoing activism and engagement to overcome environmental, economic, and social inequalities and injustice on many fronts, and the ability to transcend local boundaries and become part of global movements is both a challenge and an opportunity. The growth of the activist movement against gender-based violence is an example of the opportunities for local activism to translate into global action and policy change. In communities across the globe, activists have worked to raise awareness about gender-based violence and to create and strengthen local resources to both support victims and prevent further violence against women and girls. The 16 Days of Activism campaign against gender violence is an example of a global network of community activists. This campaign originated with local activists who came together at the 1991 Women's Global Leadership Institute. An outcome of this event was the creation of the 16 Days campaign, anchored by November 25, International Day for the Elimination of Violence Against Women, and December 10, International Human Rights Day, and the symbolical linking of gender-based violence and the violation of human rights. As part of the early 16 Days campaigns, local activists circulated petitions and collected signatures that were instrumental in shaping the agenda of the 1993 World Conference on Human Rights in Vienna. In recent years, 16 Days campaign activists have focused on the intersections of HIV/AIDS and gender-based violence (Center for Women's Global Leadership, n.d.; The Joint United Nations Programme on HIV and AIDS [UNAIDS], 2006). Another example of transnational activism is the anti-sweatshop movement linking students, community residents, workers, and labor activists, in the United States and other countries. These activists work concomitantly to change the working conditions of workers, most of whom are women, and the creation of sweat-free business policies and practices in cities and campuses (Student Labor Action Coalition, n.d.; United Students against Sweatshops, n.d.).

Advances and expansion of communication technologies have enabled community activists to reach untapped audiences and disseminate interactive media. Components of online activism include public awareness and online advocacy, organization, mobilization, and action and reaction (Vegh, 2003). Activists have used a variety of Internet-based media, from email and blogs to YouTube, Twitter, Facebook, and mobile-based apps (e.g., Snapchat, Instagram) that allow users to share and embed pictures and video on social networking sites. The use of social media subverts traditional means of activism by creating a space for protest that can be difficult for those in authority to control or suppress. In an increasingly globalized world, activists from these virtual communities use social media to provide real-time access to events of political significance, enabling rapid and more synchronous mobilization and action. Although the accessibility of Internet-based media may be democratizing, it also has the potential for risks and negative outcomes. For example, law enforcement used one of numerous social media monitoring firms to monitor protestors' locations and activities in the aftermath of a 2014 police shooting in Ferguson, Missouri, using information scraped from Instagram, Twitter, and Facebook posts (Cagle, 2016; Leetaru, 2016). Additionally, dissemination of information via social media may have unintended consequences if that information is incorrect, and communities may coalesce around erroneous or inaccurate information. For nurses and health professionals, understanding the public health implications of social medial use is imperative. Consider, for example, the ramifications of increased infectious disease transmission associated with parents of young children basing the decision not to vaccinate their children on information gathered through social media (Salathé & Khandelwal, 2011).

Media literacy can be both the means and an end in community activism. Duncan-Andrade (2006) described how engaging youth in critical production of media texts can serve as a site for critique and analysis of urban social inequalities as well as a site of production for social change. A recent initiative of the Hesperian Foundation, the Community Action for Women's Health and Empowerment, combines the traditional print resource of a book with a web-based tool that will include examples of action strategies and community-based organizational tools from groups around the world with expertise in particular areas of women's health (Hesperian Foundation, 2009). Beyond employing information technology as a tool, another challenge global health activists face is to create access to appropriate technology, such as renewable energy sources (e.g., solar, wind) for remote rural health care clinics in developing countries. Of course, technology does not come without costs and challenges, which range from the investment costs, upkeep and maintenance, updates, and the costs of personnel and training. Ensuring intergenerational continuity of community work is another ongoing challenge among community activism movements (Naples, 1998). Thus, the work of successful community activists also includes encouraging, mentoring, and empowering new activists.

NURSES AS COMMUNITY ACTIVISTS

Nurses and other health professionals may be involved in activist endeavors as members of their local communities and in conjunction with their professional roles. The involvement of nurses in community activism is not surprising, given the shared ethics of care and social justice and the activism of early nursing leaders such as Florence Nightingale, Lillian Wald, and Lavinia Dock (Andrist, 2006; Drevdahl, 2006). In today's increasingly digital and global contexts, nurses around the world use a wide range of tools as they engage in grassroots to global activism to promote social, environmental, cultural, and health systems change (Beck, Dossey & Rushton, 2013; Digital and Online Activism, n.d.). As environmental health activists, nurses have led efforts to implement smoke-free workplace policies, create physical-activity–friendly neighborhood environments, establish and monitor standards for clean air and water, and mobilize communities impacted by environmental toxins and pollutants. Nurses have also joined in grassroots campaigns such as fire sprinkler mandates to promote public safety through legislation (Pertschuk et al., 2013). Within the women's health arena, examples of nurse-led activism include the establishment of community-based maternity care for underserved populations, implementation of hospital breastfeeding policies and practices, and advocacy and policy work in the areas of reproductive health and human trafficking. Nurse activists can be an important force for change within the health care system, as evidenced by recent efforts to implement policy and practice changes in the areas of patient safety, workplace injury prevention, and health care reform. The professional expectation that nurses be involved in policy development, implementation, and evaluation will require more nurses to develop an activist skill set in the future. As each new generation of nurses comes into practice, they must balance the need to sustain existing activist endeavors while addressing new challenges as they arise.

Opportunities for activism and social justice work exist across all types and configurations of communities. Every community faces the ongoing challenge of renewing the call to action, encouraging and empowering its members to engage and participate actively in the processes and institutions that shape their social and economic lives, their health, and their well-being.

DISCUSSION QUESTIONS

1. What are the aims of community activism? Give some examples of social, economic, environmental, or cultural changes that have resulted from local community activism.

2. What are the key concepts underlying community activism? Give examples of how each of these concepts applies to a specific context.

3. What are the characteristics of successful community activist movements? Using a specific activist movement as an example, illustrate these various processes.

4. What are the opportunities and challenges community activists face in an increasingly globalized and technological world?

REFERENCES

Andrist, L.C. (2006). The history of the relationship between feminism and nursing. In L. C. Andrist, P. K. Nicholas, & K. A. Wolf (Eds.), *A history of nursing ideas* (pp. 5–22). Sudbury, MA: Jones and Bartlett.

Beck, D., Dossey, B.M., & Rushton, C.H. (2013). Building the Nightingale Initiative for Global Health—NIGH: Can we engage and empower the public voices of nurses worldwide? *Nursing Science Quarterly, 26*(4), 336–371.

Blythe, A. (July 23, 2013). Moral Monday demonstrators focus on voter rights, education cuts. *Raleigh News & Observer.* Retrieved from www.newsobserver.com/2013/07/23/3049031_moral-monday-demonstrators-focus.html?rh=1.

Braveman, P. (2006). Health disparities and health equity: Concepts and measurement. *Annual Review of Public Health, 27,* 167–194.

Brewer, P.R., & Ley, B.L., (2011). Multiple exposures: Scientific controversy, the media, and public responses to bisphenol A. *Science Communication, 33*(1), 76–97.

Cagle, M. (2016). *Facebook, Instagram, and Twitter provided data access for a surveillance product marketed to target activists of color.* Retrieved from www.aclunc.org/blog/facebook-instagram-and-twitter-provided-data-access-surveillance-product-marketed-target.

Center for Women's Global Leadership. (n.d.). *About the 16 Days: What is the 16 Days of Activism Against Gender-Based Violence Campaign?* Retrieved from https://16dayscampaign.org/wp-content/uploads/2019/10/2019-Global-16-Days-Campaign-Guide-Final.pdf.

Cohen, D., de la Vega, R., & Watson, G. (2001). *Advocacy for social justice: A global action and reflection guide.* Bloomfield, CT: Kumarian Press.

Dale, A., & Newman, L. (2010). Social capital: A necessary and sufficient condition for sustainable community development? *Community Development Journal, 45*(1), 5–21.

Digital and Online Activism. (n.d.). Retrieved from https://en.reset.org/knowledge/digital-and-online-activism.

Drevdahl, D.J. (2006). The concept of community in nursing history: Its narrative stream. In L. C. Andrist, P. K. Nicholas, & K. A. Wolf (Eds.), *A history of nursing ideas* (pp. 83–96). Sudbury, MA: Jones and Bartlett.

Duncan-Andrade, J. (2006). Urban youth, media literacy, and increased critical civic participation. In S. Ginwright, P. Noguera, & J. Cammarota (Eds.), *Beyond resistance! Youth activism and community change: New democratic possibilities for* practice and policy for America's youth (pp. 149–169). New York: Routledge.

Freelon, D., McIlwain, C. & Clark, M. (2016). *Beyond the hashtags: #Ferguson, #Blacklivesmatter, and the online struggle for offline justice.* Center for Media and Social Impact, American University. Available at https://ssrn.com/abstract=2747066 or http://dx.doi.org/10.2139/ssrn.2747066.

Freire, P. (1970/1997). *Pedagogy of the oppressed* (20th anniversary ed.). Trans. Myra Bergman Ramos. New York: Continuum.

Freire, P. (1973/1993). *Education for critical consciousness.* Trans. Myra Bergman Ramos. New York: Continuum.

Gulaid, L.A., & Kiragu, K. (2012). Lessons learnt from promising practices in community engagement for the elimination of new HIV infections in children by 2015 and keeping their mothers alive: Summary of a desk review. *Journal of the International AIDS Society, 15*(Suppl 2), 1–8.

Hesperian Foundation. (2009). *Community action for women's health and empowerment.* Retrieved from www.hesperian.org/projects_inProgress_womensactionguide.php.

Hesse-Biber, S.N. (2007). Feminist research: Exploring the interconnections of epistemology, methodology, and method. In S. N. Hesse-Biber (Ed.), *Handbook of feminist research: Theory and praxis* (pp. 1–26). Thousand Oaks, CA: Sage.

Ivashkavich, O., Hilfinger Messias, D.K., Soltani, N., & Cayir, E. (2018). Mapping social and gender inequalities: An analysis of art and new media work created by adolescent girls in a juvenile arbitration program. In K.L. Morgaine & M. Capous-Desyllas (Eds.) *Creating social change through creativity: Anti-oppressive arts-based research methodologies* (pp. 151–170). Newbury Park, CA: Sage Publications.

Jennings, L., Hardee, S., & Messias, D.K.H. (2010). Addressing oppressive discourses and images of youth: Sites of possibility. In L.B. Jennings, P.C. Jewett, T.T. Laman, M.V. Souto-Manning, & J.L. Wilson (Eds.), *Sites of possibility: Critical dialogue across educational settings* (pp. 39–67). Cresskill, NJ: Hampton Press.

Jennings, L.B., Parra-Medina, D., Messias, D.K.H., & McLoughlin, K. (2006). Toward a theory of critical social youth empowerment. *Journal of Community Practice, 14*(1/2), 29–54.

The Joint United Nations Programme on HIV and AIDS. (2006). *Stop violence against women; stop HIV.* Retrieved from www.unaids.org/en/KnowledgeCentre/Resources/FeatureStories/archive/2006/20061127_Women_violence_en.asp.

Kaleem, J., & Agrawal, N. (February 23, 2018). These are the Florida students behind the movement to end gun violence. *Los Angeles Times.* Retrieved from www.latimes.com/nation/la-na-parkland-student-activists-20180223-htmlstory.html.

Larsen, S.C. (2004). Place, activism, and development politics in the Southwest Georgia United Empowerment Zone. *Journal of Cultural Geography, 22*(1), 27–49.

Leetaru, K. (2016). Geofeedia is just the tip of the iceberg: The era of social surveillance. *Forbes.* Retrieved from www.forbes.com/sites/kalevleetaru/2016/10/12/geofeedia-is-just-the-tip-of-the-iceberg-the-era-of-social-surveillance/#4d64d3245b90.

Lewis-Charp, H., Yu, H.C., & Soukamneuth, S. (2006). Civic activist approaches for engaging youth in social justice. In

S. Ginwright, P. Noguera, & J. Cammarota (Eds.), *Beyond resistance! Youth activism and community change: New democratic possibilities for practice and policy for America's youth* (pp. 21–35). New York: Routledge.

Lightfoot, J.D. (2008). Separate is inherently unequal: Rethinking commonly held wisdom. In A.H. Normore (Ed.), *Leadership for social justice: Promoting equity and excellence through inquiry and reflective practice.* (pp. 37–59). Charlotte, NC: Information Age Publishing.

Marcolongo, M. (2002). The good mothers: Romania's HIV/AIDS activists are mostly poor mothers of thousands of children who contracted the disease due to poor medical practices under the Ceausescu regime. *Alternatives Journal, 28*(2), 23–25.

Martin, D.G., Hanson, S., & Fontaine, D. (2007). What counts as activism? The role of individuals in creating change. *Women's Studies Quarterly, 35*(3–4), 78–94.

Messias, D.K.H., McLoughlin, K., Fore, E., Jennings, L., & Parra-Medina, D. (2008). Images of youth: Representations and interpretations by youth actively engaged in their communities. *International Journal of Qualitative Issues in Education, 21*(2), 159–178.

Mitra, D. L. (2008). Student voice or empowerment? Examining the role of school-based youth-adult partnerships as an avenue toward focusing on social justice. In A.H. Normore (Ed.), *Leadership for social justice: Promoting equity and excellence through inquiry and reflective practice* (pp. 195–214). Charlotte, NC: Information Age Publishing.

Montlake, S. (2009). People making a difference: After her husband disappeared, housewife Angkhana Neelepaichit became a human rights activist. *Christian Science Monitor, 101*(86), 47.

Nam, C. (2012). Implications of community activism among urban minority young people for education for engaged and critical citizenship. *International Journal of Progressive Education, 8*(3), 62–76.

Naples, N.A. (1998). *Grassroots warriors: Activist mothering, community work, and the War on Poverty.* New York: Routledge.

Pertschuk, M., Hobart, R., Paloma, M., Larkin, M.A., & Balbach, E.D. (2013). Grassroots movement building and preemption in the campaign for residential fire sprinklers. *American Journal of Public Health, 103*(10), 1780–1787.

Piot, P. (2006). *Diverse voices, common ground: Uniting the world against AIDS.* Speech at Georgetown University, Washington D.C. March 7, 2006. Retrieved from www.unaids.org/en/media/unaids/contentassets/dataimport/pub/speechexd/2006/20060307_sp_piot_georgetownuniversity_en.pdf.

Ralston, M., & Keeble, E. (2009). *Reluctant bedfellows: Feminism, activism, and prostitution in the Philippines.* Sterling, VA: Kumarian Press.

Ransby, B. (2003). *Ella Baker and the Black freedom movement: A radical democratic vision.* Chapel Hill: University of North Carolina Press.

Reichert, E. (2007). *Challenges in human rights: A social work perspective.* New York: Columbia University.

Salathé, M., & Khandelwal, S. (2011). Assessing vaccination sentiments with online social media: Implications for infectious disease dynamics and control. *PLoS Computational Biology, 7*(10), e1002199.

Sattler, B. (2018). *Why are nurses suing the EPA?* Retrieved from https://www.wsna.org/news/2018/why-are-nurses-suing-the-epa.

Sherrod, L.R. (2006). Promoting citizenship and activism in today's youth. In S. Ginwright, P. Noguera, & J. Cammarota (Eds.), *Beyond resistance! Youth activism and community change: New democratic possibilities for practice and policy for America's youth* (pp. 287–299). New York: Routledge.

Smith, R., & Lourie, B. (2009). *Slow death by rubber duck.* Berkeley, CA: Counterpoint.

Stovall, D. (2006). From hunger strike to high school: Youth development, social justice, and school formation. In S. Ginwright, P. Noguera, & J. Cammarota (Eds.), *Beyond resistance! Youth activism and community change: New democratic possibilities for practice and policy for America's youth* (pp. 97–109). New York: Routledge.

Student Labor Action Coalition. (n.d.). Retrieved from slacuw.com.

Tufekci, Z., & Wilson, C. (2012). Social media and the decision to participate in political protest: observations from Tahrir Square. *Journal of Communication, 62*(2), 363–379.

United Students Against Sweatshops. (n.d.). Retrieved from usas.org/tag/nike/.

Whiteman, D. (2003). Reel impact: How nonprofits harness the power of documentary film. *Stanford Social Innovation Review, 1*(1), 60–63.

Vegh, S. (2003). Classifying forms of online activism: The case of cyberprotests against the World Bank. In M. McCaughey & M.D. Ayers (Eds.), *Cyberactivism: Online activism in theory and practice* (pp. 71–96). New York: Routledge.

Wallerstein, N., Sanchez-Merki, V., & Verlade, L. (2005). Freirian praxis in health education and community organizing: A case study of an adolescent prevention program. In M. Minkler (Ed.), *Community organizing and community building for health* (2nd ed., pp. 218–239). New Brunswick, NJ: Rutgers University Press.

Whiteman, D. (2009). Documentary film as policy analysis: The impact of Yes, In My Backyard on activists, agendas, and policy. *Mass Communication and Society, 12*(4), 457–477.

Witt, E. (2018). "We're not your pawns": Parkland's Never Again movement meets the lawmakers. *The New Yorker.* Retrieved from www.newyorker.com/news/news-desk/were-not-your-pawns-parklands-never-again-movement-meets-the-lawmakers.

World Health Organization. (n.d.). *Backgrounder 3: Key concepts: Health inequity.* Retrieved from www.who.int/social_determinants/final_report/key_concepts_en.pdf.

ONLINE RESOURCES

The Body: HIV/AIDS Activist Central
www.thebody.com/index/govt/activist.html
GBV Prevention Network
www.preventgbvafrica.org
Race Forward
www.raceforward.org/?arc=1
Resilience—Building a World of Resilient Communities
www.resilience.org/about
16 Days of Activism Against Gender-Based Violence Campaign
www.cwgl.rutgers.edu/16days/home.html
Soul of the City
www.ellabakercenter.org/index.php?p=sotc

75

TAKING ACTION: From Sewage Problems to the Statehouse: Serving Communities

Mary L. Behrens

"All politics is local."

Thomas P. "Tip" O'Neill, former Speaker of the U.S. House of Representatives

I have practiced as a family nurse practitioner, pediatric clinical specialist, nurse educator, and staff nurse. Running for political office was not one of my career goals. However, my father was a good role model, as he served on our local school board for 12 years. I attended college in the 1960s during a period of student activism and protests; that experience influenced me also. But it was a problem in my town that sparked my work in politics.

SEWAGE CHANGED MY LIFE

My leap into the political arena came because of a call from an upset friend who lived on property along the river that ran through our community. She told me there was raw sewage on her lawn that was washing up from the river. She had called the health department. They told her to call the state Department of Environmental Quality. That state department referred her to the health department. Out of frustration, she called me.

SEEING IS BELIEVING

I drove to my friend's neighborhood and saw the raw sewage on people's lawns. My friend told me that it appeared like clockwork when everyone flushed their toilets and used their dishwashers in the morning and evening. I decided to take action. I contacted local daycare centers and learned that they had noticed an increase in diarrhea in the children. I then called the two local TV stations and three radio stations. I informed them of a serious problem on the river, and I gave them the time and location of a press conference I was planning.

At the press conference, I stated that I was a nurse and was concerned about the sewage being a serious health threat to citizens in our town. I discussed the increased diarrhea in children reported by local daycare centers. The news media representatives who attended my press conference could see the raw sewage and captured images with their cameras. The train was moving down the track! The city, the health department, and the state Department of Environmental Quality had to deal with the calls from the press and the citizens. Our local city government and the state had to provide funds to connect this housing development to city water and sewer to stop the pollution.

MY CAMPAIGNS

As I took action on the sewage problem, I attended several city council meetings. When I observed the city council in action, I thought to myself, "I can do this and bring a perspective to the council as a nurse, mother, and concerned citizen." At the next election, I ran for city council in my ward along with 13 other candidates. With the large field of candidates, I knew I had to run a strategic campaign to win. I had a good neighbor who had been involved in other campaigns and was eager to help me. We ran a strong grassroots campaign. I walked door to door every free minute I had. I accepted every invitation to speak to various organizations, filled out questionnaires from interest groups, and looked for opportunities to meet with the press. I used a simple one-page flyer discussing my leadership skills. This helped keep expenses down. At Halloween we handed out balloons that said, "Vote for Mary."

I won! Since 1983, I have held three elected offices: city councilor and mayor, chair of the county commission, and representative in the state legislature.

Being involved in my professional associations was important to these successes. Professional membership allows you to meet other nurses around your state, encouraging leadership development, visibility, and confidence. Many nursing organizations encourage political involvement and mentoring. I have served as president of the Wyoming Nurses Association and as second vice president and first vice president of the American Nurses Association (ANA). I also served as chair of the ANA Political Action Committee (PAC) and am the Wyoming representative for the American Association of Nurses Practitioners.

THE VALUE OF POLITICAL ACTIVITY IN YOUR COMMUNITY

At the local level, you have the opportunity to help address problems that affect people's lives. For example, a citizen came to a city council meeting one evening and said he wanted passing lanes on a street in the community. He had a persuasive personality and a reputation for getting what he wanted. His initial presentation was very convincing to other council members. But I lived in this neighborhood and was concerned about the safety implications of this proposal. Part of this street abutted a park where children played. Parents parked along the street to watch or pick up their children. If passing lanes were established in this area, speeds would increase, and the potential risk of a serious accident would rise. As a fellow council member, I asked every councilperson to visit the area, particularly in the late afternoon. All of the members voted against establishing passing lanes on the street.

AN OPPORTUNITY TO LEARN THE ROPES

The local community is an excellent starting place if you want to run for higher office. You can gain experience, confidence, name recognition, and respect. I had the chance to testify before the Federal Energy Regulatory Commission in Washington, DC about the high natural gas prices we were paying in our community. Because I was the only mayor to testify (the others providing testimony were senators, representatives, or governors), I was quoted and praised for bringing a refreshing perspective to the commission.

NETWORKING

As mayor, I worked with citizens, state legislators, and our state's congressional delegation in Washington, DC.

Richard B. (Dick) Cheney was our only representative in Congress when I served as mayor of Casper, Wyoming. I formed an important connection with him because of my mayoral service. This type of connection was an important part of my network when I decided to run for the state legislature and an international nursing endeavor.

Some of my work bridged both local and state-level work. I had joined the Seatbelt Coalition in Wyoming before running for the legislature. The coalition's mission was to educate Wyoming citizens about the need for seatbelt legislation and develop a model law for the Wyoming legislature to enact. As a freshman legislator, I cosponsored the first seatbelt legislation aimed at reducing fatalities on Wyoming highways. I also sponsored several pieces of legislation to help communities with high natural gas prices. My experience on the city council prepared me to hit the ground running with issues like this when I arrived at the Wyoming statehouse.

LEADERSHIP IN THE INTERNATIONAL COMMUNITY

I had traveled 12 times to do humanitarian work in Vietnam and had attended International Council of Nursing conferences. I was concerned about the nursing shortage, not just in the United States but also in the developing world. In 2006, I sent a one-page note to then–Vice President Cheney discussing how I might contribute to the World Health Assembly that meets annually in Geneva, Switzerland. I did not specify a year but rather how my experiences at the ANA and in Vietnam could add to the discussion for a future appointment.

I was invited to meet with the Vice President but had health issues that caused me to cancel. (I could not believe I had to do that!) I was so disappointed to have missed out on this opportunity but was surprised a few weeks later when I answered the phone.

Someone said, "This is the White House." I grabbed my chair. My mind raced: "Am I dreaming this?" The Vice President had recommended that I be part of the U.S. delegation to the World Health Assembly in 3 weeks. I notified the ANA and planned to work with Barbara Blakeney, then-ANA president, who would be attending also.

Soon I was involved in phone calls with staff on logistics and schedule. Before I knew it, I arrived in Geneva for the first meeting with the U.S. Secretary of Health and Human Services Michael Leavitt. I told staff I wanted to testify on behalf of the international nursing shortage (Fig. 75.1).

Representatives of several countries had testified before me and had discussed their struggle to find nurses to provide basic services. When it was my turn, I shared my concern about the lack of nurses worldwide, especially in

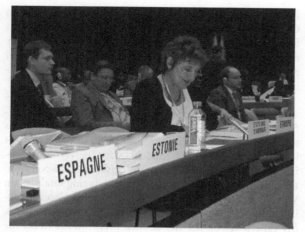

Fig. 75.1 Mary Behrens testifying at the World Health Assembly in Geneva, Switzerland.

countries in Africa. Several nurses came up to me afterward to thank me for my remarks.

MENTORING OTHER NURSES FOR POLITICAL ADVOCACY

In 2009 the ANA launched the first American Nurses Advocacy Institute, an annual year-long mentored program investing in growing nurses' competence in advocacy. Each year, state nurses' associations identify qualify candidates based upon previous grassroots experience and willingness to engage in either a project or series of activities designed to advance an initiative that pertains to the state nurses' association's legislative and regulatory agenda.

The program content resulted from dialogue by an ANA steering committee composed of members: nurse leaders/advocates. Face-to-face interactive sessions kick off the learning experience, followed by conference calls held every other month that permit continued engagement with ANA faculty and mentors. The calls provide member updates as well as an opportunity to delve more deeply into an advocacy tool or strategy. Examples of topics explored during the calls include: conducting a political environmental scan, bill analysis, preparing and delivering testimony, networking and coalition building, and communicating the value of a PAC.

Graduates of the program are also called upon to respond to federal initiatives, such as testimony delivered before the Senate Committee on Rural Health. Toni Decklever from the Wyoming Nurses Association graduated from the first ANA Institute and was invited to share the problems of access to primary care: 30 Million Patients and 11 Months to

Go: Who Will Provide Their Primary Care? (Watch the hearing at https://bit.ly/2Fr0hZp.) Toni is also a lobbyist for the Wyoming Nurses Association in the capitol in Cheyenne. It is important to mentor new young nursing leaders if nursing is to continue to have a strong political voice.

RECOMMENDATIONS FOR BECOMING INVOLVED IN POLITICS

Join a Political Party

You do not have to agree with every part of a party's political platform, but joining a political party is an important step in learning the ropes. Organized political parties provide support and guidance on how to get started with a political campaign. They can provide you with the opportunity to gain experience by working on someone's campaign before actually running yourself. You can learn the steps for running a grassroots campaign; for example, how much money you need to raise; what forms are required; how to organize a campaign committee; and how to access mailing lists, voter registration, and past precinct results. The parties also raise money, which is used to support the total slate of offices in that particular party. The party can help you to get your message out and reach all voters, especially those who might cross party lines.

Connect With Other Nurses

Nursing colleagues and associations can be extremely helpful in a political campaign. A group of nurses can send a powerful message of support when they back a candidate. Many state nurses associations have PACs to assist with endorsements and financial assistance.

Learn from Others in Your Community

Another helpful activity is to join the League of Women Voters. The name is derived from the women's suffrage movement, but currently membership is open to women and men. Local leagues will often hold public forums on various issues such as health care. It is a wonderful opportunity to contribute to the dialogue and make connections. The League of Women Voters is also concerned about getting the vote out and what motivates people to go to the polls.

Consider Serving on a Board

The *Future of Nursing: Campaign for Action,* formed with AARP and the Robert Wood Johnson Foundation, was instrumental in forming the Nurses on Boards Coalition (http://Nursesonboardscoalition.org), with the aim of getting 10,000 nurses on boards, commissions, task forces, and other health-related entities by 2020. This is an excellent way for you to gain leadership skills for public office, gain name recognition, and help your community to become healthier.

Develop Cost-Effective Campaign Strategies

When you are a candidate, you cannot be afraid to ask for money, and you need to take advantage of free and low-cost opportunities to get your message out. Flyers, mailing labels (usually the party you have joined will provide this at a bulk price), newspaper and radio advertisements, yard signs, and billboards all cost money. Press releases, letters to the editor, speaking at meetings and forums, meetings at neighborhood cafes, and news coverage are free. My least expensive campaign was my first race for city council. We produced a one-page flyer and distributed it door-to-door. Whenever you choose a strategy like this, it is important to be aware of laws and regulations so that you and your campaign staff do not run into problems. For example, you cannot leave flyers in a mailbox because it is a federal offense. If no one is at home, leaving a personal note stating "Sorry I missed you" can be an effective alternative. My husband made the political signs in our garage. It took a table saw, some nails, and stiff cardboard with my name and logo on it.

Get the Message Out

Getting out your message is critical to success. You must reach the voters. It does help to get some media training to help frame your messages. The press wants a good story and good sound bites, so your words should be carefully selected. Do not say anything you would not want to see in print or on TV. The press may not fully understand an issue, and you can help to frame the story with your nursing knowledge. If you provide accurate information, members of the media will look forward to contacting you again. I have learned from my experience. Do not be afraid to tell the TV crew that you want a head and chest only shot of you because you did not have time to change your clothes.

Serving as an elected official can be a very rewarding experience and a great opportunity for advocating for community health improvements. We need nurses serving at all levels of government. We need nurses working for safe schools and safe drinking water at the local level, working for safe highways and seatbelt use at the state level, and working for health care reform and funding for nursing education at the federal level.

You can view me talking more about my experience as a leader in policy in a YouTube video produced by the University of Wyoming, located at https://bit.ly/2Pvwotq.

76

TAKING ACTION: Contaminated Water and Elevated Blood Lead Levels in Flint

Loretta Jackson Brown[a]

"We're paying a pound of cure for things that an ounce of prevention would address."

Josh Simon

NURSES CALL TO ACTION IN LEAD CASE MANAGEMENT

I received a request asking nurses to help with case management for children with elevated blood lead levels (EBLLs) related to water contamination in Flint, Michigan. I thought to myself, "How is that even possible? Aren't there laws and regulations that govern water quality to prevent anything like this from happening?" After all,

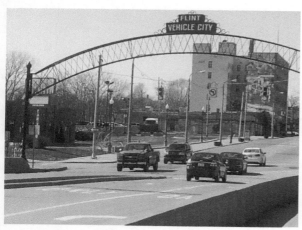

Downtown, Flint, Michigan.

---

[a]The findings and conclusions in this chapter are those of the author and do not necessarily represent the views of the Centers for Disease Control and Prevention and the Agency for Toxic Substances and Disease Registry.

having worked as a nephrology nurse, I was familiar with water quality standards. If I dialyzed my patients with contaminated water, I could kill them. I understood that responsibility and carried out my duties with the ethical code to do my patients no harm. This was not the case for the citizens of Flint. Instead, public officials contrived a plan to provide lower-quality water to some of the poorest populations through policies that gave them authority to do so. This decision resulted in a public health emergency that required federal resources, including deployment of nurses, to assist with health surveillance and patient education.

FLINT'S RICHES TO RAGS STORY

People told me that Flint was a food desert where the majority of the population lived in poor housing and were unemployed. Flint enjoyed a profitable place in the transportation industry for carriage manufacturing in the late 19th century to automobile production (General Motors was founded in Flint) in the 20th century, hence earning the nickname vehicle city. When the automobile industry sank during the recession in the 1980s, it sucked the wind out of Flint. The city in its postindustrial garb was deflated, having lost 77% of its manufacturing employment and 41% of employment overall since 1980 (Jacobs, 2009). This state of depression was palpable in childhood poverty, unemployment, violent crime, infant mortality, and overall poor health outcomes (University of Wisconsin Population Health Institute, 2016). No longer the automobile manufacturing hub, Flint had fallen on hard times and was deep in debt.

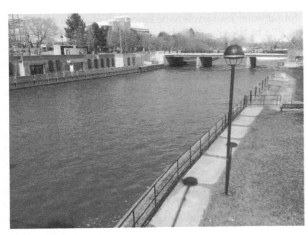

The Flint River.

STATE AND CITY FISCAL CHALLENGES

So how does deindustrialized, racially segregated Flint with its outdated infrastructure and impoverished communities generate enough revenue to provide essential public services while decreasing fiscal debt? I learned fiscal austerity is one approach state governments use to stabilize cash-strapped cities—they raise taxes, fees, or service costs for public amenities or trim spending (Peck, 2012). Moreover, when cities are severely fiscally strained, states can take action under emergency management laws by categorizing budget shortfalls as financial emergencies (Lee et al., 2016). In 2011, Michigan's governor used this approach to strip elected officials of their sovereignty, and granted it to an emergency manager (EM)—a non-elected, state-appointed authority who had no accountability to the citizens. The use of such policies to curtail spending in distressed, impoverished cities can further marginalize citizens and limit their ability to influence polices that impact their safety and well-being (Krings, Kornberg, & Lane, 2018).

DRINKING FROM THE LAKES AND THE RIVERS THAT YOU ARE USED TO

Since 1967, Flint received its water from Lake Huron via a Detroit water line. However, in April 2013, Flint's EM and other city leaders agreed to join the Karegnondi Water Authority (KWA), a group of local communities who collaborated to build a new water pipeline to Lake Huron as an economic savings. Unfortunately, Flint's contract with Detroit would expire two years before the completion of the KWA pipeline; therefore the EM recommended not renewing the Detroit contract and instead using the Flint River as a water source. In April 2014, Flint citizens began drinking water from the Flint River. Had the decision to use the Flint River been opened to public comments, residents most likely would have voted it down given the widespread belief that the river was an above ground cesspool.

What was it about the Flint River that made people fear it and was the trepidation legitimate? According to the 2003 water quality report (Sweat, Jodoin, Ross, & Brogren, 2003), the river had a high potential to breed contaminants and the city's water management system would need $25 million in upgrades to produce clean, safe water. Instead of investing dollars upfront to bring the water plant up to standards, the EM only allocated $3.8 million toward improvements. In hindsight, the water treatment preparation phase was woefully underfunded and would prove to be more costly in the end.

Shortly after switching water sources Flint began experiencing uncalculated consequences that would set off a domino effect impacting every household in the city. When the iron pipes were exposed to the highly corrosive water, the pipes corroded and released iron. The free iron reacted with chlorine that was added to destroy bacteria, hence making the chlorine unavailable to kill microorganisms. This resulted in elevated levels of bacteria. As bacteria counts climbed, water treatment experts added more chlorine disinfectant. This action led to elevated levels of trihalomethanes, a disinfection byproduct and carcinogen (Olson, 2016). Flint was cited by the Michigan Department of Environmental Quality for total coliform, *Escherichia coli*, and trihalomethanes violations (City of Flint, 2014). Moreover, one step in surface water treatment that Flint chose not to initiate was the addition of corrosion inhibitors. The decision would save Flint about $140 per day—or so they thought. Flint would soon learn the ramification of this penny wise, dollar foolish compromise.

Unaware of what was occurring at the water treatment plant, Flint residents began to complain that their tap water smelled, looked, and tasted bad. The EM dismissed their complaints and informed them that the water met quality standards, including the U.S. Environmental Protection Agency (EPA) Safe Drinking Water Act Lead and Copper Rule (Code of Federal Regulation, n.d.). Established in 1991, the rule regulates lead and copper in drinking water and, in essence, are an upstream approach to prevent a water contamination crisis. Water treatment plants are required by regulation to monitor these levels at the customer's end tap. When lead exceeds 15 parts per billion or copper exceeds 1.3 parts per million in more than 10% of samples, the city must take corrective actions to control corrosion, including notifying and educating the public. We would later learn that Flint violated this rule on several counts.

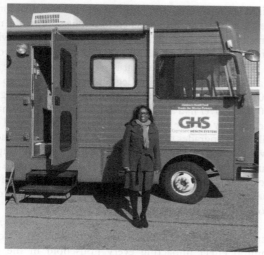
Loretta Jackson Brown at a community outreach event.

PUBLIC HEALTH AND CLINICAL CARE LINKAGE

Arriving in Flint, I quickly refreshed my knowledge of why lead was removed from so many products, what federal policies regulate environmental lead, and how levels are monitored and tested in children. Lead is a potent neurotoxin, and exposure to lead during early childhood can result in neurological and biological developmental disorders. Lead in drinking water is readily absorbed by the human body, particularly in children (40% to 50%) (Agency for Toxic Substances and Diseases Registry, 2007). In addition, lead is associated with spontaneous abortion and preterm birth in pregnant women and is linked to low birth rates and fetal death (Edwards, 2013; Sen et al., 2015).

There is no safe blood lead level, yet there are half a million U.S. children ages 1 to 5 with EBLL above 5 mcg/dL (Harvey, 2002). The children of Flint are among the most susceptible. Many reside in old, dilapidated housing, are from low-income families, and are members of racial/ethnic minority groups. When families learned how lead was affecting their children, it sparked a change in policy.

A PEDIATRICIAN'S OBSERVATION FORCES THE RETURN TO DETROIT WATER

Flint's mayor, EM, and other officials continued to deny there was a water quality problem. They even refused to give credibility to Virginia Tech University researchers who found water lead levels to be twice as high as those reported to EPA by the city (Pieper et al., 2018). However, a study led by Dr. Mona Hanna-Attisha, the director of Flint's Hurley Medical Center Pediatric Residency Program, showed a statistically significant difference in blood lead levels before (2.4%) and after (4.9%) Flint water switch. (Hanna-Attisha, LaChance, Sadler, & Champney Schnepp, 2016). Even more astounding was the increase in the number of children with EBLL (up from 4.0% to 10.6%) who resided in areas found to have high water lead levels by Virginia Tech University researchers (as high as 13,200 ppb). Flint officials could no longer refute the claims that Flint water was contaminated. On October 1, 2015, the Michigan Department of Health and Human Services announced that blood lead levels in children had spiked since Flint began using the river as a water source. The city returned to Detroit water on October 16, 2015.

COMMUNICATING LEAD HEALTH PROTECTIVE BEHAVIORS IN A COMMUNITY WHEN TRUST IS ERODED

Shortly before I deployed to Flint in March 2016, it was revealed that lead and *E. coli* were not the only contaminants lurking in Flint's water—*Legionella pneumophila*, a pneumonia-causing bacterium, was also present (Schwake, Garner, Strom, Pruden, & Edwards, 2016). In January 2016, it was revealed that the increase in Legionnaires disease, totaling 91 cases with 11 deaths from June 2014 to October 2015, was associated with contaminated water from the Flint River. What also became known was that the city's water specialist intentionally flushed pipes in residents' homes before collecting water samples, a clear violation of the EPA's protocol.

I arrived in Flint under a shroud of finger pointing and cover-ups. I immediately sensed feelings of mistrust between many groups. I knew I was an outsider in this community and if I wanted to help, I would first have to prove that I was trustworthy. To do this, I relied on the position that nurses held in the public's eye, one of the most trusted professional groups. My initial introduction when calling upon family included an opening sentence that said, "I'm a nurse." Using principles of emergency risk communication, I expressed empathy when interacting with local public health professionals and with families. In addition, I established rapport by keeping the local public health nurses informed about what I was doing, shared data on home visits with them daily, and sought out their advice for the best way to approach contact-tracing obstacles. By showing respect to families who allowed me to visit their homes, I was able to share lead prevention education with them.

FLINT FORWARD

The Flint water fiasco is a modern-day tragedy of people, politics, and polluted water for which the full impact will not be known for decades. In an attempt to get Flint financially fit, policies devised in times of austerity decapitated the voice of the people, disarmed city council members, and empowered EMs to make decisions about the people yet without the people. This public health injustice and conspiracy of silence resulted in criminal charges against 15 people, including a former Michigan state health and human services director for his connection with the deaths from the Legionnaires outbreak (Brush & Winowiecki, 2017). Numerous groups have filed lawsuits against public officials and public agencies. Flint citizens were on a bottled water program for almost 30 months, and hundreds of millions of federal and private dollars will be spent on plumbing infrastructure upgrades.

CALLING ALL NURSES: POWER OF THE PRACTITIONER

In the end, had it not been for a mother's intuition, a researcher's investigation, and a pediatrician's observations, the forgotten city of Flint might have just perished without anyone even caring. The Flint water crisis rung the bell to remind us not to sleep on policies. Although policy informs practice, it should have never been the sole driver. The people's voice and the practitioner's assessment are essential to the process of deciding what policies protect the health of a community. There are many cities across the United States at risk for environmental injustice. Public health nurses and clinical nurses can work together to improve health equity by helping to create systems whereby population data, social determinants of health, and clinical trends are examined and shared. By using data to drive change, nurses can better influence policies that affect the safety, well-being, and health of a community.

▌ DISCUSSION QUESTIONS

1. The water crisis in Flint resulted from failures in federal, state, and local polices. How should a checks-and-balances system be structured to better safeguard the health of a community when emergency management laws are enacted?
2. A U.S. public law established the World Trade Center (WTC) Health Program to provide free medical care for responders and survivors at the WTC, Pentagon, and Shanksville, PA. Should the United States create a similar program for the citizens of Flint?

REFERENCES

Agency for Toxic Substances and Diseases Registry. (2007). *Toxicological profile for lead*. Retrieved from www.atsdr.cdc.gov/toxprofiles/tp13.pdf.

Brush. M., & Winowiecki, E. (June 16, 2017). These are the 15 people charged for their connection to the Flint water crisis. *Michigan Radio*. Retrieved from www.michiganradio.org/post/update-these-are-15-people-charged-their-connection-flint-water-crisis.

City of Flint. (2014). *Annual water quality report*. Retrieved from www.cityofflint.com/wp-content/uploads/CCR-2014.pdf.

Code of Federal Regulation. (n.d.). *Title 40 protection of environment: Part 141 national primary drinking water regulations*. Retrieved from www.ecfr.gov/cgi-bin/text-idx?SID=531617f923c3de2cbf5d12ae4663f56d&mc=true&node=sp40.23.141.i&rgn=div6.

Edwards, M. (2013). Fetal death and reduced birth rates associated with exposure to lead-contaminated drinking water. *Environmental Science & Technology, 48*(1), 739-746.

Hanna-Attisha, M., LaChance, J., Sadler, R. C., & Champney Schnepp, A. (2016). Elevated blood lead levels in children associated with the Flint drinking water crisis: A spatial analysis of risk and public health response. *American Journal of Public Health, 106*(2), 283-290.

Harvey, B. (2002). *Managing elevated blood lead levels among young children: Recommendations from the Advisory Committee on Childhood Lead Poisoning Prevention*. Atlanta: Centers for Disease Control and Prevention.

Jacobs, A.J. (2009). The impacts of variations in development context on employment growth: A comparison of central cities in Michigan and Ontario, 1980-2006. *Economic Development Quarterly, 23*(4), 351-371.

Krings, A., Kornberg, D., & Lane, E. (2018). Organizing under austerity: How residents' concerns became the Flint water crisis. *Critical Sociology*. Retrieved from doi:0896920518757053.

Lee, S.J., Krings, A., Rose, S., Dover, K., Ayoub, S., & Salman, F (2016). Racial inequality and the implementation of emergency manager laws in economically distressed urban areas. *Children and Youth Services Review, 70,* 1–7.

Olson, T. (2016). The science behind the Flint water crisis: Corrosion of pipes, erosion of trust. *The Conversation*. Retrieved from https://theconversation.com/the-science-behind-the-flint-water-crisis-corrosion-of-pipes-erosion-of-trust-53776.

Peck, J. (2012). Austerity urbanism: American cities under extreme economy. *City, 16*(6), 626-655.

Pieper, K., Martin, R.L., Tang, M., Walters, L., Parks, J., Roy, S., ... & Edwards, M.A. (2018). Evaluating water lead levels during the Flint water crisis. *Environmental Science & Technology, 52,* 8124−8132.

Schwake, D.O., Garner, E., Strom, O.R., Pruden, A., & Edwards, M.A. (2016). Legionella DNA markers in tap water coincident with a spike in Legionnaires' disease in Flint, MI. *Environmental Science & Technology Letters, 3*(9), 311-315.

Sen, A., Heredia, N., Senut, M. C., Land, S., Hollocher, K., Lu, X, ,... & Ruden, D. M. (2015). Multigenerational epigenetic inheritance in humans: DNA methylation changes associated with maternal exposure to lead can be transmitted to the grandchildren. *Scientific Reports, 5*, 14466.

Sweat, M.J., Jodoin, R.S., Ross T.A., & Brogren, B.B. (2003). *The Michigan Source-Water Assessment Program: Methods used for the assessment of surface-water supplies.* Water-Resources Investigations Report 03-4134. U.S. Geological Survey. Retrieved from https://pubs.usgs.gov/wri/2003/4134/report.pdf.

University of Wisconsin Population Health Institute. (2016). *County health rankings and roadmaps: Building a culture of health, county by county.* [Data file]. Retrieved from www.countyhealthrankings.org/app/michigan/2016/overview.

ONLINE RESOURCES

American Academy of Pediatrics: Lead Exposure and Lead Poisoning
www.aap.org/en-us/advocacy-and-policy/aap-health-initiatives/lead-exposure/Pages/default.aspx

Centers for Disease Control and Prevention: Childhood Lead Poisoning Prevention
www.cdc.gov/nceh/lead/acclpp/blood_lead_levels.htm

Low Level Lead Exposure Harms Children: A Renewed Call for Primary Prevention: Report of the Advisory Committee on Childhood Lead Poisoning Prevention
www.cdc.gov/nceh/lead/acclpp/final_document_030712.pdf

U.S. Environmental Protection Agency: Lead Policy and Guidance
www.epa.gov/lead/lead-policy-and-guidance

77

Creating a Culture of Health and Working With Communities

Clair Millet and Renee S. Frauendienst

"The day may soon dawn when we Americans can enjoy a measure of life and health that is consistent with our extraordinary resources and the intelligence of our people. The pioneers have begun their work; it is far from finished. New fields, new enterprises, are visible. The times call for the high spirit of the courageous pioneers among physicians, scientists, and nurses."

Lillian Wald

HEALTH CARE IN THE UNITED STATES

The United States has a very unique and complex health care delivery system that is unlike any other health care system in the world. It is comprised of a governmental and nongovernmental system of care with a multitude of organizations and providers involved in the delivery of preventive, primary, acute, and rehabilitative care to individuals, families, groups, and communities. The structure of the health care system is derived from the influence of policy that continues to shape the health care delivery system. The focus of health care is generally on access, quality of care, equity, cost effectiveness, and population health.

The U.S. health care system, although described as one of the best systems in the world, exhibits several problems such as high costs, health disparities, high uninsured rates, and quality concerns. The United States pales in comparison to other similar high-income countries regarding measures of health outcomes and life expectancy. As U.S. life expectancy increases, so does the incidence of chronic illness and comorbidities. This vast array of problems has led to numerous reform policies and calls to action for change.

The United States has made significant progress during the past century in improving the health and longevity of its population. Smoking prevalence rates and the proportion of people without health insurance have been considerably reduced. Health reform has improved health care quality and the growth rate of health care-related costs has slowed. However, this success falls short of ensuring that everyone can achieve an optimal and equitable level of health.

INTEGRATED CARE

Defined models of care are integral to optimal health and resilience. Integrated service delivery is "the organization and management of health services so that people get the care they need, when they need it, in ways that are user-friendly, achieve the desired results and provide value for money." (World Health Organization, 2008). Integrated care is best seen as a continuum as opposed to being integrated or not integrated. It involves considerations about the arrangement and linkage of various desirable tasks which need to be achieved in order to provide a population with quality health services. Integrated care can look disparate at different service levels and there can be and are many possible variations from one community to another. For the consumer, integration means health care that is seamless and easy to navigate which contributes to better compliance and outcomes. The significant challenge is to be unambiguous about what integrated services look like in different settings and how integration can contribute to the intended aim of people getting the care they need. Health services and systems need to be better integrated to deliver high-quality care. Subsequently, communities must create the conditions that promote health and equity, and collaborations must occur across sectors and must be focused on improving well-being.

CULTURE OF HEALTH

Health begins where we are—in our homes, schools, workplaces, places of worship, neighborhoods, and communities. In 2014, the Robert Wood Johnson Foundation (RWJF) implemented a vision to engage all Americans in a national movement to build a Culture of Health that gives all members of our society the opportunity to lead healthier lives (Plough, 2014). A Culture of Health means that everyone has an opportunity to be healthier. This initiative requires addressing the social determinants of health and removing obstacles that affect the health and well-being of individuals. The social determinants include poverty, discrimination, and their consequences, including powerlessness and lack of access to good jobs with fair pay, quality education, housing, safe environments, and health care (U.S. Department of Health and Human Services [HHS], Healthy People 2020, 2013).

RWJF's Culture of Health is essentially an action framework that focuses on well-being and equity with the goal of empowering and supporting people to lead healthier lives now and in generations to come (Plough, Chandra, Leviton, Miller, Orleans, Trujillo, & Yeung, 2015). The overall goal of the Culture of Health initiative is to improve the nation's population health, well-being, and equity through activities in four different action areas: (1) making health a shared value; (2) fostering cross-sector collaboration to improve well-being; (3) creating healthier, more equitable communities; and (4) strengthening integration of health services and systems (Plough, Chandra, Leviton, Miller, Orleans, Trujillo, & Yeung, 2015).

Each of these four action areas includes a number of "drivers," which are the factors to advance a Culture of Health. RWJF describes these drivers as a set of investment priorities that are deemed important areas for activity in the action area, which are required for sustained health improvement and well-being (Chandra et al., 2016). For example, within the action area of "making health a shared value," the drivers include mindset and expectations, sense of community, and civic engagement. Each of the action areas also includes a set of measures against which Culture of Health–related outcomes can be followed.

ROLE OF NURSES IN CULTURE OF HEALTH

Implementing a Culture of Health will require new roles for nurses. Building a Culture of Health is consistent with the nursing profession's vital role in the health care system and nurses' contributions to wellness, health promotion, and disease prevention. Nurses must apply a holistic approach toward treating patients within the context of their communities. Nurses play a significant role in health at the individual, family, and population levels. They often work where people live, work, play, and learn. Nurses can be ambassadors leading a Culture of Health. Typically, nurses are fully immersed in their patients' lives and care and guide them in innovative ways to improved health. Nurses must better understand their unique role in a Culture of Health and how it intersects and integrates with the current state of communities and their capabilities.

WORKING WITH COMMUNITIES TO TRANSFORM HEALTH CARE

Health care in the United States has been on a transformation journey for many years. The Triple Aim for Healthcare frames the need for change in terms of impacting cost, patient experience, and population health. In addition, current pressures from regulators, such as government and payers, are influencing care within the four walls of a facility in the form of financial incentives, regulatory constraints, and performance improvement activities (Bohmer, 2016).

Research also elucidates that at least 80% of what makes a person healthy does not happen in a building, but rather outside through social and economic factors, physical environment, and health behaviors (Minnesota Department of Health, 2014). The Centers for Medicare and Medicaid Services (CMS) describes these factors that negatively impact well-being as unmet social and economic needs such as food insecurity and inadequate or unstable housing. They go on to state that these factors may increase risks of chronic disease, reduce a person's inability to manage health conditions, increase costs, and lead to avoidable health care usage (CMS, 2017). In order for true reform and positive movement toward healthier communities to happen, these two drivers need to come together.

In the RWJF Culture of Health framework, not only is cross-sector collaboration one of the four action areas in the structure, the Future of Nursing Campaign for Action places nursing in the forefront to making these changes happen. With nurses being the largest profession in health care and one of the most trusted occupations in the society, where better should nurses lead the way than between the intersect of care and community.

These nurse-led efforts are being seen in health care today across the United States in both rural and urban settings. The growing number of collaborative efforts highlights the impact and effectiveness of community-based interventions. Health care teams made up of nurse practitioners, community health workers, and physician consultants have successfully reduced blood pressure in some African American communities. Community nurses are working in the school settings to combat human immunodeficiency virus (HIV) infection through risk reduction interventions, and nurse-managed health care centers (NMHC) care for millions of at-risk persons across the United States. These types of interdisciplinary collaborative efforts in medically underserved areas help create lasting and trusting relationships which ultimately leads to change (Montalvo, Torrisi, Hanson-Turton & Birch, 2011).

HOSPITAL PARTNERSHIPS AND TRANSITIONS OF CARE

Now more than ever nurses practice in a wide variety of settings and are increasingly performing a broad range of tasks. They serve in the roles of care coordination, chronic disease management, and care transition inside health care settings but also lead and support other efforts that impact the health outcomes outside of facilities (private and public) such as community care, home visitation, and population health management efforts. Effective transitions in care may help to reduce health care expenditures, improve patient outcomes, and increase patient satisfaction. When transitions in care are managed, the outcome for patients is improving quality of life and ultimately decreasing readmissions (Lovelace et al., 2016). Bringing this menagerie of complex activities together is challenging (Martsolf, Gordon, May, Mason, Sullivan & Villarruel, 2016).

Subsequently, innovative models of care that blend community and nurses together begin to address this massive need for coordinated change and focus on creating a culture of health that helps to answer the future question on how to improve the health of the community. The American Academy of Nursing's Edge Runner Program distinguishes nurses who have designed innovative models of care to address today's health care challenges and unmet needs. These models typically demonstrate positive clinical and financial outcomes and will be necessary for creating a Culture of Health and working with communities.

Examples of such models are those such as Sharon Rising's Centering Pregnancy model or Sandee McClowry's INSIGHTS model. The Centering Pregnancy model is a nurse-designed care model that integrates prenatal care, social support, and education in group visits for women due at the same time in a group setting (Martzolf et al., 2016, p. 18). The model provided for a reduction in preterm birth, higher patient satisfaction with increased breastfeeding rates, and improved knowledge and readiness for birth and parenting. It also demonstrated significant cost reductions (Mason, Jones, Roy, Sullivan & Wood, 2015).

The INSIGHTS model of care is an evidence-based intervention with teacher, parent, and classroom programs that work synergistically to support children's social emotional development and academic learning. It is an evidence-based intervention that is a temperament-based, social-emotional learning intervention aimed at improving

academic achievement by reducing disruptive behaviors and enhancing children's self-regulation (Martzolf et al., 2016). Both models are nurse-designed and contribute to a Culture of Health.

A 2016 qualitative review of 39 American Academy of Nursing Edge Runner innovative care models determined that not only were they able to meet the established criteria for designation, but almost all (87%) also focused on activities related to least one aspect of the four action areas set forth by RWJF's Culture of Health. The review also found that strengthening integration of health services and systems appeared in 87% of these care models. Programs that focus on wellness in businesses, senior wellness, telemedicine, breastfeeding, and access to care in rural settings include community-based locations, multidisciplinary team members, and nurse leadership at some level (Martzolf et al., 2016).

Sometimes these partnerships seem outside of health's realm and yet when looked at more closely, the connections between health and the social factors in a community are clearly there. For example, community development, historically focusing on affordable housing, economic development, and community facilities, may be a prolific collaboration. Several examples of connections between community development, health care, and public health have shown impactful results. Everything from nonprofit affordable housing to economic growth addressing food deserts to funding and developing transportation investments can work toward addressing the determinants of health that impact special populations or locations (Erickson & Andrews, 2011).

DETERMINANTS OF COMMUNITY HEALTH ASSESSMENT TOOLS AND RESOURCES

In the passage of the Patient Protection and Affordable Care Act (ACA), not-for-profit hospitals are required to complete a Community Health Needs Assessment (CHNA) every 3 years and then develop strategies to address those needs (Artiga & Hinton 2018). These assessments require broad input from partners, both public and private, in the community including those with community/public health knowledge or expertise. Community health assessment may also elucidate not only available resources but also scarce or needed resources necessary for health and resilience.

Other initiatives and strategic partnerships that seek to improve health should also be examined and implemented where appropriate. In October 2016, the Office of the Assistant Secretary for Health released a set of recommendations to achieve Public Health 3.0, which is a paradigm for public health transformation that calls on local public health infrastructure to ensure the conditions in which everyone can be healthy (HHS Office of the Assistant Secretary, 2016). Changes to policies, systems, and environments most often begin with local actions. Communities must engage new partners and occasionally introduce innovative methodologies to improve health.

At the same time, governmental public health agencies, either as outlined in state statute or as a result of Public Health Accreditation, are required to participate in or lead a collaborative process in a comprehensive community health assessment, identify trends, and develop recommendations for policy, programs, processes, or interventions (Public Health Accreditation Board [PHAB], 2013).

The joining of these initiatives not only reduces duplication of efforts, but can create a synergy within communities that sets the health agenda to be addressed. The North Carolina Public Health/Hospital Collaborative is an exemplar that promotes effective community coordination. Goals of the partnership include creating common understanding, models of effective collaboration, and developing a national model between local public health, hospitals, and other partners (Association of State and Territorial Health Officials [ASTHO], 2013). With Registered nurses still the largest single profession within the public health workforce (National Association of County and City Health Officials [NACCHO], 2011), leadership of these initiatives by nurses can really make a difference in setting both the public and private health agendas.

BUILDING A SENSE OF COMMUNITY AND CIVIC ENGAGEMENT TO ADDRESS POPULATION HEALTH IN TRANSFORMING HEALTH CARE

Health is much more than access to medical care. Health starts in those places where we live, work, play, and learn (HHS, Healthy People 2020, 2013). That means that not only do nurses and other partners in the community need to be engaged in creating change, but the average citizen must also participate in solutions. Individuals must have a sense that he or she has a personal connection to the community, that the community matters to him or her, and that the shared experiences with others are critical for their own well-being (Chandra et al., 2016). There is greater cohesion and the ability to mobilize to communal action with a robust sense of community. RWJF Culture of Health identifies this as the first of the four action areas where communities not only view health as a priority but also are engaged in improving health (Marztsolf et al., 2016).

Notably, in order for ordinary citizens to be involved in change, there needs to be a paradigm shift in sense of community and civic engagement. This shift needs to include understanding citizens and citizenship; the role of professionals in not only engaging the community in the work being done, but as professionals being engaged; the nature of government; and the meaning of democracy (Boyte, 2008). Civic engagement is a very important component of the shared value of health because actions such as community mobilization can influence the importance that people place on investments in health and well-being (Chandra et al., 2016). In a recent RWJF Culture of Health Public Health Nurse Leader project, five students from two local Minnesota nursing programs completing internships at the CentraCare facility of the St. Cloud Hospital were engaged in a project attempting to develop a sense of community and civic engagement in nurses bound for the bedside. The goals of the project included building a foundation around health equity and the determinants of health by activating their own sense of empowerment for change through civic engagement and building a sense of community in their practice. A curriculum was designed to attempt to impact these nursing students by teaching key concepts around personal values, health equity, determinants of health, personal and public narratives, and civic skills that create civic agencies (Boyte, 2008). These concepts were taught using a teaching cycle of content, activity, and reflection with the intent of influencing not only how nurses function at the bedside, but also to instill action through civic engagement in the community both professionally and personally. Successful civic engagement requires both individual and organizational involvement.

ADVOCACY AND POLICY DEVELOPMENT TO STRENGTHEN CULTURE OF HEALTH

Policy can serve as a vehicle for progress in nursing practice and health. Regrettably, many nurses allow policy to happen around them and do not get involved in the process. Nurses possess knowledge, skills, and experience to influence the development of policy and can assume many roles in the policymaking process. Policy must become a means to not only enhance nursing practice, but an effective mechanism to assist in meeting the health care needs of our communities. It is the only way to be an effective advocate as advocacy requires working through decision makers to achieve desirable outcomes. It is crucial that nurses understand the political process both individually and through their professional organizations, as this can have a direct influence at the local, regional, state, or national levels.

CONCLUSION

Health in all policies should be considered as a strategy for addressing the complex factors that influence health and equity. It is extremely evident that transformation of health care and innovation is critically needed. Nurses are champions in community health improvement. In order for transformation to be meaningful and impactful, nurses and communities need to come together. When that happens, we will see the ability of ordinary people to be agents and architects of their own lives and communities working together on common challenges for the good of all with nurses leading the way.

DISCUSSION QUESTIONS

1. What are ways that nurses can transcend the four walls of an institution to engage at the community level?
2. What are the ways in which a population health focus might be applied in transforming the health care delivery system?
3. How can nurses and policy impact the development of a Culture of Health?

REFERENCES

Artiga, S., & Hinton, E. (May 10, 2018). *Beyond health care: The role of social determinants in promoting health and health equity. [Issue brief]*. Henry J. Kaiser Family Foundation. Retrieved from www.kff.org/disparities-policy/issue-brief/beyond-health-care-the-role-of-social-determinants-in-promoting-health-and-health-equity/.

Association of State and Territorial Health Officials. (2013). *North Carolina public health/hospital collaborative members work to promote effective community collaboration.* Retrieved from www.astho.org/North-Carolina-CHNA-Case-Study/.

Bohmer, R.M.J. (2016). The hard work of health care transformation. *New England Journal of Medicine, 375*(8), 709-711.

Boyte, H.C. (2008). *The citizen solution.* Minnesota Historical Society. St. Paul, MN: Kettering Foundation.

Centers for Medicare and Medicaid Services. (2017). *Accountable health communities (AHC) model assistant and alignment tracks participant selection.* Retrieved from www.cms.gove/Newsroom/MediaReleaseDatabase/Fact-sheets/2017-Fact-Sheet-items/2017-04-06.html.

Chandra, A., Acosta, J., Carmean, K.G., Debowitz, T., Leviton, L., Martin, L.T., ... & Plough, A.L. (2017). Building a national culture of health: Background, action framework, measures and next steps. *Rand Health Quarterly, 6*(2), 6.

Chandra, A., Miller, C., Acosta, J., Weilant, S., Trujillo, M. & Plough, A. (November, 2016). Drivers of health as a shared value: Mindset, expectations, sense of community, and civic engagement. *Health Affairs, 35*(11), 1959-1963.

Erickson, D., & Andrews, N. (November, 2011). Partnerships among community development, public health, and health care could improve the well-being of low-income people. *Health Affairs, 30*(11), 2056-2063.

Lovelace, D., Hancock, D., Hughes, S., Wyche, P., Jenkins, C., & Logan, C. (2016). A patient-centered transitional care case management program: Taking case management to the streets and beyond. *Professional Case Management, 21,* 277-290.

Martzolf, G.R., Gordon, T., May, L.W., Mason, D., Sullivan, C., & Villarruel, A. (2016). Innovative nursing care models and culture of health: Early evidence. *Nursing Outlook, 64,* 367-376.

Mason, D.J., Jones, D.A., Roy, C., Sullivan, C.G., & Wood, L. (October, 2015). Commonalities of nurse-designed models of health care. *Nursing Outlook, 63*(5), 540-553.

Minnesota Department of Health. (2014). *Advancing health equity in Minnesota: Report to the legislature.* Retrieved from www.health.state.mn.us/divs/che/reports/ahe_leg_report_020114.pdf.

Montalvo, W., Torrisi, D., Hanson-Turton, T., & Birch, S., (2011). Nurses close the gap in community health. In *The future of nursing: Leading change, advancing health* (pp. 428-431). Institute of Medicine of the National Academies. Washington, DC: National Academies Press.

National Association of County and City Health Officials (2011). *Local public health workforce benchmarks.* Retrieved from www.naccho.org/uploads/downloadable-resouces/local-public-health-workforce-staffing-benchmarks.pdf.

Plough, A., Chandra, A., Leviton, L., Miller, C., Orleans C.T., Trujillo, M., & Yeung D. (2015). *From vision to action: A framework and measures to mobilize a Culture of Health.* Princeton, NJ: Robert Wood Johnson Foundation.

Plough, A.L. (2014). Building a culture of health: Challenges for the public health workforce. *American Journal of Preventive Medicine, 47*(5S3), S388-S390.

Public Health Accreditation Board. (2013). *Public Health Accreditation Board standards: An overview.* Retrieved from www.phaboard.org/wp-content/uploads/StandardsOverview1.5_Brochure.pdf.

U.S. Department of Health and Human Services, Healthy People 2020. (2013). *Improving the health of Americans.* Retrieved from http://healtypeople.gov.

U.S. Department of Health and Human Services, Office of the Assistant Secretary for Health. (2016). *Public health 3.0: A call to action to create a 21st century public health infrastructure.* Retrieved from www.healthypeople.gov/ph3.

78

TAKING ACTION: Activism: A Community Rises

Lucia Judith Alfano

"You must do the thing you think you cannot do."

Eleanor Roosevelt

In graduate school in the spring of 2013, I was given an assignment to read the Institute of Medicine (2011) report, *The Future of Nursing: Leading Change, Advancing Health*. I read it three times and decided that this would be my guide for how I would advocate for nursing and for all people for the rest of my days. This experience was comparable to one I experienced in 1998 when I read the book of Matthew in the Holy Bible. The apostle Matthew quotes Jesus on life lessons and details the purpose of one's existence on earth.

What happened in 1998 and 2013 to me were pivotal moments in my life. Both these periods, in different forms, ignited and propelled me to move forward an agenda of advocacy for social justice, finding ways to help people improve their lives. In 1998, I was leading a church program that helped those who were unemployed or did not speak English and needed translation of important documents. In 2001, I was in nursing school and served as president of the student nurses association, when I determined it was unjust for nursing students not to have mentoring and tutoring. So, I implemented a detailed, successful mentoring and tutoring program that would expand to be state of the art today.

But my advocacy continued as a nurse. During my first nursing job on an oncology-medical unit, I realized that the family members of patients I cared for did not have support groups. We had an outpatient oncology clinic, and I made it my mission to initiate the hospital's first support group for oncology patients' family members. I volunteered for this, as the institution did not find value or need for it, but I definitely did.

Years of practice as a public health nurse has helped me understand the value of education—for myself, for patients, and for other nurses. Advocacy, however, has served as a powerful tool to help me promote equity. I advocated for nurses who did not have a voice or were terrified to speak up. I was never afraid to speak up for what was right, so I served as an unflinching union delegate for nurses. This did bring me some negative consequences, such as not being liked or not considered for promotion—but it never stopped me. There was a time when I had to make a choice—do I choose moving up in my career or advocate for better work conditions for nurses? I chose to fight for better work conditions and represent nurses who would not speak up for themselves. I knew if I fought hard enough, if I spoke up, showed evidence and helped come up with solutions, nurses would benefit.

It was exhilarating for me to get nurses the pay they deserved for their services and support them as they grew as savvy and confident clinicians. One year, I represented Susan, a novice nurse who came to me because she was working 60 to 70 hours/week and only getting paid for 37 hours. This had been going on for several months for Susan and she only gathered enough courage to seek help when she was about to quit. I met with Susan various times to uncover the details and learn about her work style. Together, we gathered evidence and prepared to meet with administration to present the issue along with solutions. Susan received retroactive pay, her case load was decreased, and her territory was modified—all of which helped her succeed in her job. We were successful because Susan had the courage to seek help and we presented the issues at hand, the data to support our position, and solutions for the administration to consider.

FROM ADVOCACY TO SERVICE

After I transitioned to academia, I knew that the "service" component of my faculty role would be important to build. Thus far, I had advocated for patients, families, nurses, and myself, but I felt there was much more to do. With the lessons of *The Future of Nursing* at the forefront of every service project I got involved with, two concepts rose to the top: (1) interprofessional collaboration and (2) health equity. I thought to myself, how could I bring together my current role as educator and advocate for students, my passion for community, and an agenda that would be interprofessional and address health equity?

Serving the Hispanic Community Through Nursing

I grew up in a household where our Hispanic identity and culture were not celebrated. I recall my mother coaching me to lie about where we were born. In second grade, my teacher changed my ethnic name to an American nickname which was much easier to pronounce: "Lucy." There were times I would deny that I knew how to speak Spanish. I was not proud to be a Latina. My Hispanic heritage did not influence my career path—or so I believed. In fact, the help I provided to Hispanic communities was merely by chance and not intentional until recent years.

It was another late night at the office, I was taking the elevator to leave the building, and as I stood there peeling off a dried-up napkin to unveil the morning Danish I never got to eat, a soft voice said, "We are having a great meeting upstairs, and there is dinner there. Forget that Danish." I was being guided by a smiling colleague to my very first meeting of the National Association of Hispanic Nurses (NAHN)! It was a pivotal moment of reclaiming my heritage. Co-mingling with other Hispanic clinicians made me realize that being Hispanic could play a role in my desire to advocate for the public.

As I began to understand NAHN's mission better, I began to learn about my own Hispanic heritage. I looked at population statistics on health, graduation rates, and other factors, all of which raised my awareness of the help Hispanics needed locally and nationally. I found out that Hispanics are the largest minority population in my New York region. Hispanics graduate high school and college the least when compared to other groups, and have higher rates of unemployment. The big shocker was the great disparity that I uncovered about Hispanics in nursing. Although the Hispanic/Latino population continues to rise and is estimated to grow to about 30% of the total population by 2020, only 4% to 5% of the total nursing population identify as Hispanic/Latino (Health Resources and Services Administration [HRSA], 2010).

All of this was so eye-opening to me. I felt overwhelmed with the need to do something and do it quickly to help alleviate the disparities I had discovered for Hispanic populations. I began to understand that my public health expertise, passion for advocating, and NAHNs mission could help me embrace my Hispanic identity.

Community Engagement for Social Justice

I was committed to building a network of stakeholders who would work with me to address the needs of Hispanics in my community of Yonkers, NY. I uncovered that Yonkers has the highest percentage of Hispanics in the state, including more than New York City (NYC 29% in a population of 8,600,700; Yonkers, 36% in a population of 200,000) (U.S. Census Bureau, 2017). After about 6 months of research, reading, and networking with local Hispanic groups, I had enough evidence to justify a need to further address Hispanic health disparities in Yonkers.

I began with a meeting with the mayor at which I presented my findings and how I wanted to address this with the launch of a NAHN chapter in Westchester, the county in which Yonkers is located. I explained to Mayor Spano the NAHN mission, the way we could work collaboratively with his office, and the vision that I had for all Hispanics in Yonkers and Westchester to live to their greatest potential. It was an exciting meeting. He was engaged and seemed excited. He also noted that Hispanic teen pregnancy was an issue of concern that he wanted nurses' help to address. We also talked about Hispanics not reaching out to the already established resources such as educational programs, parenting workshops, or food pantries. That led us to discuss the importance of culturally congruent care, appropriate literacy levels, potential language barriers, and other possible reasons for folks not reaping the benefits of available resources.

Because of our meeting, I was connected to the Hispanic advisory board of Yonkers and was given access to office space for NAHN-Westchester to meet. The Mayor also gave me access to his media personnel and a representative from his office to make sure I had all I needed to launch NAHN-Westchester.

This kind of support encouraged me to get involved with other policymakers. I soon approached my local NY State Assembly member, Shelley Mayer, who was to become one of my greatest allies and mentors. At the time, Shelley served on the Assembly Health Committee and had a passion for improving health. With NAHN-Westchester, she found a vehicle for her advocacy as well. We both knew we were a well-suited pair.

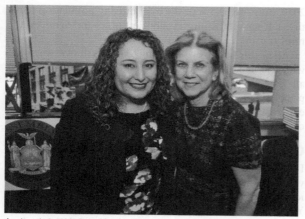

Author Lucia J. Alfano *(left)* and Shelley Mayer, New York State Assemblywoman representing the 37th Senate District. Senator Mayer is honoring Lucia during Women's History Month in 2018 for her outstanding community service.

In May 2015, NAHN-Westchester was ready to launch! It had been almost two years of planning. Among the greatest challenges were finding the right people to serve as board directors. I was relentless—going out to nursing events, nursing meetings, making new friends and calling old ones—in my efforts to help establish a good founding board.

During this time, I was a member of the New York State Action Coalition (NYSAC), which works on implementing the recommendations of the *Future of Nursing* report in New York. Its Diversity Committee was aligned perfectly with NAHN's mission, so I pursued becoming a member to capitalize on statewide and national resources. This was part of why NAHN-Westchester became a household name overnight. We were all over the radio, news, TV, internet, and social media venues. NYSAC's media connections had gotten us the publicity we needed to help us launch and succeed.

Following the launch, we received over $20,000 in grants and donations. We had over 15 community partners willing to work with us on education, health, mentoring, art, and leadership projects that would enrich Hispanic populations in Yonkers and throughout Westchester County. Organizations focused on our priority disparities opened their doors wide for us and wanted to plan health fairs and outreach programs using our voices and expertise. The most challenging part of this work was time, as this was volunteer work for all of us.

Health Equity for Hispanic Communities

NAHN-Westchester's mission is three pronged: (1) to address health disparities in Hispanic communities, (2) to support and develop leadership for current nurses, and (3) to

recruit and support the next generation of nurses. It offers nurses the opportunity to become mentors to other nurses and nursing students. Members are given opportunities to lead change in their native language, surrounded by people with similar traditions. Parent and children groups emerged with nurse liaisons who served as both a resource and a mentor to the parents. Nurses are building their leadership repertoire as they hold meetings, create budgets, apply for grants, or negotiate contracts. And nursing students are attending meetings, volunteering, asking questions, seeking mentoring, and growing as clinicians before our eyes. These are some ways in which NAHN-Westchester helps address equity in Hispanic communities.

NAHN-Westchester has become an integral part of the Yonkers community. Most of the public schools in Yonkers have a high percentage of Hispanic students. The schools host career fairs and have been eager to have NAHN's participation and the organization does so regularly by promoting nursing as a future career for middle school students.

NAHN-Westchester has also successfully addressed equity for Hispanics with interprofessional and intersectoral collaborative strategies. To date, NAHN has raised over $35,000 for scholarships, sponsorships, and leadership development. With the help of various partners, such as the local chapter of the American Heart Association, we have been able to perform heart health screenings in the community. So far, NAHN has reached over 10,000 community members for either health education or screenings, with most of them Hispanic.

CONCLUSION

My involvement in the community as an advocate and activist has made me realize that I need to be where policy is created, supported, and enacted. Besides NAHN, I am heavily involved in local politics. My mentor, Senator Shelley Mayer, has helped me learn about policymaking and politics, and I have helped her engage the Hispanic community.

Hispanics in our city were the least involved in politics, not registered to vote, and not voting. For this reason, Shelley and I have hosted various voter registration drives combined with health outreach. We also recently founded a political action committee (PAC) that focuses on supporting community leaders to run for local office, educating the public about the political process, and raising funds for political action. And in 2018, we hosted a dental drive. We both identified a community in need of toothbrushes and in need of dental care, so we used our network and resources and eventually collected over 400 beautiful electric toothbrushes, making several hundred children very happy. Our advocacy continues.

REFERENCES

Health Resources and Services Administration, Bureau of Health Professions. (2010). *Findings from the 2008 National Sample Survey of Registered Nurses*. Retrieved from https://bhw.hrsa.gov/sites/default/files/bhw/nchwa/rnsurveyfinal.pdf.

U.S. Census Bureau. (2017). *QuickFacts: New York City, New York*. Retrieved from www.census.gov/quickfacts/fact/table/yonkerscitynewyork,newyorkcitynewyork,ny/PST0452177.

79

Family and Sexual Violence, Nursing, and U.S. Policy

Kathryn Laughon and Angela Amar

"I raise up my voice not so I can shout but so that those without a voice can be heard … We cannot succeed when half of us are held back."

Malala Yousafzai

Our society is steeped in violence. In the most recent national statistics, more than 20 per 1000 people aged 12 or older will be the victims of a violent crime (Morgan & Kena, 2017). Most of our violence prevention strategies prepare potential victims to ward off violent attacks from strangers; yet, most violence against women, children, and the older population is perpetrated by someone known to the victim (Catalano, Smith, Snyder, & Rand 2009). The intimate nature of this violence, often perpetrated behind closed doors, has made these forms of violence less visible. However, the toll of violence on individuals and societies is substantial. The World Health Organization (WHO) has framed violence as a significant *public health* problem (Krug, Mercy, Dahlberg, & Zwi, 2002). A public health approach suggests an interdisciplinary, science-based approach with an emphasis on prevention. Effective strategies draw on resources in many fields, including nursing, medicine, criminal justice, epidemiology, and other social sciences.

The purpose of this chapter is to provide an overview of state, federal, and health sector policies regarding violence against women in the United States, briefly discuss policies related to violence against children and the older population, and outline the resulting implications for nurses and directions for future work.

INTIMATE PARTNER AND SEXUAL VIOLENCE AGAINST WOMEN

Intimate partner violence (IPV) is physical, sexual, or psychological harm inflicted by a current or former partner (same sex or not) or a current or former spouse (Black et al., 2011). Almost one-third of American women experience being hit, slapped, or pushed by an intimate partner, and nearly

one-quarter will experience serious forms of IPV during their lifetimes. In addition, nearly one in five women will experience a completed or attempted rape in their lifetimes (Tjaden & Thoennes, 2000). Men experience IPV and rape as well, although at far lower rates than do women. Approximately one-fourth of men will experience IPV (approximately 12% serious forms of violence) and nearly 1.5% a completed or attempted rape. Although more than half of women reporting rape report that the assailant was an intimate partner and 40% that the assailant was an acquaintance, men report that half of rapes were by acquaintances and 15% by strangers—the number raped by an intimate partner was too small to estimate.

The health effects of IPV and sexual violence are substantial, and costing as much as $8.3 billion in health care and mental health services for victims (Max, Rice, Finkelstein, Bardwell, & Leadbetter, 2004). Violence is associated with a wide range of health problems, including chronic pain recurring central nervous system symptoms, vaginal and sexually transmitted infections and other gynecological symptoms, and diagnosed gastrointestinal symptoms and disorders (Black et al., 2011). Mental health symptoms include depression, anxiety, posttraumatic stress disorder (PTSD), and alcohol and drug use (Black et al., 2011; Campbell, 2002).

STATE LAWS REGARDING INTIMATE PARTNER AND SEXUAL VIOLENCE

State laws address a number of issues important for nurses to understand. Crimes of IPV and sexual violence are addressed most frequently through state laws. Most, although not all, states have laws specifically providing enhanced penalties for assault and battery that occurs between intimate partners. (It is worth noting that most laws refer to "domestic violence" or "family abuse" rather than IPV.) For example, at least 23 states have some form of mandatory arrest for IPV (Hirschel, 2008). Research findings are mixed on whether mandatory arrest laws reduce reassault (Felson, Ackerman, & Gallagher, 2005; Hirschel, Buzawa, Pattavina, & Faggiani, 2007), although several recent studies find no relationship between arrest and subsequent violence (Hirschel, McCormack, & Buzawa, 2017; Ward-Lasher, Messing, Cimino, & Campbell, 2018). Researchers did find a relationship between contacting the police and subsequence decrease in violent victimization (Hirschel, McCormack, & Buzawa, 2017) and higher scores on standardized homicide risk assessment instruments and likelihood of later violence (Ward-Lasher, Messing, Cimino, & Campbell, 2018). These suggest that for some victims, at least, there may be some benefit in contacting the police, particularly if they are trained to use risk assessment tools. In addition, states may have enhanced penalties, such as escalating third offenses to felonies.

Until 1975, all states provided what is called the "marital rape exemption," under which it was legally impossible to commit rape against one's wife. Beginning in the mid-1970s, based in part on nursing research, these laws began to change (Campbell & Alford, 1989). Although all states currently recognize marital rape as a crime, in some states it is still treated differently than rape by a nonspouse, either by requiring greater force to be proven in the case of rape of a spouse or by providing lesser punishment (Prachar, 2010).

Nonlethal strangulation of women is a significant but often overlooked threat to public safety. Most (80%) strangulations of women are committed by intimate partners (Shields, Corey, Weakley-Jones, & Steward, 2010). They can result in significant physical health problems for victims (Taliaferro, Hawley, McClane, & Strack, 2009) and substantially increases risk of later lethal violence (Glass et al., 2008). These cases can be difficult to charge and prosecute commensurate with the severity of the crime (Laughon, Glass, & Worrell, 2009); therefore a growing number of states have strengthened laws related to strangulation.

All states provide for civil protective orders in cases where victims have a reasonable fear of violence from an assailant (Carroll, 2007). However, states vary widely in who is eligible to obtain an order and how the orders are obtained. For example, in some states, minors or dating partners may not be able to obtain orders of protection. Most states provide for civil protection orders against assailants who are accused of sexual assault, but the procedures may be different than for protective orders against intimate partners. Studies of the effectiveness of these orders are mixed (Prachar, 2010; Logan & Walker, 2009). However, what does appear certain is that in states where protective orders are robustly association with firearm removal, rates of intimate partner homicide are lower (Vigdor & Mercy, 2006; Zeoli et al., 2018).

In addition to these criminal justice remedies, state laws may address other issues related to IPV and sexual violence. As of 2013, 32 states had established intimate partner fatality review teams (Durborow, Lizdas, O'Flaherty, & Marjavi, 2013). Fatality review teams use a multidisciplinary, public health approach to reviewing fatalities and identifying risk factors (Wilson & Websdale, 2006). A handful of states require health care providers to report domestic violence against competent adults. It is important to understand that in most states, IPV and sexual assault are not mandatory reporters unless there are other factors present.

FEDERAL LAWS RELATED TO INTIMATE PARTNER AND SEXUAL VIOLENCE

There are two significant federal laws that address violence against women. The Family Violence Prevention and Services Act was first authorized in 1984. In 2010, it was authorized through 2015 but has not been reauthorized. It was most recently authorized through 2015 rec (P.L. 111-320 42 U.S.C. 10401, et. seq.). It is the primary federal funding source for domestic violence shelters and service program in the United States. This law also funds the work of state coalitions on domestic violence, community-based violence prevention efforts, and a number of smaller training and assistance programs.

The Violence Against Women Act (VAWA) was first authorized in 1994 (Title IV, sec. 40001-40703 of the Violent Crime Control and Law Enforcement Act of 1994, H.R. 3355, signed as Pub.L. 103–322). As states began creating the protective order and criminal statutes discussed earlier, the limitations of this patchwork of remedies became apparent. VAWA was therefore created to address the gaps in state laws, create federal laws against domestic violence, including protections for immigrant women and enhance gun control provisions, and fund a variety of violence-related training and other local programs (Valente, Hart, Zeya, & Malefyt, 2009). The law originally included a provision making crimes motivated by gender a civil rights offense. However, this provision was found unconstitutional in 2000 (*Brzonkala vs. Morrison*, 2000).

VAWA represented a significant turning point in public policy related to violence against women. Previously, women who received a protective order might find that violations that occurred in other states could not be enforced. The full faith and credit provision of VAWA requires that protective orders be recognized and enforced across jurisdictional, state, and tribal boundaries within the United States. Likewise, by creating federal crimes of domestic violence and stalking, criminal acts that cross jurisdictional boundaries can currently be more easily charged and prosecuted. Under VAWA, it is illegal for individuals subject to certain kinds of protective orders or convicted of even misdemeanor domestic violence offenses to possess a firearm. Given that risk of intimate partner homicide increases dramatically when firearms are available to the assailant, this represents an important safeguard for women (Campbell et al., 2003). VAWA addressed the significant hardships faced by both legal and illegal immigrant women experiencing abuse from their partners. VAWA additionally funds a wide range of victim advocacy and training programs, with the goal of ensuring that victims of violence receive consistent, competent services in all communities.

Each subsequent renewal of VAWA has strengthened these provisions. The latest renewal in 2013 expanded its definitions to explicitly include gay, lesbian, and transgender victims; expanded the safeguards available to women assaulted in tribal territories; expanded housing provisions to prohibit discrimination against victims of IPV in all forms of subsidized public housing; strengthened protections for immigrant women; and, for the first time, specifically addressed violence on college campuses (VAWA, 2013).

HEALTH POLICIES RELATED TO INTIMATE PARTNER AND SEXUAL VIOLENCE

As discussed earlier, the health consequences of violence are significant for women. In addition, women who have experienced violence have significantly higher health care costs than do women without a victimization history (Bonomi, Anderson, Rivara, & Thompson, 2009; National Center for Injury Prevention and Control, 2003). There is currently a consensus that health care settings offer a unique opportunity to identify and support women living with the effects of violence (Family Violence Prevention Fund [FVPF], 2002; WHO, 2013).

The U.S. Preventative Services Taskforce recommends that "clinicians screen women of childbearing age for IPV such as domestic violence, and provide or refer women who screen positive to intervention services." The National Academy of Medicine, formerly known as the Institute of Medicine, identified screening and brief counseling for interpersonal violence as an essential and evidence-based practice necessary to ensure the well-being of women (National Research Council, 2011). A wide variety of medical and nursing professional organizations also recommend routine screening for violence (Amar, Laughon, Sharps, & Campbell, 2013). Significant evidence currently exists for safety planning strategies to prevent homicide for women in abusive relationships. For example, the Danger Assessment instrument has been shown to have good predictive value and can assist women with making a realistic

appraisal of their likelihood of experiencing lethal violence (Campbell, Webster, & Glass, 2008). Online tools are showing great promise and may reduce the burden on health care providers. For example, a tool that embeds the Danger Assessment instrument has been demonstrated to be effective (Eden et al., 2015). In addition to providing appropriate assessments, health care institutions should also have the capacity to provide care to women in the acute period after a physical or sexual assault (WHO, 2013).

Nurses and other health professionals have a role to play in community responses to violence. Many localities have created Sexual Assault Response Teams (SARTs). These interdisciplinary teams work to ensure consistent, trauma-informed, and effective care for victims of sexual assault. Despite scant research on the effectiveness of these teams, they are a promising practice (Greeson & Campbell, 2013). Likewise, intimate partner/domestic violence fatality review teams review cases of intimate partner homicide with a public health approach. As with SARTs, we have little data on the effectiveness of these teams that have also been labeled a promising practice (Wilson & Websdale, 2006).

CHILD MALTREATMENT

Child maltreatment includes physical, sexual, and emotional abuse, as well as neglect. Actual prevalence of maltreatment is unknown, but there are more than 3 million referrals for more than 6 million children to child protective agencies annually, with nearly a quarter of these cases substantiated. A large review of meta-analyses provided clear evidence that child maltreatment is substantially underreported (Stoltenborgh, Bakermans-Kranenburg, Alink, & van Ijzendoorn, 2015). Nationally, in 2016 the rate of child fatalities was 2.36 deaths per 100,000 children. It is important to note that this is a source of substantial health disparity, with fatalities among African American children occurring at a rate 2.2 times higher than the rate for White children (U.S. Department of Health and Human Services, 2018). The estimated annual cost of child abuse and neglect in the United States for 2008 was $124 billion (Fang, Brown, Florence, & Mercy, 2012). Child maltreatment results in lifelong adverse physical and mental health consequences such as PTSD, increased risk of chronic disease, lasting impacts or disability from physical injury, and reduced health related quality of life (Corso, Edwards, Fang, & Mercy, 2008).

State and Federal Policies Related to Child Maltreatment

Because minors are considered to need additional protection due to their age, states not only have laws making the acts of abuse and neglect criminal offenses, but also laws requiring that certain adults must report suspected maltreatment to appropriate authorities. In some states, all adults are mandated reporters. In most states, specific professionals—teachers, health care professionals, social workers, law enforcement personnel, and others—are mandated reporters (Child Welfare Information Gateway, 2011). At the federal level, the Child Abuse Prevention and Treatment Act (CAPTA) provides funding to states to support prevention, assessment, investigation, prosecution, and treatment activities related to child maltreatment and funding for research activities (Child Welfare Information Gateway, 2011).

Health Policies Related to Child Maltreatment

Children's Advocacy Centers (CACs) coordinate investigation and intervention services for maltreated children by bringing together social work, legal, health care, and other professionals, and agencies in a multidisciplinary team to create a child-focused approach to child abuse cases. CACs have been shown to improve prosecution (Smith, Witte, & Fricker-Elhai, 2006), but there is little evidence to date to show that they improve health outcomes for children and their caregivers (Herbert & Bromfield, 2016). Home visitation is another strategy that shows promise for improving child health and preventing child maltreatment, although the results across interventions are mixed (Chen & Chan, 2016).

Elder Maltreatment

Each year, approximately 8% to 10% of Americans aged 60 or older experience physical, sexual, emotional, or financial abuse or neglect (Lachs & Pillemer, 2015). Precise numbers are not available due to differences in definitions of abuse, lack of a comprehensive national data system, and different state system reporting and data collection. Furthermore, only a small fraction of abuse comes to the attention of Adult Protective Services (Dong & Simon, 2011). Despite the rapid aging of the U.S. population—with projections for individuals 65 and older to increase from 40.2 million in 2010 to 54.8 million in 2020 and to 72.1 million in 2030 (Dong, n.d.)—research on elder abuse and neglect is decades behind research on gender violence and child maltreatment (Lachs & Pillemer, 2015).

State and Federal Legislation Related to Elder Maltreatment

As with child maltreatment, state laws provide for criminal charges related to the abuse of the older population (the definition of which varies from state to state but may be as young as 55 years of age). Most (but not all) states define certain individuals as mandated reporters of abuse of the older population, as well. At the federal level, the Older American Act (OAA) of 2006 developed and operates the National Center on Elder Abuse which provides funding for prevention activities, research, data collection, and long-term planning for elder justice. The Elder Justice Act (EJA) of 2010, which was part of the Patient Protection and Affordable Care Act, is the first comprehensive strategy to address elder abuse, neglect, and exploitation. Little funding has been authorized, and most of the provisions of the act have not been carried out (Collelo, 2017). Funding for elder maltreatment is significantly less than for other types of violence, and a national database analogous to the database for child maltreatment has yet to be established.

Health Care Policies Related to Elder Maltreatment

Recent efforts have focused on using the primary care setting to identify and respond to elder abuse (Perel-Levin, 2008). Multiple brief screen instruments exist and should be used in health care settings to identify those at risk (Dong, 2015). Case management strategies can be effective in providing consistency in monitoring of adult patient and caregiver behavior (Choi & Mayer, 2000). Use of multidisciplinary teams (including nurses) should be strongly considered as a first-line intervention (Pillemer, Burnes, Riffin, & Lachs, 2016). Research on effective intervention strategies in this area lags behind that of other areas of violence and is an area where nursing can make an impact.

Opportunity for Nursing

Nurses have the skills and education to take a leadership role in addressing violence and abuse on multiple levels—as providers, researchers, policy analysts, educators, and advocates. Efforts to address violence against children, women, and the older population have met with impressive successes over the past decades. These forms of violence—seen as largely justifiable and perhaps even necessary in the past—are currently recognized as both crimes and important public health problems. The evidence base for interventions to prevent these forms of violence, end them when they start, and mitigate the related health consequences is growing. However, it is clear that we still have important gaps in our understanding of both effective violence interventions and policies. While we work to address these gaps in knowledge, however, we can continue to move forward on numerous fronts. Educators should ensure that curriculums at all levels include content on violence and abuse. Given the high rates and significant health effects of violence, all nurses should have basic clinical knowledge of how to assess for, competently respond to, and appropriately refer all patients with a history of violence or abuse. Nurses can serve as powerful advocates for victims of violence, ensuring that state and federal laws meet the highest standards.

Violence and crime unite two powerful systems, health care and criminal justice, and involve multiple professionals, including physicians, nurses, social services, police, lawyers, and judges. Prevention and intervention strategies require efforts on the individual, community, institutional, and public policy levels. Nurses can have a significant voice in ensuring the best possible prevention and advocacy services at the local, state, and federal levels. Nursing research and the testimony of nurses have been foundational for federal and state laws and resulting public policy related to violence.

DISCUSSION QUESTIONS

1. Consider the differences in the treatment of violence across states and what federal provisions might be advantageous to address the discrepancies.
2. How might nursing research help to fill the gaps in the knowledge?
3. It is apparent in the chapter that different strategies exist for violence against women, child maltreatment, and elder abuse. Could the same strategies work across populations and abuse types? What might be the advantages/disadvantages to having similar strategies?

REFERENCES

Amar, A., Laughon, K., Sharps, P., & Campbell, J. (2013). Screening and counseling for violence against women in primary care settings. *Nursing Outlook, 61*(3), 187-191.

American Bar Association Commission on Domestic and Sexual Violence. (2016). Domestic violence civil protection orders. Retrieved from www.americanbar.org/content/dam/aba/administrative/domestic_violence1/Charts/migrated_charts/2016%20CPO%20Availability%20Chart.pdf.

Avellar, S.A., & Supplee, L.H. (2013) Effectiveness of home visiting in improving child health and reducing child maltreatment. *Pediatrics, 132*(10, Suppl 2), S90-S99.

Barata, P. C., & Schneider, F. (2004). Battered women add their voices to the debate about the merits of mandatory arrest. *Women's Studies Quarterly, 32*, 148.

Black, M.C., Basile, K.C., Breiding, M.J., Smith, S.G., Walters, M.L., Merrick, M.T., ... & Stevens, M.R. (2011). *The National Intimate Partner and Sexual Violence Survey (NISVS): 2010 Summary repor*t. Atlanta: National Center for Injury Prevention and Control, Centers for Disease Control and Prevention.

Bonomi, A.E., Anderson, M.L., Rivara, F.P., & Thompson, R.S. (2009). Health care utilization and costs associated with physical and nonphysical-only intimate partner violence. *Health Services Research, 44*(3), 1052-1067.

Burston, G.R. (1975). Granny-battering. *British Medical Journal, 3*, 592.

Brzonkala v. Morrison, 529 U.S. 598, 627 (2000).

Campbell, J.C. (2002). Health consequences of intimate partner violence. *The Lancet, 359*(9314), 1331-1336

Campbell, J.C., & Alford, P. (1989). The dark consequences of marital rape. *American Journal of Nursing, 89*(7), 946-949.

Campbell, J.C., Webster, D.W., & Glass, N. (2008). The danger assessment: Validation of a lethality risk assessment instrument for intimate partner femicide. *Journal of Interpersonal Violence, 24*(4), 653-674.

Campbell, J.C., Webster, D., Koziol-McLain, J., Block, C., Campbell, D., Curry, M.A., ... & Laughon, K. (2003). Risk factors for femicide in abusive relationships: Results from a multisite case control study. *American Journal of Public Health, 93*(7), 1089-1097.

Carroll, C.A. (2007). *Sexual assault civil protection orders (CPOs) by state*. Washington, DC: American Bar Association Commission on Domestic and Sexual Violence.

Catalano, S., Smith, E., Snyder, H., & Rand, M. (2009). *Female victims of violence*. Report NCJ228356. Washington, DC: Bureau of Justice Statistics. Retrieved from www.bjs.gov/content/pub/pdf/fvv.pdf.

Chen, M., & Chan, K.L. (2016). Effects of parenting programs on child maltreatment prevention: A meta-analysis. *Trauma, Violence, & Abuse, 17*(1), 88-104.

Child Welfare Information Gateway. (2011). *About CAPTA: A legislative history*. Washington, DC: U.S. Department of Health and Human Services, Children's Bureau.

Child Welfare Information Gateway. (2013). *Long-term consequences of child abuse and neglect*. Washington, DC: U.S. Department of Health and Human Services. Retrieved from www.childwelfare.gov/pubs/factsheets/long_term_consequences.cfm.

Choi, N.G., & Mayer, J. (2000). Elder abuse, neglect, and exploitation: Risk factors and prevention strategies. *Journal of Gerontological Social Work, 33*(2), 5-25.

Colello, K.J. (2017). The Elder Justice Act: Background and issues for Congress. Congressional Research Service, 7-5700, R43707. Retrieved from https://fas.org/sgp/crs/misc/R43707.pdf.

Corso, P.S., Edwards, V.J., Fang, X., & Mercy, J.A. (2008). Health-related quality of life among adults who experienced maltreatment during childhood. *American Journal of Public Health, 98*, 1094–1100.

Dong, X. (2015). Screening for elder abuse in healthcare settings: Why should we care, and is it a missed quality indicator?. *Journal of the American Geriatrics Society, 63*(8), 1686-1692.

Dong, X.Q., & Simon, M.A. (2011). Enhancing national policy and programs to address elder abuse. *JAMA, 305*(23), 2460-2461.

Duggan, A., McFarlane, E., Fuddy, L., Burrell, L., Higman, S.M., Windham, A., & Sia, C. (2004). Randomized trial of a statewide home visiting program: Impact in preventing child abuse and neglect. *Child Abuse & Neglect, 28*(6), 597-622.

Durborow, N., Lizdas, K.C., O'Flaherty, A., & Marjavi, A. (2013). *Compendium of state statutes and policies on domestic violence and health care*. San Francisco: Family Violence Prevention Fund.

Eden, K.B., Perrin, N.A., Hanson, G.C., Messing, J.T., Bloom, T.L., Campbell, J.C., & Glass, N.E. (2015). Use of online safety decision aid by abused women: effect on decisional conflict in a randomized controlled trial. *American Journal of Preventive Medicine, 48*(4), 372-383.

Fang, X., Brown, D.S., Florence, C.S., & Mercy, J.A. (2012). The economic burden of child maltreatment in the United States and implications for prevention. *Child Abuse & Neglect, 36*(2), 156-165.

Felson, R.B., Ackerman, J.M., & Gallagher, C.A. (2005). Police intervention and the repeat of domestic assault. *Criminology, 43*(3), 563-588.

Glass, N., Laughon, K., Campbell, J., Block, C.R., Hanson, G., Sharps, P.W., & Taliaferro, E. (2008). Non-fatal strangulation is an important risk factor for homicide for women. *Journal of Emergency Medicine, 35*(3), 329-335.

Greeson, M.R., & Campbell, R. (2013). Sexual assault response teams (SARTs): An empirical review of their effectiveness and challenges to successful implementation. *Trauma, Violence, & Abuse, 14*(2), 83-95.

Herbert, J.L., & Bromfield, L. (2016). Evidence for the efficacy of the Child Advocacy Center model: A systematic review. *Trauma, Violence, & Abuse, 17*(3), 341-357.

Hirschel, D. (2008). *Domestic violence cases: What research shows about arrest and dual arrest rates.* Washington, DC: National Institute for Justice.

Hirschel, D., Buzawa, E., Pattavina, A., & Faggiani, D. (2007). Domestic violence and mandatory arrest laws: To what extent do they influence police arrest decisions? *Journal of Criminal Law & Criminolog, 98*, 255.

Hirschel, D., McCormack, P.D., & Buzawa, E. (2017). A 10-year study of the impact of intimate partner violence primary aggressor laws on single and dual arrest. *Journal of Interpersonal Violence*, 1-35.

Jogerst, G.J., Daly, J.M., Brinig, M.F., Dawson, J.D., Schmuch, G.A., & Ingram, J.G. (2003). Domestic elder abuse and the law. *American Journal of Public Health, 93*(12), 2131-2136.

Krug, E.G., Mercy, J.A., Dahlberg, L.L., & Zwi, A.B. (2002). *World report on violence and health.* Geneva: World Health Organization.

Lachs, M.S., & Pillemer, K.A. (2015). Elder abuse. *New England Journal of Medicine, 373*(20), 1947-1956.

Laughon, K., Glass, N., & Worrell, C. (2009). Review and analysis of laws related to strangulation in 50 states. *Sage Pub, 33*(4), 358-369.

Logan, T., & Walker, R. (2009). Civil protective order outcomes: Violations and perceptions of effectiveness. *Journal of Interpersonal Violence, 24*(4), 675-692.

MacMillan, H.L., Thomas, B.H., Jamieson, E., Walsh, C.A., Boyle, M.H., Shannon, H.S., & Gafni, A. (2005). Effectiveness of home visitation by public-health nurses in prevention of the recurrence of child physical abuse and neglect: A randomised controlled trial. *The Lancet, 365*(9473), 1786-1793.

Max, W., Rice, D.P., Finkelstein, E., Bardwell, R.A., & Leadbetter, S. (2004). The economic toll of intimate partner violence against women in the United States. *Violence and Victims, 19*(3), 259-272.

Messing J.T., Campbell J.C., Webster D.W., Brown, S., Patchell, B., & Wilson, J.S. (2015). The Oklahoma Lethality Assessment Study: A quasi-experimental evaluation of the Lethality Assessment Program. *Social Service Review, 89*(3), 499–530.

Morgan, R.E., & Kena, G. (2017). *Criminal victimization, 2016.* No. NCJ 251150. Washington, DC: US Department of Justice, Office of Justice Programs, Bureau of Justice Statistics.

National Center on Aging, (2005). *Fact sheet: Elder abuse prevalence and incidence.* Washington, DC: National Center of Elder Abuse.

National Research Council. (2011). *Clinical preventive services for women: Closing the gaps.* Washington, DC: The National Academies Press.

Patient Protection and Affordable Care Act, 42 U.S.C. § 18001 (2010).

Perel-Levin, S. (2008). *Discussing screening for elder abuse at the primary health care level.* Geneva: World Health Organization.

Pillemer, K., Burnes, D., Riffin, C., & Lachs, M.S. (2016). Elder abuse: Global situation, risk factors, and prevention strategies. *The Gerontologist, 56*(Suppl 2), S194-S205.

Prachar, M. (2010). The marital rape exemption: A violation of a woman's right of privacy. *Golden Gate University Law Review, 11*, 717.

Rubin, D.M., Curtis, M.L., & Matone, M. (2014). Child abuse prevention and child home visitation: Making sure we get it right. *JAMA Pediatrics, 168*(1), 5-6.

Selph, S.S., Bougatsos, C., Blazina, I., & Nelson, H.D. (2013). Behavioral interventions and counseling to prevent child abuse and neglect: A systematic review to update the U.S. preventive services task force recommendation, *Annals of Internal Medicine, 158*, 179-190.

Shields, L.B., Corey, T.S., Weakley-Jones, B., & Steward, D. (2010). Living victims of strangulation: A 10-year review of cases in a metropolitan community. *American Journal of Forensic Medicine and Pathology, 31*, 320-325.

Smith, D.W., Witte, T.H., & Fricker-Elhai, A.E. (2006). Service outcomes in physical and sexual abuse cases: A comparison of child advocacy center-based and standard services. *Child Maltreatment, 11*(4), 354-360.

Stoltenborgh, M., Bakermans-Kranenburg, M.J., Alink, L.R., & van Ijzendoorn, M.H. (2015). The prevalence of child maltreatment across the globe: Review of a series of meta-analyses. *Child Abuse Review, 24*(1), 37-50.

Taliaferro E., Hawley, D., McClane, G., & Strack, G.B. (2009). Strangulation in intimate partner violence. In C. Mitchell & D. Anglin (Eds.), *Intimate partner violence: A health-based perspective* (pp. 217-325). New York: Oxford University Press.

Tjaden, P., & Thoennes, N. (2000). Extent, nature, and consequences of intimate partner violence. Washington, DC: National Institute of Justice and the Centers for Disease Control.

U.S. Department of Health & Human Services, Administration for Children and Families, Administration on Children, Youth and Families, Children's Bureau. (2018). Child maltreatment 2016. Available from https://www.acf.hhs.gov/cb/research-data-technology/statistics-research/child-maltreatment.

U.S. Government Accountability Office. (2011). *Child maltreatment: Strengthening national data on child fatalities could aid in prevention.* GAO-11-599. Retrieved from www.gao.gov/products/GAO-11-599.

Valente, R.L., Hart, B.J., Zeya, S., & Malefyt, M. (2001279). The Violence Against Women Act of 1994: The federal commitment to ending domestic violence, sexual assault, stalking, and gender-based crimes of violence. In C. M. Renzetti, J. L. Edelson, & R. L. Bergen (Eds.), *Sourcebook on violence against women.* Newbury Park, CA: Sage Publishing.

Vigdor, E.R., & Mercy, J.A. (2006). Do laws restricting access to firearms by domestic violence offenders prevent intimate partner homicide? *Evaluation Review, 30*(3), 313–346.

The Violence Against Women Act, Pub. L. 113–4.

Violence Against Women Reauthorization Act of 2013. (2013).

Ward-Lasher, A., Messing, J.T., Cimino, A.N., & Campbell, J.C. (2018). The association between homicide risk and intimate partner violence arrest. *Policing: A Journal of Policy and Practice.* Retrieved from https://academic.oup.com/policing/advance-article-abstract/doi/10.1093/police/4883358.

Wilson, J.S., & Websdale, N. (2006). Domestic violence fatality review teams: An interprofessional model to reduce deaths. *Journal of Interprofessional Care, 20*(5), 535–544.

World Health Organization. (2013). *Responding to intimate partner violence and sexual violence against women WHO clinical and policy guidelines.* Geneva: Author.

Zeoli, A.M., McCourt, A., Buggs, S., Frattaroli, S., Lilley, D., & Webster, D.W. (2018). Analysis of the strength of legal firearms restrictions for perpetrators of domestic violence and their associations with intimate partner homicide. *American Journal of Epidemiology. 187*(7), 1449–1455.

ONLINE RESOURCES

Child Welfare Information Gateway
www.childwelfare.gov
Futures Without Violence
www.futureswithoutviolence.org
National Center of Elder Abuse
www.ncea.aoa.gov
Rape, Abuse & Incest National Network
www.rainn.org

80

Human Trafficking: The Need for Nursing Advocacy

Donna Sabella

> *"Every day I was held against my will was hell, and I prayed for my death daily to set me free."*
>
> **Clarice S., human trafficking survivor**

Gisella appeared in the Emergency Department (ED), visibly distraught and complaining of stomach pain. The 25-year-old woman also had bruises on both her wrists and the imprint of a hand on her left cheek, indicating that she had possibly been recently slapped in the face by someone. She was accompanied by an older woman who stated that she was Gisella's aunt. Both women reported that the injuries were a result of a beating that Gisella had received at the hands of her former boyfriend. Several days prior to this, the same nurses had provided care for Leonard, a 53-year-old man who stated that he worked on a nearby farm. Leonard presented with respiratory problems, a rash on his chest, and pain upon urinating. Although alert, he appeared mildly confused and had trouble answering questions about person, place, and time.

Although diagnosing and treating patients' medical issues are what health care providers do well and successfully in most cases, what can prove more difficult is knowing whom they are treating. In both of the aforementioned cases, the patients could also have been victims of human trafficking (HT). Was Gisella really a victim of her ex-boyfriend who was being supported by her aunt, or is she a victim of sexual exploitation who was beaten by a violent john during a sexual encounter? Is that really her aunt, or is the aunt Gisella's pimp? Is Leonard a victim of labor trafficking who does not know where he is because he is moved from place to place for work by his traffickers, or is his confusion a result of a urinary tract infection (UTI)? Do his rash and respiratory issues stem from being exposed to various chemicals and living in close quarters with others forced to work the farm, or could there be another reason for his medical problems? Treating patients

for medical problems in any context, not just in the ED, without properly identifying potential HT victims is not enough. To provide the best care to patients and be able to advocate for HT victims, it is important that nurses increase their knowledge of what HT is and become aware of the tools available to them to successfully advocate on behalf of suspected or actual HT victims.

WHAT IS HUMAN TRAFFICKING?

HT, often referred to as modern day slavery, is a universal phenomenon that happens in every country. It is a crime and is presently considered a public health issue (Chisolm-Straker & Stoklosa, 2017). It can occur in rural and urban areas and in basically any setting imaginable, as well as to any individual regardless of age, gender, socioeconomic status, ethnicity, or level of education. Although the term *trafficking* might imply that victims need to be moved from place to place, that is not always the case. Certainly, victims can be moved from location to location, but they can also remain in one place while being trafficked (Administration of Children and Families, 2017a).

There are a number of definitions of HT, but the following is viewed as the worldwide standard and the template for numerous nations' domestic HT laws (Hepburn & Simon, 2013). Article 3, paragraph (a) of the Protocol to Prevent, Suppress and Punish Trafficking in Persons (United Nations, 2000) defines Trafficking in Persons (TIP) as:

> the recruitment, transportation, transfer, harbouring or receipt of persons, by means of the threat or use of force or other forms of coercion, of abduction, of fraud, of deception, of the abuse of power or of a position of vulnerability or of

the giving or receiving of payments or benefits to achieve the consent of a person having control over another person, for the purpose of exploitation. Exploitation shall include, at a minimum, the exploitation of the prostitution of others or other forms of sexual exploitation, forced labour or services, slavery or practices similar to slavery, servitude or the removal of organs. (p. 3)

The two major divisions of HT are sex and labor trafficking. Sex trafficking is defined as "the recruitment, harboring, transportation, provision, or obtaining of a person for the purpose of a commercial sex act" (U.S. Congress, 2000. Public Law 106-386. Victims of trafficking and violence protection act of 2000). Such an act is considered severe when the victim is under the age of 18 and when force, fraud, or coercion are involved (U.S. Department of Health and Human Services, 2017; U.S. Congress, 2000). *Labor trafficking* is defined as the " recruitment, harboring, transportation, provision, or obtaining of a person for labor or services, through the use of force, fraud or coercion

for the purpose of subjection to involuntary servitude, peonage, debt bondage, or slavery" (U.S. Congress, 2000; U.S. Department of Health and Human Services, 2017).

HT, which can be broken down into actions, means and purposes, occurs whenever any adult or minor is exploited for sex, forced labor, organ removal, and/or child soldiering and typically involves some measure of force, fraud, and/or coercion against the person being trafficked. Variations on these practices can include debt bondage, forced marriage, and domestic servitude—and it is possible to be trafficked in more than one category, such as when a child soldier is also exploited sexually (U.S. Department of State, 2016). Table 80.1 illustrates the concepts of action, means, and purpose as they relate to HT (Administration for Children and Families, 2017b).

Although exact numbers of HT victims worldwide are difficult to come by and agreed upon (Fedina, 2014), it is estimated that approximately 14,500 to 17,000 people are trafficked into the United States yearly (U.S. Department

---

TABLE 80.1   Action, Means, and Purpose Model of Human Trafficking

Actions	Means Does Not Need to Be Present in Sex Trafficking of Minors	Purpose
Recruiting includes proactive targeting of vulnerability and grooming behaviors. **Harboring** includes isolation, confinement, and monitoring. **Transporting** includes movement and arranging travel. **Providing** includes giving to another individual. **Obtaining** includes forcibly taking or exchanging something for ability to control. *****Soliciting** includes offering something of value. *****Patronizing** includes receiving something of value.	**Force** includes physical restraint, physical harm, sexual assault, and beatings. Monitoring and confinement are often used to control victims, especially during early stages of victimization to break down the victim's resistance. **Fraud** includes false promises regarding employment, wages, working conditions, love, marriage, or better life. Over time, there may be unexpected changes in work conditions, compensation or debt agreements, or nature of relationship. **Coercion** includes threats of serious harm to or physical restraint against any person, psychological manipulation, document confiscation, and shame and fear-inducing threats to share information or pictures with others or report to authorities.	**Commercial Sex Act** is any sex act on account of anything of value given to or received by any person. **Involuntary Servitude** is any scheme, plan, or pattern intended to cause a person to believe that, if the person did not enter into or continue in such condition, that person or another person would suffer serious harm or physical restraint; or the abuse or threatened abuse of the legal process. **Debt Bondage** includes a pledge of services by the debtor or someone under debtor's control to pay down known or unknown charges (e.g., fees for transportation, boarding, food, and other incidentals; interest, fines for missing quotas, and charges for "bad behavior"). The length and nature of those services are not respectively limited and defined, where an individual is trapped in a cycle of debt that he or she can never pay down. **Peonage** is a status or condition of involuntary servitude based on real or alleged indebtedness. **Slavery** is the state of being under the ownership or control of someone where a person is forced to work for another.

Source: Polaris Project and the National Human Trafficking Resource Center. (2012). Retrieved from https://humantraffickinghotline.org/resources/actions-means-purpose-amp-model.
*Only for sex trafficking.

of State, 2004) and that 40.3 million people were trafficked worldwide in 2016 (International Labour Office, 2017).

In the United States, although the number is believed to be higher, 7623 cases of potential HT were reported in calls made to the National Human Trafficking Hotline in 2016 (National Human Trafficking Resource Center, 2017). Sex trafficking tends to be the form of trafficking most people are familiar with, the one that receives the most attention in the media, and the most common form identified by U.S. citizens (Hepburn & Simon, 2013); however, labor trafficking occurs here as well. According to the U.S. Department of State (2010 & 2011), 55% of foreign adults and 62% of foreign children brought into the country in 2010 were victims of labor trafficking.

No one volunteers to be trafficked, yet certain circumstances can increase the risk factors for becoming a victim. Some common factors include poverty and economic hardship, lack of education and/or job skills, social and civil conflict and unrest, natural disasters, drug addiction, and refugee status. Some victims are forced into their situation by traffickers using various means such as kidnapping, blackmailing, or physical restraint, whereas others end up being trafficked by fraudulent practices such as being recruited for a job at a factory only to find there is no factory job and they are then forced into labor or sex work to repay the cost of getting them to the given location. Traffickers can be male or female, young or old, strangers or known individuals, and in some cases even parents who either unknowingly send their children off in what they hope is a better situation, unaware of the future their children face, or who knowingly send their children off to be sexually and/or physically exploited in exchange for being able to send money home to help support the family (Sabella, 2013).

Regardless of where or how the victimization takes place, the consequences can be devastating and lifelong. Victims are at risk for a multitude of physical, medical, and psychological problems, including posttraumatic stress disorder (PTSD), tuberculosis (TB), sexually transmitted infections (STIs), respiratory and skin problems, substance use disorders (SUDs), and reproductive issues (Richards, 2014; Sabella, 2011, 2013) for which they may seek health care. Violence against those who are trafficked is not unheard of, so we can also expect to see various indications of physical trauma such as broken bones, bite marks, and cigarette burns (Sabella, 2011, 2013). Of great importance is knowing what to look for to assess whether someone you are caring for might possibly be a victim of HT. A number of signs and symptoms commonly identified as possible indicators are provided in Box 80.1 (Polaris, 2018c).

BOX 80.1 Common Possible Indicators of Human Trafficking

Common Work and Living Conditions
- Is not free to leave or come and go as he/she wishes
- Is in the commercial sex industry and has a pimp/manager
- Is unpaid, paid very little, or paid only through tips
- Works excessively long and/or unusual hours
- Is not allowed breaks or suffers under unusual restrictions at work
- Owes a large debt and is unable to pay it off
- Was recruited through false promises concerning the nature and conditions of his/her work
- High security measures exist in the work and/or living locations (e.g., opaque windows, boarded up windows, bars on windows, barbed wire, security cameras, etc.)

Poor Mental Health or Abnormal Behavior
- Is fearful, anxious, depressed, submissive, tense, or nervous/paranoid
- Exhibits unusually fearful or anxious behavior after bringing up law enforcement
- Avoids eye contact

Poor Physical Health
- Lacks medical care and/or is denied medical services by employer

- Appears malnourished or shows signs of repeated exposure to harmful chemicals
- Shows signs of physical and/or sexual abuse, physical restraint, confinement, or torture

Lack of Control
- Has few or no personal possessions
- Is not in control of his/her own money and/or no financial records or bank account
- Is not in control of his/her own identification documents (ID or passport)
- Is not allowed or able to speak for themselves (a third party may insist on being present and/or translating)

Other
- Claims of just visiting and inability to clarify where he/she is staying/address
- Lack of knowledge of whereabouts and/or of what city he/she is in
- Loss of sense of time
- Has numerous inconsistencies in his/her story

GLOBAL SCOPE OF HUMAN TRAFFICKING: OVERVIEW OF UNIVERSAL ISSUES AND IMPACT

As mentioned previously, HT occurs everywhere in the world. It is important to distinguish between HT and prostitution. Although not everyone agrees that the two are all that different, typically prostitution is viewed as any sexual encounter that occurs between two willing and consenting adults in exchange for either money or some other goods. Furthermore, prostitution is legal in some locations, including several counties in Nevada and in countries such as Belgium, Colombia, Australia, and Germany (100 Countries, 2018); however, HT of any type, including sex trafficking as opposed to prostitution, is considered a crime. Sex trafficking involves some measure of fraud, force, and/or coercion, resulting in sex acts that are not entered into voluntarily. In keeping an eye on HT across the globe, the U.S. government collects self-reported data from more than 100 countries regarding the types of trafficking that occur in each country and whether that country is a source, transit, or destination country. The information is then published every June in the Trafficking in Person's report, also known as the TIP report (U.S. Department of State, 2018).

Based on the information revealed, each country is assigned a tier ranking indicating the level of effort expended to combat HT. Countries receiving a tier 1 designation are those most aligned with and which fully meet the minimum standards of the Trafficking Victims Protection Act (TVPA) for combating HT. Those with a tier 2 or 2a designation are believed to be making an effort to meet those standards, and those with a tier 3 classification fail to meet the standards even minimally and are viewed as lacking significant effort to do so (U.S. Department of State Tier Placement, 2017).

U.S. RESPONSES TO COMBATING HUMAN TRAFFICKING: POLICIES, LAWS, AND CONSEQUENCES

One of the earliest pieces of legislation to combat HT in the United States is known as the Victims of Trafficking and Violence Prevention Act (VTVPA). Signed into law in 2000 by then–President Clinton, the act is considered the cornerstone of federal HT-related legislation (Polaris, 2018a). The act made HT a federal crime and focused on what is referred to as the 3 Ps: preventing HT, prosecuting traffickers, and protecting HT victims. The act also served to create the Office to Monitor and Combat Trafficking in Persons, making the annual publication of the aforementioned

TIP a requirement (Polaris, 2018a). The 2000 VTVPA has been followed by Trafficking Victims Protection Reauthorization Acts of 2003, 2005, 2008, and 2013. Each reauthorization enacted various initiatives and provided specific measures that were felt to be important in the ongoing battle against HT. Examples include establishing the rights of victims to sue their traffickers in the 2003 reauthorization; providing means to fight sex tourism in the 2005 reauthorization; and enhancing criminal sanctions against traffickers and establishing programs to prevent U.S. citizens' purchase of goods made by HT victims on the 2008 and 2013 reauthorizations, respectively (Polaris, 2018a). Each reenactment is an attempt to stay current with what authorities believe is important to keep up with in the ever-changing nature of HT and the criminal behaviors of those involved in it.

More recently a number of other bills have been introduced for approval. As per aforementioned where reauthorizations are enacted to keep up with the ever-changing characteristics of this phenomenon and the need to keep up with the tactics used by those guilty of perpetuating this crime, numerous other laws, bills, and acts are put forth to provide those combating HT the legal means to do so. The TVPA of 2017, S. 1312, was passed in the U.S. Senate in September 2017 but, as of January 2018, had not become law (Congress.gov, n.d.; TVPA, 2017). Two other bills were introduced in 2017 that would reauthorize the TVPA, either in whole or in part: H.R. 2200, the Frederick Douglass Trafficking Victims Prevention and Protection Reauthorization Act of 2017 and S. 1311, the Abolish Human Trafficking Act of 2017 (Polaris, 2018b).

Aside from the aforementioned, there are a number of other laws or acts related to HT, including the Prosecutorial Remedies and Other Tools to End the Exploitation of Children Today Act of 2003 (PROTECT) and the more recent Survivors of Human Trafficking Empowerment Act 2015 (U.S. Department of State, U.S. Laws, n.d.). Some may ask why so many different laws exist. Although there are no easy answers, it is probably safe to say that because HT is a crime, the belief, which some say is misguided, is that we can stop HT if we have enough laws against it and against those who take part in any aspect of this crime. (See Todres [2011] for a discussion on why laws are not the answer.)

In addition to federal laws, there are also state laws against HT. In 2003 Washington became the first state to criminalize HT. Although laws vary from state to state, every state has enacted laws that criminalize HT and prosecute those involved in the trafficking of human beings (National Conference of State Legislatures [NCSL], n.d.). Polaris (2018d) and Shared Hope International (2018) offer information regarding various state laws and how well each state combats HT. Prosecution and conviction for any aspect of the act of HT can result in jail time and fines.

NURSING ADVOCACY, POLICY, AND PRACTICE

Trafficking in persons has often been referred to as the fastest growing criminal industry in the world nowadays and one of the most lucrative forms of criminal activity, as well (U.S. Department of Health and Human Services, n.d.). A drug can be used only once, whereas human beings can be repeatedly exploited, thereby making the selling and buying of human beings an extremely profitable endeavor. Those working in the health care field, especially nurses, need to be aware of what trafficking is, the extent to which trafficking occurs, and how to identify, support, and treat trafficking victims. The odds are likely that at some point we will or already have come across trafficking victims, many of whom are often hidden right in front of us in plain sight. As nurses, we are in a position to help make a difference in the lives of trafficking victims at several points, from the initial encounter and identification to their rescue and restoration to health.

Yet often such opportunities are missed. In a study of 21 survivors of HT in the San Francisco, Los Angeles, and Atlanta areas, researchers found that, although 28% had come into contact with health care providers in a variety of settings during their captivity, the providers did not realize their patients were being trafficked (Family Violence Prevention Fund, 2005). There is no question that we need to serve as advocates and be more active on both an individual and professional level. My personal experience in being involved in this area for more than 10 years is that nursing lags behind other disciplines, especially social work and even law enforcement and legal services, when it comes to educating, advocating, and delivering HT-related services. To increase our advocacy on behalf of victims, we need to become more knowledgeable about HT, as well as more knowledgeable about how to identify and support possible or actual victims. We need to become involved in creating HT-related policy at our places of employment and in our professional organizations, and we need to become more active in local and/or national anti-HT efforts.

NURSING ORGANIZATIONS

In the past several years, more and more nursing organizations such as the International Association of Forensic Nurses (www.forensicnurses.org), the Emergency Nurses Association (www.ena.org), and the American Psychiatric Nurses Association (www.apna.org) have posted information about HT on their websites and/or sponsored or included presentations on HT at their annual conferences. The Association of Women's Health, Obstetric and Neonatal Nurses has actually developed a position statement regarding HT (2016), as did the Emergency Nurses Association (2015). More recently the American Academy of Nursing issued a policy brief on the nursing response to HT (Speck, Mitchell, Ekroos, Sanchez, & Hilfinger, 2018).

Although some nursing organizations specifically address HT in one way or another, other organizations do not. The American Nurses Association (ANA) Code of Ethics Provisions 8 and 9, although not specifically mentioning HT, calls for nurses to collaborate with others to protect human rights, reduce health disparities, and integrate principles of social justice into nursing and health policy (2015). ANA also offers information from nonnursing sources about HT on its website (www.nursingworld.org/practice-policy/nursing-excellence/ethics/ethics-topics-and-articles/). Likewise in its 2016 position statement regarding the nurse's role in ethics and human rights, references are made to social justice, human dignity, and human rights, all of which are violated in HT, but no mention is specifically made about HT (ANA). A search of an ANA position statement page (n.d.) revealed no HT-related policy statements. Similarly, an online search of postings of the International Council of Nurses revealed nothing specifically addressing HT. Owing to the growing awareness of HT and the belief espoused by many working in the field that it has reached the level of being a public health issue, now would be a good time for all professional nursing organizations to come forth with a formal statement or policy regarding HT.

EDUCATION

Signs and symptoms of HT can manifest themselves in patients in almost every area where nurses work, making it all the more crucial that those of us in charge of the classrooms and curricula to advocate for some measure of formal classroom instruction or training for our students. Yet those schools and programs that tend to integrate content on HT are the exception and not the rule. In places where I have either worked or was being considered for a faculty position, as many schools turned down my request to teach a course on HT as permitted me to do so. I commend Drexel University and former Dean of the College of Nursing and Health Professions Gloria Donnelly for supporting my request and efforts to offer not only a course in HT, but a certificate as well in the College of Nursing and Health Professions—with the certificate open to anyone, not just nurses. Although not every program might have room in the curriculum for a required course, other options could include making it an elective or independent study, having students attend a 1-day presentation for which they could earn credit toward their clinical experience, sitting in on a webinar, or using a board-approved resource such as NetCE to learn about HT while also receiving continuing education credits (CEs) if they are already licensed.

Likewise, it is just as important that those already on the job receive some measure of training or education about HT through their employer or as a condition of licensure renewal. I was involved with conducting an informal survey of State Boards of Nursing in 2017 with staff from the McCain Institute, and we found that none of the boards that responded to our emails required any CEs in HT for nursing licensure renewal. Although not a requirement for licensure/relicensure, some states have taken the initiative to require education about HT. According to one study (Atkinson, Curnin, & Hanson, 2016), 13 states have laws that address HT education for health care providers and other professionals, with 10 making the education voluntary and 3 states making it mandatory. Thankfully, there is the option of learning about HT on our own through various online resources and readings—or through online or in person trainings, webinars, conferences, and talks offered locally and nationally.

THE WORKPLACE

I have conducted numerous trainings on HT for nurses and health care organizations. After reviewing what HT is, common signs and symptoms of HT victims, what behaviors and appearances to look for in those who present for care that could be indicative of possible victimization, and what to do and not to do when HT is suspected, the next question I usually ask is what one would do if they suspected they were caring for a victim. What is the process and protocol for next steps in their organization or facility? In more instances than not, the answers are not clear. The time to learn how to swim is not when one is drowning. It is not enough that the nurse knows what to do if her employer does not have a plan. Therefore nurses need to work with their administrators and other key personnel in developing a plan and policy regarding the appropriate actions and next steps to take once an HT victim has been identified. The National Human Trafficking Resource Center (2016) has developed a framework for developing an HT protocol in the health care setting that could prove useful to those wishing to develop such a protocol. There are also a number of articles detailing how others went about developing policies for their health care settings that offer good suggestions (DIGNITY Health, 2017: Schwarz, Unruh, Cronin, Evans-Simpson, Britton, & Ramaswamy, 2016). Refer to Box 80.2 for some possible physical signs of

BOX 80.2 Possible Physical Signs of Human Trafficking

Genital injuries are present, such as vaginal and rectal tears, abrasions, swelling, and lacerations

Urinary tract infections

Evidence of sexual assault with a foreign object

Vaginal fistulas, lacerations, and perforations

Venereal and sexually transmitted infections, including trichomoniasis; hepatitis A, B, and C; syphilis; gonorrhea; human papillomavirus (HPV); genital herpes; chlamydia; human immunodeficiency virus (HIV); acquired immunodeficiency syndrome (AIDS); and pelvic inflammatory disease (PID)

Evidence of repeated abortions

Injuries such as broken bones, missing teeth, sprains and bruises, stab wounds, and burns related to being beaten and/or tortured

Bite marks

Hearing loss from being beaten about the head

Temporal mandibular joint disease from providing oral sex

Dermatologic problems such as scabies, lice, rashes, and various infections

Gunshot wounds

Tattoos and brandings indicating being the property of the pimp or trafficker

Bald spots related to hair being pulled

Backaches related to wearing high heels

Dental problems

Indications of addiction, such as track marks

Gastrointestinal and nutritional problems and eating disorders

Headaches

Respiratory infections, including pneumonia

Sources: De Chesnay & Greenbaum, 2013; Sabella, 2011, 2013, 2015; Taylor & Blake, 2013.

HT (De Chesnay & Greenbaum, 2013; Sabella, 2011, 2013, 2015; Taylor & Blake, 2013).

CONCLUSION

Every nurse can be an agent of change. You can start or join a local coalition, volunteer with programs that serve HT victims, or donate funds to local or national HT organizations such as Polaris, Covenant House, or Shared Hope International. One can contact local politicians to increase efforts to address HT and support bills that provide services to victims. If you are a member in a professional organization that would benefit from increased focus and awareness raising regarding HT, be the person who gets the ball rolling to spread awareness. Once you feel that you have mastered the basics of HT, be the person who shares your knowledge by offering trainings and arranging for presentations in your community or among your colleagues or at your agency. Do not feel that as one person you are unable to make a difference. I took it upon myself to use the power I have as a nurse to invite myself into a program in Phoenix, AZ to research the needs and issues facing HT victims—information I brought back to Philadelphia with me to collaborate with others to create Dawn's Place, a residential program for trafficked women.

DISCUSSION QUESTIONS

1. Based on the earlier information regarding Gisella and Leonard, what are some possible signs that they might be victims of HT, and what could indicate that they are not?

2. The ED where Gisella and Leonard presented had no policy in place regarding encounters with possible HT victims. You have been charged with heading a task force to develop a policy directed to all health care providers in the facility. What elements and criteria would you include and why?

3. Most of the services/support provided for HT victims come after they have been trafficked and can be considered as secondary interventions. Review some of the possible risk factors associated with becoming an HT victim, and discuss some possible primary interventions that could serve to help prevent or reduce HT.

4. You have been asked to develop a short 2- to 3-hour training session for nursing colleagues at your organization. What content would you include in the training, and how would your training address nursing advocacy?

REFERENCES

Administration for Children and Families, Office of Trafficking in Persons. (2017a). *Myths and 265 facts about human trafficking*. Retrieved from www.acf.hhs.gov/otip/about/266 myths-facts-human-trafficking.

Administration for Children and Families, Office of Trafficking in Persons. (2017b). *Fact sheet*. Retrieved from www.acf.hhs. gov/sites/default/files/otip/fact_sheet_human_trafficking_ fy18.pdf.

American Nurses Association. (2015). *Code of ethics for nurses with interpretive statements*. Silver Spring, MD: Author.

American Nurses Association. (2016). *Position statement: The nurse's role in ethics and human rights: Protecting and promoting individual worth, dignity, and human rights in practice settings*. Retrieved from www.nursingworld.org/~4af078/globalassets/ docs/ana/ethics/ethics-and-human-rights-protecting-and- promoting-final-formatted-20161130.pdf.

American Nurses Association. (n.d.) *ANA official position statements*. Retrieved from www.nursingworld.org/practice- policy/nursing-excellence/official-position-statements/.

Association of Women's Health, Obstetric and Neonatal Nurses. (2016). *AWHONN position statement*. Retrieved from www.jognn.org/article/S0884-2175(16)30149-6/pdf? code=jogn-site.

Atkinson, H.G., Curnin, K.J., & Hanson, N.C. (2016) U.S. state laws addressing human trafficking: Education of and mandatory reporting by health care providers and other professionals, *Journal of Human Trafficking, 2*(2), 111-138.

Chisolm-Straker, M., & Stoklosa H. (2017). *Human trafficking as a public health issue: A paradigm expansion into the United States*. Cham, Switzerland: Springer International.

Congress.gov. (n.d.). *S.1312. Trafficking Victims Protection Act 2017*. Retrieved from www.congress.gov/bill/115th-congress/ senate-bill/1312.

De Chesnay, M., & Greenbaum, J. (2013). Physical trauma. In M. De Chesnay (Ed.), *Sex trafficking: A clinical guide for nurses* (pp. 263-280). New York: Springer.

Dignity Health Human Trafficking Response Program shared learnings manual. (2017). Retrieved from www.dignityhealth. org/-/media/cm/media/documents/Human-Trafficking/ Dignity%20Health_HTRP_SharedLearningsManual_170512. ashx?la=en&hash=C510A6D1D187D537147B3C0837F029 20C7687896.

Emergency Nurses Association. (2015). *Position statement: Human trafficking patient awareness in the emergency setting*. Retrieved from www.ena.org/docs/default-source/resource-library/ practice-resources/position-statements/humantraffickingpa tientawareness.pdf?sfvrsn=cd0ad835_14.

Family Violence Prevention Fund. (2005). *Turning pain into power: Trafficking survivors' perspectives on early intervention strategies*. Retrieved from www.futureswithoutviolence.org/ userfiles/file/ImmigrantWomen/Turning%20Pain%20into Power.pdf.

Fedina, L. (2014). The use and misuse of research in books on sex trafficking: Implications for interdisciplinary researchers, practitioners, and advocates. *Trauma, Violence & Abuse, 16*(2), 1-12.

Hepburn, S., & Simon, R.J. (2013). *Human trafficking around the world: Hidden in plain sight*. New York: Columbia University Press.

International Labour Office. (2017).*Global estimates of modern slavery: Forced labour and forced marriage*. Retrieved from www.ilo.org/wcmsp5/groups/public/@dgreports/dcomm/ documents/publication/wcms_575479.pdf.

National Conference of State Legislatures. (n.d.). *Human trafficking state laws*. Retrieved from www.ncsl.org/research/ civil-and-criminal-justice/human-trafficking-laws.aspx.

National Human Trafficking Resource Center. (2016). *Framework for a human trafficking protocol in healthcare settings*. Retrieved from https://humantraffickinghotline.org/resources/framework- human-trafficking-protocol-healthcare-settings.

National Human Trafficking Resource Center: Hotline statistics. (n.d.). Retrieved from https://humantraffickinghotline.org/ sites/default/files/2016%20National%20Report.pdf.

100 Countries and their prostitution policies. (2018). ProCon.org. Retrieved from https://prostitution.procon.org/view.resource. php?resourceID=000772.

Polaris. (2018a). *Current federal laws.* Retrieved from https:// polarisproject.org/current-federal-laws.

Polaris. (2018b). *Reauthorizing the Trafficking Victims Protection Act.* [Blog.]. Retrieved from https://polarisproject.org/blog/2017/ 06/29/reauthorizing-trafficking-victims-protection-act.

Polaris. (2018c). *Recognize the signs.* Retrieved from https:// polarisproject.org/human-trafficking/recognize-signs.

Polaris. (2018d). *2014 State ratings on human trafficking laws.* Retrieved from https://polarisproject.org/resources/2014- state-ratings-human-trafficking-laws.

Richards, T. (2014). Health implications of human trafficking. *Nursing for Women's Health, 18*(2), 155-162.

Sabella, D. (2011). The role of the nurse in combatting human trafficking. *American Journal of Nursing, 111*(2), 28-37.

Sabella, D. (2013). Health issues and interactions with adult survivors. In M. De Chesnay (Ed.), *Sex trafficking: A clinical guide for nurses* (pp. 151-166). New York: Springer.

Sabella, D. (2015). Chapter 6B: Emerging issues: Human trafficking. In B. Price & K. Maguire (Eds.), *Core curriculum for forensic nursing* (pp. 200-220). New York: Wolters Kluwer.

Schwarz, C., Unruh, E., Cronin, K., Evans-Simpson, S., Britton, H., & Ramaswamy, M. (2016). Human trafficking identification and service provision in the medical and social service sector. *Health and Human Rights, 18*(1), 181-192.

Shared Hope International (2018). *State grades 2017.* Retrieved from https://sharedhope.org/what-we-do/bring-justice/ reportcards/.

Speck, P.M., Mitchel, S.A., Ekroos, R.A., Sanchez, R.V., & Hilfinger, D.K. (2018). Policy brief on the nursing response to human trafficking. *Nursing Outlook, 66*(4), 407-411.

Taylor, G., & Blake, B. (2013). Sexually transmitted infections. In M. De Chesnay (Ed.), *Sex trafficking: A clinical guide for nurses* (pp. 239-262). New York: Springer.

Todres, J. (2011). Moving upstream: The merits of a public health law approach to human trafficking. *North Carolina Law Review, 89*(2), 447. Georgia State University College of Law, Legal Studies Research Paper No. 2011-02. Retrieved from https:// papers.ssrn.com/sol3/papers.cfm?abstract_id=1742953.

Trafficking Victims Protection Act 2017. (n.d.). Retrieved from www.grassley.senate.gov/sites/default/files/constituents/ TVPRAOnePager7June2017.pdf

United Nations Office on Drugs and Crime. (2000). *Opening statement of Pino Arlacchi, Under-Secretary-General, Director-General to the International Seminar on Trafficking in Human Beings.* Retrieved from www.unodc.org/unodc/en/about-unodc/speeches/speech_2000-11-28_1.html.

U.S. Congress. (2000). *Victims of Trafficking and Violence Protection Act of 2000.* Public Law 106-386. Retrieved from www. state.gov/documents/organization/10492.pdf.

U.S. Department of Health and Human Services. (2017). *Fact sheet: Human trafficking.* Retrieved from www.acf.hhs. gov/sites/default/files/otip/fact_sheet_human_trafficking_ fy18.pdf

U.S. Department of Health and Human Services, Administration for Children and Families, Campaign to Rescue and Restore Victims of Human (n.d.). *Trafficking: Human trafficking fact sheet.* Retrieved from www.acf.hhs.gov/trafficking/about/ fact_human.html.

U.S. Department of State. (2010). *Trafficking in persons report.* Retrieved from www.state.gov/j/tip/rls/tiprpt/2010/.

U.S. Department of State. (2011). *Trafficking in persons report.* Retrieved from www.state.gov/j/tip/rls/tiprpt/2011/.

U.S. Department of State. (2016). *Trafficking in persons report 2016.* Retrieved from the DOS website: www.state.gov/docu- ments/organization/258876.pdf)

U.S Departmentof State. (2017). *Tier placements.* Retrieved from https://2009-2017.state.gov/j/tip/rls/tiprpt/2016/258696.htm.

U.S. Department of State. (2018). *Trafficking in persons report.* Retrieved from www.state.gov/j/tip/rls/tiprpt/2018/index. htm.

U.S. Department of State. (n.d.). *U.S. laws on trafficking in persons.* Retrieved from www.state.gov/j/tip/laws/.

U.S. Department of State, Office to Monitor and Combat Trafficking in Persons. (2004). *Trafficking in persons report 2004.*Washington, DC. Retrieved from www.state.gov/ documents/organization/34158.pdf.

ONLINE RESOURCES

Covenant House
www.covenanthouse.org

Dawn's Place
http://ahomefordawn.org

Girls Educational and Mentoring Services (GEMS)
www.gems-girls.org

International Justice Mission
www.ijm.org

Polaris/Polaris Project
https://polarisproject.org

The Salvation Army
www.salvationarmyusa.org/usn/fight-human-trafficking/

Shared Hope International
https://sharedhope.org

United Nations Office on Drugs and Crime
www.unodc.org/unodc/en/human-trafficking/what-is-human- trafficking.html

U.S. Department of Health and Human Services
www.acf.hhs.gov/trafficking

81

TAKING ACTION: Policy, Politics, and Advocating for Medicinal Cannabis Use

Carey S. Clark

"Awareness of one's own beliefs and attitudes about any therapeutic intervention is vital, as nurses are expected to provide patient care without personal judgment of patients. Although medical cannabis legislation is evolving and more jurisdictions are adopting Medical Marijuana Programs, social acceptance may not be evolving at the same pace."

The National Council of State Boards of Nursing (NCSBN), 2018

HISTORY OF PROHIBITION OF CANNABIS

How did cannabis go from being a healing herb to an illegal drug? As we know from written documents and archeological artifacts, plant medicines have been used by humans throughout time to support health, healing, and wellness and to treat disease and illness (Petrovska, 2012). *Cannabis sativa* is one such healing plant that has been used for thousands of years. A very brief history of the plant from medicinal value through prohibition is provided in Table 81.1.

Since the late 1990s, the landscape around cannabis legalization has changed rapidly. The majority of states currently have some medicinal or adult, recreational cannabis laws in place (Petrovska, 2012), with individual states ending cannabis prohibition via legislative acts or voter referendums. At the time of this writing, current federal laws prohibiting the use of cannabis as a schedule I drug under the Controlled Substances Act (U.S. Drug Enforcement Agency, n.d.). The scheduling of cannabis impacts many things: researching the effects of cannabis; addressing critical social justice issues, such as incarceration for possession of cannabis and cannabis products; and accessing cannabis for health care and medical treatment.

GLOBAL ISSUES

Cannabis is the most used "illicit substance" globally, yet it is produced in nearly every country (National Institute of Drug Abuse, 2018). Cannabis and hemp have a long history of medicinal use, as a sacred herb in religious ceremonies, and for everyday products such as paper, rope, and sailcloth (Bewly-Taylor, Blickman, & Jelsma, 2014). In 1961 the United Nations passed the "Single Convention on Narcotic Drugs" treaty limiting cannabis use to medicinal and scientific purposes only. Despite protests from countries, such as India where cannabis was part of traditional medicinal practices, cannabis was banned at the international level, due to its psychoactivity and lack of perceived medicinal value (Bewly-Taylor, Blickman, & Jelsma, 2014). The U.S. federal government continues to comply with this and other treaties, at the same time supporting states' rights to legalize cannabis use and sale.

ENVIRONMENTAL IMPACT

The environmental impact of cannabis is concerning, as illegal growth can have a negative, uncontrollable impact on the environment. With legalization, cannabis' environmental impact can be more closely regulated and monitored to minimize negative effects (Scientific America, 2016).

Hemp has a history of being a sustainable and environmentally friendly product. Generally grown without pesticides, hemp's deep root systems can benefit soil quality, removing large amounts of carbon through photosynthesis while clearing the soil of heavy metals and materials (Canadian Hemp Trade Alliance [CHTA], 2018). Hemp products can be reused and recycled, and are 100% biodegradable; hemp

TABLE 81.1	Cannabis Timeline
1500 BC	Cannabis included in Chinese Pharmacopeia
1213 BC	Ancient Egyptians use cannabis to treat glaucoma
200 BC	Greeks treat infections and inflammation with cannabis
1600s–1700s	U.S. founding fathers grew *cannabis sativa* and hemp (a plant variety with lower levels of tetrahydrocannabinol [THC]); cannabis is mandated to be grown for industrial purposes
1850	Cannabis added to *U.S. Pharmacopeia*
1889	Cannabis found to ease opium withdrawal symptoms
1911	Massachusetts becomes first state to outlaw cannabis related to moral concerns
1915	The Harrison Act of 1915 required all U.S. physicians to use a serial number obtained via Internal Revenue Service to prescribe opium; sets stage for future federal drug regulation efforts
1916–1931	29 states outlawed use of cannabis
1937	Marijuana Tax Act essentially bans cannabis use nationwide despite American Medical Association opposition to the legislation
1930s	Creation of the Federal Bureau of Narcotics; William Randolph Hearst's supports cannabis prohibition; *Reefer Madness* movie release; first conviction for personal sale of cannabis in Denver, Colorado
1942	Cannabis removed from the *U.S. Pharmacopeia*

Sources: Boire & Fenney, 2007; Denver Public Library, 2014; Russo, 2007; Terry, 1915; Woodward, 1937.

is a renewable source (replacing wood-based products and synthetic products like plastics and clothing materials) and an energy source (hemp biodiesel) (CHTA, 2018).

SOCIAL JUSTICE AND HUMAN ISSUES

There are important social justice issues related to cannabis that are centered around racial, economic, and access concerns, including incarceration for possession and trafficking, and drug-related violence. Half of all drug arrests in the United States are related to cannabis; 88% of these arrests being for simple possession of cannabis (American Civil Liberties Union, 2013). Women are the fastest growing segment of the U.S. prison population: 25% of incarcerated women in state prisons are serving time for drug-related offenses (vs. 15% of men), and 61% of women in federal prison (vs. 50% of men) (Drug Policy Alliance, 2018; Dumont, Brockman, Dickman, Alexander, & Rich, 2012). Although drug use occurs equally across the racial spectrum, Black women are twice as likely and Latina women are 20% more likely to be incarcerated for drugs than are White women (Drug Policy Alliance, 2018; Dumont et al., 2012). The war on drugs has done nothing to change the rate of drug use, but it has served to increase the U.S. prison population (Dumont et al., 2012).

As of the time of the writing, one's zip code can determine the ability to legally access cannabis, making access to cannabinoids an ethical concern. In 2014, when Colorado first legalized cannabis for recreational use, many "medical marijuana refugees" flocked to the state, hoping to legally access cannabis (CNN, 2014). However, many others in

need of legal access to cannabis remained in states prohibiting their use. Although children are often the medical refugees, entire families are impacted (CNN, 2014).

The medicinal use of cannabis is related to many economic issues. Individuals pay out of pocket for medical cannabis as it is not covered under health insurance. From a business point of view, women and people of color are underrepresented within the cannabis industry, a field dominated by White males. The Massachusetts Cannabis Control Commission (2017), in preparation for legalization, developed a "Social Equity Program" to address such disparities within the cannabis industry.

MY JOURNEY

From 2003 to 2010, I lived in western Sonoma County in Northern California, where cannabis was grown throughout my neighborhood. During that time, many medicinal cannabis patients would share space for their crops. In the early fall, the *terpenes*, or aromatic essential oils from the cannabis plants, would fill the air. Cannabis was an accepted part of the culture in that area. In 2010 when I moved to Maine, I knew there was a medicinal cannabis program, and Maine had the second largest number of cannabis users per capita in the country, behind California. However, I was surprised the culture was much more "closeted" and less evident in everyday life.

My curiosity about medicinal cannabis use peaked when Dr. Dustin Sulak, a well-known Maine cannabis-recommending physician, came to speak with our university's holistic nursing students. We learned about the endocannabinoid system (ECS), the largest, cellular membrane receptor system in the body, that produces cannabis-like substances called *endocannabinoids*, namely anadamide and 2-AG (Clark, 2018). When deficient in endocannabinoids, one can fall out of homeostasis and become ill. Our bodies make and break down endocannabinoids on demand, so they are not stored in the body. The ECS helps to regulate the entire body, including the inflammatory and immune responses. The use of phytocannabinoids, such as cannabis, can be effective at supporting healing for different illnesses; a lack of one's own cannabinoids may contribute to illness. Supplementation with phytocannabinoids strives to enhance the tone of the ECS and can help to support the healing process.

I continued to learn about the science behind the ECS and the use of cannabis for healing through self-study and attending scientific conferences focused on medicinal cannabis. I became a member of the American Cannabis Nurses Association (ACNA) and served on the board of directors. In 2016, I connected with the Marijuana Policy Project and the Maine "Yes on 1" cannabis policy campaign movement to legalize cannabis use for all adults, support increased access to medicinal cannabis, and address social justice issues. I faced many challenges around my public support of legalizing cannabis, including lack of support and animosity in my workplace setting. Without having received full tenure from my university in the spring of 2016, I would not have felt as secure in taking a very public stance around the legalization movement.

As President of the ACNA (2018–19), I present to national and local nursing audiences about the ECS, how cannabis addresses specific health issues, and defining the nurse's role with patients. I developed the Scope and Standards of Cannabis Nurse Practice (Clark, 2017) defining how cannabis nurses interact with patients from a caring-holistic stance and using coaching tools. I work every day to end the sigma around the use of cannabis and to educate the nursing profession about the ECS. Although we have known about the ECS since the 1990s, our nursing textbooks and curricula have failed to educate nurses in any meaningful way. The ACNA has developed a resolution to include the ECS in nursing curricula, and the National Council of State Boards of Nursing (NCSBN) (2018) has made a similar nationally recognized call.

EDUCATING NURSES

Nurses need to learn basic physiologic functions of the ECS; implications of ECS deficiency (NCSBN, 2018); and how diet, stress management, exercise, and incorporation of holistic modalities (yoga, acupuncture, osteopathy,

massage) can regulate the ECS (McPartland, Guy, & DiMarzzo, 2014). As more states legalize the use of cannabis, it is imperative for nurses caring for patients using cannabis to understand cannabis laws and restrictions in their respective states. Nurses can also use a holistic approach when working with cannabis patients, discussing past and current use, incorporating motivational interviewing, and remaining patient centered when setting goals for medicinal and palliative use of cannabis (Clark, 2017; 2018). Although cannabis currently cannot be prescribed due to federal prohibition, patients may need support when receiving their medicinal cannabis recommendation, determining how they will access and pay for the medicine, and addressing safety and legal concerns (NCSBN, 2018).

As one of the few medicines needing self-titration for proper palliation of symptoms, dosing of cannabis can be challenging. Feel "high" or euphoric is not needed to feel palliation of symptoms (Clark, 2018). Cannabis strains low in tetrahydrocannabinol (THC) can help patients avoid the euphoric sensation and common side effects (dry mouth, dry eyes, anxiety, perception of time slowing down, fatigue or sleepiness). Using whole-plant medicine that is absent of pesticides, fungus, and molds with a wide variety of cannabinoids and terpenes will facilitate the ECS response (MacCallum & Russo, 2018). Consumption of cannabis can include smoking, vaporizing, oral tinctures, edible food products, rectal suppositories, transdermal, and topical application.

Differentiating between medical and recreational use of cannabis can be challenging. In general, medicinal cannabis use involves the intention to heal or palliate physical and/or mental symptoms, with less concern over obtaining a feeling of euphoria. Recreational use of cannabis focuses on obtaining the sense of high, or euphoria. As a recreational drug, cannabis is safer to use than many other drugs that can cause harm or death (Melamede, 2005). Alcohol, heroin, crack, and tobacco are the most harmful substances when it comes to addiction; cannabis is far less addictive and harmful (Lachenmeier & Rehm, 2015).

PUBLIC HEALTH–RELATED ISSUES

As we move toward greater use of cannabis, there are legitimate, public health concerns needing consideration. Using cannabis or mixing alcohol or other intoxicant medicines with cannabis increases the risks of impaired driving. THC stays in the body from weeks to months post ingestion, making testing for cannabis difficult and controversial, because the ability to accurately measure acute intoxication is limited (Hartman & Huestis, 2014). Secondhand smoke from smoking cannabis and the impact of cannabis-related substance use disorder are all serious public health concerns as cannabis use grows.

Efforts to address these concerns must be balanced with the knowledge that cannabis is far less dangerous than alcohol or other drugs. The social stigma related to cannabis use can prevent people from accessing the medicine they need. Nurses can advocate for an end to mandatory drug-sentencing guidelines and support anti-prohibition efforts.

Lastly, ensuring that patients have access to cannabis that is safe and pesticide-free is critical. Contamination from pesticides and the excess energy used for growing cannabis indoors can also have tremendous public health and environmental impacts.

REFERENCES

American Civil Liberties Union. (2013). *The war on drugs in black and white*. Retrieved from www.aclu.org/report/report-war-marijuana-black-and-white?redirect=criminal-law-reform/war-marijuana-black-and-white.

Bewly-Taylor, D., Blickman, T., & Jelsma, M. (2014). *The rise and decline of cannabis prohibition: The history of cannabis in the UN drug control system and options for reform*. Amsterdam: Transnational Institute.

Boire, R.G., & Feeney, K. (2007). *Medical marijuana law*. Oakland, CA: Ronin Publishing.

Canadian Hemp Trade Alliance. (2018). *Background: Hemp's environmental impact*. Retrieved from www.hemptrade.ca/eguide/background/hemps-environmental-impact.

Cannabis Control Commission, Commonwealth of Massachusetts. (2017). *Guidance for equity provisions*. Retrieved from https://mass-cannabis-control.com/wp-content/uploads/2018/04/FINAL-Social-Provisions-Guidance-1PGR-1.pdf.

Clark, C.S. (2017). *Scope and standards of practice for cannabis nurses*. American Cannabis Nurses Association. Retrieved from https://cannabisnurses.org/Scope-of-Practice-for-Cannabis-Nurses.

Clark, C.S. (2018). Medical cannabis: The oncology nurse's role in patient education about the effects of marijuana on cancer palliation. *Clinical Journal of Oncology Nursing, 22*(1), E-1–E-6.

CNN.com. (2014). *Medical marijuana refuges: "This was our only hope."* Retrieved from www.cnn.com/2014/03/10/health/medical-marijuana-refugees/index.html.

Denver Public Library. (2014). *Denver's other marijuana first*. Retrieved from https://history.denverlibrary.org/news/denvers-other-marijuana-first.

Drug Policy Alliance. (2018). *Women, prison and the drug war*. Retrieved from www.drugpolicy.org/resource/women-prison-and-drug-war-englishspanish.

Dumont, D.M., Brockmann, B., Dickman, S., Alexander, N., & Rich, J.D. (2012). Public health and the epidemic of incarceration. *Annual Review of Public Health, 33*, 325-339.

Hartman, R.L., & Huestis, M.A. (2014). Cannabis effects on driving skills. *Clinical Chemistry, 59*(3), 478-492.

Lachenmeier, D. W., & Rehm, J. (2015). Comparative risk assessment of alcohol, tobacco, cannabis and other illicit drugs using the margin of exposure approach. *Scientific Reports, 5*, 8126.

MacCallum, C.A., & Russo, E.B. (2018). Practical considerations in medical cannabis administration and dosing. *European Journal of Internal Medicine, 49*, 12–19.

McPartland, J.M., Guy, G.W., & Di Marzo, V. (2014). Care and feeding of the endocannabinoid system: A systematic review of potential clinical interventions that upregulate the endocannabinoid system. *Plos One, 9*(3), 1-21.

Melamede, R. (2005). Harm reduction: The cannabis paradox. *Harm Reduction Journal, 22*(2), 17.

National Institute of Drug Abuse. (2018). *What is marijuana?* Retrieved from www.drugabuse.gov/publications/drugfacts/marijuana.

Petrovska, B.B. (2012). Historical review of medicinal plants' usage. *Pharmacology Review, 6*(11), 1-5.

National Academies of Science, Engineering, and Medicine. (2017). *The health effects of cannabis and cannabinoids: The current state of evidence and recommendations for research*. Washington, DC: National Academies Press.

National Council of State Boards of Nursing. (2018). The NCSBN national nursing guidelines for medical marijuana. *Journal of Nursing Regulation, 9*(2, Suppl), S1-S58.

Russo, E. (2007). History of cannabis and its preparations in saga, science, and sobriquet. *Chemistry & Biodiversity, 4*(8), 1614-1648.

Terry, C.E. (1915). The Harrison Anti-Narcotic Act. *American Journal of Public Health, 5*(6), 518.

U.S. Drug Enforcement Agency. (n.d.). *Drug scheduling*. Retrieved from www.dea.gov/drug-scheduling.

Woodward, W.C. (1937). *Letter from the American medical association*. RE: HR 6906. Retrieved from http://druglibrary.net/schaffer/hemp/taxact/t8.htm.

82

Think Globally, Act Locally: Nursing and Global Health

Jane E. Salvage and Jill F. White

> *"'Global nursing' is not defined by working internationally or participating in mission trips, but requires a shift in consciousness and an evolving awareness regarding how our work contributes to outcomes not only in health sectors, but also in policy, education, economic relations, and environmental activism."*
>
> **William Rosa**

As health professionals committed to our local community, county, and country, it is tempting to look no further than our own backyard. There is always so much there about which we care deeply. Yet this solely local focus is not only ostrich-like but also dangerous: global health is inseparable from local and national health concerns. For example, infectious diseases do not recognize borders, and a mingling of germs and genes results in communicable diseases with the potential for rapid global spread. Compare the 36 hours it takes for some diseases to spread worldwide with the 4 years it took the medieval plague to cross Europe.

This chapter aims to inspire you to look beyond your backyard and to understand how what happens in distant places affects the health and health care of your community, your family, and yourself—just as what happens in your backyard affects people you will never meet. "Think globally, act locally!" as the environmental slogan says. Thinking globally is not an academic exercise but a way of seeing that enriches perspectives, increases knowledge, and makes nurses more motivated and effective as practitioners, managers, teachers, researchers, policymakers, and activists.

WHAT IS "GLOBAL HEALTH"?

A growing number of governments and organizations are adopting "global health" as a key policy theme, but the concept did not really exist even 20 years ago. The common term *international health* refers mainly to health work in low-income countries on issues such as infectious diseases and mother and child health, often tackled through "technical assistance" from visiting experts.

Nursing students and nurse volunteers from high-income countries such as the United States may work or study in lower-income countries and say they are "doing global health." International volunteering has both positives and pitfalls (Lasker, 2016), and these "bilateral" partnerships need careful management (Salvage, 2007). Such experiences may be mutually beneficial, but they are not "doing global health," which is a broader, deeper, more complex concept that engages with all countries and indeed with the health of the planet itself (Rosa, 2017).

A global view leads nurses to more informed and thoughtful decisions; Oulton (2016) says: "It begins with understanding the policies and politics of globalization, the growing interdependence of the world's people, (which) means that national policy and action are increasingly shaped by international forces along with other aspects of our lives" (p. 703). It also recognizes that health is interdependent and interconnected: the policies that most affect health are often not health policies, so cross-sectoral collaboration is critical.

THE WEALTH OF A NATION IS ITS PEOPLE

We live in challenging times for the health of the planet, nations, and communities. From halting infectious disease epidemics to reducing mother and child deaths, tackling and mitigating the effects of climate change, and caring for older people, the challenges have major implications for nursing as a global profession of some 23 million women and men. Consider the implications of the rising global need for continuous care and support for people with multiple long-term conditions. Older people are the fastest-growing age group worldwide; by 2050 nearly one in four people will be older than 60 years, and more than 80% will have little or no help to age well. The need for expert nursing is already acute.

Inequalities among groups of people, and within and between countries and regions, are key to understanding these challenges. There is a mass of evidence of the interaction between health and wealth at all levels, whether individual, family, community, or country. Nurses know that their patients' ways of life and the conditions in which they live and work strongly influence their health and longevity. This challenges us to complement biomedical with social models of health care and focus much more on prevention and public health.

Since the 1990s, the growing understanding of the interaction between health and poverty, and the need for cooperation and collaboration on a global scale to combat its consequences for health and for economies, has encouraged many organizations to play a larger role in global health. The United Nations (UN) responded with a visionary global agenda that set targets called the Millennium Development Goals (MDGs), 2000–2015. It promoted collaboration between public, private, and nongovernmental organizations (NGOs) concerned about health and poverty and the centrality of a healthy population to economic growth and well-being (Sridhar et al, 2017).

The three health-related MDG goals—reduce child mortality, improve maternal health, and combat human immunodeficiency virus (HIV)/acquired immunodeficiency syndrome (AIDS), malaria, and other diseases—had the greatest success in achieving or approaching the targets (World Health Organization [WHO], 2015). The MDG movement also secured global agreement on the need for a common framework to tackle the big health issues. This led to a burgeoning of global health partnerships through multisectoral, multifunded agencies.

Progress was made, but the MDGs were not fully achieved, and in 2015 the UN followed up with another ambitious proposition. *Transforming Our World: The 2030 Agenda for Sustainable Development* is a plan of action for people, planet, and prosperity to be implemented in partnership by all countries and all stakeholders (UN, 2015). Eradicating poverty in all its forms and dimensions, it says, is the greatest global challenge: "bold and transformative steps . . . are urgently needed to shift the world onto a sustainable and resilient path."

The action framework for these bold and transformative steps is the 17 Sustainable Development Goals (SDGs) 2016–2030. You can review an attractive free package (International Council of Nurses [ICN], 2018) and an invaluable primer (Rosa, 2017). The SDGs are inextricably interwoven; health is inherent in all goals and influenced by all goals, and there is one overt health goal: #3, *Ensure healthy lives and promote well-being for all at all ages*. This has goals within the goal: advancing the three existing foci of the MDGs (mothers, babies, and infectious diseases); and addressing noncommunicable diseases (NCDs), substance abuse, road traffic accidents, universal health coverage, reproductive health, and the health effects of pollution and contamination. There is also a focus on the process issues of research, financing, capacity-building, and international regulations.

IDEALS TO GOALS TO ACTIONS

The vision-based SDGs provide an overarching global framework for health policy and practice that drives the work of WHO and other organizations. The global health landscape is complex and ever changing, but WHO remains primary and pivotal. Established by the UN in 1948, it provides international leadership in technical support, monitoring health risks, surveillance of emerging communicable diseases, controlling and preventing NCDs, strengthening health systems, and emergency preparedness. WHO works in partnership with member states' governments, health systems, and universities; other UN agencies; NGOs; and business. It is constituted by the 193 UN member states, who meet annually at the World Health Assembly. In its Geneva headquarters, 6 regional offices, and more than 150 country offices, WHO directs the work of more than 7000 staff and many more consultants.

Another major player is the World Bank Group, the world's largest development institution, with 189 member countries. Its very powerful group of organizations provide financial and technical assistance to developing countries through loans and grants. Its growing awareness of the poverty/health nexus has led it to become a major funder of global health agencies such as the Global Fund and WHO itself (Sridhar et al, 2017). Its relationships are primarily with ministers of finance, who often have markedly different priorities from ministers of health.

The SDGs have also spurred the development of new global organizations, including initiatives funded by three influential philanthropic foundations whose immense wealth derives from commerce: Bloomberg Philanthropies, the Chan Zuckerberg Initiative, and the Bill and Melinda Gates Foundation. Such support is invaluable, but there are serious concerns about the governance of such donors, accountable mainly to themselves, and how their wealth and power shape decisions about priorities and ways of working.

Financial aid and technical assistance from individual high-income countries and regional groups of countries make them additional major global health players. For example, the European Union funds research and development projects in health within and beyond its member states, costing millions of dollars. The U.S. government, working with UN agencies and its own programs, makes major contributions, such as the work of the Centers for Disease Control and Prevention, in more than 60 countries. These forms of support—who the recipients are, how they are helped, and what issues are tackled—are also politically charged decisions.

GLOBAL NURSING ORGANIZATIONS

In addition to these major players, there are thousands of organizations of all types, sizes, and ambitions active in global health, making it a highly complex, often competitive, and politically contested terrain. The nursing profession actually has a much longer global presence than the UN or WHO. ICN was founded in 1899, predating WHO by nearly 50 years, and funded the first WHO nursing position. A federation of more than 130 national nursing associations, ICN has three primary functions: to represent nursing worldwide, to advance the profession, and to influence health policy. Located in Geneva close to WHO and other international organizations, it remains the major global voice of nursing, although its ambitions are hindered by lack of funds and the difficulties of modernizing and leading with such a diverse group of members.

Before 2000, ICN focused on three profession-focused pillars—nurses' socioeconomic welfare, regulation, and advancing professional practice. It has relatively recently taken a more overtly collaborative, interprofessional, and intersectoral approach and is seeking greater influence on health and health care, including through expanded influence at the policy level. It is complementing its traditional focus on advancement of the profession with a newer focus on the nursing contribution to better health. This means wider engagement with other organizations, moving beyond the "nursing bubble" in which nurses speak only to each other (Shamian, 2015).

Many more nursing organizations and networks are active in global health, including the global network of WHO Collaborating Centres in Nursing and Midwifery, Sigma Theta Tau International, and the *Nursing Now* campaign. These nursing entities regularly engage with each other informally and formally. There are many other global nursing players, including organizations and networks on specific nursing concerns and specialties ranging from primary health care to cancer nursing to climate change. NGOs, health services, and universities throughout the world also have a rich diversity of intercountry bilateral and multilateral relationships and projects that contribute to the global health and nursing agenda. Thousands of nurses meet regularly at international congresses across the globe, sharing ideas and research (Box 82.1).

BOX 82.1 Exemplar: Phindi From South Africa

Phindi always wanted to be a nurse, like her mother. Her parents died of AIDS, and the Florence Nightingale International Foundation funded her schooling through its Girl Child Education Fund. After she qualified as a nurse, the government sent her to work in the community. Some medical and nursing colleagues resented this obligation because they wanted to work in big hospitals, but Phindi enjoys the challenge and is passionately committed to helping her community.

The work is very difficult. People live in poverty and are generally unhealthy; there are too few health workers; and she travels long distances to rural clinics where there may be no clean water, electricity, medical equipment, or supplies. She often has to do the work of a doctor, pharmacist, and lab technician as well, but she feels she makes a difference, especially now that she has been trained to screen people for HIV/AIDS and tuberculosis.

She refers those she thinks are at risk to doctors for diagnosis and initial prescribing of treatment and then treats and monitors them herself.

Nurse-led screening and caseload management resulted in patients being managed as effectively as in physician-led programs—findings that Phindi described at a conference. Nurses from Botswana then told her about their work in a successful program giving antiretroviral treatment to HIV-infected children—nurse-led care again proving equally effective.

She worries about how she will raise her children and give them good quality housing and education in this village. But she says, "If I work in South Africa under difficult conditions it is not that I can't sell my labour somewhere else, but because I feel I have to assist my own country. It goes to the level of where you need to find yourself as a human being."

From All-Party Parliamentary Group on Global Health. (2016). *Triple impact: How developing nursing will improve health, promote gender equality and support economic growth.* Retrieved from www.appg-globalhealth.org.uk.

Note: The nurse's name in this exemplar has been changed.

Nurse-led organizations, comparatively weak and lacking in influence, are not yet major players. In addition, nursing is seriously underrepresented in the major global health organizations. This lack of a strong global nursing voice is part and parcel of structural global inequalities related to gender, wealth, race, and status. These inequalities also underlie the lack of attention paid to voices from low-income countries, indigenous peoples, and other disadvantaged groups, an omission that has a large and generally unrecognized negative impact on global health.

GLOBAL POLITICS AND POLICY

Many nurses make naive assumptions about health and health care and do not view these issues through a sociopolitical lens (White, 2014). Yet we can see the influence of policy and politics all around us every day, in our health and nursing priorities, in the funding of our health systems, and in the health challenges we tackle. We need to understand some history and politics if we want to be leaders of change, rather than its servants.

Neoliberalism, the market-based political and social philosophy that swept the world in the 1980s, and continues to dominate it, has a profound effect on global health and global health politics. This form of capitalism derives from an economic approach that aims to increase the role of the private sector in the economy and society through policies such as privatization, austerity, deregulation, free trade, and reductions in government spending. Its impacts include widening inequalities within and between countries; competition between health service providers; and commercialization of health services. The World Bank became increasingly influential as it tied many of the key performance indicators of its loans to health system reform along these lines, often with disastrous effects (Abbasi, 1999). These negative consequences were recognized, and a changed policy direction currently requires evidence of health systems strengthening in proposals.

The powerful influence of vested commercial interests, including the groups of huge corporations known as Big Tobacco and Big Sugar, cannot be underestimated. The traditional but often covert strength and tactics of the tobacco companies have become apparent as countries fight for plain packaging and bans on advertising. Big Sugar's influence is becoming more visible in the battle against NCDs, undermining healthy public policies to reduce sugar consumption and tax high-sugar beverages.

Action on climate change is another policy battleground. WHO predicts that between 2030 and 2050 it will cause approximately 250,000 additional deaths per year, from malnutrition, malaria, diarrhea, and heat stress. The response of governments to climate change and the science

explaining it is a further example of the intensely political nature of global health policy, strongly influenced by national politics. National changes in political philosophy can quickly change the global health policy and funding environment. A recent example is the Trump administration's withdrawal from the 2015 Paris Agreement on climate change and the rollback of other U.S. environmental protections. Political arguments along party lines in countries have consequences not just locally, but for global warming, reproductive health, and many other contested areas that have serious health consequences.

Radical Alternatives

The politics of health, then, is fraught with vested interests and contested priorities. The big question is what impact this has on a global level. The disastrous initial response to the Ebola virus disease epidemic and crisis in West Africa from 2014 to 2016 demonstrated clearly the problems with imposing external thinking and processes on local conditions. Development ultimately has to happen in the country, and by the country, and led by the people of the country; it cannot be done to them, but by them, facilitated by the international community (Ravelo, 2015): "It is the job of the outside world to take stock of that point, and adapt to local contexts rather than hope that local contexts will adapt to the solutions that we're bringing."

The imposition of programs on unstable health systems, without recognition or consideration of the limited numbers of health professionals, is another example. In Mali, the rollout of vaccination, drug supplementation, and malaria programs resulted in senior nursing staff being absent from the hospital for over half their time, with a consequent decrease in the quality and safety of in-patient care (Coulibaly et al, 2008).

Such developments have generated growing criticism of the global health establishment and the rise of grassroots social movements addressing the social, environmental, and economic determinants of health. One example is the People's Health Movement, a global network with a presence in approximately 70 countries that brings together health activists, civil society organizations, and academic institutions, particularly from low- and middle-income countries (People's Health Movement, n.d.). It calls for a more people-centered approach that highlights social justice and magnifies the voices of the poor and vulnerable, addressing the unfair economic structures that lock people into poverty and poor health.

Policy, Politics, and Nursing

Nurses are the largest group in the global health workforce by a significant margin and are often the only health care providers available. In many places they play advanced roles to fill in the missing pieces of care. Key to ensuring that all people and communities receive all the health services they need without financial hardship, nurses occupy a special position as the interface between the health system and the community. We see, hear, and experience how policy affects people and their communities, and we should be feeding that knowledge into policymaking (Box 82.2). You might think this would be welcomed with open arms by policymakers, yet it has been very difficult for nurses at all levels to make an impact on policy, for a variety of reasons. Although nurses are acknowledged as key policy implementers, they are rarely central to health and social policy development (White, 2014).

Nurses have become increasingly knowledgeable, skilled, and well educated, but this has not been matched with a significant growth in influence and status. Ninety percent of nurses worldwide are women, which helps to explain senior nurses' continuing exclusion from leadership positions in health organizations at all levels. Even within nursing, men occupy a disproportionately high number of leadership roles, and the very existence of such roles is under threat. The profession often challenges this, and sometimes makes headway, but has to fight the battle all over again when health employers decide they no longer need a nurse director or when governments do not replace their chief nurse. Even in countries that have traditionally provided global nursing leadership, the government chief nurse role has been abolished, downgraded, or never existed.

As another glaring example, WHO's commitment to nursing has waxed and waned over the decades, a story not told in its own upbeat history (WHO, 2017). There are no accurate figures, but the number of nurses employed in nursing posts fell from the late 1960s (Caughley, 2009) and was regularly tracked by ICN. The number of nurses employed in WHO programs but not in nursing-specific roles is not known but has been extremely small; for example, the number working in the large WHO headquarters department for HIV/AIDS prevention, control, and care in 2004 was zero.

The chief nurses at the WHO headquarters and in the six WHO regional offices used to have much larger teams and budgets, although never commensurate with the importance of nursing. Their declining scope and influence, attributable partly to cuts in WHO budgets, was also due to long-standing reluctance by the physician-dominated organization to recognize nursing's value. This has long been a bone of contention between WHO and other organizations, primarily ICN.

It took the election of the first ever nonphysician director-general of WHO in 2017 to make the difference. Public health expert Tedros Adhanom Ghebreyesus, who had recognized and promoted the key role of nurses in achieving universal health coverage when he was a government minister in Ethiopia, was shocked by the absence of nurses when he took up his new role at WHO. His appointment of Elizabeth Iro from the Cook Islands as chief nursing officer, reporting directly to him, is the first time in its 70-year history that a nurse has sat at the WHO's top table. He also commissioned its first ever *State of the World's Nursing* report—the first in 70 years! These are important gains, symbolically at least, but just the beginning. Nurses and their organizations need to continue to be vigilant and vocal, holding global and national leaders to account.

BOX 82.2 Exemplar: Effectiveness in Global Health Work

Australian nurse Amanda McClelland identified a critical nursing role when she engaged in high-level global health work as the Senior Officer, Emergency Health Unit, International Federation of Red Cross and Red Crescent Societies. Her role required her to bring information from the field into high-level meetings, explain the complexities and difficulties of actually implementing programs, and then interpret the science or recommendations from these meetings back to the field teams in a way that could be translated into action.

"How am I going to explain this to the volunteers and how will they explain it to the community?" she wondered. "That's great, but the community would never accept it. That's great, but we won't be able to implement the programme in that way. We're going to need to consider weather/culture/religious factors when rolling this out. I added a social mobilisation and community aspect to global strategy discussions."

From McClelland, A. (2017). *Emergencies only.* Crow's Nest, Australia: Allen & Unwin.

UNDERSTANDING POLICYMAKING

Even nurses who occupy senior positions may not be influential, for a range of reasons ranging from gender discrimination to lack of status. Many have little or no preparation for these roles and do not know how to influence and shape policy. Moreover, "political space is finite... Organised medicine knows when and how to present a united front... Nursing is far less politically accomplished and far less assertive" (Lewis, 2010).

Nursing history in many countries and at regional and international levels is strewn with evidence-based policy reviews and reports making excellent recommendations—largely unheeded. Compounded by structural inequalities related to gender, ethnicity, and social class, nurses' attempts to push for reform have not gained enough traction, and change has not happened fast enough or far enough.

Sometimes the political timing is poor. For example, an independent commission in England produced a report widely welcomed by the professions, but its impact was limited (The Prime Minister's Commission on the Future of Nursing and Midwifery, 2010). Released only a month before the Labour government lost a general election, the incoming Conservative government ignored it. Similarly, a National Expert Commission report from Canada with a strong primary health care focus was released at a time when this philosophy was not in favor with the government (Canadian Nurses Association, 2012). The United States had much greater success with the *Future of Nursing* initiative, which was generously funded and had detailed implementation and reporting requirements, promoted with great political and policy savvy (Institute of Medicine, 2011).

The Window of Opportunity

Recommendations on nursing that fail to have traction, policies that ignore or undermine nursing, and nurses' absence from policymaking—this gloomy pattern is finally starting to change for the better. Nursing is moving along the political development spectrum (Box 82.3) from self-interest to political sophistication (Cohen et al., 1996). More nurses are becoming policy entrepreneurs, that is, leaders who position themselves to influence policy; who bring together problems, policies, and politics into a novel amalgamate—new policy; and who soften up the system by presenting participants in the network (visible and invisible) with alternative representations of their realities. This leads to the opening of a window of opportunity—the potential for a truly new policy perspective (Kingdon, 2011).

That window is now opening, as the demand grows worldwide for solutions to acute problems, including current and future health worker shortages, the rising need for expert care of older people, the importance of investment in health as a public good, and greater public interest in nursing. Global awareness is growing of nurses' actual and potential contributions to improving health, creating gender equality, and strengthening economies. Meanwhile more nurses and midwives are finding the courage to become "silence breakers" and join the worldwide wave of protests against violence, sexual harassment, and other abusive behavior against women (WHO 2016; Salvage & Stilwell, 2018).

The window was pushed a little further open by a call for action from the United Kingdom All Party Parliamentary Group (APPG) on Global Health (APPG, 2016). It produced an influential report that was bipartisan and cross-disciplinary, connected national and global issues, and described the social and economic impact of nursing. Advocating greater investment in nursing to bring rich returns for global health, it highlighted the "triple impact" of nursing worldwide; namely better health, greater gender equality, and stronger economies. Building on the positive impact of these new ways of thinking about nursing, the recommendations were taken up by a 3-year global campaign, *Nursing Now*. Significantly, it is recruiting champions who are not nurses, including politicians and global health leaders. Partnering with WHO and ICN, it aims to match action at global policy level with local campaigns, as a social movement and a vehicle through which global and local energy can be harnessed.

Nursing Now works with ICN and WHO to ensure that experienced nurse leaders are available in the right places and right roles, to help nursing deliver its potential and include the nursing perspective in policymaking and decision making. It advocates creating and strengthening nursing leadership in all countries to review, improve, develop, and implement policy and strategies. This focus on policy has been the missing piece in nursing leadership programs, with the rare exception of the ICN Global Nursing Leadership Institute (GNLI). Since 2009, GNLI developed and inspired 30 nurse leaders each year from round the world—but we need not just 30 a year or 300, but 30,000 policy-competent nurse leaders.

A NEW STORY OF NURSING

The major shifts necessary to transform nursing will not emerge through a continuing series of piecemeal policy initiatives. Deep-rooted, sustainable change will depend on reaching honest, shared understanding of the barriers to change and the structural inequalities and issues that maintain them, as well as tackling the root causes and underlying drivers. This is the moment for nurses to shift the paradigm—making alliances with social movements and

---

BOX 82.3   Nursing's Four Stages of Political Development

Stage 1: Buy-in
Stage 2: Self-interest
Stage 3: Political sophistication
Stage 4: Leading the way

From Cohen, S., Mason, D., Kovner, C., Leavitt, J., Pulcini, J., & Sochalski, J. (1996). Stages of nursing's political development: Where we've been and where we ought to go. *Nursing Outlook, 44*, 259–266.

considering radical alternatives, as well as trying to gain influence at the top tables. All this could lead us to a new story of health and health care, with nurses as leading actors at the heart of sustainable health systems that meet individual and population needs.

"Doing global health" does not have to mean traveling beyond your backyard. It may mean working with a local disadvantaged and vulnerable community. It may mean political action to achieve clean air and water. It may mean policy pressure to achieve social justice and universal health coverage. "Thinking globally and acting locally" is old wisdom but never more needed of nurses and nursing than now.

DISCUSSION QUESTIONS

1. Think of a current health challenge that you are or could be tackling in your own backyard. Consider how the possible solutions you have explored might contribute to or demonstrate the "triple impact" of nursing: better health, greater gender equality, and a stronger local economy.
2. What are the global health issues of most concern to you? What evidence can you find that nursing organizations and/or WHO are addressing them?
3. Go to the websites of ICN (www.icn.ch) or Nursing Now (www.nursingnow.org). What work do you see there that is relevant to your everyday issues and concerns as a nurse?

REFERENCES

Abbasi, K. (1999). The World Bank and world health: Changing sides. *British Medical Journal, 318*, 865-869.

All-Party Parliamentary Group on Global Health. (2016). *Triple impact: How developing nursing will improve health, promote gender equality and support economic growth*. Retrieved from www.appg-globalhealth.org.uk.

Canadian Nurses Association. (2012). *A nursing call to action*. Retrieved from www.cna-aiic.ca/~/media/cna/files/en/nec_report_e.pdf.

Caughley, J. (2009). *60 Years of collaboration: The International Council of Nurses and the World Health Organization: A growing and fruitful partnership*. Geneva: International Council of Nurses.

Cohen, S., Mason, D., Kovner, C., Leavitt, J., Pulcini, J., & Sochalski, J. (1996). Stages of nursing's political development: Where we've been and where we ought to go. *Nursing Outlook, 44*, 259-266.

Coulibaly, Y., Cavalli, A., van Dormael, M., Polman, K., & Kegels, G. (2008). Programme activities: A major burden for district health systems. *Tropical Medicine and International Health, 13*(12), 1430-1432.

International Council of Nurses. (2018). *Nurses: A voice to lead*. Retrieved from www.icnvoicetolead.com.

Institute of Medicine. (2011). *The future of nursing: Leading change, advancing health*. Washington DC: The National Academic Press.

Kingdon, J. (2011). *Agendas, alternatives, and public policies* (updated 2nd ed.). New York: Longman.

Lasker, J. (2016). *Hoping to help: The promises and pitfalls of global health volunteering*. Ithaca, NY: Cornell University Press

Lewis, S. (2010). So many voices, so little voice. *The Canadian Nurse, 106*(8), 40.

McClelland, A. (2017). *Emergencies only*. Crow's Nest, Australia: Allen & Unwin.

Oulton, J. (2016). International health and nursing policy and politics today: A snapshot. In D.J. Mason, D. Gardner, F. Outlaw, & E. O'Grady (Eds). *Policy and politics in nursing and health care* (7th ed.). St. Louis: Elsevier.

People's Health Movement. (n.d.). *History*. Retrieved from https://phm-na.org/usa/history/

The Prime Minister's Commission on the Future of Nursing and Midwifery. (2010). *Front line care: Report by the Prime Minister's Commission on the Future of Nursing and Midwifery in England 2010*. Retrieved from http://webarchive.nationalarchives.gov.uk/20100331110400/http://cnm.independent.gov.uk/.

Ravelo, J. (2015). *Help row, not steer: Lessons from the Ebola crisis response. Inside Development*. Retrieved from www.devex.com/news/help-row-not-steer-lessons-from-the-ebola-crisis-response-86451

Rosa. W. (2017). The Sustainable Development Goals: A primer. In W. Rosa (Ed.), *A new era in global health*. New York: Springer.

Salvage, J. (2007). Two to tango—The pleasure and pain of international collaboration. In S. Weinstein & A. Brooks (Eds). *Nursing without borders*. Indianapolis: Sigma Theta Tau International.

Salvage, J., & Stilwell, B. (2018). Breaking the silence: A new story of nursing. *Journal of Clinical Nursing, 27*(7-8), 1295-1721.

Shamian, J. (2015). Global voice, strategic leadership and policy impact: Global citizens, global nursing. *International Nursing Review, 62*(1), 4.

Sridhar, D., Winters, J., & Strong, E. (2017). World Bank's financing, priorities, and lending structures for global health. *British Medical Journal, 358*, j3339.

United Nations. (2015). *Transforming our world: The 2030 Agenda for Sustainable Development*. Retrieved from https://sustainabledevelopment.un.org/post2015/transformingourworld.

White, J. (2014). Through a socio-political lens: The relationship of practice, education, research and policy to social justice. In P. Kagan, M. Smith, & P. Chinn (Eds). *Philosophies and practices of emancipatory nursing: Social justice as praxis*. New York: Routledge.

World Health Organization. (2015). *Health in 2015 from MDGs to SDGs*. Geneva: Author. Retrieved from http://apps.who.int/iris/bitstream/handle/10665/200009/9789241565110_eng.pdf;jsessionid=92FEA47674B715961E3A32A438E6A2E4?sequence=1.

World Health Organization. (2016). *Midwives' voices, midwives' realities report 2016.* Retrieved from www.who.int/maternal_child_adolescent/documents/midwives-voices-realities/en/.

World Health Organization. (2017). *Nursing and midwifery in the history of the World Health Organization 1948–2017.* Retrieved from www.who.int/hrh/resources/Nursing-and-Midwifery-in-History-of-WHO/en/.

ONLINE RESOURCES

International Council of Nurses
www.icn.ch
Nursing Now
www.nursingnow.org
World Health Organization
www.who.int/topics/nursing/en/

83

Infectious Disease in a Highly Connected World: Nurses' Role to Prevent, Detect, Respond

Catherine M. Dentinger and Amy R. Kolwaite

"With Ebola back in the Democratic Republic of the Congo, this year's World Health Assembly sees the threat of pandemic diseases and the fragility of global health security once again at the forefront of the global health leaders' minds."

71st World Health Assembly, May 21, 2018 (retrieved from www.devex.com/ news/what-to-watch-at-this-year-s-world-health-assembly-92787)

Not long ago, infectious diseases were thought to be well controlled through hygiene measures, vaccines, and antimicrobial medications, but that perspective has shifted. In the past 35 years, we have experienced infectious disease outbreaks in which global spread of severe infections has occurred due to an increasingly interconnected world. Timely detection of and efficient response to these events is key to limiting their magnitude and duration; this requires sustained attention, international engagement and coordination, and reliable resources. Nurses, the largest sector of the global health care workforce, are integral to preventing, detecting, and responding to these infectious disease threats.

CONTEXT

"Vaccines and antibiotics have made many infectious diseases a thing of the past; we've come to expect that public health and modern science can conquer all microbes. But nature is a formidable adversary."

Dr. Tom Frieden, Centers for Disease Control and Prevention (CDC), February 2016

By the 1960s, advances in public sanitation, immunizations, and antimicrobials led to large declines in morbidity and mortality from infectious diseases in some countries and toward what was thought to be their eventual elimination as a human health concern (Burnet, 1962). However, just 20 years later, the human immunodeficiency virus (HIV) pandemic challenged that perspective. Since the first cases of what would become known as acquired immunodeficiency syndrome (AIDS) were described in the United States in 1981 (CDC, 1981), HIV infection has become endemic in most countries. An estimated 36.9 million people are infected worldwide, and 1.7 million new infections occurred in 2016 (Joint United Nations Programme on HIV/AIDS [UNAIDS], 2019). Across the subsequent decades, viruses including Zika, West Nile, Monkeypox, Chikungunya, Nipah, Ebola, and Dengue have become endemic or caused transmission in areas where they had not previously circulated (Hennessey, Fischer, & Staples, 2016; Parola et al., 2006; Reed et al., 2004; CDC, 1999a, 1999b, 2000, 2003, 2010; World Health Organization [WHO], 2014). During the 2002–2003 severe acute respiratory syndrome (SARS) coronavirus outbreak, we learned just how quickly a respiratory virus causing severe disease could spread across the world (Ruan, 2006). Resurgences of disease caused by measles virus, vaccine-derived poliovirus, and *Vibrio cholera* have occurred following natural disasters, migration, political conflict, and declines in vaccination rates (Cerda & Lee, 2013; Gardner et al., 2018; Macdonald & Hebert, 2010; CDC, 2013b). In addition, the prevalence of multidrug-resistant pathogens has increased due to many factors, including insufficient infection control and inappropriate antimicrobial use for human therapeutic interventions and as growth promoters in animal feed (Bronzwaer et al., 2002; Davies & Davies, 2010; Smith, Harris, Johnson, Silbergeld, & Morris, 2002; CDC, 2013a, 2013d; van Panhuis et al., 2013). Influenza viruses, which frequently mutate during replication and occasionally exchange entire genes, continue to cause substantial annual global mortality and intermittent pandemics (Dawood et al., 2009; Shinde et al., 2009; Subbarao et al., 1998). In short, the era of hubris with respect to infectious disease control was brief.

Pathogen introduction, transmission, and adaptation in human populations result from a complex interaction of host, agent, and environment and the adaption of microorganisms to pressures that are not completely understood (Enright et al., 2002; Jones et al., 2008; Wolfe, Dunavan, & Diamond, 2007). Lederberg et al. coined the term *emerging infectious disease* (EID) in 1992 to name this process and to expand the efforts needed to understand and respond to it (Lederberg, 1992; CDC, 1994). Conditions identified to date that facilitate the emergence of novel pathogens or the reemergence of infections that had been well controlled include population growth, urbanization, displacement, and poverty; climate change and ecosystem alterations; rapid global travel and commerce; and widespread use of antimicrobials. In addition, the intentional release of infectious pathogens also remains a concern (Arguin, Marano, & Freedman, 2009; Hollingsworth, Ferguson, & Anderson, 2007).

Population Growth, Urbanization, Displacement, and Poverty

"Annawadi itself was nothing special in the context of the slums of Mumbai. Every house was off-kilter, so less off-kilter looked like straight. Sewage and sickness looked like life."

Katherine Boo, Behind the Beautiful Forevers: Life, Death, and Hope in a Mumbai Undercity

The United Nations (UN) estimates that 55% of the world's growing population live in urban areas compared with 30% in 1950; most of this growth and urbanization is occurring in Asia and Africa (UN, 2018b). Migration of rural populations, often those in search of economic opportunity, has resulted in rapid growth of communities that have minimal social or health services, and inadequate housing and sanitation. These densely populated, poorly serviced areas pose challenges for preventing, identifying, and controlling infectious diseases (Afsana & Wahid, 2013). As human populations expand into new habitats and ecosystems, or closer to livestock and live animal markets, the potential for zoonotic disease transmission increases (Finucane & Spencer, 2013; Weaver, 2013; Yang, Utzinger, & Zhou, 2015). This is thought to have played a

role in pathogen introduction into human populations including novel influenza viruses, HIV, Ebola virus, hantavirus, and tick-borne organisms such as those that cause ehrlichiosis and Lyme disease (Muehlenbein, 2012). Natural disasters, including those related to climate changes, and violent conflict also force rapid and unanticipated population movement (Haines, Kovats, Campbell-Lendrum, & Corvalan, 2006; McMichael, Woodruff, & Hales, 2006; Rajabali, Moin, Ansari, Khanani, & Ali, 2009). In June 2016, the United Nations High Commission on Refugees (UNHCR) estimated that 65.5 million people have been forcibly displaced (UN, 2018a). Displaced persons often relocate into haphazardly formed communities with limited access to basic services and may have poor baseline health and nutritional status and low vaccination rates. These characteristics may increase their risk of acquiring disease having poor outcomes and facilitating disease transmission (Gayer, Legros, Formenty, & Connolly, 2007; Henke-Gendo et al., 2009; Possas, 2016). Furthermore, in these communities, the public health infrastructure needed to respond to a threat is often lacking resulting in outbreaks that can rapidly escalate. For example, in refugee camps in the South Sudan, an outbreak of hepatitis E virus infection related to poor sanitation and contaminated drinking water sickened more than 5000 individuals and caused several deaths among pregnant women (CDC, 2013c). Outbreaks of diseases that were once eliminated or controlled can quickly resurface. The Syrian Arab Republic, which had been poliomyelitis free since 1999, experienced outbreaks of vaccine-derived poliomyelitis following the interruption of vaccination programs because of civil war (Mbaeyi et al., 2018; WHO, 2013). In contrast, when pathogens with epidemic potential are introduced in areas with a strong public health infrastructure, the outbreak can be effectively controlled. When individuals with cholera arrived in New York City from the island of Hispaniola, they were quickly identified and treated, and public health officials were immediately notified and could begin investigations; no secondary cases occurred (Newton et al., 2011).

Climate Change and Ecosystem Alteration

"Everything we do has microbial consequence."

Nicholas Ashbolt, PhD, School of Public Health, University of Alberta, 2013

As environmental conditions change, the distribution of microorganisms and their vectors may be altered, resulting in new exposures to pathogens. Climatic changes favoring wider distribution of the vector, *Aedes aegypti* and *Aedes albopictus* mosquitoes, for example, combined with rapid urbanization, may play a role in facilitating dengue virus infections (Colon-Gonzalez, Fezzi, Lake, & Hunter, 2013; Morin, Comrie, & Ernst, 2013). As the distribution of these mosquitoes has expanded, viral transmission is no longer limited to tropical and subtropical areas (WHO, 2012). Vector expansion can result in pathogen exposures in populations with no underlying immunity, potentially resulting in high rates of disease and new clinical presentations. Introduction of Zika virus into an immunologically naive population in rural Brazil in 2016 may have played a role in the high numbers of Zika virus congenital syndrome in their population (Possas, 2016).

Global Travel and Commerce

Globally, air travel has increased dramatically; the International Air Transport Association estimates that 3.8 billion individuals traveled by air in 2016 and that this number will nearly double by 2035 (International Air Transport Association, 2016). Humans travel for work and family obligations, to obtain health care services, and for leisure and may contribute importantly to the spread of disease (Hollingsworth et al., 2007). The 2002–2003 SARS epidemic highlighted just how quickly this can happen for respiratory pathogens, but travel can play a role in the transmission of other pathogens as well. In 2005, carbapenem-resistant *Enterobacteriaceae* (CRE) was isolated from a person hospitalized in France who had recently been hospitalized in the United States (Naas, Nordmann, Vedel, & Poyart, 2005). In 2008, a novel CRE isolate was cultured from a Swedish traveler who had recently been hospitalized in India (D. Yong et al., 2009).

Global commerce also influences the introduction of pathogens into populations. For example, much of the global food supply is grown, processed, and distributed via multinational networks that connect livestock and agricultural enterprises to processing, packaging, and distribution centers worldwide. The complexity and massive volume of these operations create opportunities for the introduction and rapid spread of pathogens and make detecting and controlling them challenging (Leibler et al., 2009). Products contaminated with microbial pathogens may be consumed far from their origin, resulting in widespread and difficult-to-trace outbreaks. In 2011 an outbreak of *Listeria monocytogenes* associated with cantaloupe from one U.S. farm sickened at least 147 individuals in 28 states, 33 of whom died (Cartwright et al., 2013; McCollum et al., 2013). In Europe, the same year, a novel strain of *Escherichia coli* that sickened nearly 4000 people and caused 53 deaths was eventually linked to seeds imported from Egypt, sprouted on a farm in Germany, and consumed throughout Europe (Buchholz et al., 2011). A single factory may process the same food item under different brand names, complicating investigations and recalls. In 2011, salmonella-contaminated peanut butter from a single processing plant sickened people in 20 U.S. states. Although only one brand of peanut butter was associated with illness, the plant produced peanut butter under different brand names (CDC, 2013e).

These are just a few examples of recent disease outbreaks that illustrate the complexities of human pathogen ecology. They also highlight the need to develop collaborative global partnerships that support timely and effective responses.

GLOBAL CONCERN, GLOBAL ACTION

International Health Regulations

International cooperation to control infectious disease threats has a long history. The dawn of the modern era of these efforts is perhaps the International Sanitary Conference that was held in Paris in 1851 to address a cholera pandemic; these efforts continued as steamship use accelerated the introduction of plague, yellow fever, and cholera in ports around the world (Howard-Jones, 1974). Across the decades, as health threats changed, the rate of travel increased multifold, and gaps in control became apparent, efforts have had to be updated. The WHO, founded in 1948, has generally served as the coordinating body for these efforts.

After the 2002–2003 SARS coronavirus outbreak, the WHO adopted revised International Health Regulations (IHRs) in 2007. The IHRs are legally binding on WHO member states (Tappero et al., 2017; WHO, 2007). These regulations include goals for global surveillance for specific diseases as well as for responding to public health events of international concern (PHEIC). All member states are required to develop, strengthen, and maintain core surveillance and response capacities, facilitate cross-border cooperation, and provide logistic and financial support to improve capacity for these activities (WHO, 2007). The IHRs also promote improved coordination between different sectors, including agricultural authorities such as the Food and Agriculture Organization and the World Organization for Animal Health to reduce the potential for outbreaks from food, livestock, and wild animal sources (Newell et al., 2010; Pavlin, Schloegel, & Daszak, 2009).

Achieving the goals of the revised IHRs has been challenging, particularly in low-resource countries or those facing political instability and conflict. These areas are often the most at-risk for an infectious disease threat and least able to implement and sustain core activities (Guha-Spair, Hoyois, Wallemacq, & Below, 2016). Furthermore, the IHRs have not addressed the underlying health infrastructure weaknesses or the limited access to care and goods in many of these areas, both of which affect IHR adherence (Heymann et al., 2015). In addition, the revised IHRs have not adequately addressed appropriate global governance. For example, when Indonesia was unable to obtain influenza vaccine developed based on a strain they submitted for required surveillance, they stopped submitting strains altogether (Fidler, 2008). This left an important gap in global avian influenza surveillance; more importantly, it revealed inadequacies in governance and health rights. In response, pandemic influenza preparedness policies were updated to include a doctrine of equal benefits from equal sharing (WHO pandemic flu prep sharing viruses, 2007) (Fidler & Gostin, 2011).

More recent outbreaks, including the 2009 influenza A (H1N1) pandemic, the 2012 emergence of Middle East Respiratory Syndrome Coronavirus (MERS-CoV), and the 2014 Ebola virus disease (EVD) outbreak in West Africa, further highlighted the limited adherence to the IHRs in some areas (Bialek et al., 2014; WHO, 2018). The West Africa EVD outbreak, in particular, reinforced the need for *sustained* global support for IHRs and a recognition that shifting priorities away from these efforts may have contributed to the delayed and inadequate response (Fink S, 2014). It also forced a revisit of the connection between individual and collective health security: global health security is threatened when individuals do not have access to affordable essential health services, technologies, and medicines (Abramowitz, Hipgrave, Witchard, & Heymann, 2018; Heymann et al., 2015). In short, these events revealed that the revised IHRs require ongoing attention, review, and dedicated resources.

Global Health Security Agenda

In response to the West Africa EVD outbreak, and to support countries to achieve core IHR capacities, the Global Health Security Agenda (GHSA), a partnership of nearly 50 nations, international organizations, and nongovernmental stakeholders, was launched in February 2014 (Frieden, Damon, Bell, Kenyon, & Nichol, 2014). The GHSA supports multilateral and multisector collaborations to strengthen national and international capacity to prevent, detect, and respond to infectious diseases threats resulting from naturally occurring, deliberate, or accidental events. Activities to strengthen these capacities, outlined in 11 action packages, have been agreed upon by all GHSA partners. Prevention activities focus on the systems, policies, and procedures to avoid outbreaks from antimicrobial resistant organisms, zoonotic, and vaccine-preventable diseases. Detection activities target strengthening national laboratory systems capable of accurate, timely surveillance, and reporting; and creating a workforce (e.g., clinicians,

veterinarians, epidemiologists, laboratorians, administrators) who can meet relevant IHR core competencies. Response activities include developing Emergency Operations Centers; creating linkages between public health and other sectors; and training rapid response teams to engage international partners during public health emergencies (Frieden et al., 2014).

ROLE OF NURSES TO PREVENT, DETECT, AND RESPOND TO PUBLIC HEALTH THREATS

Nurses at all levels of health care systems are vital to the success of the GHSA and to IHR adherence. Across the world, nurses are key to effective prevention activities in settings ranging from intensive care units to areas that lack health facilities altogether. In these settings, they also often serve as the first line of detection (International Council of Nurses, 2011). It was a New York City school nurse who identified a large cluster of students presenting with influenza-like illness to her clinic and alerted public health authorities in the early stages of the 2009 influenza A (H1N1) pandemic (Balter, Gupta, Lim, Fu, & Perlman, 2010; Buehler, 2012; Hartocollis, 2009). Nurses are frequently cited as the most trusted professionals and as such may be uniquely positioned to work with individuals and communities to learn detailed histories, including potential exposures, and hidden concerns that may advance our understanding of transmission risks and reduce stigma that prevent individuals from seeking care (McCarthy N, 2019). Nurses may also be the first to initiate response activities once unusual events are detected. After the first case of EVD presented at her health center in Conakry, Guinea, (before it was widely recognized that the epidemic had moved into the capital), Nurse Koroma, who helped care for the patient, immediately implemented response activities. These activities included reporting the suspected EVD case to the response team in her district, initiating strict infection control at the health center, monitoring those who cared for the case, establishing careful triage of all patients at the clinic entrance, and conducting surveillance and monitoring for suspect EVD cases at the center. Although that first patient, a pregnant woman and her fetus, succumbed to the infection, as did the attending obstetrician and a medical student, no additional cases of health care–associated EVD occurred at that institution during the epidemic (personal communication, Nurse Koroma, Conakry, Guinea, February 2015).

Nurses serve as epidemiologists coordinating with clinicians and laboratorians to confirm diagnoses, investigate cases, trace contacts, administer prophylaxis, conduct outreach to identify additional cases, collect specimens, provide comfort, advocate for resources, manage and analyze data, report results, and use results to design, implement, and test prevention measures (Ho & Parker, 2006). Nurses are also partners in research activities such as during the Ebola vaccine trials in West Africa (Edem-Hotah et al., 2018) and as evidenced in their long-term participation in the Nurses' Health Study (Morabia, 2016). They serve as health communicators to prepare accurate, effective messages for individuals, families, health systems, and communities and as infection control practitioners to identify, manage, and mitigate health care–associated infections (Baltzell, McLemore, Shattell, & Rankin, 2017; MacIntyre, Chughtai, Seale, Richards, & Davidson, 2014). Nurses also serve as leaders and administrators in health care systems to design and evaluate policies, and they serve on national and international rapid response teams for public health emergencies. Finally, nurses are scientists testing hypotheses to advance knowledge in many areas of health (Grady & Adams, 2015; Hamilton, 2016).

Nurses play a critical role in GHSA prevention activities, as evidenced by their involvement in efforts to reduce the burden of infections caused by antimicrobial resistant organisms (Edwards, Drumright, Kiernan, & Holmes, 2011). Antimicrobial stewardship involves coordinated interventions to improve and measure the prudent use of antimicrobials by promoting the appropriate therapeutic regimen, including right drug, right dose, right duration, and right route of administration. Stewardship and infection control programs are an essential element in improving patient outcomes, reducing antimicrobial resistance, decreasing the spread of multidrug resistant organisms, limiting costs, and preventing the need for additional medications. Nurses are well poised to participate in patient education, assess for adverse drug reaction history, and ensure clinicians are obtaining cultures prior to antibiotic administration. Given their important role, the inclusion of nurses as members of the antimicrobial stewardship team has been endorsed by the CDC, the American Nurses Association (ANA), the American Academy of Nursing, the National Institute of Nursing Research, the International Council of Nurses, and accrediting agencies (International Council of Nurses, 2017; Monsees, Popejoy, Jackson, Lee, & Goldman, 2018).

Nurses often serve as frontline health care workers (HCWs) and as such are key to detection activities. In many areas of the world, including those with fragile health systems, nurses often serve as first line clinicians. In these areas, nurses also serve as trainers to develop and support a workforce, such as community health workers (CHWs), capable of providing basic health and prevention services in their communities. When well trained and supported, these CHWs help to monitor rural communities for unusual infectious events, as they did during the 2017 pneumonic plague outbreak in Madagascar (Razafindrakoto, Kapesa, Andriamihamina, & Dentinger, 2018). Shortages of nurses in much of the world is a great concern for global health security; increasing and supporting these workers is a potential solution to strengthening GHSA and adherence to IHRs (Edmonson, 2015; Edmonson, McCarthy, Trent-Adams, McCain, & Marshall, 2017).

Nurses have been, and will continue to be, critical to responding to infectious disease outbreaks globally. Because nurses are usually involved in local response efforts including patient care, infection prevention and control (IPC), contact management and reporting, they are key to controlling these outbreaks locally and preventing their spread. In 1976, in Zaire (currently the Democratic Republic of the Congo), nurses cared for the first identified EVD patients, became the first cases of health care–associated EVD, and were instrumental in limiting transmission of the virus beyond their community (WHO, 1978). Similarly, in 1997, Hong Kong nurses participated in investigation and response activities to the first known case of human influenza A (H5N1) infection, and during the 2002 monkeypox outbreak in the United States, nurses from the CDC along with their colleagues from affected state and local health departments participated in all aspects of response efforts (CDC, 1998) (C. Dentinger, CDC personal communication).

CASE STUDY: EBOLA VIRUS DISEASE OUTBREAK: WEST AFRICA, 2014

In December 2013, cases of EVD appeared in a village of Guinea, West Africa that bordered Sierra Leone and Liberia (Baize et al., 2014). EVD, one of several viral hemorrhagic diseases, has a high fatality rate and, at the time, no known treatment or vaccine (CDC, 2018). Although EVD outbreaks had occurred in Central and Eastern African countries (e.g., Democratic Republic of the Congo, Gabon, Uganda, Sudan), this was the first identified EVD outbreak in West Africa. It was thought that this cluster would be contained in the remote region of Guinea where it began, as had occurred in previous outbreaks. Instead, for reasons not entirely understood but thought to be related to human movement between the rural areas of Guinea, Sierra Leone, and Liberia and into the urban areas of these countries, cases of EVD began to increase (Gatherer, 2014). The increase in cases quickly overwhelmed the fragile health infrastructure and limited public resources of these countries, some of the poorest in the world. In July 2014, when EVD was diagnosed in a traveler from Liberia in Lagos, Nigeria and subsequently in several of his contacts and care providers, the severity of the outbreak was understood by even those beyond the public health community (Shuaib et al., 2014). This was reinforced when an American physician and an aid worker became infected after caring for patients in Liberia and were transported to the United States for care (Blinder & Grady, 2014).

The EVD outbreak in West Africa highlighted how transmission occurring in health care settings can quickly amplify an outbreak—early in the epidemic, Ebola virus transmission to HCWs occurred in health care facilities that were not Ebola treatment units (ETUs) (Hageman et al., 2016). HCWs had one of the highest rates of EVD in the outbreak, with infection 21 to 32 times more likely than in the general adult population (Olu et al., 2015; WHO, 2015). Assessments conducted early in the outbreak identified substantial lapses in IPC as a main driver for health care–associated transmission (Hageman et al., 2016).

Nurses were a critical part of response teams formed by staff from the affected countries, WHO, government health and development agencies from several countries, military medical units, and nongovernmental organizations. Some of these nurses formed teams to develop and deliver IPC trainings for HCWs at facilities throughout the region. These trainings included general and Ebola-specific IPC and techniques for effective screening and identification of EVD cases at the entry point of health care facilities. In addition, in Sierra Leone, nurses supported the Ministry of Health and Sanitation to establish a National IPC Program, complete with policies and guidelines. As part of this program, the chief nurse officer of the Sierra Leone Ministry of Health and Sanitation appointed IPC specialists at each of the government hospitals. These specialists, many of them nurses, were responsible for overseeing IPC at their appointed health care facilities. In 2018, these IPC positions remain at Sierra Leone government hospitals, contributing to a strong National IPC Program, equipped and ready to respond in the event of another infectious disease outbreak.

Nurses in the United States and around the world also participated in activities in their home countries. In September 2014, nurses at Emory University Hospital provided care to the first cases of EVD treated in the United States (Lyon et al., 2014). Emory University had a treatment unit designed to manage diseases such as EVD; staff there had trained and practiced responding, and they had 48 hours of warning that two individuals with EVD would be arriving in their unit. Regardless, caring safely for these two individuals was so challenging; it surprised even these well-trained nurses (Ribner, keynote speaker, Infectious Disease Society of America [IDSA] annual meeting, October 2015, Philadelphia, PA). When the nurses in a Dallas hospital cared for the first U.S.-diagnosed case of EVD, they had had none of this preparation; when two of them acquired EVD after caring for

the patient, the risks associated with providing care even in well-resourced settings became apparent (Chevalier et al., 2014). In response to the Dallas cases, the ANA, together with the CDC, quickly organized a webinar to share best practices. Nurses and nurse leaders across the country participated in that webinar and then led their communities and institutions to prepare for preventing health care–associated EVD infections; since then, the ANA and CDC have partnered with several organizations to develop the Nursing Infection Control Education Network (ANA, 2019).

In cities such as New York, with large numbers of global travelers, nurses participated on teams to establish four Ebola units where EVD patients could safely be treated, and they provided care in one of those units for the first New York City case of EVD. New York City nurses also screened and monitored travelers returning from Ebola-affected countries, developed tools to reduce stigma, and reassure the population and conducted IPC trainings at clinics and hospitals across the city.

The response to the 2014 Ebola outbreak ultimately included all nurses in Guinea, Sierra Leone, Liberia, and Nigeria, and neighboring countries; those who left their home countries to assist with the response, and those who prepared for potential cases in their home countries. An infectious global public health threat requires nurses from all countries at all levels of the health care system. We will need to share practices that worked and improve those that did not. We will need nurse researchers to rigorously test hypotheses based on observation and collected data.

CONCLUSION

As human-pathogen interactions evolve in response to population growth and displacement, increased global travel and commerce, environmental changes, and pressure from antimicrobial use, we can expect to encounter increasingly complex webs of infectious disease exposures and transmission. Preventing, detecting, and responding to these events requires multinational, multisector collaboration. Governments, nongovernmental organizations, academic institutions, health care professionals, private industry, and communities must leverage resources to develop effective policies and practices to improve public health infrastructure to prevent, detect, and respond rapidly to infectious threats. Effective prevention strategies, universal access to affordable essential health care, sensitive surveillance systems, and coordinated rapid response must be strengthened globally. Furthermore, nurses' knowledge, experience, and expertise must be more completely captured to design effective solutions (McGillis Hall & Kashin, 2016).

We face these challenges in a global political atmosphere that poses threats to international cooperation, yet pathogens are unlikely to heed isolationist policies. As noted by journalist Ed Yong, natural disasters may result in communities uniting, but infectious disease outbreaks can cause communities to divide (Yong, 2018). These divisions can result in infections going undetected, allowing them to flourish. Under the most collaborative of times, it takes extraordinary efforts during epidemics to calm the public and engage cooperation. Calls for isolationism will happen, but they must not happen among health care leaders, including among nurses; rather these professionals must responsibly and effectively guide their populations to limit the duration and magnitude of these events, and to prevent human suffering. Ultimately, engagement in global health is not only a humanitarian concern but also a priority for our collective well-being, efficient use of limited resources, and protecting our future. Irrespective of national borders, nursing leadership at every level and in every country is needed to address these challenges.

DISCUSSION QUESTIONS

1. How might nurses and nursing organizations improve policies to encourage the judicious use of antibiotics?
2. How can nurses and nursing organizations engage their communities in constructive ways when public health threats are imminent?
3. How can nurses and nursing organizations respond to the global shortage of primary care providers?

REFERENCES

Abramowitz, S.A., Hipgrave, D.B., Witchard, A., & Heymann, D.L. (2018). Lessons from the West Africa Ebola epidemic: A systematic review of epidemiological and social and behavioral science research priorities. *Journal of Infectious Diseases, 218*(11), 1730–1738.

Afsana, K., & Wahid, S.S. (2013). Health care for poor people in the urban slums of Bangladesh. *The Lancet, 382*(9910), 2049-2051.

American Nurses Association. (December 6, 2019). *Infection prevention and control: Nursing Infection Control Education Network.* Retrieved from www.nursingworld.org/practice-policy/work-environment/health-safety/infection-prevention/.

Arguin, P. M., Marano, N., & Freedman, D. O. (2009). Globally mobile populations and the spread of emerging pathogens. *Emerging Infectious Diseases, 15*(11), 1713-1714.

Baize, S., Pannetier, D., Oestereich, L., Rieger, T., Koivogui, L., Magassouba, N., . . . & Gunther, S. (2014). Emergence of Zaire Ebola virus disease in Guinea. *New England Journal of Medicine, 371*(15), 1418-1425.

Balter, S., Gupta, L.S., Lim, S., Fu, J., & Perlman, S.E. (2010). Pandemic (H1N1) 2009 surveillance for severe illness and response, New York, New York, USA, April-July 2009. *Emerging Infectious Diseases, 16*(8), 1259-1264.

Baltzell, K., McLemore, M., Shattell, M., & Rankin, S. (2017). Impacts on global health from nursing research. *American Journal of Tropical Medicine and Hygiene, 96*(4), 765-766.

Bialek, S.R., Allen, D., Alvarado-Ramy, F., Arthur, R., Balajee, A., Bell, D., . . . & Watson, J. (2014). First confirmed cases of Middle East respiratory syndrome coronavirus (MERS-CoV) infection in the United States, updated information on the epidemiology of MERS-CoV infection, and guidance for the public, clinicians, and public health authorities—May 2014. *Morbidity and Mortality Weekly Report, 63*(19), 431-436.

Blinder A., & Grady D. (2014, August 2, 2018). American doctor with Ebola Arrives in U.S. for treatment. *New York Times.* Retrieved from www.nytimes.com/2014/08/03/us/kent-brantley-nancy-writebol-ebola-treatment-atlanta.html?_r=0.

Bronzwaer, S.L., Cars, O., Buchholz, U., Molstad, S., Goettsch, W., Veldhuijzen, I.K., . . . & Degener, J.E. (2002). A European study on the relationship between antimicrobial use and antimicrobial resistance. *Emerging Infectious Diseases, 8*(3), 278-282.

Buchholz, U., Bernard, H., Werber, D., Bohmer, M.M., Remschmidt, C., Wilking, H., . . . & Kuhne, M. (2011). German outbreak of *Escherichia coli* O104:H4 associated with sprouts. *New England Journal of Medicine, 365*(19), 1763-1770.

Buehler, J.W. (2012). CDC's vision for public health surveillance in the 21st century. Introduction. *Morbidity and Mortality Weekly Report Supplement, 61*(3), 1-2.

Burnet, F. M. (1962). *Natural history of infectious disease* (3rd ed.). Cambridge, England: Cambridge University Press.

Cartwright, E.J., Jackson, K.A., Johnson, S.D., Graves, L.M., Silk, B.J., & Mahon, B.E. (2013). Listeriosis outbreaks and associated food vehicles, United States, 1998-2008. *Emerging Infectious Diseases, 19*(1), 1-9; quiz 184.

Centers for Disease Control and Prevention. (1981). Pneumocystis pneumonia—Los Angeles. *Morbidity and Mortality Weekly Report, 30*(21), 250-252.

Centers for Disease Control and Prevention. (1994). *Addressing emerging infectious disease threats: A prevention strategy for the United States.* Atlanta: Author.

Centers for Disease Control and Prevention. (1998). Update: Isolation of avian influenza A (H5N1) viruses from humans—Hong Kong, 1997-1998. *Morbidity and Mortality Weekly Report, 46*(52-53), 1245-1247.

Centers for Disease Control and Prevention. (1999a). Outbreak of Hendra-like virus—Malaysia and Singapore, 1998-1999. *Morbidity and Mortality Weekly Report, 48*(13), 265-269.

Centers for Disease Control and Prevention. (1999b). Update: Outbreak of Nipah virus—Malaysia and Singapore, 1999. *Morbidity and Mortality Weekly Report, 48*(16), 335-337.

Centers for Disease Control and Prevention. (2000). West Nile virus activity—New York and New Jersey, 2000. *Morbidity and Mortality Weekly Report, 49*(28), 640-642.

Centers for Disease Control and Prevention. (2003). Multistate outbreak of monkeypox—Illinois, Indiana, and Wisconsin, 2003. *Morbidity and Mortality Weekly Report, 52*(23), 537-540.

Centers for Disease Control and Prevention. (2010). Locally acquired dengue—Key West, Florida, 2009-2010. *Morbidity and Mortality Weekly Report, 59*(19), 577-581.

Centers for Disease Control and Prevention. (2013a). *Antibiotic resistance threats in the United States, 2013*. Atlanta: Author.

Centers for Disease Control and Prevention. (2013b). Global control and regional elimination of measles, 2000-2011. *Morbidity and Mortality Weekly Report, 62*(2), 27-31.

Centers for Disease Control and Prevention. (2013c). Investigation of hepatitis E outbreak among refugees—Upper Nile, South Sudan, 2012-2013. *Morbidity and Mortality Weekly Report, 62*(29), 581-586.

Centers for Disease Control and Prevention. (2013d). Multidrug-resistant *Bacteroides fragilis*—Seattle, Washington, 2013. *Morbidity and Mortality Weekly Report, 62*(34), 694-696.

Centers for Disease Control and Prevention. (2013e). Notes from the field: *Salmonella* Bredeney infections linked to a brand of peanut butter—United States, 2012. *Morbidity and Mortality Weekly Report, 62*(6), 107.

Centers for Disease Control and Prevention. (2018). *Ebola (Ebola virus disease)*. Retrieved from www.cdc.gov/vhf/ebola/index.html

Cerda, R., & Lee, P.T. (2013). Modern cholera in the Americas: An opportunistic societal infection. *American Journal of Public Health, 103* (11), 1934-1937.

Chevalier, M.S., Chung, W., Smith, J., Weil, L.M., Hughes, S.M., Joyner, S.N., . . . & Lakey, D.L. (2014). Ebola virus disease cluster in the United States—Dallas County, Texas, 2014. *Morbidity and Mortality Weekly Report, 63*(46), 1087-1088.

Colon-Gonzalez, F.J., Fezzi, C., Lake, I.R., & Hunter, P.R. (2013). The effects of weather and climate change on dengue. *PLOS Neglected Tropical Diseases, 7*(11), e2503.

Davies, J., & Davies, D. (2010). Origins and evolution of antibiotic resistance. *Microbiology and Molecular Biology Reviews, 74*(3), 417-433.

Dawood, F.S., Jain, S., Finelli, L., Shaw, M.W., Lindstrom, S., Garten, R.J., . . . & Uyeki, T.M. (2009). Emergence of a novel swine-origin influenza A (H1N1) virus in humans. *New England Journal of Medicine, 360*(25), 2605-2615.

Edem-Hotah, J., McDonald, W., Abu, P.M., Luman, E.T., Carter, R.J., Koker, A., & Goldstein, S.T. (2018). Utilizing nurses to staff an Ebola vaccine clinical trial in Sierra Leone during the Ebola outbreak. *Journal of Infectious Diseases, 217*(Suppl 1), S60-s64.

Edmonson, C. (2015). Strengthening moral courage among nurse leaders. *Online Journal of Issues in Nursing, 20*(2), 9.

Edmonson, C., McCarthy, C., Trent-Adams, S., McCain, C., & Marshall, J. (2017). Emerging global health issues: A nurse's role. *Online Journal of Issues in Nursing, 22*(1), 2.

Edwards, R., Drumright, L., Kiernan, M., & Holmes, A. (2011). Covering more territory to fight resistance: Considering nurses' role in antimicrobial stewardship. *Journal of Infection Prevention, 12*(1), 6-10.

Enright, M.C., Robinson, D.A., Randle, G., Feil, E.J., Grundmann, H., & Spratt, B.G. (2002). The evolutionary history of methicillin-resistant *Staphylococcus aureus* (MRSA). *Proceedings of the National Academy of Sciences of the United States of America, 99*(11), 7687-7692.

Fidler, D.P. (2008). Influenza virus samples, international law, and global health diplomacy. *Emerging Infectious Diseases, 14*(1), 88-94.

Fidler, D.P., & Gostin, L.O. (2011). The WHO pandemic influenza preparedness framework: A milestone in global governance for health. *Journal of the American Medical Association, 306*(2), 200-201.

Fink, S. (September 3, 2014). Cuts to WHO hurt response to Ebola. *New York Times*. Retrieved from www.nytimes.com/2014/09/04/world/africa/cuts-at-who-hurt-response-to-ebola-crisis.html?searchResultPosition=1.

Finucane, M.P., & Spencer, J.H.P. (Writers). (2013). *Rapid urbanization and infectious disease outbreaks: The case of avian influenza in Vietnam*. Recorded at the East-West Center office in Washington, DC, September 17, 2013. Producer: East-West Center, Honolulu, HI.

Frieden, T.R., Damon, I., Bell, B.P., Kenyon, T., & Nichol, S. (2014). Ebola 2014—New challenges, new global response and responsibility. *New England Journal of Medicine, 371*(13), 1177-1180.

Gardner, T.J., Diop, O.M., Jorba, J., Chavan, S., Ahmed, J., & Anand, A. (2018). Surveillance to track progress toward polio eradication—Worldwide, 2016-2017. *Morbidity and Mortality Weekly Report, 67*(14), 418-423.

Gatherer, D. (2014). The 2014 Ebola virus disease outbreak in West Africa. *Journal of General Virology, 95*(Pt 8), 1619-1624.

Gayer, M., Legros, D., Formenty, P., & Connolly, M.A. (2007). Conflict and emerging infectious diseases. *Emerging Infectious Diseases, 13*(11), 1625-1631.

Grady, P.A., & Adams, M.H. (2015). NINR/NLN co-sponsor 2015 National Nursing Research Roundtable: The nexus of practice, research, and education for the health of the nation. *Nursing Education Perspectives, 36*(4), 267-270.

Guha-Spair D., Hoyois, P., Wallemacq, P., & Below, R. (2016). *Annual disaster statistical review 2016*. Retrieved from www.emdat.be/sites/default/files/adsr_2016.pdf.

Hageman, J.C., Hazim, C., Wilson, K., Malpiedi, P., Gupta, N., Bennett, S., . . . & Park, B.J. (2016). Infection prevention and control for Ebola in health care settings—West Africa and United States. *Morbidity and Mortality Weekly Report Supplement, 65*(3), 50-56.

Haines, A., Kovats, R.S., Campbell-Lendrum, D., & Corvalan, C. (2006). Climate change and human health: Impacts, vulnerability, and mitigation. *The Lancet, 367*(9528), 2101-2109.

Hamilton, N. (October 19, 2016). Nurses are caretakers, not scientists, right? Wrong. *Scientific American*. Retrieved from https://blogs.scientificamerican.com/guest-blog/nurses-are-caretakers-not-scientists-right-wrong/.

Hartocollis, A. (2009). Seeing warning signs of outbreak, school nurse set response in motion. *New York Times*. Retrieved from www.nytimes.com/2009/04/27/nyregion/27response.html?pagewanted=all&_r=0.

Henke-Gendo, C., Harste, G., Juergens-Saathoff, B., Mattner, F., Deppe, H., & Heim, A. (2009). New real-time PCR detects prolonged norovirus excretion in highly immunosuppressed patients and children. *Journal of Clinical Microbiology, 47*(9), 2855-2862.

Hennessey, M., Fischer, M., & Staples, J.E. (2016). Zika virus spreads to new areas—Region of the Americas, May 2015–January 2016. *Morbidity and Mortality Weekly Report, 65*(3), 55-58.

Heymann, D.L., Chen, L., Takemi, K., Fidler, D.P., Tappero, J.W., Thomas, M.J., . . . & Rannan-Eliya, R.P. (2015). Global health security: The wider lessons from the West African Ebola virus disease epidemic. *The Lancet, 385*(9980), 1884-1901.

Ho, G., & Parker, J. (2006). Avian influenza: Risk, preparedness and the roles of public health nurses in Hong Kong. *Nursing Inquiry, 13*(1), 2-6.

Hollingsworth, T.D., Ferguson, N.M., & Anderson, R.M. (2007). Frequent travelers and rate of spread of epidemics. *Emerging Infectious Diseases, 13*(9), 1288-1294.

Howard-Jones, N. (1974). The scientific background of the International Sanitary Conferences, 1851-1938. 6. *WHO Chronicle, 28*(11), 495-508.

International Air Transport Association. (2016). *IATA forecasts passenger demand to double over 20 years.* Retrieved from www.iata.org/pressroom/pr/Pages/2016-10-18-02.aspx.

International Council of Nurses. (2017). *Position statement on antimicrobial resistance.* Retrieved from www.icn.ch/sites/default/files/inline-files/PS_A_Antimicrobial_resistance_0.pdf.

Joint United Nations Programme on HIV/AIDS. (2019). *Global HIV and AIDS statistics, 2019.* Retrieved from www.unaids.org/en/resources/fact-sheet.

Jones, K.E., Patel, N.G., Levy, M.A., Storeygard, A., Balk, D., Gittleman, J.L., & Daszak, P. (2008). Global trends in emerging infectious diseases. *Nature, 451*(7181), 990-993.

Lederberg, J. (1992). The interface of science and medicine. *Mount Sinai Journal of Medicine, 59*(5), 380-383.

Leibler, J.H., Otte, J., Roland-Holst, D., Pfeiffer, D.U., Soares Magalhaes, R., Rushton, J., . . . & Silbergeld, E.K. (2009). Industrial food animal production and global health risks: Exploring the ecosystems and economics of avian influenza. *Ecohealth, 6*(1), 58-70.

Lyon, G.M., Mehta, A.K., Varkey, J.B., Brantly, K., Plyler, L., McElroy, A.K., . . . & Ribner, B.S. (2014). Clinical care of two patients with Ebola virus disease in the United States. *New England Journal of Medicine, 371*(25), 2402-2409.

Macdonald, N., & Hebert, P.C. (2010). Polio outbreak in Tajikistan is cause for alarm. *Canadian Medical Association Journal, 182*(10), 1013.

MacIntyre, C.R., Chughtai, A.A., Seale, H., Richards, G.A., & Davidson, P.M. (2014). Respiratory protection for healthcare workers treating Ebola virus disease (EVD): Are facemasks sufficient to meet occupational health and safety obligations? *International Journal of Nursing Studies, 51*(11), 1421-1426.

Mbaeyi, C., Wadood, Z.M., Moran, T., Ather, F., Stehling-Ariza, T., Nikulin, J., . . . & Sharaf, M. (2018). Strategic response to an outbreak of circulating vaccine-derived poliovirus type 2—Syria, 2017-2018. *Morbidity and Mortality Weekly Report, 67*(24), 690-694.

McCarthy, N. (2019). America's most and least trusted professions. [Infographic]. Retrieved from www.statista.com/chart/12420/americas-most-and-least-trusted-professions/.

McCollum, J.T., Cronquist, A.B., Silk, B.J., Jackson, K.A., O'Connor, K.A., Cosgrove, S., . . . & Mahon, B.E. (2013). Multistate outbreak of listeriosis associated with cantaloupe. *New England Journal of Medicine, 369*(10), 944-953.

McGillis Hall, L., & Kashin, J. (2016). Public understanding of the role of nurses during Ebola. *Journal of Nursing Scholarship, 48*(1), 91-97.

McMichael, A.J., Woodruff, R.E., & Hales, S. (2006). Climate change and human health: present and future risks. *The Lancet, 367*(9513), 859-869.

Monsees, E., Popejoy, L., Jackson, M.A., Lee, B., & Goldman, J. (2018). Integrating staff nurses in antibiotic stewardship: Opportunities and barriers. *American Journal of Infection Control, 46*(7), 737-742.

Morin, C.W., Comrie, A.C., & Ernst, K. (2013). Climate and dengue transmission: Evidence and implications. *Environmental Health Perspectives, 121*(11-12), 1264-1272.

Muehlenbein, M. (2012). Human-wildlife interactious and emerging infectious diseases. In E. Brondízio, & E. Moran (Eds.), *Human-environment interactions: Current and future directions.* London: Springer.

Naas, T., Nordmann, P., Vedel, G., & Poyart, C. (2005). Plasmid-mediated carbapenem-hydrolyzing beta-lactamase KPC in a *Klebsiella pneumoniae* isolate from France. *Antimicrobial Agents and Chemotherapy, 49*(10), 4423-4424.

Newell, D.G., Koopmans, M., Verhoef, L., Duizer, E., Aidara-Kane, A., Sprong, H., . . . & Kruse, H. (2010). Food-borne diseases - the challenges of 20 years ago still persist while new ones continue to emerge. *International Journal of Food Microbiology, 139*(Suppl 1), S3-S15.

Newton, A.E., Heiman, K.E., Schmitz, A., Torok, T., Apostolou, A., Hanson, H., . . . & Mintz, E.D. (2011). Cholera in United States associated with epidemic in Hispaniola. *Emerging Infectious Diseases, 17*(11), 2166-2168.

Olu, O., Kargbo, B., Kamara, S., Wurie, A.H., Amone, J., Ganda, L., . . . & Kasolo, F. (2015). Epidemiology of Ebola virus disease transmission among health care workers in Sierra Leone, May to December 2014: A retrospective descriptive study. *BMC Infectious Diseases, 15*, 416.

Parola, P., de Lamballerie, X., Jourdan, J., Rovery, C., Vaillant, V., Minodier, P., . . . & Charrel, R.N. (2006). Novel chikungunya virus variant in travelers returning from Indian Ocean islands. *Emerging Infectious Diseases, 12*(10), 1493-1499.

Pavlin, B.I., Schloegel, L.M., & Daszak, P. (2009). Risk of importing zoonotic diseases through wildlife trade, United States. *Emerging Infectious Diseases, 15*(11), 1721-1726.

Possas, C. (2016). Zika: What we do and do not know based on the experiences of Brazil. *Epidemiology and Health, 38*, e2016023.

Rajabali, A., Moin, O., Ansari, A.S., Khanani, M.R., & Ali, S.H. (2009). Communicable disease among displaced Afghans: Refuge without shelter. *Nature Reviews Microbiology, 7*(8), 609-614.

Razafindrakoto, J., Kapesa, L., Andriamihamina, J., & Dentinger, C. (2018). *President's malaria initiative staff respond to a pneumonic plague outbreak.* Paper presented at the American Society of Tropical Medicine and Hygiene, New Orleans, LA.

Reed, K.D., Melski, J.W., Graham, M.B., Regnery, R.L., Sotir, M.J., Wegner, M.V., . . . & Damon, I.K. (2004). The detection of monkeypox in humans in the Western Hemisphere. *New England Journal of Medicine, 350*(4), 342-350.

Ruan, S.W., Wang, W., & Levin, S. (2006). The effect of global travel on the spread of SARS. *Mathematical Biosciences and Engineering, 3*(1), 2005-2018.

Shinde, V., Bridges, C.B., Uyeki, T.M., Shu, B., Balish, A., Xu, X., . . . & Finelli, L. (2009). Triple-reassortant swine influenza A (H1) in humans in the United States, 2005-2009. *New England Journal of Medicine, 360*(25), 2616-2625.

Shuaib, F., Gunnala, R., Musa, E.O., Mahoney, F.J., Oguntimehin, O., Nguku, P.M., . . . & Vertefeuille, J.F. (2014). Ebola virus disease outbreak—Nigeria, July-September 2014. *Morbidity and Mortality Weekly Report, 63*(39), 867-872.

Smith, D.L., Harris, A.D., Johnson, J.A., Silbergeld, E.K., & Morris, J.G. (2002). Animal antibiotic use has an early but important impact on the emergence of antibiotic resistance in human commensal bacteria. *Proceedings of the National Academy of Science, 99*(9), 6434-6439

Subbarao, K., Klimov, A., Katz, J., Regnery, H., Lim, W., Hall, H., . . . & Cox, N. (1998). Characterization of an avian influenza A (H5N1) virus isolated from a child with a fatal respiratory illness. *Science, 279*(5349), 393-396.

Tappero, J.W., Cassell, C.H., Bunnell, R.E., Angulo, F.J., Craig, A., Pesik, N., . . . & Martin, R. (2017). US Centers for Disease Control and Prevention and its partners' contributions to global health security. *Emerging Infectious Diseases, 23*(13, Suppl).

United Nations. (2018a). *UNHCR figures at a glance.* Retrieved from www.unhcr.org/figures-at-a-glance.html.

United Nations. (2018b). *World urbanization prospectus.* Retrieved from https://esa.un.org/unpd/wup/.

van Panhuis, W.G., Grefenstette, J., Jung, S.Y., Chok, N.S., Cross, A., Eng, H., . . . & Burke, D.S. (2013). Contagious diseases in the United States from 1888 to the present. *New England Journal of Medicine, 369*(22), 2152-2158.

Weaver, S.C. (2013). Urbanization and geographic expansion of zoonotic arboviral diseases: mechanisms and potential strategies for prevention. *Trends in Microbiology, 21*(8), 360-363.

Wolfe, N.D., Dunavan, C.P., & Diamond, J. (2007). Origins of major human infectious diseases. *Nature, 447*(7142), 279-283.

World Health Organization. (1978). Ebola haemorrhagic fever in Zaire, 1976. *Bulletin of the World Health Organization, 56*(2), 271-293.

World Health Organization. (2007). *International Health Regulations (2005).* Retrieved from www.who.int/ihr/publications/9789241596664/en/index.html.

World Health Organization. (2012). *Global strategy for dengue prevention and control, 2012–2020.* Retrieved from www.who.int/denguecontrol/9789241504034/en/.

World Health Organization. (2013). *Polio in the Syrian Arab Republic.* Retrieved from www.who.int/csr/don/2013_10_29/en/index.html.

World Health Organization. (2014). *Global alert and response: Ebola virus disease (EVD).* Geneva: Author.

World Health Organization. (2015). *Health worker Ebola infections in Guinea, Liberia and Sierra Leone: Preliminary report.* Retrieved from www.who.int/csr/resources/publications/ebola/health-worker-infections/en/.

World Health Organization. (2018). *Strengthening health security by implementing the International Health Regulations (2005).* Retrieved from www.who.int/ihr/en/.

Yang, G.J., Utzinger, J., & Zhou, X.N. (2015). Interplay between environment, agriculture and infectious diseases of poverty: case studies in China. *Acta Tropica, 141*(Pt B), 399-406.

Yong, D., Toleman, M.A., Giske, C.G., Cho, H.S., Sundman, K., Lee, K., & Walsh, T.R. (2009). Characterization of a new metallo-beta-lactamase gene, bla(NDM-1), and a novel erythromycin esterase gene carried on a unique genetic structure in *Klebsiella pneumoniae* sequence type 14 from India. *Antimicrobial Agents and Chemotherapy, 53*(12), 5046-5054.

Yong, E. (2018). Is America ready for a global pandemic? *The Atlantic.* Retrieved from www.theatlantic.com/magazine/archive/2018/07/when-the-next-plague-hits/561734/.

ONLINE RESOURCES

Careful Use of Antibiotics
www.cdc.gov/getsmart/index.html
Center for Infectious Disease Research and Policy
www.cidrap.unm.edu
Centers for Disease Control and Prevention
www.cdc.org
Global Health Security Agenda
www.ghsagenda.org
International Health Regulations
www.who.int/ihr/en/
National Institute of Nursing Research
www.ninr.nih.gov
One Health
www.onehealthinitiative.com
World Health Organization
www.who.int

Page numbers followed by *f, t,* or *b* indicate figures, tables, or boxes, respectively.

635